Canine Sports Medicine and Surgery

CANINE
SPORTS MEDICINE
AND SURGERY

EDITORS:

Mark S. Bloomberg, DVM, MS, Diplomate ACVS

Late Chairman, Department of Small Animal Clinical Sciences
College of Veterinary Medicine
University of Florida
Gainesville, Florida

Jon F. Dee, DVM, MS, Diplomate ACVS

Chief of Surgery, Hollywood Animal Hospital
Hollywood, Florida
Adjunct Assistant Professor, Department of Clinical Sciences
Ohio State University
Columbus, Ohio
and University of Florida
Gainesville, Florida

Robert A. Taylor, DVM, MS, Diplomate ACVS

Staff Surgeon, Alameda East Veterinary Hospital, Denver
Co-Director, Bel-Rea Institute of Animal Technology, Denver
Clinical Affiliate, Veterinary Teaching Hospital
Colorado State University
Fort Collins, Colorado

ASSOCIATE EDITOR:

James R. Gannon, BVSc, FAVSc, MRCVS

Sandown Veterinary Clinic
Springvale, Victoria, Australia

W.B. SAUNDERS COMPANY
A Division of Harcourt Brace & Company
Philadelphia   London   Toronto   Montreal   Sydney   Tokyo

W.B. SAUNDERS COMPANY
A Division of Harcourt Brace & Company

The Curtis Center
Independence Square West
Philadelphia, Pennsylvania 19106

Library of Congress Cataloging-in-Publication Data

Canine sports medicine and surgery / editors, Mark S. Bloomberg, Jon F. Dee, Robert A. Taylor; associate editor, James R. Gannon.

p.   cm.

ISBN 0–7216–5022–8

1. Canine sports medicine.   I. Bloomberg, Mark S.   II. Dee, Jon F.
III. Taylor, Robert A. (Robert Augustus)   [DNLM: 1. Dog Diseases.
2. Dogs—physiology.   3. Dogs—injuries.   4. Dogs—surgery.
5. Physical Conditioning, Animal.   6. Wounds and Injuries—veterinary.
SF 991 C2235 1998]

SF991.6.C36   1998   636.7′08971027—dc20

DNLM/DLC   96–24186

CANINE SPORTS MEDICINE AND SURGERY   ISBN 0–7216–5022–8

Printed in the United States of America.

Last digit is the print number: 9   8   7   6   5   4   3   2   1

We wish to dedicate this book
in memory of Mark Bloomberg.
He was a great friend, teacher, surgeon, and leader.
He is sorely missed

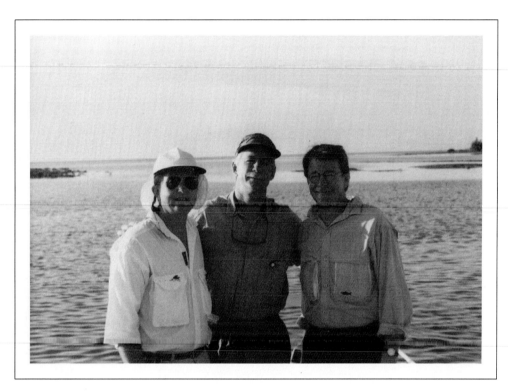

Left to right: Mark S. Bloomberg, Robert A. Taylor, Jon F. Dee

CONTRIBUTORS

NEAL C. ANDELMAN, VMD
Hospital Director, Westbridge Veterinary Hospital, West Bridgewater, Massachusetts
Dermatology

STEVEN PAUL ARNOCZKY, DVM
Wade O. Brinker Chair of Veterinary Surgery and Director, Laboratory for Comparative Orthopaedic Research, College of Veterinary Medicine, Michigan State University, East Lansing, Michigan
Stifle Injuries

BRIAN S. BEALE, DVM, DACVS
Adjunct Assistant Professor, Texas A and M University College of Veterinary Medicine; Staff Surgeon, Gulf Coast Veterinary Specialists, Houston, Texas
Arthropathies

MARK S. BLOOMBERG, DVM, MS, DACVS†
Chairman, Department of Small Animal Clinical Sciences, College of Veterinary Medicine, University of Florida, Gainesville, Florida
Osteochondrosis of Sporting and Working Dogs \ Greyhound Racing Injuries: Racetrack Injury Survey \ Bandages and Splints

LINDA BLYTHE, DVM, PhD
Associate Dean, Student and Academic Affairs, Oregon State University College of Veterinary Medicine; Consulting Neurologist, Oregon State Veterinary Teaching Hospital, Corvallis, Oregon
Neurological Dysfunction in Sporting and Working Dogs

CHRISTOPHER M. BOEMO, BVSc (Hons)
Part-time Lecturer in Greyhound Surgery, University of Melbourne Faculty of Veterinary Science; Principal, Keysborough Veterinary Practice, Keysborough, Victoria, Australia
Genitourinary Diseases in the Canine Athlete \ Injuries of the Metacarpus and Metatarsus

S. GARY BROWN, DVM, DACVS
Surgeon, Veterinary Orthopedic and Surgery Service, Fremont, California
Unique Veterinary Problems of Coursing Dogs

PETER D. CONSTABLE, BVSc, MS, PhD
Assistant Professor and Section Head, Food Animal Medicine and Surgery, Department of Veterinary Clinical Medicine, University of Illinois, Urbana, Illinois
Veterinary Problems of Racing Sled Dogs

A. MORRIE CRAIG, PhD
Professor in Toxicology, College of Veterinary Medicine, Oregon State University, Corvallis, Oregon
Drug Testing in Sporting Dogs

DONALD CUDDY
Tarneit, Victoria, Australia
Whelping, Raising, and Training of Racing Greyhounds

PATRICK DALTON
Clogherlea, County Tipperary, Ireland
Whelping, Raising, and Training of Racing Greyhounds

PHILLIP E. DAVIS, MVSc (Syd), MRCVS
Senior Lecturer, Veterinary Clinical Sciences, The University of Sydney, Sydney, New South Wales, Australia
Racing Performance in Greyhounds: Manipulation, Traction, Tissue Mobilization, and Sustained Stretch Exercises

JON F. DEE, DVM, MS, DACVS
Chief of Surgery, Hollywood Animal Hospital, Hollywood, Florida; Adjunct Assistant Professor, Department of Clinical Sciences, Ohio State University, Columbus, Ohio and University of Florida, Gainesville, Florida
Tarsal Injuries \ Long-Bone Fractures in the Racing Greyhound \ Glossary

LARRY G. DEE, DVM
Adjunct Faculty Member, College of Veterinary Medicine, University of Florida, Gainesville; Hollywood Animal Hospital, Hollywood, Florida
Racing Greyhound Adoption Programs

LOÏC M. DEJARDIN, DVM, MS
Research Associate, Laboratory for Comparative Orthopaedic Research, Michigan State University, College of Veterinary Medicine, East Lansing, Michigan
Stifle Injuries

KEITH DILLON
Greyhound Breeder, Olathe, Kansas
Artificial Lures

MICHAEL W. DRYDEN, DVM, PhD
Associate Professor of Veterinary Parasitology, College of Veterinary Medicine, Kansas State University, Manhattan, Kansas
Gastrointestinal Parasites and Kennel Management \ External Parasites

†Deceased.

WILLIAM W. DUGGER, BSA, DVM
Palm Beach Kennel Club, West Palm Beach, Florida
Greyhound Racing Injuries: Racetrack Injury Survey

RICHARD D. EATON-WELLS, BVSc, MACVSc, MRCVS
Director, West Chermside Veterinary Specialists, Brisbane,
Queensland, Australia
*Muscle Injuries in the Racing Greyhound \ Injuries of the
Digits and Pads \ Long-Bone Fractures in the Racing
Greyhound*

DESMOND P. FEGAN, MVB (Dublin)
Principal, Sandown Veterinary Clinic, Springvale, Victoria,
Australia
*First Aid and Track Care of Racing Greyhounds and Other
Sporting Breeds \ Natural Breeding*

RAY G. FERGUSON, BVSc
Part-Time Lecturer in Greyhound Medicine, University of
Melbourne Faculty of Veterinary Science; Head Clinician,
Monash Veterinary Clinic, Clayton, Victoria, Australia
Genitourinary Diseases in the Canine Athlete

JAMES R. FREEMAN, JR., DVM
Staff Veterinarian, Merial Limited, Athens, Georgia
Veterinary Problems Unique to Security and Detector Dogs

KATHRYN J. FROST, MSc
Adjunct Faculty, University of Alaska Fairbanks and University
of Alaska Anchorage; Marine Mammals Biologist, Alaska
Department of Fish and Game, Fairbanks, Alaska
Training Sled Dogs

JAMES R. GANNON, BVSc, FACVSc, MRCVS
Guest Lecturer in Greyhound Elective, Murdoch University, Perth;
Consulting Veterinarian, Greyhound Racing Control Board,
Victoria; National Coursing Association, Victoria; Australian and
New Zealand Greyhound Association, and Sandown Veterinary
Clinic Hospital, Springvale, Victoria, Australia
*Soundness Examination of the Sporting Canid \ Diseases of
the Muscles \ Physical Therapy in Canine Sporting
Breeds \ Drug Control Programs in Canine Sports
Medicine \ Glossary*

DOMINIQUE GRANDJEAN, DVM, PhD
Professor, Unité de Medecine de L'Elevage et du Sport, Ecole
Nationale Veterinaire D'Alfort, Maisons–Alfort, France
*Origin and History of the Sled Dog \ Nutrition for Sled
Dogs \ Veterinary Problems of Racing Sled Dogs*

GARY GUCCIONE
Executive Director, National Greyhound Association, Abilene,
Kansas
Origin and History of the Racing Greyhound and Coursing Dogs

KENNETH W. HINCHCLIFF, BVSc, PhD
Associate Professor, Veterinary Clinical Sciences, College of
Veterinary Medicine, The Ohio State University, Columbus, Ohio
Veterinary Problems of Racing Sled Dogs

STEVEN A. HOLLOWAY, BVSc, MVS, MACVSc, DACVS
Research Associate, The University of Melbourne School of
Veterinary Science, Parkville, Victoria, Australia
Stress- and Performance-Related Illness in Sporting Dogs

BEDE W. IRELAND, ASTC, Civil Eng
Fellow, Institution of Engineers, Castle Hill, New South Wales,
Australia
Race Track Biomechanics and Design

PAUL B. JENNINGS, JR., VMD, MMedSci
Veterinary Surgeon, Gore Hybrid Technologies, Inc., Flagstaff,
Arizona
*Origins and History of Security and Detector
Dogs \ Veterinary Problems Unique to Security and Detector
Dogs*

KENNETH A. JOHNSON, MVSc, PhD, FACVSc, MRCVS
Professor of Companion Animal Studies and Head, Division of
Companion Animals, University of Bristol, Department of
Clinical Veterinary Science, Bristol, United Kingdom
Carpal Injuries

ROBERT L. JOHNSON, MD
Associate Director, Maternal Fetal Medicine, Good Samaritan
Regional Medical Center, Chairman, Department of Obstetrics and
Gynecology, Desert Samaritan Hospital, Mesa, Arizona
Canine Insemination: Artificial, Chilled, and Frozen

FRANK R. JORDAN, DVM
Staff, Abilene Animal Hospital, P.A., Abilene, Kansas
Management of Pregnancy and Parturition

ROBERT R. KING, DVM, PhD
Assistant Professor, Department of Small Animal Clinical
Sciences, College of Veterinary Medicine, University of Florida,
Gainesville, Florida
Pulmonary Diseases of Working and Sporting Dogs

HERB "DUTCH" KOERNER
Greyhound Breeder and Kennel Owner, Hayes, Kansas
Raising, Training, and Conditioning the Racing Greyhound

JOHN R. KOHNKE, BVSc, RDA
Technical Director, Vetsearch International Pty Ltd, Sydney, New
South Wales, Australia
Nutrition for the Racing Greyhound

MERRY LESTER, BSPT
Affiliate Faculty, Regis University, Denver, Colorado
Physical Therapy in Canine Sporting Breeds

DANIEL D. LEWIS, DVM, DACVS
Associate Professor of Small Animal Surgery, Department of
Small Animal Clinical Sciences, College of Veterinary Medicine,
University of Florida, Gainesville, Florida
Osteochondrosis of Sporting and Working Dogs

ESTHER McCARTNEY
Field Trialer Extraordinare, Cheyenne, Wyoming
History of Competitive Upland Game Bird and Retriever Dogs

KEN McCARTNEY, BS, JD
Field Trialer; Past President of the National Amateur Retriever Club, Cheyenne, Wyoming
History of Competitive Upland Game Bird and Retriever Dogs

C. WAYNE McILWRAITH, BVSc, PhD, FRCVS, DACVS
Professor of Surgery and Director of Equine Sciences, College of Veterinary Medicine and Biomedical Sciences, Colorado State University, Fort Collins, Colorado
What's New on the Horizon for Comparative Orthopedic Sports Medicine

STUART NELSON
Iditarod Trail Committee, Wasilla, Alaska
Veterinary Problems of Racing Sled Dogs

JEAN A. NEMZEK, DVM, MS, DACVS
Postdoctoral Scholar, Unit for Laboratory Animal Medicine, University of Michigan, Animal Research Facility, Ann Arbor; Surgeon, Veterinary Care Specialists, Milford, Michigan
Stifle Injuries

RICHARD D. PARK, DVM, PhD
Professor, Department of Radiological Health Sciences, College of Veterinary Medicine and Biomedical Sciences, Colorado State University; Chief of Radiology Section, Veterinary Teaching Hospital, Colorado State University, Ft. Collins, Colorado
Imaging Techniques and Radiographic Examination of the Appendicular Skeletal System

ROBERT B. PARKER, DVM, DACVS
Chairman and Head, Department of Surgery, The Animal Medical Center, New York, New York
Physeal Injuries

NIGEL R. PERKINS, BVSc (Hons), MS, DACT
Senior Lecturer, Department of Veterinary Clinical Sciences, Massey University, Palmeston North, New Zealand
Breeding Soundness Examination of the Working Dog

RICHARD A. READ, BVSc, PhD, FACVSc
Associate Professor, School of Veterinary Studies, Murdoch University, Murdoch, Western Australia, Australia
Diseases of the Sesamoid Bones

GREGORY A. REINHART, BS, MS, PhD
Director, Strategic Research, Research and Development, The Iams Company, Lewisburg, Ohio
Nutrition for Sporting Dogs

ROBERT K. RIDLEY, DVM, PhD
Professor of Veterinary Parasitology, College of Veterinary Medicine, Kansas State University, Manhattan, Kansas
Gastrointestinal Parasites and Kennel Management \ External Parasites

GEOFFREY M. ROBINS, BVet Med, MRCVS, FACVSc
Specialist, Small Animal Surgeon, West Chermside Veterinary Clinic, Queensland, Australia
Diseases of the Sesamoid Bones

WILLIAM G. RODKEY, DVM, DACVS
Director, Basic Science Research, Vice President, Scientific Affairs, Steadman Hawkins Sports Medicine Foundation, ReGen Biologics, Vail, Colorado
What's New on the Horizon for Comparative Orthopedic Sports Medicine

SIMON C. ROE, BVSc, PhD
Associate Professor of Small Animal Orthopaedic Surgery, Department of Companion Animal and Special Species Medicine, North Carolina State University, Raleigh, North Carolina
Injury and Diseases of Tendons

KARIN A. SCHMIDT, DVM
Bering Sea Animal Clinic, Anchorage, Alaska
Veterinary Problems of Racing Sled Dogs

ROBERT SEPT, DVM
Bering Sea Animal Clinic, Anchorage, Alaska
Veterinary Problems of Racing Sled Dogs

KATHERINE S. SETTLE, DVM
Partner/Owner of Sanford Animal Hospital and All Animals Veterinary Hospital, Mesa, Arizona
Canine Insemination: Artificial, Chilled, and Frozen

VICTOR M. SHILLE, DVM, PhD, DACT
Professor Emeritus, College of Veterinary Medicine, University of Florida, Gainesville, Florida
Suppression or Prevention of Estrus in Racing and Sporting Dogs

ROSS V. STAADEN, BVSc, PhD
Clinician and Surgeon, Applecross Veterinary Centre, Karawara, Australia
The Exercise Physiology of Sporting Dogs

ALICE J. STANLEY
Consultant on Search and Rescue Matters, Spotsylvania County, Virginia
Origin, History, Training, and Utilization of Search, Rescue, and Tracking Dogs

J. RICHARD STEADMAN, MD, DABOS
Adjunct Clinical Professor, University of Texas Southwestern, Dallas, Texas; Orthopaedic Surgeon and Principal Chairman, Medical Group, U.S. Ski Team; Steadman Hawkins Clinic and Steadman Hawkins Sports Medicine Foundation, Vail, Colorado
What's New on the Horizon for Comparative Orthopedic Sports Medicine

JOHN R. STEPHENS, BSc(Ed), FAICD
Sandown Greyhound Racing Club, Springvale, Victoria, Australia
Racing and Training Greyhounds

ROBERT A. TAYLOR, DVM, MS, DACVS
Staff Surgeon, Alameda East Veterinary Hospital, Denver; Co-Director, Bel-Rea Institute of Animal Technology, Denver; Clinical Affiliate, Veterinary Teaching Hospital, Colorado State University, Ft. Collins, Colorado
Physical Therapy in Canine Sporting Breeds \ Bandages and Splints \ Glossary

PHILIP G. A. THOMAS, BVSc (Hons), PhD, DACT
Visiting Lecturer, University of Queensland and University of
Sydney; Staff Theriogenologist, West Chermside Veterinary
Clinic, Brisbane, Queensland, Australia
Breeding Soundness Examination of the Working Dog

ALBERT S. TOWNSHEND, AB, DVM
Owner of Eastern Shore Animal Hospital, Charter Secretary/
Treasurer, International Sled Dog Veterinary Medical Association,
Chestertown, Maryland
Veterinary Problems of Racing Sled Dogs

HENRI VAN BREE, DVM, PhD, Diplomate ECVS, ECVDI
Professor, Department of Medical Imaging, Faculty of Veterinary
Medicine, University of Ghent, Merelbeke, Belgium
Diagnostic and Surgical Arthroscopy in Small Animals

BERNADETTE VAN RYSSEN, DVM, PhD
Assistant, Department of Medical Imaging, Faculty of Veterinary
Medicine, University of Ghent, Merelbeke, Belgium
Diagnostic and Surgical Arthroscopy in Small Animals

KIRK L. WENDELBURG, DVM, DACVS
Hospital Director, Animal Specialty Group, Los Angeles,
California
*Disorders of the Hip Joint in the Canine
Athlete* \ *Lumbosacral Stenosis in the Sporting Dog*

PREFACE

This book arose from a need to collect the knowledge and ideas of those with a special interest in the working dog. While many of us were first challenged by the greyhound breed, we soon learned to admire and marvel at the many working breeds and their unique injuries and problems. There is a strong international interest in the injuries and conditions unique to the canine athlete. We are pleased to have assembled international experts to present current methods regarding their areas of expertise. The text is intended for veterinarians, veterinary students, animal technicians, owners, breeders, trainers, and handlers with an interest in the canine athlete. We are especially indebted to Dr. Jim Gannon, who served as associate editor and provided leadership in Australia.

Each chapter is written by an acknowledged authority and represents contemporary thoughts and practices. We are delighted in the exceptional quality of the chapters contributed by these invited authors.

We want to thank our editor, Ray Kersey, Senior Developmental Editor David Kilmer, and the rest of the W.B. Saunders editorial staff. We wish to thank Linda Lee and Maureen Homersham for their writing efforts and their ability to expedite chapter correspondence.

JON F. DEE
ROBERT A. TAYLOR

Contents

SECTION I

ORIGIN AND HISTORY OF SPORTING AND WORKING DOGS

CHAPTER 1

ORIGIN AND HISTORY OF THE RACING GREYHOUND AND COURSING DOGS

GARY GUCCIONE

Greyhounds have been the speed dogs of the world since antiquity. They and their close cousins lay claim as the oldest purebreed canine family still in existence, with origins deeply rooted in the lands that cradled the earliest civilization of humankind. The greyhound's history is heaped in richness and tradition, marked by both splendor and tragedy. The greyhound is the subject of art and literature that have endured over the centuries and is continually the focus of unswerving honor and praise from its human masters.

A member of the gazehound or sighthound family, the greyhound is easily recognized for its distinct sleekness and deceiving fragility but is most characterized by its speed, grace, and agility. Its sense of smell has never been well developed; it relies instead on exceptionally keen eyesight and an acute sense of hearing. During the hunt, greyhounds do not stop to dig and seldom cry out or bark. The greyhound's conformation allows for perfect balance and control and the ability to change direction without hesitation, difficulty, or risk. Clarke wrote that "It (the greyhound) represents Nature's most perfect example of streamlining for speed in animal form. What the swallow and the swift are to birds, what the shark and the mackerel are to fishes, so, too, is the greyhound to other dogs."

Some creditable authorities have claimed that the fastest of greyhounds are capable of speeds beyond 50 mph, although most accounts safely place that speed somewhere between 44 and 47 mph. No doubt the fastest speeds are registered by today's fleet professional canine athletes that compete on the best commercial racetracks throughout the world. Their ultimate speeds are attained in the first straightaway of a race, shortly after leaving the starting box en route to the first turn. For pure speed at a short distance, few land animals and no other canine breed can match the greyhound. In the gazehound category, the breeds that follow the greyhound in terms of speed (in descending order) are the whippet, saluki, borzoi, Scottish deerhound, Afghan hound and Irish wolf-

hound. Average speeds for the last five of these range from about 28 mph to 34 mph.

The wolf is the true ancestor of all domestic dogs, and it is sound speculation that the greyhound and all members of the gazehound family descended from the pale-footed wolf. Murals and paintings suggest that dogs strikingly similar to the greyhounds and salukis of today were around between 8000 and 4000 BC. The Mideast region of the world—likely in the regions of Arabia and Egypt—was the stage of this early development. If not rough coated, many of the dogs were at least "feathered," much like today's saluki.

The greyhound evolved in a countryside of few hills or woods where it hunted and relied on speed to escape enemies. In plentiful supply were hares, antelope, desert fox, wolves, and gazelle—ideal game for the greyhound with its swiftness and agility. Primitive man needed to hunt for food but was without modern weapons to overcome game. Hence, for many the greyhound was the means of sustaining life. Little wonder that reverence for the greyhound began at the very dawn of civilized time.

The desert's isolation from the rest of the world allowed the breed to maintain a degree of purity. Owners, desiring better hunters, continually bred their fastest to their fastest, generation after generation, until eventually the breed was firmly established and the type fixed—so much so that the original type has changed very little up to the present. Even with the inevitable migration of the breed to other lands, where it was then crossed with each area's native stock, the greyhound type was so dominant and pure through centuries of inbreeding that the breed's distinct characteristics—long thin neck, tucked-up loins, sweeping quarters—always managed to prevail.

The original Arab greyhounds, as hunters and the source of sport, won the admiration and respect of their owners. They were

1

even permitted to ride their owners' camels and shared the luxuries of their masters' tents—a courtesy afforded no other dog of that time. The birth of a greyhound in early Arabian culture was second only in importance to the birth of a son. It was believed that by wearing beads and amulets, the greyhound could ward off evil spirits. Greyhounds were frequently depicted in Egyptian murals, and their likeness was occasionally found on the tombs of the pharaohs. Cleopatra reputedly was a greyhound fancier.

Is it any surprise that the greyhound is the only canine breed specifically mentioned in the Bible? In Proverbs 30:29–31, King Solomon displays his wisdom by speaking glowingly of the breed: "There be three things which go well, yea, are comely in going. . . . A greyhound, and a goat also, and a king against whom there is no rising up."

Eventually the desert was no longer isolated from the rest of the world, and the Arab greyhound found its way to other civilizations. Persians believed they were the only dogs allowed in the next world and privileged enough to give information and evidence against humankind. The Tartars brought the greyhound to Russia, where it was later crossed with local dogs, giving rise to the borzoi branch of the gazehound family. The greyhound arrived in Afghanistan (taken there possibly by Syrians), where when crossed with the local breeds it became the ancestor of the Afghan hound. With its heavy coat and strength, the Afghan hound was well suited for this cold and hilly terrain. Salukis, prominent in Egypt, probably became the ancestors of the Southern European greyhound.

The ancient Greeks became caretakers of the greyhound centuries preceding the birth of Christ. In fact, the breed became known as Greekhound, then, through careless use, grakehound—very possibly the origins for the name greyhound. (Another theory is that the word stems from the writings of Caius, who claimed: "The greyhound hath his name of this word 'gre,' which soundeth 'gradus' in Latine, in English 'degree,' because, among all dogges these are the most principal, occupying the chiefest place, and being simply and absolutely the best of the gentle kinds of houndes.") According to English author Adair Dighton, the Greeks were so intent on keeping the breed pure that they exercised the precaution of "having sharp spikes worked into the body clothing of certain breeds to prevent promiscuous connection." Greyhounds show up on the designs of Athenian water vases and Grecian urns, dating back to 600 BC. Greek coins and gems (ranging from 500 BC to AD 200) found in the Aegean Sea depict a breed with no feathered tails and no saluki muzzles—dogs that were much like the modern greyhound (Fig. 1–1). The Greek writer Flavius Arrianus wrote of the practice of hunting with greyhounds about AD 200; his description of the hounds of his time is similar to that of the greyhound of today. It was Arrianus, in fact, who laid out the first primitive rules of coursing with greyhounds.

The Roman Empire was no less impressed by greyhounds, making them the subject of much art. In the British Museum, for example, is a statue of two Roman greyhounds from the first century AD. The greyhounds—a dog and a bitch—are smooth skinned and very similar to today's greyhounds.

Through the early portion of the Dark Ages, the greyhound migrated throughout the European continent. There is clear evidence that greyhounds were used in France and Germany in the ninth century to course hares, deer, wolves, and wild pigs.

A major progression in the breed's development occurred when the greyhound migrated with Gallic and Celtic tribes to England. There is documentation that greyhounds were in England as far back as 3500 years ago, and a 1959 uncovering of the Averbury Stone Circle, Europe's largest prehistoric monument, revealed a skeleton of a greyhound-like dog. The Celtic hound of the second century was clearly a greyhound type. When the Gallic tribes were driven out of England to Ireland, they took their greyhounds with them and managed to keep the breed pure and smooth coated. St.

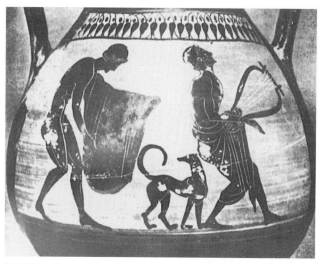

FIGURE 1–1. Predecessors of the modern greyhound were often depicted on Greek coins, urns, and other artifacts, as seen on this sixth century BC Greek amphora. (From Ash EC: The Book of the Greyhound. London, Hutchinson & Co. Ltd., 1933, p. 41.)

Patrick, on his escape from slavery, traveled in a boat in which the principal cargo was greyhounds, which were being exported for use in the Roman arena. An old Welsh proverb proclaimed that you might know a gentleman by his horse, his hawk, and his greyhound. Saxon tribal chiefs often were given greyhounds among state gifts of honor. In the tenth and eleventh centuries the price was the same for a greyhound, a hawk, and a man servant (Fig. 1–2).

Greyhounds even became implicated in military politics. When King Richard II was captured in the Castle of Flint, his pet greyhound, Mathe, immediately ran to Richard's bitter rival, the Earl of Lancaster (later Henry IV), and licked his hand in a gesture of betrayal. King John accepted greyhounds in lieu of fines; Henry II was also a fan of the breed. Henry VII had so many greyhounds roaming his palace that he ordered the household to bar any more dogs from his court except by his own royal command.

The darkest chapter of the greyhound's history unfolded in medieval times, when in the year 1014 Canute (a Dane) became King of England and shortly thereafter enacted the Forest Laws. The woods and fields at that time were alive with game, and often the hunting by poor villagers would come into conflict with the hunting by the king and chiefs. To remedy that, the Forest Laws included a statute that said only noblemen could own and hunt with greyhounds. Merry Olde England was hardly merry for the poor commoner who had relied on game caught by his greyhounds to feed his family. So of necessity, many commoners hunted anyway. Every 40 days violators were brought to special courts where they were fined or, if they refused to snitch on neighbors, flogged and tortured. Sometimes a peasant's silence cost him a hand or a foot at the chopping block. His greyhounds were then either mutilated so they could no longer hunt or, if of royal color (white or predominantly so), given to the nobility.

It was clearly a war against the greyhound itself, and mutilation of many greyhounds was only one of various ways this detestable law affected the breed. While a brindle and a black coat aided concealment—especially for night hunting—white pups were of no use to poachers, and so were almost always immediately destroyed at birth. Conversely, white greyhounds were greatly valued by the court and nobles. In Ireland, France, and England, white suggested purity and was viewed with a certain respectful awe by everyone, including the downtrodden.

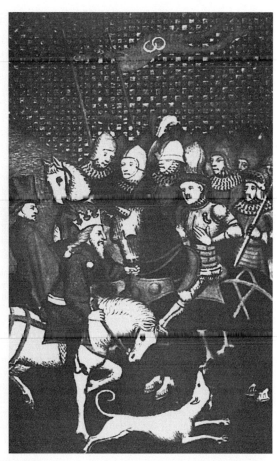

FIGURE 1–2. By the eleventh century in England, greyhounds had become a symbol of royalty, similar to falcons and horses. Kings and nobles enjoyed nothing more than hunting with or coursing their greyhounds. (From Ash EC: The Book of the Greyhound. London, Hutchinson & Co. Ltd., 1933, p. 76.)

Tragically this war on greyhounds went on for at least four centuries—all because royalty felt compelled to curb the nuisance of common people hunting with their greyhounds! Some of the sections of the Forest Laws were not abolished until the 1500s, by Queen Elizabeth I—herself a die-hard fan of the breed who would later order Lord Norfolk to draft the first formal rules of greyhound coursing. Small wonder that greyhound racing, championed in its fundamental forms of hunting and coursing by such female royalty as Cleopatra and Queen Elizabeth, would become known as the sport of queens.

Greyhounds were unarguably the fashionable dogs of England in the sixteenth century. It was a regular practice for lords and ladies to go hawking and coursing with their greyhounds. The greyhound was often presented as a token of esteem to foreign potentates. It was considered one of the most generous of gifts—especially among the Irish.

By Queen Elizabeth's time, the greyhound had evolved into two distinct types. The first was the larger, rougher deerhound, utilized for hunting bigger game. The second was the smaller greyhound type, which was used for hunting hare and other small quarry.

It is indisputable that greyhounds were first used as hunters for the purpose of putting food on the family table. However, eventually the element of recreation and sport became popular—probably more than 2000 years ago. In 1776, the Earl of Orford, a zealous greyhound owner and advocate, organized the first coursing club

in England, the Swaffham Coursing Society. Other clubs would soon spring up in England (and eventually other greyhound countries), including the Altcar Society. Founded in 1825, the Altcar Society gave birth to the world's most renowned coursing prize, the Waterloo Cup. In 1858, the National Coursing Club was founded as the supreme authority on coursing matters in England.

Lord Orford's contribution to greyhound racing went far beyond his role with the Swaffham Coursing Society. A keeper of a large kennel (perhaps as many as 100 dogs), Lord Orford experimented with crossing the greyhound with other breeds. By at least one account, many greyhounds at that time were rough coated and narrow muzzled; Lord Orford's intention was to get a faster, more tenacious, and better-skinned greyhound. Initial experiments with lurchers and deerhounds proved unsuccessful. He then tried crossing the greyhound with the English bulldog (which then was more like today's bull terrier), and although the first efforts were not very successful, subsequent generations yielded a more competitive, more courageous pup with finer skin and a finer tail. According to Ash, it took seven generations before Lord Orford obtained greyhounds with "small ears, rat tails and skins almost without hair, together with the innate courage found in the Bulldog breed that never gives in . . . rather to die than relinquish the chase." Lord Orford's greyhounds were destined to become the ancestors of modern-day greyhounds.

Lord Orford's spectacular death may well have been exactly the way the eccentric (some claimed insane) greyhound breeder would have wanted it. In his latter years, Lord Orford had become a prisoner in his own house, watched over by hired help who were determined to protect him, largely from his own compulsions. They would not allow him to attend coursing meets, and this irritated him to no end. Then on a cold November day in 1797 his Lordship's great greyhound Czarina was matched against another heralded racer, Maria. Lord Orford, unable to bear being held captive any longer, escaped from his attendants, and not wearing hat, gloves, or coat, rode after the two greyhounds in the midst of their course. Friends ran toward him and tried to persuade him to return, but he ignored them and continued riding alongside Czarina and Maria. Moments after Czarina was declared the winner, a jubilant Lord Orford fell off his horse onto his head and died before attendees could reach him. For devotion and contributions to the sport and breed, Thomas Goodlake suggested in his 1828 *Courser's Manual* that the "memory of the Earl of Orford, therefore, may with propriety be introduced as a toast at every coursing meeting, as the father of its sport."

Greyhounds were first imported into America in the nineteenth century, primarily out of necessity. Millions of pesky jackrabbits, with appetites bigger than the Midwestern breadbasket they scourged, were ruining crops and the lives of many farmers. Ireland and England exported all the four-legged exterminators the farms needed, and the greyhound quickly (true to its nature) took its rightful place in American history by helping tame the West. This was no ordinary dog called upon to rescue the American farmer—this canine hunter, which was sent from the British Isles, refined through centuries of selective breeding that made it ideally suited for the purpose. Even this new terrain—the semi-arid, wide-open prairies of America's western heartland—resembled to some degree the very desert countryside in which the greyhound breed was born. The situation in Australia was not altogether different, and with the mass migration of Europeans to the island continent, the pattern of calling on greyhounds for hunting and coursing purposes was repeated. Like America, Australia would see coursing evolve into the modern-day phenomenon of greyhound track racing.

In commenting on the exportation of greyhounds to America, Clarke wrote: "To the settlers of English and Irish stock, the emigrants from Lancashire and Lincolnshire, from Kerry and Kildare, with a heritage of hunting and coursing in their blood, what more natural than they arrange for later immigrants to bring out with them the dog whose whole history and breeding had been designed to cope with and master the hares and jackrabbits that hitherto had met no rivals for pace on the native prairies?"

General George A. Custer was a greyhound enthusiast, famous also among deerhound fanciers for having owned and hunted with that breed in the West. Two years after Custer and the 7th Cavalry were wiped out at the Little Big Horn, one of his former orderlies, Major James H. (Hound Dog) Kelly—who had been indoctrinated by Custer on the intricacies of breeding and training—set a record for running down antelope with greyhounds.

In 1886 the first formal coursing meet in America was staged at Cheyenne Bottoms, near Great Bend, Kansas. Coursing clubs soon sprang up throughout the Midwest. Eight years after Cheyenne Bottoms, the American Coursing Board was founded, a counterpart to England's National Coursing Club. The American Coursing Board would be the parent organization of the National Coursing Association, founded in 1906, at Friend, Nebraska, which in turn evolved into the National Greyhound Association, headquartered since 1945 in Abilene, Kansas.

In 1919, modern know-how and this marvelous ancient breed joined to give rise to a brand new sport when an engineer named O. P. Smith invented a mechanical lure and successfully demonstrated it at Emeryville, California. Skeptics said the greyhound would never adapt to chasing an artificial lure around an oval track, but Smith, considered the father of American greyhound racing, proved them wrong. A year later, the first successful greyhound meet at a racetrack was held in Tulsa, Oklahoma, paving the way for scores of tracks to open at a wide variety of locations in the ensuing decade. Running races at night kept the sport free from competition with horse racing and secured its popularity with Americans as a spectator sport. The new sport of track racing soon caught on in other countries. In America, the ancient sport of coursing was finally phased out as a public event in 1978, but Americans have still been able to enjoy the speed and grace of the greyhound at more than 55 pari-mutuel racetracks located in 18 states (as of 1993). Throughout most of the 80s and early 90s, greyhound racing attracted upward of 25 million fans a year and has been ranked as high as sixth in terms of attendance among American spectator sports.

Greyhound racing continues to be a major sport in other countries of the world, including England, Ireland, Australia, and New Zealand. The sport is also enjoyed on a lesser scale in numerous European countries, as well as Macao, Mexico, and Indonesia.

As for the breed itself, England, Ireland, Australia, and the United States remain the major producers of champion racing

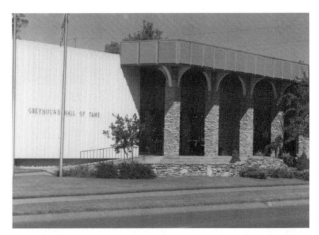

FIGURE 1–3. The Greyhound Hall Of Fame in Abilene, Kansas, pays tribute to the history of the greyhound—the only museum of its type in the world.

stock. The registries in all four countries operate under strict guidelines that maintain the integrity and purity of the breed; however, the frequent exchange of breeding stock among these countries has clearly proven beneficial to the quality of the breed worldwide.

The age-old practice of breeding the fastest or best of the breed for the sake of getting "better hunters" (now racers) persists among greyhound lovers of today, just as it did in ancient times. It should guarantee the preservation of a wonderful and noble breed whose history has enriched humankind beyond measure. All the reverence and adulation man has given the greyhound breed has been more than richly deserved and has been repaid manyfold (Fig. 1–3).

Suggested Reading

American Greyhound Track Operators Association: American Greyhound Racing Encyclopedia. Miami, 1963.
Ash EC: The Book of the Greyhound. London, Hutchinson & Co. Ltd., 1933.
Clarke HE: The Greyhound. London, Popular Dogs Publishing Co Ltd, 1965.
Dighton A: The Greyhound and Coursing. London, Grant Richards Ltd, 1921.
Goodlake T: The Courser's Manual or Stud Book. Harris & Co, 1828.
Hoffman CT: This Is Greyhound Racing. Miami, Carl T. Hoffman, 1972.
Salmon MH: Gazehounds and Coursing. St. Cloud, MN, North Star Press, 1977.

CHAPTER 2

ORIGIN AND HISTORY OF THE SLED DOG

DOMINIQUE GRANDJEAN

The heritage of the sled dog is a long and proud one, stretching back thousands of years. The people of the North depended on them for protection, companionship, hunting, trapping, and most of all, transportation. Sled dogs enabled explorers such as Byrd, Peary, and Amundsen to explore the frozen wastelands of two continents and played a vital role in bringing civilization to the snowbound areas of the world.

As early as 1873 the Royal Canadian Mounted Police was bringing order to northern frontiers with dog team patrols. Throughout Alaska and Canada, mail teams delivered the news to outlying settlements. One of the proudest chapters in sled dog history was written in 1925. In January of that year, a case of diphtheria was discovered in Nome, Alaska, and the supply of antitoxin in that city was inadequate to stave off an epidemic. A relay of 22 native and mail teams forged through the rough interior of Alaska and across the Bering Sea ice to bring the serum to the grateful citizens.

In New York City's Central Park, a statue of Balto, who led one of the relay teams, commemorates the Nome serum run. The inscription reads: "Dedicated to the indomitable spirit of the sled dogs that relayed the antitoxin 600 miles over rough ice, treacherous waters, through arctic blizzards from Nenana to the relief of stricken Nome in the winter of 1925. Endurance. Fidelité. Intelligence."

Few of the inhabitants of the Far North are dependent on dogs for basic survival today. However, the same intimate relationship between human and dog still exists and is evidenced through the sport of sled dog racing.

The sled dog sport has existed as a recognized sport only since the beginning of our century. At that time, especially during the gold rush in Alaska, groups of people decided to compare the qualities of the dog teams they were using to carry their equipment. Nothing else was needed for the sled dog sport to be born.

FIRST RACES IN ALASKA

After many discussions between dog team owners, it was decided in Nome, in 1907, to build the famous Nome Kennel Club. The aim was simple: to be able to organize "official" races, with clear rules and a real organization. One year later, a lawyer from Nome, Albert Fink, wrote the first racing rules of the very first official sled dog race—the All Alaska Sweepstake.

- All drivers will be members of the Nome Kennel Club.
- All dogs will be registered by the Nome Kennel Club.
- Drivers can use as many dogs as they wish, but all dogs starting the race must cross the finish line, in the team or in the basket of the sled.
- All dogs will be marked before the start, so that no substitution is possible during the race.
- If two teams are close together, one following the other, the one caught up must give way by immediately stopping and stay for "a certain time" before starting again.

With these first and very simple rules, the "mushers" started the race, a 408-mile trail from Nome to Candle and back. The word *musher* is used for the driver of a dog team; in fact, it comes from the French word *marche* (literally, "walk"), a term that was utilized by French Canadians to make their teams go.

Five days after the start of the race, the first finishers were back in Nome. A new legend was born!

On this trail covering mountains, frozen rivers, tundras, forests and glaciers, a young Norwegian immigrant, Leonhard Seppala, became forever the biggest name in the entire sled dog sport. With teams of Siberian huskies, Leonhard Seppala won the All Alaska Sweepstake in 1915, 1916, and 1917 (Table 2–1).[1]

Between 1908 and 1915 the dogs changed; the first huskies were imported from Siberia, and with the musher "Iron Man" John Johnson broke the record in 1910 (74 hours 14 minutes, and 37 seconds). In 1909 Scotty Allan won the race with a team of "crossed Alaskans" (malamutes mixed with setters) in about 80 hours racing in a windy storm. Another great name of the sled dog sport, Scotty Allan raced eight sweepstakes: He won three, finished in second place three times, and finished in third place twice.

In 1917 the first race ever held in the "lower 40" was staged in Ashton, Idaho. The sport was briefly interrupted during the two World Wars as dogs and drivers were pressed into the service of their countries.

But the one who helped to increase the performances of sled dogs is a veterinarian, "Doc" Roland Lombard. By bringing his knowledge to competitions, he won more titles at the Anchorage Fur Rendez-vous World Championship than anybody else and became the first president of the International Sled Dog Racing Association (ISDRA).

Among all these figures of growing sport, one must also name

TABLE 2–1. Results of First 10 Editions of the All Alaska Sweepstake

Year	Winner	Breed	Average Speed (miles per hour)
1908	John Hagness	Crossed malamutes	3.51
1909	Scotty Allan	Crossed malamutes	4.97
1910	John Johnson	Siberian huskies	5.58
1911	Scotty Allan	Crossed malamutes	5.05
1912	Scotty Allan	Crossed malamutes	5.05
1913	Fay Delzene	Crossed malamutes	5.39
1914	John Johnson	Siberian huskies	5.04
1915	Leonhard Seppala	Siberian huskies	5.18
1916	Leonhard Seppala	Siberian huskies	5.06
1917	Leonhard Seppala	Siberian huskies	5.21

Data from Grandjean D. Le sport de traîneau à chien et ski-pulka. Rec Med Vet 167:589–593, 1991.

George Attla, an Athabascan Indian born in Huslia, Alaska, who won everything and published *Everything I Know About Training and Racing Sled Dogs,* a book that for years has been the bible of mushing.

EVOLUTION OF THE SPORT

North America

Since the beginning of the century, the number of races in the United States and Canada has continually increased. After Alaska, a second main spot for the sport has been in New England, with the founding of the New England Sled Dog Club in 1924. In 1932, sled dog racing became part of the Olympic Games at Lake Placid as an official demonstration sport. The development of competition stopped during World War II and did not resume until the late 1960s. In 1971 the state of Alaska made sled dog racing a national sport. Of the current North American races, the main ones are:

- Fur Rendez-vous World Championship (Anchorage, Alaska)
- World Championship Sled Dog Derby (Laconia, New Hampshire)
- World Championship Dog Derby (La Pas, Manitoba)
- North American Championship (Fairbanks, Alaska)
- Alaska State Championship (Kenaï-Soldotna, Alaska)
- Race of Champions (Tok, Alaska)
- Surdough Rendez-vous (Whitehorse, Yukon Territory)
- US Pacific Coast Championship (Priest Lake, Idaho)
- All American Championship (Ely, Minnesota)
- Midwest International (Kalkaska, Michigan)
- Quebec International Course de Chiens (Quebec City, Quebec)
- Triple Couronne Canadienne (Mastigouche, Quebec)

All races are annual events attended by thousands of spectators. They include three heats (15 to 40 miles each, depending on the category) raced on Friday, Saturday, and Sunday, sometimes downtown. Long or ultra-long distance races are also popular, such as the John Beargrease Sled Dog Marathon (500 miles; Minnesota); the Iditarod (the ''Last Great Race on Earth''; 1049 miles; Alaska); the Yukon Quest (1000 miles; Canada and Alaska).

New legends were born, with mushers such as Jo Redington (creator of the Iditarod), Rick Swenson (five times Iditarod winner), Susan Butcher (four times champion), and Libby Riddles (first woman to win the Iditarod).

In 1995 the first long distance stage race, the Nenana Come Back Race, a concept developed in Europe in 1988, was held in the Fairbanks area.

Scandinavia

Scandinavia (Denmark, Norway, Sweden, Finland) is another home for sled dog sports, but with a different evolution because of the existence of pulka racing. One to four dogs pull a small sled called a *pulka,* followed by a cross-country skier. Even the dogs are different (German shorthair, pointers). The reasons for choosing these dogs are: history; the ability of these dogs to run faster than sled dogs for shorter distances (5 to 8 miles); and the behavior patterns of the dogs and their desire to run alone. Scandinavians have organized official competitions for 60 years, and pulka is one of the main sports in Norway, although sled dog competitions are important. The 1994 Olympics officially hosted sprint races and dedicated a long distance race (Femundlopet). Pulka and sled dog sports are now among the most important sports in Norway and are growing in popularity in Sweden, Finland, and Denmark.

Central Europe

In Europe, the first sled dog race was organized in Switzerland in 1965. The sport has grown, with racing circuits in Switzerland, Germany, and France. In each country, official structures were built, using racing rules from the ISDRA, and starting in 1983, from the European Sled Dog Racing Association (ESDRA). The first European Championships were organized in 1984 in St. Moritz, Switzerland, and are now held annually.

The Alpirod International Sled Dog Race, which originated in 1988, was the biggest yearly event for sled dogs in Europe. It was the first stage race ever organized, with an average of 14 heats, held in four different countries (France, Italy, Switzerland, Austria). The total length of the race was more than 100 km. There were more than 50 teams representing 12 to 15 nationalities, a clear indication that the sport really is international, and there were approximately 700 dogs. The first four editions were won by Alaskans; between 1992 and 1994 the winner was a French musher, Jacques Philip, and in 1995, Roger Leegard from Norway.

INTERNATIONAL FEDERATION FOR SLED DOG SPORT

The International Federation for Sled Dog Sport (IFSS) was founded in 1989, as result of dog sports competitions expanding beyond their regional and national boundaries. The IFSS has the responsibility of standardizing racing rules and creating an international structure.

Early in 1995, 39 national federations from five continents were members of IFSS. The organization has been officially recognized by the Assemblée Générale des Fédérations Internationales Sportives (AGFIS) and is now awaiting recognition by the International Olympic Committee (IOC). The first official sprint world championship was organized in Saint Moritz, Switzerland, in 1990 and has been held each year since (alternating between Europe and North America). The sport has continued to grow worldwide (Fig. 2–1),[2] with the number of sled dog teams competing in official races being greater than 50,000. The IFSS provides the worldwide organizational structure of national sled dog sport federations; structured with several committees (including an Animal Welfare Committee covering veterinary organizations and doping regulations), IFSS now meets all the requirements for Olympic recognition. Actual members of IFSS are regrouped in Table 2–2.

RACING SLED DOGS

Brief History

Some 4000 years ago, the nomadic tribes north of Lake Baikal, in south central Siberia, were the first to hitch a dog to a sled. Over the centuries the art of driving sled dogs reached a peak with the Siberian peoples known as the Chukchi and the Samoyed. These tribes used their dogs as companions, guards, pets, hunters, reindeer herders, and sled dogs. The Chukchi people were the first to depend seriously on the ability of their dogs to pull loaded sleds. In a recent booklet printed by Friends of Northern Dogs (FOND)[3] Robert Crane, a Russian scholar and a Siberian husky fancier, wrote that the combination of climatic changes and displacement of the Chukchi people by a more powerful southern people forced the Chukchi to base their economy on sled dog transportation and to journey long distances over the vast, irregular tundra and ice shelf.

By 1800 BC there were Eskimos on the Alaskan shores of the

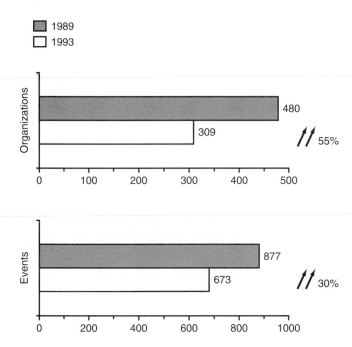

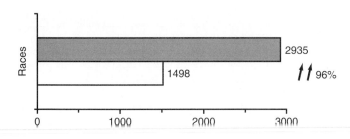

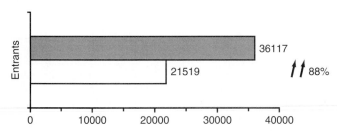

FIGURE 2–1. Increases in sled dog sports from 1989 to 1993. (From Levorsen B: 1992–1993 Sled Dog sport survey. IFSS ed. Pocatello, Idaho, 1994, p 6.)

Arctic Ocean. There is evidence that they used sled dogs to pull toboggans, harnessing three or four dogs in tandem, one behind the other. When the renowned Norwegian explorer Fridtjof Nansen observed North American Eskimos some 37 centuries later, what he saw them doing must not have been too different from all they had done before. History's first records on the use of sled dogs in the Siberian subarctic appear in Arabian literature of the tenth century, in writings of Marco Polo in the thirteenth century, and in those of Francesco da Vollo in the sixteenth.

The original sled dog was basically a hunter, descended perhaps from domestic dogs from southern latitudes, dogs that had accompanied their hunting masters north many generations earlier. The

dogs that survived in the rigorous climate of Siberia were large, furry, and wolf-like, the ancestors of today's northern breeds. Not only were their coats thick but also they developed undercoats for further protection against biting winds and bitter cold. Their ears were short, to minimize heat loss, and could be pricked upright to maximize their efficiency. The ears were filled with soft, insulating hair. The pads on their feet were tough to withstand the miles of tracking and hunting on frozen jagged terrain.

The first mushers were the explorers, hunters, and trappers who moved into arctic latitudes and found the best way to travel overland in winter was by the same method as the natives: by dog sled. The most popular mushers were the ones carrying mail packets for the Hudson's Bay Company.[3] John Beargrease, a Chippewa Indian in Minnesota, carried mail up and down the north shore of Lake Superior. The mail in Alaska went from Seward to Nome and back, with stops at Knik, Iditarod, and Ruby. In 1963 the US Post Office honored the last mail driver, Chester Noongwook of Savoonga on St. Lawrence Island in the Bering Sea. The last official patrol of the Royal Canadian Mounted Police was in March 1969, a 500-mile round trip from Old Crow to Fort MacPherson and back.

Evolution of the Dogs

Isolation of Arctic peoples like the Koryaks, the Samoyeds, or natives from the Kamchatka Peninsula explains the kind of "pure breed" of arctic dog, almost unchanged since that period.

At the beginning, selection was very primitive. Only the most

TABLE 2–2. Members of IFSS (International Federation for Sled Dog Sport)

Countries	Organizations	Members	Events	Races	Teams
Austria	9	600	12	66	1151
Belgium	3	250	6	24	480
Czech Republic	1	480	10	28	345
Denmark	2	130	16	75	460
England	7	550	16	52	1084
Finland	26	1000	14	37	464
France	60	1600	15	69	1744
Germany	5	2400	48	284	3161
Hungary	1	30	2	2	20
Ireland	1	3	0	0	3
Italy	5	400	30	137	2390
Luxembourg	1	20	1	6	44
Holland	5	200	6	30	481
Norway	80	800	90	193	1966
Scotland	4	120	6	24	381
Spain	5	250	4	26	220
Andorra	1	5	1	2	4
Wales	3	25	5	13	178
Sweden	56	5000	89	289	3977
Switzerland	3	175	9	49	671
Ukraine	1	5	1	1	5
Russia	3	80	4	8	70
Slovenia	1	30	1	3	25
United States	122	11500	330	1097	10525
Canada	63	6200	122	321	4591
Japan	7	345	7	47	1329
Australia	4	200	15	22	152
New Zealand	5	127	11	49	336
South Africa	1	100	10	10	82
Argentina	1	27	1	1	18
Chile	1	13	1	1	8

From Levorsen B: 1992–1993 Sled Dog Sport Survey. IFSS ed. Pocatello, Idaho, 1994.

intelligent lead dogs and the strongest males were kept for reproduction. Other males were castrated, and no other breed was included until the end of the nineteenth century.

The *Siberian husky* originated in the Kamchatka peninsula region of Siberia. It is an ancient breed developed over centuries by the Chukchi people as a sled dog. The animals were first imported from Siberia to Alaska by a Russian trader in 1909, specifically to race in the second running of the All Alaska Sweepstake. The Siberian husky is a medium-sized dog, weighing from 35 to 60 pounds, females being an inch shorter and weighing 10 or more pounds less than males. They may be any color, from solid black to pure white (even spotted); the eyes may also be any color. The coat is double, a thick downy undercoat and a medium-length straight and somewhat soft outercoat that sheds ice and snow. There are very tough, thick pads on their feet; these have evolved for travel over ice and snow for great distances. Quick and light on its feet, the Siberian husky is a very athletic dog that can travel at speeds of 12 to 15 miles per hour for long distances, but it is also able to reach 20 miles an hour for a few miles.

The *Alaskan malamute,* so named because of the Inuit peoples they served, the Mahlemutes, is a draft animal. When used to pull freight, males weigh about 85 pounds and stand 25 inches or more at the shoulder; females stand about 23 inches at the shoulder and weigh 75 pounds. They are substantial dogs, with deep chests and heavy double coats. Malamutes have brown eyes, coats ranging from light gray to black, and white legs and bellies.

The *Samoyed,* named for the tribe from northwestern Siberia, is a solid white dog. The breed developed isolated from outside influence, hence the relative dissimilarities to other arctic breeds. They are medium-sized, weighing 40 to 60 pounds, with the females slightly smaller, and were designed by nature to cover great distances pulling heavier loads. The coat is double, with a thick downy undercoat and a very harsh, long outer coat that sheds ice and snow.

Spectators attending their first sled dog race often are astonished by the variety of dogs now used in racing teams. The average spectator not only sees pure arctic breeds pulling sleds but also other purebreds such as Irish setters, Dalmatians, and American coon and fox hounds.

Although not a pure breed, the most popular and fastest dog in the sport today is the *Alaskan husky,* a breed that is essentially a mixture of arctic dogs. The breed was developed over the last 40 years specifically for sled dog competition. It is a blend of breeds that may include very fast dogs such as whippets or greyhounds, and double-coated dogs such as the native village dogs, Indian dogs, Eskimo dogs, Siberian huskies, and malamutes. Alaskan huskies can be any color, and their coats vary in length and texture, depending on where they live and their ancestry. Their eyes may be any color, and they are generally medium sized, weighing between 35 and 70 pounds. Other special crossbreeds developed for racing purposes are the Targhee hound (a cross between a staghound and Irish setter) and the Quebec hound, a cross between various hounds and dogs native to the Province of Quebec.

In Europe, German shorthaired pointers are the most successful pulka racing dogs, and Norwegians are developing new crossbreeds more adapted to the race conditions in the Alps.

While sled dogs vary considerably in appearance, they share certain characteristics. Whether hound or husky, the top performers on today's racing teams have a strong slightly roached back, well-angled shoulders, and a deep chest denoting good lung capacity. Compact, tough feet and a protective coat of hair aid team dogs in performing their tasks. Size is an important factor, and contemporary racing dogs are relatively small, averaging 24 inches at the shoulder and weighing less than 50 pounds.

Optimal Conformation of a Racing Sled Dog

Until recently the optimal conformation of a racing sled dog was mainly determined by the practical experience of a musher. The first serious morphometric study concerning sled dogs competing at an international level was published in 1989.[4] By systematic measurements conducted for an 8-year period on hundreds of dogs, Gilchrist established a conformation database describing the skeletal efficiency of a racing sled dog. The first data to consider are the global balance of the dog. In an ideal dog, scapula, pelvis, humerus, and femur must have the same length; the average length of these four bones is called the constant (c) and is considered as a referral point for all the other parameters. Therefore, the following data pertaining to conformation will be given as a percentage of the constant:[5]

- The height at shoulder must be around 200 per cent of c.
- Distance between the elbow and the ground must be around 160 per cent of c.
- Tarsus to ground must be around 90 per cent of c.

Gilchrist also considers a few important points, such as the following:

- The length of the dog must be superior to his height by about 10 per cent.
- Angulation of the scapula must be between 32 and 34 degrees, and angulation of the pelvis around 30 degrees.

These results allow us to correlate some morphometric data to the biochemical potential of the dogs.

More recently, Fuhrer et al[5] demonstrated that a complete conformational study of the dog could be done while it was running on a treadmill, but without providing more information than the global method.

Finally, in 1994, Rooks[6] wrote about his results considering statistics from the 1994 Iditarod teams. For this author, skeletal efficiency becomes highly important as the correlation of increased stress placed on the biomechanical system as a result of the high speeds and long distances incurred in a race. An efficient skeleton will give the dog better "mileage" and fewer breakdowns. For Rooks, in measuring a dog, it is best to compare it with itself, and the dog's constant measurement is taken by averaging the four major bones—scapula, humerus, pelvis, and femur. The four major bones should be close to equal in length. Occasionally the scapula and pelvis will tend to be shorter than the humerus and femur. Marked differences in bone length can cause unequal biochemical stress on joints and probable orthopedic problems. Furthermore, the various classes of racing dogs may yield differences in ideal conformation; as a group the unlimited sprint class dogs tend to be smaller than the ones running in limited sprints.

Balance is the comparison of the measurements of the tibia/fibula (stifle to hock) and radius/ulna (elbow to carpus). Without balance of bone length, a dog may exhibit a "cow-hocked" stance and resultant imbalance in muscling. Vertical distance from the elbow to the ground is usually longer than the constant measurement; although the hock to ground distance is usually about 10 per cent shorter than the constant, the proportion of length to height is important.

From his 1994 Iditarod teams' statistics, Rooks also considers that the top team's dogs are taller and longer than all other competitors' (Table 2–3). The top line of the dog should be smooth, with a natural fall-away arch at the hindquarters, creating increased potential for speed. A swayback appearance indicates poor muscle tone and/or muscle quality. If a natural arch of the back is positioned too far forward (humpback), the result is a decrease in speed capacity.

TABLE 2–3. Symmetry/Conformation Measurements (in cm), 1994 Iditarod

Team Finishing Status	Height Front Leg	Height Back Leg	Back Length	Scapula	Front Leg Extension	Chest Circum.
1–5	61.5	60.5	35.7	8.0	63.1	63.0
6–10	59.6	58.3	35.7	7.7	61.1	63.8
11–15	61.5	59.4	34.9	8.3	62.2	65.4
16–20	57.9	57.5	34.6	8.0	59.9	62.7
Midpack	58.2	56.3	35.3	8.4	59.9	67.3
Backpack	56.5	55.1	34.4	8.1	58.6	65.9

From Rooks RL: Creating a winning team. Vet Check 1(3):4–7, 1994.

Flexion and range of motion are also highly important for racing sled dogs. An increased range of motion results in increased stride and less work over long distances; it takes fewer steps for these dogs to reach the finish line. Additionally, dogs with increased range of motion have fewer chances of injury. Too straight a leg (creating a shortened stride and increased work over long distances) leads to an increase in potential for cartilage trauma and orthopedic problems and impedes speed as well. More research needs to be done concerning the biomechanics of the racing sled dog and the precise determination of its optimal conformation, but some scientific work has started, and the future will see veterinarians able to provide more precise information to the mushers.

Sled dogs are now part of a sport in which men and women compete on an equal basis and in which women have claimed victories in both national and international events. Age is also not a deterrent to the sport, and victory is as sweet to the 3-year-old one-dog driver as it is to the 60-year-old big team driver. The whole sled dog sport now awaits its appearance in the Olympics.

References

1. Grandjean D: Le sport de traîneau à chien et ski-pulka. Rec Med Vet 167:589–593, 1991.
2. Levorsen B: 1992–1993 Sled Dog Sport Survey. IFSS ed. Pocatello, Id, 1994, p 6.
3. Friends of Northern Dogs (FOND): The Northern Dog. FOND. Elkhorn, Wis, 1994, p. 31.
4. Gilchrist L: Skeletal efficiency of racing sled dogs. Howl 12(3):20–28, 1989.
5. Fuhrer L, Dunlap H, Reynolds A: Evolution morphologique du chien de traîneau; conséquences biomécaniques. Rec Med Vet 167:659–665, 1991.
6. Rooks RL: Creating a winning team. Vet Check 1(3):4–7, 1994.

CHAPTER 3

HISTORY OF COMPETITIVE UPLAND GAME BIRD AND RETRIEVER DOGS

ESTHER McCARTNEY \ KEN McCARTNEY

Gun dogs in America come under three general classifications: pointing breeds, spaniels, and retrievers. While each breed has its own brief recorded history and more or less suspected origin, the parallels of development after registration begins are remarkable. The consequences of registration and formal competitions are such for each breed that a detailed look at the development of competition with emphasis on the most popular of the current breeds, its culture, and its direction helps understand the enthusiasm for gun dogs today.

For a student of history, the chronology of events that culminate in the modern retrieving breeds* parallels the increase in leisure time in the United States. In recent years, Labrador retrievers have gone to the top of the list of total breedings registered each year by the American Kennel Club.

There is little reliable ancient history for sporting dogs. For instance, there is no recognized connection with the name Labrador and the country of the same name. See reference 1 for a description of researching dog breed names. The source of the name is not known. In the early 1880s pure black water dogs were exported from Newfoundland. Trade wars between England and Newfoundland before 1830 limited exportation. It may have been during this era that the ancestors of the modern Labrador became Anglo-Saxon, although no recognized treaties commit to the origin for certain. The recorded history of dog breeds stems only to the formal breed clubs of England and America. As with most purebred dogs, the formality of registration for gun dogs began in the last century.

*Labrador retrievers, Chesapeake Bay retrievers, golden retrievers, flat coated retrievers, curly coated retrievers, and Irish water spaniels, as recognized for competition by the American Kennel Club for field trial competitions.

Clubs that provide for and register dog breeds have had a positive effect on preserving sought-after characteristics while pressuring less desirable genetics. Evolution continues both with the breed characteristics and working ability of the field dogs. It is more so with the animals' field work than with the basics of appearance. So many external variables contribute to success in the field that little or no scientific study has been employed to reveal patterns of success in field competitions. One thing common to the winners today is a great deal of hard work. Some pedigree or training techniques are found that make for better chances, but the odds are remarkably high against winning a National Retriever Club Field Trial no matter how the sport is approached. Before explaining what that level of competition involves, consider the development of the dogs, the clubs, and the competitions themselves.

THE CLUBS

Early breeders in both England and America were motivated to impress standards of conformity on recognized dog breeds. For animals with field-working potential, this promptly led to competitions. The registering organizations became involved with structuring competition. It was paramount that conforming animals be of classic proportion, finely coated, and able to meet certain field-working standards. What is a retriever without the ability to retrieve a shot bird?

The conformity competitions expanded slightly at first to recognize working traits, but soon field competition took on a following all its own.* Enlightened breeders in America attempted to breed dual-quality champion animals, dual quality meaning classic retriever looks with hardy, blocky bodies (eg, bench champions) and stylish retrieving skills (eg, FC, AFC, NFC).† To the credit of many fine breeding programs, several dual champions were made in the early years of competitions, and occasionally dual champions are still made.

Satellite competition–sanctioning organizations have come and gone, but none maintains the preeminence of the American Kennel Club. Nearly 20 per cent of the American Kennel Club members are field trial clubs.[2]

In addition to the old line clubs, the old line breeders responsible for the clubs had a healthy effect on the breed and were responsible for the cliquishness of the early sport. Unfortunately the stabilizing effect offered by the classic big name kennels of the past, where conscious multigeneration decisions were made in the breed's best interest, which actually impacted the gene pool significantly, is largely gone today. A "successful" individual stud dog can have a remarkable effect on the breed. The large number of breedings occurring indicates much less emphasis on planning the lineage. Neighbors or competitors are likely to get together and plan one litter or discuss a stud dog's potential with a gun dog bitch on a one-time basis. Gone are the documented several-generation programs.

REGISTERING

The earliest efforts to bring order to that element of the canine population that evidenced a willingness to retrieve occurred in

England in the late 1880s. It was a full and proper endeavor most appropriately reserved to the nobility, for whom leisure time existed.

The English Kennel Club listed the Labrador as a represented breed by 1904. The first English Labrador club was organized in 1916. In 1931 the interest of wealthy American breeders resulted in the breed being recognized by the New York Corporation that today dominates registered dogs—the American Kennel Club. As with all show breeds, emphasis was placed on body shape and coat, and only a slight measure of retrieving performance was required by the original standard. It was not unheard of for the landed gentry to "compete" their retrievers in the field. As early as 1899 there were recorded competitions for retrieving dogs in England. The breed took on a new direction in the United States in 1931, when on Long Island, New York, the first American field trial took place. In the nearly 70 years since, competitions for retrieving dogs have expanded steadily in the form of dog versus dog in AKC licensed field trials, and since the late 1980s, in the form of dog versus test in Hunting tests.

The trend in field dogs is away from the classic body style. Working-dog owners tend to have an unholy deference to the looks of the breed. Many of today's field champions would be listed as "part lab" if they turned up at the local dog pound. The rigors of the field have generally downsized the successful field trial dog. To hold up over a long time of competition, athletic ability is far more important than a shiny coat, blocky head, or other definition.

HISTORY OF COMPETITION

Given a baseball, a bat, and a glove, it is not necessary to play the game of baseball, but the temptation is astronomical. Yet only a small percentage of the baseball players in the world make it to the big leagues. For a summary of trials held and dogs entered, see reference 3. It is not necessary to take a retrieving puppy to a hunting dog test or field trial, but what goes on there, naturally, sets a standard of performance and accomplishment that is emulated throughout retrieverdom. A good hunting dog needs to be able to do a blind retrieve, respond to a whistle, come when it is called, wait to be released to retrieve, sit quietly for oncoming game, respect another working dog, and generally adhere to the "conditions observed in the average day's hunt," which give rise to the AKC's standard for non-slip retriever trials.

To understand the dogs in competition today, it helps to be aware that the flavor of the sport has evolved from its aristocratic inception. Until 1939, no amateur won an open field trial competition. The early trials were run by hired professional dog trainers and handlers for the benefit of dog breeders—to share vicariously in their dogs' accomplishments. It was not until 1951 that competitions were sanctioned by the AKC for amateur handlers. Professionals began "national" competitions (for dogs that qualify in local trials) in 1941. Amateurs did not enjoy this same striving for excellence until 1957.

World War II had a significant effect on the sport. Many professional retriever trainers were enrolled in the K9 Corps of the US Army. Not surprisingly, retriever competition records for years after reflect many of their names. As in England, trainers working for American kennels considered their station and traveled, ate, and drank separately from their employers. It was not until the late 1950s that their "Mister" and "Sir" relationship began to erode.

Professional trainers have made the transition from servant to educator. The quality of the amateur trainers and handlers has understandably improved. The sport has taken a remarkable hands-on turn. Although, in the early years, large kennel names dominated the retriever breed, now the number of breedings has skyrocketed.

---

*The American Kennel Club registering of purebred retrievers allows affixing certain titles to the mane of accomplished retrievers.

†AFC-Amateur Field Champion, FC-Field Champion, NFC-National Field Champion, NAFC-National Amateur Field Champion, CFC-Canadian Field Champion, CAFC-Canadian Amateur Field Champion (also CNFC and CANFC).

The stakes run 42 weekends each year by 207 AKC trial holding clubs, including two National All-Age Championship Stakes.

Nearly every community has AKC-registered retrieving puppies for sale from time to time.

The professional trainers and handlers for owners with substantial resources still dominate the sport. Retrievers travel well. They can ride in a vehicle, confined in a small space with minimal daily exercise. Many opportunistic professionals travel with 24 or more competitive animals for weeks of competitions in a row.

PRICE OF COMPETITION

The investment required to have a competitive retriever continually escalates. To begin with, a successful competitor requires a special animal. The desire to retrieve has to be higher than average, and the willingness to train with discipline has to match the trainer's tendencies. It is also necessary to have good eyesight and sound physical characteristics, as the average champion begins training at the age of 6 months and can be expected to title at or around the age of 6 years. While there are several washout stages, an animal on the fast track can be sold to a field trial home at any stage in the process. Field trial competitive retrievers sold in the early 1990s at prices ranging as high as $50,000, which is best appreciated when one considers that the life expectancy of a finished competitor is probably less than 6 years.

The average sportsman can expect a registered puppy to cost from $300 to $800. Professional training to a quality hunting stage usually costs $900 to $1800. Many field trial washouts sell in the range of $1500 to $1800. With modern dog food costing more than $1.00 a day, and routine vet service, absentee care, and normal living accommodation costs factored in, a sporting dog is certainly no small investment. For most owners, the return is well worth the cost.

Unfortunately the success rate of puppy selection from a litter of eight (on average), in the absence of any known scientific method, is as low as the numerical probability at best. Seldom do more than one or two puppies in a litter become accomplished field trial competitors.

After selection, the training process is expensive and/or very time consuming. Beginning when the dog is around 6 months of age, basic vocabulary has to be taught, forced, and reinforced, all the while combining plenty of field retrieving, which is best done with live birds to maintain style and desire. Training is complicated by the animal's short interest span. Seldom can a training session exceed 10 to 15 minutes. Boarding, training fees including live birds, ammunition, and travel to and from ideal training locations can cost over $750 monthly in 1997.

The cost of competition is not insignificant and is compounded by the AKC prohibition against cash prizes. A retriever is recognized with points, championships, qualifying to compete in national competitions, in puppy price, or stud fees, or perhaps in sale price, but not in terms of dollars won. Competition entry fees approach $50 per stake per weekend, and dogs run by professionals are normally charged at least the price of the entry by the handler. Many trial dogs run 20 to 25 competitions each year, their owners hoping to qualify them for both the open and amateur national trials, as well as an occasional Canadian weekend when the American registered dogs are welcome.

COMPETITIONS

Early American field trials were organized by men and women of great affluence and lofty social position. Many gained experience traveling to Scotland for the aristocratic pheasant drives and patterned their shooting after the preserves and gamekeepers of the old country.

TABLE 3–1. NRC 1992 National Championship Statistics

Dogs Qualified		Dogs Entered		Dogs Scratched	
97		97		2	
Starters by Breed and Sex					
Black Lab males	55		Black Lab females		24
Yellow Lab males	4		Yellow Lab females		1
Golden males	1		Golden females		0
Chesapeake males	0		Chesapeake females		0
No chocolate Labs were qualified					
Oldest Dog		**Youngest Dog**		**Average Age**	
3/6/82		10/29/89		6.8 years	
Dogs Handled by Men			**Dogs Handled by Women**		
74			11		
Dogs Handled by Pros			**Dogs Handled by Amateurs**		
46			39		

From Retriever Field Trial News, vol 28, no 9, p 12, January 1993.

This influence caused testing the dogs on land to predominate the early competitions. A different approach began almost from the start with Chesapeake Bay retrievers. This breed was recognized as far back as 1880, and the American Breed Club dates from 1918. These animals traditionally sought game birds in the icy waters of the Chesapeake Bay and were reported early to have been assisted by hand signals.

In the mid 1930s a growing number of all-breed retriever trials forced the Labrador trainers and others to concentrate more energy on water work to keep up with the Chesapeake. During the late 1930s and early 1940s, the traditional Scottish land drive format gave way to a format modeled after that used at first by the Chesapeake clubs. It is this format that has evolved to the modern field trial (Tables 3–1 and 3–2).[4, 5]

Instead of the hidden Scottish gunners and all freshly shot flying birds, today's competitions allow for exposed official gunners, usually in pairs, standing clearly visible in the field. They throw birds so that each competing dog watches the fall. This allows for the use of dead birds and offers uniformity for the increased

TABLE 3–2. NARC 1993 National Amateur Statistics

Dogs Qualified	Dogs Entered	Dogs Qual/NE	Dogs Scratched
130	95	34	1 (1 after no. 5)
Starters by Breed and Sex			
Black Lab males	59	Black Lab females	26
Yellow Lab males	8	Yellow Lab females	0
Golden males	2	Golden females	0
No Chesapeake or chocolate Labs entered			
Oldest Dog	**Youngest Dog**		**Average Age**
4/14/82	5/14/90		6.47 years
Men Handlers			**Women Handlers**
71			24

NE, not entered.
From Retriever Field Trial News, vol 29, no 5, p 7, August/September 1993.

number of entries. Gone are the time-consuming tests involving questing for a crippled fall.

As the dog skill level has grown through better breeding and better training, judges have devised multiple marked retrieves, often using separate sets of guns at much longer distances than would exemplify traditional hunting conditions. "Blind" retrieves have become much more difficult and demand extremes of discipline and willingness to perform. The popularity of the electric dog training collar has grown in the last dozen or so years to the point where it is the norm rather than the exception, and as a result, there seems to be no limit to the number of whistles a modern retriever will accept and to which a meaningful response can be anticipated.

While the standard still describes a field trial in terms of the average day's hunt, in practice the trials have drifted away from typical hunting situations. While field trial dogs make fine hunting companions and, in fact, partially trained field trial washouts are hotly sought after by the average hunter, much more precision and discipline at far greater distances are required of the competitor than the hunter. Field trial tests can easily range over 300 yards for both marks and blind retrieves. Crippled birds, for instance, are generally called "no birds" and a more uniform situation substituted for the classic dog opportunity they represent.

A current criticism for the modern field trial has given rise to a new form of competition. It is frequently said that licensed AKC field trial competition is too intense. Field trial dogs, required to place number 1 in a field of 100 good dogs, are necessarily too mechanical, too well trained, and completely unnatural. Instincts are ignored, and discipline is substituted for desire. To this end a new form of competition has arisen in the last half dozen years—hunting tests. It is here that retrievers are challenged to complete the judges' setup test, rather than to be compared to the other dogs doing the same work. Successfully completing certain tests warrants titles: junior hunter, senior hunter, master hunter, etc. Some overlap is inevitable into and out of both forms of competition. Numbers of competitors in this form of field competition are rising steadily.

References

1. Maxwell BC: The Truth About Sporting Dogs. New York, Howel Book House, Inc., 1972.
2. Retriever Field Trial News, vol 27, no 6, p 7, October 1991.
3. Retriever Field Trial News, vol 28, no 10, p 6, February/March 1993.
4. Retriever Field Trial News, vol 28, no 9, p 12, January 1993.
5. Retriever Field Trial News, vol 29, no 5, p 7, August/September 1993.

CHAPTER 4

ORIGIN, HISTORY, TRAINING, AND UTILIZATION OF SEARCH, RESCUE, AND TRACKING DOGS

ALICE J. STANLEY

In our long relationship with dogs, it has been their keen scenting ability that has proven useful time and again to provide early warning of an intruder, to aid in the hunt for food, and even to search for lost humans. In the last instance, the dog's ability to discriminate human scent from all others has been applied for both criminal and humanitarian purposes. It is the humanitarian aspect, the use of dogs trained for search and rescue (SAR), in which perhaps the phrase "man's (or woman's) best friend," is most applicable. Dogs trained for this work are special animals in a job with equally special demands and hazards.

When one is considering the health and safety of SAR dogs, a basic knowledge of training, scent theory, and the unusual situations and hazards they face is essential. While a discussion of specific injuries and illnesses will be covered in later chapters, it is prudent to briefly state here both the more common and the more unusual as each is determined by the type of mission being performed by the dog. Veterinarians knowledgeable in the history, training, and use of SAR dogs will be prepared for the prevention or treatment of injuries and illnesses the dogs may encounter. They will be able to instruct handlers in first aid and help assemble emergency field first aid kits for those occasions when the immediate assistance of

a veterinarian is not available. Veterinarians who practice in the area where a search is occurring, whether they commonly encounter SAR dogs or not, will also be able to respond with the added benefit of understanding the work and training of these dogs.

Before a discussion of the use of dogs in search and rescue, a definition of terms is required. There are two primary descriptions of scent work in SAR: tracking and airscenting.

TRACKING DOGS

The origin of the use of tracking dogs to search for both game and humans is lost in antiquity, although the modern concept and training methods began in Europe and spread to the United States in the mid 1900s. American Kennel Club (AKC) Tracking Tests began in 1936 and, in the 1950s, the Baltimore Police Department became the first to utilize tracking dogs in law enforcement work.[1] Today, tracking remains a vital aspect of law enforcement canine training for both criminal and SAR work.

There are technically two definitions that fall under the term *tracking*. The first, the word *tracking* itself, generally refers to a dog that works with its nose to the ground, following precisely where the person walked. There is continuing debate whether the dog actually follows "human scent" or follows the scent of disturbed and crushed vegetation left by the movement of the person through the area. In all probability it is both. However, because we can only speculate what "scent" is to the dog, that debate is better left to other sources. It is important only to realize that the dog can follow a person's "track" and can discriminate between ground scents left by two or more people.

The second definition is of the "trailing" dog. This dog will frequently move to a fence line, ditch, or similar "collecting" point several feet from the track, where it is assumed human scent has been blown by the wind. Often the trailing dog works with its nose several inches above the ground, moving back and forth, searching for what is essentially scent residue. This dog is undoubtedly following human scent, since there obviously would be no crushed vegetation away from the missing person's actual path of travel.

Because many tracking dogs also "trail," both are usually referred to as tracking dogs and encounter the same problem of track destruction by time, weather, and/or contamination by other people. Tracks are basically bacterial in nature and subject to a limited lifespan. The longer the time lapse, the less the scent strength, and the less likely the dog is to successfully complete the track. Extreme exposure to heat and sunlight, extended time lapse, and trampling of the area by others will eventually destroy the missing person's scent. Because of the track's relatively fragile nature, these dogs are most successful in criminal cases in which law enforcement officers can seal off the area to prevent inadvertent contamination by others. Also, law enforcement agencies are contacted immediately after committing of a crime, and the dog, normally handled by a member of the department, can arrive on the scene quickly while the track scent is still strong. Under these conditions, tracking dogs prove highly useful not only in leading officers to the subject but also in placing a subject at the crime scene (scent discrimination) and in locating evidence discarded as the criminal left the scene.

Tracking dogs are also utilized by private citizens for search and rescue, and the AKC offers titles for both Tracking Dog (TD) and Tracking Dog Excellent (TDX). While many dogs achieving the AKC titles may not be applied in actual search situations, they can encounter the same hazards and problems as working dogs.

Training these dogs begins with working fresh, minutes-old tracks, normally of people they know, and progresses over a period of weeks or months to tracks of strangers that are allowed to "age" for several hours. The reward system varies, depending upon the dog's use (law enforcement or civilian) and the handler's preference. Civilian dogs are usually rewarded with food, praise, or play. Police dogs are generally rewarded in training with a "bite" of the "victim," who is protected either by a heavily padded sleeve or by a full body suit, although they are trained not to bite on actual missions unless the handler is endangered. Most tracking dogs are worked on-leash, which is particularly crucial in criminal cases when the person sought may be dangerous and the dog must remain within sight and control of the handler at all times. This by no means guarantees the dog's safety, however, because the dog works in rugged wooded terrain where it may encounter snakes, ticks, and natural hazards that can result in sprains, strains, fractures, bites, and similar injuries.

These dogs are often very focused and, unless watched closely by the handler, may literally run themselves into exhaustion. They tend to track with their mouths closed, thereby inhibiting the natural cooling process of panting, and heatstroke must be a major concern. For this reason, handlers must be prepared to physically stop the dog and offer it water frequently.

One unique injury associated with police tracking dogs is, of course, potential bullet wounds. On more than one occasion, the dog and handler have run up on a criminal who responded by opening fire. For safety purposes, another armed officer usually accompanies the handler, who is busy watching the dog, but the possibility always exists for such an injury.

The use of tracking dogs also requires careful attention to the proper harness. Because the dog pulls strongly when on the track, the use of collars is extremely dangerous; choke collars are never used, and even leather collars can severely damage the dog's throat or neck. For this reason, special nonrestrictive harnesses are preferred. These harnesses are normally of the figure-8 type, which consists of leather straps around the dog's neck and middle, with connecting straps that run down the back of the neck and between the front legs. Such harnesses do not place any strain on the dog's shoulders and balance the pull between the back and chest.

As with all SAR dogs, tracking dogs represent months, even years, of training and must frequently work under the most trying conditions. Annual physical examinations, coupled with appropriate vaccinations and heartworm prophylaxis, are crucial to both their work and their well-being.

AIRSCENTING DOGS

The second type of SAR work involves the airscenting dog; this work is based on a principle entirely different from tracking. Airscenting dogs do not seek where the person *has* been (the track), but rather where the person *is* at the moment. This is accomplished by the dog working with its nose high in the air, much like a bird dog, seeking the airborne human scent. The airscenting concept had its American origins in Seattle when Bill and Jean Syrotuck began training dogs for search work in the early 1960s.[2] The Syrotucks trained their German shepherd dogs for tracking, but soon found this method too limited for most search situations. Family and friends of missing people often conducted their own search before calling authorities, which so contaminated the surrounding area that any track was virtually destroyed. Although the dogs were trained in scent discrimination, this relied upon a "pure" scent article belonging to the victim, one untouched by others. All too frequently, another family member would carry the article to the handler, thereby contaminating it with his or her own scent. In addition, the person may have been missing for many hours or days before "outside" help was called in, further limiting the potential success of traditional tracking dogs.

The Syrotucks learned of a method employed by the US Coast Guard during World War II in which dogs were trained to locate downed aircraft by seeking the airborne scent of aircraft fuel. Reasoning that dogs could be taught to seek airborne human scent (composed of the dead skin cells shed by humans, called rafts), they began a program of research and training to prove their theory. Experimentation by the Syrotucks showed this scent could travel for long distances, could be funneled by terrain features such as drainages, would rise or fall with the hot or cool air, was filtered or hindered by dense vegetation, and was constantly produced by all humans, living or dead. Using this knowledge, they developed search strategies that always placed the dog downwind so the scent would be blown to the dog as it worked across the wind, back and forth in wide sweeps, until the entire area had been covered. After proving the airscenting concept a viable alternative to tracking, the Syrotucks began developing training methods for both dogs and handlers.

Because the scent traveled such long distances and the slower handler could hamper the dog's enthusiasm and ability to follow the scent, they trained the dogs to work off-leash, which, in turn, led to yet another discovery: After making a find, the dog would excitedly return to the handler, looking for its reward. Using this natural enthusiasm, they created the "refind"—the dog returns to the handler, indicates a "find" with body language, then turns and leads the handler back to the victim.

One of the most crucial lessons learned was the importance of motivation. The dog would be asked to work long hours, day after day, in the worst terrain and weather. To actively, eagerly search for a stranger, it would need a strong, consistent reward system. Praise was not enough, because the dog had little interest in praise from a stranger. Food was ineffective, because the dog might not be hungry at the moment of the find (often the case in extreme heat), or it might be asked to work disaster areas strewn with food (a distraction, to say the least). By observing which dogs were the better workers, the Syrotucks found that play with a tangible object, such as a stick or ball, provided that crucial motivation. Dogs with a strong play drive were by far the most enthusiastic and reliable workers, making that drive one of the most important in selecting potential search dogs.

Once the basics of training were established, the Syrotucks developed standards of performance for both dogs and handlers. Handlers had to become experts in first aid, map and compass, victim behavior, terrain analysis, and a myriad of wilderness skills. Dogs had to be completely obedient, agile enough to handle the most rugged terrain, and sociable enough to safely endure crowds of people, including small children. The Syrotucks found the German shepherd dog to be ideal for the work, and to this day the organization they founded, the American Rescue Dog Association (ARDA), requires the use of German shepherds.

Other attributes determined to be requirements for the working search dog include: large enough to handle any type of terrain, yet small enough so that three or four fit into an Army helicopter; a double coat that provides natural insulation against weather extremes; a structural build that enables it to work tirelessly hour after hour, day after day, in all terrain; the temperament to be an enthusiastic searcher, yet calm enough to handle even the most unusual situations; and, a proven scenting ability.

In addition, the dog needs a certain amount of independence to range off-leash ahead of the handler and to work scent to its source without direction, possibly over hundreds of feet, then return to the handler on a refind and lead the handler to the victim. That independence has also been shown in instances in which these most highly trained dogs have ignored a handler's commands because the dog knew if it obeyed the command it would miss the victim. SAR work requires the handler's utmost trust in his or her dog and is one of the most impressive arenas for demonstrating the dog's intelligence. Clearly the dog's ability to handle search work rests not only on scenting ability but also on its rapport with its handler. This rapport is developed by a combination of search, obedience, and agility training.

Search training begins as short, simple problems with the dog finding its handler, and progresses over several months to working longer hours to find a stranger. Each find is rewarded by an exciting play session, with both the handler and the "victim" participating. In obedience the dogs are expected to be under complete control at all times, on- and off-leash, and must know the normal commands, such as heel, sit, and down. They also must immediately "drop" to a down position when given a hand signal by the handler (critical in a noisy or distance situation in which the dogs must be stopped but the handler might not be heard giving a verbal command) and to come or stop instantly when their course would take them into danger, as on a busy highway or the edge of a cliff.

Agility, achieved by work on an obstacle course, is also an extremely critical part of the dog's training. Many injuries can be prevented if the dog has developed, through proper obedience and agility training, the instant control and self-assurance needed to handle rough terrain. Search dogs are required to climb ladders, walk narrow planks, cross teeter-totters (unstable footing), scale ramps, crawl through narrow spaces, and overcome other similar obstacles, all while under the handler's total voice control. When the dog is working, that training is proven time and again when the handler is able to watch the dog safely negotiate shaky footing or can stop the dog with one word if it approaches what seems to be a bottomless chasm.

After establishing these performance standards and training requirements, the Syrotucks founded ARDA in 1972, with five units spread across the country. Today, ARDA has more than doubled in size and the overall use of search dogs has grown rapidly, with more than 100 units now providing this service at various levels of skill and experience. The Syrotucks' development of airscenting dogs introduced a versatile element to SAR work, ranging from wilderness missions to disasters to drownings. All of these applications, whether they involve tracking or airscenting dogs, entail hazards peculiar to each type of mission, and the following breakdown sets out situations encountered by working SAR dogs.

TYPES OF SAR MISSIONS

Wilderness. These usually involve heavily wooded terrain, ranging from mountains to swamps.

Search dogs working wilderness missions encounter a variety of hazards, including insect stings, snakebite (Fig. 4–1), fractures, shock, hypothermia or hyperthermia, temporary disability from skunk spray (which can destroy the dog's scenting ability for an extended time as well as irritate the eyes), and gastric torsion. An important precaution for search dogs is maintenance on heartworm medication year round, because they may be called to work areas in which heartworms are endemic.

Disasters. These missions may involve searching collapsed structures after earthquakes, volcanic eruptions, tornadoes, hurricanes, and other natural disasters, as well as buildings destroyed by explosions. American dogs have been used on missions ranging from the 1980 Mount Saint Helen's eruption to the 1994 Los Angeles earthquake (Fig. 4–2) and the 1995 Oklahoma City bombing.

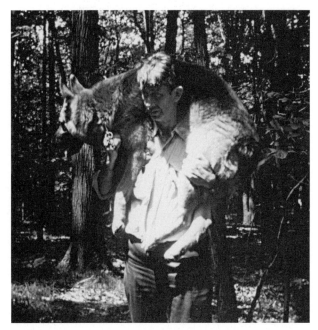

FIGURE 4–1. Field first aid can be critical; handler carries dog bitten by rattlesnake. (Photo courtesy of American Rescue Dog Association.)

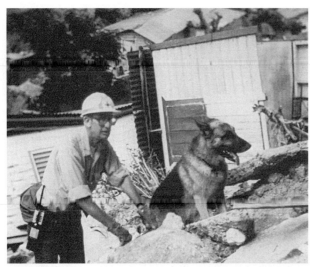

FIGURE 4–2. An ARDA team searches for victims amid the rubble of the Puerto Rican mudslides, 1985. (Photo courtesy of American Rescue Dog Association.)

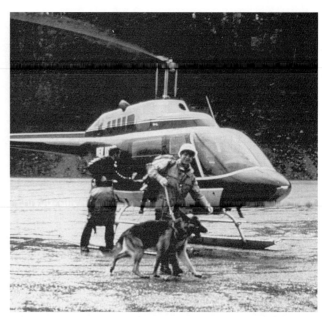

FIGURE 4–3. Search dogs are frequently transported by helicopter (note turning rotor blades). (Photo courtesy of American Rescue Dog Association.)

Disaster missions share many hazards common to wilderness work, including insect bites and hypothermia. However, disasters may be in a part of the United States different from the one in which the dog commonly works, or even in a foreign country. A handler accustomed to the Midwest, for instance, may not be prepared for scorpion stings the dog suffers while working the scene of a tornado in the Southwest. Again, the assistance of a veterinarian can be invaluable for briefing handlers on a much broader range of first aid than normally required for "local" wilderness missions.

The stress level for disaster work is often high, since the dog may be quartered in cramped tents thousands of miles from home, with different water, limited supplies, and the pressure of hours spent working in hazardous conditions. Additionally, transport to remote areas may require the use of helicopters or military transport aircraft, which, to save both time and fuel, load and unload the dogs without shutting down the engines, thereby submitting them to an incredible amount of noise and further stress (Fig. 4–3).

On-scene hazards range from the possibility of collapse of a weakened structure on the dog during an earthquake aftershock to a fall down an unseen elevator shaft. Chemical and poisonous gases may be leaking, and propane explosions can occur. Footing is extremely insecure over shifting rubble (booties are rarely worn because the dog loses its feel and its ability to grip with its toes). Objects wait to impale the unsuspecting dog, including reinforcing steel bars ("rebar") that protrude from broken concrete, shards of glass, nails, and countless other items that can pierce the dog's foot, chest, or eye.

Most disaster sites are remote, with normal transportation lines severed, and handlers who have some knowledge of critical-care first aid will be better prepared to handle these situations. A detailed first aid kit, its use well understood by the handlers, is mandatory, particularly when responding to foreign countries.

Drownings. Dogs may be used to locate victims partially or totally submerged in water; these searches may be conducted either from a boat or from the shore.

Another unique application of airscenting dogs, also developed by an ARDA unit (Virginia), is their use in locating drowning victims. It is believed the dog picks up scent carried to the surface by oxygen bubbles rising in the water, and that this scent is probably a combination of skin cells and body gases. Dogs have indicated the location of drowning victims as long as a month after the incident and in depths of up to 100 feet.

Heatstroke is a continuing concern for dogs working drownings, since the dogs often ride in the open bow of a boat, where the sun's heat is made worse by its reflection off the water. Dogs must be offered water frequently and watched closely for signs of hyperthermia (Fig. 4–4).

Although all search dogs should be taught to swim, water searches carry with them the possibility of drowning if the dog becomes trapped in swift currents or by other obstacles. For this reason, handlers must be instructed in CPR, as veterinary assistance

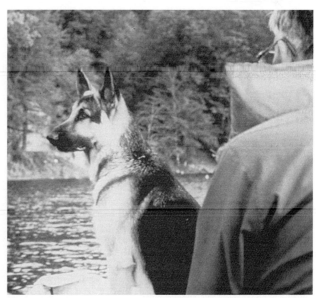

FIGURE 4–4. Drowning searches expose dogs to heatstroke as they ride in the open bow of a boat. (Photo courtesy of American Rescue Dog Association.)

would rarely be timely enough to ensure the dog's survival. The danger of propellers is also a problem, although most handlers work the dogs on-leash so they can be ''reeled'' back into the boat should they fall overboard. Searches of the shoreline entail the same hazards as any wilderness search.

Cadaver Searches. Normally these are conducted under wilderness conditions, searching for the remains of a subject suspected or known to be deceased (Fig. 4–5).

Although some believe the dog must be specially trained to find cadavers, ARDA units have successfully found bodies months after death with no special training other than the normal use of live volunteers at regular unit training sessions. These dogs react to bodies the same as to live victims, with strong ''alerts'' (indications of human scent by body language), ''close-ins'' (leaves the handler, works the scent in to its source), and refinds. The hazards faced during these searches are the same as for any wilderness mission.

Avalanches. The dog may be used to locate victims buried beneath snow and ice.

In 1969, Jean Syrotuck's dog made the first find of an avalanche victim by an American-trained dog, and today the use of dogs on these missions is common. Obviously the greatest hazard is from subsequent avalanches, and although avalanche areas are carefully regulated so emergency evacuation can be accomplished rapidly, the possibility of a dog and handler being trapped under snow and ice remains a very real danger.

Search dogs, whether tracking or airscenting, must be maintained as any other dog, with annual physical examinations and vaccinations. However, they are susceptible to problems occurring far from any professional assistance. Because of this, veterinarians familiar with the work they do can be of invaluable assistance to handlers by ensuring that those handlers are well prepared to cope with field emergencies to keep the dog alive until it can be taken to the hospital. Above all, it must be remembered the well-being and survival of a search dog may mean the well-being and survival of a human.

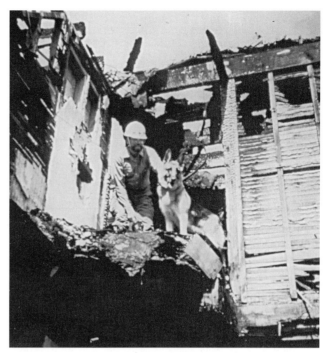

FIGURE 4–5. Dog/handler team searches for victim on second floor of a burned-out house. (Photo courtesy of American Rescue Dog Association.)

References

1. Davis W: Go Find. 2nd printing. New York, Howell Book House, 1974, pp 12, 18–19.
2. American Rescue Dog Association: Search and Rescue Dogs: Training Methods. New York, Howell Book House, 1991, pp 1–11.

CHAPTER 5

ORIGINS AND HISTORY OF SECURITY AND DETECTOR DOGS

PAUL B. JENNINGS, Jr.

The origins of security and detector dogs lie in the protective role dogs have fulfilled for humans since the beginning of time. History is replete with examples of dogs as guards for primitive peoples, their use as attack dogs by Assyrians, Egyptians, Romans, Middle Age armies, and even Napoleon's famous dog, ''Moustache.''[1] The dog's sentry and scouting capabilities were recognized early and used by such diverse groups as North American Indians and the nineteenth century armies of Germany, Russia, and France.[2] The Germans introduced dogs for law enforcement in the late 1880s and by 1911 had 500 police stations using dogs, primarily German

shepherds and Doberman pinschers.[3] The city of Ghent, Belgium, was the first to establish a school for police dogs, in 1889.[4] Soon thereafter, police dogs began to appear in the cities of the United States, with New York City initiating its program in 1907.[5]

Although police needs prompted canine use, war and the threat of war frequently have provided the impetus for military uses of dogs. In the 1880s the German army began to train dogs to perform scout duty with infantry patrols and rifle batallions and to carry messages between the front and headquarters.[2] Sentry dogs also were assigned to jaeger batallions. Dogs were used for sentry and scout duty in the Russo-Japanese War in 1904–1905, the Italo-Turkish War in 1911, and the Balkan Wars in 1912–1913.[6]

When World War I began, the nucleus of military dog use was in place for the German, British, French, Italian, and Belgian armies. Duties included transporting people, goods, and weapons; guarding ammunition dumps, prisoners, and food supplies; doing sentry duty in the trenches; delivering messages; pulling sleds in the Alps; and being first-aid dogs. This was the largest use of working dogs in history, with estimates of 30,000 dogs being used by the Germans and 5000 each by France, Great Britain, and Italy.[1, 2, 6] The British and Belgians lent some trained dogs to the American Expeditionary Forces later in the war; however, the United States did not train dogs of its own during this conflict.[7]

Between world wars, Germany opened a large dog training school in Frankfurt, but the only American military interest in working dogs was for sled dogs in Alaska.[6]

When the United States entered World War II, no formal military dog program yet existed. Through the determined efforts of American dog fanciers and some interested Army officers, a group of major dog clubs formed an organization called Dogs for Defense to promote dog use by the military for the war effort.[2] This group voluntarily acquired and trained dogs that were used primarily in sentry work at war plants and quartermaster installations (Fig. 5–1). The Remount Branch of the Office of the Army Quartermaster General then took over administration of the program, plus training and shipment of dogs for all services, while Dogs for Defense continued to procure the dogs, most of which were donated by patriotic Americans. Initial dog use was for sentry duty along the East, West, and Gulf coasts and munitions factories inland. Eventually, training facilities were constructed at Front Royal, Virginia (messenger dogs), Fort Robinson, Nebraska (attack dogs), San Carlos, California (attack, scout, messenger dogs), Camp Rimini, Montana (sled dogs), Beltsville, Maryland (attack, scout, first aid, messenger), and Cat Island, Mississippi (jungle warfare) (Fig. 5–2). The first six scout and two messenger dogs, which were sent to the Pacific Theater in the spring of 1943 as part of a test program, worked well[8] (Fig. 5–3). The scout dogs warned patrols of the presence of the Japanese within a range of up to 1000 yards. Because the messenger dogs did not work as well under combat conditions, their use was curtailed. Between December 1944 and June 1945, 15 Infantry Scout Dog platoons were organized and shipped overseas, seven to Europe and eight to the Pacific. The

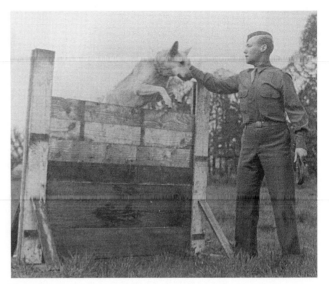

FIGURE 5–2. World War II dog "Duchess" jumping over hurdle at K-9 Training Camp, 1943. (Photo courtesy of United States Army.)

Marines also made successful use of scout dogs in the Pacific Theater.

When the Germans and Italians began using nonmetallic land mines in North Africa, the first canine mine detector unit was activated by the Allies in 1943. The dogs were taught to indicate the position of a buried mine by sitting down near it. When the dog encountered a trip wire, it was trained to halt or refuse to advance. The two mine detector units sent to North Africa proved

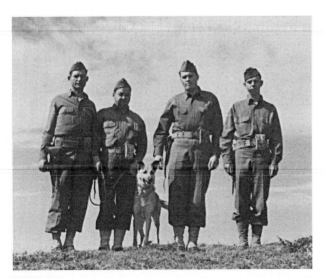

FIGURE 5–1. World War II sentry dog "Pal" with trainers and handlers in Newfoundland, 1942. (Photo courtesy of United States Army.)

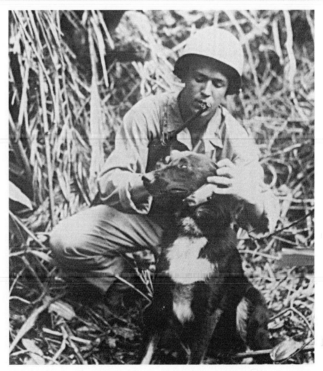

FIGURE 5–3. Pouch being placed on neck of messenger dog "Teddy" by his handler, a member of the 26th Quartermaster War Dog Platoon, Aitape, New Guinea, 1944. (Photo courtesy of United States Army.)

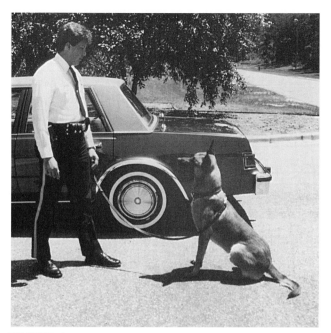

FIGURE 5–4. United States Secret Service dog training to detect explosives in a vehicle. (Photo courtesy of United States Secret Service.)

to be ineffective under battle conditions, and further training of mine detector dogs was abandoned.

The US Army trained a total of 10,425 dogs during World War II; 8531 were issued in the United States and 1894 were shipped overseas.[8] Additional dogs were issued to the Navy, Marines, and Coast Guard.

Following World War II, many military dogs were deprogrammed and returned to their owners. Although several dog breeds had been tried and used during the war, the German shepherd finally was selected as the one breed for the military, because of temperament, size, strength, availability, and adaptability to all climates.[8]

Before the outbreak of war in Korea, the United States Army was using more than 100 dogs for sentry duty. Only the 26th Infantry Scout Dog Platoon from Fort Riley, Kansas, saw active duty in Korea, although five additional scout dog platoons were trained.[9] Following Korea, only the 26th Infantry Scout Dog Platoon was retained. The military dog program was transferred to the United States Air Force in 1958, and a training center was established at Lackland Air Force Base, San Antonio, Texas.[10]

Beginning in the late 1950s, use of dogs in civilian police work expanded, and by 1961, police departments in 120 cities had dogs, primarily German shepherds.[11] These dogs were used as a psychological deterrent, for searching, and in defense of the handler, in tracking, and in crowd control.[12]

Between the Korean War and in the United States involvement in Vietnam, the military showed little interest in the use of dogs. The French forces in Algeria and Vietnam and the British in Malaysia continued to use dogs in scout, tracker, and sentry duty. In 1960 the US Military Assistance Advisory Group, Vietnam, suggested that military dogs be used by the South Vietnamese Army to combat Vietcong terrorism. An Army of the Republic of Vietnam (ARVN) Scout and Sentry Dog Program was established and, by September 1962, 327 dogs were assigned to the ARVN forces.[13]

US forces first brought working dogs to Vietnam in 1965 with the Military Police. The first Scout Dog platoon arrived in 1966,

and at the end of that year, 673 US dogs were in Vietnam. By August 1969, the US Army had 601 scout dogs, 302 sentry dogs, and 26 tracker dogs; the US Marines had 66 scout dogs and 59 sentry dogs; the US Navy had 35 sentry dogs; the US Air Force had 450 sentry and patrol dogs; and the ARVN had another 450 dogs. Only a few mine and tunnel dogs were sent to Vietnam, and reports of their effectiveness were mixed.[13]

Following Vietnam the infantry abolished the scout and tracker program. Procurement and training of dogs for all of the military services was again centralized with the Air Force in Texas. Sentry dog training was eliminated in favor of the use of patrol dogs, which are more manageable, have some scouting capability, and can work in crowds, both on- and off-leash.[7, 10] Henceforth, only Military Police units would be authorized to use dogs.

In the late 1960s and early 1970s, illegal drug use became a major problem among young people in the United States and among service personnel in Vietnam. Drug detector dogs were developed for the military services, and domestic canine drug deterrent programs mushroomed. Today, many state and local police forces have narcotic detector dogs, and many such dogs—plus military dog teams—are aiding the US Border Patrol and the US Customs Service.[14–17]

In the 1960s, a few federal law enforcement agencies saw the need for a bomb detection program. In 1971, under the auspices of the US Army Land Warfare School at Aberdeen, Maryland, dogs were tested and found capable of detecting dynamite and plastic explosives. The Federal Aviation Administration (FAA) began using bomb dogs in 1972. In March of that year, a German shepherd dog and its handler found a bomb in a briefcase at John F. Kennedy Airport in New York.[18] The FAA henceforth implemented a K-9 Explosive Detector Team Program, in which dogs are procured by the Department of Defense, and handlers and dogs are trained at Lackland Air Force Base for use at most major international airports.[10]

The US Secret Service also has bomb detector dogs for protection of the President and other leaders (Fig. 5–4).

Relatively recently, explosive detector dogs have been used in Afghanistan to clear roads mined by the Russians (who left in 1989). A US-supported program has trained dogs and mujahideen handlers to open mined roads so that refugees can return to their homes.[19, 20]

A dog that can perform more than one task saves handlers, reduces needs for kennels, and provides maximum utilization of dog and handler time. Early attempts in the 1960s to cross-train scout and sentry dogs were unsuccessful.[13] Dual training has been effective with patrol-explosive and patrol-drug dogs. These dual-

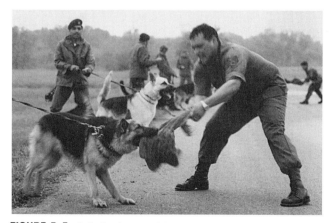

FIGURE 5–5. Agitation is part of the controlled aggression training of a patrol dog. (Photo courtesy of United States Air Force.)

trained dogs can detect and can protect their handlers if challenged. Not all dogs are suitable for this combined training. Under the present program, detector training comes first. If the dog completes detector training successfully but does not pass the patrol training portion, it can be reclassified as a straight "contraband" dog (Fig. 5–5).

At present the Department of Defense procures, trains, and transports certified dogs for all the military services, plus providing explosive detector dogs for the FAA. The FAA needs nonaggressive breeds because of the need to use dogs in crowds, at airports, and with world leaders. Sporting breeds—especially Labrador and Golden retrievers—have been used effectively by this agency.

As can be seen from this overview, the interest in dog use by the US military has been sporadic, whereas police requirements have been fairly consistent when a need has been identified. It has always been difficult to convince military commanders that a dog can do anything better than their own high-tech sensor devices. It is only when the US has become involved in situations in which only a dog can locate and track the enemy, guard the facilities, or detect drugs and explosives that an urgent call has come to "Give us some dogs." The European military, however, although having some of the same skepticism as the Americans, has consistently kept its dog units active. I have visited the Swiss, German, Austrian, and British military forces and have seen firsthand how they have continued to use dogs effectively. The British, for example, have used tracker and bomb detector dogs very effectively in Northern Ireland.[21]

We have not seen the end of dog use by military forces. Dogs with military skills (especially detector) are being used effectively to guard our borders, airports, and seaports and are actively participating in the war on drugs and terrorism. In the event of future conflict, these unique canine skills can be adapted readily for military duty.

References

1. Trew CG: The Story of the Dog and His Uses to Mankind. New York, EP Dutton & Co., 1939, pp 88–101.
2. Downey F: Dogs for Defense: American Dogs in the Second World War. New York, DP McDonald, 1955, pp 1–12.
3. Judy W: Training the Dog. Chicago, Judy Publishing Co., 1948, pp 130–135.
4. Brockwell D: The Police Dog. New York, GH Watt, 1924.
5. Wright R: Police dogs; how a versatile program can survive budget cuts. Police Chief 51(1):18, 1984.
6. Stauffer AP: The War Dog Program. Historical Section, General Administrative Services Division, Office of the Quartermaster General, Washington, 1943, pp 1–14.
7. Tietjen SB: The other soldier; military working dogs. Pure-Bred Dogs/American Kennel Gazette 99(9):35, 1982.
8. Dogs and National Defense. Department of the Army, Office of the Quartermaster General, Washington, 1958.
9. Haggerty AJ: Dogs in war; a special collection. Pure-Bred Dogs/American Kennel Gazette 108(6):71, 1991.
10. Military Working Dogs. US Air Force Fact Sheet, Lackland Air Force Base, Texas, 1992.
11. Leonard VA: The Police of the 20th Century. Brooklyn, The Foundation Press, Inc, 1964, p 49.
12. Leonard VA: Police Patrol Organization. Springfield, Ill, Charles C Thomas, 1970, pp 75–79.
13. Clark WHH: The History of the United States Army Veterinary Corps in Vietnam, 1962–1973. Roswell, Ga, WH Wolfe Assoc, 1991.
14. Ross K: K-9 narcotics detection training. Police Chief 55(5):53, 1988.
15. Suthard RL: Law enforcement's best friends. Police Chief 58(1):50, 1991.
16. Francis C: Border Patrol's star "sniffers" lead drug war. Dog World 73(7):16, 1988.
17. Francis C: Are drug dogs fighting both sides? Dog World 78(1):37, 1993.
18. Berluti FF: Connecticut's explosive-detecting canines. Police Chief 58(10):59, 1991.
19. Francis C: Sniffers in Afghanistan. Dog World 76(5):13, 1991.
20. Francis C: Mine-detecting dogs secure Afghanistan. Dog World 76(6):14, 1991.
21. Durrant GR, Director, Royal Army Veterinary Corps and Remount Services: Personal communication, 1990.

SECTION II

PHYSICAL EXAMINATION

CHAPTER 6

SOUNDNESS EXAMINATION OF THE SPORTING CANID

JAMES R. GANNON

Sporting activities such as greyhound racing, game retrieval, and sled dog racing result in many types of injuries. However, the same general principles of examination are involved, whether it is conducted by a veterinarian only or by the owner, trainer, or breeder, with added clinical appraisal by a veterinarian.

The purpose of the procedure is to detect any problem or abnormality that may affect the performance of the subject and to determine whether the aberration is temporary or permanent in any animal intended for sale, lease, sporting performance, or breeding. The guiding principle of a thorough soundness examination is to take a comprehensive approach rather than to restrict the procedure to one or two body systems. In effect, the examiner will investigate the musculoskeletal, circulatory, respiratory, and nervous systems, and will perform a selected clinical pathology scan.

MUSCULOSKELETAL EXAMINATION

This includes an assessment of stance, superficial musculature, and joint mobility using simple observation, manipulation, and palpation, respectively. These procedures may be undertaken competently and efficiently with or without veterinary assistance. However, the detection of an area of concern or of gross abnormality would signal the need for definitive diagnosis and therapy by a veterinarian.

The following steps should be included in the examination procedure or at least considered a foundation upon which to build a more specific protocol: observation of the stance and gait; assessment of the range of flexion and extension of the joints of the trunk and limbs; palpation of the superficial musculature; cardiorespiratory examination; and a complete blood count plus biochemical profile.

Observation and Palpation
Step 1

The investigator should stand directly in front of the subject and make the observations. Squatting or sitting directly in front of the

animal permits greater precision. Note whether the nails, nail beds, joints, and toe angulation—including the dew claws—show any abnormality. This is a time to detect split or broken nails, infected nail beds, sprung toes, dislocated toes, swollen sprained toes, dropped toes, knocked-up toes, all of which are considered in Chapter 27. Any injury to a *limb* will usually result in a redistribution of body weight and consequent uneven stance; for example, an inflamed, painful wrist will be larger and carry less weight than the normal injury-free joint.

The *elbows* should be located close to the body; elbows held out from the body indicate joint or muscle injuries leading to impaired action when the weight comes down on the affected limb. At the same time, observe the *chest* for any variation in shape and size, as injuries to these muscles affect stability during performance because of inability to hold the forelimb close to the body. Both *shoulders* normally have the same shape and contour, although injuries to the muscles, bones, and joints of the shoulder area may be associated with swelling, atrophy, or changes in weight-bearing capacity. These lead to shape and contour changes, obvious when both sides are compared simultaneously, but which may not be obvious when each is viewed separately from the side.

The *head* is carried squarely without rotation or sideways deflection unless the dog has sustained injuries to the neck vertebrae or muscles, which usually results in some degree of head or neck displacement. Check the *lips* for any signs of brown rusty "lip-lick" stain. This discoloration is frequently associated with infection of the sheath in the male or vaginal infection in the female, dental tartar, gingivitis, or tonsillitis and may persist for 4–6 weeks after correction of the initial problem. The *ears* sit evenly unless they sustain damage to their tips and margins or are producing a waxy discharge. Chilblains and fly worry (see glossary) will cause cracking and bleeding of the tips and margins. Ear discharges are associated with bacterial and fungal infections, parasitic infestations (fleas and mites), or foreign bodies (grass seeds) in the ear canal, all of which may affect ear carriage. Finally, observe the *eyes* for size, symmetry, pupil size, corneal changes (such as cloudiness, pannus), or discharges.

Step 1 should normally take about 1 full minute if no abnormalities are detected that require further detailed examination.

Step 2

The subject should be standing squarely, with the weight evenly distributed on all four legs. The examiner should move to the rear of the subject, squatting or sitting at arm's length from the hindquarters and make the following assessment: The weight should be distributed evenly on each *hindlimb*. Limbs with an injury will carry less weight. Mild injury results in lifting of the hip and thigh, while severe injury causes lowering of the hip and thigh of the affected limb.

Common *calcaneal tendon* injury results in swelling either locally or along the full length of the tendon, and any such changes are readily observable at this stage of the examination process.

Check for any evidence of "track leg" ("Jacks") along the inside edge of the *shin bone* on either side. Jacks or track leg is a swelling varying from soft to firm consistency, occurring on the inside edge of the tibia (shin bone) caused by striking this area of the bone on the outside of the elbow or forearm when the hindlimb sweeps past the forelimb during each stride. It occurs most commonly on the left hindlimb but may occur on the right or both hindlimbs. The outside border of the shin bone, where the large vein (lateral saphenous) crosses, is a common site for fracture of the fibula, also characterized by a firm swelling just above or below the prominent vein. Moving up to the calf area, one can inspect for any difference in the size or shape of the gastrocnemius and superficial digital flexor muscles. Increased thickness occurs with tearing of the muscle tendon junction, while decreased thickness (disuse atrophy) follows reduced muscle use associated with bone, joint, or local muscle injury of the lower limb.

The size or contour of the muscles of the inside of the *thigh*—especially at the distal end of the gracilis muscle—requires special attention, as changes in shape in this area are associated with tearing of the muscle fibers or muscle sheath, either of which can seriously impair performance. Also, observe for any difference in the size or contour of the muscles on the outside of the thigh, especially the largest—the biceps femoris—because ripples, corrugations, or deep splits in the sheath of the outer thigh muscles will impair performance if not given prolonged and intensive therapy.

Shape changes about the *hips* and hip-thigh junctions may be due to deformity of the ilium (dropped hip) or to tearing of the sheath or fibers of the hip muscles—tensor fasciae latae and gluteal muscles. The *tail* should be straight and carried close to the body. Tail kinks result from fractures and dislocations, and tail elevation is associated with infection of the vagina and/or infection of the anal sacs. Swelling of the base of the tail, associated with pain on manipulation, and elevated carriage may be due to fracture, sprain, or dislocation at the tail base subsequent to local trauma. In the male, both testes should be fully descended. In the female, any abnormal vulval swelling, discharge, or skin lesion should be noted.

Step 3

The dog should be standing with the weight evenly distributed with the examiner directly behind the dog, enabling the following observation: The *head* must be carried squarely, without rotation or deflection to one side, and the ears will appear normal and matching. The *neck* should be straight, with the muscles on each side of even shape, size, and contour. Any deflections suggest major structural damage, while dimples and ripples in musculature indicate muscle sheath or fiber tearing. The shape, size, and contour of the muscles of the *shoulders* call for careful inspection. Marked

deformities may be associated with tears of the triceps muscle or the supraspinatus or infraspinatus muscles of the shoulder blade. Recent injury is accompanied by inflammation and swelling—old injury with fibrosis and contracture. Similarly, the shoulder blades (scapulae) should be symmetrical, without variations resulting from previous fracture.

In the *saddle area* (trapezius and thoracic rhomboid muscles), any dimpling, withering, or tearing of the muscles results in a distinct depression, whereas normally the back should be straight and level with the top of the shoulder blades and flowing smoothly into the muscles of the neck. When examining the *rib cage* from above, look for small changes that may be due to fracture or other rib injury, or marked changes that may be associated with lung damage. Examine the muscles along the *backline* for changes in size or contour. Irregularities here may be due to muscle sheath or fiber tears, atrophy from previous rhabdomyolysis, or damage to the spinal vertebrae. Inspection of the *hips* for matching size and contour complements the inspection made in Step 2.

Step 4

The examiner sits or squats on the left side of the dog at arm's length and observes the toes, including the nails, nail beds, the joints, and position of each toe, checking for sprung toes, dislocated toes, knocked up toes, and dropped toes.

The *metacarpals* require close attention, particularly the middle third of the left fifth metacarpal and the proximal third of the right second metacarpal, as these are the specific sections of the metacarpals most subject to stress in the greyhound running at speed in a counterclockwise direction on the turns of the track. If the normal remodeling process is unable to cope with the stresses imposed by the racing and training program, the dog sustains injury ranging from periostitis to cortical bone fissure fractures to full shaft fractures—all characterized by dorsal aspect changes. Swelling or enlargements on the palmar aspect of the fifth metacarpal usually indicate injury to the abductor digiti quinti or flexor tendon. While swelling on the dorsal aspect of the *wrist* is readily apparent, similar changes in the palmar region require closer inspection. Tearing of the insertion of the flexor carpi ulnaris muscle causes swelling around and above the accessory carpal bone (stopper bone), whereas chip and full fractures of the latter result in more swelling around and below the bone. Examine the *feet* for bilateral symmetry and weight distribution.

Observe the *elbow* for any conformation abnormalities or swellings. Round fluid swellings on the point of the elbow (olecranon) and over the bony prominence at the side of the elbow indicate bursitis. This is an inflammation of the lubricant envelope (bursa) interposed between the skin and the bony prominences. Pressure from lying on hard surfaces, or knocks and bruising to these locations, results in distention and swelling of the bursae. In the *shoulder* area, look carefully for any swellings due to torn muscles. These are most commonly seen over the upper portion of the long head of the triceps muscle and over the muscles lying immediately behind and parallel to the bony ridge running down the middle of the scapula or shoulder blade (the infraspinatus and deltoideus muscles). Attention should also be paid to atrophy, contracture, or change of contour of the muscles of the shoulder area. Inspect the *chest* for fluid accumulation under the skin at the bottom of the chest along the breast bone. Such swellings usually indicate chest or shoulder muscle tears, in which bleeding and inflammatory fluids from the injury gravitate downward to the chest area. Note any excessive arching of the back or shape changes to the backline muscles. Excessive arching is most commonly due to abdominal discomfort or spinal strains or displacements.

Observe for any change in shape or swelling at the *hips* and top of the *thigh*. Of major concern is the triangular muscle (tensor fasciae latae) at the top of the thigh just under the hip bone, where serious tears resulting in swelling and discomfort are relatively common. The thigh is inspected for any ripples or irregularities in shape indicating splits and tears in the muscle sheaths. The *stifle* joint may be swollen, puffy, or unduly flexed as a result of sprain or injury within the joint or to the associated support tissues. The common calcaneus tendon and its muscles behind the stifle are inspected for obvious swelling, withering, or other shape change. The tibia is now checked for swelling on the outside of the bone in the area of the lateral saphenous vein. Swelling here is due to a fracture of the fibula bone, as noted in Step 3. Now look carefully at the *hock* for any swelling. Soft fluid or doughy swelling is due to sprains or to bleeding following fractures. Firm hard swellings indicate healing callus from previous injury.

Swellings in the front of the *metatarsus* are caused by tendon strain of the cranial tibialis and/or digital extensor muscles or from stress fractures of the metatarsal (quarter) bones, particularly in the area of the upper half of the fifth metatarsal and the top of the second and third metatarsals. Swelling behind the metatarsals at the upper end just near the hock may be due to an avulsion fracture of the fifth metatarsal bone or to a condition called *curb*, which is a strain of the superficial digital flexor tendon in this area. The foot and toes are observed in the same way as the front foot.

By lifting the dog's left hind limb, the examiner has a clear view of the abdomen and the inside of the opposite hind limb. In this area the skin is so thin that one can see through it and observe the underlying muscles and veins. Look for swelling and discoloration due to bruising and bleeding, usually due to tearing or severe strain of the underlying muscles, especially the pectineus muscle and the gracilis muscle at the rear half of the inside of the thigh. Note also the sheath of the male and check for excessive discharge. On the female check for enlargement of the mammary glands owing to milk formation following an estrous cycle.

Step 5

This examination is also undertaken with the subject standing squarely with the weight distributed evenly on all four legs. The observer squats or sits facing the right side of the animal at arm's length and makes precisely the same observations as those carried out on the left side. This also will take up to 1 minute to perform, giving a total of up to 5 minutes spent on a simple but thorough observation of the subject.

Step 6

This step consists of observation of the *gait or limb movements* as the dog walks on various surfaces. In most cases this can be more readily carried out during the normal morning and evening exercise period. For dogs exercised in the poor light of early morning and late evening, and for those exercised mainly on walking machines, it may be worthwhile to conduct this brief

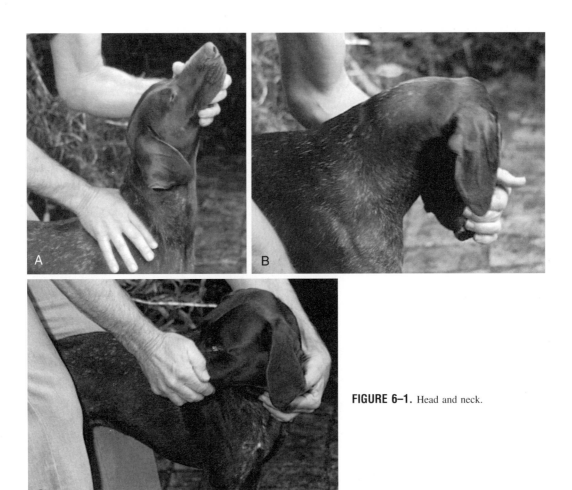

FIGURE 6–1. Head and neck.

examination. With the dog on a loose lead, the examiner walks in front of, behind, and to the side to observe any dipping, limping, or scuffing of the nails of any of the feet. Make sure that the action of each limb is checked on different surfaces, eg, grass, asphalt, or concrete, and then on gravel, as some lamenesses are not apparent on some surfaces.

All trainers are capable of conducting this simple observation procedure. It takes less than 6 minutes and can be done at any convenient time or location. Once a routine is developed, the examination time can be shortened even more, but it is time well spent as it yields a great deal of helpful information.

Manipulation Procedure

A hands-on examination of the limb joints is used to assess flexibility and detect injury to joints and associated structures resulting in discomfort on flexion or extension. The procedure is detailed in a video from the American Greyhound Council (see Suggested Readings).

Stand the subject squarely with the weight evenly distributed. The trainer stands astride the subject so that it is positioned comfortably between the legs, facing the same direction. The examination is conducted as follows:

Head and Neck (Fig. 6–1)

1. With the hand under the animal's chin, elevate its nose so that the head and neck point vertically upward.
2. With the hand on the nasal bones, gently push the head downward to bring the tip of the nose to the front of the chest.

3. With the hand on the side of the face, bend the head and neck around slowly and gently to bring the tip of the nose close to the ribs, first on one side of the body and then on the other.

Result

Any pain or resentment shown by the subject indicates injury to the muscles, vertebrae, joints, or ligaments of the head and neck region and will require veterinary investigation.

Left Forelimb—Elbow and Shoulder (Fig. 6–2)

1. With the hand grasping the middle of the dog's forearm, flex the elbow joint as fully as possible. Release the limb.
2. With the hand grasping the metacarpal region of the foot, draw the limb backward and upward until the elbow is level with the spine and the toes approach the hip. This fully flexes the shoulder joint and partly extends the elbow joint.
3. With the hand behind the elbow, raise the forelimb upward and forward until the front leg is parallel with the ground. This fully extends the shoulder, elbow, and wrist joints.

Result

1. If the subject forcibly resists full flexion of the elbow, there is a strong possibility of an injury in the elbow joint, of the ulna immediately distal to the olecranon, in the biceps or triceps muscles, or in the shoulder joint.
2. If the subject shows pain on flexion or extension or both of the shoulder joint, there is a strong suspicion of injury within that joint (osteochondritis dissecans) or to the supraspinatus, infraspinatus, deltoideus, or biceps brachii muscles.

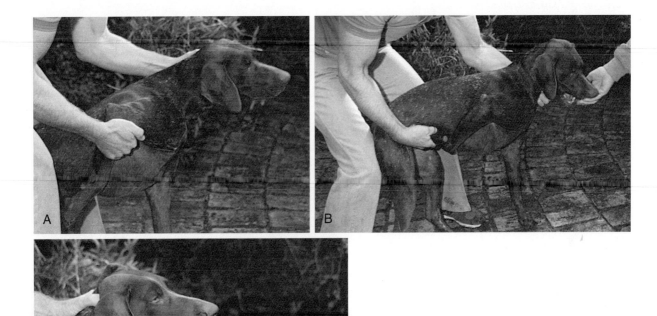

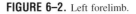

FIGURE 6–2. Left forelimb.

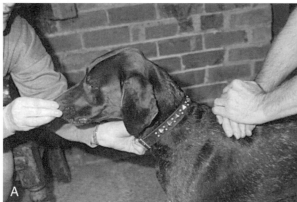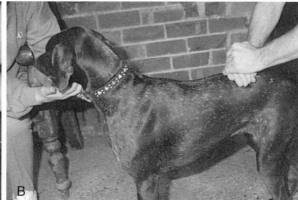

FIGURE 6–3. The back.

3. When the foot is drawn upward and backward to fully flex the shoulder, it will be noted that the elbow joint locks in a 90-degree position. If the elbow straightens out instead of staying in the 90-degree position, there may be tearing of the biceps brachii muscle or injury to the transverse ligament holding it in the bicipital groove of the humerus.
4. If the wrist fails to extend and the foot hangs down when the elbow is lifted upward and forward, there has been tearing of one or both of the tendons on the front of the forelimb (extensor carpi radialis and/or the common digital extensor).

Right Forelimb—Elbow and Shoulder

Repeat the procedures outlined for the left forelimb.

Back (Fig. 6–3)

1. Press firmly with the fingers on the muscles of the dog's saddle area (thoracic rhomboid).
2. With the palm of the hand on the bony vertebral spine, apply firm, sharp, downward pressure along the whole of the spine from the shoulder blades to the hip bones.
3. With the hands under the chest, lift the forefeet 10 to 20 cm from the ground, noting any discomfort or resistance by the animal.

Result
1. Pain in the saddle muscles may indicate exertional rhabdomyolysis.
2. Discomfort on spinal upward or downward pressure indicates spinal displacement.

Left Hindlimb: Hip, Stifle, and Hock (Fig. 6–4)

1. With the left hand on the front of the stifle and the right hand on the right hip of the subject to maintain balance, draw the left hindlimb backward until the fully extended limb is parallel with the ground.
2. Grasping the metatarsal bones below the hock joint, lift the foot upward and forward until the toes reach the level of the shoulder joint.
3. With the pads of the foot in the left hand, and the right hand on top of the stifle, firmly flex both hock and stifle. Note the distance between the toes and the stifle joint when the limb is in the fully flexed position. When the same procedure is carried out on the right hindlimb, note whether the distance from the toes to the stifle joint is the same on each side.

Result
1. Pain or resistance by the animal on fully extending the leg backward often reflects injury in the hip joint or the thigh or groin muscles.
2. Pain or resistance on drawing the foot toward the shoulder may indicate fracture of the hock or metatarsal bones, sprain of the hock joint ligaments, or injury to the common calcaneus tendon or its muscles of origin.

Right Hindlimb—Hip, Stifle, Hock

Repeat the procedures outlined for the left hindlimb.

Left Hind Foot (Fig. 6–5)

With the right hand supporting the metatarsal area, use the left hand to fully flex and extend each of the phalangeal and metatarsophalangeal joints and the tarsal joint. Rotate the metatarsus medially and laterally.

Result

Discomfort on movement of the phalangeal joints may reveal arthritis, sprung joint (sprain), dislocation, or torn dorsal elastic ligaments. Pain or reduced range of movement at the metatarsophalangeal joint is usually associated with sesamoid bone fracture, ligament sprain, dislocation, or distal epiphyseal fracture of a metatarsal. Resistance on straightening of the hock suggests injury to the joint ligaments, tendon insertion of the cranial tibial muscle, or possibly periostitis or a stress fracture of a metatarsal bone. Discomfort on rotation of the foot may be the result of tarsal ligament sprain or stress fracture of a metatarsal or hock bone.

Right Hind Foot

The manipulative examination of fully flexing, extending, and rotating is performed in the same manner as that used to examine the left hind foot.

Left Front Foot (Fig. 6–6)

Fully flex and extend each of the dog's phalangeal and metacarpophalangeal joints and the carpal joint. Rotate the metacarpus medially and laterally, and then with the thumb apply upward and downward pressure on the accessory carpal bone.

Results

Discomfort on fully flexing and extending each of the three toe joints reveals the same problems outlined in the examination of the

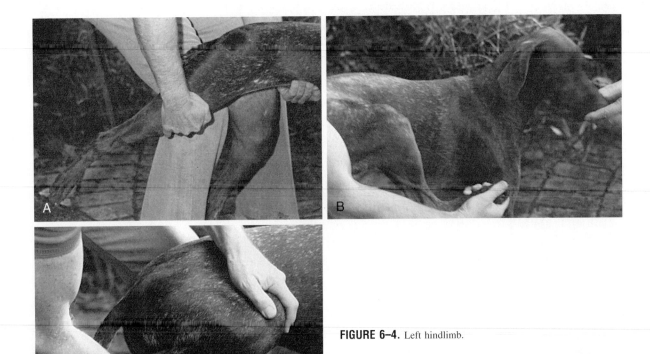

FIGURE 6–4. Left hindlimb.

hind foot. Pain on full flexion of the wrist has a range of possible causes, eg, metacarpal periostitis or hairline fracture, arthritis within the wrist, damaged insertion of the extensor tendon (extensor carpi radialis), sprain of the accessory carpal bone (stopper bone) ligaments, or avulsion fracture of the accessory carpal bone. Discomfort on outward rotation of the wrist indicates injury to the muscles and ligaments beside and below the accessory carpal bone (abductor digiti quinti and distal accessory carpal ligaments). Discomfort on inward rotation of the wrist indicates strain of the flexor tendons and the ligaments at the back of the wrist. Pain on accessory carpal bone pressure suggests avulsion or full fractures, sprain of the accessory carpal bone ligaments, or injury to the insertion

of the flexor carpi ulnaris muscle on the upper border of the accessory carpal bone.

Right Front Foot

The examination procedure parallels that used for examination of the left front foot.

Summary

Manipulation of each joint is quite a rapid procedure; the entire examination can be completed in 3 to 5 minutes. Each joint is

FIGURE 6–5. Left hind foot.

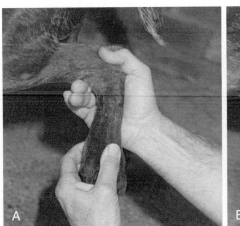
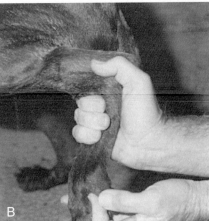

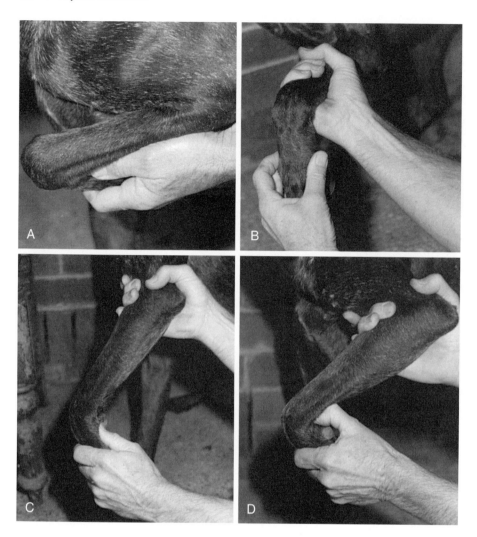

FIGURE 6–6. Left front foot.

moved through its full range of movements three to five times at each examination. This will indicate any reduction in mobility as well as any injury or abnormality.

The loosening of the joints also relaxes tense and tight muscles associated with normal joint movement. Thus, trainers will find that free swinging and manipulation of the limbs and the joints becomes a form of physiotherapy with diagnostic and relaxing values.

Palpation

This section of the examination is more time consuming than the other two parts and requires an appreciation of the superficial anatomy of the sporting canid. Palpation utilizes the thumb and tips of the fingers to examine the periphery and then the belly of each of the readily palpable muscles of the forelimbs, hindlimbs, and trunk. The aim is to detect muscular defects, ie, fascial tears, fibrosis, inflammatory swelling, changes in texture due to bruising or exudates, and areas of increased sensitivity resulting from mild to severe trauma. Digital pressure is firm enough to produce a distinct sense of recognition of muscle tone and the above discernible changes without causing pain or discomfort to the normal musculature.

CIRCULATORY EXAMINATION

Sporting canids exhibiting postexercise ataxia, cyanosis, prolonged recovery, and exercise distress should undergo a pre-exer-

cise and postexercise assessment of the circulatory system by a veterinarian.

RESPIRATORY EXAMINATION

Clinical history is of particular importance. A nonproductive husky cough of short duration (1 to 6 hours), occurring only after exercise, is indicative of exercise-induced bronchoconstriction similar to exercise-induced asthma of humans. A persistent productive cough is more commonly associated with lung and respiratory infection, suggesting a need for microbiological culture and sensitivity testing and parasitic investigation of the respiratory exudates. While standard stethoscopic and radiological procedures will suffice in most appraisals, bronchoscopic inspection of the airways may be required to ascertain the cause of respiratory embarrassment.

Chapter 12 deals with these and related problems in more detail.

NERVOUS SYSTEM EXAMINATION

The sporting dog undergoing a soundness examination will rarely be found to have a major neurological problem because of the impact this has on performance. However, determination of suspected spinal disorders may require sampling of cerebrospinal fluid, with plain or contrast media radiology in addition to physical examination, to obtain a likely prognosis. See Chapter 10 for further information on neurological disorders.

CLINICAL PATHOLOGY EXAMINATION

The *complete blood count* will reveal any anemia, bacterial and some viral infections, acute allergic responses, and excessive stress as reflected in hyperadrenocortical changes.

Serum biochemistry will indicate liver and kidney damage, electrolyte disturbances, mineral imbalances, bone pathology, heart and skeletal muscle damage, endocrine disorders such as thyroid deficit, and digestive enzyme aberrations.

Full use should also be made of *microbiological studies*, including culture and sensitivity testing of swabs taken from the respiratory, digestive, and reproductive systems, particularly when chronic, recurrent, or nonresponsive episodes are experienced.

Suggested Readings

Blythe L, Gannon JR, Craig M: Care of the Racing Greyhound. American Greyhound Council, 1994.

Gannon JR: Soundness Examination of the Racing Greyhound. Video tape, American Greyhound Council, 1994.

Hungerford JG (Ed): Proceedings 122—Greyhound Medicine and Surgery. Sydney, Post Graduate Committee in Veterinary Science, University of Sydney, 1989.

Miller ME, Christensen GC, Evans HE (Eds): Anatomy of the Dog. Philadelphia, WB Saunders Company, 1964.

SECTION III

MEDICAL PROBLEMS

CHAPTER 7

STRESS- AND PERFORMANCE-RELATED ILLNESS IN SPORTING DOGS

STEVEN A. HOLLOWAY

WHAT IS STRESS?

Stress is any stimulus, as fear or pain, that disturbs or interferes with the normal physiological equilibrium of an organism.[1] It may also be defined as physical, mental, or emotional strain or tension. Both of these definitions are applicable to the effect of stress on the performance of canine athletes because both physical and emotional stresses may result in physiological changes that reduce athletic potential. It is well known from physiological studies in humans and rats that almost any type of physical or mental stress can lead within minutes to greatly enhanced secretion of adrenocorticotropic hormone (ACTH) and, consequently, cortisol.[2] Comparatively little has been published in the scientific literature about the effects of stress on the pituitary-adrenal axis in the racing greyhound, and even less scientific information is available on the effects of stress on performance of the various sporting breeds. Despite these limitations, many veterinarians are familiar with common "stress-related" clinical syndromes in racing dogs. The purpose of this chapter is to describe stress-related diseases in sporting dogs and apply knowledge from physiological studies in other species to describe the pathogenesis, diagnosis, treatment, and prevention of stress-related diseases.

PERFORMANCE PHYSIOLOGY AND THE EFFECTS OF STRESS

A dog's athletic ability depends on a variety of physiological variables, including cardiac output, red blood cell number and volume, respiratory oxygen extraction, and muscle mass and fiber type. Additionally, the desire to chase a lure may be just as important in greyhound racing as the physical characteristics of a dog. There are no other normal stresses to which the body is exposed that even nearly approach the extreme stresses of heavy exercise. In fact, if some of the extreme stresses were continued for prolonged periods, they would be lethal. For example, during a 400-meter race a greyhound's temperature may increase to 105° F (42° C), packed cell volume may increase to over 70 per cent, blood pH may decline to less than 7.0, and cardiac output may increase up to several times normal.[3] To race successfully, athletic dogs must maintain a constant metabolic environment that is closely adjusted by the neuroendocrine system. Stress factors such as injuries, poor nutrition, or infections result in disturbance of the normal homeostatic mechanisms. It is not surprising then that even small stresses can alter the normal physiological characteristics of a canine athlete and can cause marked reductions in athletic performance. In greyhound racing a few tenths of a second can separate first from last place. For this reason the effects of a diverse range of even minor stressful stimuli need to be considered when an athletic dog is investigated for the problem of losing performance.

Typically, stressful stimuli result in a stereotyped and nonspecific neuroendocrine response mediated through the sympathetic nervous system and hypothalamic–pituitary axis. Almost any form of stress produces immediate changes within the pituitary–adrenal axis.[2] In humans, mental stress has been shown to lead to a rapid increase in ACTH secretion and cortisol production resulting from increased limbic system activity transmitting signals to the posteriomedial hypothalamus.[4] Physical stress in the form of infection, inflammation, or tissue damage stimulates the release of humoral factors from the body's mononuclear phagocyte system (monokines). During strenuous exercise, eccentric muscle contraction (ie, involving contraction of muscles as they are lengthened) increases the production of the monokines interleukin-1 (IL-1) and tumor necrosis factor-α (TNF-α).[5] IL-1 and TNF-α act on the hypothalamic region of the brain to initiate a neuroendocrine response that increases the production of glucocorticoids (cortisol), catecholamines (epinephrine), and glucagon. These factors alter normal tissue metabolism in such a way as to meet the body's immediate needs. In the short term the hormonal stress response may be beneficial, allowing rapid mobilization of amino acids and fats from their cellular stores. This in turn supplies both energy and substrate for the synthesis of other compounds, including glucose, needed by the different tissues of the body. Amino acids become available to be used to synthesize intracellular substances such as purines, pyrimidines, and creatine phosphate that are necessary for reproduction of new cells.[4] Additionally, cortisol has potent anti-inflammatory effects that may be beneficial in the short term in some diseases.

Although the initial neuroendocrine response to stress is beneficial, continued response results in development of physiological exhaustion. Under conditions of continued stress the production of cortisol would be expected to ultimately result in development of hyperadrenocorticism (Cushing's disease). Fortunately, the rising plasma concentrations of glucocorticoids limit their own production by inhibiting pituitary ACTH release in a process known as *negative feedback*. Despite this regulation, during severe and prolonged stress the secretory spike frequency of ACTH increases, and glucocorticoid levels rise and continue to rise at high concentrations over extended periods.[6] Although overt hyperadrenocorticism does not develop, it is now becoming clear that effects of prolonged stress can lead to a variety of physiological changes (including immune suppression and tissue catabolism) that are deleterious to the animal.

The exact nature of the immunosuppressive effects of glucocorticoids in dogs with chronic stress is not known. This is because most of the research on the immunosuppressive effects of glucocorticoids has been largely done in the glucocorticoid-sensitive species such as rats and rabbits, and the results may not be directly applicable to dogs.[7] However, clinical observation would suggest that a similar pattern of immunosuppression occurs in dogs exposed to exogenous or endogenous glucocorticoids. With severe stress, endogenous cortisol production is sufficient to cause overt changes in the leukogram. Characteristic glucocorticoid-induced changes include leukocytosis with neutrophilia, monocytosis, lymphopenia, and eosinopenia. Glucocorticoids decrease neutrophil adherence and tissue migration and predispose the body to infection. Decreased macrophage phagocytic ability and ability to process antigens may also occur with increased exposure to glucocorticoids. Glucocorticoids also decrease circulation of T lymphocytes, suppress lymphocyte activation, decrease response to mitogens, and reduce antigen recognition and cytotoxic ability.[7]

Exercise itself should be regarded as a stress factor affecting the immune system. Studies in humans suggest that exercise induces a cascade of coordinated hormonal responses that influence the behavior of immune cells.[5] Although acute time-limited exercise produces increases in glucocorticoid production, it is unlikely that this is solely responsible for the immunomodulation occurring with exercise. During exercise the release of epinephrine, glucocorticoids, monokines, and β-endorphins influences both the blood flow and function of the immune organs. Despite variations in the type, duration, and intensity of exercise, there are consistent patterns that emerge regarding the effects of exercise on the leukocyte subpopulations of the blood.[5] With acute time-limited exercise, neutrophil populations increase in the period during and after exercise. Natural killer (NK) cells, B cells and T cells are all recruited to the blood during exercise, and the total lymphocyte count increases. T-Helper cells decrease and cytotoxic T cells increase. However, with severe chronic exercise stress, blood lymphocyte counts fall below normal, and serum immunoglobulin levels decrease. The duration of this suppression depends on the intensity and duration of the exercise.[5] Taken together, these findings suggest that acute intermittent exercise may actually be beneficial, particularly for the innate immune mechanisms, involving NK cells and macrophages. However, chronic exercise stress observed during training and high-performance athletic competition may actually cause immunosuppression.[5] Low-grade inflammatory foci may result in a plethora of adverse metabolic effects resulting in anemia, increased bone marrow iron storage, tissue catabolism, increased

endogenous corticosteroid production, and the acute phase protein production. Infections can increase metabolic rate, decrease lean body mass, and reduce the ability of peripheral tissues to extract oxygen from the blood.[8] Increased metabolic rate may be mediated by IL-1, TNF-β, or bacterial endotoxins and subsequently increases cortisol, catecholamines, and glucagon production, resulting in the breakdown of tissue to provide energy substrate, the overall effect being to increase tissue catabolism and reduce athletic performance.

The presence of concurrent stressful illness can have a profound effect on basal thyroid hormone levels. In humans this syndrome is described as the *sick euthyroid syndrome* and, although less well characterized in dogs, probably occurs in a similar manner.[9] Studies in euthyroid humans with acute and chronic illnesses have revealed decreased basal levels of thyroxine (T_4) and triiodothyronine (T_3) and increased reverse T_3 levels. In the dog, depressed serum T_4 and T_3 concentrations have been reported in various nonthyroidal illnesses such as diabetes mellitus, chronic renal failure, hepatic disease, and a variety of other medical illnesses.[9] The effects of the normal stresses involved in canine training and racing upon thyroid hormone metabolism are unknown, and studies of the endocrine changes that occur with greyhound racing are very few.[10, 11] However, it would seem likely that stress-related diseases in dogs may produce similar changes in thyroid hormone metabolism as in other species.

In studies of humans and rats the synthesis of sodium, potassium, ATPase (Na$^+$, K$^+$-ATPase) pumps in skeletal muscle is to a major extent controlled by thyroid hormones.[12] This is of considerable significance in view of the fact that potassium efflux from skeletal muscle is crucial in the control of skeletal muscle blood flow during exercise. The Na$^+$, K$^+$-ATPase pumps restore intracellular potassium concentration during exercise, and recently it has been proposed that the development of fatigue might be partly explained by muscle cell inexcitability due to accumulation of potassium ions in the extracellular space.[12] Studies in humans suggest that the major endocrine factor stimulating synthesis of the Na$^+$, K$^+$-ATPase pumps is thyroid hormone, and the concentration of Na$^+$, K$^+$-ATPase pump varies with thyroid status. In diabetes or during starvation, when plasma T_3 is reduced, the concentration of the Na$^+$, K$^+$-ATPase pumps is decreased.[12] This represents a possible mechanism whereby chronic stressful illness, by reducing thyroid hormones values, might result in poor performance.

CAUSES OF STRESS IN SPORTING DOGS

The major causes of stress can be divided into two categories—environmental and emotional—although the causes are often interrelated. Environmental stress includes all the factors that contribute to the housing, training, transport, and racing of sporting dogs. Extremes of temperature, humidity, overcrowding, dirty kennels, and exposure to infectious agents and parasites are all common problems in the rearing and training of sporting dogs (Table 7–1).

Stressful conditions such as overcrowding, poor sanitation, ineffective parasite control, feeding raw, poorly inspected meat products, and drinking contaminated water all contribute to an increased incidence of enteric disease in racing dogs. Additionally, the immune suppressive effects of chronic exercise stress probably exacerbate other infectious disease processes. In many instances the cumulative effects of several minor stressful factors may lead to increased susceptibility to infection. In the warmer and more humid areas of the world, parasitism and gastrointestinal infectious diseases are major problems. In particular, infestation with large numbers of *Ancylostoma caninum* (hookworms) can cause severe anemia, loss of performance, and death. Other parasites such as *Trichuris vulpis* (whipworms), coccidia species, and *Giardia lam-*

TABLE 7–1. Causes of Stress in the Racing Greyhound

Environmental	Emotional
Overcrowding	Fighting
Poor sanitation	Prerace excitement
Intestinal parasites	Transport
Infectious diseases	Competition for food
Giardia	Need for exercise
Ehrlichia	Sexual competition
Babesia	Overwork
Lyme disease	
Heartworm	
Poor nutrition	
Poor vaccination practices	
Poor quarantine practices	
Poor husbandry techniques	
Racing injuries	
Temperature and humidity	
Poorly maintained kennels	
Iatrogenic injury	

blia often cause chronic diarrhea, ill health, and poor performance in greyhounds. Ill thrift caused by bacterial gastroenteritis is a common illness in racing greyhounds. Infection with *Salmonella* sp., enteropathogenic *Escherichia coli*, and other pathogenic bacteria may cause diarrhea, dehydration, and poor condition in greyhounds.

Similarly, tick-borne diseases, including Lyme disease, ehrlichiosis and babesiosis may be causes of anemia, ill thrift, and poor performance in sporting dogs. Ticks may be so difficult to eradicate in some kennels that prophylactic tetracycline therapy is required to prevent ehrlichiosis and/or Lyme disease. Ehrlichiosis and Lyme disease both cause polyarticular lameness, which may be clinical or subclinical. The effects of subclinical disease are impossible to determine, but probably the disease significantly affects performance. Certainly, chronic ehrlichiosis and babesiosis are both causes of anemia, and chronic ehrlichiosis may cause irreversible bone marrow failure.

In those areas of the world where *Dirofilaria immitis* (heartworms) is endemic, failure to provide effective prophylaxis is a major cause of infection and lost performance. Heartworm disease is a common cardiac disease of racing dogs.[13] Even small heartworm burdens can be expected to affect racing performance and probably cause sufficient damage to limit a dog's racing career. A predisposition to respiratory disease is a result of inadequate vaccination, overcrowded conditions, poor ventilation, cold or damp kennels, and a lack of effective quarantine procedures. A major cause of the dissemination of infectious tracheobronchitis (kennel cough) is the introduction of asymptomatic carrier dogs.[14]

Nutritional deficiencies are probably more common than anticipated in racing greyhounds. A major cause of nutrition sporting deficiency in dogs is the content of "home-made" diets. Several good references outlining the nutritional requirements of sporting dogs are now available.[15–18] Careful questioning of owners about content and analysis of such diets is required to determine if a nutritional deficiency exists. In particular, careful attention to protein requirements, vitamins, and use of electrolyte supplements is important. The soft nature of many greyhound diets leads to excessive tartar build-up and severe periodontal disease. Low-grade chronic bacteremia may result from infected teeth, causing poor condition and racing performance. The unavailability of drinking water may also be crucial in the pathogenesis of recurrent dehydration problems in racing greyhounds. Greyhounds often fail to drink enough water in the post-race period despite loss of considerable quantities of water in saliva associated with panting.

The effects of competition and aggression between dogs include injuries, poor nutrition, and chronic stress. Both emotional and physical stress may result from overcrowded kennel facilities. Other physical causes of stress include racing injuries, fighting between dogs, administration of treatments by veterinarians, and training techniques. Many injuries in greyhound racing are soft tissue injuries.[19] Because of this, minor injuries are not easily detected by veterinarians, and considerable experience is required to detect minor injuries that may be decreasing performance. Dogs that continue to race with injuries may develop a chronic pain syndrome, which apart from direct performance-reducing effects of the injury, may induce physiological effects of stress. For instance, one author has concluded that injuries resulting in chronic high-intensity pain may induce potassium and bicarbonate deficits in racing greyhounds.[20] Although clinical data supporting this hypothesis are lacking, the effects of chronic injuries on the overall health of canine athletes should not be ignored and deserve further investigation. In many instances, greyhounds may actually be suffering from several medical problems, one of which is a soft tissue injury.

The assessment of training techniques is of paramount importance in determining the cause of chronic injuries in greyhounds. Training techniques overly emphasizing endurance work or involving too little work to adequately strengthen muscles and tendons may result in injury or decrease in performance. Excessive work in hot or humid conditions may predispose to dehydration or potassium deficiency, both of which may result in poor racing performance.[20] A full description of greyhound training techniques is beyond the scope of this chapter, but several good references are now available that outline successful training programs for greyhound racing.[19, 21] Emotional stress that occurs prior to racing, often during transport and placement in holding pens, may have devastating effects on racing performance. Nervousness prior to racing results in increased production of epinephrine and glucocorticoids, which depletes muscle glycogen stores and energy. Salivation and uncontrollable panting may result in dehydration and respiratory alkalosis, both of which can potentially diminish athletic performance.[20, 22]

The use of pharmaceutical aids by trainers and veterinarians can also be a cause of physical stress in greyhounds. Corticosteroids, anabolic steroids, vitamins and minerals, antibiotics, and other medications are commonly administered to racing greyhounds. In the case of anabolic steroids (which in many places may be illegal), the benefits of improved muscle mass must be weighed against the risk of possible adverse physical effects. The anti-inflammatory effects of glucocorticoids must be weighed against their numerous deleterious effects on the musculoskeletal and immune systems. Overuse of the potent nonsteroidal anti-inflammatory agents such as meclofenamic acid (Arquel) and flunixin meglumine (Banamine or Finadyne) may cause severe gastrointestinal ulceration and blood loss. Poor injection technique resulting in deep-seated myositis, cellulitis, or abscess formation is frequent in greyhound practice and may also result in poor performance. In my experience this is particularly common with the use of intramuscular injections of iron or oil-based pharmaceuticals by lay people. Widespread abuse of broad-spectrum antibiotics may predispose to resistant bacterial infections and increased susceptibility to enteric pathogens such as *Salmonella* sp.[23]

DIAGNOSIS OF THE CAUSES OF POOR PERFORMANCE

Veterinary attention is most frequently sought for sporting dogs when their racing performance falls below par. In many cases a thorough musculoskeletal examination will determine that an orthopedic or soft tissue injury is the cause of the dog's lost performance. However, in others, injury will not be detected on physical examination, and the clinician must determine if an underlying cause exists. In such circumstances, veterinarians are presented with a diagnostic challenge to determine if an underlying stress disorder is affecting the performance physiology of the dog. Perhaps the foremost question is, "Was the dog ever performing well?" It is very important to differentiate between a dog that is losing performance and a dog that is inherently a poor athlete but physiologically normal.

In greyhound practice it is important to compare a dog's current racing times to its previous racing times to determine if a pattern of substandard performance exists. In such instances, the age, previous grade, and best times at different tracks are important. Similarly, a dog's running style may give the clinician a clue to the nature of the underlying problem. For example, lack of stamina may indicate a medical problem, whereas problems with cornering might indicate a muscular problem. One should be aware that poor performance may be related to one or a number of stressful events. A thorough history, physical examination, and appropriate laboratory tests are required to determine the underlying etiology and pathogenesis of lost performance. A complete list of all of the causes of poor performance is covered elsewhere in this book. An excellent consultation format for examining racing greyhounds has been provided by Ferguson.[13] In this chapter we will outline several specifically stress-related clinical syndromes of greyhounds commonly associated with poor performance.

SPECIFIC STRESS-RELATED SYNDROMES IN RACING GREYHOUNDS

Evaluation of poor performance in greyhounds frequently may show several clinical signs indicative of severe physical or environmental stress. Such animals often develop dry seborrhea, dehydration, polyuria and polydipsia, exertional rhabdomyolysis, nonregenerative anemia, and a loss of body fat and muscle mass. Although a variety of underlying stress factors may be involved, these clinical signs should be considered indicative of a chronically stressed animal. In many cases a number of intercurrent illnesses such as tracheobronchitis, pneumonia, diarrhea, parasitism, urinary infections, and muscle injuries may be detected, each contributing to the poor health of the animal. In such instances, a vicious circle of stress, immune suppression, infections, and catabolism resulting in more stress seems to occur. Although endocrine data are lacking to support the physiological mechanisms involved, and clinical case reports are largely anecdotal, the presenting characteristics of such animals are well reported by many veterinarians familiar with greyhound practice. In such cases, a complete evaluation includes the history (all racing history, training techniques, and husbandry), physical examination, and laboratory tests to determine and correct all underlying stress factors. It is unfortunate that the most severely affected animals may be euthanatized if a previously poor racing career does not justify the expense of treatment.

A syndrome commonly associated with the effects of stress is so called *water diabetes syndrome* (WDS).[19, 21, 22] WDS is characterized by polyuria, polydipsia, metabolic acidosis, hyposthenuria, dehydration, and loss of performance. Additionally, many of these dogs have concomitant exertional rhabdomyolysis.[22] They appear to have a form of acquired diabetes insipidus since a number of them respond to rest and treatment with antidiuretic hormone (ADH). However, some dogs respond poorly to treatment with ADH, indicating perhaps that ADH deficiency is not the cause of the syndrome. Suggestions for the cause of WDS have included stress-associated hyperadrenocorticism, bacterial infections, and overuse of electrolyte supplements.[19, 21, 22] Although cortisol levels are increased with stress, true hyperadrenocorticism (ie, Cushing's disease) does not exist because the negative feedback mechanism is still intact. This compares with the situation in pituitary-dependent or adrenal dependent hyperadrenocorticism in which autonomously secreting tumors cause marked elevations in cortisol production independent of the negative feedback mechanism. Also, typical laboratory findings associated with hyperadrenocorticism are absent in dogs with WDS. It is my opinion that the stress-associated hypercortisolemia alone is unlikely to be sufficient to be responsible for the marked polyuria and polydipsia often seen with WDS.

Another possible explanation for renal unresponsiveness to ADH is the effects of low-grade bacteremia and endotoxemia in a syndrome analogous to polyuria associated with pyometra in bitches.[22] The finding that a number of these dogs have mild to severe hypokalemia suggests the possibility that an acquired form of renal unresponsiveness to ADH may be involved. As a result, WDS may represent a form of hypokalemic nephropathy and the addition of potassium to the diet may be beneficial. A possible precedent for this is that hypokalemia in cats may cause nephropathy that manifests as inability to concentrate urine.[24] In cats with hypokalemia the degree of concentration impairment is a function of the duration and severity of the potassium deficit. If a similar pathogenesis exists in greyhounds with WDS, this would in part explain the observation that some dogs respond to ADH and others do not. Hypokalemia may impair renal tubular cell function and therefore may disturb the accumulation of solute in the renal medulla, impairing the ability of the renal collecting duct to respond to ADH (medullary washout). Additionally, hypokalemia may also decrease the release of ADH. In cats, most cases of potassium depletion nephropathy can be corrected by addition of potassium to the diet, providing irreversible renal tubular damage has not occurred. With prolonged potassium deficiency, irreversible renal tubular damage may occur. If a similar situation exists in dogs, this may explain the responsiveness of some dogs to therapy with ADH and potassium.

The cause of the potassium deficit in WDS is unknown. Although dietary deficiency is a possibility, it is difficult experimentally to induce hypokalemia in healthy dogs by feeding a potassium-deficient diet. Other potential causes might include gastrointestinal loss through vomiting or diarrhea, or urinary loss through renal tubular acidosis or polyuric renal failure. In cats, persistent metabolic acidosis with renal failure is associated with abnormally high excretion indices for urinary potassium. In turn, potassium depletion may induce metabolic acidosis, which in turn may cause further potassium depletion, and so on, with a vicious circle ensuing.[25] Whether this occurs in greyhounds with WDS is speculative. However, most reports suggest that both hypokalemia and metabolic acidosis occur commonly in WDS.[20–22] Unfortunately, data on urinary potassium excretion indices or ADH levels have not been recorded for greyhounds with WDS, and the syndrome is poorly defined. Future research should center on defining the presence of hypokalemia as the causal agent and the possible involvement of bacterial toxins in the pathogenesis of WDS. If hypokalemic nephropathy is the cause of WDS, research into the relationship among urinary potassium loss, chronic stress, and causes of metabolic acidosis is warranted.

Another disease that has been associated with stress is the *balding thigh syndrome* (BTS), a term used to describe a pattern of alopecia over the caudal thigh region that is frequently seen in racing greyhounds. Occasionally the alopecia may extend to the ventral abdominal skin and the elbow regions of affected dogs. Many of the greyhounds exhibiting BTS have a history of good performance when first introduced to training, but begin to lose performance and race poorly thereafter.[26] Additionally, some dogs may develop dehydration and recover slowly after racing.[26] Typically, BTS is characterized by absence of inflammation, and there is minimal pruritus associated with the condition. In some cases there is hyperpigmentation, although this should not be confused with natural pigmentation areas that are visible because of alopecia developing. The epidermis in BTS is usually of normal thickness when compared with that of unaffected greyhounds.

BTS has been attributed to the development of hyperadrenocorticism and/or hypothyroidism as a result of stress associated with racing.[26, 27] Although clinically many of the dogs with BTS are in training and subsequently may be undergoing stress, I have also seen dogs that developed BTS that were not in training at all. Currently there are no published scientific data to support hyperadrenocorticism as the cause of BTS. Although a marked increase in cortisol may occur in stressed animals, this should not be defined as hyperadrenocorticism, which is typically associated with the presence of pituitary or adrenal tumors in the dog. Furthermore, although the syndrome appears to be associated with the stresses of training and racing, attributing hair loss to hypercortisolemia may be incorrect. In further support of this view, most affected dogs lack the dermatological signs of hyperadrenocorticism such as thin skin, comedones, and poor healing. Other typical findings in dogs affected with hyperadrenocorticism such as polyuria, polydipsia, hepatomegaly, and increased liver enzymes are also absent in BTS.

BTS has also been attributed to hypothyroidism,[27] and many cases have been treated with replacement doses of L-thyroxine based on laboratory findings of a low resting T_4 value. Because many of the affected dogs have other stressful illnesses, assessment of the thyroid status should be carefully interpreted, and diagnosis of hypothyroidism should be based only on a lack of significant increase in serum T_4 following a thyroid-stimulating hormone (TSH) test. Additionally, normal T_4 values may be lower in greyhounds than in other breeds of dogs.[28] Moreover, in another study of racing greyhounds there was no statistical correlation between basal thyroid hormone concentrations or TSH response and racing performance.[10] The fact that some dogs respond to replacement doses of L-thyroxine should not be interpreted as positive evidence that hypothyroidism is the cause of the alopecia. L-Thyroxine has a general trophic effect upon hair growth and may have mood-modifying behavior, both of which may explain the improvement noted in BTS. Currently the cause of BTS in greyhounds is unknown. Based on clinical observations, a stress association is likely, but a definitive pathogenesis has not yet been proven.

Definitive tests to determine the etiopathogenesis of BTS should include skin biopsy to better define the pathological changes involved. Similarly, attributing the cause to endocrine abnormalities should be carefully based on the results of appropriate laboratory tests. For hypothyroidism an appropriate test is the TSH stimulation test, and for hyperadrenocorticism the ACTH response test or low-dose dexamethasone response test is recommended.

It is my opinion that BTS is not a typical endocrine dermopathy, and several other possible causes may exist. One is that BTS is a form of localized telogen effluvium associated with stress or that the hairs are being removed by the dog in a syndrome analogous to psychogenic alopecia of cats. The finding that some dogs develop bald thighs without any work or apparent stress may indicate there is a genetic potential for developing BTS. Clearly, more investigation is required to better define the cause of BTS in racing greyhounds.

LABORATORY ASSESSMENT OF STRESS

The myriad of endocrine changes associated with stress in greyhounds makes scientific quantification of the effects of stress difficult. The most commonly measured parameter of a dog's ability to mount a stress response is the cortisol level. Unfortunately, the measurement of a single plasma cortisol concentration is often misleading because of the random fluctuations that occur during the day in normal animals.[6]

In humans, there is a diurnal variation in cortisol, with higher circulating cortisol in the early morning hours and low levels in the evening. The daily rhythm is superimposed on episodic secretion of cortisol. In dogs, a diurnal variation in plasma cortisol has been difficult to confirm.[29] Cortisol levels reflect "bursts" of ACTH, and the plasma cortisol concentration at any given sampling time is dependent on the timing of the pituitary burst of ACTH and the adrenocortical response. Furthermore, ACTH secretion in response to stress is also episodic. The average spike frequency of ACTH increases under stress, and average spike frequency in the morning and the evening is statistically lower under nonstressed conditions.[30] One report of basal resting cortisol in the racing greyhound concentrations suggests a lack of a diurnal variation of plasma cortisol.[11] However, a study of Hennesey suggested that a diurnal pattern similar to that occurring in humans occurs in greyhounds also.[31] Further studies by Hennesey investigated the adrenal response of greyhounds to transportation to the race track and the effects of racing on pre- and post-race cortisol values.[31] A substantial increase in cortisol values was associated with transportation to the track and with racing itself. A criticism of the study is that post-race cortisol values were not adjusted for the intracellular fluid shifts associated with exercise, which have been shown to be quite substantial in greyhounds following racing.[3] Nevertheless, these results indicate a substantial stress response by the pituitary-adrenal axis associated with transport and exercise in greyhounds.

It is unclear what effect an individual's ability to respond to stress has on the ability to perform athletically. Studies conducted in greyhounds and other species suggest that individuals may vary in their adrenal responsiveness to stress and that the type of response is repeatable for each individual.[31] In the short term, a marked adrenal response to stress may be beneficial in providing increased blood glucose for energy. However, in the longer term, animals that develop marked adrenal responsiveness to stress may be more susceptible to the detrimental effects of long-term stressful situations. Whether the ability to determine an individual's stress response is of predictive value in determining racing performance or the likelihood of developing a stress-related illness is unknown. Until more information becomes available, measurement of plasma cortisol (basal or ACTH response test) should not be used as an individual assay to quantitate the adverse effects of stress in racing greyhounds. Rather, these tests should be interpreted in relation to the presence of clinical signs indicative of a stress-related illness.

Although there are no quantitative tests that measure the amount of stress in a racing dog's life, there are several laboratory tests that may indicate that a dog is suffering the adverse effects of stress.[32] In particular, a decline in red blood cell parameters or the presence of a stress or inflammatory leukogram may indicate an underlying stressful disease and should prompt further investigation. Increases in plasma creatinine phosphokinase (CK) values may indicate an underlying muscle injury or low-grade exertional rhabdomyolysis. Similarly, trace myoglobinuria on urinalysis may also indicate recent muscle injury. It is of importance for the clinician interpreting laboratory results in greyhounds to be aware of the normal variations in hematology and biochemistry (Table 7–2). The interested reader is referred to an excellent review by Lording.[32]

TREATMENT OF STRESS-RELATED SYNDROMES IN SPORTING DOGS

The treatment of any of the stress-related diseases in sporting dogs depends on the correct identification of causative agent(s). As stated previously, considerable experience is required to identify

TABLE 7–2. Hematology and Biochemistry of Greyhounds and Other Sporting Dogs*

Parameter	Greyhounds	Sporting Dogs	Greyhounds	Sporting Dogs
	US Units		SI Units	
Hemoglobin gm/dl	19.0–21.5	12.0–18.0	Same values gm/dl	
PCV %	55–65	37–55	0.55–0.65	0.37–0.55 l/l
White cells × 10³/μl	5.5–6.5	6.0–17.0	Same values × 10⁹/L	
Neutrophils × 10³/μl	2.0–4.5	3.0–11.5	Same values × 10⁹/L	
Bands × 10³/μl	10–0.3	0–0.3	Same values × 10⁹/L	
Lymphocytes × 10³/μl	0.8–1.9	1.0–4.8	Same values × 10⁹/L	
Monocytes × 10³/μl	0.2–0.8	0.2–1.4	Same values × 10⁹/L	
Eosinophils × 10³/μl	0.1–1.3	0.1–1.6	Same values × 10⁹/L	
Basophils × 10³/μl	rare	rare	Same values × 10⁹/L	
Platelets × 10³/μl	200–500	200–500	Same values × 10⁹/L	
MCV fL	65–78	60–77	Same values	
MCHC gm/dl	32–37	32–36	Same values	
Total solids gm/dl	48–65	60–80	4.8–6.5	6–8.0 gm/L
Sodium mEq/L	138–158	145–155	Same values in mmol/L	
Potassium mEq/L	3.8–5.8	2.7–5.0	Same values in mmol/L	
Chloride mEq/L	100–115	96–122	Same values in mmol/L	
Bicarbonate mEq/L	22–28	18–22	Same values in mmol/L	
Calcium mg/dl	7.6–10.4	9.0–11.4	1.9–2.6	2.25–2.85 mmol/L
Phosphate mg/dl	2.7–6.5	5.5–7.7	0.9–2.1	1.8–2.5 mmol/L
Urea mg/dl	0.6–1.7	0.5–1.8	3.6–10.4	3.0–10.7 mmol/L
Creatinine mg/dl	3.6–10.2	4.8–10.20	0.17–6	0.08–0.17 mmol/L
Glucose mg/dl	59–120	67–126	3.3–6.7	3.0–7.0 mmol/L
Cholesterol mg/dl	109–241	140–330	2.8–6.2	3.6–9.0 mmol/L
Bilirubin mg/dl	0.12–0.84	0–0.56	2–15.0	0–10.0 mmol/L
ALT U/L	5–80	5–95	Same values	
AP U/L	10–120	40–100	Same values	
AST U/L	10–80	<75	Same values	
CPK U/L	50–400	<300	Same values	
Total Protein gm/dl	4.5–6.2	5.4–7.4	45–62	54–74 gm/L
Albumin gm/dl	2.3–3.9	2.9–3.9	23–34	29–39 gm/L
Globulins gm/dl	2.1–3.2	2.5–3.5	21–32	25–35 gm/L

*Normal values for greyhounds and other sporting dogs as used at the University of Melbourne Veterinary Clinic and Hospital.
Normal values that vary between greyhounds and sporting dogs are shown in bold type.

underlying muscle injuries, infections, poor nutrition, or poor husbandry techniques. In each case, treatment should be designed to be curative for the clinical disease as well as to identify any underlying management technique that predisposes the dog to recurrence. For example, a respiratory infection may require antibiotic treatment, but is there an underlying problem of overcrowding, poor quarantine, or poor immunity due to poor nutrition or parasitism? Treatment of stress-related diseases in sporting dogs should consider the whole practice of racing, training, and management. Careful attention to vaccination, appropriate nutrition, kenneling, and training techniques is crucial. Treatment of the specific stress syndromes in greyhounds is covered below.

Severe dehydration associated with WDS should be treated as an emergency. Initial treatment with a balanced isotonic electrolyte solution is favored and the calculated body water deficit replaced over a period of 4 hours. A baseline urinalysis should be obtained as well as measurement of blood urea nitrogen (BUN), creatinine, and serum electrolytes. A full chemistry profile and complete blood count may also be beneficial in determining the presence of related disease problems. Because many dogs will be hypokalemic, potassium replacement is required. Potassium may be administered by parenteral or oral routes. However, administration of potassium in intravenous fluids should be monitored, as rates exceeding 0.5 mEq/kg/hr may induce cardiac arrhythmias or phlebitis. Furthermore, when there is excessive renal loss of potassium, administration of intravenous fluids may result in increasing distal renal tubular potassium loss. For this reason, supplementation with oral potassium gluconate (Tumil-K) may be superior to parenteral therapy. Dogs with severe hypokalemia should receive 5 to 10 mEq/kg/day orally in two divided doses.

Once initial dehydration and electrolyte abnormalities are corrected, daily maintenance and ongoing losses should be replaced intravenously because many dogs will fail to drink sufficient water to replace urinary losses. Standard therapy in veterinary medicine for diabetes insipidus has been parenteral administration of vasopressin tannate (Pitressin tannate in oil) given as 3 to 5 units IM to dogs every 24 to 72 hours.[33] A similar treatment is commonly used for WDS in greyhounds. The product, however, is now discontinued. The synthetic analogue, desmopressin acetate (DDAVP), may be superior to ADH and more readily available. DDAVP is currently available as an injectable or an intranasal formulation for humans. The injectable form is given as 0.2 μg IM twice daily, while the intranasal form can be administered into the conjunctival sac at a rate of 2 to 4 drops twice daily. As stated previously, WDS in greyhounds appears to be an acquired form of diabetes insipidus, and the response to ADH therapy may be variable. Following initial treatment with ADH or DDAVP urine specific gravity and water intake should be monitored daily; if no improvement in urine specific gravity and water intake has occurred over the first 3 days and hypokalemia has been corrected, then renal medullary solute washout should be considered to have occurred. Renal medullary solute washout is treated by gradual water deprivation of 5 to 10 per cent per day of the previously measured unrestricted water intake. Dehydration should be avoided, and it is advisable to weigh the dog daily to check for dehydration. Treatment with ADH or DDAVP and supplementation with a balanced potassium-rich electrolyte solution should continue during this time. Recovery in severely affected dogs may take several weeks, and nearly all dogs will require rest from exercise for several weeks to months.

Until the exact pathophysiology of this disorder is known, effective prophylaxis should consist of identifying susceptible dogs and removing all possible contributing stress factors. In frequently dehydrated dogs, supplementation with intravenous fluids and oral potassium-rich electrolyte solutions may also be beneficial. Dogs with severe weight loss, infections, dehydration, and multiple illnesses often require extended hospitalization and treatment for multiple problems. In many cases the economic worth of a racing dog may preclude long and expensive treatment and the animal will be euthanatized. In those dogs in which treatment is undertaken, it is essential that all underlying diseases be treated; in particular, intestinal parasites, heartworm disease, ehrlichiosis, and babesiosis may be present. Heartworm disease and the chronic form of ehrlichiosis carry a poor prognosis for future racing. Bacterial pneumonia is particularly common in racing greyhounds and should be treated with appropriate antibiotics based on the results of a culture and sensitivity test. The tractable nature of most greyhounds makes them readily amenable to transtracheal wash to obtain bronchial fluid samples.

In addition to treatment of any underlying diseases, providing adequate nutrition is important to prevent continuing tissue catabolism. In many cases, enteral feeding techniques may be beneficial in the initial recovery phase when a dog is not eating. Anabolic steroids are widely advocated but should be used with caution when there is a possibility of a positive drug test occurring. Similarly, the use of iron supplements, vitamins, and other hematinics to treat anemia is controversial but unlikely to be harmful if the cause of the anemia is identified.

References

1. Webster's Encyclopedic Unabridged Dictionary of the English Language. Avenal, NJ, Gramercy, 1994.
2. Guyton AC: The adrenocortical hormones. *In* Guyton A (ed): Textbook of Medical Physiology. Philadelphia, WB Saunders Company, 1992, pp 851–852.
3. Rose RJ, Bloomberg MS: Responses to sprint exercise in the racing greyhound. Res Vet Sci 47:212–218, 1989.
4. Guyton AC: The adrenocortical hormones. *In* Guyton AC (ed): Textbook of Medical Physiology. Philadelphia, WB Saunders Company, 1992, p 848.
5. Hoffmann-Goetz BM, Pederson BK: Exercise and the immune system: A model of the stress response? Immunol Today 15:382–387, 1994.
6. Peterson ME: Adrenal gland diseases. *In* Ettinger SJ (ed): Textbook of Veterinary Internal Medicine. Philadelphia, WB Saunders Company, 1989, pp 1723–1724.
7. Papich MG, Davis LE: Glucocorticoid therapy. *In* Kirk RW (ed): Current Veterinary Therapy X. Philadelphia, WB Saunders Company, 1989, pp 54–63.
8. Bilbrey SA, Buffington CT: Metabolism and nutrition in the surgical patient. *In* Bojrab MJ, Bloomberg MS (eds): Disease Mechanisms in Small Animal Surgery. Philadelphia, Lea & Febiger, 1993, pp 49–53.
9. Feldman EC, Nelson RW: Canine and Feline Endocrinology and Reproduction. Philadelphia, WB Saunders Company, 1987, pp 67–70.
10. Beale KM, Bloomberg MS, et al: Correlation of racing and reproductive performance in greyhounds with response to thyroid function testing. J Am Anim Hosp Assoc 28:263–269, 1992.
11. Taylor J, Hauler AD: Endocrinology. University of Sydney Refresher Course for Veterinarians, Proceedings 64. University of Sydney, 1983, pp 449–466.
12. Klaus TC, Everts MA: Regulation of the Na K-potassium pump in skeletal muscle. Kidney Int 35:1–13, 1989.
13. Courtney CH, Sundlof SF, et al: Impact of filariasis on the racing greyhound. J Am Anim Hosp Assoc 21:421–425, 1985.
14. Ford RB, Vaaden SL: Canine infectious tracheobronchitis. *In* Greene CE (ed): Infectious Diseases of the Dog and Cat. Philadelphia, WB Saunders Company, 1990, pp 259–265.
15. Grandjean D, Paragon BM: Nutrition of racing and working dogs. Part 1. Comp Cont Education 14:1608–1615, 1992.
16. Grandjean D, Paragon BM: Nutrition of racing and working dogs. Part 2. Comp Cont Education 15:45–47, 1993.
17. Grandjean D, Paragon BM: Nutrition of racing and working dogs. Part 3. Comp Cont Education 15:203–211, 1993.
18. Kohnke J: Feeds and feeding greyhounds. University of Sydney Refresher Course for Veterinarians, Proceedings 122. University of Sydney, 1989, pp 421–467.
19. Ferguson RG: A consultation format for greyhounds. University of Sydney Refresher Course for Veterinarians, Proceedings 122. University of Sydney, 1989, pp 323–339.
20. Hauler AD: Electrolyte metabolism in greyhounds. University of Sydney Refresher Course for Veterinarians, Proceedings 122. University of Sydney, 1989, pp 393–404.
21. Murray JW: Some aspects of greyhound training. University of Sydney Refresher Course for Veterinarians, Proceedings 122. University of Sydney, 1989, pp 207–211.
22. Gannon JR: Exertional rhabdomyolysis in the racing greyhound. *In* Kirk RW (ed): Current Veterinary Therapy VII. Philadelphia, WB Saunders Company, 1982, pp 783–787.
23. Greene CE: Salmonellosis. *In* Greene CE (ed): Infectious Diseases of the Dog and Cat. Philadelphia, WB Saunders Company, 1990, pp 542–549.
24. Dow SW, LeCouteur R: Hypokalemic polymyopathy of cats. *In* Kirk RW (ed): Current Veterinary Therapy X. Philadelphia, WB Saunders Company, 1989, pp 812–815.
25. Dow SF, Fettman MJ: Renal disease in cats, the potassium connection. *In* Bonagura J (ed): Current Veterinary Therapy XI. Philadelphia, WB Saunders Company, 1992, pp 820–822.
26. Gannon JR: Metabolic diseases of greyhounds. *In* Blythe LL, Gannon JR, et al (eds): Care of the Racing Greyhound. Birmingham, American Greyhound Council, Inc., 1994, pp 274–275.
27. Gannon JR: Medical diseases of greyhounds. University of Sydney Refresher Course for Veterinarians, Proceedings 64. University of Sydney, 1977, pp 267–269.
28. Rosychuk RAW, Freshman JL, et al: Serum concentrations of thyroxine and 3,5,3'-triiodothyronine in dogs before and after administration of freshly reconstituted or previously refrozen thyrotrophin-releasing hormone. Am J Vet Res 49:1722–1725, 1988.
29. Kempainen RJ: Evidence for episodic but not circadian activity in plasma concentrations of adrenocorticotrophin, cortisol and thyroxine in dogs. Endocrinology 103:219–226, 1984.
30. Feldman EC, Nelson RW: Canine and Feline Endocrinology and Reproduction. Philadelphia, WB Saunders Company, 1987, p 138.
31. Hennesey DP: Stress and performance in greyhounds. University of Sydney Refresher Course for Veterinarians, Proceedings 122. University of Sydney, 1989, pp 343–350.
32. Lording PM: Interpretation of clinical pathology laboratory profiles. University of Sydney Refresher Course for Veterinarians, Proceedings 122. University of Sydney, 1989, pp 343–350.
33. Nichols R: Diabetes insipidus. *In* Kirk RW (ed): Current Veterinary Therapy X. Philadelphia, WB Saunders Company, 1989, pp 973–978.

CHAPTER 8

DERMATOLOGY

NEAL C. ANDELMAN

It is not the purpose of this chapter to present a complete discourse on the topic of canine dermatology. There are some excellent textbooks devoted to this topic. Instead, this chapter presents and discusses some of the dermatological problems that have unique presentations in the sporting breeds.

Sporting dogs are probably no more predisposed to skin lesions than other breeds, but their opportunities to acquire skin lesions are certainly greater than with their "nonworking" counterparts because of their "occupational" exposure. This is particularly true of lesions involving the feet. In most breeds, skin disorders are a nuisance for both the dog and its owners, but in sporting breeds they can seriously affect performance and are therefore of greater importance. Because the feet of sporting dogs are so significant to their function, we will begin our discussion of dermatological disorders from the ground up.

PODODERMATITIS

Pododermatitis is an inflammation of the skin of the paw (Fig. 8–1). In particular, the interdigital skin is of concern. Because sporting breeds are often exposed to harsher environmental conditions than are most other breeds, it is not surprising that pododermatitis is commonly encountered. Trauma is probably the most common cause of pododermatitis in sporting dogs. The trauma in hunting dogs is often related to rough terrain over which they run. Additionally, some dogs are housed in runs or turn-out areas with gravel or other rough footing materials. Greyhounds are subject to other sources of trauma leading to pododermatitis. The sand used

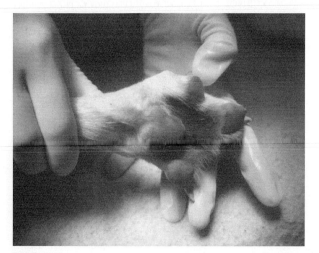

FIGURE 8–1. Pododermatitis. The ventral surface of the paw is inflamed. This dog was pruritic and lapped frequently at the paw.

to form the racing surface is composed of many different-sized particles. The actual mixture used depends on local climatic conditions. Large particles provide excellent drainage, which is important in areas of high rainfall. Smaller particles (technically silt and clay) retain moisture but tend to clump when allowed to dry. If the track surface is not kept at its ideal moisture level and groomed in a proper manner, racing greyhounds may suffer traumatic pododermatitis as the foot slides forward in its normal racing stride. This may be caused either by contact with clumped portions of track or the sharp edges of loose sand particles. Splinters, thorns, awns (bristle-like ends of spikelets of plants such as foxtails), and other vegetative matter are fairly common sources of foreign bodies in hunting dogs that can cause pododermatitis. Most geographic areas have some specific plant material that can cause pododermatitis.

While hypothyroidism is listed as a possible cause of pododermatitis, it is an uncommon situation in greyhounds despite the fact that hypothyroidism is seen in the breed (see Bald Thigh Syndrome). In some retrievers, however, hypothyroidism has been diagnosed when only the interdigital skin is involved (not the trunk). These dogs may develop secondary pyodermas.

Primary infections or infections secondary to irritants or foreign bodies are seen in all dogs. Hunting dogs, however, are more prone to fungal infections because of their exposure to these organisms in wooded areas in which they may work. Penetrating interdigital wounds can introduce fungal spores beneath the skin surface. Either "intermediate" types of infections, such as sporotrichosis, or "deep" types, such as blastomycosis, are possible (see Sporotrichosis). Bacterial infections are an unusual primary cause of pododermatitis in sporting breeds but commonly produce secondary infection.

Parasitic infections are another potential cause of pododermatitis. Again, there is a regional difference in the incidence, partly depending on annual temperature ranges. Demodectic or sarcoptic mites can be seen in any breed. Because of the number of dogs using a limited-size exercise area, sporting breeds may be more likely than other breeds to be exposed to helminth parasitic dermatitis. Hookworm larvae (*Ancylostoma* species and *Uncinaria* species) can cause pododermatitis in dogs in warmer climates, particularly if sanitation practices are lax or if the dogs spend much time on dirt surfaces. *Pelodera strongyloides* is another parasite in this category.

NAIL AND NAIL BED DISORDERS

The health and integrity of the nails and nail beds are crucial to the performance of sporting dogs. While lesions of pododermatitis and the foot pads are often obvious, nail lesions can be very subtle. Careful examination of the nails and nail beds is often necessary to identify them as the cause of the clinical signs. Trauma to the nail is more likely to occur as the nail grows longer. The trauma can be blunt as with objects falling onto the foot or the foot

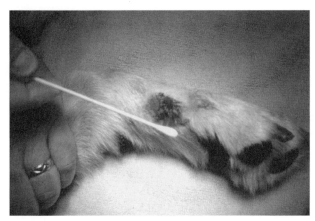

FIGURE 8–2. Broken nail on P1 (dew claw) caused by trauma. In this photograph taken 2 days after the injury paronychia is seen. The wound was extremely painful. Treatment could be medical (antibiotic therapy after removal of the nail "shell") or surgical (amputation of the nail). In racing greyhounds the latter is recommended when front dew claws are present to prevent recurrence of the same injury.

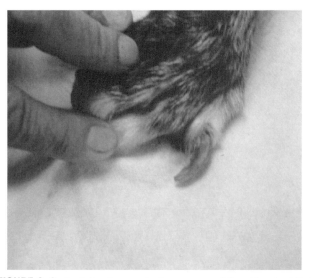

FIGURE 8–4. Sand abrasions on the inner aspect of the nail and nail bed on a racing greyhound.

bumping into an immovable object. The trauma can be local or general. In extreme cases the nail can be torn from the underlying soft tissues, but more commonly the nail cracks (Fig. 8–2). The resulting opening often results in secondary bacterial infection (paronychia) if not promptly treated. Paronychia may be defined as an infection or inflammation of the nail bed (claw fold) (Fig. 8–3).

Greyhounds also may suffer trauma to the nail beds if the joint between the second and third phalanges is injured or the nail itself is dislocated during racing. In some cases the nail may appear uninjured, but the ungual crest area is damaged, causing the nail to grow in an abnormal direction and resulting in interference with an abutting toe, thereby affecting performance. Racing greyhounds are subject to unusual trauma of the nail beds if the surface of the track is dry. When the greyhound's foot strikes the surface it slides forward for a short distance before beginning the "push-off" start of the stride. If the surface is dry, the foot slides forward more

than normal, and abrasions of the nail beds can result (Fig. 8–4). Because the toes spread slightly during this sliding phase, the typical pattern of inflammation involves the medial aspect of the fifth digit and the lateral aspect of the second digit. If greyhounds from diverse kennels at a track have similar abrasive inflammation of the nail beds, then the track surface should be considered a possible cause.

Chemical irritation (rock salt, fertilizers, petroleum products, and many others) and thermal injury are causes of paronychia, starting as an inflammatory lesion but later developing secondary bacterial

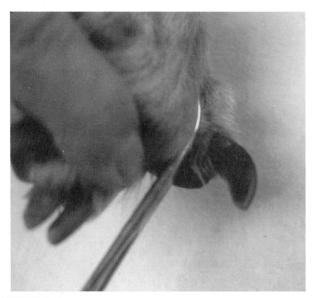

FIGURE 8–3. Paronychia. Note the swelling and inflammation in the nail bed.

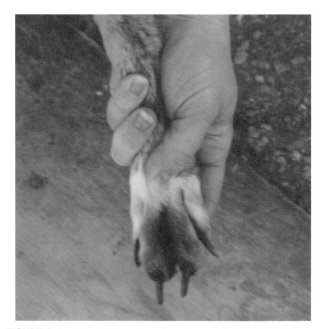

FIGURE 8–5. This racing greyhound was frequently exercised in a turnout pen with poor drainage and a strong odor of ammonia. All four feet were involved. Note swelling at the nail bed (paronychia) and inflammation, which has advanced proximally. Marked improvement occurred when the feet were soaked in a povidone-iodine solution and the dog was placed in an environment in which the turnout pens were clean and dry.

infection. Greyhounds may also develop a form of chemical irritation from chronic exposure to organic compounds in turnout pens when urea and fecal matter are allowed to accumulate (Fig. 8–5).

Bacterial infections of the nail beds secondary to traumatic or chemical irritation of the nail are usually associated with a single nail. When multiple nails are involved, systemic conditions such as hypothyroidism should be considered unless it can be demonstrated that all the nails received some local insult.

Fungal or yeast infections of the nails and nail beds occasionally occur, most commonly in hunting dogs that work in areas in which the soil is warm and moist. Greyhounds that exercise in turnout pens that never dry out completely may also develop paronychia. Cultures of exudate from these dogs may reveal a mixed infection with combinations of bacterial and yeast organisms and, less commonly, fungal infections.

Immune-mediated disorders can occur in all breeds of dogs and affect the nails or nail beds. I have seen a few cases of pemphigus foliaceus in retired greyhounds in which the primary signs were pain and brittle, twisted nails. (Onychodystrophy refers to abnormal nail formation and onychalgia refers to painful nails) (Fig. 8–6). The diagnosis is best confirmed with biopsy, but care must be taken not to scrub the tissues too vigorously in the preoperative preparation. Trauma to the nail area can disrupt the delicate vesicles that pathologists use as part of the diagnostic criteria for identification. Peroxidase-antiperoxidase (PAP) technique should also be requested if pemphigus foliaceus is suspected.

Greyhound trainers and sporting dog handlers differ in their opinions regarding optimal nail length, but most agree that the nails should be trimmed to a point where they fall just short of the ground when the dog is standing and the paw is flat. Extremes should be avoided. Nails kept very short may result in pain for the dog if the nail is further abraded during work. Long nails increase the overall length of the toe as a whole, which dramatically increases the pressure transmitted to the joints above. This is also the explanation for the logic in amputating (permanently) a nail on a toe when a joint above the nail is calcified or otherwise damaged. Relieving the "stress" on the injured joint may return the dog to function.

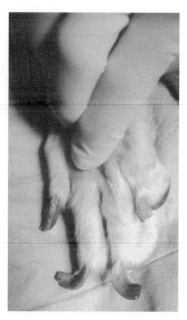

FIGURE 8–6. Pemphigus foliaceus. Note the onychodystrophy. This dog was a retired greyhound that developed lesions at 5 years of age. The nails were extremely painful (onychalgia). This dog rapidly improved on a regimen of corticosteroid therapy; normal nails were maintained with low-dose medication twice a week.

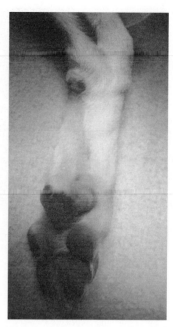

FIGURE 8–7. This 2-year-old racing greyhound developed multiple "corns" on all four feet—some within the pads, some interdigital, and a few on the pad margins (note the 1-cm diameter papilloma on the edge of the main carpal pad). Histopathologic study confirmed viral papilloma. Note the pododermatitis that was induced when the trainer "expressed" the interdigital corns. Several dogs from this Kansas farm developed similar lesions at the same time.

PADS

Many of the agents that damage the nails and interdigital skin can damage the foot pads also. Hunting dogs are often exposed to rough terrain that can bruise or lacerate pads. Some greyhound trainers will "truck-walk" dogs for exercise. If this practice takes place over a paved surface, the greyhound's foot pads are subject to abrasions and lacerations (from surface debris). In extreme cases the pad may be abraded away, causing permanent damage to the surface. Similar lesions may be caused by exercising on hard-packed sand, particularly in hot climates, where the pads may blister.

Most greyhound trainers will attempt to express a "corn" (Fig. 8–7) by soaking the foot and then applying manual pressure to the pad, a procedure that is seldom appreciated by the greyhound. Corns that do not respond to this treatment are usually surgically removed. Some dogs suffer from sporadic bouts of viral papillomas, while others will experience only a single episode. Once the lesion is treated there is usually a rapid return to function.

Most kennels use disinfectants regularly in an effort to stop pathogenic organisms from spreading. When used according to label directions, most chemical disinfectants are safe and cause no irritation to the feet. However, in many kennel situations the chemicals are not carefully diluted, and the resulting solutions either may be ineffective or too concentrated and may irritate the feet. The latter is more likely to result when a kennel or a neighboring kennel experiences a disease outbreak. The "more-is-better" philosophy is sometimes utilized to ensure "killing" more germs. Foot pads exposed to chemical irritants may swell, lose pigmentation (particularly noticeable with chlorine disinfectants such as bleach), blister, or become hyperkeratotic (Fig. 8–8). Affected dogs may be unable to perform for extended periods.

Another chemical irritation can be seen in northern climates where rock salt is used to melt snow from walks and driveways. If

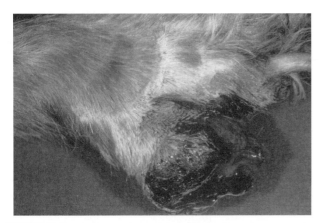

FIGURE 8–8. Hyperkeratosis can be confused with melanomas such as the one depicted here. A biopsy should be done on nonresponsive lesions to confirm a diagnosis.

rock salt is wedged between toes, the water from melting snow can mix with the rock salt to form hydrochloric acid and result in a severe chemical burn. Dogs that work in areas where these chemicals are used should have their feet carefully checked when returning to the kennel.

A few greyhound tracks have used petroleum products such as diesel oil on the surface of the track during the winter racing to keep the surface from freezing. Greyhounds racing over such a surface are prone to paronychia and interdigital inflammation. Even careful washing of the feet with a detergent to remove the oil has not prevented some greyhounds from developing chronic inflammations. Most of the tracks in climates where the winter temperatures fall below freezing have subsurface heating elements that eliminate the need for surface oil.

Greyhound tracks, particularly older ones, often have turnout pens in which it is difficult to remove the sand. It is common practice in these pens to periodically add more sand on top of the old. The result of this practice is that organic wastes, including urea, build to levels high enough to cause inflammation of the pads and nail beds.

It is particularly important to wash the feet of greyhounds exposed to these conditions. Many of the newer tracks in the United States have turnout pens designed so that the old sand can be removed periodically and fresh sand substituted.

Although the reader is referred to the sections in this book dealing with sled racing dogs of the north, a specific foot pad condition of Siberian huskies, malamutes, and huskies applies here. Although zinc-responsive dermatoses occur in many breeds as an acquired disorder, evidence suggests a genetic basis in the Northern breeds mentioned. Foot pad (and facial) lesions may include hyperkeratosis and crusting. Less commonly, ulcers may develop. The genetic condition may also lead to dwarfism if untreated by supplementation with zinc.

Autoimmune diseases such as systemic lupus erythematosus, discoid lupus, or pemphigus foliaceus may affect the foot pads but do not occur with greater frequency in sporting breeds than in other types of dogs. The importance of the condition of the foot pads in sporting dogs cannot be overemphasized. Dogs with infections or inflammations of the pads simply cannot perform near their optimal level.

Many techniques are available for surgical correction of pad lesions, ranging from simple suturing of pad lacerations to sophisticated procedures involving transplantation of tissues to fill in pad defects. Basic techniques are discussed here, but Swaim and others have described in detail techniques for reconstructive surgery of

the pads. Since lacerations and other wounds of the pads are so common in sporting breeds, a discussion of suggested technique follows. In addition, pad problems following amputation of a greyhound toe are discussed. Suturing of the pads following a laceration is not a procedure that should be treated lightly. Breakdown of a pad incision or infection in the pad can have disastrous results in any sporting dog. Complete and thorough cleansing of the wound and surrounding tissues is essential. Sand or other small foreign particles are easily trapped inside the pad and should be removed with aggressive cleansing and flushing with saline or other physiological solution. Many disinfecting scrub solutions will reduce bacterial counts without damaging tissue.

Following surgical preparation of the wound, a nonabsorbable suture material is applied in a simple interrupted pattern with the sutures placed approximately 2 to 3 mm from the wound edges. Swaim has suggested that the sutures be placed the full depth of the wound to close all dead space and immobilize the deeper tissues. It is important that the knots be tied with enough tension to hold the tissues together, but not so tight as to cause strangulation of the deeper (dermal) tissues. These deeper tissues contain a high percentage of adipose tissue that is easily damaged. I have found that monofilament sutures cause minimal discomfort for patients; however, many other materials have been successfully used. Skin staples are a poor choice for pad wounds as they do not allow comfortable ambulation for the patient and do not extend into the deeper tissues of the pad.

Postoperatively, the wound will heal more rapidly if the patient is kept as inactive as possible. While there is some disagreement on the advisability of bandaging skin lacerations, pad lacerations should always be covered with a dressing after suturing. I prefer a dry dressing with a nonadhering material covering the incision. If the wound is deep or extensive, additional support with external fixation is also indicated. Dressings protect the suture materials from abrading and weakening. They also prevent the natural flattening of the pad that occurs during ambulation. This flattening puts tension on the pad sutures, and without a dressing there is more likelihood of dehiscence. Dressings are usually changed 5 to 7 days postoperatively with suture removal 10 to 14 days after surgery. If the dressing has been allowed to become moist, the pad tissues may take even longer to heal. Swaim recommends always using a metal splint.

Amputation of a digit on a greyhound toe is common. The pad should always be preserved with as much of the adipose tissue as possible to protect the "stump." Occasionally the pad in a postoperative patient will be found in a position that is not protecting the remaining bony tissues, usually in a dorsal position on the cranial aspect. This may be corrected by removing a wedge of skin on the caudoventral aspect (equal in size to the amount the pad is to slide) and, with gentle dissection, repositioning the pad in a more ventral position by pulling it distal and caudal. Suturing the wound holds the pad in its new position. Note that the sutures will not be in the pad itself but rather in the adjacent skin.

As mentioned previously, some dermatological problems of the sporting breeds are either unique to them or of special importance or with unusual presentations. Discussion of these conditions follows.

IDIOPATHIC CUTANEOUS AND RENAL GLOMERULAR VASCULOPATHY OF GREYHOUNDS

In 1985 a previously unreported disease syndrome in greyhounds was recognized. Signs included multifocal cutaneous lesions, including erythema, ulceration, and distal limb edema, sometimes associated with other clinical signs. Because the first recognized outbreak occurred at the Greentrack Racing Park in Alabama, the terms *Alabama rot* and *Greentrack disease* are used by greyhound trainers and veterinarians. Within 1 year of the initial reports, similar cases were reported in Florida, Colorado, and New England. The syndrome has now been recognized at most of the greyhound racing tracks across the country. The syndrome has not been reported outside of the continental United States.

When the first reports of the disease were discussed by veterinarians anecdotally, the consensus was that staphylococcal organisms were the etiological agents. Despite evidence refuting this hypothesis, a widespread belief persists that staphylococcal bacteria cause the syndrome and that antimicrobial therapy will treat it. Neither of these statements is true (see Treatment).

Clinical Signs. The disease has been recognized only in greyhounds. Both males and females are affected similarly. While the primary age group affected coincides with the age of racing (15 to 48 months of age), the syndrome is also seen in pups on breeding farms as well as in breeding bitches.

The skin lesions in affected greyhounds are distinctive. The first sign to appear is a cutaneous and erythematous swelling, often on a distal limb but occasionally on the ventral thorax or groin. The swollen area is often tender. Tarsus, stifle, and medial thigh (in that order) are the most commonly affected sites, but forelimb lesions are also seen. Since the initial report of this disease was published, I have seen two histologically confirmed cases of the syndrome on the muzzle of greyhounds, but this presentation is unusual.

The areas involved are usually from a few millimeters up to 10 cm (Fig. 8–9). If the ventral chest area is involved, then even larger amounts of tissues may be affected. Within 1 to 2 days the swollen tissue ulcerates and discharges a serosanguineous fluid. A significant feature in early recognition of the syndrome is that the skin ulcers are very sharply demarcated and involve the entire depth of the dermal tissues.

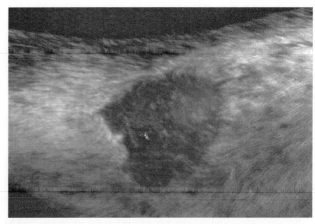

FIGURE 8–10. An ulcer that had opened 4 days previously. Only gentle topical application of an aqueous antibiotic solution was utilized.

Lymph nodes in affected areas are not palpably involved, and unless there is renal involvement, the ulcers begin to heal within a few days. The healing time is partially dependent upon the size of the initial lesion, but most ulcers are covered with a cicatrix in 10 to 30 days, providing the wound is kept clean with a topical aqueous solution of an antimicrobial agent (Figs. 8–10 and 8–11). Povodine-iodine has been used successfully for this purpose. The most striking external manifestation of this disease is the cutaneous lesions; however, some greyhounds will also have renal involvement (44 of the 168 reported in the first published article describing

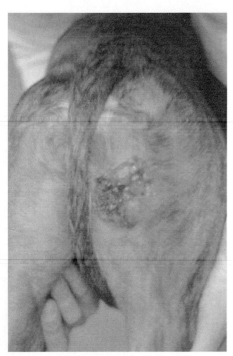

FIGURE 8–9. A typical fresh ulcer. Note the sharply demarcated borders. A serosanguineous fluid drained from this lesion a few hours before this photograph was taken.

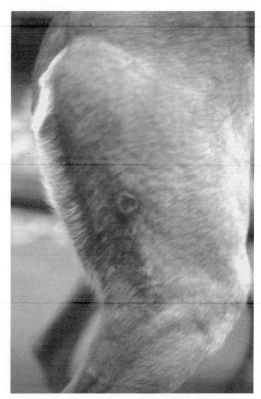

FIGURE 8–11. A small ulcer that is almost healed. Note the cicatrix formation at the periphery of the lesion. Again, only topical treatment was used.

this condition). In greyhounds that develop them, renal lesions may occur before, concurrently with, or after the development of skin lesions. The most common presentation, however, is for both lesions to develop concomitantly. Such greyhounds develop fevers (temperature 39.2 to 40° C) and lethargy at the time the skin lesions develop. Distal limb edema (most often hind leg) develops within a few days, along with rapid onset of azotemia. Typical signs of renal failure appear, including polyuria, polydipsia, tarry stools, and vomiting. In a second manifestation of the skin and renal syndrome, the kidney lesions appear approximately 10 days after the skin lesions develop. This form is seen less often than the concurrent development of lesions. A third manifestation of the combined skin and renal syndrome is also seen but, again, less commonly than the coincidental form. In this pattern the azotemia develops before the cutaneous ulceration.

Clinical Laboratory Findings. When the disease was first reported, many veterinarians cultured the wounds and *Staphylococcus* species were frequently reported. However, extensive culturing in many affected greyhounds found no consistent pattern of bacterial organisms in the ulcers. *S. aureus, S. epidermidis,* and *Proteus* organisms were the most likely to be seen. Anaerobic bacterial cultures are routinely negative. Recently, affected greyhounds have been tested for Rocky Mountain spotted fever, *Ehrlichia* species, *Borrelia burgdorferi,* and *Leptospira* species. None of these tests have identified the etiological agent. Electron microscopy has likewise failed to demonstrate any evidence of the etiology. No microorganisms, immune complexes, or cryoglobulin crystals have been found.

In greyhounds displaying renal lesions as well as cutaneous lesions, there are of course significant changes in the blood chemistry. Azotemia and serum creatinine are consistently elevated. Some patients die before changes are noted in serum electrolyte levels. In patients surviving more than 48 hours, typical signs of renal insufficiency may develop, including hypocalcemia, hyperphosphatemia, and hyperkalemia. In addition, most of these greyhounds display slight elevations in the white blood cell (WBC) counts (10,000 to 15,000). (While a WBC count in this range may be normal for most breeds, it is an elevation in the racing greyhound.) A moderate decrease in platelet counts (50,000 to 125,000) is often noted. Fenwick et al, noted that a severe decrease in platelets to below 100,000 may be the best indicator of potential renal complications.

Urinalysis in renal failure patients usually reveals low specific gravity (1.010 to 1.020) despite proteinuria and hematuria. The sediment almost always contains red blood cells (RBC). If the affected greyhound survives for more than 24 hours, casts appear in the urine, and the specific gravity begins to rise.

In summary, the greyhounds exhibiting only cutaneous lesions usually have normal clinical laboratory findings. Fenwick et al stated that ''It is likely that all greyhounds that develop skin lesions also have some kidney damage. In many cases the damage to the kidneys is not severe enough to cause clinically evident disease or even biochemical abnormalities.'' Those dogs showing both cutaneous and renal lesions have clinical laboratory signs of peracute renal failure; however, the clinical laboratory tests are not specifically diagnostic for this syndrome. Only histopathology can confirm the diagnosis. This is significant, since trainers and veterinarians may lump any greyhound skin ulcer under the general heading of Alabama rot.

Gross and Histopathology Findings. The cutaneous lesions seen in this syndrome are consistent regardless of the presence of renal lesions. Grossly the skin ulcers have sharply demarcated borders that should alert the veterinary practitioner to the syndrome. Typical findings include hemorrhage and edema in the area of the ulcer. At sites in which the ulcers are small and superficial, micro-

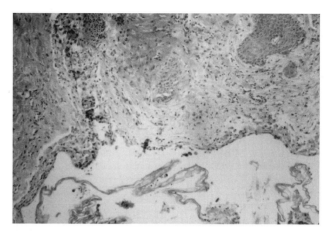

FIGURE 8–12. Histopathological study (H&E stain) illustrating blood vessel occlusion with resulting localized infarct of the dermis.

scopic examination reveals thrombosis of arterioles, venules, and capillaries. The result of the blood vessel occlusion is that the dermis is either necrotic or absent, having sloughed (Fig. 8–12). If the deep dermal or subcutaneous arteries are thrombosed, a deeper infarct develops with necrosis of entire pilosebaceous units, extensive hemorrhage, and edema with variable fibrosis in the dermis and subcutis. Older ulcers are usually covered by a purulent exudate that often contains cocci. This finding explains the frequent reports of *Staphylococcus* infections as a causative agent.

Affected subcutaneous and deep dermal arteries undergo changes ranging from mild to severe. In the most severe cases the arteries undergo fibrinoid necrosis (Fig. 8–13). The lesions are vascular lesions, and the pathological changes are the result of compromised blood supply.

In the renal manifestations of this syndrome, the kidneys are swollen and congested. Pale cortical petechiae can be seen in an irregular pattern. Microscopically the primary vascular lesions occur in the afferent arterioles at the glomerular vascular pole. Mural fibrin deposits are commonly seen. While the efferent arterioles are usually not necrotic, they often contain thrombi. Veins and arteries larger than the afferent arterioles appear normal. Because the blood supply to the glomeruli is compromised, many glomeruli will become ischemic and die (Fig. 8–14). Many tubules will show hypoxic changes and often contain a variety of casts.

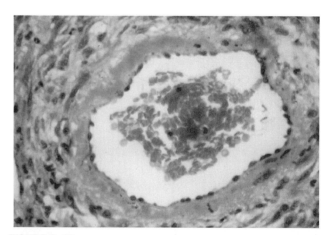

FIGURE 8–13. Histopathological study (H&E stain) illustrating fibrinoid necrosis of a subcutaneous artery.

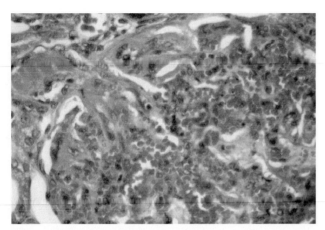

FIGURE 8–14. Histopathological study (H&E stain) illustrating a renal glomerulus that contains thrombi, hemorrhage, and necrosis. These lesions are due to compromised renal afferent arteriole blood flow.

Treatment. In greyhounds exhibiting only cutaneous lesions it is not necessary to institute extensive treatment regimens. Simple cleansing of the wounds with water-soluble antimicrobials at least three times a day will usually allow them to heal. In those cases in which skin ulcers are extensive (usually on the ventral thorax and abdomen), more vigorous therapy is indicated. Fluid loss from these wounds is comparable to thermal injuries and requires fluid replacement and systemic antimicrobial therapy. No single antibiotic has proven most effective.

In those dogs displaying the renal and cutaneous forms of the disease, treatment of heroic proportions must be rapidly instituted if the patient is to survive. Intravenous fluids, electrolytes, vitamins, and parenteral alimentation are necessary. During the first 1 to 3 days the fluid intake must be matched with the outflow to avoid overhydrating patients with poor renal function or absence of it. Once kidney function improves, increased fluid administration will help to lower the BUN and serum creatinine levels. If the patient survives more than a few days, gastrointestinal uremic ulcers are common. Sucralfate therapy is indicated.

Prognosis. If the skin lesions are the only manifestation and the ulcers are not extensive, the prognosis for returning to racing is good. Dogs with more extensive skin lesions may recover clinically but may not return to race at their previous level. It is hypothesized that extensive cicatrix formation in these dogs may limit their full stride.

Despite the severity of the peracute renal failure in dogs with kidney involvement, many do survive with intensive treatment. The resultant weight loss (some of which is loss of muscle mass) and general debilitation dramatically reduce the chances of these patients returning to race at their previous form. At best, it will be many months before these patients can resume training.

Discussion. The cause of the vasculopathy is not known; however, several hypotheses have been advanced. The fact that only greyhounds have been involved suggests that the breed has a specific genetically inherited syndrome or that there is a genetically inherited susceptibility to a specific etiological agent.

Investigators at several sites are currently researching this syndrome. Fenwick et al at Kansas State University have been conducting ongoing research on the pathogenesis of the syndrome and have focused their attention on the Shiga-like toxin–producing bacteria (eg, *Escherichia coli O157:H7*), which may be found in raw meat. These toxins are associated with hemolytic–uremic syndrome (HUS) seen in humans.

HUS renal lesions and the renal lesions associated with the greyhound vasculopathy are similar. Microangiopathic hemolytic anemia, thrombocytopenia, fever, and renal failure are hallmarks of HUS. In HUS the thrombosis may be restricted to the kidneys, occurs primarily in infancy, and is not associated with neurological signs. A genetic predisposition is suspected in HUS because of the occurrence of the syndrome in multiple family members, but there is no evidence to support this theory. There have been reports of HUS in nonrelated human patients following exposure (in fast-food restaurants) to undercooked beef containing a specific *E. coli* toxin. Since greyhounds are frequently fed either 3-D or 4-D beef that is uncooked, the similarity between the two syndromes suggests *E. coli* toxins as the etiological factor in the syndrome in greyhounds.

BALD THIGH SYNDROME

One of the most common dermatological syndromes in retired greyhounds is the bald thigh syndrome. Veterinarians unfamiliar with this condition sometimes assume that the symmetrical alopecia on the thighs of affected dogs is due to pressure wear from lying in cages all day. This is rarely the case. The underlying cause of bald thigh syndrome is hormonal (hypothyroid).

SPOROTRICHOSIS

While fungal infections were mentioned as a possible cause of pododermatitis or pad infections, Sporotrichosis deserves special attention because of the greater risk of infection faced by hunting dogs. The disease is caused by *Sporothrix schenckii*, an organism that exists in mycelial form in the environment and in yeast form in the body. Temperatures above 25° C are required for the organism to survive in soils, particularly soils with high organic content. Puncture wounds from splinters and thorns are possible entry sources for the sporothrix organisms.

Although in dogs the disease most often is disseminated and multinodular, localized lesions are possible. Some of the lesions ulcerate and drain while others may crust. Regional lymphadenopathy is usually present. (Cats with sporotrichosis have infective organisms within the draining fluid that can cause the condition in humans. This is not the case with dogs because the exudate is not infective.) Sporotrichosis should be included in the differential diagnosis in cases of suspected pyoderma when there is no response to antibiotic therapy and the dog lives or works in an environment in which the disease may exist. In dogs the exudate from draining lesions is unlikely to contain fungal organisms (unlike in cats). Diagnostic procedures may include culture (tissue and exudate), histopathology, and fluorescent antibody tests.

Potassium chloride is currently considered the most reliable treatment; however, ketoconazole therapy is being investigated and appears likely to become the treatment of choice.

HYGROMAS

Hygromas are a form of bursitis that develops in areas where the hard bone of a joint lies in proximity to the skin, ie, there is little padding. Elbow joints are the most commonly involved, but on occasion hygroma may develop in hock joints. In these areas of little padding the bursa becomes inflamed after repeated trauma. The bursa's response to inflammation is to produce fluid. Lying on hard surfaces is the most likely cause; thus, dogs that spend much time in cages are more susceptible. I have seen hygromas develop in several litters. It is uncertain if some dogs are genetically prone to this condition or if all of the dogs were subjected to harsh cage conditions.

Controversy exists as to the best method of treatment. Most veterinarians agree that small hygromas are best managed conservatively with either no treatment or with hydrotherapy (cold water). Increasing the padding in the cage area is always a good idea. For larger hygromas some veterinarians aspirate the fluid and then inject corticosteroids into the shrunken cavity. Others treat by opening drainage holes and suturing in Penrose drains, which stay in place for 10 to 14 days. In either case the hygroma may not completely disappear; however, the remaining thickened bursal tissues rarely interfere with function.

STAPHYLOCOCCUS

All dogs are susceptible to *Staphylococcus* species infections of the skin, but only those that are of particular importance to sporting dogs are mentioned in this section. Dermatologists often try to identify the specific *Staphylococcus* species that is causing skin disease. It is beyond the scope of this section to discuss specific pathogens; rather, the group is combined under the general heading of *Staphylococcus* organisms.

Superficial Staphylococcal Pyoderma

This group of bacterial skin infections includes two major syndromes of importance to the sporting breeds. The first is folliculitis, which is seen in all dogs and therefore is not discussed in detail. *Staphylococcus* organisms are the most frequent etiological agents cultured. The syndrome is often secondary. Demodicosis or poor sanitary conditions that allow dirt and debris to remain on the hair coat are both examples of primary conditions with secondary folliculitis. Both pruritic and nonpruritic syndromes occur, and dermatologists argue whether these are two different diseases or two forms of the same disease. Except for the pruritus, the lesions are identical. Many practitioners diagnose the condition when "bulls-eye" lesions are seen, but while this sign suggests folliculitis, it is not pathognomonic. The pustular infection of folliculitis always involves a hair follicle.

The second syndrome is sometimes called puppy pyoderma, puppy staph, or impetigo, the name that will be used in this section. Although impetigo is seen in all breeds, it is of particular importance in kennels where large numbers of dogs are raised. The etiological agent is often a *Staphylococcus* organism, but other pathogens may be present. Pups are usually less than 6 months old when affected. Sometimes impetigo is secondary to skin mites, inadequate nutrition, systemic infections with either bacteria or viruses, or poor sanitation. Primary immune-mediated diseases may also be involved, but more commonly impetigo occurs when passively received maternal antibody levels within a pup's body fall below protective levels against staphylococcal organisms. Impetigo-affected pups usually have superficial pustules that often contain a pale yellow exudate and occur independently of the hair follicles. The pustules often have a zone of erythema surrounding them. Groin and axillae are frequent sites of lesions, but other areas may be affected. In some pups the pustules may be large (bullous), but the lesions are similar except for size. Most practitioners diagnose the condition on the basis of clinical appearance and history. Culture of the pustules should reveal a *Staphylococcus* infection.

Treatment is usually determined by the severity of the signs; however, topical therapy is usually sufficient. Each practitioner has a favorite therapy, which might include antibacterial shampoos or topical astringents. The use of antibiotics should be limited to resistant cases that do not clear with topical therapy. Pups that do not respond to conservative therapy or have persistent recurrence should be reevaluated for other primary diseases.

In kennel situations, the importance of good sanitation cannot be overemphasized. Pups chronically exposed to urine and feces are prone to impetigo and a host of other problems.

Deep Staphylococcal Pyoderma

Deep skin infections can seriously affect the performance of sporting dogs. Several syndromes are recognized in many breeds of dogs, including some called hot spots (pyotraumatic folliculitis), nasal pyodermas, canine acne, German shepherd pyoderma, and pododermatitis. (Shar pei pyodermas would fill a separate textbook!) Again, these are discussed in detail in general dermatology texts. This section is concerned with the deep staphylococcal pyoderma that may occur as the initial clinical presentation or may follow one of the superficial infections mentioned above.

Many of the same predisposing primary conditions for superficial *Staphylococcus* infections are present in deep pyodermas. Ectoparasites, poor nutrition, and allergic disease are examples of predisposing factors for deep infections (Fig. 8–15). Poor sanitation may be another contributing factor. Skin that is chronically wet (in frequent contact with spilled water or urine) macerates and allows penetration of pathological organisms. This is of particular concern to greyhounds that may be "crate wetters" (Fig. 8–16). The seborrheic skin deposits of hypothyroid dogs encourage *Staphylococcus* growth and may play a role in deep infections. Immune-mediated diseases should also be considered in chronic deep pyodermas. The immune problems may be primary or secondary to stress. Hunting dogs and racing greyhounds are prone to more stress than most other breeds. Genetics plays a role, as some sporting breeds are more prone than others to particular types of deep staphylococcal infections. German short-haired pointers, for example, are more prone to canine acne than some other dogs.

In some greyhounds there is a unique predisposing factor related to the muzzles worn during turnout periods, training, and racing. The dorsal skin of the greyhound may be affected by the plastic or leather muzzle rubbing against the skin. The skin on the sides of the face under the attaching straps may also be affected. Plastic muzzles seem less likely to cause the problem than leather ones. Poorly fitted muzzles, unclean muzzles, and wearing of muzzles for a long time in warm, humid weather may all be factors.

Culture (and sensitivity testing) of deep pyodermas is a logical diagnostic procedure because therapy may be long term, and no

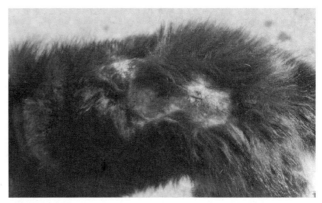

FIGURE 8–15. Immature dog (husky) with sarcoptic mange and deep *Staphylococcus* pyoderma. The pyoderma was recognized and treated with antimicrobial therapy. The pustules dried and scabbed, as shown here, but the alopecia and pruritus persisted until the mites were recognized and then treated.

one antibiotic is going to be lethal to all pathogens. While *Staphylococcus* species should be isolated from these lesions, there may well be other opportunistic organisms present such as *Pseudomonas, E. coli,* or *Proteus* species. Bovier states that if a coagulase positive *Staphylococcus* has not been isolated, the primary pathogen has been missed.

Clinical signs vary greatly with deep *Staphylococcus* infections (Fig. 8–17). In the hunting dog that has a penetrating "fox-tail," for example, the pyoderma will be localized. In the greyhound pup with generalized demodectic mange, the deep pyoderma may be generalized (see Fig. 8–15). When the hair follicles are involved (folliculitis), progression of signs may lead to rupture of the follicle (furunculosis) with hair and keratin coming into contact with the subcutaneous tissues. The result of this process may be tissue eosinophilia (see Staphylococcal Hypersensitivity).

Affected areas have deep pustules that eventually will rupture (see Fig. 8–16). A small number of lesions scab over as they heal. Deeper or widespread areas may have combinations of draining lesions and healing lesions. In extreme cases, cellulitis and abscesses may develop.

Any underlying primary disease must be treated if the condition is to be cured and recurrence avoided. One of the more frequent causes of treatment failure is insufficient duration of antibiotic therapy. Many dermatologists recommend treating at least 10 days beyond the time when all clinical signs have disappeared. In some cases, 8 to 10 weeks of therapy may be necessary. This is significant in racing greyhounds, because the antibiotics will be detected

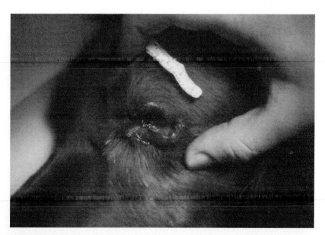

FIGURE 8–17. Deep pyoderma of the eyelids. Note the pustules and swelling. Deep pyodermas can develop on any part of the skin. This pyoderma of the lids is not to be confused with the staphylococcal hypersensitivity reaction that sometimes can be noted as a ring of alopecia around the eye(s), even though the infection is at a more distant site.

in post-race sampling. Trainers and owners are often eager to end therapy as quickly as possible so that the patient may resume racing. In cases of deep *Staphylococcus* pyoderma the result of inadequate therapy is usually the prolongation of treatment and loss of racing days. Antibiotic therapy should be guided by culture results.

Antibacterial shampoos (benzoyl peroxide, povidone-iodine, and chlorhexidine) are valuable in superficial infections, but they are not likely to be effective by themselves. Bacterins and staph phage lysates have also been used successfully in cases that do not respond to antibiotic and topical therapy.

STAPHYLOCOCCAL HYPERSENSITIVITY

Staphylococcus organisms produce a variety of antigenic toxins that may cause reactions. It is difficult in some cases to determine if lesions are due to *Staphylococcus* infections, to toxins, or to combinations of both. Intense pruritus is always present, and surface erythema is noted. The appearance is often that of a bulls-eye or target lesion, as noted in the section on *Staphylococcus* pyodermas. Alopecia may develop, and lesions may coalesce so that large areas of skin are involved.

At least one cell-wall antigen, *Staphylococcus* protein A, has been demonstrated to bind with IgE in the surface of mast cells, causing degranulation. Tissue edema and erythema result in the clinical signs frequently seen with *Staphylococcus* hypersensitivity. It is also thought that *Staphylococcus* toxins may directly increase the permeability of the skin and allow additional organisms to penetrate. Undoubtedly the hypersensitivity reaction is a complex one and probably involves multiple pathways. This is an active area of dermatological research.

Diagnosis of the *Staphylococcus* hypersensitivity reaction is, in part, diagnosis by exclusion. Other hypersensitivities such as flea bite and food reactions must be eliminated. Immune-mediated diseases must also be ruled out. Lack of response to corticosteroids and rapid response to appropriate antibiotic therapy should give rise to a strong suspicion of *Staphylococcus* hypersensitivity. Biopsy and intradermal skin testing help provide more definitive information.

Some patients have recurrences of clinical signs even after long-term therapy. While long-term treatment can be instituted in most

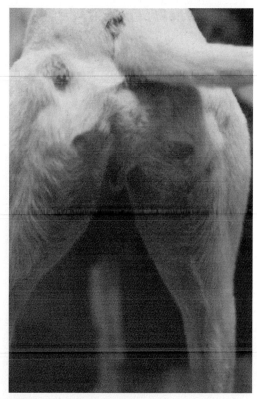

FIGURE 8–16. A racing greyhound that was a "crate wetter." The symmetrical nature of the lesions on the inner thighs suggests either an allergic or hormonal etiology; however, the condition improved with antimicrobial therapy alone and remained cleared when the dog was kept in a drier environment. Note also the more typical lesions of inflammation and alopecia around the tail base. This photograph was taken after therapy was instituted, and many of the lesions have dried and formed scabs.

breeds, this would be impossible in the racing greyhound, which, under current racing rules, cannot perform while taking systemic medications.

References

Blythe L, Gannon JR, Craig M: Care of the Racing Greyhound. Portland, OR, American Greyhound Council, 1994.

Ettinger SJ, Feldman EC: Textbook of Veterinary Internal Medicine, 4th ed. Philadelphia, WB Saunders Company, 1995.

Evans HE: Miller's Anatomy of the Dog, 3rd ed. Philadelphia, WB Saunders Company, 1993.

Evans HE, deLahunta A: Miller's Guide to the Dissection of the Dog, 4th ed. Philadelphia, WB Saunders Company, 1995.

Kronfeld E: Vitamin and Mineral Supplementation for Dog. Santa Barbara, Calif, Veterinary Practice Publishing Company, 1989.

Scott DW, Miller WH Jr, Griffin CE: Muller and Kirk's Small Animal Dermatology, 5th ed. Philadelphia, WB Saunders Company, 1995.

Smith HA, Jones TC, Hunt RD: Veterinary Pathology. Philadelphia, Lea & Febiger, 1972.

Swaim SF: Surgery of Traumatized Skin. Philadelphia, WB Saunders Company, 1980.

Suggested Readings

Bevier DE: Canine staphyloccal pyoderma. Vet Med Rep 2:288–291, 1990.

Carpenter JL, Andelman NC: Idiopathic Cutaneous and Renal Glomerular Vasculopathy of Greyhounds. Vet Pathol 25:401–407, 1988.

Codner EC, Thatcher CD: Nutritional management of skin disease. Comp Cont Ed 15:411–424, 1993.

DeBoer DJ: Canine staphylococcal pyoderma. Vet Med Rep 2:254–266, 1990.

Fenwick B, Hertzke D, Cowan L: Alabama Rot: Almost the Complete Story. Eleventh Annual International Canine Sports Medicine Symposium pp 15–22, 1995.

Fox SM, et al: Management of thermal burns—III. Comp Cont Ed 8:439–444, 1986.

Halliwell REW: Rational use of shampoos in veterinary dermatology. J Small Anim Pract 32:401–407, 1991.

Herron MR: Nails. Current Techniques in Small Animal Surgery, 2nd ed. WB Saunders Company, 1980.

Hill PB, Moriello KA: Canine pyoderma. JAVMA 204:334–340, 1994.

Ihrke PJ, et al: Pemphigus foliaceus of the footpads in three dogs. JAVMA 186:67–69, 1985.

Ihrke PJ: The management of canine pyodermas. Curr Vet Ther 8:505–517, 1983.

Lloyd DH: Therapy for canine pyoderma. Curr Vet Ther 11:540–544, 1992.

Mason IS, Lloyd DH: The role of allergy in the development of canine pyoderma. J Small Anim Pract 30:216–218, 1989.

Medleau L, et al: Frequency and antimicrobial susceptibility of *Staphylococcus* species isolated from canine pyodermas. Am J Vet Res 47:229, 1986.

Reedy LM: The role of staphyloccal bacteria in canine dermatology. AAHA Scientific Proceedings, 1981.

Rosser EI: Sporotrichosis and public health. Curr Vet Ther 10:633–634, 1989.

Scott DW, Miller WH: Disorders of the claw and clawbed in dogs. Compend Cont Educ 14:1448–1458, 1992.

Scott DW, MacDonald JM, Schultz RD: Staphylococcal hypersensitivity in the dog. JAMAH 14:766–779, 1978.

Swaim SF, et al: Evaluation of surgical scrub and antiseptic solutions for surgical preparation of canine paws. JAVMA 198(11):1941–1945, 1991.

Swaim SF, Angarano DW: Chronic problem wounds of dog limbs. Clin Dermatol 8:175–186, 1990.

CHAPTER 9

Genitourinary Diseases in the Canine Athlete

RAY G. FERGUSON \ CHRISTOPHER M. BOEMO

The same genitourinary tract conditions that affect other canines affect racing and sporting dogs. Stress-related problems such as the water diabetes syndrome, and post-racing dysuria present a challenge to veterinarians. Veterinarians need to understand all factors involved in the etiology of these conditions to correct or eliminate them. Although some myths still exist concerning medical treatment of sporting dogs, they respond to medications in exactly the same manner as do other canines. Caution needs to be exercised when using corticosteroid therapy with the greyhound because of the animal's apparent sensitivity to the drug and the potential to induce the water diabetes syndrome.

MALE GENITOURINARY DISEASES

Posthitis

Posthitis, a purulent discharge present at the preputial orifice and dried on the surrounding hairs, is common in most male dogs. The amount of discharge varies, but it is of no significance to the dog's health. Trainers often regard posthitis as a potential focus of infection, especially if the dog licks the region excessively. Severe posthitis may be caused by bacterial or fungal infections, foreign bodies, neoplastic growths, urine scalding secondary to phimosis,[1] or overly zealous treatments with irritant or concentrated antiseptics.

If a marked purulent discharge is present, the prepuce should be carefully examined for foreign bodies, especially grass seed awns, neoplastic growths on the penis or prepuce, and penile ulceration. In the absence of foreign bodies or neoplastic growths, the prepuce should be flushed with 20 ml of a warm 0.1 per cent chlorhexidine solution twice a day for 7 days. If this fails to resolve the condition, an antimicrobial and corticosteroid ointment (1 ml) should be applied twice a day. Swabbing and culture should be carried out in refractory cases, and appropriate antibiotic therapy instituted on the basis of sensitivity results.

Prostatitis

Bacterial prostatitis may occur in the young canine sporting dog, although it is observed commonly in older entire male dogs, and usually results from an ascending urinary tract infection. *Escherichia coli, Proteus* species, *Staphylococcus* species, and *Streptococcus* species are commonly isolated.[2] The infection causes nonspecific systemic signs of depression, malaise, fever, a straddling stiff hind gait, cautious movement, and, occasionally, tenesmus. Blood or blood-stained exudate may drip from the penis. On rectal palpation, the gland is spongy and painful. Urinalysis reveals the presence of red blood cells and inflammatory cells. Prostatic washes also reveal inflammatory cells and bacteria. Culture and sensitivity tests should be carried out on prostatic washes.

Bacterial prostatitis responds quickly to antibiotic therapy. Inadequately treated cases may progress to a more chronic prostatitis with irregular hypertrophy of the gland with or without abscesses.[2, 3]

Prostatic Hypertrophy

Prostatic hypertrophy is rare in young dogs. Its occurrence increases with ongoing exposure of the gland to androgens.[3] The gland enlarges symmetrically, with or without the presence of cystic cavities. Dogs with prostatic hypertrophy have an increased tendency to develop bacterial prostatitis. Chronic prostatitis can lead to hyperplasia. Prostatic washes, cytologic and ultrasonographic examinations and/or biopsy are indicated in cases of prostatic enlargement to differentiate among chronic prostatitis, benign prostatic hyperplasia, and prostatic neoplasia. Benign hypertrophy may be present asymptomatically or may result in impairment of defecation with increased straining, incomplete bowel emptying, production of thin, pencil-like stools, and/or dysuria. Cystitis may be a secondary complication due to incomplete bladder emptying.[3]

Treatment of prostatic hypertrophy involves the use of progestogens, such as medroxyprogesterone acetate (5 mg/kg injected subcutaneously and repeated at 5- to 6-monthly intervals as needed to control symptoms) or castration. Medical treatment has only a relatively temporary effect and must be provided on an ongoing basis, so that castration is the treatment of choice. However, the breeding potential of the dog needs to be considered. Subtotal intracapsular prostatectomy[4] and total prostatectomy[5] procedures have been described for the treatments of prostatic hyperplasia and neoplasia, respectively, but they are not without complications. In our experience, valuable stud dogs may be treated with progestogens without total loss of fertility; however, semen collected from these dogs does not freeze satisfactorily.

Cryptorchidism

Cryptorchidism is common in sporting dogs in spite of the fact that cryptorchid dogs are rarely used at stud. The inheritance pattern of the condition is not fully defined. Autosomal recessive genes may be involved in some breeds, and this makes the condition difficult to eliminate.[1, 6] Cryptorchidism may be bilateral or unilateral. The testes may be within the abdomen or easily palpable just outside the inguinal ring. Dogs with bilateral intra-abdominal cryptorchidism are sterile. Before any surgery is contemplated, the dog's athletic ability must be assessed. Dogs with little athletic ability are usually retired from competition, and a bilateral orchidectomy should be carried out. If the dog has athletic potential and both testes are intra-abdominal, they are best left in situ until the end of the dog's athletic career and then removed. This should happen before 5 years of age to minimize the risk of testicular neoplasia. If one testis is intra-abdominal and the other is in the inguinal region, the dog may continue racing and be castrated at the end of its competitive life. If there is any concern about the

risk of testicular neoplasia or testicular torsion, the intra-abdominal testis should be removed. Undescended testicles have a higher incidence of neoplasia and torsion than normally descended testes.[3, 6, 7] In the racing greyhound it is relatively routine to remove inguinal testicles at 6 to 12 months of age, before the animal's initial education or early in its racing career. This is because of the tendency (albeit subjective) for these testes to interfere with the animal's ability to negotiate bends.[7] If the dog runs wide when cornering or has an abnormal gait during exercise and no musculoskeletal abnormalities can be found that could be attributed to this abnormality, the inguinal testis can be implicated, because it probably becomes entrapped during running. This testis should be removed.

Bilateral orchidectomy should not be carried out with any dog destined for racing. In our experience, castrated dogs, in general, do not race well and need regular anabolic hormone therapy.[8] Two greyhounds have, however, raced well after castration. One dog received 25 mg methyltestosterone every second day, while the other was given monthly injections of depot testosterone.[7, 8]

Orchitis

Orchitis is rare in sporting dogs. Bacterial causes include *Staphylococcus, Streptococcus, E. coli, Proteus* species, and *Brucella canis.* Because of the close association of the epididymis and the testis, orchiepididymitis is commonly encountered.[3] Foreign bodies such as grass seed awns may also cause orchitis. The condition is usually unilateral, but complications may occur in the contralateral testis as a result of local or systemic hyperthermia.

The affected testis is usually swollen, firm, warm, and painful to touch. There may also be systemic signs of malaise and pyrexia. Commonly the epididymis is also enlarged, and the serosal cavity may be distended and tense with accumulated fluid. Atrophy and irregular fibrosis are common in chronic cases. Abscess, spermatocoele, and granuloma formation may occur. If there are no draining sinus tracts, antibiotic therapy is indicated. If there is a draining tract, then an abscess or a foreign body should be suspected, and careful surgical exploration is indicated. Antibiotic selection should be, when possible, on the basis of sensitivity testing. Scrotal cooling is an important adjunct to therapy to minimize thermal damage to spermatogenesis, which may be permanent, even with resolution of the acute disease. Unilateral orchidectomy may be indicated if there is severe damage to the testicular tissue. Replacement anabolic therapy is not required after unilateral orchidectomy.

Testicular Torsion

Testicular torsion is a rare condition in racing dogs. It occurs most commonly in undescended testes and is almost invariably secondary to neoplastic changes in intra-abdominal testes.[7, 9] Intrascrotal torsion of normal testicles has also been reported.[10] Whereas it is apparent how uneven, unbalanced growth of an intra-abdominal testicular neoplasm would predispose to torsion, the etiology of testicular torsion in normal testes remains uncertain; vigorous exercise has been proposed.[7] Caudal abdominal pain and hindlimb stiffness are the most common presenting signs in acute intra-abdominal testicular torsion. Scrotal pain and swelling are seen in torsions of descended testes. There may also be reluctance to stand or move about, general malaise, anorexia, and mild pyrexia. Unilateral orchidectomy is indicated and is usually straightforward in cases of both intra-abdominal and scrotal testicular torsions. Replacement anabolic therapy is not required.

Congenital Abnormalities

Congenital abnormalities of the male urogenital tract are very rare. A case of hypospadias (failure of ventral fusion of the urethra and prepuce along part of its length) has been observed by one of us (CMB) in a greyhound pup. This condition may occur in both genetic males and intersexes and is treated by amputation of the distal penile structures.[3] Aplasia of the epididymis and associated parts of the vas deferens has been described in various breeds of dog[11] and should be included in the differential diagnosis of the aspermic dog. The persistence of the penile frenulum (a band of tissue joining the penis to the prepuce ventrally) has also been noted and is associated with pubertal or postpubertal clinical signs of sudden sitting down and crying out because of discomfort experienced with intermittent penile engorgement.[12] Surgical resection of the fibrous band results in resolution of the signs.

FEMALE GENITOURINARY DISEASES

Vaginitis

Infantile vaginitis is common in prepubertal bitches. A slight creamy to yellow discharge is evident at the vulva; the bitch usually shows no sign of discomfort. Treatment is not usually indicated, although the use of an antimicrobial and anti-inflammatory ointment or cream may relieve the signs of the condition and the anxiety of the owner.

Bacterial and fungal infections, foreign bodies such as grass seed awns, and structural abnormalities such as partitioning or pouching of the vagina, vestibulovaginal junctional strictures, and the presence of remnants of the müllerian ducts can result in vaginitis.[3, 13] Vaginal examination under general anaesthesia should be carried out to diagnose any abnormalities, and persistent or recurrent vaginitis warrants culture and sensitivity testing.

Clinical signs of vaginitis include purulent vulval discharge with crusts on the adjacent surface of the tail. Affected bitches are often dysuric with frequent micturition and may flick their tail agitatedly. Cystitis due to ascending infection may be a secondary complication.

Treatment of vaginitis involves infusion of 1 ml of an antimicrobial and corticosteroid preparation three times a day. Many bitches, however, resent vaginal infusions, and systemic antibiotics based on culture and sensitivity may be required to effect a cure. Any structural abnormalities of the vagina should be treated surgically. Foreign bodies are surgically removed.

Clitoral Hypertrophy

Clitoral hypertrophy is a common condition seen as a sequel to the androgenic effect of administration of anabolic hormones to suppress estrus.[14] Although the extent of hypertrophy depends on the type and amount of anabolic steroid preparation used, some bitches would seem to be more susceptible to the development of hypertrophy than others. In most cases of clitoral hypertrophy, the clitoris is usually quite prominent, but it may not be visible unless the vulval lips are parted. Often the tail hairs irritate the hypertrophied clitoris. There may be significant purulent vaginal discharge. Bitches affected by this condition may race poorly and commonly have a sullen demeanor. Treatment involves stopping administration of the anabolic hormone and applying a topical antimicrobial and corticosteroid cream three times a day. Regression of the hypertrophy takes months after administration of the anabolic hormone is stopped. In some cases, regression never occurs.

Endometritis

Endometritis is a rare condition in young sporting dogs but a common condition of entire bitches older than 6 years.[15] Endometritis occurs in diestrous bitches because of repeated high progester-one levels. High progesterone levels stimulate cystic endometrial hyperplasia, which is the first phase in the development of endometritis. The most commonly isolated pathogen is *E. coli*, but *Streptococcus, Staphylococcus,* and *Pseudomonas* can also be isolated.[16]

One of us (CMB) has observed one case of endometritis involving an 11-month-old diestrous greyhound bitch. The animal had become acutely ill with vomiting, depression, and inappetence. There was a slight mucoid vaginal discharge; abdominal palpation was resented with muscle guarding. Treatment consisted of ovariohysterectomy, and recovery was uneventful.

RACING SYNDROMES

Post-Racing Dysuria

Post-racing dysuria is a syndrome observed only in males. It occurs mainly in young dogs that have a nervous excitable nature. It is commonly related to stressful conditions such as schooling, long waits at trialing tracks, and long periods of kenneling on race nights. Dysuria may be a sign associated with the polydipsia and polyuria of water diabetes syndrome, the hindlimb incoordination and toenail scuffing associated with postexercise electrolyte imbalances and muscle cramping, or it may be the only sign noted in the greyhound. The syndrome has been described in the literature[17] and relatively recently was classified into three stages of increasing severity.[18]

The control of urination is a complex process with somatic, sympathetic, and parasympathetic interaction.[18, 19] The bladder is under sympathetic dominance during the filling phase with alpha-adrenergic stimulation of the trigone and smooth muscle of the proximal urethra increasing outflow resistance.[18, 20] Normal urination results with a change to parasympathetic dominance and inhibition of somatic and sympathetic activity.[18, 19] Elevation of cortical awareness in anticipation of, or in response to, racing or kenneling increases the sympathetic tone of the autonomic nervous system, reduces parasympathetic activity, and reduces inhibition of motor impulses to the urethral striated muscle. Alpha-adrenergic stimulation of the trigone and smooth muscle of the proximal urethra increases the resistance to outflow. Reduced parasympathetic tone results in lower detrusor muscle activity, reduction in the degree of bladder neck widening, and increased outflow resistence. These alterations to normal function are usually not absolute but are relative, resulting in varying degrees of dysfunction.[20] With high tone in the urethra and reduction in detrusor tone, urine can be voided only in a fine stream, and bladder emptying may be incomplete.

The clinical signs of postexertional dysuria may be divided into three categories of increasing severity:

Stage 1. Dysuria occurs 2 to 48 hours after a run. Affected animals stand as if to begin urination, but the onset is delayed by 10 to 20 seconds. When the passage of urine occurs, it is passed as a finer than usual stream occasionally with a discernible pulsed flow, especially toward the end of micturition.

Stage 2. The delay in beginning of urination is more prolonged than in stage 1, and there is evidence of much greater resistance to outflow; a fine, pulsed stream of urine or a only few short squirts of urine are produced. Abdominal palpation may reveal a tense distended bladder, and attempts at bladder emptying are usually incomplete. Urinalysis often is not unusual in stage 1 and stage 2 dysuria, unless dysuria is present in addition to water diabetes syndrome or exertional rhabdomyolysis.

Stage 3. There is total inability to urinate. The dog repeatedly attempts to urinate without success, and marked discomfort is observed. Bladder hyperdistention occurs, and severe abdominal discomfort is present. Urine from stage 3 dysuric dogs is often dark brown because of hemoglobinuria and hematuria. Bladder atony is a potential complication. The principles of treatment are to reduce the outflow resistance, to increase the intravesical pressure, and to achieve bladder emptying. The extent of treatment required depends upon the severity of the dysuria and urine retention.

Stage 1 cases may be treated simply by reducing and/or avoiding stress. As long as there is sufficient urine flow to empty the bladder and the dog is not distressed, most cases will resolve over 24 to 48 hours. Stage 2 cases require medical therapy with alpha-adrenergic blocking agents. Phenoxybenzamine at a dose rate of 10 to 20 mg orally three times a day provides good urethral relaxation and is usually sufficient to establish urine flow.[18] Diazepam at a dose rate of 5 to 10 mg orally three times a day may also be used in conjunction with phenoxybenzamine to help relax the urethra. Prazosin HCl, 1 to 5 mg twice a day, has been recommended as an alternative to phenoxybenzamine,[21] but we have not used it for this purpose. The presently unavailable guanethidine sulfate used at a dose of 5 to 10 mg twice a day provided excellent clinical response.[17] Once urethral relaxation has occurred, parasympathomimetics such as bethanechol, 10 to 20 mg orally three times a day can be used to increase detrusor muscle tone.

Stage 3 cases require sedation and urethral catheterization. The bladder is evacuated, and if atony is suspected, the catheter should be secured in place for 2 to 3 days. Phenoxybenzamine, diazepam, and bethanacol are prescribed as above, and the patient is closely monitored for efficient voiding of urine. Prophylactic antibiotic cover is indicated, especially if there is gross hematuria or if the catheter is to be indwelling for several days. Once recovered, affected dogs should have their level of training reduced with attempts made to avoid any stressful situation. Anabolic steroids may be given where permitted by racing regulations to reduce the adverse effects of stress.[18]

Prognosis is very good. With modification of the animal's training program, it adapts to the stresses of racing, and recurrences of the problem are infrequent. Some patients, however, do require ongoing postexertional alpha-adrenergic blocker therapy.

Post-Race Myoglobinuria

Myoglobinuria is a common finding in most dogs after any major physical activity.[22] The myoglobinuria may discolor the urine, or it may be detectable only with laboratory tests. It usually persists for up to 24 hours. The myoglobin originates from muscle injury and breakdown of muscle fibers during exertion. Grade 1 or 2 muscle injuries are detectable during post-run musculoskeletal examination of the dog. We have found mild elevations in creatine phosphokinase (CPK) of up to 400 IU for 24 to 36 hours post racing. These levels fall to less than 100 IU within 48 hours after exercise. If the dog is alert and in good health, the myoglobinuria and CPK levels are of no significance to its health and performance. Caution needs to be observed when a myoglobin hemoglobin test is found to be positive by means of urinary dipsticks. The commonly used urinary dipsticks cannot differentiate among hemoglobinuria, hematuria, and myoglobinuria. Urine sediment examination is indicated for the presence of erythrocytes, inflammatory cells, renal casts, and leukocytes to differentiate myoglobinuria from hemoglobinuria and hematuria.[22] The presence of myoglobinuria and CPK levels greater than 400 IU 48 hours after exercise indicate marked muscle injury, and a very careful musculoskeletal examination should be carried out to define the extent of the injury.

Post-racing myoglobinuria may also be observed in dogs that have canine exertional rhabdomyolysis (CER). Affected dogs are dehydrated and commonly show pain when moving. Pain is readily elicited on palpation of the affected muscle groups, usually the thoracic and lumbar paravertebral muscles.

Pre-Race Myoglobinuria

Pre-race myoglobinuria may occur in excitable and nervous dogs that have been kenneled for long periods. It may also be observed in those animals that have waited for prolonged periods at trial tracks while being stimulated by the sight and sound of the lure. These dogs may lose up to 0.5 kg body weight because of fluid loss from panting and salivation. If the dog is already in a mild state of dehydration on arrival at the track, further fluid loss reduces tissue perfusion. Tissue hypoxia then occurs, and muscle cell damage ensues. Myoglobin and other proteins leak into the circulation. Some of the myoglobin is eliminated via the urine. This condition may predispose to CER.

Cystitis

Cystitis is a relatively common condition in sporting dogs.[23] Both sexes can be affected, but females are more prone to it. Cystitis is usually the result of an ascending infection from the lower urinary tract with *E. coli, Proteus* species, *Pseudomonas* species, *Staphylococcus* species, *Streptococcus* species, and *Klebsiella* species.[24] Rarely does cystitis result from hematogenous spread of bacterial organisms. Animals with cystitis exhibit varying degrees of stranguria and increased frequency of urination. Frequent attempts at urination with production of only a small volume of urine on each occasion are common.[25]

The animals are usually active and alert and afebrile. Urine examination by means of dipsticks reveals hematuria, proteinuria, and pyuria. Should uroliths be present, obstruction and inability to pass urine may occur.

Treatment of cystitis involves systemic antibiotics, based on culture and sensitivity, in conjunction with urinary antiseptics and urinary acidifiers.[26] Initial treatment with trimethoprim/sulfadiazine or clavulanic acid-augmented amoxicillin should be continued until culture and sensitivity results are obtained. Affected dogs should avoid any strenuous activity until the condition has resolved.

Nephritis

Infectious nephritis is not common in sporting dogs. Young dogs on rearing and schooling establishments are often affected. The source of infection is usually hematogenous, with *Escherichia coli* being commonly isolated on culture.[26] Infection by *Leptospira icterohaemorrhagiae* also is not infrequent and is usually confirmed by serological studies.[27] Clinical signs include depression, poor athletic form, rough coat, fever, and pain on renal palpation. Leptospirosis commonly occurs with the additional signs of inappetence, vomiting, diarrhea, conjunctival vascular congestion, severe dehydration, and jaundice. Hematological findings are variable, with leukocytosis often present. Liver enzymes, urea, and creatinine show marked elevation in leptospiral infections. Urinalysis in dogs with nephritis shows pyuria, hematuria, and bacteria. Leptospires may be found in darkfield examination of urine. Differential diagnosis of nephritis in dogs includes postexertional myoglobinuria and cystitis.

Treatment of mild nephritis involves rest from racing, removal from all sources of stress, and antibiotic therapy based on culture and sensitivity. Penicillin, streptomycin, and tetracyclines are effective against *Leptospira* serotypes, but full supportive therapy to counteract dehydration, electrolyte imbalances, and blood loss is indicated. Control of recurrent urinary tract infections may need pulsed treatments with antibiotics or urinary antiseptics such as hexamine hippurate. Pulsed treatments with antibiotics involves the administration of twice the normal dosage of antibiotic given once weekly. Urinary antiseptics are given twice a day for 2 days after strenuous exercise.

References

1. Allen WE: Surgery of the urinogenital tract. *In* Bedford PGC (ed): Atlas of Canine Surgical Techniques. Oxford, Blackwell Scientific Publications, 1984, p 123.
2. Robertson JJ: Surgical management of prostatic disease. *In* Bojrab MJ (ed): Current Techniques in Small Animal Surgery, 3rd ed. Philadelphia, Lea & Febiger, 1990, p 393.
3. Jones DE, Joshua JO: The male. *In* Reproductive Clinical Problems in the Dog. Bristol, Eng, Wright, 1982, p 122.
4. Robertson JJ, Bojrab MJ: Subtotal intracapsular prostatectomy—results in normal dogs. Vet Surg 13(2):6, 1984.
5. Christie TR: Prostate. *In* Bojrab MJ (ed): Current Therapy in Small Animal Surgery. 2nd ed. Philadelphia, Lea & Febiger, 1983.
6. Johnson SD: Reproduction. *In* Proc Post-Grad C'tee Vet Sci Univ Syd 108:202, 1988.
7. Boemo CM: Torsion of an intra-abdominal testicle in a greyhound pup: A case study. *In* Proc Post Grad C'tee Vet Sci Univ Syd 122:313, 1989.
8. Ferguson RG: 1998 in print.
9. Pearson H, Kelly DF: Testicular torsion in the dog: A review of 13 cases. Vet Rec 97:200, 1975.
10. Young ACB: Two cases of intra-scrotal torsion of a normal testicle. J Small Anim Pract 20:229, 1979.
11. Copland MD, MacLachlin NL: Aplasia of epididymis and vas deferens in the dog. J Small Anim Pract 17:443, 1976.
12. Joshua JO: Persistence of the penile frenulum in a dog. Vet Rec 74:1550, 1962.
13. Holt PE, Sayle B: Congenital vestibulo-vaginal stenosis in the bitch. J Small Anim Pract 22:67, 1981.
14. Murray JW: Anabolics and their relationship to greyhound performance. *In* Proc Post-Grad C'tee Vet Sci Univ Syd 64:341, 1983.
15. Johnson SD: Disease of the uterus and oviducts. *In* Proc Post-Grad C'tee Vet Sci Uni Syd 108:142, 1988.
16. Parry BW: Clinical pathology of canine and feline reproductive disorders. *In* Proc Post-Grad C'tee Vet Sci Uni Syd 108:356, 1988.
17. Gannon JR: Fitness and stress related problems in the racing greyhound. *In* Proc Aust Greyhound Vet Assoc Conf 1985. Melbourne.
18. Boemo CM: Dysuria in the racing greyhound. *In* Proc Aust Greyhound Vet Assoc Conf 1994. Canberra.
19. De Lahunta A: Lower motor neuron–general visceral efferent system. *In* Veterinary Neuroanatomy and Clinical Neurology. Philadelphia, WB Saunders Company, 1977, p 110.
20. Bovee KC: Dysfunction of urine voiding. In Proc Post-Grad C'tee Vet Sci Uni Syd 61:371, 1982.
21. Irwin PJ: Personal communication.
22. Ferguson RG: A consultation format. *In* Proc Post-Grad C'tee Vet Sci Uni Syd 122:323, 1989.
23. Hauler AD: Electrolyte metabolism. *In* Proc Post-Grad C'tee Vet Sci Uni Syd 122:393, 1989.
24. Hirsh DC: Multiple antimicrobial resistance in Escherichia coli isolated from the urine of dogs and cats with cystitis. JAVMA 162:885, 1973.
25. Greene RW, Scott RC: Lower urinary tract disease. *In* Ettinger SJ (ed): Textbook of Veterinary Internal Medicine vol 2. Philadelphia, WB Saunders Company, 1975, p 1541.
26. Bovee KC: Infections of the urinary tract—small animals. *In* Proc Post-Grad C'tee Vet Sci Uni Syd 61:343, 1982.
27. Lording PM: Interpretation of clinical pathology profiles. *In* Proc Post-Grad C'tee Vet Sci Uni Syd 122:369, 1989.

CHAPTER 10

NEUROLOGICAL DYSFUNCTION IN SPORTING AND WORKING DOGS

LINDA BLYTHE

The nervous system of the dog consists of the brain, spinal cord, and cranial and peripheral nerves. The last two connect with both sensory receptors and motor units. The nervous system monitors the environment and allows the animal to respond to it by initiating motor responses and by regulating all other functional systems in the body. Dysfunction of the nervous system, from whatever cause, can often render the dog incapable of athletic performance.

ASSESSMENT OF THE NERVOUS SYSTEM WITH LOCALIZATION OF LESION

Assessment of the nervous system and localization of lesions is a problematic endeavor that requires knowledge of basic neuroanatomy and neurophysiology as well as testable functional components such as proprioception (knowledge of where the body is in space), postural and protective reflexes, perception of touch and pain, and gait. Dysfunction of other systems can share some of the same clinical signs as those of a nervous system disorder and can cause confusion in evaluation. For example, motor weakness can be a neurological dysfunction, a result of a primary metabolic disorder, eg, hypoglycemia, or the result of a primary muscle problem. A complete physical and neurological examination is the key in differentiating between the possible origins of the dysfunction and in establishing a diagnosis, prognosis, and therapy.

A neurological examination tests the integrity of the central nervous system by systematically evaluating seven functional subdivisions of it (Fig. 10–1) and the peripheral nerves. The following will be a brief overview of localization of a neurological lesion, and the reader is referred to neurological texts for in-depth explanations.[1–3]

Brain

Lesions in the brain are frequently associated with one or more of the following: changes in behavior; alterations in level of consciousness, eg, depression, mania; history or occurrence of seizures; gait deficits; and cranial nerve deficits. Observation of deficits in function of any of the 12 pair of cranial nerves is the most reliable

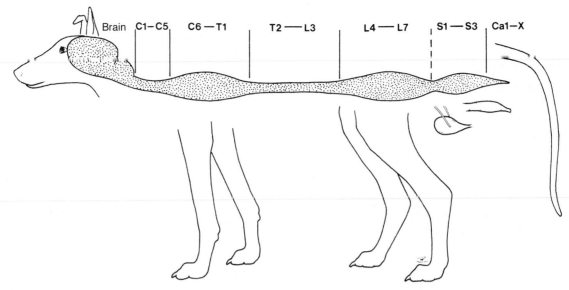

FIGURE 10–1. The seven major subdivisions of the central nervous system. These include the (1) brain; (2) upper cervical spinal cord segments (C1–C5) that carry sensory and motor information to and from the brain and supply some of the neck muscles; (3) caudal cervical and cranial thoracic spinal cord segments (C6–T1) that comprise the brachial enlargement and control the muscles to the forelimbs; (4) thoracic and cranial lumbar spinal cord segments (T2–L3) supplying the intercostal muscles; (5) lumbar spinal cord segments (L4–L7) with part of sacral segments S1 and S2 supplying the pelvic enlargement that innervates the muscles of the rear limbs; (6) sacral spinal cord segments (S1–S3) supplying the bladder, rectum, and anus; and (7) Ca1 to a variable number of caudal spinal cord segments that innervate the tail muscles.

indicator of primary brain dysfunction, and all 12 should be tested in any suspected neurological condition. A vestibular deficit often will include head tilt, nystagmus, leaning or rolling to one side, and reluctance to move. Cerebellar deficits due to congenital, developmental, or traumatic lesion are often characterized by a hypermetric gait, intact but inappropriate proprioception responses (hypometric or hypermetric), intention tremors especially evident in the head during movement, and loss of the menace response. Evaluation of the palpebral, corneal, cough, gag, and jaw tone reflexes, the perception of touch and pain over the face, and the function and size of the muscles of the head (masseter, temporalis, facial muscles) and neck (cleidomastoideus and cleidocervicalis portions of the brachiocephalicus, omotransversarius, sternocephalicus, and trapezius) are necessary to determine and localize a neurological lesion of the brain.

Spinal Cord

Spinal cord damage can be determined and localized to the various functional segments seen in Figure 10–1 utilizing the concept of upper motor neuron (UMN) disease and lower motor neuron (LMN) disease. The LMN are those neurons in the brain (cranial nerve nuclei that have motor function, ie, cranial nerves III, IV, V, VI, VII, IX, X, XI, and XII) and in the spinal cord (ventral horn neurons) whose axons directly innervate skeletal muscles. On the other hand, UMNs are those neurons in the brain that initiate voluntary movement by subsequently activating the LMNs when the animal wishes to move. Reflexes are "hard wired" in neural pathways between a sensory neuron and an LMN (+/− spinal cord- or brain-connecting interneurons) whereby an appropriate stimulus, such as a pinch to the toe or a tap on a tendon, will result in direct muscle movement without any involvement of the brain or the UMNs. Table 10–1 compares and contrasts the similarities and differences in clinically testable functions relative to disease affecting LMNs and UMNs. In brief, the loss of any of the reflexes within one of the spinal cord segments (see Fig. 10–1) localizes

the lesion to that cord segment(s). Exaggerated reflexes indicate that the lesion is cranial to the reflex arc or neural circuit.

With the localization of a lesion to one or more parts of the nervous system, a list of differential diagnoses can be made relative to the findings. For example, finding deficits relative to the brain, eg, cranial nerve deficits or seizures, would localize a lesion to within the head. However, those same clinical signs coupled with LMN signs of loss of withdrawal and patellar reflexes in the pelvic

TABLE 10–1. Comparison of Clinical Signs Present with Lower Motor Neuron (LMN) and Upper Motor Neuron (UMN) Disease

	LMN Signs	UMN Signs
Voluntary movement	Paresis to Paralysis	
Sensory perception	Loss of Proprioception ↓ Hypalgesia ↓ Analgesia	
Reflexes	Hyporeflexia→Areflexia	Normal→Hyperreflexia
Muscles	Hypotonic	Hypertonic
	Marked neurogenic atrophy	Mild disuse atrophy
	EMG abnormalities (after 5 days)	No EMG changes

limbs would indicate a diffuse or multifocal disease, such as canine distemper.

CONGENITAL, GENETIC, AND PROGRESSIVE DEGENERATIVE NEUROLOGICAL DISEASES

A large number of rare breed–specific neurological disorders have been reported in sporting and working dogs. In-depth reviews of these conditions can be found in texts by Braund and Chrisman.[1, 2] Some disorders are present at birth and thus are congenital, and may or may not have a genetic basis. Other degenerative disease processes can occur primarily in juvenile and/or adult sporting dogs. A brief summary of these diseases follows.

Deafness

Congenital deafness may not be recognized until the puppies are several weeks to 3 months of age. Loss of hearing may be a result of malformation of the structures of the inner ear, exposure of the bitch to ototoxic agents, or possible viral infection. An autosomal recessive deficit has been reported or suggested for bull terriers, Doberman pinschers, rottweilers, and pointers. Congenital deafness has also been reported to occur in other terriers, including the smooth fox terriers, Staffordshire, Shropshire, Sealyham, West Highland white, and Scottish terriers, as well as greyhounds, Ibizan hounds, border collies, Shetland sheep dogs, and the Walker American foxhound. Dogs with blue eyes and white-hair coats related to the gene for merle color, which would include the Australian heeler, Australian shepherd, and the Dalmatian, can have familial deafness present at birth. Congenital deafness may be unilateral or bilateral and is often a permanent nontreatable condition.

Vestibular Disease

Vestibular disease is manifested by head tilt, circling, weakness of ipsilateral extensor muscles resulting in gait abnormalities, reluctance to rise, and leaning or falling to one side. Nystagmus is often absent in dogs with congenital disease. These signs may be present at the time of initial ambulation or up to 3 months of age and be present for life. Smooth fox terriers and Tibetan terriers have been reported with this condition. Combined congenital deafness and vestibular dysfunction has been reported in Doberman pinscher puppies owing to an autosomal-recessive genetic disorder.

Cerebellar Dysfunction

There are three classic clinical signs of cerebellar dysfunction that are used to localize a lesion to this part of the brain. These are dysmetria of the limbs, head tremors, and lack of a menace response. The dysmetria is characterized by jerky uncoordinated movements with hypermetria most commonly evidenced. The decrease or absence of a menace response is difficult to evaluate in puppies less than 6 to 8 weeks of age since it is a learned visual response.

Congenital cerebellar malformation has been reported in bull and fox terriers and Irish setters with the initiating cause unknown. In these animals, signs are usually noted when the animals first start to ambulate. The syndrome is not progressive, and some improvement in gait and head control may occur in time. Progressive cerebellar dysfunction is another group of known or suspected genetic disorders that has been reported in a number of breeds of sporting dogs including Labrador retrievers, Australian kelpies (autosomal recessive), rough-coated collies (autosomal recessive),

border collies, Kerry blue terriers (autosomal recessive), Cairn and fox terriers, Samoyeds, Airedale terriers, golden retrievers, Great Danes, and German shepherds. In general, clinical signs of cerebellar dysfunction start at 2 to 4 months of age, and prognosis is often poor because of the progressive nature of the signs and the lack of any effective therapy. Late-onset, slow progressive cerebellar disease has been reported in mature Brittanys ranging in age from 7 to 13 years and in Gordon setters (autosomal recessive) between 6 and 30 months of age. Both have a similar poor prognosis because of the progressive nature of the disease.

Hydrocephalus

Hydrocephalus is probably the most common congenital neurological disorder in dogs and may have a teratogenic, genetic, or infectious etiology. The last etiology may also cause adult onset of hydrocephalus. Clinical signs range from notable disfiguration of the skull and marked neurological deficits in neonatal pups to seizures, gait abnormalities, and cerebral hemisphere deficits in dogs with normal skull anatomy. Any breed of dog can be affected, but small breeds have been documented to be at higher risk. The prognosis is poor.

Epilepsy and Seizures

Seizures are abnormal electrical events in the brain that result in either a loss of consciousness and tonic/clonic convulsions or in focal motor seizures in which a specific group of muscles undergo uncontrolled intermittent contraction. Prodromal signs may include behavior changes, vomiting, and excessive salivation prior to the seizure, with postictal signs of blindness, depression, disorientation, polyphagia, and polydipsia. There are a number of extracranial as well as intracranial causes of seizures. The latter include idiopathic epilepsy, which occurs in young dogs, usually before 3 years of age, and is believed to have a higher incidence and thus a possible genetic predisposition in some breeds of dogs. These include German shepherds, keeshondes, cocker spaniels, Labrador retrievers, golden retrievers, and Saint Bernards. Seizuring dogs require a thorough medical and neurological work-up to differentiate between and rule out the multiple causes before a diagnosis of idiopathic epilepsy can be made. Therapy in this latter disorder or trauma-induced seizure activity consists of daily medication with barbiturates or other antiseizure medication to suppress the seizure activity.[4] Greyhounds and sled dogs in sanctioned events are not allowed to race under this medication, and other sporting and working dogs may have their performance altered by these CNS altering medications.

Narcolepsy

Narcolepsy in dogs is most commonly seen as a sudden onset of cataplexy resulting in collapse and flaccid paralysis for a period of a few seconds to 20 minutes. Often some environmental stimulus such as food, exercise, sexual activity, or presence of another dog triggers the onset of an attack, and multiple attacks can occur within a day. The pathogenesis is unknown, and a genetic component has been shown in some breeds and is suspected in others. These breeds include rottweilers, Doberman pinschers (autosomal recessive), Labrador retrievers (known genetic predisposition), Saint Bernards, malamutes, springer spaniels, and Australian shepherd mixes. Medication to reduce or eliminate clinical signs of the disorder include oral imipramine hydrochloride (0.5 to 1.5 mg/kg two or three times a day) or oral methylphenidate hydrochloride (0.25 mg/kg once or twice a day). The prognosis for a working or sporting dog is guarded because exercise can induce the clinical signs and greyhounds, and sled dogs are required to race medication-free.

Hypomyelination

Hypomyelination is a deficiency of myelin, primarily affecting the CNS of dogs. There is one report of peripheral nerve myelin being defective in two Golden retriever litter mates. Clinical signs of CNS hypomyelination are first seen when the puppies begin to ambulate and consist of motor weakness, wide-based stance, tremors that disappear at rest or during sleep, and a dancing or bouncing movement when standing. Samoyed, Lutcher hound, and Weimaraner are breeds of dogs in which this disease syndrome has been reported. In time, most affected animals gradually improve. The causative factor relative to the hypomyelination is not known. In addition, there is a more clinically severe hypomyelination syndrome occurring in springer spaniels that is believed to be an X-linked recessive trait. In this breed, the clinical signs are progressive and may include seizure activity. The prognosis for recovery with hypomyelination in springer spaniels is poor.

Spinal Dysplasia or Dysraphism

This condition is a congenital malformation of the spinal cord seen most commonly in Weimaraners as a genetic defect of a codominant gene with reduced penetrance and variable expression. This condition has also occasionally been diagnosed in Dalmatians and rottweilers. Clinical signs are evident when the puppies first begin ambulating and can be correlated to the varying parts of the spinal cord affected, most commonly the thoracic and upper lumbar segments. Severity of signs varies between animals but remains static within an animal for life.

Bone Disorders (with secondary neurological signs)

Congenital and developmental abnormal bone formation can result in secondary compressive lesions to the spinal cord or brain in sporting or working dogs. Clinical signs may be acute due to a fracture or subluxation or may be insidious with chronic progressive bone malformation. Radiographs are the optimum diagnostic test. Therapeutic measures, such as surgery, may result in survival and functional ability as a pet, but with a very guarded prognosis for a sporting dog.

Hemivertebra. Hemivertebra is a malformation of one or more vertebra. It is often present without any clinical evidence of dysfunction; however, it is the most common congenital anomaly associated with corresponding neurological problems. A sporting or racing dog with a hemivertebra may be more susceptible to injury during running and jumping, and the subsequent neurological damage is often career limiting. Thoracic hemivertebra has been reported to be autosomal recessive in some families of German short-haired pointers.

Atlantoaxial Luxation. Atlantoaxial luxation is a condition in which the atlas and the axis articulation is unstable, leading to trauma to and compression of the cervical spinal cord during flexion. Although it is most often thought to be a disease of small dogs, there are reports of rottweilers and Doberman pinschers having congenital lesions resulting in neurological dysfunction.

Wobbler Syndrome. The *wobbler syndrome* is a common term for a developmental cervical vertebral malformation and malarticulation with secondary spinal cord compression. Great Danes less than 2 years of age and Doberman pinschers greater that 2 years of age comprise the majority of cases (ie, approximately 80 per cent in one reference),[2] but the condition has occurred in German shepherds, rottweilers, Labrador retrievers, fox terriers, Weimaraners, golden retrievers, Rhodesian ridgebacks, Irish wolfhounds and setters, and Pyrenean mountain dogs. In this latter group, the compressive spinal cord lesion was more commonly at the midcervical region. Clinical signs of ataxia and motor weakness may be insidious and progressive or acute as a result of trauma to the neck. Diagnosis is made on the basis of radiographic and myelographic studies of the cervical spine. Prognosis is dependent on the breed, severity, and rate of neurological degeneration. Surgery may be indicated to keep the dog a functional pet. This lesion carries a guarded to poor prognosis for an active sporting or working dog.

Neuromuscular Disease

There are multiple neuromuscular disorders that occur in working or sporting dogs.[1, 2] Some have a breed-specific known or suspected genetic basis, while others remain sporadic, often idiopathic diseases in these animals.

Myasthenia Gravis. This is a rare disease of the neuromuscular junction that causes episodic motor weakness that is precipitated by exercise and reversed with rest. There are two forms of myasthenia gravis in dogs, a congenital form and an acquired form. In both forms, there is a paucity of acetylcholine receptors on the skeletal muscles. Congenital forms have been reported in Jack Russell terriers, springer spaniels, and smooth-haired fox terriers and are usually more severe and progressive in the young 6- to 8-week-old pups. Acquired myasthenia gravis with antibody production and immune-mediated destruction of the acetylcholine receptors is most common in middle- to large-sized adult dogs, and especially overrepresented are Labrador retrievers, golden retrievers, and German shepherds. Detection of the serum acetylcholine receptor antibodies is the definitive diagnostic assay only for the acquired form. Treatment with anticholinesterase drugs may reduce clinical signs, but the prognosis for a full functioning working or sporting dog is guarded to poor. Some spontaneous recovery of the acquired form has been reported.

Dancing Doberman Disease. This is a rare, chronic, progressive neuromuscular disease of Doberman pinschers in which the early clinical signs consist of inadvertent flexion of one or both pelvic limbs while the dog is simply standing, thus mimicking dancing. In time, neurological dysfunction progresses to include paresis, ataxia, and muscle wasting, especially of the gastrocnemius muscle. There is no treatment, and while the slow progression often allows these animals to be acceptable pets, they are not able to be athletes.

Hereditary Myopathy. There are a number of rare hereditary myopathies in breeds of working and sporting dogs that severely limit the athletic ability of a dog.

Labrador retriever hereditary myopathy is an autosomal recessive trait in both black- and yellow-coated Labrador retrievers. Clinical signs of gait and posture abnormalities, muscular weakness during exercise, and muscle atrophy may be evident at 6 to 8 weeks or appear later at 6 to 7 months. No neurological deficits are evident, and clinical signs stabilize within the first year with affected animals functioning as pets at best.

Familial reflex myoclonus is another idiopathic disease of skeletal muscle in Labrador retrievers that may be genetically predisposed in certain lines of dogs. The clinical signs of muscle spasms and progressive muscle stiffness are first evident at 3 weeks of age and are progressive. Prognosis is poor to guarded, and no treatment has been found to be curative.

Muscular dystrophy is a primary X-linked, genetically determined skeletal muscle disease that has been best studied in golden retrievers, but has also been reported in Samoyeds, rottweilers, and Irish terriers. Clinical signs of weakness with exercise intolerance, gait stiffness, and muscle atrophy are first seen in male pups between 6 and 8 weeks of age with progression until about 6 months, at which time the signs remain static. Prognosis is poor as currently there is no treatment.

Mitochondrial myopathy, a disease of muscles of young Clumber and Sussex spaniels, is believed to be due to abnormalities in the muscle mitochondria. Exercise intolerance is the predominant clinical sign, and metabolic acidosis occurs concurrently. Prognosis is poor as there is no current therapy.

Megaesophagus can be seen in a congenital form in German shepherds, Great Danes, Irish setters, Newfoundlands, and greyhounds, while acquired megaesophagus can occur in any breed. Clinical signs of regurgitating recently eaten food coupled with radiographic findings of a dilated esophagus indicate this disease. Prognosis for the congenital form is guarded since the condition in some dogs remains static, while in others, becomes normal with maturity.

Malignant hyperthermia is a condition that is seen most commonly in racing greyhounds, but also in pointers, spaniels, border collies and Doberman pinscher crossbreds. Manifestation of the disease can be life threatening when these animals are put under general anesthesia with halothane or enflurane gas. The primary defect is in calcium channels of the skeletal muscle, which are triggered by exposure to caffeine, the aforementioned gas anesthetics, and stressors such as excitement and exercise. The prognosis in a racing animal in which exercise incites clinical signs is guarded since medications such as dantrolene are not permitted.

Degenerative Neuropathies

Progressive degenerative diseases are rare but pose severe limitations to a dog undertaking work or athletic competition. Recognition that these syndromes exist and the breeds in which they have been reported assists a veterinarian in establishing a differential diagnosis and prognosis.[1,2]

Degenerative Myelopathy. Degenerative myelopathy is the most common degenerative neurological condition that affects large dogs. Most common in German shepherd dogs over 5 years of age, it has been reported in younger dogs of this breed as well as in other breeds of dogs, such as Siberian huskies, collie and collie crosses, Chesapeake Bay retrievers, Labrador retrievers, and Kerry blue terriers. Deficiencies of vitamins E and B₁₂, immune-mediated degeneration, and vascular disorder have all been postulated as causative factors. Affecting the long tracts of white matter predominantly in the thoracic spinal cord, the insidious and progressive disease starts with pelvic limb ataxia and paresis with further development of depressed reflexes and truncal ataxia. Treatment with a combination of exercise, vitamins B and E, and oral epsilon-aminocaproic acid (EACA) at 500 mg/day may slow the progression of the disease, but prognosis is poor for return to normal sport or working proficiency.

Hound Ataxia. Adult foxhounds, harrier hounds, and beagles in the United Kingdom have degenerative clinically progressive disease primarily of the CNS—hound ataxia—that has been associated with the feeding of ruminant stomach parts. Clinical signs are limited to weakness and paresis of the pelvic limbs that interfere with work in these adult dogs. There is no treatment and a change of diet is recommended.

Giant Axonal Neuropathy. Affecting only German shepherds, giant axonal neuropathy is a rare autosomal recessive trait that results in progressive degeneration of the peripheral and central nervous systems that starts at 14 to 16 months of age. From initial signs of proprioceptive loss, motor weakness, decreased reflexes primarily in the pelvic limbs, the disease results in tetraparesis, loss of bark, and megaesophagus by 18 to 24 months. Accumulation of neurofilaments in the distal axons is the characteristic pathological finding. Prognosis is poor as there is no effective therapy.

Spinal Muscular Atrophy. Spinal muscular atrophy is a pro-

gressive degenerative disease of the brain and spinal cord neurons. It has been reported in Brittany spaniels (autosomal dominant), English pointers, German shepherds, rottweilers, Swedish Lapland dogs, Cairn terriers, and crossbred Great Danes. Clinical signs of motor weakness, tremors, muscle atrophy, and decreased reflexes are evident between 4 weeks and 5 months and progress to tetraparesis in many of the dogs. The definitive diagnosis is made by histopathological study. Prognosis is poor as there is no effective therapy.

Degenerative Sensory Neuropathy. Degenerative sensory neuropathies are rare and involve only the sensory side of the peripheral and central nervous systems. Clinical signs of proprioceptive deficits with ataxia but no motor weakness, absence of or depressed reflexes, facial hypalgesia or paresthesia, hearing loss, and occasionally self-mutilation have developed in mature dogs of the following breeds: Brittany, Siberian husky, Doberman pinscher, whippet, golden retriever, and Scotch collie. Pathologically it is a sensory neuropathy, clinical signs are slowly progressive over months to years, and there is no therapy. A progressive sensory neuropathy of young (approximately 2 months of age) Boxer dogs has been reported to be an inherited autosomal recessive trait in some families. Loss of pain perception and acral mutilation in 3- to 8-month-old English pointer and Czechoslovakian short-haired pointer dogs has been reported as an autosomal recessive trait. Clinical signs become evident when the dogs begin incessant licking and biting their paws. There is no therapy, and prognosis is poor. Idiopathic self-mutilation (acral lick dermatitis, lick granuloma, and neurodermatitis) relative to degenerative changes in sensory and mixed peripheral nerves has been reported in Doberman pinschers, German shepherds, Irish setters, and Great Danes. Treatment with tricyclic antidepressant drugs may reduce the licking behavior, suggesting some abnormal behavioral basis for the condition.

Distal Symmetrical Polyneuropathy. Distal symmetrical polyneuropathy has been reported in young adult Great Danes, Chesapeake bay retrievers, Saint Bernards, rottweilers, Labrador retrievers, collies, and Newfoundlands. The disease is characterized by slow chronic hindlimb paresis that progresses to lower motor neuron (LMN) disease involving the forelimbs and masseter muscles of the head. Diagnosis is based on clinical signs and biopsy evidence of loss of large-diameter fibers and demyelination limited to peripheral nerves. There is no treatment of this idiopathic disease, and prognosis is poor.

Laryngeal Paralysis. Hereditary, acquired, and idiopathic forms of laryngeal paralysis have been reported.[2] The hereditary form has been identified in purebred and crossbred Siberian huskies and Dalmatians, while the idiopathic forms are primarily in adult large breeds such as Chesapeake Bay retrievers, Irish setters, and Saint Bernards. Clinical signs of inspiratory distress, loss of endurance, voice changes, and collapse due to air obstruction may be seen as solo signs or with other neurological abnormalities such as motor weakness and LMN signs in limb and head musculature, starting at 4 to 6 months of age. The prognosis in dogs with the idiopathic or acquired forms of laryngeal paralysis with surgical intervention is good, which is in contrast to that for dogs with the hereditary condition.

Idiopathic Facial Paralysis. An acute onset of idiopathic facial paralysis unrelated to middle ear disease has been reported to occur and have a genetic predisposition in cocker spaniels, English setters, and boxers. Degeneration of the facial nerve(s) is evident on biopsy. Clinical signs of facial nerve dysfunction are evident and may improve over a period of weeks to months or remain static. Although this idiopathic form is responsible for a high percentage of sole facial nerve paralyses, ruling out other causative factors such as otitis media/interna and trauma is necessary before the diagnosis of this condition. Treatment is empirical and aimed primarily at protecting the eyes from desiccation.

Storage Disease Syndrome. There are a number of breeds in which rare storage disease syndromes have been reported. A lysosomal storage disease, gangliosidosis, is an autosomal-recessive defect causing accumulation of ganglioside in neurons and neuroglial cells in both the CNS and peripheral nervous system of English springer spaniels, German short-haired pointers, and Japanese pointers. Progressive ataxia, head tremors, visual impairment, and marked mental changes are the clinical signs relative to the condition. Ceroid lipofuscinosis results in accumulation of lipofuscin in the cells of the CNS and occurs as an autosomal recessive trait in English setters, Border collies, and Tibetan terriers. Sporadic cases have been reported in cocker spaniels, salukis, Japanese retrievers, blue heelers, Yugoslavian sheepdogs, and Dalmatians. Clinical signs usually are not apparent until the dogs are mature, ie, 1 to 9 years of age, but often 2-year-old affected dogs have clinical evidence of the disease. Fucosidosis, a deficiency of alpha-L-fucosidase, has been reported in English springer spaniels as an autosomal-recessive trait and is characterized by progressive motor and mental deterioration starting at 6 to 12 months of age. Glycogenosis, a glycogen storage disease, has been reported in Lapland dogs, German shepherds, Akitas, and English springers (autosomal recessive) in which progressive weakness becomes apparent between 2 and 6 months of age. In all of these diseases, diagnosis is made by premortem biopsy or postmortem evaluation of the CNS.[2] Prognosis is poor as no treatment is available.

INFECTIOUS DISEASES AFFECTING THE NERVOUS SYSTEM

Bacterial Diseases

Discospondylitis. This is an infectious process located within or between vertebrae and is most common in large dogs. German shepherds, Great Danes, Doberman pinschers, and Labrador retrievers were most commonly reported to be afflicted with this condition.[5] It has been hypothesized that immunosuppression may be a factor in the increased incidence in German shepherds and Airedale terriers. Prevalence of the disease in large male dogs has also been suggested to be related to trauma and the stresses placed on the spine due to large size and increased activity. The source of bacteria may be from hematogenous spread from a preexisting gastrointestinal, urinary, or skin infection or from a migrating foreign body. Foxtails and other plant awns may also be a causative factor. Radiography is most helpful in making this diagnosis; the prognosis varies, depending on the severity of the spinal cord and vertebral involvement. Aggressive long-term antibiotic therapy can result in complete recovery if vertebral stability is intact.

Migrating Plant Awns and Meningomyelitis or Meningoencephalitis. Field dogs are invariably exposed to various plant awns during their work and commonly develop one or two sequelae to migrating awns: discospondylitis when the entry point is in the feet or infection of the brain when the entry point is through the nose or ear. Prognosis depends on surgical localization and removal of the awn and the degree of neurological damage, with brain involvement having a more guarded prognosis.

Tetanus. Tetanus is a nervous system disease caused by the toxin of *Clostridium botulinum*. Sporting dogs in field conditions are often likely to be under circumstances that expose them to this condition. Anaerobic wounds, such as a puncture caused by a nail, can become contaminated with this bacterium and result in clinical signs 5 to 10 days post infection. These signs consist of stiffness of gait, reluctance to move, spasms of facial muscles (sardonic grin) and those of the limbs (sawhorse stance), all of which increase with sensory stimulation. Localized tetanus in one limb may be

seen initially. Prognosis is usually favorable with high therapeutic doses of penicillin, tetanus antitoxin, and wound cleansing, but full recovery may take several months.

Viral Diseases

Canine Distemper. Canine distemper is the most common and serious of the neurological diseases of sporting and working dogs. The neurotropic virus can invade and affect any part of the CNS, with clinical signs relative to the area affected. Dogs with some degree of immunosuppression due to the stresses of training and work, crowding, high environmental temperatures, poor nutrition, or high parasite loads may not have appropriate responses to regular vaccination programs. However, "properly" vaccinated dogs have been known to develop the disease. Devastating outbreaks in greyhound kennels have been reported. Neurological signs may occur without any sign of systemic disease or may be a sequela to respiratory or gastrointestinal disease caused by this virus. Prognosis for return to full working abilities is guarded to poor.

Rabies. Rabies is a viral disease of all warm-blooded mammals. It is most often transmitted by the bite of an infected animal, but wound contamination from infected saliva or urine, or the ingestion of an infected animal, may be a source of the virus for sporting dogs. With current state requirements for vaccination, most dogs are immune. Many racing jurisdictions and race tracks are now requiring rabies vaccination for greyhounds. Clinical signs vary from early nonspecific signs of inappetence, vomiting, and mental anxiousness to later stages of either the dumb or furious forms of encephalitis. The former is more common, with progressive paresis to paralysis of the muscles of the head and body with terminal respiratory failure 3 to 6 days after initial clinical signs. The furious form is characterized by aggressive and restless behaviors with occasional seizures. Death follows in 4 to 8 days. The prognosis is poor to hopeless, as there is no effective therapy, spontaneous recoveries are rare, and infected dogs present a zoonotic threat to humans.

OTHER SPORADIC NONPROGRESSIVE ACQUIRED NEUROLOGICAL OR NEUROMUSCULAR DISEASES

Muscle Cramping. Greyhounds are the most common breed to be affected with muscle cramping, although the condition has been reported to occur in young Dalmatian dogs and in field-trial English springer spaniels with hereditary phosphofructokinase deficiency. In greyhounds, multiple causes can cause a post-race prolonged, painful, involuntary contraction of a single muscle or group of synergistic muscles. Suggested causes include dehydration, calcium deficiency, metabolic disorders, and circulatory and nervous system dysfunctions.[6] Prognosis for return to racing in greyhounds is favorable when the causative factor can be determined and appropriately treated. Cramping in the aforementioned other two breeds has a poorer prognosis because of primary metabolic muscle dysfunction.

Coonhound Paralysis. Coonhound paralysis is a result of polyradiculoneuritis and was first described in raccoon-hunting dogs. Since then, injection of raccoon saliva has been shown to produce the disease in some dogs. Sporadic cases of polyradiculoneuritis have also been reported in many other dogs that have had no exposure to raccoons. The pathophysiology is believed to be a triggering of the immune system to attack the peripheral nervous system, producing acute onset of progressive flaccid paralysis of skeletal muscle over a period of 12 to 48 hours. Hyperesthesia to touch may be present. Complete recovery may occur within days with good nursing care, but in some dogs, the paralysis persists for weeks to months. In these latter cases, marked muscle atrophy occurs, and this musculature may not completely regenerate. The prognosis for return to work is dependent on the severity of the disease and the level of recovery. Dogs affected with this disease are more susceptible to repeat episodes.

Botulism. Botulism is a toxic disease caused by the eating of carrion or food contaminated with *Clostridium botulinum* and its neurotoxin. Hunting and field dogs may be affected because of their having greater access to spoiled carcasses. Type C toxin affects dogs on rare occasions, causing rapid, progressive, flaccid paralysis (lower motor neuron [LMN] disease) of the skeletal muscles of the limbs and head. A definitive diagnosis is difficult to make and is based on the history of possible exposure, clinical signs, ruling out tick paralysis (see below), and electrodiagnostic findings of decreases in nerve conduction velocities and abnormal electromyographic potentials in the muscles. The only treatment is supportive care, and the prognosis in dogs is usually favorable for return to function.

Tick Paralysis. Field trial and hunting dogs are exposed to greater opportunities to acquire ticks from the environment. *Dermacentor variabilis,* the common wood tick, and *Dermacentor andersoni,* the Rocky Mountain wood tick, are most commonly the source of the paralysis. A neurotoxin produced by the ticks and injected during a bite blocks the release of acetylcholine from the presynaptic membrane and interferes with the propagation of action potentials along the axons. Progressive motor weakness, noted as incoordination plus altered quality of the bark, dysphagia, and cough are the early signs of toxicosis. Progression of the neurological signs occurs over 12 to 24 hours, with paralysis and loss of reflexes. If the early clinical signs are not detected, death from respiratory muscle paralysis can occur. Diagnosis is made on discovery of one or more ticks and clinical evidence of LMN signs of all four limbs and the head. Therapy consists of tick removal and/or an insecticide dip and good nursing care until recovery occurs. The prognosis for recovery is good. Tick paralysis in Australia is a more serious clinical condition, with more aggressive therapy required. The condition of the dogs may worsen for a few days after tick removal, and the prognosis is more guarded in these dogs.

Toad Paralysis. Bufotoxins are formed in some species of toads such as the Colorado River toad (*Bufo alvarius*) and the marine toad (*Bufo marinus*). In the southern United States, field trial and working dogs experience the most problems with this toxicity. Once the dog has mouthed or bitten a poisonous toad, excessive

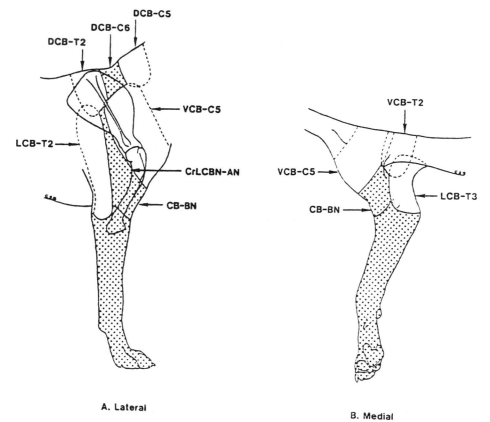

A. Lateral

B. Medial

FIGURE 10–2. Pattern of cutaneous anesthesia expected with complete brachial plexus avulsion. The area of anesthesia is stippled. The adjacent cutaneous areas are outlined by dashed lines. Note the anesthetized cutaneous areas of the dorsal cutaneous branch of C6 (DCB-C6), the cranial lateral cutaneous branch of the axillary nerve (CrLCBN-AN), and the cutaneous branch of the brachiocephalicus nerve (CB-BN). Loss of sensation of the skin supplied by the dorsal cutaneous branch of C6 indicates that spinal rootlet avulsion has occurred with a poor prognosis for return to function. In the lateral view, the anesthetized area distal to the elbow consists of the autonomous zones or cutaneous areas of the cranial cutaneous antebrachial nerve of the axillary nerve and the cutaneous branches of the radial and ulnar nerves. The anesthetized area distal to the elbow in the medial view consists of the autonomous zones or cutaneous areas of the cranial cutaneous antebrachial nerve of the axillary nerve and the cutaneous branches of the musculocutaneous, median, radial, and ulnar nerves. DCB-T2 = dorsal cutaneous branch of T2; DCB-C5 = dorsal cutaneous branch of C5; VCB-C5 = ventral cutaneous branch of C5; LCB-T2 = lateral cutaneous branch of T2; VCB-T2 = ventral cutaneous branch of T2; LCB-T3 = lateral cutaneous branch of T3. These sensory areas can be used to determine the extent and severity of forelimb nerve damage and to monitor response to therapy. (From Bailey CS: Patterns of cutaneous anesthesia associated with brachial plexus avulsions in the dog. JAVMA 185:889–899, 1984.)

drooling, head shaking, incoordination, vomiting, hemorrhagic diarrhea, increased respiratory rate, and seizures are the progressive clinical signs, with death in severe cases occurring within 30 minutes. Therapy consists of removing any remaining toxin by washing out the mouth, administration of seizure medications, such as intravenous diazepam or pentobarbital to effect, intravenous atropine (0.04 mg/kg), and propranolol (5 mg/kg with repeat dose in 20 min if needed) if signs of heart dysfunction occur. Prognosis is good when the toxicity is detected and treated early. Seizuring dogs have a more guarded prognosis.

TRAUMATIC INJURIES TO THE NERVOUS SYSTEM

Acute Traumatic Injuries

Trauma to the Peripheral Nervous System. Traumatic injuries, such as falls or impact with solid objects including other dogs, eg, greyhounds running into each other when the lure is retracted on the rail at the end of a race, are the most common source of injuries to the peripheral nervous system. Bone fractures and abnormal extreme stretching, eg, abduction of a limb, can also cause damage to peripheral nerves. The forelimb nerves and the brachial plexus are more commonly affected than the nerves of the rear limb. When injury occurs, the full extent of the damage may be evident immediately or may develop over the next 12 hours as a result of swelling and edema of and around the nerves. Clinical signs of both motor and sensory losses depend on the severity of the trauma and the number and location of the nerves.[3] Figure 10–2 is a diagram of the loss of cutaneous sensation of both touch and pain when complete avulsion of the brachial plexus roots occurs. The key area to test when this lesion is suspected is the skin over the top of the scapula, designated DCB-C6 in Figure 10–2. Loss of sensation in this area carries a grave prognosis. Guides to determination of the varying degrees and extent of peripheral nerve damage to the nerves of the forelimb have been published.[7, 8] Veterinarians who map the sensory losses and record them can follow the effects of their therapy by repeat testing of these areas of sensory loss. It is known that pain perception is carried on the smallest nerve fibers and that recovery of pain perception, followed by recovery of perception of touch to an area, is a good prognostic indicator and precedes the return of the corresponding motor function of the damaged mixed nerve. With moderate to severe trauma to the brachial plexus, partial or total neurogenic muscle atrophy will occur over 2 to 3 weeks, facilitating diagnosis of peripheral nerve lesions (Fig. 10–3). Treatment consists of corticosteroids, whirlpool baths, and cage rest. Nerves that have been severed may require surgical intervention to rejoin the cut ends. In all cases when the axon has died or been transected, the regrowth rate is estimated to be 1 to 3 mm per day. The prognosis for sporting or working dogs is guarded with most moderate to severe peripheral nerve injuries.

Three other conditions have been reported or are believed to occur relative to damage to peripheral nerves.

"*Limber tail*" has been described by owners and veterinarians as a clinical condition in hunting and field trial dogs. Characterized by acute onset of a flaccid tail, the condition usually reverses itself spontaneously in 3 to 5 days, and always within a week's time. In a survey conducted by faculty at Auburn University, it was found that three different circumstances were associated just before, ie, 12 to 24 hours, the onset of the flaccid tail (Dr. Jan Steiss, personal communication). These were confinement in a small kennel for long periods (eg, in traveling), overworking a dog in early stages of training, and spending an evening outside with cold environmental temperatures. No other clinical neurological abnormalities are associated with this idiopathic syndrome, and the pathophysiology remains to be determined.

Trauma to the suprascapular nerve ("*sweeney*") due to a blow to the point of the shoulder where this nerve courses around the neck of the scapula. This nerve innervates the supraspinatus and the infraspinatus muscles, and its dysfunction results in a gait in which the shoulder abducts during the weight-bearing phase. Medical therapy as described above may assist in the restoration of nerve function, but surgery may be required to free a scar-bound nerve post recovery.

Pinched cervical nerves at the base of the neck in sled dogs have been thought by some veterinarians to be a clinical syndrome that is related to the pressures of the pulling harness over long runs. However, scientific investigations and documentation of this condition as a true pressure peripheral neuropathy need to be verified with electromyographic and pathological studies.

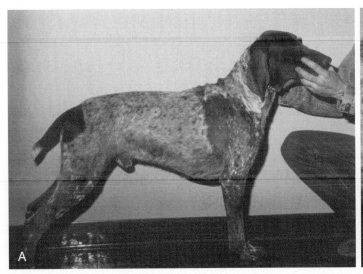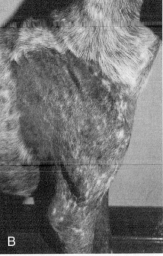

FIGURE 10–3. *A*, Two-year-old male German Short Hair that had brachial plexus trauma 6 months previously. Atrophy of the muscles supplied by the suprascapular, radial, musculocutaneous, cranial, pectoral, and axillary nerves is evident *(B)*, but was improved from that present 4 months earlier. EMG abnormalities were documented in all of the muscles supplied by the brachial plexus.

Trauma to the Head and Spine. Traumatic injuries to the cranial vault and the vertebral spine and the neurological components within are not uncommon and are often devastating. Localization of the neurological lesion by means of the neurological examination with radiographs is the best diagnostic tool in acute cases. Dogs with head or spinal cord trauma must be monitored frequently to detect deterioration of the nervous system.

Therapy with corticosteroids, dimethylsulfoxide (DMSO), or mannitol and antibiotics if a fracture is suspected, should be aggressively instituted. The prognosis is guarded, especially if the animal is severely paretic or paralyzed, and is dependent on the degree of damage. Residual deficits post recovery may limit the dog's usefulness as a racing or sporting athlete.

Chronic, Progressive, Traumatic Induced Lesions

Cauda Equina Syndrome/Lumbosacral Instability. In my surveys of veterinarians working with field trial and hunting dogs, this disease was the number one concern for neurological dysfunction in these dogs. This condition is covered in depth in Chapter 23. The resultant neurological dysfunctions include hindlimb weakness, ataxia, muscle atrophy, flaccid tail, and hypotonia of the anal sphincter with fecal and urinary incontinence, all of which indicate LMN signs of the cauda equina. Electromyography can identify which muscles have loss of innervation. Complete testing should be done on all muscles supplied by each of the major motor nerves in the rear limbs, as well as select muscles of the forelimb and head to rule out conditions with polyneuropathy. Dogs with cauda equina syndrome should have abnormal EMG changes only in the muscles supplied by the sixth and seventh lumbar, sacral, and caudal nerves. Surgical decompression with dorsal laminectomy can provide relief with some restoration of function, but the prognosis has to be guarded in a sporting or working dog.

Spondylosis Deformans. Spondylosis deformans is a ventral and lateral exostosis of vertebra reflecting vertebral instability. The bony lesion most commonly causes back pain and stiffness and rarely progresses to compress nervous tissue. However, in the lumbosacral region, this exostosis may affect the caudal spinal cord and nerve roots, contributing to the aforementioned syndrome of cauda equina.

STRESS-INDUCED METABOLIC DISEASES AFFECTING THE NERVOUS SYSTEM OR BEHAVIOR

All mammalian species react to stressful events by a number of normal nervous and hormonal responses. When these stresses are intermittent and not excessive, the responses they invoke assist the animal's body in responding to the increased demands that competition in an event requires. Prolonged or excessive stress can result in deleterious effects to both the animal's general health and

its performance. In greyhounds, undesirable behavior of restlessness, barking, increased aggression, or physiological alterations, manifested by excessive salivation, rapid bounding heart rate, prolonged rapid panting, diarrhea, increased muscle tension, and quivering, may occur before a race; difficulty in passing urine, coughing for 1 to 2 hours, and excessive water intake may occur after a race. All are related to excessive activation of the nervous system, especially the sympathetic and parasympathetic nervous system, as a result of stress. Stress-induced diarrhea on the long races is also a common problem of sled dogs. Dogs differ in their ability to handle stressful events, and those that do not adapt well may be able to undergo behavior modification. In many cases they are often retired from work or athletic performance.

Long-term excessive stress or inappropriate responses to stress can also cause chronic metabolic problems. These will be covered in other sections of the text, but include hyperadrenocorticism, hypothyroidism, bald thigh syndrome, and water diabetes syndrome in racing greyhounds, and chronic dehydration. In addition, problems with slow-healing wounds and frequent minor infections such as cystitis, tonsillitis, sheath or vaginal infections, and nail bed infections are seen with long-term inappropriate responses to the effects of stress on the immune system. Maximal exercise has been documented to temporarily suppress the immune system. Trainers need to be sure that optimal environmental conditions are in place, such as housing with appropriate temperatures and airflow and soft bedding. They also need to make sure that the health of the dog is optimized by reduction of parasite loads and good nutrition. Finally, trainers need to know their individual dogs and adjust their training and work to reduce these responses as well as using appropriate training methods that minimize unnecessary stresses.

Visual dysfunctions of sporting and working dogs also involve the nervous system but will be covered in depth in other chapters. Hearing deficits not of congenital origin, as previously described, are most often secondary to otitis media or interna. Dogs with pendulous ears are especially prone to chronic infections. Migrating plant awns have been described and can also result in deafness.

References

1. Braund KG: Clinical Syndromes in Veterinary Neurology, 2nd ed. St. Louis, Mosby-Year Book, Inc, 1994.
2. Chrisman CL: Problems in Small Animal Neurology, 2nd ed. Philadelphia, Lea & Febiger, 1991.
3. Oliver JE, Lorenz MD, Kornegay JN. Handbook of Veterinary Neurology. Philadelphia, WB Saunders Company, 1987.
4. Thomas WB: Managing the epileptic dog. Compendium 12:1573–1579, 1994.
5. Kornegay JN: Discospondylitis. *In* Textbook of Small Animal Surgery, 2nd ed. Philadelphia, WB Saunders Company, 1993, vol 1, pp 1087–1094.
6. Blythe LL, Gannon JR, Craig AM: Care of the Racing Greyhound. Abilene, American Greyhound Council, 1994, pp 271–274.
7. Bailey CS: Patterns of cutaneous anesthesia associated with brachial plexus avulsions in the dog. JAVMA 185:889–899, 1984.
8. Bailey CS, Kitchell BL: Clinical evaluation of the cutaneous innervation of the canine thoracic limb. J Am Anim Hosp Assoc 20:939–950, 1984.

CHAPTER 11

PULMONARY DISEASES OF WORKING AND SPORTING DOGS

ROBERT R. KING

Despite the number of racing greyhounds and other working breed dogs, few common or unique pulmonary diseases and problems have been described to date. This chapter's discussion is divided into noninfectious respiratory problems (nasal bone fractures, elongated soft palate, segmental airway collapse, tracheobronchial foreign bodies, exercise-induced bronchoconstriction, exercise-induced intrabronchial hemorrhage, and pneumothorax) and infectious respiratory problems (rhinitis, tonsillitis, tracheobronchitis, and bacterial pneumonia).

Animals with pulmonary disorders commonly have coughing, cyanosis, exercise intolerance, or increased respiratory effort as the primary clinical sign(s). The correct approach to determine the diagnosis for the presenting problem(s) includes a detailed history and a complete physical examination. Following acquisition of this information, additional diagnostic procedures are usually necessary to confirm the diagnosis before appropriate treatment(s) can be prescribed.[1–4] Response to therapy is another means of establishing a tentative diagnosis, but when the correct diagnosis is missed because of limited testing, rational alternative therapies may be overlooked and inappropriate or detrimental treatments can be administered.

NONINFECTIOUS RESPIRATORY PROBLEMS

Nasal Bone Fractures

Trauma can occur secondary to the dog's striking the racing muzzle against the front of the starting box before it is released at the start of the race. This can result in fractures of the incisive, maxillary, or nasal bones 0.3 to 0.5 cm dorsal and caudal to the external nares.[5] The presence of blood in the starting box, epistaxis, or blood in the oral cavity and on the racing muzzle suggests fracture of nasal bones. Ice packing of the nose and cage rest are often sufficient to control minor bleeding. Pressure packing the nasal cavity with gauze sponges with the dog under anesthesia may be necessary with severe epistaxis. Clotting defects should be considered and appropriate tests done when bleeding is prolonged.[6, 7] Radiographic examination of the nasal cavity is usually unnecessary, and healing of uncomplicated fractures should be complete in 2 to 3 weeks. Complicated fractures with displacement of incisive, maxillary, or nasal bones causing nasal cavity obstruction should be evaluated radiographically and the fractures repaired or the bone fragments removed.

Elongated Soft Palate

Soft palate elongation is the most common airway obstructive problem in brachycephalic breeds;[8–10] it also occurs in nonbrachycephalic dogs,[9–11] including greyhounds.[12] In affected animals the posterior portion of the soft palate extends beyond the tip of the epiglottis, interfering with laryngeal function. During exercise or increased inspiratory effort, the caudal portion of the soft palate is sucked into the glottis, obstructing the airway. The level of respiratory distress depends on the degree of soft palate elongation and the amount of edema and inflammation.[9, 10, 12] Secondary changes (not reported in greyhounds or other sporting and working dogs) include tonsillar enlargement, laryngeal saccule eversion, and laryngeal or tracheal collapse due to the chronic increase in negative pressure generated during inspiration.[9,10]

A typical history in affected greyhounds includes noisy breathing or snoring while sleeping and a grunting or roaring inspiratory noise during trials and races.[12] Recovery time to normal breathing is prolonged after running, and animals should be closely observed for signs of hyperthermia (tachypnea and dyspnea, followed by anxiety, excitement, and respiratory collapse). Animals showing these signs should be cooled immediately to prevent death.

A tentative diagnosis of elongated soft palate can be made on the basis of history and an oral examination without sedation or anesthesia. However, the possibility of other pharyngeal or laryngeal problems warrants a thorough examination under general anesthesia. Confirmation of the diagnosis is made when the soft palate is noted to extend beyond the epiglottis, obstructing the laryngeal opening.[8–10, 12] Anesthetic protocols and surgical techniques have been described with the goal of resection to shorten the soft palate so that its caudal border lies slightly rostral to the tip of the epiglottis.[8–12] Corticosteroids—specifically prednisolone (0.5 to 1.0 mg/kg just before surgery and every 8 hours for three doses)—are recommended to reduce edema following soft palate resection.[10]

Segmental Airway Collapse

Tracheomalacia is a rare congenital malformation resulting in segmental tracheal collapse secondary to inadequate supporting cartilaginous and myoelastic structures.[13–18] If the defect is extrathoracic, as described in young greyhounds,[13] partial airway obstruction is present during inspiration. The condition can be divided into primary (congenital) and secondary (acquired) subgroups.[14, 18] Primary tracheomalacia is probably due to immaturity of the tracheobronchial cartilage[13, 14, 18] and is usually self-limiting in humans, generally resolving within the first 2 years of life.[14, 18] Secondary tracheomalacia is due to degeneration of previously normal tracheobronchial cartilage caused by chronic inflammation or vascular compression.[14–18] This condition, described in small mature dogs as *acquired tracheal collapse,* is caused by deficiencies in chondroitin sulfate and calcium resulting in focal hypocellularity of cartilage and areas of replacement by fibrocartilage or fibrous tissue.[19]

Clinical signs in racing greyhounds are usually inapparent at rest and during walking exercise. However, during and following training, respirations become progressively noisy and respiratory rate increases. Finally, if the tracheal defect is severe, inspiratory stridor and dyspnea may result in cyanosis and ataxia.[13] Palpation of the trachea may induce coughing and reveal abnormal tracheal cartilages. Confirmatory diagnosis can be made with radiographs or tracheobronchoscopy. A number of surgical procedures including tracheal resection and external and internal stent devices have been described,[20–22] but none has been used in racing greyhounds.[13]

Tracheobronchial Foreign Bodies

Aspiration of solid foreign bodies into the tracheobronchial tree occurs most often in working or sporting dogs between 2 and 8 years of age.[23–26] Medium- to large-sized hunting dogs that are the best trained and fastest are over-represented. Most cases occur during the dry summer months when animals are hunted in high standing pastures or grasslands.

Coughing is the predominant clinical sign, and most owners can precisely identify when it began.[24–26] The severity of respiratory distress and dyspnea depends on the degree of airway obstruction. Particles of plant origin (foxtails or grass awns), because of the well-developed terminal barbs, project proximally toward the larger airways, causing the barbs to migrate farther and farther into the lung periphery. Failure to remove the aspirated foreign material in a timely manner, especially if it is of plant origin, often results in purulent tracheobronchitis, abscess formation, bronchopleural fistula, or empyema.[23–26] Migration may be so extensive that the foxtail traverses the pleural space and is eventually extruded through the skin.[23] Continued signs of coughing, dyspnea, and stridor in the absence of a known cause are definite indications for radiography of the thorax and possibly bronchoscopic examination of the airways.[24–27]

Intratracheal foreign bodies are usually easy to detect radiographically, but location, size, and radiodensity are important factors affecting visualization.[27] Ideally the intraluminal location of the obstructive mass is seen as air surrounding the obstruction except for its attachment at the mucosa. Distal intrabronchial obstruction with smaller foreign bodies initially causes no radiographic abnormality because of collateral ventilation of the lung segment. Only after accumulation of lung secretions distal to the bronchial occlusion may focal consolidation become visible.[24–27] In cases in which the inhaled foreign body is not clearly identified radiographically, tracheal instillation of a bronchographic contrast medium or bronchoscopy is indicated. The latter procedure is often the preferred method for localization of the foreign body because extraction can often be accomplished at the same time as diagnosis.[24–27] Foreign body removal via a flexible fiberoptic bronchoscope is not without risk. Faulty judgment or operator inexperience can lead to serious complications including (1) trauma to the airway, resulting in bleeding, infection, or perforation; (2) displacement of the foreign body to a more unfavorable or peripheral location; (3) fracture or disintegration of the material or object into smaller pieces; and (4) hypoxemia. If bronchoscopic examination is not possible or removal of the foreign body is unsuccessful, exploratory thoracotomy is indicated.[27, 28]

Exercise-Induced Bronchospasm

Exercise-induced bronchospasm is a clinical syndrome characterized by transient airflow obstruction in both asthmatic and nonasthmatic humans.[29–32] Experimental studies in dogs suggest a similar, if not identical, syndrome;[33–45] however, recognition of this condition in working or sporting dogs is poorly documented.[46] In humans, exertion for at least 12 minutes usually causes bronchodilation during strenuous activity, whereas short, intense periods of exercise (4 to 10 minutes) can trigger bronchial smooth muscle constriction 5 to 15 minutes following activity.[29–32] Spontaneous return to normal airflows occurs within 20 to 60 minutes. Similar findings have been reported in experimental dogs exposed to high flows of low-humidity air,[34–45] and some believe it occurs in racing greyhounds.[46] Symptoms of exercise-induced bronchospasm in humans include chest tightness, breathlessness, coughing, or wheezing, either during or soon after completion of exercise.[31, 32] Greyhounds suspected of having exercise-induced bronchoconstriction show marked loss of stamina 300 to 400 meters into a race and either maintain a steady pace or progressively slow down during the race.[46] A dry, nonproductive cough is typically heard in both humans and greyhounds immediately after strenuous exercise[30–32, 46] and is believed by some to be a reliable indicator of significant bronchoconstriction.[30, 46] Studies indicate that several factors tend to exacerbate the severity of the bronchospasm, including nasal obstruction (sinusitis and rhinitis),[31, 32] exercise conditions (dry, cold air),[30–32, 36] underlying bronchial hyperreactivity,[31, 32, 47] intensity of exercise,[30–32] and interval since last episode of exercise-induced bronchospasm.[30]

Diagnosis in humans is based on history, symptoms, and pulmonary function testing.[29–32] The syndrome has been identified in nearly 90 per cent of individuals with chronic asthma and 35 to 40 per cent of nonasthmatics. History and clinical signs, in addition to tests of lung function, are considered diagnostic standards for nonhuman subjects suspected of having naturally occurring or experimentally induced bronchospasm,[34–45, 47] but there are no reports of treadmill testing or evaluations immediately after strenuous exercise.[46] These types of studies need to be done to document the presence of this syndrome in greyhounds.

The initiating stimulus for exercise-induced bronchospasm is thought to be associated with airway cooling and drying,[29–32, 34–45] which results in the release of a number of chemical mediators from mast cells, including histamine, leukotrienes, prostaglandins, thromboxanes, and platelet-activating factor. This process creates the observed rapid bronchoconstriction and attendant increase in airway secretions and vascular permeability. Concurrent stimulation of afferent irritant receptors may also trigger reflex cholinergic bronchospasm.[32, 33]

Management of exercise-induced bronchospasm includes both pharmacological and nonpharmacological treatments. The therapy of choice for preventing or treating clinically significant signs is the inhalation of beta$_2$-adrenergic agonists.[29, 31, 32, 46, 48–50] Inhaled albuterol, bitolterol, metaproterenol, pirbuterol, and terbutaline are all approved adrenergic medications for international athletic competition and have no ergogenic effect on maximal exercise performance.[31] Similarly, clenbuterol, salbutamol, and terbutaline have demonstrated efficacy in dogs.[46, 48, 50] Inhaled corticosteroids, because of their effects on reducing airway inflammation and bronchial reactivity, also can be used alone or with beta$_2$-adrenergic agonists.[29, 31, 32] Oral theophylline, some antihistamines, and inhaled anticholinergic drugs are recommended alternative medications.[31, 32, 49]

Nonpharmacological treatments include prolonged warm-up periods prior to strenuous exercise and choosing optimal exercise conditions.[29–32] Warm-up periods of 15 to 30 minutes followed by 15 minutes of rest before competition seem to induce a 2- to 4-hour refractory period in which exercise does not cause further bronchoconstriction in humans. The mechanism for this induced refractory period is poorly understood, but it is thought to be related to depletion of mast cell mediators.[32] Finally, strenuous exercise in warm, humid environments is quite effective in diminishing the severity of bronchospasm in some athletes.[29–32] The use and effectiveness of nonpharmacological therapy for exercise-induced bronchospasm have not been reported in working or sporting dogs.

Exercise-Induced Intrabronchial Hemorrhage

Exercise-induced intrabronchial hemorrhage is a common problem in the competitive race horse industry, affecting at least 75 per cent of all Thoroughbreds following strenuous exercise.[51–55] The effect of bleeding into the airways on racing performance is still somewhat unclear, but some racetracks prohibit horses that bleed from further racing. Studies in greyhounds indicate that intrabronchial hemorrhage also occurs following running, with intrabronchial red cell numbers being increased in all dogs examined; however, the frequency of visible bleeding into the airways was only 10 to 15 per cent.[56, 57]

Possible causes of exercise-induced intrabronchial hemorrhage in horses have included asphyxia, blood-borne pathogens, chronic lung disease, coagulation defects, parasitic infections, recurrent laryngeal neuropathy, small airway disease, and uneven mechanical stresses on the lung parenchyma during exercise.[53] Recently, marked increases in pulmonary vascular pressures during strenuous exercise have been shown to cause stress failure of pulmonary capillaries leading to intrabronchial bleeding in horses.[58] Similar hemodynamic changes leading to stress failure of pulmonary capillaries also would seem likely to occur in strenuously exercising dogs;[59] however, studies have yet to address this possibility.

Many therapeutic regimens have been advocated to prevent exercise-induced intrabronchial hemorrhage in horses, but few medications have proven efficacy.[53] Furosemide is used extensively at racetracks where it is permitted, and there is evidence that it reduces pulmonary arterial, right atrial, and capillary pressures in exercising horses.[60–62] Additionally, diuretic and venodilator effects may also be beneficial in reducing pulmonary vascular pressures.[60] Without more information on the pathogenesis and effect of intrabronchial hemorrhage in racing greyhounds, therapeutic intervention seems unwarranted.

Pneumothorax

The presence of air within the pleural space, or pneumothorax, occurs most frequently in racing greyhounds following collisions with other dogs at speed or falls while running.[63] Classified as a traumatic form of pneumothorax, it can result from either nonpenetrating or penetrating chest injury.[64, 65] Radiographic evidence of rib fracture is not always present, in which circumstance the likely pathogenesis is an abrupt increase in intrathoracic pressure that results in alveolar rupture, interstitial emphysema, and dissection of air toward the visceral pleura or the mediastinum.[65] This explanation also provides rationale for the occurrence of pneumomediastinum and subcutaneous emphysema, conditions that often accompany pneumothorax in these circumstances.[63, 65, 66] When rib fracture(s) are present, the likely mechanism is laceration of the visceral pleura by rib fragments; in such circumstances hemothorax also may be present.[64, 65] In racing greyhounds with pneumothorax secondary to nonpenetrating trauma, there have been no associated rib fractures.[63, 66]

Clinical signs depend on the magnitude of the pneumothorax and the volume and pressure of mediastinal air. Typically, greyhounds show marked reductions in racing performance and respiratory distress following moderate exertion along with subcutaneous emphysema at the base of the neck;[63, 66] however, some may be relatively asymptomatic.[66] Auscultation may reveal absence of or diminished breath sounds and a chest wall that is hyperresonant on percussion.[64, 65] Once the dog's condition is stabilized, radiographs should be taken to confirm the diagnosis. Underlying pulmonary diseases, such as bullae or cysts, diaphragmatic hernias, heartworm infection, lung abscessation, pleural effusion, and pneumonia must be ruled out;[64, 65] however, no associated problems have been reported in greyhounds.[63, 66]

Management of traumatic pneumothorax varies, depending on the clinical signs in addition to the volume and progression of air accumulation in the pleural space. Minor pneumothoraces with small leaks and volumes of accumulated air (less than 20 to 30 per

cent) and minimal signs of respiratory discomfort can usually be managed by cage rest or repeated needle thoracocentesis.[63–66] If air slowly reaccumulates, several additional aspirations may be necessary before the leak ceases. Signs of severe respiratory distress associated with rapid or continued accumulations of air in the pleural space (not reported in greyhounds to date) should be treated with tube thoracostomy and water seal drainage.[64, 65] This procedure decreases the risk of lung laceration associated with repeated thoracocentesis while providing constant evacuation of pleural air and rapid re-expansion of the lung. Concurrent use of antibiotics without evidence of infection is advocated by some[63] but seems unwarranted. The chest tube(s) should remain in place until less than 10 cc of air can be evacuated over a 12-hour period.[64, 65] If accumulations of air continue for more than 48 hours along with clinical signs of dyspnea, or if the source of air leakage can be seen radiographically, thoracotomy should be done.[65, 67] Kennel confinement and a 6- to 8-week break from training are recommended following resolution of traumatic pneumothorax, regardless of the treatment method.[63, 66]

INFECTIOUS RESPIRATORY PROBLEMS

Rhinitis

The effect of rhinitis on racing or hunting performance in dogs is undocumented, whereas in human athletes inflammation or obstruction of the nasal passages is known to intensify exercise-induced bronchospasm by diminishing nasal filtration, heating, and humidification.[32] Potential causes of infectious rhinitis in young working and sporting breed dogs include bacterial, mycotic, parasitic, and viral infections;[68] only parasitic infections caused by *Eucoleus aerophilus* (*Capillaria aerophila*) and *E. boehmi* have been reported.[69, 70] It is not known how dogs become infected with *Eucoleus,* but earthworms have been suggested as likely intermediate hosts.[71] Clinical signs may include face rubbing, sneezing, epistaxis and mucopurulent nasal discharge,[69] although many dogs appear normal.[70] Diagnosis is easily accomplished by demonstrating characteristic eggs in nasal discharges, swabs, or flushing; eggs are also easily recovered by fecal flotation. In chronic cases, skull radiographs show increased soft tissue densities of the nasal cavity and ethmoid region. Tissue samples from the nasal mucosa also can be used to histopathologically diagnose these infections.[69] Treatment with invermectin (0.2 mg/kg once orally) or fenbendazole (50 mg/kg orally once daily for 10 days) has been recommended, but reinfection or temporary suppression of egg production is likely. Cleanup of contaminated housing and exercising areas is recommended because *Eucoleus* eggs persist in the environment.

Tonsillitis

Primary tonsillitis can be acute or chronic and usually occurs in juvenile dogs.[72–77] Clinical signs of coughing, retching, fever, and inappetence are caused by inflammation of the pharyngeal mucosa, with or without tonsillar enlargement.[73–77] Diagnosis is based on history and physical examination findings. Acutely inflamed tonsils appear reddish with small punctate hemorrhages and may have white or yellowish plaques of inflammatory exudate. Bacterial culture and sensitivity testing is usually not indicated before treatment because of the similarity of organisms found in health and tonsillar infection.[72, 78] Treatment with amoxicillin (11 to 22 mg/kg orally, two or three times daily for 7 days) or other broad-spectrum antibiotic usually results in clinical improvement, although tonsillar enlargement, when present, may persist for several weeks.[73–78] Chronic or recurrent tonsillitis has been suggested by some to be part of the normal maturation process of cellular and humoral immunity.[72, 74–76, 78] Others believe that persistent or chronic tonsillar infections may lead to the development of autoimmune disorders.[72] In adult dogs, chronic vomiting or regurgitation, upper or lower respiratory tract infections, periodontal disease, open-mouth breathing, and the licking of mucocutaneous regions or infected skin are potential causes of secondary tonsillitis.[74–78]

Treatment of these patients should be directed at the source of the infection, and bacterial culture and sensitivity testing of samples from the tonsillar area is probably indicated.

Tonsillectomy is occasionally warranted, particularly in dogs with chronic or recurrent tonsillitis that is unresponsive to antibiotic therapy or in cases in which tonsillar enlargement results in upper air-flow obstruction.[73–77, 79] The latter condition, described in racing greyhounds,[79] apparently causes no loss of appetite or difficulty in swallowing. Upper airway noise or stridor is not present at rest, during walking, or with mild exercise; however, strenuous running of greater than 400 meters results in loud, forceful, stridorous breathing and reduction in racing performance. Procedures for the removal of tonsils are described in veterinary textbooks.[74, 75, 79] General anesthesia and endotracheal intubation are essential. To prevent aspiration of blood, moistened gauze sponges should be placed in the pharynx around the endotracheal tube before the tonsils are removed. Bleeding can be controlled by blood vessel ligation or electrocoagulation. Patients should be closely monitored following recovery from surgery because aspiration of blood or saliva may lead to respiratory compromise. Food should not be provided for 24 hours. Corticosteroids are recommended if pharyngeal edema occurs after surgery, in addition to broad-spectrum antibiotics for 7 days. Soft foods can be given after 24 hours and should be continued for 2 weeks. Complete healing occurs by 10 to 14 days, but training with a lure is not recommended for 8 weeks.[79]

Tracheobronchitis
Parasitic Lung Infections

Filaroides (Oslerus) osleri is the only pulmonary parasite documented as a cause of significant clinical disease in working and sporting dogs.[80–84] Infections occur worldwide, but there is little information on prevalence. Two surveys of greyhounds from England indicated incidences of 18 percent,[80, 81] but there are no data from the United States or elsewhere substantiating these findings.[85] Some investigators believe *F. osleri* infections are becoming more common,[86] but case reports or reviews of this disease in working and sporting dogs over the last 10 years have been infrequent.[83]

Filaroides osleri is unlike other metastrongyloids because an intermediate host is not required to complete the life cycle.[84, 87, 88] Adult worms reside in submucosal nodules or plaques that project into the lumen of the trachea near its bifurcation into right and left principal bronchi.[84, 87–89] Thin-walled eggs, released by ovoviviparous female worms, contain first-stage larvae that are coughed up, swallowed, and passed as infective larvae in the feces.[87–89] It is postulated that transmission of *F. osleri* larvae occurs directly from bitches to their pups by salivary contamination during licking or by the ingestion of fresh larvae-infected feces from the bitch (or littermates).[87–89] Following ingestion, first-stage larvae migrate through the wall of the small intestine to the lungs via the hepatic portal circulation or the mesenteric lymphatics.[87, 88] Small nodules, containing immature worms, appear in the trachea 2 months after infection.[84, 88] Clinical signs consist of paroxysmal coughing and respiratory distress, particularly after exercise; severe cases are usually seen in young dogs.[82–84, 86, 88]

Diagnosis can be difficult. First-stage larvae are found infrequently by fecal examination with either flotation or Baermann techniques.[88] Samples of pharyngeal mucus can be used to demonstrate larvae, but intermittent shedding of eggs by female worms makes repeated sampling likely.[88] Bronchoscopic examination of the airways is considered the most reliable procedure for establishing a diagnosis, because it allows visualization of the size and location of the parasitic nodules in addition to collection of airway mucus for confirmatory examination of eggs and larvae.[83, 86, 88] Thoracic radiography may be of diagnostic benefit in long-standing cases. Evidence for successful treatment is conflicting. Amelioration of clinical signs reportedly occurs following prolonged treatment with thiacetarsamide and several of the benzimidazoles, such as albendazole, fenbendazole, oxfendazole, and thiabendazole, at increased dosages.[13, 87, 88] However, consistent evidence of therapeutic success is lacking.[87, 88] This represents a significant problem because there are no effective treatments for dogs infected with *F. osleri,* and infections often occur early in puppyhood. Therefore, current recommendations when *F. osleri* infections are identified in a kennel or elsewhere include elimination of infected dogs (by euthanasia or transfer off the premises) or delivery of pups from infected bitches by cesarean section followed by raising them artificially or by placing them on a nurse-bitch in an area away from all infected dogs.[87, 88]

Viral/Bacterial Infections

Several viruses, bacteria, and mycoplasmas have been implicated as causative agents of infectious tracheobronchitis (kennel cough).[90–99] Viral infections most frequently contributing to this syndrome include parainfluenza type 2 and canine adenovirus type 2.[90, 92–94, 97–99] Canine adenovirus 1, distemper virus, herpesvirus, and reoviruses also have been isolated, but they play a less significant role in this disease.[93] *Bordetella bronchiseptica* is the most commonly recovered and important primary or secondary bacterial species identified from dogs with infectious tracheobronchitis.[90–94, 96, 97] *Mycoplasma cynos* has also been recovered from the respiratory tract of dogs with pulmonary disease; however, its role as a primary pathogen in infectious tracheobronchitis is still uncertain.[90, 91, 93, 95] Evidence indicates that sequential or simultaneous infections with two or more pathogens (particularly when *B. bronchiseptica* is present) results in much greater respiratory debilitation than infection with a single agent.[90, 91, 93, 98, 99–101]

Canine Parainfluenza Virus Type 2. Canine parainfluenza virus type 2, also known as simian virus 5, is a relatively large (150 to 250 nm) RNA virus with a lipoprotein envelope containing three proteins.[102, 103] One glycoprotein has hemagglutinin and neuraminidase activities (the latter exposes receptors for virus attachment); the second glycoprotein is responsible for the virion's cell fusion activity and hemolytic function, while the third envelope protein (nonglycosylated) forms the inner envelope layer that maintains the virion structure and integrity.[102, 103] It is a relatively unstable virus, losing most of its infectivity within 4 hours at room temperature. Organic solvents or surface-active agents rapidly inactivate the virus because the viral envelope has a high lipid content.[102]

Canine parainfluenza virus type 2 is the most common viral isolate from dogs with infectious tracheobronchitis.[90, 94, 97] Experimental infections using intratracheal or aerosol methods of virus inoculation result in replication of the virus in epithelial cells of the nasal mucosa, trachea, bronchi, bronchioli, and peribronchial lymph nodes.[90, 98, 101] Clinical signs of uncomplicated parainfluenza infection (serous nasal discharge and cough) develop 7 to 9 days after virus exposure and last 3 to 5 days.[90, 96, 98–101] Persistence of viral infection has not been demonstrated, but rapid spread of the virus from dog to dog lasts for up to 9 days.[90, 104] Positive antibody titers are present 8 to 10 days after virus exposure.[99, 101] Lesions are those of tracheobronchitis and bronchiolitis (lymphocytic, plasmacytic, and neutrophilic infiltration in the submucosa) in addition to squamous metaplasia and loss of cilia in the large airways.[90, 98,

[99, 101] Cellular infiltrates consisting of lymphocytes, plasma cells, and histiocytes are present in greater than 50 per cent of the small nonrespiratory bronchioles.[98, 99, 101]

Canine Adenovirus Type 2. Canine adenovirus type 2 is a medium-sized (70 to 90 nm) DNA virus without a lipoprotein envelope.[105, 106] Viral particles have a dense central core and an outer coat or capsid. Attachment to host cells occurs when glycoprotein fibers, projecting from outer capsid pentamers, contact an appropriate cell surface receptor.[105, 106] Virions enter the cell via clathrin-coated pits.[106] Pentamers are removed in the cytoplasm, and the core migrates to the nucleus where viral replication occurs. Intranuclear inclusion bodies, a hallmark of adenovirus infections, represent accumulations of unassembled viral components.[105, 106] Agglutination of red blood cells, a characteristic of adenovirus type 2, occurs when tips of the glycoprotein fiber bind to erythrocyte receptors. Stability of adenovirus type 2 in the environment is relatively long, based on evidence that no loss of infectivity occurs after 20 days at room temperature.[105] However, inactivation of the virus occurs rapidly at 56° C.

Canine adenovirus type 2, although less frequently isolated from dogs with infectious tracheobronchitis,[90, 94, 97] typically produces a more severe respiratory disease than parainfluenza virus.[90, 100, 107] Experimental infections using intranasal, intratracheal, or aerosol routes of virus inoculation have been used to more clearly delineate the pathogenesis of adenovirus type 2 respiratory tract infections. Following virus exposure, replication takes place in the nasal mucosa, tonsils, pharynx, trachea, and lungs.[90, 107–109] Clinical signs of uncomplicated adenovirus 2 infection include coughing, lethargy, increased breathing effort, and wheezing (due to bronchial hyperresponsiveness)[107, 108] as early as 1 day following exposure.[107–109] Temperature elevations (up to 40° C) in addition to ocular and nasal discharges are noted after 4 to 6 days. Resolution of infection may take 2 to 3 weeks,[100, 107] depending on the pathogenicity of the strain and degree of impairment of host defenses at the time of virus exposure. Latent infections occur; however, spread of the infection to other dogs is restricted to the first 10 days after exposure.[90, 107] Positive antibody titers are present 12 to 14 days following virus exposure.[107] Viral replication in the airways is associated with necrotizing and proliferative bronchitis and bronchiolitis and the presence of large, amphophilic, intranuclear inclusions in swollen nuclei of degenerating bronchiolar epithelial cells.[107–109]

Bordetella bronchiseptica. Bordetellae are small aerobic, gram-negative rods or coccobacilli that localize to the cilia of respiratory epithelium.[110, 111] These microorganisms synthesize at least one lipopolysaccharide toxin that is similar both chemically and biologically to the lipopolysaccharide toxins of other gram-negative bacteria.[110] Virulent strains produce fimbriae (pili) and an extracellular enzyme, adenylate cyclase.[111] Proteinaceous fimbrial adhesins bind the bacteria to each other and to host cilia, whereas tracheal cytotoxin, which is probably a bacterial peptidoglycan fragment specifically toxic to ciliated respiratory epithelial cells,[112] causes ciliostasis.[111] Adenylate cyclase increases intracellular cyclic adenosine monophosphate, which reduces the phagocytic activity of neutrophils and macrophages and stimulates secretory cell function via increasing chloride flux through the tracheal mucosa.[111, 113, 114] *Bordetella bronchiseptica* also produces a highly lethal toxin (formerly called *dermonecrotic toxin*) that is thought to cause inflammation in areas adjacent to the organism.[111, 115, 116] Additional products including proteases, hemagglutinins, and a hemolysin may also play a part in the pathogenesis of respiratory infections.[111, 117]

Although *B. bronchiseptica* is considered to be part of the normal bacterial flora of the nasopharynx,[118] it is also a primary respiratory pathogen.[91, 94, 101, 119–121] Dogs of all ages are susceptible, but isolation rates are usually higher in young animals, particularly those kept in close confinement.[90–92, 94, 96, 110, 119, 120] Information on the

pathogenesis of *B. bronchiseptica*–induced respiratory disease in dogs primarily comes from experimental infections.[47, 101, 120, 121] Initial clinical signs of coughing and nasal discharge occur 2 to 10 days after aerosol[120, 121] or intratracheal[47, 101] inoculation. Coughing and wheezing (associated with bronchial hyperresponsiveness)[47, 101] is exacerbated by excitement or exercise.[92, 120, 121] Rectal temperatures and white blood cell counts are seldom increased. Infection is readily transmitted to susceptible dogs by aerosol and direct contact.[111, 119] Recovery can be expected in 1 to 2 weeks; however, clearance of *B. bronchiseptica* from the respiratory tract may take up to 14 weeks.[120] Positive antibody titers are present 7 to 10 days after bacterial infection.[101, 120, 121]

Pulmonary lesions associated with *B. bronchiseptica* infection are limited primarily to the ciliated epithelial mucosa.[101, 120, 121] Extensive neutrophilic infiltration of the ciliated epithelium occurs during the first day of infection and becomes more intense over the next 2 weeks.[120, 121] Bacteria are present only on ciliated epithelial cells.[120, 121] Cell structure remains intact for the first 3 to 5 days of the infection, but this is followed by epithelial cell necrosis, loss of cilia, and plugging of bronchi and bronchioles with a cellular exudate composed of alveolar macrophages and neutrophils.[47, 101, 120, 121] Alveolar involvement is minimal.[120, 121] With resolution of the infection, usually by 6 to 14 weeks,[120] tracheobronchial and bronchiolar lesions resolve.[121]

Clinical Findings

Clinical signs of tracheobronchitis are more severe (coughing, fever, inappetence, respiratory distress, mucopurulent oculonasal discharges, and wheezing) and of longer duration when *B. bronchiseptica* infections occur concurrently with other agents (adenovirus, distemper virus, parainfluenza virus, or mycoplasma) or when animals have poor vaccination histories.[90, 91, 101] Signs can last from a few days to several weeks, depending on the rate and extent of bacterial proliferation, the quantity of toxins released, the virulence of the strain of organism, and the degree of impairment of host defenses. Secondary complications in otherwise healthy dogs are rare, the most serious being bacterial bronchopneumonia due to *B. bronchiseptica* (largely related to its capacity to impair ciliary function[111, 112] and to produce adenylate cyclase,[111, 114] which diminishes the bactericidal activity of alveolar macrophages and neutrophils) in inadequately treated or untreated animals.

Diagnosis of Infection

Clinical diagnosis of infectious tracheobronchitis is usually made on the basis of the history, physical examination, and clinical signs. Complete blood counts, serum biochemical profiles, and thoracic radiographs are not unusual, with the exception of complicated infections in which bronchopneumonia is present.[90–94, 96, 97] Diagnostic confirmation of infection can be accomplished by obtaining respiratory tract secretions for cytological examination and bacterial culture, virus isolation from nasopharyngeal swabs, or serological confirmation of viral exposure with paired serum antibody titers.[47, 90, 91, 97–101, 107, 119, 120]

Treatment

Antimicrobial Agents. Despite the role that viruses play in this disease and the belief that many *B. bronchiseptica* infections are self-limiting, antimicrobial therapy is recommended, particularly if clinical signs are severe or last longer than 14 days.[90, 91, 93, 122–124] Selection of antimicrobial drugs should be based on results of in vitro culture and sensitivity tests of respiratory tract secretions or percutaneous fine-needle aspiration specimens from the lung.[1, 4] Antibiotics reported to have in vitro sensitivity against most isolates include most of the aminoglycosides (amikacin, gentamicin, kanamycin, neomycin, tobramycin), chloramphenicol, the macrolides, the extended-spectrum penicillins (carbenicillin, ticarcillin), the polymyxins, the quinolones (ciprofloxacin, enrofloxacin), the tetracyclines (doxycycline, minocycline), and the trimethoprim-sulfonamides.[122, 125–127] It is noteworthy that potentially effective antimicrobials far outnumber those that have demonstrated efficacy in experimental[123] and natural infections.[124, 128] Only trimethoprim-sulfadiazine consistently reduced *B. bronchiseptica* numbers when given orally at 15 mg/kg orally, twice daily for 14 days.[124, 128] Other recommendations include ampicillin or amoxicillin at 11 to 22 mg/kg orally, twice to three times daily for 14 days,[92] and tetracycline at 22 mg/kg orally, three times daily for a minimum of 7 days.[93]

Besides altering the immune status, adenylate cyclase[111] and tracheal cytotoxin[112] produced by *B. bronchiseptica* may be partially responsible for the disparity observed between in vitro antibiotic sensitivities and clinical response.[90, 122] Recently, antimicrobial agents capable of penetrating phagocytes have been proposed as a means of increasing antibiotic deposition in the upper airways and lung.[129, 130] The majority of antimicrobials capable of concentrating within alveolar macrophages and neutrophils are lipid soluble and include chloramphenicol, the macrolides (clarithromycin, erythromycin), the quinolones (ciprofloxacin, enrofloxacin), the tetracyclines (doxycycline, minocycline), and trimethoprim-sulfonamide combinations.[129, 130]

Levels of antibiotics in sinus secretions and bronchial fluids may also be important in the treatment of patients with *B. bronchiseptica* infections. Erythromycin, the quinolones, the tetracyclines, and the trimethoprim-sulfonamide combinations have demonstrated the best sinus secretion and bronchial fluid penetration.[130] The aminoglycosides penetrate nasal secretions and bronchial fluid poorly.[130] Penetration of antibiotics into lung tissues, while more important in parenchymal lung infections than tracheobronchial infections, may still have some bearing on the resolution of *B. bronchiseptica* infections. Data indicate that ciprofloxacin, erythromycin, the tetracyclines, and trimethoprim-sulfonamide combinations penetrate lung tissue well and achieve concentrations that exceed serum levels.[130] In light of this information, it is not surprising that studies evaluating the efficacy of ciprofloxacin[131] and trimethoprim-sulfadiazine[124, 128] in *B. bronchiseptica* infections have been encouraging. Why the macrolides and the tetracyclines have been relatively ineffective antimicrobial agents against infectious tracheobronchitis associated with *B. bronchiseptica* is not known. However, resistance to these classes of antibiotics is usually plasmid mediated[130] and at least one report demonstrated that *B. bronchiseptica* isolates develop R plasmid antibiotic resistance.[132]

From the preceding information, the most effective antibiotic choices for the treatment of infectious tracheobronchitis caused by *B. bronchiseptica* appear to be ciprofloxacin (5 to 15 mg/kg),[133] enrofloxacin (2.5 to 7.5 mg/kg),[133] and the trimethoprim-sulfonamide combinations (15 to 30 mg/kg)[133] administered orally (enrofloxacin and the trimethoprim-sulfonamides can also be given by injection), twice daily for 14 days. The trimethoprim-sulfonamides would be the best choice for young dogs less than 30 weeks old because of detrimental effects on cartilage development caused by the quinolone antibiotics.[134]

An alternative approach recommended for treating infectious tracheobronchitis is the use of aerosolized or intratracheally administered antimicrobial drugs.[135, 136] Studies reported in the veterinary literature have suggested encouraging results;[122, 137, 138] however, the techniques have not been adopted by veterinary clinicians as evidenced by the paucity of references on their use in treating bronchopneumonias over the past 5 years. Nevertheless, aerosol or intratracheal treatments provide a means of more safely administering drugs like the aminoglycosides or polymyxins, which have demonstrated in vitro sensitivity to *B. bronchiseptica,* but are

poorly absorbed from mucosal surfaces and relatively toxic when administered parenterally. Aerosol treatment with gentamicin, kanamycin, and polymyxin B (50 mg, 250 mg, and 166,666 IU, respectively, nebulized from 3 ml suspensions for 10 minutes twice daily for 3 days) reduced clinical signs and colony counts of *B. bronchiseptica* in the tracheas of experimentally infected dogs.[122] Although clinical cures were not demonstrated, additional blinded or placebo-controlled studies with this therapeutic regimen as well as intratracheal treatments seem warranted, particularly since endotracheal instillations of antibiotics have been shown to reduce morbidity and mortality in human patients with bronchopneumonia.[136] Another advantage of these treatment methods would seem to be increased hydration of airway secretions, which should improve movement of bacteria and cellular debris out of the airways via the mucociliary clearance mechanism. Intratracheal administration of antibiotics and corticosteroids, although recommended in several references,[137, 138] has no proven advantage over antibiotics alone. Therefore, until controlled studies show beneficial effects with aerosol or intratracheal instillation of antibiotic-steroid combinations, their use cannot be recommended. Potential adverse effects of aerosolized and intratracheally administered antimicrobial agents include bronchial irritation (primarily with polymyxins, unlikely with the aminoglycosides), resorption of the antibiotic from the airway lumen into the blood (serum levels of aminoglycosides are very low, often less than 1 μg/ml in patients with normal renal function; however, potentially toxic levels may occur with impaired renal function), and emergence of resistant microorganisms (predominantly a problem in the setting of prophylactic rather than therapeutic local administration).[136]

Antiviral Agents. Aerosolization of antiviral agents, particularly ribavirin, which has in vitro activity against the parainfluenza viruses, has not been evaluated as a treatment for infectious canine tracheobronchitis, although reports of clinical improvement in human patients with influenza, parainfluenza, and respiratory syncytial virus pneumonias following ribavirin treatment have been published.[136] Studies to determine the efficacy of this antiviral drug in dogs infected with parainfluenza virus are needed.

Bronchodilators. Bronchodilators seem warranted in the treatment of infectious tracheobronchitis based on documentation of bronchial hyperresponsiveness with *B. bronchiseptica*[47, 101] and canine parainfluenza virus type 2 and adenovirus type 2[107, 108] infections, alone or in combination.[99–101] Albuterol (0.02 to 0.05 mg/kg orally two to four times daily), metaproterenol (0.325 to 0.65 mg/kg orally four to six times daily), and terbutaline (1.25 to 5.0 mg total, orally two to three times daily) are beta$_2$-selective agonists that produce effective bronchodilation.[139] Common side effects include skeletal muscle tremors and restlessness, which usually subside within 5 days. Stimulation of airway mucus secretion also occurs, resulting in a less viscous secretion. Long-term use of these drugs can result in refractoriness as a result of down-regulation of beta-receptors. The methylxanthines include the immediate-release products such as aminophylline (as the salt) (11 mg/kg, orally four times daily) and theophylline (9 mg/kg, orally four times daily), plus the sustained-release products such as Theo-Dur tablets (20 mg/kg, orally twice daily), Slo-bid Gyrocaps (20 to 25 mg/kg, orally twice daily), and Choledyl SA tablets (as the salt) (39 to 47 mg/kg, orally twice daily).[139] They are equally effective in relaxing large and small airway smooth muscle (similar to the beta$_2$-agonists), and they may improve airway function by increasing mucociliary transport rates and preventing microvascular leakage. Common adverse effects include central nervous system excitation (manifested as restlessness, tremors, seizures), gastrointestinal upset (nausea, vomiting), diuresis, and tachycardia.[139] Dogs given quinolone antibiotics concurrently with any of the methylxanthines should be closely monitored because metabolism of the bronchodilator drugs may be reduced, leading to signs of toxicity.[130]

Cough Suppressants. Cough suppressants, alone or in combination with bronchodilators, are recommended for treatment of nonproductive coughing.[90, 93] The bronchodilators, described previously, may be considered peripheral antitussives because of their effect on airway caliber.[139] It is thought that bronchodilation relieves irritant receptor stimulation (suggested as a reason for the bronchial hyperresponsiveness seen in dogs with infectious tracheobronchitis)[47, 100, 101, 107, 108] induced by inflammation or mechanical deformation of the bronchial wall during bronchoconstriction. Centrally acting antitussives include both narcotic and non-narcotic drugs.[139] Narcotic cough suppressants act on the cough center to depress its sensitivity to afferent stimuli. Hydrocodone (0.22 mg/kg, orally twice to four times daily) is more potent and causes less respiratory depression than codeine (1 to 2 mg/kg, orally three times daily).[170] Common side effects include analgesia, constipation, and sedation. Butorphanol tartrate (0.5 to 1.0 mg/kg, orally twice to four times daily, or 0.055 to 0.11 mg/kg, subcutaneously/intramuscularly as needed), a narcotic agonist/antagonist, is a potent antitussive that has mild respiratory and central nervous system depressive side effects.[139] An advantage of this preparation is that it is not a controlled drug. Dextromethorphan hydrobromide (1 to 2 mg/kg, orally three to four times daily) is a non-narcotic opioid, available as an alcohol-based syrup without prescription.[139] Its antitussive efficacy is reportedly equal to codeine, and studies in humans have shown that the combination of dextromethorphan with a beta$_2$-selective agonist bronchodilator is superior to dextromethorphan alone.[140] Excessive use of any of these products may compromise ventilation, in addition to predisposing the patient to retention of airway secretions. Suppression of coughing in patients with infectious tracheobronchitis complicated by bacterial pneumonia is not recommended.

Prevention and Control. A comprehensive vaccination program against the agents causing infectious tracheobronchitis is the best method of reducing the prevalence and severity of respiratory disease in the individual animal as well as among animals within a kennel environment. In selection of a vaccination program that will provide protection against infectious tracheobronchitis, vaccination with the following antigens is recommended: *B. bronchiseptica,* canine adenovirus type 2, canine distemper virus, and canine parainfluenza virus type 2.[90–93] Each of these antigens is commercially available as monovalent and multivalent products for parenteral administration; however, these vaccines are likely to be neutralized by maternal antibodies if administered to puppies less than 12 weeks of age.[90] Therefore, puppies vaccinated before 12 weeks of age should receive multiple injections, 2 to 4 weeks apart until 16 weeks of age. The parenterally administered vaccines produce high antibody titers lasting up to 12 months, but vaccination does not necessarily prevent infection.[90, 91, 93] Parenteral vaccination against canine adenovirus type 2 protects susceptible dogs against disease as well as infection; canine parainfluenza virus type 2, against disease but not infection. Vaccination may not be effective against virulent strains of *B. bronchiseptica.*[90, 93]

Alternatively, intranasal vaccination with live avirulent *B. bronchiseptica* combined with modified live canine parainfluenza virus type 2 may be used. Administration of this product appears to be a better choice than parenteral injections since intranasal vaccines do not interfere with maternal antibodies, are safe when administered to pregnant bitches, elicit significant local immunity as early as 4 days after inoculation,[141] and reduce both clinical disease and duration of *B. bronchiseptica* shedding.[142–144] Vaccination of puppies can begin as early as 3 weeks of age with revaccination recommended annually.[91, 93] A small percentage of dogs may develop a cough and have nasal discharge following intranasal vaccination[141, 143] that may require antimicrobial treatment.[145]

Kennels experiencing frequent outbreaks of infectious tracheobronchitis can reduce epidemic respiratory disease by minimizing

population density, maximizing ventilation by providing at least 12 air changes per hour, and maintaining humidity below 50 per cent.[93] Isolation of infected dogs and dogs believed to have been exposed from the "normal" population for 1 or 2 weeks is critical to resolving the outbreak.[90] Personnel handling coughing dogs should wear clean, disposable clothing and gloves. Contaminated facilities, cages, and metal eating utensils should be disinfected with household bleach (5.6 per cent sodium hypochlorite) diluted with water by adding 1 part bleach to 30 parts water. The solution is effective, inexpensive, and virucidal.[90, 93] Other useful disinfectants include benzalkonium chloride (Roccal-D) and chlorhexidine (Nolvasan).[90] Ideally, isolation facilities should be available for dogs with clinical signs of infection.

Bacterial Pneumonia

Bacterial pneumonia is an important clinical problem in working and sporting breed dogs,[146] having been identified as a frequent cause of poor performance in greyhounds from Kansas.[78] Case reports suggest that the most common microorganism isolated from greyhounds with pneumonia is *Streptococcus equi* subsp. *zooepidemicus.*[147, 148]

Streptococci are small, facultatively anaerobic, gram-positive cocci that occur in pairs or chains and account for between 20 and 47 per cent of cases of canine pneumonia.[125, 149, 151] Types of hemolytic reactions observed on blood agar plates are used to differentiate streptococci into alpha, beta, and gamma groups.[152] Beta-hemolytic streptococci are further divided into immunological (Lancefield) groups A through O based on specific cell wall polysaccharides.[152] Most pathogenic strains causing pneumonia in dogs belong to groups C and G,[125, 147–151] whereas human infections are predominantly group A.[152, 153] Intracellular and extracellular products are created by both alpha- and beta-hemolytic streptococci, with the alpha-hemolytic respiratory pathogen *S. pneumoniae* considered to be of particular pathogenic significance in humans.[152–154]

Important virulence factors for hemolytic streptococci include: (1) capsular polysaccharide, which acts to restrict phagocytosis;[155] (2) surface protein A;[156] (3) pneumolysin (a cytoplasmic toxin), which inhibits the beating of cilia on respiratory epithelium,[157] disrupts the alveolar-capillary barrier,[158] inhibits neutrophil bactericidal activity (by reducing chemotaxis, phagocytosis, and the respiratory burst),[159] and inhibits lymphocyte proliferation in response to mitogens and synthesis of all immunoglobulin classes;[160] and (4) autolysin, which is a cell wall–associated enzyme that mediates the release of cytoplasmic proteins (neuraminidase and pneumolysin) and other cell wall fragments.[161]

Nonvirulence products include (1) neuraminidase (a cytoplasmic protein), which exposes receptors for *Streptococcus* species attachment;[162] (2) immunoglobulin A1-specific protease, which may act to compromise host defenses at the mucosal surface;[163] (3) a protein-like adhesin molecule, which mediates the attachment of streptococcal organisms to the target receptor on respiratory epithelial cells;[164] (4) erythrogenic toxin, which is responsible for pyrogenicity and enhancement of the action of gram-negative endotoxins;[152] (5) hyaluronidase, which depolymerizes hyaluronic acid and is thought to play a role in the spread of streptococci in tissues;[154] (6) streptokinases, which may prevent formation of effective fibrin barriers at the periphery of streptococcal lesions;[152] and (7) streptolysin O (a hemolysin), which is a cell membrane–damaging toxin.[165]

Very little is known about the toxins of beta-hemolytic groups C and G and their potential role in disease pathogenesis; however, some strains elaborate extracellular and intracellular toxins resembling those of *S. pneumoniae* and beta-hemolytic group A streptococci.[152, 166–170]

Other alpha-hemolytic streptococci (not *S. pneumoniae*) are often referred to as the viridans group, which normally colonize the upper respiratory tract.[152] They are considered to have a low degree of pathogenicity compared to beta-hemolytic streptococci.[152] Non-hemolytic streptococci also are generally of low pathogenicity.[152] In circumstances in which virulence is low, the magnitude of the bacterial challenge is crucial. There may be a critical or threshold inoculum size, beyond which the normal clearance mechanisms may be surpassed. Continued elimination of the initial inoculum is inadequate, bacterial multiplication occurs, and pneumonia ensues.[171, 172] Finally, abnormalities in host defenses may influence bacterial-host interaction in favor of bacterial invasion and result in pneumonia.[171]

The most likely sequence for colonization of the lower respiratory tract by streptococci in dogs seems to be microaspiration of organisms from the oropharyngeal region following a viral (canine adenovirus type 2 or canine parainfluenza virus type 2) respiratory tract infection. After establishment of infection in the alveoli, a characteristic sequence takes place in the development of streptococcal pneumonia based primarily on the virulence of the organism.[173–175] First, bacterial invasion by the encapsulated streptococci causes vascular leakage and edema mediated in part by the release of hyaluronidase and pneumolysin.[154, 156] This fluid serves as a vehicle for carrying streptococcal organisms into the terminal bronchioles and alveoli. Inspiratory movements also aid the spread of infection toward the lung periphery. Neutrophils soon enter the infected area and reach sufficient numbers to fill the alveoli completely, producing consolidation.[173–175] At this stage, released C3a and C5a from complement activation stimulate phagocytosis by neutrophils even though type-specific opsonizing capsular antibodies have not yet appeared.[173] Such early phagocytosis follows the trapping of streptococcal organisms against alveolar walls or other neutrophils. Nonspecific heat-labile opsonins contribute to the effectiveness of this early phagocytic process and subsequent killing of streptococcal organisms. After several days, monospecific anticapsular antibody appears. By neutralizing the antiphagocytic properties of the capsular polysaccharide, this antibody considerably enhances phagocytosis and intracellular killing. Once most of the organisms have been ingested, alveolar macrophages derived from monocytes of the blood enter the lesion and increase in numbers.[174, 175] This change in cellularity to a dominance by macrophages is associated with clearance of bacteria and leukocytic debris and thinning of the exudate.

In low-virulence streptococcal infections, damage in the alveolar regions is restricted to type I epithelial cells.[174] Unaffected type II epithelial cells proliferate, transform into elongated pneumocytes of intermediate morphology, and then undermine and strip off damaged type I epithelial cells from the basement membrane.[174] Thereafter the intermediate type pneumocytes differentiate into type I epithelial cells, completing the repair process.[174] In contrast, more virulent streptococcal infections cause early damage to type I epithelial cells that progresses to necrosis, leaving areas of denuded alveolar basement membrane.[175] Accompanying the degeneration and necrosis of type I epithelial cells, alveolar epithelial repair by proliferation and transformation of type II cells to type I cells is inhibited.[175] Hypertrophic and hyperplastic foci of type II pneumocytes may persist following the initial inflammatory response, followed by emigration and proliferation of fibroblasts in defects in the epithelium with resultant fibrosis.[175] Thus the outcome of streptococcal pneumonia seems related to the pathogenicity of the infecting organism.

Case reports of severe streptococcal pneumonias in greyhound dogs caused by beta-hemolytic *S. equi* subsp. *zooepidemicus* (Lancefield group C)[147, 148] were documented or strongly suspected to have been associated with concurrent viral respiratory infections similar to human cases in which streptococcal pneumonias frequently occur after respiratory infections with neuraminidase-pro-

ducing viruses.[154] All dogs in these reports had severe infections, and several died, with evidence at autopsy of hematogenous spread of the infection to the heart, brain, kidneys, adrenal glands, spleen, and lymph nodes.[147, 148] In animals recovering from these complications, permanent lung damage can be expected and may result in reduced performance.[146]

Clinical Findings

Most bacterial infections of the lower respiratory tract have an acute onset manifested by exercise intolerance, depression, fever, inappetence, productive cough, varying severity of respiratory distress, and serous or mucopurulent nasal discharge. Lung sounds are usually increased with crackles and wheezes audible over variable regions of the chest. Animals with mild disease may not have obvious signs of pulmonary infection.[146–151, 176]

Diagnosis of Infection

A diagnosis of bacterial pneumonia can usually be confirmed after evaluation of information obtained from thoracic radiographs, a complete blood count, and the examination of airway fluids obtained by transtracheal aspiration, fiberoptic bronchoscopy, or transthoracic lung aspiration.[1, 4, 176]

Early radiographic signs of infection include focal to widespread interstitial and sometimes peribronchial densities. As the infection progresses, areas of alveolar consolidation develop, particularly in the cranioventral lung lobes. An early, diffuse interstitial pattern is likely a response to viral infection.[1, 4, 176] Radiographs should be carefully examined for evidence of hilar infiltrates or lymphadenopathy, pulmonary artery enlargement, and mass lesions, which are characteristic for other diseases but can be hidden by overlying alveolar densities.[1, 4]

Neutrophilic leukocytosis with a left shift and monocytosis is often present on the complete blood count; however, a normal or stress leukogram is not uncommon.[149–151, 176] The serum biochemical panel should be normal.

Airway fluids, obtained by transtracheal aspiration, potentially contain essential information for establishing a definitive diagnosis of bacterial pneumonia because airways below the level of the larynx are normally sterile.[1, 4, 125, 176, 177] Thus, specimens collected with this procedure can be expected to be uncontaminated by oral flora. Samples of airway secretions should be rapidly processed for culture and cytological examination since delay may result in false-negative culture results.[1] Cytological examination of Wright-Giemsa–stained smears of aspirated material typically reveals septic inflammation with a predominance of degenerate neutrophils.[1, 4, 125, 149–151, 176, 177] However, bacteria are not always demonstrable, and their absence in cytological specimens does not rule out bacterial pneumonia.[1, 176, 177] Nonseptic neutrophilic inflammation is likely to be present if antibiotics have been administered in the past few days.[1] Rational medical management, including selection of antibiotics, can be carried out based on cytological findings while awaiting culture and antibiotic sensitivity testing results.[1, 125, 176, 177]

Transtracheal aspiration should be the initial procedure to obtain diagnostic information from the patient suspected of having bacterial pneumonia.[1, 4, 149–151] Alternative diagnostic procedures with greater sensitivity (recovery of organisms responsible for disease) and specificity (lack of contaminant organisms), such as fiberoptic bronchoscopy (using a catheter-sheathed brush system), transthoracic lung aspiration, or open lung biopsy, should be considered when transtracheal aspiration is not diagnostic or following unsuccessful resolution of previously diagnosed pneumonia.[1, 4, 176, 177]

Treatment

Antimicrobial Agents. Antibiotics reported to have in vitro sensitivity against most streptococcal isolates include chloramphenicol, the cephalosporins, some of the penicillins (ampicillin, amoxicillin), the quinolones and the trimethoprim-sulfonamides.[125, 151, 176] The best choices, based on penetration of bronchial fluid and lung tissue, are the quinolones and the trimethoprim sulfonamide combinations.[130] Case reports suggest the cephalosporins may be efficacious;[149] however, the penicillins may not.[148] Dosage recommendations are as follows: cephalexin, 10 to 30 mg/kg orally, three to four times daily and ciprofloxacin (5 to 15 mg/kg), enrofloxacin (2.5 to 7.5 mg/kg), and the trimethoprim-sulfonamide combinations (15 to 30 mg/kg) orally, twice daily for 14 days.[133] These antibiotics can also be administered by injection, with the exception of cephalexin. Cephalothin sodium, 10 to 30 mg/kg intramuscularly or intravenously, is the parenteral equivalent of cephalexin. The cephalosporins or the trimethoprim-sulfonamides would be the best choices for young dogs less than 30 weeks of age because of detrimental effects on cartilage development caused by quinolone antibiotics.[134]

Mobilization of Airway Secretions. Maintenance of hydration, nebulization with saline, mild activity, and coupage of the chest are important therapeutic measures that should be considered in addition to antibiotic therapy.

Dehydration hinders mucociliary clearance of bacteria and respiratory secretions; however, overhydration may exacerbate the degree of respiratory compromise because of increased interstitial and alveolar fluid accumulation.[176]

Nebulization of saline increases the moisture content of airway fluids and has additional mucolytic properties. Although time consuming, administration of nebulized saline is easily performed and quite helpful in resolving bacterial infections of the lung. A face mask or placement of the animal in an enclosed chamber or oxygen cage is the usual method of aerosol administration.[176] Nebulization should be performed for 10 to 30 minutes, several times daily. Observation of the dog is important since bronchoconstriction can occur, making the degree of respiratory distress more severe. Pretreatment with a bronchodilator such as aminophylline (as the salt) (11 mg/kg, intramuscularly or intravenously)[139] 15 to 20 minutes before the procedure is helpful.

Mild activity combined with coupage is particularly helpful in mechanically stimulating the cough reflex. The palm of the hand is used to strike the chest in a clapping motion over the areas of the lung. The procedure should be done for 3 to 5 minutes, several times daily.[176]

Additional Therapy. Routine use of bronchodilator drugs is controversial. If there is evidence of bronchial hyperresponsiveness, such as wheezing, use of terbutaline (1.25 to 5.0 mg total, orally two to three times daily) or aminophylline (as the salt) (11 mg/kg, orally four times daily) may be beneficial.[139] Corticosteroids and cough suppressants should not be administered since they interfere with the normal defense mechanisms of the lung. Animals with severe respiratory compromise as evidenced by dyspnea, tachypnea, or marked hypoxemia ($PaO_2 < 60$ torr) need oxygen therapy.[4, 176]

Once a therapeutic plan is established, the patient should be monitored for 48 to 72 hours to evaluate response to therapy. If no improvement in clinical signs is noted, treatment(s) should be reevaluated. If improvement is observed, treatment(s) should continue for a minimum of 7 days beyond resolution of all clinical signs (including radiographic changes). Treatment duration of 3 to 6 weeks is common.

References

1. Schaer M, Ackerman N, King RR: Clinical approach to the patient with respiratory disease. In Ettinger SJ (ed): Textbook of Veterinary Internal Medicine, 3rd ed. Philadelphia, WB Saunders Company, 1989, vol 1, pp 752–766.
2. King LG, Hendricks JC: Clinical pulmonary function tests. In Ettinger SJ, Feldman EC (eds): Textbook of Veterinary Internal Medicine, 4th ed. Philadelphia, WB Saunders Company, 1995, vol 1, pp 738–754.
3. Hawkins EC: Diagnostic tests for the nasal cavity and paranasal sinuses. In Nelson RW, Couto CG (eds): Essentials of Small Animal Internal Medicine. St Louis, Mosby–Year Book, 1992, pp 157–162.
4. Hawkins EC: Diagnostic tests for the lower respiratory tract. In Nelson RW, Couto CG (eds): Essentials of Small Animal Internal Medicine. St Louis, Mosby–Year Book, 1992, pp 185–206.
5. Burley DR: Nasal bone fractures in greyhounds [letter] JAVMA 194:1005, 1989.
6. Green RA, Thomas JS: Hemostatic disorders: Coagulopathies and thrombosis. In Ettinger SJ, Feldman EC (eds): Textbook of Veterinary Internal Medicine, 4th ed. Philadelphia, WB Saunders Company, 1995, vol 2, pp 1946–1963.
7. Reagan WJ, Rebar AH: Platelet disorders. In Ettinger SJ, Feldman EC (eds): Textbook of Veterinary Internal Medicine, 4th ed. Philadelphia, WB Saunders Company, 1995, vol 2, pp 1964–1976.
8. Bright RM: Pharynx: Shortening of the elongated soft palate. In Bojrab MJ, Brichard SJ, Tomlinson Jr JL (eds): Current Techniques in Small Animal Surgery, 3rd ed. Philadelphia, Lea & Febiger, 1990, pp 186–187.
9. Bright RM, Wheaton LG: A modified surgical technique for elongated soft palate in dogs. J Am Anim Hosp Assoc 19:288–292, 1983.
10. Harvey CE: Soft palate resection in brachycephalic dogs. J Am Anim Hosp Assoc 18:538–544, 1982.
11. Clark GN, Sinibaldi KR: Use of a carbon dioxide laser for treatment of elongated soft palate in dogs. JAVMA 204:1779–1781, 1994.
12. Blythe LL, Gannon JR, Craig AM: Respiratory system: Excessive soft palate. In Blythe LL, Gannon JR, Craig AM (eds): Care of the Racing Greyhound, A Guide for Trainers, Breeders and Veterinarians. Portland, American Greyhound Council Inc, 1994, p 61.
13. Blythe LL, Gannon JR, Craig AM: Respiratory system: Collapsing tracheal rings. In Blythe LL, Gannon JR, Craig AM (eds): Care of the Racing Greyhound, A Guide for Trainers, Breeders and Veterinarians. Portland, American Greyhound Council Inc, 1994, pp 61—62.
14. Chen JC, Holinger LD: Congenital tracheal anomalies: Pathology study using serial macrosections and review of the literature. Pediatr Pathol 14:513–537, 1994.
15. Coghill TH, Moore EA, Accurso FJ, et al.: Primary tracheomalacia. Ann Thorac Surg 35:538–541, 1983.
16. Dungworth DL: The respiratory system: Larynx and trachea. In Jubb KVF, Kennedy PC, Palmer N (eds): Pathology of Domestic Animals, 4th ed. San Diego, Academic Press Inc, 1993, vol 2, p 566.
17. Ettinger SJ, Ticer JW: Diseases of the trachea: Collapsed trachea. In Ettinger SJ (ed): Textbook of Veterinary Internal Medicine, 3rd ed. Philadelphia, WB Saunders Company, 1989, vol 1, pp 799–804.
18. Messineo A, Filler RM: Tracheomalacia. Semin Pediatr Surg 3:253–258, 1994.
19. Dallman MJ, McClure RC, Brown EM: Histochemical study of normal and collapsed tracheas in dogs. Am J Vet Res 49:2117–2125, 1988.
20. Dumon J-F: A dedicated tracheobronchial stent. Chest 97:328–332, 1990.
21. Fingland RB: Trachea: Tracheal collapse. In Bojrab MJ, Birchard SJ, Tomlinson Jr JL (eds): Current Techniques in Small Animal Surgery, 3rd ed. Philadelphia, Lea & Febiger, 1990, pp 342–352.
22. Nelson AW: Lower respiratory system: Diseases of the trachea and bronchi. In Slatter D (ed): Textbook of Small Animal Surgery, 2nd ed. Philadelphia, WB Saunders Company, 1993, vol 1, pp 777–780.
23. Brennan KE, Ihrke PJ: Grass awn migration in dogs and cats: A retrospective study of 182 cases. JAVMA 182:1201–1204, 1983.
24. Dobbie GR, Darke PGG, Head KW: Intrabronchial foreign bodies in dogs. J Small Anim Pract 27:227–230, 1986.
25. Jones BD, Roudebush P: The use of fiberoptic endoscopy in the diagnosis and treatment of tracheobronchial foreign bodies. J Am Anim Hosp Assoc 20:497–504, 1984.
26. Lotti U, Niebauer GW: Tracheobronchial foreign bodies of plant origin in 153 hunting dogs. Compend Contin Educ Pract Vet 14:900–904, 1992.
27. Ettinger SJ, Ticer JW: Diseases of the trachea: Obstructive tracheal disease and foreign bodies. In Ettinger SJ (ed): Textbook of Veterinary Internal Medicine, 3rd ed. Philadelphia, WB Saunders Company, 1989, vol 1, pp 808–810.
28. Nelson AW: Lower respiratory system: Foreign body of trachea and

bronchi. *In* Slatter D (ed): Textbook of Small Animal Surgery, 2nd ed. Philadelphia, WB Saunders Company, 1993, vol 2, pp 782–783.

29. Brusasco V, Crimi E: Allergy and sports: Exercise-induced asthma. Int J Sports Med 15(Suppl 3): S184–S186, 1994.

30. Kyle JM, Walker RB, Hanshaw SL, et al: Exercise-induced bronchospasm in the young athlete: Guidelines for routine screening and initial management. Med Sci Sports Exerc 24:856–859, 1992.

31. Mahler DA: Exercise-induced asthma. Med Sci Sports Exerc 25:554–561,1993.

32. Virant FS: Exercise-induced bronchospasm: Epidemiology, pathophysiology, and therapy. Med Sci Sports Exerc 24:851–855, 1992.

33. Davis B, Roberts AM, Coleridge HM, et al: Reflex tracheal gland secretion evoked by stimulation of bronchial C-fibers in dogs. J Appl Physiol 53:985–991, 1982.

34. Freed AN: Regional and temporal variation in canine peripheral lung responses to dry air. J Appl Physiol 67:1727–1733, 1989.

35. Freed AN, Adkinson Jr NF: Dry air-induced late phase responses in the canine lung periphery. Eur Respir J 3:434–440, 1990.

36. Freed AN, Bromberger-Barnea B, Menkes HA: Dry air-induced constriction in the lung periphery: A canine model of exercise-induced asthma. J Appl Physiol 59:1986–1990, 1985.

37. Freed AN, Fuller SD, Stream CE: Transient airway cooling modulates dry-air-induced and hypertonic aerosol-induced bronchoconstriction. Am Rev Respir Dis 144:358–362, 1991.

38. Freed AN, Kelly LJ, Menkes HA: Airflow-induced bronchospasm: Imbalance between airway cooling and airway drying? Am Rev Respir Dis 136:595–599, 1987.

39. Freed AN, Omori C, Hubbard WC, et al: Dry air- and hypertonic aerosol-induced bronchoconstriction and cellular responses in the canine lung periphery. Eur Respir J 7:1308–1316, 1994.

40. Freed AN, Omori C, Schofield BH, et al: Dry air-induced mucosal cell injury and bronchovascular leakage in canine peripheral airways. Am J Respir Cell Mol Biol 11:724–732, 1994.

41. Freed AN, Peters SP, Menkes HA: Airflow-induced bronchoconstriction: Role of epithelium and eicosanoid mediators. J Appl Physiol 62:574–581, 1987.

42. Freed AN, Stream CE: Airway cooling: Stimulus specific modulation of airway responsiveness in the canine lung periphery. Eur Respir J 4:568–574, 1991.

43. Freed AN, Yiin KT, Stream CE: Hyperosmotic-induced bronchoconstriction in the canine lung periphery. J Appl Physiol 67:2571–2578, 1989.

44. Freed AN, Wang D, Menkes HA: Dry air-induced constriction: Effects of pharmacological intervention and temperature. J Appl Physiol 62:1794–1800, 1987.

45. Tang GJ, Freed AN: The automatic nervous system modulates dry air-induced constriction in the canine lung periphery. Am Rev Respir Dis 145:1301–1305, 1992.

46. Blythe LL, Gannon JR, Craig AM: Respiratory system: Exercise-induced bronchoconstriction. *In* Blythe LL, Gannon JR, Craig AM (eds): Care of the Racing Greyhound, A Guide for Trainers, Breeders and Veterinarians, Portland, American Greyhound Council Inc, 1994, p 62.

47. Nishikata H, Kobayashi H, Sato H, et al: Induction of bronchial hyperresposiveness by *Bordetella bronchiseptica* infection in dogs. Ann Allergy 62:51–58, 1991.

48. Teeter JG, Freed AN: Effect of salbutamol on dry air and acetylcholine-induced bronchoconstriction in the canine lung periphery. Eur Respir J 4:972–978, 1991.

49. Wang D, Adkinson NF Jr, Menkes HA, et al: Aminophylline reduces air-flow-induced constriction in the canine lung periphery. Am Rev Respir Dis 137:31–37, 1988.

50. Wang D, Chen HI, Chou CL, et al.: Terbutaline acts at multiple sites to inhibit bronchoconstriction induced by dry air in canine peripheral airways. Am Rev Respir Dis 145:1295–1300, 1992.

51. Pascoa JR, Ferraro GL, Cannon JH, et al: Exercise-induced hemorrhage in racing thoroughbreds: A preliminary study. Am J Vet Res 42:703–707, 1981.

52. Raphel CF, Soma LR: Exercise-induced pulmonary hemorrhage in thoroughbreds after racing and breezing. Am J Vet Res 43:1123–1127, 1982.

53. Sweeney, CR: Exercise-induced pulmonary hemorrhage. Vet Clin North Am Equine Pract 7:93–104, 1991.

54. Sweeney CR, Humber KA, Roby KA: Cytologic findings of tracheobronchial aspirates from 66 thoroughbred racehorses. Am J Vet Res 53:1172–1175, 1992.

55. Whitwell KE, Greet TRC: Collection and evaluation of tracheobronchial washes in the horse. Equine Vet J 16:499–508, 1984.

56. King RR, Raskin RE, Rosbolt J: Exercise-induced pulmonary hemorrhage. Does it occur in racing greyhounds? *In* Proceedings of the Fifth International Racing Greyhound Symposium. Palm Beach, 1989, pp 51–52.

57. King RR, Raskin RE: Intrabronchial hemorrhage in greyhound dogs after racing. *In* Proceedings of the Seventh International Racing Greyhound Symposium, Orlando, 1991, pp 18–21.

58. West JB, Mathieu-Costello O, Jones JH, et al: Stress failure of pulmonary capillaries in racehorses with exercise-induced pulmonary hemorrhage. J Appl Physiol 75:1097–1109, 1993.

59. Elkins RC, Milnor WR: Pulmonary vascular response to exercise in the dog. Circ Res 29:591–599, 1971.

60. Olsen SC, Coyne CP, Lowe BS, et al: Influence of furosemide on hemodynamic responses during exercise in horses. Am J Vet Res 53:742–747, 1992.

61. Manohar M: Furosemide attenuates the exercise-induced increase in pulmonary artery wedge pressure in horses. Am J Vet Res 54:952–958, 1993.

62. Manohar M, Hutchens E, Coney E: Furosemide attenuates the exercise-induced rise in pulmonary capillary blood pressure in horses. Equine Vet J 26:51–54, 1994.

63. Blythe LL, Gannon JR, Craig AM: Respiratory system: Pneumothorax. *In* Blythe LL, Gannon JR, Craig AM (eds): Care of the Racing Greyhound, A Guide for Trainers, Breeders and Veterinarians. Portland, American Greyhound Council Inc, 1994, pp 62–63.

64. Bauer T, Woodfield JA: Mediastinal, pleural, and extrapleural diseases: Pneumothorax. *In* Ettinger SJ, Feldman EC (eds): Textbook of Veterinary Internal Medicine, 4th ed., vol 1, Philadelphia, WB Saunders Company, 1995, pp 829–831.

65. Kramek BA, Caywood DD: Pneumothorax. Vet Clin North Am Small Anim Pract 17:285–300, 1987.

66. Jones BR, Bath ML, Wood AKW: Spontaneous pneumomediastinum in the racing greyhound. J Small Anim Pract 16:27–32, 1975.

67. Orton EC: Pleura and pleural space: Pneumothorax. *In* Slatter D (ed): Textbook of Small Animal Surgery, 2nd ed. Philadelphia, WB Saunders Company, 1993, vol 1, pp 397–398.

68. Van Pelt DR, McKiernan BC: Pathogenesis and treatment of canine rhinitis. Vet Clin North Am Small Anim Pract 24:789–806, 1994.

69. King RR, Greiner EC, Ackerman N, et al.: Nasal capillariasis in a dog. J Am Anim Hosp Assoc 26:381–385, 1990.

70. Schoning P, Dryden MW, Gabbert NH: Identification of a nasal nematode (*Eucoleus boehmi*) in greyhounds. Vet Res Comm 17:277–281, 1993.

71. Campbell BG, Little MD: Identification of the eggs of a nematode (*Eucoleus boehmi*) from the nasal mucosa of North American dogs. JAVMA 198:1520–1523, 1991.

72. The tonsils in the pathogenesis of disease. Vet Rec 95:234, 1974.

73. Blythe LL, Gannon JR, Craig AM: Juvenile greyhounds: Tonsillitis. *In* Blythe LL, Gannon JR, Craig AM (eds): Care of the Racing Greynhound, A Guide for Trainers, Breeders and Veterinarians. Portland, American Greyhound Council Inc, 1994, p 308.

74. Dulisch ML: The tonsils. *In* Slatter D (ed): Textbook of Small Animal Surgery, 2nd ed. Philadelphia, WB Saunders Company 1993, vol 1, pp 973–977.

75. Gunn C: Lips, oral cavity, and salivary glands: The tonsils. *In* Gourley IM, Vasseur PB (eds): General Small Animal Surgery. Philadelphia, JB Lippincott Co, 1985, pp 218–220.

76. Harvey CE: Oral, dental, pharyngeal, and salivary gland disorders: Tonsillitis. *In* Ettinger SJ (ed): Textbook of Veterinary Internal Medicine, 3rd ed. Philadelphia, WB Saunders Company, 1989, vol 2, pp 1237–1238.

77. Mattson A: Pharyngeal disorders: Tonsillitis. Vet Clin North Am Small Anim Pract 24:828–830, 1994.

78. Harvey CE: Therapeutic strategies involving antimicrobial treatment of the upper respiratory tract in small animals. JAVMA 185:1159–1161, 1984.

79. Blythe LL, Gannon JR, Craig AM: Respiratory system: Tonsillar hypertrophy. *In* Blythe LL, Gannon JR, Craig AM (eds): Care of the

Racing Greyhound, A Guide for Trainers, Breeders and Veterinarians. Portland, American Greyhound Council Inc, 1994, pp 60–61.

80. Hovell GJR, Weston R: Cramp in greyhounds (letter). Vet Rec 87 (Members Inf Suppl 47):103; 1970.

81. Jacobs DE, Prole JHB: Helminth infections of British dogs: Prevalence in racing greyhounds. Vet Parasit 1:377–387, 1976.

82. Keep JM: *Filaroides (Oslerus) osleri* infestation in conjunction with a generalized infection in a greyhound. Aust Vet J 27:43–45, 1951.

83. Tyson JD: *Filaroides osleri* in a greyhound (letter). Vet Rec 121:334, 1987.

84. Urquhart GM, Jarrett WFH, O'Sullivan JG: Canine tracheobronchitis due to infection with *Filaroides osleri*. Vet Rec 66:143–145, 1954.

85. Schoning P, Cowan LA: Gross and microscopic lesions of 230 Kansas greyhounds. J Vet Diagn Invest 5:392–397, 1993.

86. Kohnke J: Respiratory diseases. *In* Kohnke J (ed): Veterinary Advice for Greyhound Owners. Letchworth, Herts, Ringpress Books Ltd, 1993, pp 120–126.

87. Bowman DD, Lynn RC: Helminths: Family Filaroididea. *In* Bowman DD, Lynn RC (eds): Georgis' Parasitology for Veterinarians, 6th ed. Philadelphia, WB Saunders Company, 1995, pp 197–201.

88. Urquhart GM, Armour J, Duncan JL, et al: Veterinary helminthology: Metastrongyles of dogs and cats. *In* Urquhart GM, Armour J, Duncan JL, et al (eds): Veterinary Parasitology. Essex, England, Longman Scientific & Technical, 1987, pp 58–60.

89. Dungworth DL: The respiratory system: Larynx and trachea. *In* Jubb KVF, Kennedy PC, Palmer N (eds): Pathology of Domestic Animals, 4th ed. San Diego, Academic Press Inc, 1993, vol 2, pp 569–570.

90. Appel MJ: Canine infectious tracheobronchitis (kennel cough). A status report. Compend Contin Educ Pract Vet 3:70–81, 1981.

91. Bemis DA: Bordetella and mycoplasma respiratory infections in dogs and cats. Vet Clin North Am Small Anim Pract 22:1173–1186, 1992.

92. Blythe LL, Gannon JR, Craig AM: The immune system, infectious diseases, and vaccination programs: Infectious diseases. *In* Blythe LL, Gannon JR, Craig AM (eds): Care of the Racing Greyhound, A Guide for Trainers, Breeders and Veterinarians. Portland, American Greyhound Council Inc, 1994, pp 89–90.

93. Ford RB: Infectious tracheobronchitis. *In* Bonagura JD (ed): Kirk's Current Veterinary Therapy XII. Philadelphia, WB Saunders Company, 1995, pp 905–908.

94. McCandlish IAP, Thompson H, Cornwell HJC, et al: A study of dogs with kennel cough. Vet Rec 102:293–301, 1978.

95. Randolph JF, Moise NS, Scarlett JM, et al: Prevalence of mycoplasmal and ureaplasmal recovery from tracheobronchial lavages and prevalence of mycoplasmal recovery from pharyngeal swab specimens in dogs with and without pulmonary disease. Am J Vet Res 54:387–391, 1993.

96. Thrusfield MV, Aitken CGG, Muirhead RH: A field investigation of kennel cough: Incubation period and clinical signs. J Small Anim Pract 32:215–220, 1991.

97. Ueland K: Serological, bacteriological and clinical observations on an outbreak of canine infectious tracheobronchitis in Norway. Vet Rec 126:481–483, 1990.

98. Wagener JS, Minnich L, Sobonya R, et al: Parainfluenza type II infection in dogs. A model for lower respiratory tract infection in humans. Am Rev Respir Dis 127:771–775, 1983.

99. Wagener JS, Sobonya R, Minnich L, et al: Role of canine parainfluenza virus and *Bordetella bronchiseptica* in kennel cough. Am J Vet Res 45:1862–1866, 1984.

100. Quan SF, Witten ML, Grad R, et al: Changes in lung mechanics and histamine responsiveness after sequential canine adenovirus 2 and canine parainfluenza 2 virus infection in beagle puppies. Pediatr Pulmonol 10:236–243, 1991.

101. Lemen RJ, Quan SF, Witten ML, et al: Canine parainfluenza type 2 bronchiolitis increases histamine responsiveness in beagle puppies. Am Rev Respir Dis 141:199–207, 1990.

102. Davis BD, Dulbecco R, Eisen HN, et al: Paramyxoviruses. *In* Davis BD, Dulbecco R, Eisen HN, et al (eds): Microbiology, 4th ed. Philadelphia, JB Lippincott Co, 1990, pp 1007–1014.

103. Fenner FJ, Gibbs EPJ, Murphy FA, et al: Paramyxoviridae. *In* Fenner FJ, Gibbs EPJ, Murphy FA, et al (eds): Veterinary Virology, 2nd ed. San Diego, Academic Press Inc, 1993, pp 471–477.

104. Binn LN, Lazar EC, Helms J, et al.: Viral antibody patterns in laboratory dogs with respiratory disease. Am J Vet Res 31:697–702, 1970.

105. Davis DB, Dulbecco R, Eisen HN, et al: Adenoviruses. *In* Davis DB, Dulbecco R, Eisen HN, et al (eds): Microbiology, 4th ed. Philadelphia, JB Lippincott Co, 1990, pp 915–927.

106. Fenner FJ, Gibbs EPJ, Murphy FA, et al: Adenoviridae. *In* Fenner FJ, Gibbs EPJ, Murphy FA, et al (eds): Veterinary Virology, 2nd ed. San Diego, Academic Press Inc, 1993, pp 329–336.

107. Quan SF, Witten ML, Grad R, et al: Acute canine adenovirus 2 infection increases histamine airway reactivity in beagle puppies. Am Rev Respir Dis 141:414–420, 1990.

108. Grad R, Sobonya RE, Witten ML, et al: Localization of inflammation and virions in canine adenovirus type 2 bronchiolitis. Am Rev Respir Dis 142:691–699, 1990.

109. Castleman WL: Bronchiolitis obliterans and pneumonia induced in young dogs by experimental adenovirus infection. Am J Pathol 119:495–504, 1985.

110. Goodnow RA: Biology of *Bordetella bronchiseptica*. Microbiol Rev 44:722–738, 1980.

111. Robbins JB, Pittman M: Bordetella. *In* Davis BD, Dulbecco R, Eisen HN, et al (eds): Microbiology, 4th ed. Philadelphia, JB Lippincott Co, 1990, pp 621–624.

112. Rosenthal RS, Nogami W, Cookson BT, et al: Major fragment of soluble peptidoglycan released from growing *Bordetella pertussis* is tracheal cytotoxin. Infect Immun 55:2117–2120, 1987.

113. Al-Bazzaz FJ: Role of cyclic AMP in regulation of chloride secretion by canine tracheal mucosa. Am Rev Respir Dis 123:295–298, 1981.

114. Novotny P, Chubb AP, Cownley K, et al: Adenylate cyclase activity of a 68,000-molecular-weight protein isolated from the outer membrane of *Bordetella bronchiseptica*. Infect Immun 50:199–206, 1985.

115. Kume K, Nakai T, Samejima Y, et al: Properties of dermonecrotic toxin prepared from sonic extracts of *Bordetella bronchiseptica*. Infect Immun 52:370–377, 1986.

116. Nakai T, Sawata A, Kume K: Intracellular locations of dermonecrotic toxins in *Pasteurella multocida* and in *Bordetella bronchiseptica*. Am J Vet Res 46:870–874, 1985.

117. Bemis DA, Plotkin BJ: Hemagglutination by *Bordetella bronchiseptica*. J Clin Microbiol 15:1120–1127, 1982.

118. McKiernan BC, Smith AR, Kissil M: Bacterial isolates from the lower trachea of clinically healthy dogs. J Am Anim Hosp Assoc 20:139–142, 1984.

119. Bemis DA, Carmichael LE, Appel MJG: Naturally occurring respiratory disease in a kennel caused by *Bordetella bronchiseptica*. Cornell Vet 67:282–293, 1977.

120. Bemis DA, Greisen HA, Appel MJG: Pathogenesis of canine bordetellosis. J Infect Dis 135:753–762, 1977.

121. Thompson H, McCandlish IAP, Wright NG: Experimental respiratory disease in dogs due to *Bordetella bronchiseptica*. Res Vet Sci 20:16–23, 1976.

122. Bemis DA, Appel MJG: Aerosol, parenteral, and oral antibiotic treatment of *Bordetella bronchiseptica* infections in dogs. JAVMA 170:1082–1086, 1977.

123. McCandlish IAP, Thompson H: Canine bordetellosis: Chemotherapy using a sulfadiazine-trimethoprim combination. Vet Rec 105:51–54, 1979.

124. Thrusfield MV, Aitken CGG, Muirhead RH: A field investigation of kennel cough: Efficacy of different treatments. J Small Anim Pract 32:455–459, 1991.

125. Hirsh DC: Bacteriology of the lower respiratory tract. *In* Kirk RW (ed): Current Veterinary Therapy IX. Philadelphia, WB Saunders Company, 1986, pp 247–250.

126. Roudebush P, Fales WH: Antibacterial susceptibility of *Bordetella bronchiseptica* isolates from companion animals with respiratory disease. J Am Anim Hosp Assoc 17:793–797, 1981.

127. Sparks SE, Jones RL, Kilgore WR: In vitro susceptibility of bacteria to a ticarcillin-clavulanic acid combination. Am J Vet Res 49:2038–2040, 1988.

128. Batey RG, Smits AF: The isolation of *Bordetella bronchiseptica* from an outbreak of canine pneumonia. Aust Vet J 52:184–186, 1976.

129. Bergogne-Berezin E, Vallee E: Pharmacokinetics of antibiotics in respiratory tissues and fluids. *In* Pennington JE (ed): Respiratory Infections: Diagnosis and Management, 3rd ed. New York, Raven Press Ltd, 1994, pp 731–732.

130. Sonnesyn SW, Gerding DN: Antimicrobials for the treatment of respiratory infections. *In* Niederman MS, Sarosi GA, Glassroth J (eds):

Respiratory Infections. Philadelphia, WB Saunders Company, 1994, pp 511–537.

131. Woolfrey BF, Moody JA: Human infections associated with *Bordetella bronchiseptica.* Clin Microbiol Rev 4:243–255, 1991.

132. Graham AC, Abruzzo GK: Occurrence and characterization of plasmids in field isolates of *Bordetella bronchiseptica.* Am J Vet Res 43:1852–1855, 1982.

133. Papich MG: Antimicrobial drugs. *In* Ettinger SJ, Feldman EC (eds): Textbook of Veterinary Internal Medicine, 4th ed. Philadelphia, WB Saunders Company, 1995, vol. 1, p 274.

134. Papich MG: Antimicrobial drugs. *In* Ettinger SJ, Feldman EC (eds): Textbook of Veterinary Internal Medicine, 4th ed. Philadelphia, WB Saunders Company, 1995, vol 1, p 283.

135. Ilowite JS: Inhaled antibiotics. *In* Neiderman MS, Sarosi GA, Glassroth J (eds): Respiratory Infections. Philadelphia, WB Saunders Company, 1994, pp 541–542.

136. Thys J-P, Aoun M, Klastersky J: Local antibiotic therapy for bronchopulmonary infections. *In* Pennington JE (ed): Respiratory Infections: Diagnosis and Management, 3rd ed. New York, Raven Press Ltd, 1994, pp 741–766.

137. Hutchison RV: Intratracheal gentamicin and dexamethasone for treatment of infectious tracheobronchitis in the dog. Vet Med Small Anim Clin 70:943–945, 1975.

138. Turner T: Intratracheal treatment for kennel cough (letter). Vet Rec 121:182–183, 1987.

139. Boothe DM, McKiernan BC: Respiratory therapeutics. Vet Clin North Am Small Anim Pract 22:1231–1258, 1992.

140. Tukiainen H, Karttunen P, Silvasti M, et al: The treatment of acute transient cough: A placebo-controlled comparison of dextromethorphan and dextromethorphan-beta$_2$-sympathomimetic combination. Eur J Respir Dis 69:95–99, 1986.

141. Bey RF, Shade FJ, Goodnow RA, et al: Intranasal vaccination of dogs with live avirulent *Bordetella bronchiseptica:* Correlation of serum agglutination titer and the formation of secretory IgA with protection against experimentally induced infectious tracheobronchitis. Am J Vet Res 42:1130–1132, 1981.

142. Chladek DW, Williams JM, Gerber DL, et al: Canine parainfluenza-*Bordetella bronchiseptica* vaccine: Immunogenicity. Am J Vet Res 42:266–270, 1981.

143. Shade FJ, Goodnow RA: Intranasal immunization of dogs against *Bordetella bronchiseptica*-induced tracheobronchitis (kennel cough) with modified live *Bordetella bronchiseptica* vaccine. Am J Vet Res 40:1241–1243, 1979.

144. Thrusfield MV, Aitken CGG, Muirhead RH: A field investigation of kennel cough: Efficacy of vaccination. J Small Anim Pract 30:550–560, 1989.

145. Ostle GN: Cough associated with canine vaccination (letter)? Vet Rec 125:446, 1989.

146. Blythe LL, Gannon JR, Craig AM: Respiratory system: Pneumonia. *In* Blythe LL, Gannon JR, Craig AM (eds): Care of the Racing Greyhound, A Guide for Trainers, Breeders and Veterinarians. Portland, American Greyhound Council Inc, 1994, p 60.

147. Drum S: Kennel cough in Wisconsin. Greyhound Rev 21:51–54, 1993.

148. Wyand DS, Sherman BA: Streptococcal septicemia in racing greyhounds. J Am Anim Hosp Assoc 14:399–401, 1978.

149. Harpster NK: The effectiveness of the cephalosporins in the treatment of bacterial pneumonias in the dog. J Am Anim Hosp Assoc 17:766–772, 1981.

150. Jameson PH, King LA, Lappin MR, et al: Comparison of clinical signs, diagnostic findings, organisms isolated, and clinical outcome in dogs with bacterial pneumonia: 93 cases (1986–1991). JAVMA 206:206–209, 1995.

151. Thayer GW, Robinson SK: Bacterial bronchopneumonia in the dog: A review of 42 cases. J Am Anim Hosp Assoc 20:731–735, 1984.

152. McCarty M: Streptococci. *In* Davis BD, Dulbecco R, Eisen HN, et al (eds): Microbiology, 4th ed. Philadelphia, JB Lippincott Co, 1990, pp 525–538.

153. Quinn PJ, Carter ME, Markey BK, et al. The streptococci and related cocci. *In* Quinn PJ, Carter ME, Markey BK, et al (eds): Clinical Veterinary Microbiology. Spain, Wolfe Publishing, 1994, pp 127–136.

154. Boulnois GJ: Pneumococcal proteins and the pathogenesis of disease caused by *Streptococcus pneumoniae.* J Gen Microbiol 138:249–259, 1992.

155. Austrian R: Pneumococcus: The first one hundred years. *In* Quie PG, Kass EH (eds): The Pneumococcus and the Pneumococcus Vaccine. Chicago, University of Chicago Press, 1982, pp 1–7.

156. Crain MJ, Waltman WD, Turner JS, et al: Pneumococcal surface protein-A (PspA) is serologically highly variable and is expressed by all clinically important serotypes of *Streptococcus pneumoniae.* Infect Immun 58:3293–3299, 1990.

157. Feldman C, Mitchell TJ, Andrew PW, et al: The effect of *Streptococcus pneumoniae* pneumolysin on human respiratory epithelium *in vitro.* Microb Pathog 9:275–284, 1990.

158. Rubins JB, Charboneau D, Paton JC, et al: Dual function of pneumolysin in the early pathogenesis of murine pneumococcal pneumonia. J Clin Invest 95:142–150, 1995.

159. Paton JC, Ferrante A: Inhibition of human polymorphonuclear leukocyte respiratory burst, bactericidal activity, and migration by pneumolysin. Infect Immun 41:1212–1216, 1983.

160. Ferrante A, Rowan-Kelly B, Paton JC: Inhibition of *in vitro* human lymphocyte response by the pneumococcal toxin pneumolysin. Infect Immun 46:585–589, 1984.

161. Berry AM, Lock RA, Hansman D, et al: Contribution of autolysin to virulence of *Streptococcus pneumoniae.* Infect Immun 57:2324–2330, 1989.

162. Krivan HC, Roberts DD, Ginsburg V: Many pulmonary pathogenic bacteria bind specifically to the carbohydrate sequence GalNAc beta 1-4-Gal found in some glycolipids. Proc Natl Acad Sci USA 85:6157–6161, 1988.

163. Mulks MH, Kornfeld SJ, Plaut AG: Specific proteolysis of human IgA by *Streptococcus pneumoniae* and *Haemophilus influenzae.* J Infect Dis 141:450–456, 1980.

164. Andersson B, Beachey EH, Tomasz A, et al: A sandwich adhesin on *Streptococcus pneumoniae* attaching to human oropharyngeal epithelial cells *in vitro.* Microb Pathog 4:267–278, 1988.

165. Kehoe MA, Miller L, Walker JA, et al: Nucleotide sequence of the streptolysin O (SLO) gene: Structural homologies between SLO and other membrane-damaging, thiol-activated toxins. Infect Immun 55:3228–3232, 1987.

166. Arditi M, Shulman ST, Davis AT, et al: Group C β-hemolytic streptococcal infections in children: Nine pediatric cases and review. Rev Infect Dis 11:34–44,1989.

167. Barnham M, Cole G, Efstratiou A, et al: Characterization of *Streptococcus zooepidemicus* (Lancefield group C) from human and selected animal infections. Epidem Inf 98:171–182, 1987.

168. Hallas G, Widdowson JP: Antibody to hyaluronidase of streptococci of Lancefield group C and G. *In* Holm SE, Christensen P (eds): Basic Concepts of Streptococci and Streptococcal Diseases. Surrey, England, Reedbooks Ltd, 1982, pp 181–183.

169. Schofield CR, Tagg JR: Bacteriocin-like activity of group B and group C streptococci of human and of animal origin. J Hyg 90:7–18, 1983.

170. Stamm AM, Cobbs CG: Group C streptococcal pneumonia: Report of a fatal case and review of the literature. Rev Infect Dis 2:889–898, 1980.

171. Pratter MR, Irwin RS: Viridans streptococcal pulmonary parenchymal infections. JAMA 243:2515–2517, 1980.

172. Sarkar TK, Murarka RS, Gilardi GL: Primary *Streptococcus viridans* pneumonia. Chest 96:831–834, 1989.

173. Johnston RB: Pathogenesis of pneumococcal pneumonia. Rev Infect Dis 13(Suppl 6):S509–S517, 1991.

174. Rhodes GC, Tapsall JW, Lykke AWJ: Alveolar epithelial responses in experimental streptococcal pneumonia. J Pathol 157:347–357, 1989.

175. Rhodes GC, Lykke AWJ, Tapsall JW, et al: Abnormal alveolar epithelial repair associated with failure of resolution in experimental streptococcal pneumonia. J Pathol 159:245–253, 1989.

176. Rodebush P: Bacterial infections of the respiratory system. *In* Greene CE (ed): Infectious Diseases of the Dog and Cat. Philadelphia, WB Saunders Company, 1990, pp 114–124.

177. Moser KM, Maurer J, Jassy L, et al: Sensitivity, specificity and risk of diagnostic procedures in a canine model of *Streptococcus pneumoniae* pneumonia. Am Rev Respir Dis 125:436–442, 1982.

CHAPTER 12

DISEASES OF THE MUSCLES

JAMES R. GANNON

Sporting activities in all athletes require periods of maximal physical exertion or endurance. At such times, severe stress is placed on the locomotor system. The most common cause of reduction in performance in the sporting canid is found in this system. Not all muscular problems are traumatic in origin. Some may have a metabolic basis; others, genetic or immunological. An appreciation of the range of disorders and the recuperative powers of voluntary muscles requires some understanding of their physiology and architecture.

REVIEW OF ANATOMY OF SKELETAL MUSCLE

For convenience, the reductionist approach may be used to divide the functioning skeletal muscle into four zones: fiber network, support network, muscle fiber (myofiber) membrane, and neuromuscular connections.

Fiber Network

The muscle mass is composed of many muscle fibers, which are extremely long cylindrical skeletal muscle cells, varying from 10 to 120 μm in diameter. The fibers may course the entire length of one muscle, or they may be shorter and connected to similar short fibers to form a continuum from the muscle origin to insertion. Thus each fiber has many nuclei, the majority of which are located peripherally. The muscle fibers are grouped into fasciculi, each myofiber being composed of many myofibrils. Each myofibril is composed of many myofilaments. Each myofilament is composed of parallel strands of actin and myosin.

Support Network

The support network combines the muscle sheath, connective tissues, and capillary bed. The whole muscle is ensheathed in a relatively thick connective tissue, the epimysium, an extension of the perimysium, which binds the myofibers into its groups to form the fasciculi. The perimysium carries the blood vessels and nerves. Within the fasciculus, the space between the muscle fibers is filled with a sparse reticular connective tissue called the *endomysium*, which carries a network of blood capillaries and terminal innervating nerve fibers.

Muscle Fiber (Myofiber) Membrane

The outer membrane of the myofiber—the cell wall—is the sarcolemma, which encloses the cytoplasm of the cell, the sarcoplasm, comprising the myofibrils, nuclei, ribosomes, and mitochondria. Two important but separate invaginating networks of tubules extend from the sarcolemma into the sarcoplasm—the centrotubules and the sarcoplasmic reticulum.

The centrotubules penetrate into the cell interior among the myofibrils. The lumina of these centrotubules communicate directly into the extracellular space. When a wave of depolarization extends from the motor end plate to initiate a contraction, the electrical changes are carried along the membranes of the centrotubular system and so reach all myofibrils in the depth of the myofiber. The sarcoplasmic reticulum is a separate, closed, membranous channel system consisting of a complex series of branching and anastomosing channels that fill most of the space between the myofibrils. The sarcoplasmic reticulum is capable of binding calcium and magnesium ions strongly to its membrane surfaces.

When depolarization occurs at the motor end plate, the electrical disturbances are carried throughout the centrotubules, which causes the release of calcium and magnesium ions from the sarcoplasmic reticulum into the adjacent myofibrils. This results in activation of the myosin-bound ATPase and consequent contraction of the muscle. As electrical stability returns to the centrotubules and the sarcolemma at the end of the contraction, calcium and magnesium ions are re-bound to the sarcoplasmic reticulum. Thus the ATPase action ceases and muscle relaxation occurs.

Neuromuscular Connections

Each myofiber receives a single terminal branch of a motor axon that finishes close to the sarcolemma at a motor end plate. When a nerve impulse passes down the axon, acetylcholine is released at the motor end plate, which causes massive rapid depolarization throughout the sarcolemma and its centrotubules with consequent release of calcium and magnesium ions from the sarcoplasmic reticulum; contraction of the myofiber now ensues. At the same time, acetylcholine released at the motor end plate is rapidly broken down by the enzyme cholinesterase. The degree of innervation of the myofibers is inversely proportional to the degree of precision of control exercised by the muscle—for example, extrinsic ocular muscles have 1 neuron to 5 myofibers, while a limb muscle may have 1 neuron to 2000 fibers.

MUSCLE TRAUMA DISORDERS

Treatment methods vary in response to the nature and degree of muscle injury. These have been classified and considered in detail for the greyhound,[1] and further explored in Chapter 21. Tenosynovitis and transverse humeral ligament rupture of the biceps brachium are discussed in Chapter 22.

POST-TRAUMA DISORDERS

These disorders take the form of contractures of collagen-laden scar tissue and ossification of encysted hematomas and associated necrotic tissue. Contractures have been reported in the infraspinatus,[2, 3] semitendinosus,[4, 5] gastrocnemius, and quadriceps[6] musculature following disruption of the muscle sheath and fibers or the musculotendinous junction. Clinical history uniformly includes prolonged gait abnormality, lameness, and atrophy of surrounding muscles. In general, fibrotic contractures of the infraspinatus muscle of the forelimb respond well to tenotomy.

Contractures of the hindlimb musculature have a poor prognosis for any sporting activity, although the literature does cite some degree of success with surgical correction of the quadriceps contraction and femoral adhesions by interposing absorbable gelatin foam between the muscle and bone.[7] However, the quadriceps abnormality appears to be regularly related to femoral fracture or prolonged hindlimb extension in casts or splints. Nevertheless, the semitendinosus and gastrocnemius contractures follow muscle disruption with subsequent healing by fibrosis. Femoral fractures sustained during sporting activities may be associated with compartmental syndrome,[8, 9] in which there is marked increase in pressure in interfascial planes predisposing to fibrosis and contracture.* Surgical correction of this post-trauma disorder, using fasciotomy and open drainage, should be prompt, both for pain relief and minimizing of subsequent fibrosis from tissue anoxia.

Clinical signs of compartmental syndrome include a swollen, painful leg with tense, painful muscle. Diminished distal nerve function and pulse compromise may also be present. A tentative diagnosis based on clinical signs may warrant compartmental fasciotomy.

Localized myositis ossificans appears most commonly in the hindlimb musculature 2 to 4 weeks following trauma.[10, 11] It is associated with local inflammatory changes, lameness, palpable firm enlargement within the muscle, and progressive stiffness and weakness. Radiographically the lesions have defined borders with a central transparency that distinguishes them from sarcoma. Surgical removal or resection has been reported as ameliorating lameness and discomfort.

METABOLIC DISORDERS

Cramp. This is a prolonged, involuntary contraction of skeletal muscle producing pain, discomfort, temporary loss of weight-bearing ability, and a pronounced change in shape, size, and texture of the affected muscle. Considering the frequency of its occurrence in the sporting canid, little definitive material has been published regarding this exercise-induced problem. It is thought to be multifactorial and may be associated with one of the following: dehydration; relative calcium deficit; faulty metabolism from lactate accumulation or impaired enzyme function due to selenium, vitamin E, or related deficiency; circulatory disturbances resulting in damage to, or spasm of, local blood supply with consequent tissue anoxia; or possibly a neurological disturbance to a local axon or the CNS from pressure related to hematomas, exudates, or trauma.[12]

Treatment of cramp is unspectacular, but needs to be prompt and vigorous, with the application of local heat, deep kneading massage, and stretching of the cramped muscle. Prevention is a greater

*Editor's Note On Compartmental Syndrome: Muscle injury in a confined space may produce an increase in pressure due to edema or hemorrhage. Four compartments have been described in the dog extremity.[8, 9] The craniolateral compartment of the crus, caudal compartment of the antebrachia, caudal compartment of the crus, and the femoral compartment are created by the normal anatomical bone and fascial barriers of the extremity. Normal compartmental pressures are reported to range from −2 to +8 mm Hg,[8] and significant necrosis of skeletal muscle occurs at pressures above 30 mm Hg if present for more than 8 hours. Compartmental pressures of 120 mm Hg can cause irreversible nerve block. Compartmental pressure can be measured with a Stryker Intracompartmental Pressure Monitor (Stryker Surgical, Kalamazoo, MI).

challenge, but benefit has been derived from use of the following regimen for dogs in training.

Inclusion of *dietary supplements* such as electrolytes in the drinking water with an additional 2 gm of potassium chloride in the main meal. Dicalcium phosphate 8 gm daily together with 4000 units of retinol vitamin A, 450 units of vitamin D, and 200 units of alpha-tocopherol (vitamin E) daily are routinely used in Australia. Trace element supplementation to ensure adequate intake of selenium and 200 mg of vitamin C as the nonacidic calcium ascorbate are included.

Medication administered to avoid or reduce the incidence of cramp includes quinine bisulfate, 300 mg, 1 to 4 hours before exercise to decrease the excitability of the motor end plate of the myofiber; peripheral vasodilators, eg, dihydroergotoxine mesylate (Hydergine) 0.5 ngn orally, 1 to 4 hours prior to exercise, or adenosine 5-monophosphate (AMP5) 200 to 400 mg intramuscularly 1 to 4 hours before exercise. In addition, for those problems revealed by blood and urine scans, specific therapy would be employed, eg, hematinics for anemia, antibiotics for infections.

Exertional Rhabdomyolysis. This metabolic disorder is common in the racing greyhound, although cases have been reported in other breeds and species following vigorous exercise.[13–16] Predisposing factors include inadequate physical fitness for the workload undertaken, being hot and excited prior to activity, a relative potassium deficiency, and fast workouts done too closely together (lactic acid accumulation). Rhabdomyolysis presents as varying degrees of inflammation of the muscles of the back (thoracic rhomboid and longissimus area), which become swollen, tense, hot, and painful to the touch.

Muscle cell breakdown leads to myoglobinuria, difficult painful movement, and highly acid urine. Mortality is quite high in untreated cases because of rapid onset of renal failure from myoglobin deposits in the nephron. Dogs with acute cases with extensive involvement of the longissimus muscles seldom return to full work capacity because of permanent loss of muscle tissue and its replacement by fibrosis. However, the prognosis for restoration of normal exercise tolerance is vastly improved with prompt diagnosis and therapy: intravenous fluids using Standard Maintenance Fluid, Ringer's solution, or 5 per cent glucose in normal saline, but avoiding Hartmann's solution because of its lactate content. To each liter of Ringer's solution add 500 ml of 4.2 per cent bicarbonate solution for the first 48 hours, then reduce this to 250 ml for the next 48 hours. Intravenous fluids are administered every 12 hours: 1.5 to 1.25 liters for 2 to 4 days, depending upon the patient's response. Anabolic steroids (nandrolone, boldenone, methandriol) will reduce the negative nitrogen balances. They are given intramuscularly: an initial dose of 25 mg, followed by 12.5 mg on alternate days for another two or three doses. Nonsteroidal anti-inflammatory therapy is essential: intravenous sodium hyaluronate 10 mg or flunixin meglumine 50 mg daily for 2 to 4 days. Less severe cases may require only oral therapy with phenylbutazone, indomethacin, ibuprofen, copper salicylate, or aspirin. Prophylactic antibiotics may be given for 5 days, together with kennel rest, warm soft bedding, and gradual return to walking or swimming exercise following a suitable convalescence.

GENETIC MUSCLE DISORDERS

Myotonia. Although it has been reported in several breeds of sporting canids, myotonia does not appear to be a problem of the greyhound.[17] Myotonia refers to the prolonged contraction of skeletal muscles following the suspension of voluntary effort or of any external stimulation. This results in a stiff stilted gait, making uphill or downhill movement, stair climbing, or obstacle scaling extremely difficult. Cold environments exacerbate the problem, while warmth and gentle exercise are beneficial. Myotonia is not relieved by anesthesia, indicating a true muscular rather than a nervous origin. The condition appears to be genetic in origin, and no successful treatment has been reported even when it has occurred in conjunction with abnormalities such as hyperadrenocorticism.

Labrador Myopathy. This is an autosomal recessive trait characterized by reduced exercise tolerance, hypotonia, and progressive muscle atrophy.[18-20] The head is carried low with the neck flexed, the gait is stilted, and the condition may progress to muscle soreness, respiratory distress, and cyanosis. Cold, excitement, and exercise aggravate the condition. Affected puppies begin to exhibit early symptoms at 3 to 4 months of age, and the myopathy tends to progress to about 12 months of age, at which stage most cases stabilize. There is no specific treatment for this genetic disorder, although diazepam 10 mg orally twice a day may be helpful. Prognosis is good for longevity, but very poor for work capacity. Diagnosis is based on clinical signs, including depression or absence of myotactic patellar and triceps reflexes, and, muscle biopsy findings of myofiber size variations, whorling, atrophy, and necrosis.

Myoclonus. This problem has also been reported in the sporting canid,[21] notably the Labrador, spaniel, and golden retriever, although chow chows and Irish terriers are also carriers of the recessive gene. Onset may be as early as 1 to 16 weeks of age, with evidence of a periodic, sustained, nonpainful, tonic muscle contraction leading to limb rigidity, opisthotonus, facial muscle contraction, and jaw clamping. Attacks in lateral recumbency result in generalized extensor rigidity resembling strychnine poisoning or tetanus. The myoclonic responses are exacerbated by external stimuli, exercise, and handling. Again, there is no specific treatment, and diazepam has no influence on the condition. Muscle biopsy findings reportedly differ from those of myotonia in that there is hydropic degeneration of the mitochondria and intermyofibrillar vacuolization.

Myasthenia Gravis. Myasthenia gravis is perhaps the most commonly reported muscular disorder of genetic origin,[22] although noninherited forms may occur secondarily to soft tissue carcinomas, osteosarcomas, or infective processes.[23-25] It is caused by a neuromuscular transmission defect resulting from the action of autoantibodies on acetylcholine at the neuromuscular junction. The inherited form is an autosomal recessive with complete penetrance. There is no sex predilection. Megaesophagus is often associated with myasthenia gravis, especially in the larger sporting breeds. Symptoms may occur at an early age, commencing in the head, neck, and forelimbs with gradual progression to the hindquarters. There are proprioceptive defects with depressed patellar and triceps reflexes. Consequently, victims exhibit periodic weakness, which is aggravated by exercise to the point of ataxia, collapse, and respiratory distress. Drooling, inappetence, and prolonged high-pitched barking are characteristic, while vomiting and regurgitation occur with any associated megaesophagus. Secondary aspiration pneumonia is seen as a complication. Diagnosis is based on clinical observations and supported by laboratory immunoassay for acetylcholine receptor antibody. Treatment with cholinesterase inhibitors is usually attended by encouraging results, eg, edrophonium chloride 1 to 2 mg intravenously and/or neostigmine or pyridostigmine 30 to 60 mg orally two to four times daily, depending on response. Atropine aids in the reduction of airway constriction and excess salivation. Care must be taken with initial therapy to avoid a cholinergic crisis and respiratory collapse. Prednisolone 2 mg/kg orally daily in divided dose is usually beneficial in the immune-mediated abnormality. (Avoid the use of aminoglycoside antibiotics (streptomycin, gentamicin, neomycin) for the treatment of secondary aspiration pneumonia or related infections because of their effect on the neuromuscular junction.) Prognosis varies with age of

onset, severity of the disorder, response to treatment, and associated complications or megaesophagus and pneumonia. Spontaneous recovery is not uncommon in younger animals, although recurrences should be anticipated.

Malignant Hyperthermia. A genetic myopathy triggered by pharmacological agents, especially halothane anaesthetic gas and succinylcholine muscle relaxant, malignant hyperthermia has been reported in most sporting breeds.[26, 27] The underlying mechanism appears to be a calcium transport defect in the sarcoplasmic reticulum resulting in a sudden increase in myoplasmic calcium induced by the chemical agents. The calcium ion overload activates the acute catabolic processes characterizing malignant hyperthermia, namely, prolonged forceful muscle contraction resulting in pronounced temperature elevation (42° C to 43° C; 107° F to 109° F), electrolyte imbalances, circulatory collapse, and hypotensive shock. The condition may be rapidly fatal even when recognized early and treated promptly with total body cooling, intravenous fluids, Dantrolene 1 mg/kg intravenously until symptoms abate, then orally.

IMMUNOLOGICAL MUSCLE DISORDERS

Eosinophilic Myositis. This is an immune–mediated acute inflammatory degeneration of the temporal and masseter muscles induced by autoantibodies against the type 2 myofibers that predominate in these locations. Initially the affected muscles are swollen, tense, and painful on palpation or stretching, causing jaw clamping, inappetence, dehydration, and weight loss due to loss of prehension.[28] Later there is pronounced atrophy of these jaw and head muscles with limitation of oral motion due largely to fibrosis of the masseter muscles. A muscle biopsy sample shows swollen eosinophilic myofibrils with hyalinization and disruption; lymphocytes and granulocytes are scattered throughout. Prednisolone orally, 2 mg/kg daily in divided dose for 14 days followed by a gradually decreasing regimen, has given beneficial responses.

A similar clinical syndrome affecting only the extraocular muscles has been reported in golden retrievers.[29] Biopsy findings revealed similar though less severe histological changes, all of which regressed with oral corticosteroid therapy.

A third similar syndrome of dermatomyositis has been reported[30] as an immune-related myositis of the temporal and masseter muscles appearing in conjunction with primary skin lesions that vary from vesicles, papules, and pustules to painful exudative skin ulcers. It is inherited as a dominant trait with variable penetrance.

INFECTIOUS MUSCLE DISORDERS

Various organisms have been recorded as causing polymyositis in sporting canids.[31-33] Clostridial infection of injection sites and deep penetrating wounds produced marked swelling, lameness, fever, and local crepitus from gas production. Appropriate antibiotic therapy combined with radical drainage and removal of necrotic tissue has been most effective.

References

1. Gannon JR: Muscle Injuries — Their Extent and Therapy in the Greyhound. The Veterinary Annual. Bristol, Stonbridge Press. 1978.
2. Bennett RR: Contracture of the infraspinatus muscle in dogs. A review of 12 cases. JAVMA 22:481–487, 1986.
3. Wright R, Windon A: Contracture of the infraspinatus muscle in a hunting dog. Vet Med/Small Anim Clin 77:1501–1504, 1982.
4. Moore RW, et al: Fibrotic myopathy of the semitendinosus muscle in four dogs. Vet Surg 10:169–174, 1981.

5. Clarke RE: Fibrosis and contracture of the semitendinosus muscle in a dog. Aust Vet J 66:259–261, 1989
6. Carberry CA, Flanders JA: Quadriceps contracture in a cat. JAVMA 198:1329, 1986.
7. Wright JR: Correction of quadriceps contraction. Calif Vet 34:7–9, 1980.
8. Bassinger RR, et al: Osteofascial compartment syndrome in the dog. Vet Surg 16: 427–434, 1987.
9. Haan JJ, Beale B: Compartment syndrome in the dog. J Am Anim Hosp Assoc 29: 134–139, 1993.
10. Braund KG: Myopathies in the dog and cat. Vet Med 81:918–928, 1986.
11. Deuland RT, et al: von Willebrand heterotopic osteochrondrofibrosis in doberman pinschers. JAVMA 197:383–387, 1990.
12. Gannon JR: Cramp—An exercise induced myopathy of greyhounds. Proc Univ of Sydney Refresher Course for Veterinarians (Proceedings 122), 19–24, Univ of Sydney, 1989.
13. Bjotvedt G: Racing induced cardiomyopathy in greyhounds. Vet Med 80:54–57, 1985.
14. Flettman MJ: Fluid and electrolyte metabolism during heat stress. Comp Cont Ed 6: 391–397, 1986.
15. Lassen ED: Effects of racing on hematologic and serum biochemical values in greyhounds. JAVMA 188:1299–1303, 1986.
16. Gannon JR: Exertional Rhabdomyolysis in the Racing Greyhound. Current Veterinary Therapy VII. Philadelphia, WB Saunders Company, 1982, pp 783–878.
17. Farrow B, Malik R: Hereditary myotonia in a chow chow. J Sm Anim Pract 22:451–465, 1981.
18. Hoskin JD, Root CR: Myopathy in a Labrador retriever. Vet Med/Small Anim Clin 73:1387–1390, 1983.
19. McKerrel RE, Braund KG: Hereditary myopathy in Labrador retrievers. J Small Anim Pract 28:479–489, 1987.
20. Blot S, et al: Hereditary myopathy in a Labrador retriever. Proc Ann ACVIM Forum 1991, p 131.
21. Wright JA, et al: Muscle hypertonicity in the cavalier King Charles spaniel — myopathic features. Vet Rec 118:511–512, 1986.
22. Braund KG: Myopathies in dogs and cats. Vet Med 81:918–928, 1986.
23. Klebanow ER: Thymoma and acquired myasthenia gravis in the dog. J Am Anim Hosp Assoc 28: 63–69, 1992.
24. Shelton GD: Acquired myasthenia gravis. J Vet Int Med 4:281–284, 1990.
25. Moore AS, et al: Osteogenic sarcoma and myasthenia gravis in a dog. JAVMA 197:226–227, 1990.
26. Wright RP: Malignant hyperthermia in a greyhound. Vet Med 82:1012–1020, 1987.
27. Rand JS, O'Brien PJ: Exercise induced malignant hyperthermia in an English springer spaniel. JAVMA 190:1012–1014, 1987.
28. Brogdon JD, et al: Diagnosing and treating masticatory myositis. Vet Med 86:1164–1170, 1991.
29. Carpenter JL, et al: Canine bilateral extraocular polymyositis. Vet Pathol 26:510–512, 1989.
30. White SD, et al: Dermatomyositis in an adult Pembroke Welsh corgi. J Am Anim Hosp Assoc 238:398–401, 1992.
31. Mane MC, et al: A putative clostridial myositis in a dog. J Sm Anim Pract 33:345–348, 1992.
32. Poonacha KB, et al: Clostridial myositis in a dog. JAVMA 194:69–70, 1989.
33. Whittington RJ, Freeman PG: Myositis due to Clostridium chauvoei in an Afghan Hound. Aust Vet Pract 16:7–8, 1986.

SECTION IV

PARASITOLOGY

CHAPTER 13

GASTROINTESTINAL PARASITES AND KENNEL MANAGEMENT

ROBERT K. RIDLEY \ MICHAEL W. DRYDEN

Although parasitism is a major concern of the racing greyhound industry, there is limited published research on gastrointestinal parasites of greyhounds in the United States.[1-5] Surveys have been conducted in Great Britain on the incidence of gastrointestinal parasites of the greyhound.[6-11] In one study conducted in Southeast England the authors reported that, depending on the age of the dog, between 25 and 42 per cent of the greyhounds were infected with *Uncinaria stenocephala*, 3 to 29 per cent were infected with *Toxocara canis*, and 2 to 5 per cent were infected with *Trichuris vulpis*.[7] Because climatic conditions in those parts of the Unites States where greyhounds are bred intensively are different from climatic conditions in England, it is difficult to extrapolate from the British studies. Not only are climatic conditions different, but the most common hookworm found in the United States, *Ancylostoma caninum*, is rarely found in the United Kingdom.[9, 11]

INCIDENCE OF PARASITISM IN GREYHOUNDS: MIDWEST UNITED STATES BREEDING FARMS

A recent report from the United States stated that 68 per cent of the greyhounds from one breeding farm in the Midwest were infected with gastrointestinal nematodes.[12] In another study,[13] parasites from 230 greyhounds necropsied at the Kansas Veterinary Diagnostic Laboratory were recovered and identified. In this population of greyhounds, 88 (40 per cent) were parasitized. *A. caninum* was the most common species (16 per cent) identified in this study. At least 42 (19 per cent) of the greyhounds were infested with tapeworms, with 27 (12 per cent) harboring *Dipylidium caninum*. The incidence of tapeworms reported in greyhounds in Great Britain has ranged from none[6] to 72 per cent.[7] The effect of infestation with *Dipylidium caninum* on the health and performance of the greyhounds is unknown, but indicates past or present flea infestation. Heartworms (*Dirofilaria immitis*) were not identified in any

of the 230 greyhounds in the aforementioned study. Two studies from race tracks in Florida reported heartworm incidence in greyhounds of 19 per cent (37/191) and 19.8 per cent (21/106).[14, 15] In New South Wales, 11 per cent of greyhounds examined were positive for *D. immitis* microfilariae.[16]

Many greyhound breeders periodically use large animal formulations of ivermectin as general dewormers at doses approximating 200 to 300 μg/kg. Although ivermectin is not effective against adult heartworms, it is a dependable heartworm preventive and microfilaricide, even at oral doses as low as 2 μg/kg once monthly or 50 μg/kg once every 2 months.[5] That, plus the fact that the prevalence of dirofilariasis is lower in Kansas than in Florida, would probably explain why no heartworms were found in the Kansas Study.

Sarcocystis sp.,[6] *Angiostrongylus vasorum*,[3, 17] and *Filaroides osleri*[7, 8] have been reported with serious consequences in greyhounds in some areas of the world. With the exception of one greyhound with *Sarcocystis* sp., those parasites were not observed in the Kansas study. Greyhound breeders usually feed diets that contain raw meat (primarily beef), but it is almost always purchased frozen, a process which destroys *Sarcocystis* sp. bradyzoites.[18]

Kenneled greyhounds have such high rates of parasitism because of contaminated environments, high somatic larval burdens in bitches resulting in transplacental and transmammary transmission, resistance of parasites to currently available anthelmintics, and postparturient immunosuppression. Except for the depressed immune response, all of these factors can probably be attributed to inappropriate use of anthelmintics.

EPIDEMIOLOGY

Studies in Australia and Great Britain showed that soil from greyhound runs was contaminated with significant numbers of *T. canis* eggs.[19, 20] In the Midwest, greyhounds generally have unrestricted access to sand or dirt exercise runs, with each run typically housing pups from the same litter. Greyhounds are exercised in dirt or sand runs 3 to 7 meters wide and 45 to 100 meters long. To acclimate them to racetrack conditions, greyhounds more than a year old are housed in indoor crates and turned out up to four times daily into large "turnout" pens. Infrequent removal of feces from runs and turnout pens results in soil contamination by parasite eggs, oocysts, and larvae, which in turn results in almost continual exposure of the greyhounds to the infective stages (eggs and larvae) of parasites.[21]

Parasite eggs and larvae recovered from soil samples taken monthly from exercise runs and turnout pens in Kansas included *T. canis*, *T. vulpis*, *Eucoleus boehmi*, and *Capillaria aerophila*. *T. canis* was the predominant parasite egg recovered and accounted for more than 95 per cent of all eggs recovered. *A. caninum* larvae were also recovered from the soil.[22]

Parasite eggs and oocysts recovered in feces deposited in the runs and pens included *T. canis*, *Toxascaris leonina*, *A. caninum*, *T. vulpis*, *E. boehmi*, *C. aerophila*, *Isospora canis*, *D. caninum*, *Taenia* sp., and *Giardia canis*. *T. canis* was also the predominant parasite egg recovered in feces. Numbers of parasite eggs recovered varies depending on the age of the animals, type of substrate (soil versus sand), management procedures (frequency of feces removal, anthelmintics used, and anthelmintic resistance. Based on the rate of parasite ova recovered from seeded soil samples, it was calculated that the top 10 cm of soil in runs from one farm housing animals 3 to 6 months of age was contaminated with 50.6 million larvated *T. canis* eggs. Removing and replacing sand from runs is not effective unless breeders are fastidious about not placing infested dogs on the clean runs. Dogs harboring intestinal helminth infections are continuously shedding eggs, so recontamination of sand occurs within 2 months.

Although the eggs of *T. canis* and *T. vulpis* are highly resistant and are reported to remain viable in soil for years,[15, 23] soil contamination is lowest during the hot, dry months. Aggressive deworming during these times would result in minimizing soil contamination by parasite eggs and larvae.

Despite intensive use of anthelmintics, which are often rotated every 2 to 4 weeks, greyhounds—especially younger animals—are often heavily parasitized and show very high quantitative egg counts and large numbers of worms at necropsy. That would indicate that environmental contamination is a major problem on greyhound breeding farms and results in frequent or almost continuous reinfection.

TRANSMAMMARY AND TRANSPLACENTAL TRANSMISSION

When dogs over 3 months of age ingest infective *T. canis* eggs, most of the larvae do not complete the tracheal migration route to become established in the intestine but instead are carried by the systemic circulation to various tissues of the body.[24] In male dogs this becomes a dead end for the larvae, but in pregnant bitches the larvae become active in the last trimester and migrate via the placenta to the neonatal liver. After the pups are born, the larvae migrate to the lungs and complete their life cycle, becoming patent within 21 to 40 days.[25, 26] Some of the reactivated larvae also migrate to the mammary tissue of the bitch and are shed in the milk, but this is a minor route of transmission of *T. canis* as compared to the transplacental route.[27, 28]

Some of the *T. canis* larvae do not become established in the gut of the pups and are ingested by the bitch when she cleans them.[29] This results in the postparturient patent *T. canis* infection seen in bitches about 4 weeks after whelping and is likely due to

immunosuppression. Within a few weeks the bitch spontaneously clears the ascarid infection after the pups are weaned.[21, 25, 29]

Transplacental and transmammary transmission of *T. canis* and *A. caninum*, respectively, from infected greyhound bitches to their pups was studied using parasite egg passage patterns in feces of preparturient and postparturient greyhounds and their pups.[21] Quantitative fecal examinations were done weekly for 20 to 27 weeks on six naturally parasitized greyhounds (four females, two males). Four greyhound bitches were bred, and, after whelping, qualitative fecal examinations were conducted on each pup once weekly for 10 weeks. Egg shedding of *T. canis* was remarkably similar for all four bitches. Quantitative fecal egg counts were negative during pregnancy and for 3 weeks postpartum, but 4 weeks after whelping all the bitches were patent for *T. canis*. Between 4 and 10 weeks postparturition all bitches stopped shedding *T. canis* eggs. This pattern was also observed by others.[25, 29] The 37 naturally infected pups from all four bitches started shedding *T. canis* eggs between 3 and 4 weeks of age and continued until dewormed 6 weeks later. Two of the bitches were bred and whelped again the following year. The same preparturient and postparturient egg shedding patterns were observed during the second pregnancies, but this time the weekly eggs per gram (EPG) were reduced between 50 and 70 per cent.

Although greyhound bitches were patent for only a few weeks after whelping, environmental contamination is significant if feces are not collected frequently. Based on average EPG, total fecal volume, and length of patency, calculations done in one study showed that a single bitch deposited 377 million *T. canis* eggs into the environment during her 9 weeks of patency.

The transmission and egg shedding patterns of *A. caninum* are different from those of *T. canis*. When infective larvae penetrate the skin or are ingested, some of the larvae become arrested within muscle tissue,[30, 31] while others migrate through the liver and lungs before completing their development in the small intestine. During pregnancy the arrested hookworm larvae become active and migrate to the mammary tissue, are passed in the milk, and infect newborn pups when they nurse.[32, 33] Transplacental (eg, prenatal) transmission apparently does not occur with *A. caninum*.[27, 28] "Leakback" occurs when arrested *A. caninum* larvae in somatic tissues migrate to the intestine and develop to egg-laying adults.[31] This leakback often occurs during pregnancy or after anthelmintic treatment of a patent hookworm infection. Following pregnancy the combination of the postparturient immune suppression and heavily contaminated environment leads to a heavy intestinal hookworm burden and the sharp rise in egg shedding. It has been shown[21] that hookworm egg numbers in bitches' feces increased gradually throughout pregnancy and then increased sharply 2 to 3 weeks postparturition. If pups are infected by ingesting larvae from the bitch's milk, *A. caninum* eggs can be found in their feces 2 to 3 weeks after birth.

It is usual for bitches to spontaneously clear *T. canis* but not *A. caninum* after whelping. It is apparent that transplacental transmission of *T. canis* is a common, if not universal, problem in greyhound kennels, and that preparturient *A. caninum* egg shedding may be an indication of potential transmammary transmission to pups.

ANTHELMINTIC RESISTANCE

The term *anthelmintic resistance* is used to describe the heritable ability of some populations of helminth parasites to survive treatment with a dose level of a given anthelmintic to which they were previously susceptible, often much less than the "label dose," "therapeutic dose," or "use level." Resistance differs from *tolerance*, which is nonresponsiveness of a consistent percentage of worms in an untreated population. Tolerance is innate in the population and does not result from selection pressure exerted by drugs. Resistance therefore occurs when a population of worms inherits the ability to resist treatment that would be effective against a different population, and tolerance was there all along. Resistance occurs under intensive management systems, where frequent deworming is necessary to prevent clinical parasitism. *Side-resistance* occurs when a population of worms does not respond to treatment because of selection by another drug with a similar mode of action. *Cross-resistance* resembles side-resistance, but involves drugs with different modes of action.[34-36]

Individual worms that survive normal therapeutic doses of antiparasitic drugs contaminate the environment with eggs or larvae. Those progeny are endowed with the parental genome and therefore are resistant to the same deworming protocol. With repeated treatments with the same anthelmintic, those resistant parasites comprise an ever-increasing population of the total parasite load, and the product becomes ineffective.[37, 38]

Specific deworming regimens vary among breeders, but most dogs are first dewormed 2 to 3 weeks after they are born. They are treated with the same or a different anthelmintic every 2 to 3 weeks thereafter until they are about 1 year old, after which time they are treated every 3 to 4 weeks for the rest of their lives. Such practices have led to benzimidazole resistance in equine cyathostomes and ovine trichostrongyles.[38, 39] Antiparasiticides as new as Ivermectin are also becoming less effective because of resistance developed by the parasites.[40, 41] Anthelmintic therapy with benzimidazoles,[42-46] thiabendazole,[46] levamisole,[45] and piperazine[43] in horses and sheep treated as infrequently as twice yearly has resulted in resistant populations of worms parasitizing host animals.

Although anthelmintic resistance is recognized as a problem in sheep, goats, horses, and to some extent in cattle, it is not usually a factor considered by veterinarians when selecting a drug for therapeutic or prophylactic use in small animals. There are reports of anthelmintic resistance in dogs and cats. A report from Australia indicated no clinical improvement in a 9-week-old greyhound treated with 100 mg pyrantel pamoate and 380 mg oxantel pamoate. The puppy was re-treated with the same dose of the same compound, and 1 week later the fecal sample contained 30,000 hookworm ova/gm (30,000 EPG).[47] Two pups from a greyhound kennel in Kansas were treated with pyrantel pamoate at the label dose of 5 mg/kg. At necropsy the worms were identified and counted. More worms were recovered from the treated pups than from untreated controls from the same litter. If the dosage of pyrantel pamoate was increased to 1.7 times the label dose (8.3 mg/kg), the fecal egg count was reduced by 99.89 per cent when compared to untreated controls.[21] It should be emphasized that these data cannot be extrapolated to *T. canis* in the general pet population.

New anthelmintics are being used to control parasites in kenneled greyhounds, but strategic deworming protocols for kenneled animals have not kept pace with those used to control ruminant parasites. We continue to depend on suppressive anthelmintic treatment but fail to understand the pharmacology of the anthelmintics we use, the limitations of their efficacy, and the consequences of substituting intensive anthelmintic use for rigorous management. Reinfection and egg shedding can occur within 16 and 30 days, respectively,[31] for *A. caninum* and *T. canis*, so while resistance is a potential problem, reinfection from contaminated environments is probably responsible for most control failures.

RECOMMENDATIONS FOR OPTIMIZING ANTHELMINTIC USAGE AND DECREASING THE PROPENSITY FOR CREATING DRUG RESISTANCE

There is little in the literature on management and control protocols for parasitic diseases in kenneled greyhounds, and no broad recommendations can be made without evaluating the efficacy of deworming programs (anthelmintics used, frequency, rotation scheme) on a given premise. Resistance is a problem of isolated populations (or kennels), and each anthelmintic used must be evaluated to determine which are effective. In the case of ruminant trichostrongyles, rapid drug rotation (less than 1 year) selects for resistance, but fewer treatments are required to prevent disease.[38]

Fecal egg reduction counts (FERC) can be used to determine which drugs are marginally effective. Resistance should be suspected in a population of worms if the FERC is less than 95 per cent 10 to 12 days following treatment at the correct dose with an otherwise effective anthelmintic.[48, 49] One should expect side-resistance, especially with benzimidazoles, and increasing the dose to achieve control increases selection pressure speeds the development of resistance. If quantitative egg counts are not reduced by appropriate levels after treatment, that anthelmintic and others in the same class should be eliminated from the deworming program. Anthelmintics are administered either in food or to individual animals, depending on management practices and the anthelmintic being used. When animals are fed in groups, some puppies will not consume the calculated dose, and the resultant underdosing in turn results in continued contamination of the premises with parasite eggs. It has been demonstrated that guessing weights often results in severe underdosing in horses and sheep,[50] so care should be taken when dosing individual animals that appropriate doses are given. Kennel owners and breeders should discuss and review deworming schedules and anthelmintics used with their veterinarians, who in turn should be fully informed of the biology of the parasites involved, and the pharmacology and safety margins of the dewormers used. Ideally, animals should be dewormed 10 to 12 days before they are sold or purchased to reduce the possibility of contaminating their new surroundings with potentially resistant parasite eggs. New dogs should be isolated for 3 to 4 weeks, and fecal examinations done before they are placed in runs that have been, or will be, used by other dogs. In the purchasing of bitches, a history of parasite deworming protocols used in the kennel of origin and a history of parasite problems might indicate the level of their somatic larval burden and the potential for transplacental and transmammary transmission of *T. canis* and *A. caninum*.

The single most effective management practice kennels can implement to aid in the control of intestinal parasites is to pick up the feces in runs daily. Soil contamination is the crucial factor in parasite transmission in greyhound kennels; only by reducing parasite contamination of the environment will effective control ever be achieved. Some kennels "salt" (with NaCl) or disc (harrow) runs with the aim of reducing parasite transmission. The effectiveness of spreading NaCl in runs to destroy parasite eggs and larvae is unknown. While discing does help to loosen the soil and reduce injuries, it probably has little effect upon parasite transmission because *T. canis* eggs can be found 15 cm below the surface. The ideal situation would be to rely less on anthelmintics and more on understanding the transmission patterns, extent of contamination, frequency of reinfection, and immunity to reinfection for parasite control. Tactical anthelmintic treatment of bitches to prevent larval transmission of *A. caninum* and *T. canis* by transmammary and transplacental transmission would be the most effective way of reducing parasite loads in their puppies. Somatic larvae are most susceptible to anthelmintics during the later stages of pregnancy, and treatments are often more effective if continued while bitches are lactating. Fenbendazole, 50 mg/kg administered daily from day 40 of gestation until 14 days postpartum, reduced *T. canis* infections in puppies by almost 100 per cent.[51] While no adverse reactions were noted in bitches, puppies from bitches treated with fenbendazole at 150 mg/kg from day 20 to day 39 of gestation were reported to have CNS disease and brain degeneration.[52] Ivermectin is effective in reducing lactogenic transmission of *A. cani-*

num. Non-greyhound bitches experimentally infected with *A. caninum* were treated with 0.5 mg/kg ivermectin 10 days pre partum and post partum. This treatment regimen reduced lactogenic transmission of *A. caninum* in pups by 100 per cent when compared to untreated controls. Toxicosis of pups or bitches was not observed.[53]

No anthelmintics are currently approved for use in pregnant greyhound bitches at the dosages needed to eliminate reactivated larvae, and the safety of such treatments has not been conclusively proved in greyhounds.

PUBLIC HEALTH ASPECTS

It is known that humans who accidentally ingest infective eggs of *T. canis* are at risk of developing visceral larva migrans (VLM) or ocular larva migrans (OLM). The parasites do not establish in the intestine, but humans effectively serve as paratenic hosts. The eggs hatch in the intestine after they are ingested, and the larvae migrate to the viscera (VLM) or the eyes (OLM). Children are especially at risk, so care should be taken to prevent contact with contaminated runs and pens. *A. caninum* can cause cutaneous larva migrans or creeping eruption (CLM) in humans when larvae penetrate the skin and migrate subcutaneously.[54–56] *A. caninum* also can establish in the human intestine and reach the adult stage, resulting in a syndrome called eosinophilic enteritis. *A. caninum* infection in humans is usually subclinical but sometimes results in sudden-onset acute abdominal pain. Hookworms do not become sexually immature in the human host, and so patent infections of humans with *A. caninum* do not occur.[57–61]

References

1. Abbitt B, Huey RL, Eugster AK, Syler J: Treatment of giardiasis in adult greyhounds using ipronidazole-medicated water. JAVMA 188:67–69, 1986.
2. Breitschwerdt EB, Malone JB, MacWilliams P, et al: Babesiosis in the greyhound. JAVMA 182:978–982, 1983.
3. Williams JF, Lindeman B, Padgett GA, Smith OL: Angiostrongylosis in a greyhound. JAVMA 186:1101–1103, 1985.
4. Williams JF, Lindsay M, Engelkirk P: Peritoneal cestodiasis in a dog. JAVMA 186:1103–1105, 1985.
5. MacCall LW, Dziminanski MT, Plue RE: Ivermectin in heartworm prophylaxis: Studies with experimentally induced and naturally acquired infections. Proceedings of the Heartworm Symposium, 1986. Washington, American Heartworm Society, 1986, pp 9–13.
6. Farmer JN, Herbert IV, Partridge M, Edwards GT: The prevalence of Sarcocystis spp in dogs and red foxes. Vet Rec 102:78–80, 1978.
7. Jacobs DE, Prole JHB: Helminth infections of British dogs: Prevalence in racing greyhounds. Vet Parasitol 1:337–387, 1976.
8. Weston R: Endoparasites in dogs supplied for laboratory use. J Inst Anim Tech 26:69–75, 1975.
9. Jacobs DE: The epidemiology of hookworm infection in dogs in the UK. Vet Ann 18:220–224, 1978.
10. Jacobs DE, Pegg EJ, Stevenson P: Observations on the epidemiology of helminth infections in greyhounds and police dog kennels. Parasitology 73:999, 1976.
11. Walker MJ, Jacobs DE: Epidemiology of Uncinaria stenocephala infections in greyhound breeding kennels. Vet Parasitol 10:317–321, 1982.
12. Veatch J: Concomitant salmonellosis and canine distemper in the kennel. Sixth Annual International Racing Greyhound Symposium Central Veterinary Conference, Kansas City, 1990.
13. Schoning P: Gross pathologic changes in greyhounds: Gastrointestinal lesions and internal parasites, Part 2. Canine Pract 19:8–11, 1994.
14. Ely ML, Courtney CH: Sensitivity and specificity of Filarochek heartworm antigen test and Dirotect heartworm antibody test for immunodiagnosis of canine dirofilariasis. J Am Anim Hosp Assoc 23:367–371, 1987.
15. Levine ND: Nematode Parasites of Domestic Animals and Man, 2nd ed. Minneapolis, Burgess, 1980, pp 256–295.
16. Martin TE, Collins GH: Prevalence of Dirofilaria immitis and Dipetalonema reconditum in greyhounds. Aust Vet J 62:159–163, 1985.
17. Jacobs DE, Prole JHB: Angiostrongylus vasorum and other nematodes in British greyhounds. Vet Rec 96:180, 1975.
18. Levine ND: Veterinary Protozoology. Ames, Iowa State University Press, 1985, pp 1–414.
19. Jacobs DE, Woodruff AW, Shah AI, Prole JHB: Toxocara infections and kennels workers. Racing Greyhound 2:38–39, 1977.
20. Collins GH, Moore J: Soil survey for eggs of Toxocara species. Ann Trop Med Parasitol 76:579–580, 1982.
21. Ridley RK, Dryden MW, Gabbert NH, Schoning P: Epidemiology and control of helminth parasites in greyhound breeding farms. Compend Contin Educ Pract Vet 16:585–599, 1994.
22. Smith HJ: Inhibited development of Ostertagia ostertagi, Cooperia oncophora, and Nematodirus helvetianus in parasite-free calves grazing fall pastures. Am J Vet Res 35:935–938, 1974.
23. Dryden MW, Gaafar S: Whipworm infection in small animals. Compan Anim Pract 2(5):17–22, 1988.
24. Sprent JFA: Observations on the development of Toxocara canis (Werner, 1782) in the dog. Parasitology 48:184–209, 1958.
25. Douglas JR, Baker NF: The chronology of experimental intrauterine infections with Toxocara canis in the dog. J Parasitol 45(suppl):43–44, 1959.
26. Noda R: On the prenatal infection of dogs with ascarids, Toxocara canis. Bulletin of the University of Osaka, Prefect Series B; Agricultural Biol 4:111–119, 1954.
27. Burke TM, Roberson EL: Prenatal and lactational transmission of Toxocara canis and Ancylostoma caninum: Experimental infection of the bitch before pregnancy. Int J Parasitol 15:71–75, 1985.
28. Burke TM, Roberson EL: Prenatal and lactational transmission of Toxocara canis and Ancylostoma caninum: Experimental infection of the bitch at midpregnancy and at parturition. Int J Parasitol 15:485–490, 1985.
29. Lloyd S, Amersinghe PH, Soulsby EJL: Periparturient immunosuppression in the bitch and its influence on infection with Toxocara canis. J Small Anim Pract 24:237–247, 1983.
30. Lee KT, Little MD, Beaver PC: Intracellular (muscle-fiber) habitat of Ancylostoma caninum in some mammalian hosts. J Parasitol 61:589–598, 1975.
31. Kalkofen UP: Hookworms of dogs and cats. Vet Clin North Am Small Anim Pract 17(6):1341–1354, 1987.
32. Stone WM, Girardeau M: Transmammary passage of Ancylostoma caninum larvae in dogs. J Parasitol 54:426–429, 1968.
33. Stone WM, Peckham JC: Infectivity of Ancylostoma caninum larvae from canine milk. Am J Vet Res 31:1693–1694, 1970.
34. Taylor MA, Hunt KR: Anthelmintic drug resistance in the UK. Vet Rec 125:143–147, 1989.
35. Roush RT: Occurrence, genetics and management of insecticide resistance. Parasitol Today 9(5):174–179, 1993.
36. Prichard RK, Hall CA, Kelly JD, et al: The problem of anthelmintic resistance in nematodes. Aust Vet J 56:239–251, 1980.
37. Coles GC, Roush RT: Slowing the spread of anthelmintic resistant nematodes of sheep and goats in the United Kingdom. Vet Rec 130:505–510, 1992.
38. Craig TM: Anthelmintic resistance. Vet Parasitol 46:121–131, 1993.
39. Wescott RB: Anthelmintics and drug resistance Vet Clin North Am Equine Pract 2(2):367–380, 1986.
40. Giordano DJ, Tritschler JP II, Coles GC: Selection of ivermectin-resistant Trichostrongylus colubriformis in lambs. Vet Parasitol 30:139–148, 1988.
41. Egerton JR, Suhayda D, Eary CH: Laboratory selection of Haemonchus contortus for resistance to ivermectin. J Parasitol 74:614–617, 1988.
42. Uhlinger C, Johnstone C: Prevalence of benzimidazole-resistant small strongyles in horses in a southeastern Pennsylvania practice. JAVMA 187:1362–1366, 1985.
43. Campos-Pereira M, Kohlek I, Campos R, et al: A field evaluation of anthelmintics for control of cyathostomes in horses in Brazil. Vet Parasitol 38:121–129, 1991.
44. Vercruysse J, Dorny P, Meurrens K: Benzimidazole resistance of nematodes in sheep in Belgium. Vet Rec 125:602–603, 1989.
45. Waller PJ, Dobson RJ, Axelsen A: Anthelmintic resistance in the field: Changes in resistance status of parasitic populations in response to anthelmintic treatment. Aust Vet J 65:376–379, 1988.

46. Drudge JH, Lyons ET, Tolliver SC: Resistance of equine strongyles to thiabendazole: Critical tests of two strains. VM/SAC 72:433–438, 1977.
47. Jackson R, Lance D, Townsend K: Isolation of anthelmintic resistant Ancylostoma caninum. NZ Vet J 35:215–216, 1987.
48. Coles GC, Tritschler JP, Giordano DJ: Larval development test for detection of anthelmintic resistant nematodes. Res Vet Sci 45:50–53, 1988.
49. Coles GC: Strategies for control of anthelmintic-resistant nematodes of ruminants. JAVMA 192:330–334, 1988.
50. Besier RB, Hopkins DL: Anthelmintic dose selection by farmers. Aust Vet J 65:193–194, 1988.
51. Burke TM, Roberson EL: Fenbendazole treatment of pregnant bitches to reduce prenatal and lactogenic infections of *Toxocara canis* and *Ancylostoma caninum* in pups. JAVMA 183:987–990, 1981.
52. Stoye M, Vorbohle HJ: Effect of fenbendazole on resting somatic larvae of Toxocara canis in the pregnant bitch. Zentralbl Veterinarmed B 32:637–651, 1985.
53. Stoye M, Meyer O, Schnieder T: The effect of ivermectin on reactivated somatic larvae of Ancylostoma caninum Ercolani 1859 (Ancylostomidae) in the pregnant dog. Zentralbl Veterinarmed B 36:271–278, 1989.
54. English PB: Zoonotic diseases transmitted by domestic companion animals in Australia. Aust Vet Practitioner 12:68–73, 1982.
55. Radcliffe CE: Creeping eruption in Iowa. *In* Diseases Common to Animals and Man. Brookings, South Dakota State University, 1970, pp 34–35.
56. Schantz P: Of worms, dogs, and human hosts: Continuing challenges for veterinarians in prevention of human disease. JAVMA 204:1023–1028, 1994.
57. Croese J, Loukas A, Opdebeeck J, Prociv P: Occult enteric infection by Ancylostoma caninum: A previously unrecognized zoonosis. Gastroenterology 106:3–12, 1994.
58. Croese J, Loukas A, Opdebeeck J, et al: Human enteric infection with canine hookworms. Ann Intern Med 120:369–374, 1994.
59. Loukas A, Croese J, Opdebeeck J, Prociv P: Detection of antibodies to secretions of Ancylostoma caninum in human eosinophilic enteritis. Trans R Soc Trop Med Hyg 86:650–653, 1992.
60. Loukas A, Opdebeeck J, Croese J, Prociv P: Immunologic incrimination of Ancylostoma caninum as a human enteric pathogen. Am J Trop Med Hyg 50:69–77, 1994.
61. Walker NI, Croese J, Clouston AD, et al: Eosinophilic enteritis in northeastern Australia: pathology, association with Ancylostoma caninum, and implications. Am J Surg Pathol 19:328–337, 1995.

CHAPTER 14

EXTERNAL PARASITES

MICHAEL W. DRYDEN \ ROBERT K. RIDLEY

FLEAS

In the United States, the cat flea *Ctenocephalides felis* is by far the most common flea infesting both dogs and cats.[1] *Ctenocephalides canis*, the dog flea, is not as common as the cat flea in North America. Other fleas that may be found infesting dogs and cats include *Pulex irritans*, the human flea, *P. simulans* and *Echidnophaga gallinacea*, the poultry sticktight flea. The flea found most commonly infesting greyhounds is the cat flea. In fact, in Kansas it is the only flea we have found infesting greyhounds.

Cat fleas are small (1/8 to 1/4 inch long), laterally compressed ectoparasitic insects of mammals and birds. Adult fleas have piercing mouthparts that enter the skin of the host for a blood meal. Fleas range in color from light brown (actively reproducing females) to very dark brown (newly emerged fleas and males on the animal). There are more than 2200 species of fleas infesting mammals and birds worldwide, but only a few species commonly infest dogs.

Like butterflies, fleas develop by complete metamorphosis. The life cycle of the flea involves an egg, larva, pupa (cocoon), and adult. Flea eggs are pearly white, oval with rounded ends, and the size of a grain of sand (less than 0.5 mm). The eggs are not sticky and easily roll off the fur of the host when laid.

Flea eggs hatch in 1 to 10 days, depending on the temperature and humidity. Newly hatched flea larvae are slender, white, segmented, and 1/8 inch long. Larvae are free living and feed on organic debris found in the environment. They also feed on adult flea feces, which is partially digested dried blood. Larvae are negatively phototropic and move under crates, bedding material, organic debris (grass, branches, leaves, soil) searching for food. Most larvae complete their development within a few inches from where they hatched, but some may move up to 3 feet.

The larval stage usually lasts 5 to 11 days, depending on the availability of food and the climatic conditions. Understanding larval habitat is critical when implementing an environmental flea control program. The temperature and humidity where flea larvae develop is crucial to their survival.[1,2] Temperature below 60° F and relative humidity below 70 per cent prolong larval development. During certain times of the year the larval stage may be prolonged up to 3 weeks because of the cooler weather.

If the humidity in developmental sites drops below 50 per cent or if temperature exceeds 95° F to 100° F for several hours, flea larvae will die.[3,4] Most flea problems are seen in the spring and fall during times of increased rainfall, higher humidity, and mild temperature. In the southeastern United States, flea problems can occur year-round because of the warm and humid climate.

Flea larvae cannot survive in shade-free areas of turnout pens or runs during summer. Once it gets hot and the sand or dirt dries out, larvae die. Flea larvae develop best outdoors in warm, moist areas out of direct sunlight.[4]

The mature larva spins a silk-like cocoon in which it will pupate. Cocoons are ovoid, about 1/4 inch long, whitish, and loosely spun.

Because the cocoon is sticky, it quickly becomes coated with debris from the environment, which helps camouflage it. Flea cocoons can be found in soil, on vegetation, in carpet, in cracks in floors, and on animal bedding. The pupae may take one to several weeks to develop, depending on environmental conditions. The time required from egg to adult usually takes from 21 to 28 days but can be extended for several months, depending upon temperature.[3, 5]

Once pupae are fully developed, the adult fleas remain inside the cocoon and usually do not emerge until stimulated by air currents, heat, physical pressure, or vibration. A small percentage of fleas residing inside cocoons can survive for several months before they emerge, making control more difficult.[6] That is why fleas reappear after apparent successful treatment.

Newly emerged fleas are attracted to their hosts by the warmth of the animal's body, movement, shadows, and exhaled carbon dioxide.[1, 7] Newly emerged fleas on kennel floors, in vegetation, or along the edges of buildings occasionally bite humans before finding their preferred hosts (dogs, cats, raccoons, opossums).[1] Newly emerged fleas can survive for 1 to 3 weeks without feeding,[1, 4] but as soon as they find a host they feed and mate, and the females start laying eggs within 36 to 48 hours.[8-10] A female cat flea can lay 25 to 40 eggs per day with a potential to produce more than 2000 eggs in her lifetime.

Female cat fleas feed voraciously, consuming up to 15 times their body weight in blood daily.[9] While feeding, fleas deposit large quantities of partially digested blood, which appears as dark reddish to black feces. The flea feces can be found in the hair coat of the dog and in the bedding, and is a necessary dietary component of flea larvae.

Adult cat fleas are permanent ectoparasites. Actively reproducing adults feed, mate, and lay eggs on the host. The immature stages are found in the host's environment.[1, 10] Cat fleas do not leave their hosts to lay eggs in cracks and crevices, but eggs will fall off the host and are deposited any place the flea-infested greyhound is taken or has access to. So if environmental conditions in a trailer or truck are suitable for survival of eggs and larvae (as described previously), an infestation could be established there. Greyhounds that are hauled in trailers or trucks where flea eggs have been deposited will become flea infested unless the conveyance is thoroughly cleaned after each trip.

Fleas can cause several problems in greyhounds. When feeding they inject saliva into the wound, which can produce an allergic reaction known as flea allergy dermatitis (FAD). The irritation will cause the dogs to scratch and rub, resulting in hair loss and skin abrasions. In heavy infestations, pups can become anemic because of blood loss. Fleas also transmit *Dipylidium caninum*, the double-pored tapeworm, the most common tapeworm found in greyhounds. Fleas acquire the tapeworms during their larval stage. Larvae eat the tapeworm eggs contained in tapeworm segments passed in the dog's feces, and the microscopic immature tapeworm develops as the flea larva develops through the pupal and then adult stages. Flea infestation causes irritation to the animal, and dogs bite and lick themselves. In so doing, they ingest some adult fleas containing the infective stages, which are released to become adult tapeworms in the small intestine of the dog.

Flea Control in Greyhound Kennels

The elimination of flea infestations should be based on the concept of integrated pest management that embraces mechanical and chemical measures for controlling and eliminating fleas. This integrated approach is directed toward both the animal and its environment. A complete flea control program must involve treatment of all infested greyhounds, in addition to thorough mechanical and chemical environmental control. An understanding of the biology and habitat of fleas is essential for any control program to succeed. Unless developing and newly emerged fleas in the environment are eliminated, it is unlikely that any control program will be successful.

The objectives of an environmental flea control program are to: (1) kill existing populations of fleas in the environment (on the kennel floor, shaded outside runs, shredded paper, blankets used for bedding, etc); (2) prevent the development of the immature stages (interrupt the life cycle by killing flea eggs and larvae); (3) provide continuing control of adult fleas in the environment (application of residual insecticides or repeated application of short-acting insecticides).

Before discussion of how to implement a successful flea control program, it is important to examine the reason most control programs fail. There are a variety of chemicals available to kill eggs, larvae, and recently emerged adult fleas, but flea pupae and adults still in the cocoon are much more resistant to insecticide application. The cocooned pupae are in cracks and crevices, under bedding material, etc, where larvae have crawled to spin their cocoons. Pupae have a low metabolic rate and are protected by a sticky cocoon that is covered with debris, so most insecticides kill less than half of the pupae.

Therefore, even after application of an insecticide, pupae continue to develop, and adults surviving in the cocoons continue to emerge for 2 to 5 weeks.[1, 11] This "pupal window" is the most common cause of treatment failure.[1] In most flea infestations treatment programs must be consistent and persist for at least 4 to 5 weeks to eliminate the problem.

Traditionally, emphasis in environmental flea control has been directed at eliminating newly emerged adult fleas. However, efforts should also be directed at preventing the development of immature life cycle stages by mechanical measures and the application of insect growth-regulating compounds.

Elimination of fleas outside can be an important aspect of flea control, but several important points must be considered. Application of insecticides in open, unshaded areas of turnout pens or runs is unnecessary because flea development is not occurring there. Only those areas protected from direct sunlight, where the soil is moist, provide conditions suitable for flea development. Insecticides should be applied along edges of fences and buildings, and when treating a yard, efforts should be concentrated in those areas around gardens, bushes, mulch, or other moist shaded areas. Spraying insecticides over the large expanse of a shade-free lawn will generally not be beneficial. Mowing and raking the yard before application of insecticides and removing organic debris from under bushes will enhance any control procedure.

Cage bedding should be cleaned out daily, and floors around and under cages should be washed weekly with a detergent solution and allowed to dry. Vehicles and trailers used to transport greyhounds must be cleaned and thoroughly dried after each trip. Flea-infested animals can be depositing eggs in the vehicles, resulting in a continuing flea cycle and a constant source of reinfestation.

Weeds growing in fence rows between runs or pens provide shade that keeps the sand damp and is an excellent habitat for developing stages. Any action that dries sand in runs and turnout pens, such as raking, harrowing, or tilling, every 2 weeks will do more to eliminate an outdoor flea problem than applying an insecticide. Refuges, such as dense vegetation that offers a damp microenvironment out of direct sunlight, should be mowed or clipped. Leaf litter and other organic debris should be removed. Opening shaded areas to sunlight creates conditions not conducive to flea development. Piles of refuse, wood, or abandoned sheds should be eliminated because they provide havens for other cat flea hosts, such as stray cats, raccoons, and opossums.

Flea infestations in housing may be controlled effectively by using an insecticide in combination with an insect growth regulator.[12]

The mist from foggers (bombs) will not penetrate under structures that are only a few inches off the floor (dog crates, stacked boxes, chairs, etc). To reach those areas, aerosols, pump sprays, or pressurized tanks can be used to direct the chemical. Remember that flea larvae are motile and seek dark, moist areas.

If it is possible, treatment of the animals and the environment should be carried out on the same day. A variety of insecticide formulations can provide effective flea control on the animal, but these products are effective only if used consistently and if the environment is treated appropriately. Products that appear to work well on greyhounds are synergized pyrethrin flea sprays and permethrin dips, spot-ons, and sprays.

Insect growth regulators (IGRs) are compounds that inhibit the development of immature stages of insects and are classified as either juvenile hormone analogues/mimics (JHAs) or chitin synthesis inhibitors (insect development inhibitors).[13] Methoprene, fenoxycarb, and pyriproxyfen mimic the activity of juvenile hormone and are classified as JHAs. The most important function of juvenile hormone is in regulating the molting process of insects.[14] When insects molt from one larval stage to the next, juvenile hormone levels are relatively high and are responsible for maintaining larval characteristics. During the last larval stage (third instar) the levels of juvenile hormone in the hemolymph of the flea larvae decrease dramatically allowing pupation to proceed. Treatment of larvae with JHAs causes abnormal development of pupae and leads to mortality.[15, 16] JHAs also have significant ovicidal activity.[16, 17] While JHAs are lethal to immature stages of insects, current data indicate that they are extremely safe for mammals. JHAs are stable when applied in the indoor environment and provide prolonged residual activity (6 to 12 months). In one study, total-release aerosols (foggers) containing synergized pyrethrins and chlorpyrifos or propetamphos plus dichlorvos failed to provide significant larvicidal activity after only 1 week when applied to carpet or cotton fabric.[11] When either fenoxycarb or methoprene was added to the foggers, development of larvae was inhibited for at least 28 weeks.[11]

Lufenuron, a benzoylphenyl urea, is classified as a chitin synthesis inhibitor or insect development inhibitor. These compounds act by inhibiting the formation of chitin, which is an essential component of the insect exoskeleton. Research with chitin synthesis inhibitors has shown that several compounds have considerable activity against developing fleas.[18, 19] Lufenuron is the only chitin synthesis inhibitor currently marketed for flea control in the United States. Lufenuron is administered orally in the food, and treated dogs maintain effective blood levels for up to a month after a single dose. Female fleas that feed on animals given a single oral dose of lufenuron laid nonviable eggs for 2 weeks.[20] As blood levels of lufenuron decline, some eggs hatch, but the larvae die for up to 44 days.[20] Adult fleas are not affected by the compound. Lufenuron is given to dogs once a month with food to prevent fleas from producing viable offspring. Lufenuron is extremely safe for dogs, and there are no known contraindications, warnings, or side effects when used at the recommended dose.

Permethrin, a synthetic pyrethroid, is an insecticide that has 1 to 2 weeks residual activity and is safe to use on or around greyhounds. Chlorpyriphos (Dursban) is another commonly used insecticide. In kennels, chlorpyriphos should be allowed to dry before returning greyhounds onto treated surfaces. Chlorpyriphos is a potent organophosphate insecticide, and while safe if used appropriately, toxicity can occur if it is applied incorrectly. Imidacloprid and fipronil are highly effective insecticides that provide flea control for about 30 days. They can be applied easily in spot-on formulations. As with all insecticides, always read and follow label recommendations and consult your veterinarian.

IGR-insecticide on-animal sprays, dips, foams, and collars have been approved for use on dogs and cats. A methoprene-pyrethrin spray has been on the market for several years for use on dogs and cats. The natural pyrethrins produce knockdown of existing fleas, while the methoprene provides 30 days of residual ovicidal activity to interrupt the development of flea eggs deposited in the hair coat.

Although use of flea shampoos on greyhounds as a routine approach to flea control is not practical, shampoos can be of benefit in those cases in which a bitch and her pups are heavily flea infested. The bitch can be shampooed with a pyrethrin flea shampoo, allowed to soak in the lather for 15 minutes to ensure that all the fleas are killed, and then thoroughly rinsed. Once a shampoo is rinsed off, there is no residual insecticide. The pups can then be combed with a fine-tooth flea comb or a mild flea powder used to rid them of fleas. The bitch can then be put back with her pups without residual insecticide causing a problem while the pups nurse. At the same time, all bedding material should be removed and cleaned.

When considering flea control products for your kennel or home, be cautious toward claims made by distributors of "nonchemical" or "natural" flea control products. There are very few data to substantiate any of the claims made by the manufacturers of such devices and compounds currently on the market. Controlled on-animal and off-animal studies have shown that ultrasonic flea collars and other ultrasonic devices do not repel fleas, affect jumping rates, interfere with reproduction, or alter development of fleas. Dogs and cats can hear the sound produced by these devices, and some animals will exhibit behavioral disturbances when exposed to the high-frequency sound. The use of brewer's yeast, B-complex vitamins, and elemental sulfur products as flea repellents is common practice. Studies have shown that these materials are not effective as flea repellents.

In conclusion, an effective flea control program combines the consistent application of on-animal flea control products and the use of a residual insecticide and an insect-growth regulator in the environment. Re-treatment may be necessary in 2 to 3 weeks as fleas continue to emerge from cocoons.

SARCOPTIC MANGE

Sarcoptes scabei var *canis*, or itch mites, are small, roughly circular mites that burrow in tunnels in the skin. The females are 330 to 600 μm in length and produce eggs that are about half as big as the adults. Males are slightly smaller, 200 to 240 μm. All the legs of adults of both sexes are short. Itch mites are easily recognized under the microscope by the presence of triangular spines on the dorsal surface.

In addition to dogs, various subspecies or strains of *S. scabei* occur worldwide, and although primarily a parasite of canines, the mite will infest all domestic animals and man. *Sarcoptes* sp found on dogs will not reproduce on humans, but will cause pruritus.

Life Cycle. The female mites burrow into skin and form tunnels in which they lay three to five eggs per day. Female mites will lay 40 to 50 eggs in their lifetime.[21] Eggs hatch in 3 to 5 days into six-legged larvae that stay in the tunnel or wander on skin. If they stay in the tunnel, they molt through two nymphal stages, which in turn make new feeding pockets. Complete development from the eggs to adults takes 17 to 21 days,[21, 22] resulting in a very rapid increase in the number of mites on a given host. Females stay in the feeding pocket (molting pocket) until they are fertilized. The females then extend the feeding pockets into a tunnel and lay eggs after 4 to 5 days. Adult *S. scabei* females are found singly.

The mites do not live very long off the host. At 68° F to 77° F they can live 5 to 6 days if humidity is above 75 per cent.[21, 23] The mites are primarily transmitted by intimate contact with other infected animals. The incubation period varies between 2 and 6 weeks, depending on site of infestation and the number of mites transmitted.

Pathology. The inflammation caused when the female mites burrow deeply in skin is likely the result of a hypersensitivity reaction against mite feces and shed exuviae. This, in concert with mechanical irritation by the mites, causes the characteristic pruritus and attendant scratching associated with itch mite infestation. Chronic infestations result in exudate that forms crusts on surface of the skin, and the skin becomes wrinkled. There is often widespread loss of hair. Pyoderma is commonly seen secondary to mite infestation.[24]

Clinical Signs. Pruritus is the cardinal sign of *S. scabei* infestation and usually develops from 10 days to 8 weeks after contact. There is no age, sex, or breed predisposition. The thin-skinned areas (ventral abdomen, chest, ears, elbows) are most often affected. The back is usually spared.[23] There are often papulocrustous lesions and excoriation. In chronic cases, the lesions can become generalized, and there may be peripheral lymphadenopathy.

Diagnosis. Diagnosis is often based on history, the rapid onset of pruritus, and the distribution of lesions as noted above. Microscopic examination of multiple skin scrapings from the edge of the lesions is indicated, but sarcoptic mange mites are difficult to demonstrate. Finding the characteristic mites, mite eggs, or even parts of mites is diagnostic. Even with multiple skin scrapings (10 to 30), the mites may be found in only 50 per cent of cases.[23] A technique we find useful is to scrape or comb seborrheic debris onto a stainless steel examining table where it can be collected into a beaker and heated in 5 per cent KOH until the debris is digested. This material is then centrifuged at $200 \times G$ for 5 minutes, the supernatant fluid discarded, and the sediment then suspended in Sheather's sugar solution. The material is then treated as a fecal flotation for parasite ova, except in this instance one is looking for mites, mite eggs, or parts of mites. A therapeutic diagnosis, ie, response to therapy, is often used as a last resort.

Treatment. Fortunately, sarcoptic mange is easily cured, but all in-contact dogs must be treated. Because of the burrowing nature of the mites and the serum exudate, it is beneficial to clip the hair and bathe the animal in an antiseborrheic/keratolytic shampoo (eg tar/sulfur) prior to topical treatment. A weekly parasiticidal dip for 3 to 5 weeks usually results in a complete cure. Although not an approved treatment, ivermectin administered orally or subcutaneously (200 to 300 μg/kg twice at 2- to 3-week intervals) is commonly used in greyhounds.[25–27] In kennels, it is also necessary to treat the environment with a residual insecticide because the mites will live off the host for a short time (2 to 3 days) and can quickly reinfect treated animals. If pyoderma is present, it must be treated with antibiotics before starting miticidal treatment.

Because scabies mites are difficult to demonstrate, mange is one of the most commonly misdiagnosed diseases and is often treated as an allergy. Untreated, sarcoptic mange may last for years. *S. scabei* will infest humans, but will not reproduce. (Some veterinarians claim to diagnose mange by the fact that they itch after handling a mangy dog). The disease in humans is generally self-limiting within 12 to 14 days.[22]

DEMODICOSIS

Demodex folliculorum var *canis* (*Demodex canis*), the etiological agent of "red mange," is best considered to be a noncontagious parasitic disease of dogs and is caused by a microscopic alligator-shaped mite that lives in hair follicles.

Life Cycle. The female mites produce eggs that develop into six-legged larvae. Protonymphs, nymphs, and adults have eight legs; the adult stage is reached in 20 to 35 days.

Newborn pups do not harbor mites, but transmission to the pups from the dam occurs while they are nursing during the first 72 hours of life. (Pups taken by cesarean section do not get mites.) *D. canis* mites are not easily transmitted to neonatal animals and this is the reason demodicosis is not considered to be contagious (vs *S. scabei*). In utero transmission has been reported but is probably not very important in the epidemiology of the disease.

Pathology. Demodicosis has long been considered to be the result of an inherited immunological defect, which is a functional abnormality associated with the cell-mediated (T cell) immune system.[23, 28, 29] Dogs with localized demodicosis have normal electrophoretic immunoglobulin patterns and normal T-cell function, whereas dogs with generalized demodicosis have severely depressed T-cell responses.[30, 31] As generalized demodicosis becomes chronic, the animal shows marked T-cell suppression.

It was formerly thought that affected animals inherited a specific T-cell defect that prevented them from mounting an immune response to *D. canis* mite, and as the number of mites increased, a humoral immunosuppressive factor was produced by, or induced by, the mites, especially the internal ones. This immunosuppressive factor was thought to induce a generalized cell-mediated immunodeficiency that further compromised the animals' ability to ward off the mites.[30–32]

More recent work has challenged some of the previous theories. In one study there was good correlation between demodicosis complicated by pyoderma and suppression of lymphocyte blastogenesis, but in dogs with uncomplicated demodicosis there was no suppression of blastogenesis.[33] Other studies have also shown that immunosuppression follows, rather than precedes, the clinical manifestations of generalized demodicosis.[34]

There is good evidence to support the hereditary predisposition for developing generalized demodicosis. The disease is common in certain breeds of purebred dogs and also within certain lines within breeds.[35] In addition, several littermates are often affected, and certain bitches may produce several affected litters.[35, 36]

The American Society of Veterinary Dermatologists recommends that dogs with generalized demodicosis not be used for breeding.[23]

Clinical Signs. Although demodicosis is usually seen in dogs less than 1 year old, it can occur in mature adult dogs. Two forms of demodicosis, localized and generalized, are recognized. *Localized demodectic mange* occurs with well-demarcated areas of alopecia, erythema, and scaling, usually confined to areas around the lips, periorbital area, and forelimbs. Localized demodectic mange is generally self-limiting and not related to immune defect or heredity. There is usually no pruritus or second-degree pyoderma. *Generalized demodectic mange* occurs when there is extensive initial involvement, or when the number of localized lesions increases, and occurs primarily in purebred dogs. Initial lesions of generalized demodicosis are similar to the localized form and involve the skin of the face and forelimb, especially the feet. Pruritus is a frequent complaint because of second-degree bacterial infection. The animals often smell rancid because of bacterial action on skin lipids. There is often marked, generalized lymphadenopathy. Animals suffering from generalized demodicosis may be febrile, anorectic, and debilitated. Approximately 10 per cent of localized cases will progress to the more serious generalized form. *Demodectic pododermatitis* is a form of generalized demodicosis localized to the feet. *Adult-onset demodicosis* is usually associated with a neoplastic process or debilitating disease (eg, malignant lymphosarcoma, malignant melanoma, hyperadrenocorticism, atopy, diabetes mellitus).

Diagnosis. In contrast to sarcoptic mange, demodectic mange is easily diagnosed by microscopic examination of deep skin scrapings (pinch up an area, and scrape deep enough to get some blood). However, demonstration of an occasional mite does not confirm a diagnosis of demodicosis. Large numbers of adults or a preponderance of immature mites indicates clinical disease. If demodicosis is suspected but no mites can be demonstrated, another skin scraping should be done.

Treatment. Because most dogs are immunologically competent, the prognosis for localized demodicosis is very good and the disease is self-limiting. However, as already noted, approximately 10 per cent of localized cases will become generalized. If the lesions are asymptomatic and the owner understands benign neglect, no treatment is usually necessary. Lesions in immunocompetent dogs resolve in 3 to 8 weeks. If, however, the lesions are pruritic, or the owner cannot understand scientific neglect, therapy should be started. Usual treatment involves benzoyl peroxide shampoo, followed by amitraz (Mitaban) dips.

The prognosis for *generalized demodicosis* always is guarded and may be poor, depending on the severity of second-degree pyoderma, which is usually due to *Staphylococcus* spp., *Proteus* sp., or *Pseudomonas* sp. Treatment for generalized demodicosis is much more complicated, and success depends on the breeder, the owner, the veterinarian, and the immune status of the animal. In dogs less than 1 year of age with generalized demodicosis, about half of cases will self-cure. However, if the breeding history shows chronic demodicosis in the kennel, self-cure is unlikely. If the disease does not spontaneously regress by 1 year of age, or if onset occurs in animals older than 1 year, specific therapy will most likely be necessary. If treatment is undertaken, owners need to understand that treatment will be expensive and prolonged. Initially the dog should be bathed with a benzoyl peroxide shampoo or some other antibacterial agent that will also serve to soften the skin and have a flushing effect on the hair follicles where the mites are found. Bactericidal antibiotics that sequester in the skin, such as erythromycin, lincomycin, or gentamicin, are also often useful prior to treatment for the mites per se.

Amitraz is the primary treatment of choice. Various treatment protocols exist with dipping schedules weekly to every 2 weeks and concentrations varying from 0.025 to 0.125 per cent.[37–41] The label protocol for treating demodicosis with amitraz is treatment every 2 weeks with a 0.025 per cent solution. Treatment success is assessed by conducting regular monthly skin scrapings, monitoring for a decrease in mite numbers. Treatment may take several months and should continue for 4 weeks after scrapings show no mites. If mite numbers do not decrease or lesions have not cleared after 20 weeks, alternative therapy should be considered.[23] Side effects of amitraz include sedation (8 per cent), pruritus (<3 per cent), ataxia, hyperexcitability, convulsions, bloat, atypical appetite, vomiting, and diarrhea. Steroids are contraindicated in any kind of demodicosis.

Alternative therapy typically consists of increasing the concentration of the amitraz dip or the frequency of treatments. Protracted (60 to 90 days) daily oral administration of milbemycin (0.5 to 1.0 mg/kg)[42] or ivermectin (0.6 mg/kg)[43–46] has proven quite effective, although with potential serious side effects. Those treatment protocols should also include antibacterial treatment for secondary pyoderma.

Although humans harbor demodectic mites, *Demodex* spp are considered to be host-specific.

OTODECTIC MANGE

Otoacariasis or ear mites is caused by *Otodectes cynotis*. Ear mites are more often seen in cats than in dogs, but are an occasional cause of otitis externa in dogs. (Rabbit ear mites are caused by *Psoroptes* sp.) Otodectic mites have tarsal suckers with unjointed pedicles on first and second pairs of legs in the female and on all four legs in males.

Life History. Ear mites spend their entire life in ears, but can also be found on the feet, face, neck, and tail head.[41] Ear mites survive off the host for several weeks, so reinfestation of treated animals is a potential problem.[23]

Pathology. Otodectic mites feed on epidermal debris; they do not pierce skin but elicit immediate and delayed hypersensitivity reactions in the host.[24, 47, 48] Secondary bacterial or yeast infection, with the concomitant pruritus and scratching, usually occurs. Most infestations occur at an early age with the development of an immune response that helps to prevent later infestations.

Clinical Signs. Dogs typically shake their heads vigorously and scratch their ears. The ears may droop and show a typical dark, oily exudate. Prolonged infestations may result in torticollis, rupture of the tympanum, and middle and inner ear infections. Floppy-eared dogs such as greyhounds often develop aural hematomas from head shaking. Ectopic infections often occur on the face and neck.

Diagnosis. Diagnosis is made by microscopic identification of mites recovered by swabbing the ears or by otoscopic examination.

Treatment. The ears should be thoroughly cleaned with a non-drying preparation before institution of miticidal treatment. There are a myriad of commercial preparations for cleaning ears. Following cleaning, a miticidal otic preparation should be used according to label directions. Although not approved, ivermectin (300 μg/kg orally or subcutaneously, repeated in 2 to 3 weeks) is effective.[23, 49–51] Because the mites "wander" out of the ears, a weekly pyrethrin shampoo, in addition to treating the ears, will increase the chances of success. If the ear will not drain, a lateral ear resection may be required. To control ear mites in kennels and breeding farms, it is necessary to treat the environment with chlorpyrifos or permethrin.

CHEYLETIELLOSIS

"Walking dandruff" is caused by the mite *Cheyletiella yasguri*. These are large, whitish mites, about 300 to 500 μm long, with characteristic protruding, hooklike mouthparts (palpal claws) and long tapering legs that extend beyond the body. The eggs are large (110 × 230 μm), three or four times as large as hookworm eggs.

Life History. The mites are widespread and spend their entire life (egg to larva to nymph to adult) on one host. It takes about 35 days from egg to adult.[41] The mites live in the keratin layer of the epidermis and are transferred from host to host by direct contact. Larvae and nymphs die in about 24 hours away from the host. Adults may survive about 10 days off the host. Young animals are more often affected.

Pathology. The mites burrow very superficially in skin and form pseudotunnels. *Cheyletiella* causes subacute to chronic nonsuppurative dermatitis.[24] In dogs, there is rapid-onset seborrhea with or without pruritus, resulting in scaling and crusting, primarily on the back, scapular area, lumbar area, neck, top of head, and nose.[41, 52] In puppies, lesions usually occur first on the rump. Some animals are asymptomatic carriers.

Diagnosis. Diagnosis is based on history (rapid onset with dorsal seborrhea with or without pruritus, recent group contacts, etc, and demonstration of the mites. A convenient method of demonstrating the mites is the use a piece of clear cellophane tape to pick up mites from the skin. The hair is parted, and the tape is pressed onto suspect areas. The mites adhere to the tape, which can be used as a coverslip to examine for mites. If desired, a little mineral oil can be used as a mounting medium. The 5 per cent KOH digest method, as described above for diagnosing sarcoptic mange, can also be used. However, the mites can often be observed moving about on the animals, especially on the forehead and face.

Treatment. All in-contact animals should be treated, since asymptomatic animals can be carriers and the disease is highly contagious. Bedding should be changed and housing treated with insecticide. Animals should be treated with a keratolytic shampoo (tar and sulfur) *plus* an insecticidal dip (carbaryl, lime/sulfur, pyrethroids, or pyrethrins) repeated at 2-week intervals for 4 to 8 weeks. Although not approved, ivermectin administered at 300 μg/kg subcutaneously or orally, repeated in 2 to 3 weeks, has been used.[53, 54]

Because the mites will survive off the host, premises should be sprayed with an organophosphate (eg, Dursban) or permethrin.

Cheyletiella sp. does affect humans, producing pustules, macules, and attendant pruritus.[55, 56] Often the diagnosis of cheyletelliosis comes from breeders complaining about itching. Human lesions are usually self-limiting after cleaning up of the environment.

References

1. Dryden M, Rust M: The cat flea—Biology, ecology and control. Vet Parasitol 52:1–19, 1994.
2. Dryden MW: Biology of the cat flea, Ctenocephalides felis felis. Comp Anim Pract 19:23–27, 1989.
3. Silverman J, Rust MK, Reierson DA: Influence of temperature and humidity on survival and development of the cat flea, Ctenocephalides felis (Siphonaptera: Pulicidae). J Med Entomol 18:78–83, 1981.
4. Silverman J, Rust MK: Some abiotic factors affecting the survival of the cat flea, Ctenocephalides felis (Siphonaptera: Pulicidae). Environ Entomol 12:490–495, 1983.
5. Dryden MW: Evaluation of certain parameters in the bionomics of Ctenocephalides felis felis (Bouche' 1835). MS Thesis, Purdue University, W. Lafayette, Ind, 1988, 115 pp.
6. Silverman J, Rust MK: Extended longevity on the preemerged adult cat flea (Siphonaptera: Pulicidae) and factors stimulating emergence from the pupal cocoon. Ann Entomol Soc Am 78:763–768, 1985.
7. Osbrink WL, Rust MK: Cat flea (Siphonaptera: Pulicidae): Factors influencing host-finding behavior in the laboratory. Ann Entomol Soc Am 78:29–34, 1985.
8. Akin DE: Relationship between feeding and reproduction in the cat flea, Ctenocephalides felis (Bouche). MS Thesis, University of Florida, Gainesville, 1984, 125 pp.
9. Dryden MW, Gaafar SM: Blood consumption by the cat flea, Ctenocephalides felis (Siphonaptera:Pulicidae). J Med Entomol 29:394–400, 1991.
10. Dryden MW: Host association, on-host longevity and egg production of Ctenocephalides felis felis. Vet Parasitol 34:117–122, 1989.
11. Osbrink WLA, Rust MK: Distribution and control of cat fleas (Siphonaptera: Pulicidae) in homes in Southern California. J Econ Entomol 79:135–140, 1986.
12. Dryden MW, Prestwood AK: Successful flea control. Comp Cont Ed Pract Vet 15:821–831, 1993.
13. Chamberlain WF: Insect growth regulating agents for the control of arthropods of medical and veterinary importance. J Med Entomol 12:385–400, 1975.
14. Jennings RC: Insect hormones and growth regulators. Pestic Sci 14:327–333, 1983.
15. El-Gazzar LM, Koehler PG, Patterson RS, Milio J: Insect growth regulators: Mode of action on the cat flea, Ctenocephalides felis (Siphonaptera: Pulicidae). J Med Entomol 23:651–654, 1986.
16. Marchiondo AA, Riner JL, Sonenshine DE, et al: Ovicidal and larvicidal modes of action of fenoxycarb against the cat flea. J Med Entomol 27:913–921, 1990.
17. Olsen A: Ovicidal effect on the cat flea, Ctenocephalides felis (Bouche') of treating fur of cats and dogs with methoprene. Int Pest Control 27:10–16, 1985.
18. El-Gazzar LM, Patterson RS, Koehler PG: Activity of chitin synthesis inhibitors on the cat flea, Ctenocephalides felis Bouche. J Agric Entomol 5:117–120, 1988.
19. Hink WF, Zakson M, Barnett S: Evaluation of a single oral dose of lufenuron to control flea infestations in dogs. Am J Vet Res 55:822–824, 1994.
20. Hink WF, Drought DC, Barnett S: Effect of an experimental systemic compound, CGA-186499, on life stages of the cat flea (Siphonaptera; Pulicidae). J Med Entomol 28:424–427, 1991.
21. Arlian LG, Vyszenski-Moher DL: Life cycle of Sarcoptes scabie var. canis. J Parasit 74:427–430, 1988.
22. Muller GH, Kirk RW, Scott DW: Small Animal Dermatology, 3rd ed. Philadelphia, WB Saunders Company, 1983.
23. Kwochka KW: Mites and related disease. Vet Clin North Am Small Anim Pract 17:1263–1284, 1987.
24. Moriello KA: Parasitic hypersensitivity. Semin Vet Med Surg 6:286–289, 1991.
25. Campbell WC: Use of ivermectin in dogs and cats. In Campbell WC (ed): Ivermectin and Abamectin. New York, Springer-Verlag, 1989, pp 245–259.
26. Scheidt VJ, Medleau L, Seward RL: An evaluation of ivermectin in the treatment of sarcoptic mange in dogs. Am J Vet Res 45:1201–1202, 1984.
27. Yazwinski TA, Pate L, Tilley W: Efficacy of ivermectin against Sarcoptes scabei and Otodectes cynotis infestations in dogs. Vet Med/Small Anim Clin 76:1749–1751, 1981.
28. Folz SD: Demodicosis (Demodex canis). Comp Cont Ed Pract Vet 5:116–124, 1983.
29. Miller WH: Canine demodicosis. Comp Cont Ed Pract Vet 2:334–344, 1980.
30. Scott DW, Farrow BRH, Schultz RD: Studies on the therapeutic and immunologic aspects of generalized demodectic mange in the dog. J Am Anim Hosp Assoc 10:233–244, 1995.
31. Scott DW, Schultz RD, Baker E: Further studies on the therapeutic and immunologic aspects of generalized demodectic mange in the dog. J Am Anim Hosp Assoc 12:203–213, 1976.
32. Muller GH, Kirk RW, Scott DW: Cutaneous parasitology. In Small Animal Dermatology, 3rd ed. Philadelphia, WB Saunders Company, 1983, pp 301–379.
33. Barta O, Waltman C, Oyekan PP: Lymphocyte transformation suppression caused by pyoderma failure to demonstrate it in uncomplicated demodectic mange. Comp Immunol Microbiol Infect Dis 6:9–18, 1983.
34. Barriga OO, Al-Khalidi S, Martin S, Wyman M: Evidence of immunosuppression by Demodex canis. Vet Immunol Immunopathol 32:37–46, 1992.
35. Scott DW: Canine demodicosis. Vet Clin North Am Small Anim Pract 9:79–92, 1979.
36. Henfrey JI: Canine demodicosis. In Pract 12:187–192, 1990.
37. Folz SD, Kratzer DD, Conklin RD, et al: Chemotherapeutic Treatment of naturally aquired gereralized demodicosis. Vet Parasitol 13:85–93, 1985.
38. Kwochka KW, Kunkle GA, O'Neill Foil C: The efficacy of amitraz for generalized demodicosis in dogs: A study of two concentrations and frequencies of application. Comp Cont Ed Pract Vet 7:8–17, 1985.
39. Bussieras J, Chermette R: Amitraz and canine demodicosis. J Am Anim Hosp Assoc 22:779–782, 1986.
40. Scott DW, Walton DK: Experience with the use of amitraz and ivermectin for the treatment of generalized demodicosis in dogs. J Am Anim Hosp Assoc 21:535–541, 1985.
41. Foley RH: Parasitic mites of dogs and cats. Comp Cont Ed Pract Vet 13:783–801, 1991.
42. Garfield RA, Reedy LM: The use of oral milbemycin oxime (Interceptor) in the treatment of chronic generalized demodicosis. Vet Dermatol 3:231–235, 1992.
43. Yathiraj S, Rai MT, Reddy NRJ, et al: Treatment of demodicosis in canines with ivermectin. Indian Vet J 68:784–786, 1991.
44. Paradis M, Laperriere E: Efficacy of daily ivermectin treatment in a dog with amitraz-resistant generalized demodicosis. Vet Dermatol 3:85–88, 1992.
45. Ristic Z: Ivermectin in the treatment of generalized demodicosis in the dog. Vet Dermatol 4:40–41, 1993.
46. Ristic Z, Medleau L, Paradis M, White-Withers NE: Ivermectin for treatment of generalized demodicosis in dogs. J Am Vet Med Assoc 207:1308–1310, 1995.
47. Powell MB, Weisbroth SH, Roth L, Wilhelmsen C: Reaginic hypersensitivity in Otodectes cynotis infestation of cats and mode of mite feeding. Am J Vet Res 41:877–882, 1980.
48. Weisbroth SH, Powell MB, Roth L: Immunology of naturally occuring Otodectes otoacariasis in the domestic cat. J Am Vet Med Assoc 165:1088–1093, 1974.
49. Fukase T, Hayashi S, Sugano R, et al: Ivermectin treatment of Otodectes cynotis infestation of dogs and cats. J Vet Med Japan 44:160–165, 1991.

50. Jeneskog T, Falk K: The effect of local ivermectin treatment on ear mite infestation in a cat breeding colony. Scand J Lab Anim Sci 17:17–19, 1990.

51. Song MD: Using ivermectin to treat feline dermatoses caused by external parasites. Vet Med 86:500–502, 1992.

52. Alexander MM, Ihrke PJ: Cheyletiella dermatitis in small animal practice: A review. Calif Vet 3:9–12, 1982.

53. Paradis M, Villeneuve A: Efficacy of ivermectin against Cheyletiella yasguri infestation in dogs. Can Vet J 29:633–635, 1988.

54. Paradis M, Scott D, Villeneuve A: Efficacy of ivermectin against Cheyletiella blakei infestation in cats. J Am Anim Hosp Assoc 26:125–128, 1990.

55. Guzman RF: A survey of cats and dogs for fleas; with particular reference to their role as intermediate hosts of Dipylidium caninum. NZ Vet J 32:71–73, 1984.

56. Beresford-Jones WP: The fleas Ctenocephalides felis felis (Bouche, 1833), Ctenocephalides canis (Curtis, 1826), and the mite Cheyletiella (Canestrini, 1886) in the dog and cat: Their transmissibility to humans. *In* Soulsby EJL (ed): Parasitic Zoonoses—Clinical and Experimental Studies. New York, Academic Press, Inc, 1974, pp 383–390.

SECTION V

MUSCULOSKELETAL SYSTEM

CHAPTER 15

MUSCLE INJURIES IN THE RACING GREYHOUND

RICHARD D. EATON-WELLS

When one is considering muscle injuries in the greyhound, it is important to remember that this dog is a complex anatomical racing structure. A greyhound can accelerate rapidly from zero to approximately 35 to 40 mph.[1] Its skeletal system is subjected to the stresses associated with sudden changes in direction and falls, and it is often involved in collisions with other dogs and stationary objects. These factors plus the will to win or the willingness to overexert result in high-energy injuries to many musculoskeletal structures. In addition, a greyhound may sustain serious injury with what appears to be minimal expenditure of energy, eg, a spiral fracture of the tibia while "dancing" on the end of the lead or a ruptured gracilis muscle while being walked.

Musculoskeletal injuries occur in all working or sporting breeds, but there are injuries that are peculiar to the racing greyhound. It is this group that is detailed here. Some injuries are difficult to diagnose because of the nature of the anatomy, eg, avulsions of the deep ventral abdominal muscles; others, because of being covered by a thick fibrous sheath, eg, disruptions of the musculotendinous junction of the gastrocnemius or longitudinal splits in the vastus lateralis. Alterations in the normal anatomy may also be used as diagnostic aids. Partial or complete rupture of the gastrocnemius muscle causes a slight "dropping" of the hock and flexion of the digits, because of the apparent shortening of the superficial digital flexor tendon. In other muscle injuries the only indication of serious muscle disruption may be discoloration of the area resulting from local hemorrhage or persistent edema distal to the injury caused by a deep hematoma. Occasionally, injured muscles may be too deep to detect by palpation; diagnosis in these cases may have to be by default or exploratory surgery. Ultrasound, using a fluid offset head, is useful in detection of early or minor changes in the muscle architecture associated with injury.

In Australasia and the United Kingdom, greyhound racing is more hobby oriented, and the majority of greyhounds are owned and trained by individuals with a limited number of dogs, whereas in the United States the dogs are housed and trained at the track in large multikennel complexes, each kennel housing 30 to 50 dogs.

Because of the time available to the hobby trainer, much more emphasis is placed on prevention of major musculoskeletal injury. Regular musculoskeletal examinations are carried out after each race or trial to check for injuries. These may be performed by a veterinarian, the owner/trainer, or a so-called muscle man—a lay person who specializes in the examination of dogs. Any injuries are treated by an appropriate method. Regular physical examinations are a major factor in prevention of serious musculoskeletal injury and subsequently in reduction in the time that a greyhound is not racing or producing income.

Diagnosis of most muscle injuries is by direct palpation. When possible, each individual muscle or group of muscles should be palpated to detect any change suggestive of injury.[2, 3] These changes vary from mild edema to gross muscle disruption. Detection of a pain focus is less diagnostic than the presence of these changes. Because the changes associated with injury may be subtle, a systematic approach to the examination is essential. Most trainers and veterinarians specializing in greyhound medicine have developed their own approach to the physical examination of the racing greyhound.

What to look for when conducting a physical examination of the musculoskeletal system:

1. Minor swelling or edema and loss of anatomical detail
2. Muscle spasm or so-called cellulome
3. Splits along the normal lines of muscle fibers, eg, the serratus ventralis, vastus lateralis, or tensor fasciae latae
4. Tears in the normal fascial sheaths. These may be acute injuries, as evidenced by edema and loss of detail, or chronic injuries that have developed a distinct fibrous scar around the edges that may be readily palpable.
5. Evidence of gross muscle disruption: (a) palpable defects in the anatomy, eg, as gracilis, long head of triceps, tensor fasciae latae or pectineus, or major ventral abdominal muscle injuries; (b) persistent edema that does not respond to conservative therapy, eg, injuries to the vastus lateralis, internal abdominal

oblique, gastrocnemius, or the shoulder muscles medial to the scapula.

Some basic philosophy with regard to the aims of treatment of muscle injuries in the greyhound: When possible, injuries should be prevented. Owners and trainers should be encouraged to perform regular muscle checks on dogs in training so that minor injuries can be detected and treated before they progress to more serious problems. Basic principles of sports medicine should be followed to reduce the amount of edema and inflammatory response following injury. Ice applied to the area as soon as possible after the injury will make the initial diagnosis easier and the response to treatment faster, and decrease the length of time the dog is away from racing. The correct use of the many types of physiotherapy equipment, such as magnetic field therapy, laser, ultrasound, and microwave is very important.

Early return to controlled physical exercise will reduce adhesions and encourage wound repair. Judicious use of nonsteroidal anti-inflammatory agents will expedite return to function.

The concept of a physiological basis for musculoskeletal conditions should not be discarded, nor should the reports of successful manipulative therapy be discounted. In the field of human athletic endeavor, these concepts are recognized and utilized in the appropriate situations. Muscle injuries are readily monitored in the racing dog, so the results of manipulative or other alternative therapy are easily followed.

It is important to recognize that a pain focus may be the result of referred pain, and treatment should be directed toward alleviating the primary cause.

There are two well-recognized pain/spinal mechanical fault syndromes of which to be aware: Pain in the cervicothoracic area and pain in the lower lumbar/sacral area.

Pain in the cervicothoracic area involves pain on palpation of the cervicothoracic dorsal spinous process or the abaxial spinal muscles, the acromial head of the deltoid, the long and lateral heads of the triceps, and upon flexion of the carpus. This pain syndrome is immediately dissipated by manipulating the lower neck.

With pain in the lower lumbar/sacral area there is resentment of deep palpation of the immediate spinal area, and there is tenderness and increased muscle tension in the gluteals, tensor fasciae latae, and the proximal third of the vastus lateralis. This is readily treated by manipulation of the lumbosacral area. Those interested in the concept that local derangements are not purely due to physical injury should read Hauler's work.[5]

We should continually strive to improve our methods of handling musculoskeletal injuries. Injuries that were considered career threatening a few years ago now can be satisfactorily repaired and the dog returned to racing. New techniques, instruments, materials, and an improved understanding of the physiology involved have resulted in improved results. Surgical expertise has also improved so that the more complex injuries are better managed. However, we should not become complacent about our ability to handle musculoskeletal injuries, as there are still injuries that are difficult to diagnose or treat.

CLASSIFICATION OF MUSCLE INJURIES

Muscle injuries have been classified into three basic types[6]: Stage 1: Mild myositis without disruption of fascia or myofibrils; stage 2: similar to stage 1 but extending to include fascial sheath tears; stage 3: disruption of muscle fibers and the sheath with hematoma formation.

TREATMENT OF MUSCLE INJURIES

In any muscle injury it is necessary to treat the primary injury and prevent excessive fibrous tissue formation during the healing phase. Immediate treatment of muscle injury should include ice packs, padded dressings when possible, and nonsteroidal anti-inflammatory agents. A better understanding of the principles of muscle injuries has resulted in changes in their treatment and improvement in results.

The minor trauma associated with *stage 1* injuries should initially be treated by application of ice to reduce the amount of local swelling. To encourage healing, one of the conservative modalities, such as massage, ultrasound, magnetic field therapy, or faradic stimulation, may be used once the acute inflammatory phase is over.

Stage 2 muscle injuries will respond to aggressive conservative therapy following the application of ice to reduce initial edema. Tensor fasciae latae injuries often result in development of severe muscle spasm that not only makes the diagnosis difficult but also delays the healing process. Local acupuncture dissipates this initial muscle spasm and greatly aids both the diagnosis and the healing process.

In *stage 3* injuries (muscle or sheath ruptures); some minor deficits in the muscle or sheath may be treated conservatively. Larger disruptions or total muscle rupture should be treated surgically. It is important to recognize that small tears may result in loss of performance. If this occurs, surgical repair of the deficit is warranted. Major muscle disruptions may need to be surgically repaired if the dog is to return to racing. In addition, a carefully planned course of physiotherapy must be initiated to strengthen the fibrous reaction that accompanies the healing process.

A comprehensive list of muscle injuries that a greyhound can sustain is almost endless, and this should be borne in mind when a racing dog is examined for musculoskeletal injury. In addition, serious deep muscle lacerations may occur after fights, even with minimal skin damage.

INJURIES TO THE CERVICAL AND THORACIC PORTIONS OF THE TRAPEZIUS AND RHOMBOID MUSCLES

These injuries may be caused by dog fights or as a result of overexertion. Acute injuries may be difficult to diagnose as they will often be masked by local swelling and edema. However, direct palpation of the area is painful. Chronic injuries are readily detectable on palpation because of a "ring" of fibrous or scar tissue. If the dog resents palpation of these fibrous rings, they are clinically significant and should be repaired surgically. The fibrous scar is excised, and primary repair of the affected muscle accomplished with single interrupted 4/0 polyglyconate sutures.

MUSCLE INJURIES OF THE FORELEG

Long Head of Triceps ("Monkey" or "Pin" Muscle)

A common injury, the treatment of which is somewhat controversial, involves partial avulsion of a small proportion of the muscle's origin, and in my opinion, once healed, has no effect on the dog's racing ability. The injury was for many years treated by injection of a sclerosing agent. Since the whole concept of modern sports medicine is to reduce the amount of inflammatory reaction and resultant scar tissue, this treatment has lost favor. Gross dissection of the triceps muscle reveals that the part of the long head that

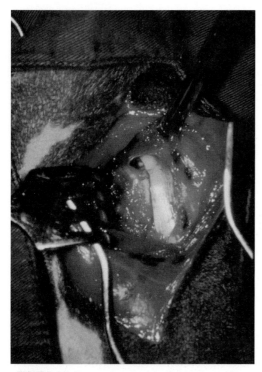

FIGURE 15–1. Exposure of the intertubercular groove.

avulses is only a small part of the whole muscle group. With this in mind, the treatment now involves the use ice packs to reduce the swelling and edema, followed by 5 to 7 days of restricted leash exercise. The dog is then allowed a week of full-leash exercise before returning to normal race training, the aim being to return the dog to the track within 4 to 6 weeks. Another school of thought, which claims that partial avulsions are more prone to recur, believes that the dog should be exercised immediately after the initial injury to ensure that all weakened tissue has avulsed. The conservative treatment protocol described above is then followed. Surgical repair of this muscle has become popular in North America. However, the end results would appear to be similar to those obtained with conservative treatment, and more time is lost before the dog is racing again.

RUPTURE/AVULSION OF THE TRANSVERSE HUMERAL LIGAMENT

The shoulder joint is a ball-and-socket joint that derives its stability from the muscles and tendons, the joint capsule, and the medial and lateral glenohumeral ligaments that traverse and surround it. The biceps brachii muscle arises, via a tendinous origin, from the supraglenoid tubercle of the scapula. It crosses the shoulder joint anteriorly and passes through the intertubercular groove on the proximomedial aspect of the humerus. The bicipital tendon is kept in this groove by the transverse humeral ligament, which extends from the greater tubercle cranially to the lesser tubercle caudally.[7] The action of the biceps brachii is to flex the elbow and to extend the shoulder. It has also been suggested that the tendon of origin draws the supraglenoid tuberosity into the intertubercular groove during extension of the shoulder joint. This acts to determine the path that the glenoid cavity describes as it articulates with the head of the humerus.[8] There are three reports in the literature of injury to the intertubercular ligament in the racing dog.[9–11] The

condition has also been reported in a German shepherd,[12] a Border Collie,[13] and an Afghan hound.[14]

Careful palpation of the craniomedial region of the proximal humerus deep to the brachiocephalicus muscle during flexion of the shoulder joint will reveal caudomedial displacement of the tendon of origin of the biceps brachii muscle and subluxation of the shoulder joint. Extension of the shoulder joint causes the tendon of origin to return to its proper location within the intertubercular groove. This movement of the tendon in and out of the groove can be readily palpated. Radiographs taken of the shoulder joint are normal. There is usually muscle atrophy in chronic cases. Treatment is surgical stabilization of the tendon within the groove.

Recommended surgical techniques are (1) use of implants to maintain the tendon in place,[9, 10] and (2) placement of a screw in both the lesser and greater trochanters so that synthetic sutures can be used to replace the transverse humeral ligament.[11] If the injury is acute, it may be possible to repair the ruptured ligament primarily, or the insertion may be reattached with a screw and spiked washer. The treatment of choice at this time appears to be the placement of screws and a synthetic ligament to maintain the ligament within the groove.

The surgical approach is with the affected leg down and the medial aspect of the shoulder joint prepared for routine surgery. A 12-cm skin incision is centered over the craniomedial aspect of the greater tubercle. The brachiocephalicus muscle is retracted caudally after the fascia is incised along its anterior border. The insertion of the superficial pectoral muscle is incised, and retraction of the muscle caudally exposes the bicipital tendon; exposure of the intertubercular ligament is achieved by cranial and caudal retraction of the supraspinatus and deep pectoral respectively (Fig. 15–1). Two screws are then placed in position and either the ligament remnants are sutured together or a suture is placed to maintain the tendon in position (Fig. 15–2). It may be necessary to partially

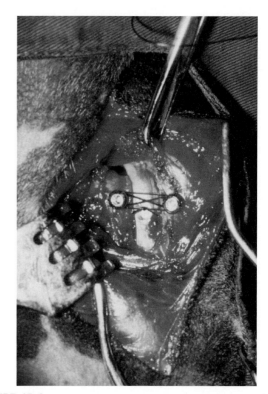

FIGURE 15–2. Placement of two screws and a polyglyconate suture to maintain the tendon in place.

incise the insertion of the deep pectoral muscle for adequate exposure of the area of the intertubercular ligament. Routine closure with 2/0 absorbable sutures is performed.

AVULSION OR RUPTURE OF THE ORIGIN OF THE BICEPS BRACHII

This injury occurs in many breeds as a result of sudden deceleration forces being transmitted through the shoulder joint. It is repaired either by reattachment of the origin to the supraglenoid tubercle or by anchoring the tendon of origin to the proximal humerus. Either repair carries a poor prognosis for return to winning form.

AVULSION OF THE BICEPS BRACHII INSERTION

Avulsion of the insertion of the radial head of this muscle occurs more commonly in racing dogs than in a rearing environment. It is has also been reported in nonsporting breeds. It is diagnosed upon physical examination. The loss of tension in the tendon of insertion is readily palpable. The area of insertion should be radiographed to check for the presence of an avulsed bone chip (Fig. 15–3). It may also be seen as a cause of chronic lameness. Repair is by reattachment of the chip with a small pin and a tension band (Fig. 15–4). The leg should be supported in an elasticized sling for 2 weeks to allow the muscle to retain its function without damaging the repair.

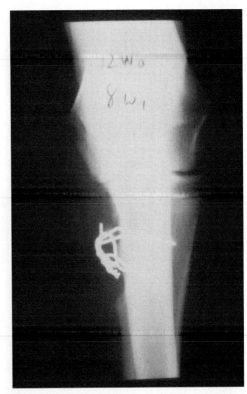

FIGURE 15–4. Postoperative radiograph showing reattachment of the bone fragments with a pin and tension band.

AVULSION OF THE ORIGIN OR INSERTION OF THE EXTENSOR CARPI RADIALIS

A common injury on rearing farms where puppies are raised in large areas is caused by collision with trees, shrubs, or wire fences while galloping. Surgical repair is successful if the muscle innervation has not been damaged. Avulsion injury of the insertion, or rupture of the tendon as it crosses the carpus, is more common in racing dogs. These injuries are rarely repaired, because the incidence of failure is high, and secondary fibrosis provides good return to function.

MUSCLE INJURIES OF THE TRUNK

Pectoral Muscle Injuries

These muscles are commonly injured either at the start of a race or when a dog is pulling up in the catching pen. Although these injuries are usually minor, stage 2 injuries of the deep pectoral can occur. Large defects in the muscle should be repaired surgically. Small defects may be treated conservatively.

Lateral Thoracic Muscle Injuries

Major tears in the serratus ventralis are detected on palpation. Acute injuries have edematous edges, and there is loss of muscle detail; the dog will resent palpation of the area. Acute injuries may be treated surgically. Chronic injuries have a distinct palpable defect, which has a fibrous periphery, in the muscle or fascia. These chronic injuries may result in low-grade pain and reduced performance. In my opinion, if they are clinically significant, they

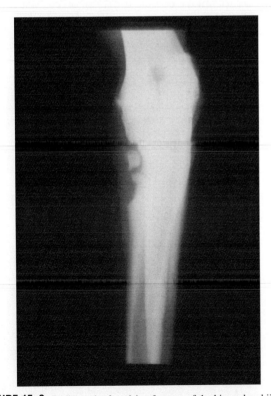

FIGURE 15–3. Radiograph of avulsion fracture of the biceps brachii insertion.

should be treated by surgical debridement of the fibrous scar and primary repair of the resulting defect. Injuries to the lateral lumbar muscles tend to present as "splits," which run parallel with the muscle fibers. These should be repaired surgically with fine absorbable sutures.

Ventral Abdominal Muscle Injuries

Small tears or gross disruption may occur in the origin or insertion of the ventral abdominal muscles. Injuries to the origin of the rectus abdominis or the external abdominal oblique are readily diagnosed on palpation; however, injuries to the insertion of the rectus abdominis, even those that involve gross disruption from the prepubic tendon, may be impossible to palpate because of the thick aponeurosis of the external abdominal oblique and the associated local swelling. The use of ultrasound will greatly aid in delineating the extent of these injuries. Once the muscle has avulsed from the prepubic tendon, both the repair and its postoperative protection are difficult, and the prognosis for full return to racing is poor. An injured external abdominal oblique is difficult to reattach because of the friable nature of the muscle and the diffuse nature of the tendon of attachment, but the prognosis is better for return to competitive racing.

MUSCLE INJURIES IN THE HIND LEG

Sartorius Muscle Injuries

Sartorius muscle injury usually involves tears in the muscle sheath, evidenced by deformation and pain on palpation. They are treated by physiotherapy with or without local acupuncture. It should be borne in mind that a branch of the lateral cutaneous femoral nerve crosses this muscle. Pain on direct palpation of this nerve should not be mistaken for injury to the muscle.

Tensor Fasciae Latae Injuries (TFL)

Injury to the TFL muscle often causes lameness in the racing dog. It may produce an area of spasm and extreme sensitivity on palpation, or the muscle may be ruptured. These ruptures can occur as (1) rupture of the origin, usually brought about by collision with some stationary object; (2) vertical splits along the line of the muscle fibers; (3) an avulsion injury involving the attachment to the fasciae latae. Misdiagnosis of injury to the TFL may result in development of a chronic muscle injury with scar formation and resultant loss of performance.

On clinical examination there is pain on extension of the hip joint. The muscle itself may be turgid and painful, or there may be a deficit on palpation. Injuries to the muscle belly are extremely painful, and it is not uncommon for a dog with such an injury to need a lameness evaluation. This lameness is brought about by either spasm or a small hematoma within the muscle belly. Muscle spasm is best treated by local acupuncture, which results in rapid reduction in the degree of pain and complete resolution within 24 hours. Reexamination can then be carried out to assess the degree of muscular injury. Occasionally a massive hematoma will develop after the muscle has ruptured, and the physical diagnosis must be presumptive and confirmed surgically.

Complete or partial avulsion injuries may be managed by either primary surgical repair or the use of 830-nm laser therapy with a power output of 30 mW. The early results using this latter technique appear to be superior to those for surgical repair. If an operation is chosen, the area is routinely prepared for aseptic surgery. A longitudinal incision is made directly over the area through the skin and subcutaneous fascia. Any hematoma is removed and the muscle

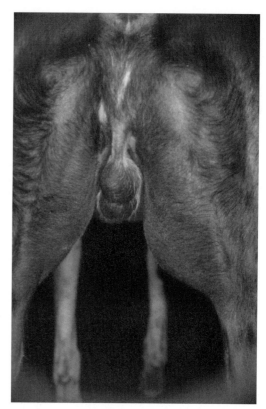

FIGURE 15–5. Ventral displacement of the origin of the gracilis muscle.

reattached to the fascia with a series of 2/0 polyglyconate "pulley" sutures. An attempt should be made to suture as much of the medial attachment of the muscle as possible. The sutures should not be placed into the vastus lateralis, as they will cause pain when the dog is exercised. This pain reaction will persist until the sutures break down, which in the case of polyglyconate sutures will be in about 6 to 8 weeks. The incision is closed routinely.

The dog is confined to leash exercise or a small yard for voiding purposes for 7 to 10 days, and then allowed increasing amounts of uncontrolled exercise over the next 4 to 6 weeks. It can then be returned to race training. The prognosis for TFL injuries is good, although there may be some loss of performance if the vastus has

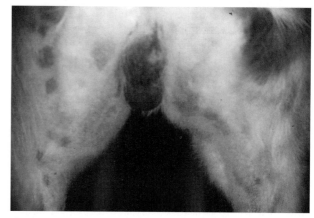

FIGURE 15–6. Dorsal displacement of the insertion of the gracilis muscle.

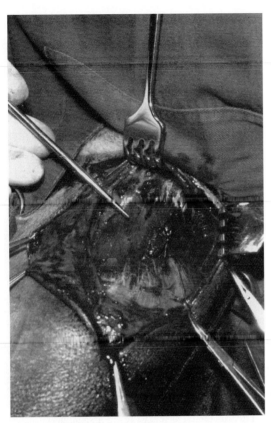

FIGURE 15–7. Ruptured gracilis origin.

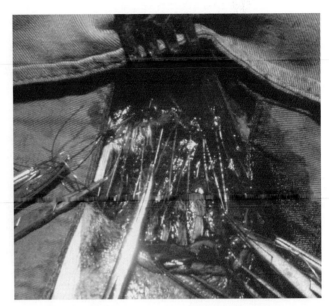

FIGURE 15–8. No. O Maxon sutures preplaced in origin.

been incorporated in the surgical repair or if the dog has not been adequately exercised during convalescence.

If laser therapy is to be used, an 830-nm, 30-mW laser acupuncture unit is necessary. The regimen consists of daily treatments locally for 10 to 14 days or until the hematoma has started to decrease; the frequency is then reduced to every second day for another 10 to 14 days and then to twice weekly for a further 10 to 14 days. The dog is allowed free galloping yard exercise during the treatment and then returned to normal race training. The decreased morbidity, the rapid return to race training, and the minimal scar tissue formation with this regimen have been encouraging.

Gracilis Muscle Injury ("Dropped Back Muscle")

Rupture of the gracilis muscle is the most common major muscle injury in the racing greyhound.[15] Gracilis muscle injury can occur at the muscular origin or the tendinous insertion in either hind leg. Unilateral injury is the most common; however, injury can occur bilaterally either concomitantly or in the previously unaffected leg when the dog is returned to work. The origin or insertion may be completely or partially injured. Partial injuries usually involve the posterior margin of the muscle. Dogs may injure both origins simultaneously. These injuries can be repaired surgically, and the dogs will return to racing; they will not, however, return to previous form.

A gracilis muscle injury usually involves either a race or a trial. The dog may have sustained an obvious injury or failed to perform to expectations. The diagnosis of gracilis muscle injury is based on careful clinical observation and palpation of the medial aspect of the thigh. With acute injury this will reveal an area of hemorrhage

and either ventral displacement of the origin (Fig. 15–5) or dorsal displacement of the insertion (Fig. 15–6). If the injury is not diagnosed at the track, the swelling and subcutaneous hemorrhage that make the injury more obvious become evident in 12 to 24 hours.

Surgical repair is the method of choice for dogs young enough and good enough to return to racing. The dog is placed in lateral recumbency with the injured leg down. Distraction of the upper leg allows the medial side of the affected leg to be prepared for aseptic surgery. A horizontal skin incision is made directly over the ruptured origin. The subcutaneous tissue is retracted to reveal the muscle injury (Fig. 15–7), and any hematoma or debris is removed.

Because of the friable nature of the muscular origin, five or six preplaced, near-far-far-near pulley sutures of 0/-polyglyconate are placed from the subpubic tendon to the muscle (Fig. 15–8) and progressively tightened to gradually overcome the natural muscle contraction (Fig. 15–9). In male dogs, care is necessary to ensure that the vascular pedicle of the testis is not included in the sutures. For insertion injuries, a longitudinal incision is made directly over the area and the subcutaneous tissue dissected to reveal the rupture

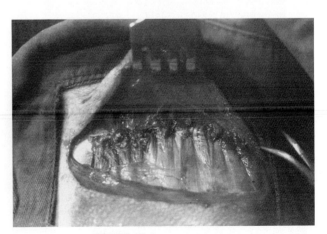

FIGURE 15–9. Sutures tightened.

(Fig. 15–10). The injury is repaired using a similar suture pattern in the muscle and its fascial attachment to the tibia (Figs. 15–11 and 15–12). Good hemostasis and careful approximation of the subcutaneous tissue is essential to prevent postoperative hematoma formation. The skin is closed routinely. Postoperative dressings for the insertion are difficult to apply but may be used.

Postoperatively the dogs are confined to a kennel for 5 to 7 days, being exercised on a leash for bladder emptying purposes three to four times daily. Dogs that are accustomed to a walking machine may begin this type of exercise for a short period (3 minutes twice a day) from day 5 for 7 to 10 days. If they are not used to this type of exercise, leash walking should be started on day 10 for 7 to 10 days. If at this time the repair feels satisfactory, the exercise is extended. Three weeks postoperatively the dogs are allowed free access to a short run, approximately 30 meters long, twice a day for 2 weeks. By 5 weeks following the operation the dogs are allowed into a long yard and encouraged to gallop freely for 2 more weeks. By this time they should be sufficiently conditioned to permit them to be returned to serious training. Using this regimen a dog can be expected to be back racing 10 to 12 weeks after repair.[16] In those dogs that do not begin regular controlled exercise soon after the operation, the rehabilitation period tends to be longer because of recurrent bouts of muscle pain and of re-injury. The prognosis for surgical repair is excellent with no loss of performance. A regimen of acupuncture similar to that used in TFL injuries has not been evaluated, but it may be a viable alternative to surgical repair.

The gracilis insertion has been depicted as a broad muscular band,[7] but this is not the case in the greyhound. There is a thin aponeurosis cranially and a thick tendon, approximately 1 cm wide, caudally that attaches to the medial aspect of the proximal tibia. Every effort should be made to repair this thick caudal portion. It has been suggested that the fascial aponeurosis from the posterior

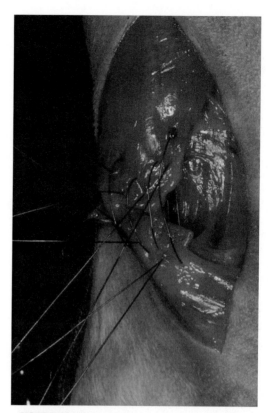

FIGURE 15–11. Preplaced sutures prior to tightening.

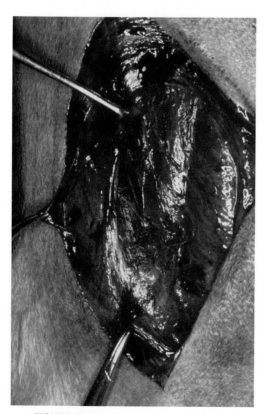

FIGURE 15–10. Ruptured tendon of insertion.

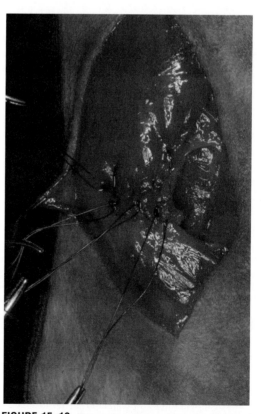

FIGURE 15–12. Sutures in tendon and insertion tightened.

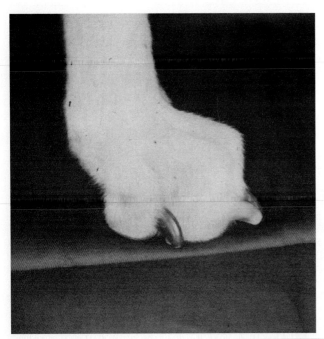

FIGURE 15–13. Characteristic flexion of the digits associated with injury to the gastrocnemius muscle.

aspect of the gracilis muscle is an important factor in the extension of the tarsus.[16] Clinical evaluation of greyhounds that rupture the tendon of insertion does not support this theory. Dogs treated conservatively did not experience problems with extension of the tarsus, nor did any of those treated surgically, when no attempt was made to reestablish this fascial attachment.[17]

Discussion

The exact etiology and predisposing factors, if any, surrounding major muscle injuries in the hind leg are not known. Sudden or excessive exercise in unfit dogs may be the cause in some cases. However, the majority of these muscle injuries occur in race-fit dogs. I have noticed that some dogs that abduct or swing a hind leg when racing or trialing may stop doing so if they sustain either a ruptured gracilis or tensor fasciae latae. This poses the question whether there may be some underlying musculoskeletal problem that is going undiagnosed. It has been stated that gracilis muscle injuries are secondary to a spinal mechanical fault rather than excess physical strain.[5] This concept is both thought provoking and difficult to substantiate.

Gastrocnemius Muscle and Tendon Injuries

Injuries to the muscular attachment and the musculotendinous junction and severance of the tendon of insertion all occur in the gastrocnemius muscle.

Injuries to the origin are usually evidenced by acute onset of lameness and severe pain on palpation of the posterior aspect of the stifle joint in the area of the muscular attachment. Injury to the musculotendinous portion of one or the other of the heads of the gastrocnemius muscle will result in marked loss of speed. Since the injury is usually only a partial rupture or injury to one belly of the muscle, the injury may be chronic by the time it is seen by the veterinarian. The dog usually has a history of marked loss in form with easing on the turns. Clinical examination may reveal thickening of the musculotendinous junction, although the thickness of the fascia may make detection of the injury and determination of its severity difficult. The characteristic sign of an injury to this area is the dropping of the hock and the flexion of the digits due to apparent shortening of the superficial digital flexor tendon. This is seen in both musculotendon and tendon injuries (Fig. 15–13). However, it does not usually occur with origin injuries.

References

1. Hill FWG: Muscle Injuries, Their Extent and Therapy in the Racing Greyhound. Post-Grad. Committee in Veterinary Science, University of Queensland, 34:298, 1972.
2. Davis PE: Examination of the greyhound for racing soundness. In Greyhounds Proceed. no. 64, Post-Grad. Committee Vet. Sci., University of Sydney, pp 601–671, 1983.
3. Davis PE: The diagnosis and treatment of muscle injuries in the racing greyhound. Aust Vet J 43:519–523, 1967.
4. Gilchrist DJ: Acupuncture as it applies to greyhound practice. In Greyhounds, Proceed. no 64, Post-Grad. Committee Vet. Sci., University of Sydney, pp 391–396, 1983.
5. Hauler AD: Aetiology of muscle injury. In Greyhounds Proceed. no. 64, Post-Grad. Committee Vet. Sci., University of Sydney, pp 407–413, 1983.
6. Gannon, JR: Some Aspects of Greyhound Practice. Proc Am Anim Hosp Assoc 49, 1974.
7. Evans HE, Christensen GC: Miller's Anatomy of the Dog, 2nd ed. Philadelphia, WB Saunders Company, 1993.
8. Craig E, Hohn RB, Anderson WD: Surgical stabilization of traumatic medial shoulder displacement. J Am Anim Hosp Assoc 16:92, 1980.
9. Goring RL, Parker RB, Dee L, Eaton-Wells RD: Medial displacement of the tendon of origin of the biceps brachii muscle in the racing greyhound. J Am Anim Hosp Assoc 20:933, 1984.
10. Fox SM, Bray JP: Surgical correction for rupture of the transverse humeral ligament in a racing greyhound. Aust Vet Practit 22:2–5, 1992.
11. Boemo CM, Eaton-Wells RD: Medial displacement of the tendon of origin of the biceps brachii muscle in 10 greyhounds. J Small Anim Pract 36:69–73, 1995.
12. Bennett D, Campbell JR: Unusual soft tissue problems in the dog. J Small Anim Pract 20:27, 1979.
13. Vaughan LC: Muscle and tendon injuries in dogs. J Small Anim Pract 20:717, 1979.
14. Brunnberg VL, Kostlin, RG, Waild H: Zue rupture des ligamentum transversum intertuberculare humen beim hund. Klientier Praxis. 26:257, 1981.
15. Vaughan LC: Gracilis muscle injury in greyhounds. J Small Anim Pract 10:363–375, 1969.
16. Frandson RD, Davis RW: "Dropped muscle" in the racing greyhound. J Am Vet Assoc 126:468–469, 1955.
17. Eaton-Wells RD: Surgical repair of acute gracilis muscle rupture in the racing greyhound. Vet Comp Orthop Trauma 5:18–21, 1992.

CHAPTER 16

INJURY AND DISEASES OF TENDONS

SIMON C. ROE

Tendons transfer shortening in muscles to more distal portions of the limb. To do this efficiently, tendons must be thin and strong, must resist lengthening, and be able to glide around joints. They also contribute to the efficiency of locomotion, particularly in the high-performance animal, by storing and subsequently releasing energy during the loading and unloading portions of the stride.

This chapter begins with a short review of the structure, function, and mechanics of tendons. It then presents the different mechanisms of injury and the healing response, with emphasis on recovery from strain injury. It concludes by addressing specific tendon injuries observed in the athletic dog, their diagnosis, and treatment alternatives.

STRUCTURE AND FUNCTION

Tendons begin inside the muscle belly to which they are attached. The fibrous backbone of muscle begins to coalesce as the tendon develops (Fig. 16–1A). The muscle cells are intimately attached to this foundation, and thus, as a contraction occurs, the shortening of these cells is transferred to the point of attachment of the tendon. In the upper portions of the limb, tendons are usually short, thick, or broad, flat structures termed *aponeuroses*. Distal in the limb, they tend to be long and thin. Muscle shortening is transferred to the far end of the limb while bulk is minimized. This results in a longer lever arm of action and more efficient use of the energy of contraction.

Tendons cross at least one joint to produce their effect. Because of the movement that occurs near their point of action and around the joints, tendons must glide relative to adjacent tissues. More distal portions are often encased in a sheath that contains a small amount of lubricating fluid. Annular ligaments hold the tendons close to the limb on the acute-angle side of joints.

On a microstructural level (Fig. 16–1B), tendon is primarily collagenous. Although present in many different sizes and shapes, tendons are consistently composed of highly organized, directionally arranged type 1 collagen. This molecule is a triple helix of a protein chain. After being produced by and extruded from a tenocyte, it forms longitudinal arrays in the extracellular space. A number of fibrils associate to produce a fiber. Fibers develop a waviness or crimp, which is important for storage of energy during initial loading. In addition to collagen, the tendon substance contains some proteoglycans, some elastin, and tenocytes.

The microstructure of tendon is altered at sites where it bends around a joint. Because the tendon experiences compression at the point of bend, there is partial transformation to a cartilaginous structure.[1] Proteoglycans in the extracellular matrix increase, and cells assume a more rounded chondrocytic morphology. This adaptation to compressive loads within a tendon also is thought to be the reason for the development of sesamoids. Important sesamoids in sporting dogs are the patella and those in the digital flexor tendons.

Macroscopically, tendon may have many forms. The classic structure involves the development of fascicles surrounded by loose fibrous tissue termed *endotendon* (Fig. 16–1C). Fascicles are packed together and contained within an outer thin fibrous layer—the *epitendon*. The vascular supply to tendon is often limited because movement of the tendon relative to the surrounding tissues prohibits extensive vascular bridging. Also, healthy tendon has little metabolic requirement. Primary sources of blood vessels are extensions from the muscle belly, from the point of insertion, and from the surrounding soft tissues. When the tendon is very mobile, vessels may enter via loose vincula within the sheaths. Vascular studies of canine digital flexor tendons have described portions that appear avascular and must receive nutrition via diffusion.[2]

The junction of the tendon to bone at the point of action is an important link in the mechanical system (Fig. 16–1D). The structure of this attachment is also specialized to provide a transition of tissue types from soft flexible tendon to hard rigid bone. The tendon flares as its outer sheath becomes continuous with the periosteum of the bone. Within the tendon substance, there is an increase in proteoglycans in the matrix and the cells appear more chondroid. This fibrocartilaginous zone then becomes mineralized and finally merges with the lamellae of the bone. Of note on examination of this junction microscopically is that collagen fibers beginning in the tendon can be identified intact across all zones, and even extending into the lamellae of the bone. This gradual transmission of tissue type may reduce concentration of stress at the junction of these two dissimilar materials.

MECHANICS OF TENDON

An appreciation of the way in which tendons respond to the loads that they must transfer is important to understanding tendon structure, function, and injury. The longitudinal arrangement and uniformity of collagen in tendon impart significant strength in tension while allowing flexibility in other directions. When a tendon is first loaded, there is a small amount of deformation (Fig. 16–2). Initially there is a less stiff region or toe region. Microscopically the crimp in the collagen molecule flattens out during this phase. As the collagen fibers resist elongation, tendon becomes more stiff and exhibits a mostly linear response. The response up to the yield point is elastic. If the load is removed, the tendon will resume its original length. Because the energy causing the elongation is efficiently stored in the collagen molecules, there is little hysteresis in the unloading curve. If the load event damages collagen molecules, the tendon begins to yield. This region of the curve is the plastic region, meaning that the tendon will have some permanent deformation after the load is removed. As the load increases, further deformation causes more damage, and failure usually occurs. It must be remembered that, in the body, neural feedback mechanisms will attempt to protect the tendon from these damaging loads.

exceeds the yield point. It must be recognized that there is a large safety factor built into tendon, and loads associated with normal physiological activities rarely extend beyond half of the elastic range. For injury to occur, either the load must be considerably in excess or the yield point of the tendon lowered. Although the former may occur and is quite catastrophic, the latter is of much more significance. Lowering of the yield point can occur by two mechanisms. Disease and other degenerative conditions can disrupt and disorganize the collagen arrangement. Of more significance in athletes is the progressive weakening of tendon from cumulative injury. Repeated high-frequency loading events may cause microfiber injury accumulation at a greater rate than can be dealt with by the repair mechanisms. The nature of tendon vasculature and the related weak response to injury are discussed in a subsequent section, but for the moment, the situation of repeated loading and compounding injury slowly lowers the yield, and failure loads of the structure must be appreciated.

High-load trauma resulting in tendon injury alone is unusual. This is because, in most instances, tendon can absorb energy more efficiently than either the muscle or bone elements of the system. Muscle tears or avulsion fractures may occur before complete failure of a tendon. It is, however, important to realize that a tendon may not be completely spared in this type of injury, and in treatment, associated incomplete disruption may need to be considered.

TENDON HEALING

Transection without Repair. Direct transection of a tendon results in separation of the ends owing to both shortening of the muscle and alteration of the range of motion. Trauma to the surrounding soft tissues and possibly tendon sheath results in their incorporation in the tendon's healing process. Because tendon and bone are both load-bearing tissues, there are many similarities to the healing cascade.[3] The structure that forms during healing may therefore be termed a *callus*. It begins as an area of profuse disorganized tissue doing its best to provide some strength and undergoes remodeling in an attempt to rebuild a functional, load-bearing unit.

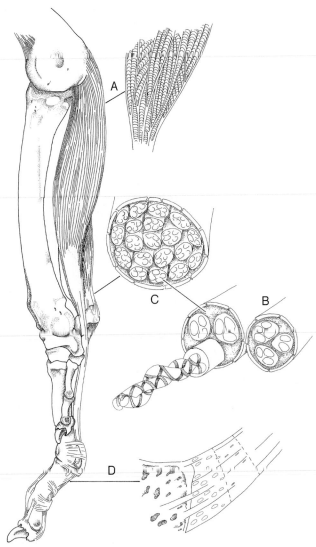

FIGURE 16–1. *A*, Musculotendinous junction. *B*, Tendon microstructure. *C*, Tendon macrostructure. *D*, Bone-tendon junction.

Two other mechanical factors must be considered when investigating how tendons behave under physiological loading. First, their stiffness and their failure load increase as the rate of loading increases. This characteristic is most beneficial to function in impact loading situations. Second, they are viscoelastic. If a load is applied and held on a tendon, it will gradually increase in length. This response progressively lessens as fluid and molecular rearrangement reach equilibrium. This type of loading occurs infrequently in nature. This viscoelastic tendency must be considered when evaluating how tendon responds when large loads are applied at high frequency, such as during racing or other prolonged athletic activities. Reduction of the viscoelastic response in tendon by frequent cycling produces a stiffer, stronger structure.

INJURY MECHANISMS

Direct trauma causing laceration either directly or via bone injury and subsequent associated soft tissue injury is the most obvious cause of tendon damage. The second mechanism of injury is strain. This damage occurs when the tensile load within the structure

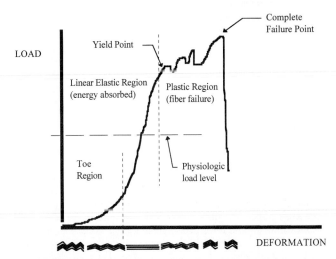

FIGURE 16–2. Graphic representation of the load vs deformation response of tendon. The state of the collagen fibers is depicted along the X axis. When unloaded, the collagen crimp and linear continuity are appreciated. As the tendon resists load, the crimp angle reduces. The stiffness of the tendon increases when the crimp is fully flattened. The response is linear in this elastic region. Yield begins as fibers break. Permanent elongation occurs in the plastic region. Complete tendon rupture soon follows.

The wound and gap fill with hematoma and the nonspecific healing cascade for fibrous tissues begins. Vascular and fibroblastic proliferation and invasion permit the formation of immature granulation tissue. As the clot is replaced and fibroplasia becomes more extensive, the gap between the retracted ends is filled with a disorganized collagen matrix. Type 3 collagen is initially deposited on the fibrinogen framework and is slowly replaced by stronger type 1 collagen. An important part of this replacement process is reorganization toward a tendon-like structure. It is believed that organization is induced by load being applied to the maturing scar by the tendon ends.[4] However, the loss of functional length of the muscle-tendon unit usually inhibits this, and the tissue filling the gap remains part of the wound scar. The ends become fixed to the scar and movement may be limited. It is unlikely that the tendon will be functional if some organized form does not develop.

Surgical Repair. Because this healing process rarely returns function to the musculotendinous unit, surgical repair is frequently warranted for fresh injuries that have resulted in gap formation. The aims of surgical and postoperative therapy are to restore function length, allow healing without stretching, and avoid development of adhesions that might limit range of motion of the tendon.

Early management of the wounds and debridement of damaged tissue helps control inflammation and limit the extensiveness of surrounding tissue involvement. Tendon ends should be identified. If there is little damage evident, primary suture may be considered. In crush wounds or when contamination or infection is present, it may be prudent to tag the tendon ends with nonabsorbable suture and delay repair. Once the wound environment is controlled and health and vascularity of involved tissues established, the tendon repair can be performed.

There are few rules in determining what suture to use and what pattern to place, but there are many exceptions. A few basic principles may be applied and adapted to specific situations. The suture material should slide easily through tissue. It should have good knot security and be nonirritant. In gliding tendons, soft braided suture, such as polyglycolic acid (Vicryl), may cause less irritation to the surrounding sheath than the less flexible monofilament types. The size of the suture is determined by the size of the structure and the density of the collagen. Because tendons may experience significant loads, the tendency is to select a large-diameter suture. However, a large suture may distort the tissue into which it is placed and not tie or loop appropriately. The strength of a repair is dictated first by the "hold" the suture has in the tendon end and then by the suture. It is often easier to obtain a secure hold with slightly smaller material and then gain more "suture" strength by placing additional strands across the repair. The decision to use an absorbable or nonabsorbable material requires consideration of the expected time until the tendon will regain sufficient strength from the healing process. The suture will be required to maintain strength of the repair for longer when the vascular supply to the tendon is poor, when the injury occurs in a gliding portion of a tendon, or when the load on the tendon is expected to be substantial throughout the healing period. As many of these factors frequently complicate tendon repair, nonabsorbable suture is often chosen.

Many suture patterns have been proposed to obtain the best strength of repair. It must be remembered that, while it is quite easy to draw a pattern on paper, creating that same pattern while placing a suture in tendon is much more difficult. Because tendon is so longitudinally arranged and the tissue between fascicles is weak, simple interrupted patterns tend to pull out easily. Because of the fragility of the tissue, the ends should be handled as little as possible. Taper-needle profiles will be sufficient in all but the most dense tendon and will cause less damage. A straight needle has some advantages for some of the patterns described below.

Patterns that pull fascicle bundles together achieve a good hold

but may squeeze the tendon and reduce the blood flow within its substance (Fig. 16–3A). The Bunnel and Bunnel-Mayer patterns are examples of this type. The Kessler pattern and its many modifications achieve hold of a tendon by forming loops that wrap around a small bundle of fascicles.[5] Both of these patterns may be placed by securing each end and tying two knots or, with materials that draw easily through the tendon, may be placed in a continuous pattern and have only one knot. In gliding tendons, the suture should be placed so that the knot is "inside" the tendon. Once the primary load-bearing suture is placed, a fine continuous or interrupted horizontal mattress suture may be placed in the epitendon to add some strength and minimize adhesion formation.

The three-loop pulley suture also has good strength in tendons when compared with a locking-loop pattern.[6] However, this is not unexpected as the three-loop pulley pattern results in six strands of suture material crossing the repair while the locking loop only has two.

Aponeuroses tend to be flat and thin. They usually are less longitudinally arranged and thus hold regular patterns more efficiently. Their thinness often requires that small-diameter suture be used, and therefore strength is gained by placing many strands across the disruption. Horizontal mattress and cruciate suture patterns hold well. I use a running continuous pattern that runs the length of the wound and then returns, overlapping the first run—sometimes termed a *baseball suture*—to repair the broad flat tendon of the deep gluteal muscle following craniolateral approach to the hip (Fig. 16–3B).

Disruption of the tendon from bone requires reattachment. A locking-loop or pulley-suture pattern is placed in the tendinous portion of the repair, and the suture ends lead through small tunnel(s) drilled through the bone (Fig. 16–4). Because these injuries often take a long time to gain strength and the suture may be subject to tearing on the bone edges, it is advisable to place more than one suture and to protect the repair with sutures from the epitendon to periosteum or surrounding soft tissues. This type of repair is often indicated at the attachment of the gastrocnemius tendon to the calcaneus. Because of the high loads expected, the repair may be augmented with synthetic materials or with fascia so that more immediate load bearing may be allowed without failure.

Although optimal suture and pattern selection will provide a strong repair, success is probably equally influenced by the postoperative care requested and provided. Bandage support is frequently employed in the first few weeks to reduce joint range of motion and tendon load. In major load-bearing tendons, such as the gastrocnemius, an external fixator is frequently selected to prevent overloading the repair. However, if the musculotendinous unit spans two joints, immobilizing just one joint may not protect the tendon completely.

Overactivity of the patient is the most likely reason for failure of tendon repairs. It may take only one loading incident—a quick twist, a slip, a lunge—to disrupt the most precise of repairs. Because of this, activity of patients undergoing tendon repair must be completely limited to minimize the opportunities for disaster. This is particularly difficult for tendon injuries, as reasonable strength may be attained in the first few weeks of healing and the patient appears clinically normal. However, it is important that the protracted time required for adequate strength to resist high loads be considered in all activity plans. It will take more than 12 weeks for dense, poorly vascularized tendon to be considered organized sufficiently for unrestrained active loading. Despite these concerns, some motion and some loading are beneficial to the healing process.[7] Fibroblasts of the forming callus align with tissue stress and deposit more organized collagen when stimulated by load. Adhesions from surrounding soft tissue must be stretched in the early healing period to maintain full range of motion. Physical therapy regimens should include application of heat followed by passive

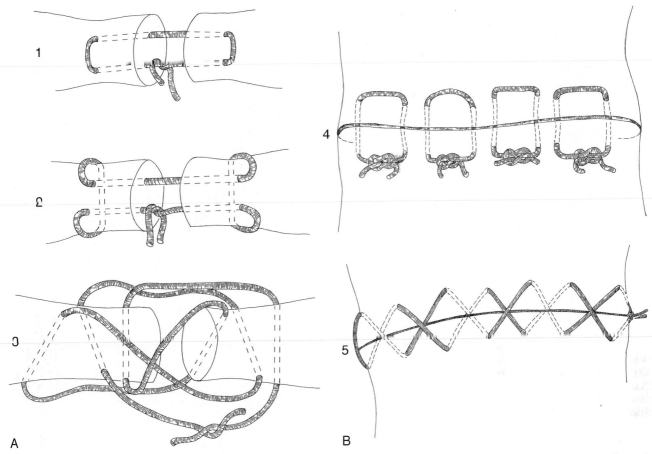

FIGURE 16–3. *A*, Suture patterns for thin, round tendons: 1. Bunnel-Mayer. 2. Locking loop. 3. Three-loop pulley. *B*, Suture patterns for tendon aponeuroses; 4. Horizontal mattress suture. 5. Baseball suture.

range-of-motion exercises. If the patient can be well controlled, walking may be instituted around 4 to 6 weeks after repair.

The most obvious indication of failure of a repair follows acute disruption and return of the impairment of function. However, failure may also be a much slower process. Sequential loss of purchase of sutures, or weakening of the suture material before healing is attained, may lead to a widening of the gap and compromise of function of the musculotendinous unit. If loading begins before the healed tissue is mature, the scar may stretch.

SHORTENING AND LENGTHENING

Tendon injury that was not treated initially, or in which treatment failed, will result in lengthening of the musculotendinous unit. In some instances, surgically shortening the tendon may reestablish function of the unit. It is best to excise the previously damaged portion of the tendon if possible so that the chances of further stretching are reduced. It the musculotendinous junction was the site of initial injury, shortening must usually be performed in the tendon and a guarded prognosis given because reinjury or continued stretching of the musculotendinous junction may recur.

Methods for shortening involve gathering the excess tendon with a suture, forcing a permanent fold in the tendon, or performing stepwise or segmental tenectomy. The tenectomy approaches are indicated in gliding tendon when extra bulk may inhibit function. Techniques that utilize all available tendon to strengthen the anastomosis are likely to be stronger. An approach used to shorten a chronically elongated gastrocnemius tendon is to transect the tendon the distance proximal to the calcaneus that will produce the required shortening. The distal stump is split and opened centrally and two small holes drilled through the calcaneus. One or two locking-loop sutures are placed in the proximal tendon end, and they are pulled through the bone tunnels and tied. The reflected distal tendon stumps are used to augment the repair by placing horizontal mattress sutures through both stumps and the proximal end. The stumps are very secure because they already have a mature junction with the calcaneus. They also provide good vascularity to the site of healing.

Lengthening of musculotendinous units with the aim of maintaining their function is rarely required. Most contracted and shortened tendons are associated with total loss of likely effectiveness of the unit. Incision to remove the restriction the shortened unit places on range of motion may be effective if followed by physical therapy to prevent healing in the same foreshortened position. Extensive disease may best be approached by total excision of the fibrotic tissue so that recurrence is less likely.

STRAIN INJURY

As discussed under mechanics of tendon, a single high load may damage fibers of a tendon (exceed the yield point) without any alteration in functional length. This single event will have little residual effect as long as the damaged fibers are repaired before another injurious load needs to be resisted. However, damage like

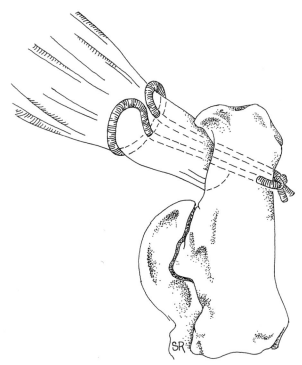

FIGURE 16–4. Reattachment of tendon avulsed from bone. The tendon is purchased with the required number of locking-loop sutures, and the ends are passed through bone tunnels at the point of tendon attachment.

this lowers the yield point for the tendon and makes it more susceptible to major injury. Important, then, in the consideration of the outcome of this type of injury is appreciation for the intrinsic ability of tendon to heal. In bone, "microcracking" may not stimulate a repair response, and cracks may be removed only during nonspecific remodeling.[8] It is unknown how much damage need occur for tenocytes to be able to sense the need for a response. A particular tendon's rate of turnover of collagen to produce removal of microfiber damage is also unknown. Because of the low metabolic activity and minimal blood supply, it is hypothesized that this process is very slow. It is therefore likely that the tendon is susceptible to cumulative injury. At some level of injury, a repair response will be stimulated. Vascular and cellular invasion lead to removal of damaged tissue and synthesis of new collagen. However, in most instances, this tissue is not as strong as, or is not well integrated into, the original structure. To account for this deficiency, extra matrix is often deposited, and thickening of the structure becomes apparent. To achieve strength, the immature, disorganized matrix must be remodeled and, as already pointed out, this process is very slow. As the injury heals, the tendon profile will slowly return to normal. It is important to realize that this process must be described in terms of months or even years, when high performance is expected.

Management of Strain Injury. In an active patient with a high threshold for pain and an enormous drive to perform, injury to a small number of fibers may cause little lameness or loss of performance. However, the scenario may be repeated many times, the number of compromised fibers increases, and the injured tendon becomes weaker and even more susceptible to catastrophic damage. In their more chronic form, mild strain injuries often cause periodic lameness that resolves with rest from strenuous activity. The site may be thickened and occasionally swollen. This too may fluctuate, depending on the current level of injury.

Strain injury at any stage is best treated with rest and time.[4] Any

events that injure the diseased tendon will inhibit the healing process. In humans, light work has been shown to be beneficial to maintain range of motion and stimulate the cells of the healing callus. However, it must be remembered that controlling veterinary patients, particularly competitive ones, is most difficult. Walking on a leash in an environment away from likely stimuli may be provided. Heat, stretching, and passive range of motion will promote healing while maintaining function. The most important realization for management of strain injury is that it will take a *long* time for the tendon to repair itself to a level that can sustain loads experienced in competition or vigorous play. A final point about tendon is that it must bear weight to remain healthy or to mature. If a tendon is completely immobilized, it will slowly atrophy. More vascular regions, such as the tendon-bone junction, appear affected first. Likewise, the fibrous callus that bridges a repaired tendon will not mature if it remains "unloaded." The need for controlled, light activity and the thin line that must be navigated to optimize healing become even more obvious.

SPECIFIC CONDITIONS

Contracture of the Infraspinatus Tendon. This condition occurs in working breeds, but the cause is unknown. It may be termed more correctly a combined muscle and tendon injury, as there is frequently significant fibrosis of the muscle belly.[9] The site that is dealt with to relieve the symptoms is the tendon, and thus it is discussed in this chapter. No specific age or breed predilection has been suggested. Most dogs have altered forelimb motion that may be confused with a limp but is usually not painful. Some dogs will have a previous history of being lame after heavy work but others will not. The condition is occasionally bilateral, although rarely are both limbs affected at the same time. The altered forelimb motion is quite characteristic. During the swing phase, there is outward rotation of the limb with the elbow adducted and the distal limb abducted. The carpus flips forward at the end of the swing phase. The length of the stride is short. Dogs may have difficulty going up stairs. Shoulder range of motion is limited. The humerus may deviate away from the body so that when the dog is in lateral recumbency with the affected leg uppermost, the forelimb cannot be lowered (Fig. 16–5). On palpation, the muscles around the shoulder are found to be atrophied, and the infraspinatus muscle may feel fibrotic. There is usually little pain.

Medical treatment and physical therapy are rarely attempted because surgical release of the fibrotic restriction is nearly always successful. A caudolateral approach to the shoulder is used to expose the fibrotic tissue that extends from behind the acromion to the greater tubercle. This tissue is transected until shoulder motion

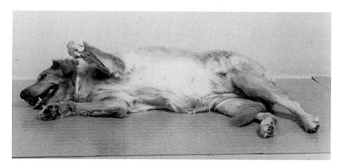

FIGURE 16–5. Golden retriever with contracture of the infraspinatus muscle. Because the fibrotic tendon, muscle, and lateral joint capsule restrict the dog's ability to adduct the distal limb, when this affected dog lay on its side, the foot remained suspended in the air.

returns to normal. In more advanced stages the joint capsule may need to be opened to complete remobilization. The fibrotic tissue can be removed to help prevent recurrence. Limited active therapy, such as walking, even in the first week after surgery will prevent the fibrous bridge from re-forming. Normal activity is allowed after 2 to 3 weeks. Prognosis for full recovery is excellent.

Tendinitis of the Origin of the Biceps Brachii. The tendon of origin of the biceps brachii muscle arises from the supraglenoid tubercle on the cranial "beak" of the scapula and runs through the shoulder joint space into a groove on the medial side of the greater tubercle of the humerus. It is surrounded by a sheath through this groove and is lubricated with synovial fluid. This bursal space around the tendon is continuous with the shoulder joint space.

Disease of the bursa and tendon in this area is identified mostly in middle-aged larger-breed dogs.[10, 11] Forelimb lameness is often gradual in onset. In the early stages, it may be evident only after hard work or play, similar to an arthritic condition. With increasing severity the lameness can become more persistent. Its presence without previous lameness is usually associated with exacerbation of subclinical changes. Affected dogs may have few findings on physical examination. Discomfort may be elicited by shoulder flexion, particularly while holding the elbow extended. The most frequent finding that suggests further investigation is tenderness or thickening or both on deep palpation on the medial side of the greater tubercle.

Early in the disease process no changes will be evident on plain radiographs. However, acute injury may involve avulsion of some or all of the supraglenoid process, with subsequent displacement of the fragment cranial and distal from the glenoid. Chronic injuries may or may not be associated with changes on plain radiographs. Osteophytes may develop around the tendon sheath and be evident as mineralized opacities "behind" the greater tubercle. High-contrast, good-quality images are necessary to distinguish these changes. Osteophytes may also alter the medial aspect of the greater tubercle on a craniocaudal projection. Enthesiophytes may be present on the supraglenoid tubercle from chronic strain injury of the tendon-bone junction. Extensive inflammation of the sheath may extend to the shoulder joint, involving it in the degenerative inflammatory process. Osteophytes may be present on the caudal lip of the glenoid and/or humeral head.

The next diagnostic step is to tap the bursa and/or shoulder for cytological examination of the synovial fluid. Evidence of inflammation or degenerative disease based on cell type and number may support the diagnosis. However, if the process is quiescent, subtle alterations of the cytological profile may be difficult to interpret. There may also be differences between the fluid from the bursa and the joint space if the process is confined. An arthrogram of the shoulder may assist in the diagnosis because it should highlight the structures of the extension of the joint capsule around the biceps tendon.[12] In the normal joint, contrast material filling this extension depicts a smooth outline of a sac that follows the line of the tendon and extends 1 to 2 cm distal from the tubercle. The diameter of the distal portion of the sac may be greater than the portion in the groove of the greater tubercle. The outline of the tendon is usually evident within the extension. With progressive proliferative changes of the bursa, there will be increasingly obvious filling defects and roughening of the bursal outline. The outline of the tendon may indicate thickening. With severe changes, the bursa may not fill. If the shoulder joint is also involved, synovial changes may be present throughout the joint.

Management of bicipital tendinitis varies with the chronicity and severity of the injury. Early in the process, a conservative approach may allow the tendon to heal and the bursal inflammation to resolve. Activity must be strictly limited and controlled. As already mentioned, enforcing such a regimen in an energetic, excitable working dog may be very difficult. The length of time of restriction must be based on an appreciation of the extent of damage in the tendon and the anticipated healing time. Even minor injury may take 2 to 3 months to repair. The difficulty of convincing both owner and patient that this length of time is necessary is exacerbated by the fact that any limp or discomfort often resolves in the first few weeks. It is important to convey the necessity for prolonged protection of injured tendon that has "clinically" healed. A single jump from an excited patient may disrupt the immature healing tissue and restimulate the inflammatory process in the bursa.

When the bursitis/tendinitis is more chronic, intrabursal injection of a long-acting corticosteroid may reduce the inflammatory process.[10] It is very important that this procedure be performed with strict attention to asepsis and absolute compliance with activity restriction instructions. Clinical response to the corticosteroids is usually quick and often complete. The corticosteroids may reduce the intensity of the healing response within the tendon, and therefore an even longer confinement period may be indicated.

Severe changes in the tendon and sheath may not be able to resolve sufficiently to eliminate clinical lameness or allow the tendon to heal sufficiently so that reinjury can be avoided. If a patient does not respond to more conservative therapy and there is evidence of severe changes in the bicipital groove, the tendon may be surgically entrapped just distal to the groove. Techniques describe both leaving the tendon attached to the scapula (to ensure shoulder stability) and excising the diseased tendon from its origin and redirecting it through a bone tunnel in the greater tubercle to establish a biological attachment for the biceps.[11]

Luxation of the Biceps Brachii Tendon. The tendon of origin of the biceps brachii muscle courses through a groove on the medial side of the greater tubercle. Injury to the transverse ligament that holds the tendon in place may allow luxation. It is thought that the transverse ligament is usually diseased and bursitis is present around the tendon and within the groove. The presentation is similar to that of bicipital bursitis/tendinitis (see above). There is mild chronic lameness, discomfort on flexion and/or extension of the shoulder, and tenderness on deep palpation of the medial area of the greater tubercle. Diagnosis is made by palpation of the luxation event as the shoulder is flexed or externally rotated.[13]

Although restriction of activity may be sufficient to achieve resolution of the lameness in nonworking dogs, if strenuous activity is required, surgical reinstatement of the transverse restraint for the tendon is indicated. Also, the depth of the groove for the tendon should be assessed and the groove deepened if necessary. A number of techniques are available for confining the tendon to the groove. A screw on either side of the groove and either nonabsorbable monofilament suture or wire connecting them is a simple method. Short bone plates and wire staples have also been used. The prognosis for return of function may relate most to the degree of bursitis/tendinitis present. In athletic animals, the chance of returning to competitive work without a great deal of careful physical therapy is fair.

Rupture of the Insertion of the Biceps Brachii Tendon. The biceps brachii tendon inserts on the proximocranial aspect of the radius. Rupture of this tendon has been identified in racing greyhounds.[14] Affected dogs have mild forelimb lameness at the walk. There may be local tenderness and pain when the elbow is extended while holding the shoulder flexed. Elbow range of motion with the shoulder flexed may also be increased. The injury is managed by surgical repair or reattachment, depending on the level involved (Fig. 16–6). The limb should be immobilized in a spica splint for 2 to 3 weeks to protect the repair and activity strictly limited for a further 4 to 6 weeks to allow maturation.

Injury to the Insertion of the Flexor Carpi Ulnaris. The flexor carpi ulnaris muscle inserts onto the accessory carpal bone via tendons from its humeral and ulnar heads. Stretching of these

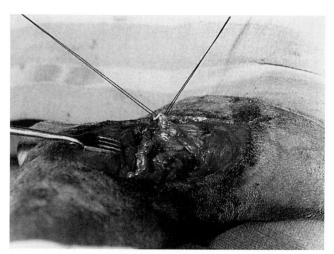

FIGURE 16–6. Intraoperative photograph of a ruptured biceps tendon of insertion in a greyhound being repaired with a locking-loop pattern.

tendons can occur if a partial strain injury is followed by continued activity and inadequate rest. Avulsion of the insertions can occur with acute overextension with lateral stress. Surgical management consists of techniques similar to those already described for severance of a tendon from bone.[14]

A syndrome involving injury to the palmar retinaculum of the accessory carpal bone may be confused with injury to the tendons of the flexor carpi ulnaris. Deep palpation just below the accessory carpal bone will reveal a horizontal tear in these retinacular tissues. This tear can be repaired via a palmar approach. A ''cruciate'' or baseball pattern using a nonabsorbable monofilament suture material is usually chosen for repair (see Fig. 16–3*B*). The carpus should be splinted in flexion for 2 to 3 weeks and activity restricted for 6 weeks.

Stretching of the Flexor Tendons. For pups to maintain normal conformation, their bones, muscle, and tendons must develop simultaneously. Stretching of the flexor tendons occurs in large-breed dogs while they are in their most active growth phase. They begin by developing ''flat'' feet as the deep and superficial flexors are often first involved. This may progress to hyperextension of the carpi, and occasionally, the hindlimbs may also collapse. The origin of this disorder is unknown. Theories based on some abnormality of the collagen molecules produced by tenocytes as tendon lengthens often incriminate nutritional imbalances that alter enzyme activity or the cross-linking process. Essential minerals and trace elements may be involved because they are often important cofactors for normal enzyme function. Management of these pups involves ensuring a balanced diet and splinting. Support is removed after 2 to 3 weeks and activity slowly increased over the next 2 weeks. Prognosis is good.

An entirely different pathophysiology is present when stretching of the superficial digital flexor tendons is seen in the elite canine athlete.[14] Repeated strain injury following the very high loads of competition and training results in chronic inflammation as the tendon attempts to heal. Elongation of the tendon structure may alter toe conformation. This syndrome is termed *bowed tendons* and has some similarities to the same condition in the equine athlete. Discomfort from the chronic injury causes a decrease in performance. Resection of the damaged portion of the tendon aims at reducing the discomfort. This will result in a ''flat toe'' at the proximal interphalangeal joint, which appears to have little clinical significance.

Laceration of the Superficial and Deep Flexor Tendons. Lac-

eration of the palmar or plantar aspect of the foot, usually in the region of the metacarpal or metatarsal pad, may involve the flexor tendons. This type of trauma occurs when the foot lands in a hole with a sharp back edge. An open can or broken glass bottle is often implicated. These lacerations are also dramatic, because bleeding from severed arteries may be profuse and difficult to control.

Involvement of the flexors in the injury is assessed by observation of digit carriage and range of motion. If the superficial extension is damaged, the P1–P2 joint will be ''dropped'' and have a greater degree of flexion on manipulation. If the deep flexor is also involved, the toenail will be well off the ground, because of inability to flex P2–P3. The joint may also have increased extension on palpation.

The wound should be cleaned and lavaged vigorously. The source of bleeding should be identified and the vessels ligated. If tendon damage is suspected, the tendon should be explored. If laceration has occurred, the ends will have retracted, and the wound will usually need to be opened to retrieve them. If the wound is fresh and able to be cleaned, primary repair may be performed. If there is contamination or infection, the ends may be tagged and repair performed once the wound is healthy.

Repair techniques for thin round tendons are described in the earlier section on Surgical Repair. The tendon ends are often difficult to handle, and passing a needle frequently causes splitting and fraying. A pattern that buries the knot inside the repair may be beneficial to reduce adhesions and sheath irritation. Because the repair is not strong, the foot should be bandaged in flexion for 2 to 3 weeks and weight bearing avoided. This may be followed by another 2 to 3 weeks of bandage support in a normal position. Once bandage support is removed, activity should be increased gradually.

Avulsion of the Long Digital Extensor Tendon. The long digital extensor muscle originates via a tendon attached to the lateral aspect of the lateral femoral condyle, just cranial to the origin of the lateral collateral ligament. After a short intra-articular course and passing through a groove on the craniolateral aspect of the tibial plateau, the tendon joins the muscle belly on the lateral aspect of the cranial tibia.

Avulsion of the tendon from the femoral condyle occurs mostly in young large-breed dogs. Most patients have chronic lameness. The stifle is often painful, and there is a lateral swelling. Radiographs may assist the diagnosis, as a bone fragment frequently remains attached to the tendon.

Reattachment of the avulsed fragment with either K-wires or a screw and washer reestablishes the origin. In chronic cases in which the fragment cannot be returned to its location on the femur, the intra-articular portion of the tendon (including the bone fragment) is excised and the remaining portion secured to the proximal tibia with screw and washer, suture, or a staple. Stifle flexion should be limited by maintaining a splint or bandage for 2 to 3 weeks. Activity should continue to be restricted for a further 4 to 6 weeks. The prognosis for normal function is good.

Injury of the Achilles Mechanism. The primary tendon of the Achilles mechanism extends from the gastrocnemius muscle to the calcaneus. Contributions are also received from the biceps femoris, semitendinosus, and gracilis muscles. The superficial digital flexor tendon also runs with these tendons but continues beyond the calcaneus. These tendons may be severed by direct trauma or be involved in varying degrees of strain injury.

Complete severance results in inability to maintain hock extension while bearing weight. The plantar aspect of the pes may contact the ground. If the superficial digital flexor is intact, the digits may still appear flexed. Surgical repair is necessary to restore function. General techniques are described earlier in this chapter. Because of the load borne by the gastrocnemius tendon, a strong repair is necessary. The repair is protected by preventing hock flexion. Because of the difficulty in maintaining a splint for the required healing time, a bilateral external fixator is often used to maintain the hock in extension. The small size of the bones distal to the tibiotarsal joint may complicate the placement of pins. One approach is to use a positive profile center-threaded pin in the proximal calcaneus and one in the mid to distal tibia. Predrilling will reduce the damage to the calcaneus. Another approach is to place two distal pins in the metatarsals and bridge the joint with either curved bars or with straight bars from one tibial pin to one metatarsal pin. In very small dogs, a screw from the calcaneus into the distal tibia may be adequate. Activity must be strictly limited, even with this solid fixation, because premature pin loosening may occur. Also, the gastrocnemius muscle has some role in assisting stifle flexion, and so load within the tendon is not completely eliminated by limiting only the hock.

Strain injury of the Achilles mechanism generally involves the gastrocnemius apparatus. It should be remembered that injury may occur anywhere from the origin to the insertion. Avulsion of the head of the gastrocnemius muscle from the distal femur may mimic lower tendon injury, although hock dysfunction is generally less, because usually only one head of the muscle is involved. On plain radiographs, one of the fabellae is displaced distal from the femur. Fracture of this sesamoid is frequently seen. Surgical reattachment to the femur using heavy monofilament suture or wire anchored around the fabellar fragment and through holes in the supracondylar tubercle of the femur is generally successful.[15]

Musculotendinous junction tears result in collapse of the hock. Frequently the site of damage is painful on deep palpation. Acutely, swelling may be evident and, more chronically, fibrosis and thickening can usually be palpated. Surgical repair requires anchoring sutures in the tendon bulk and passing them up through the muscle belly. A button or similar stent may be used to prevent the suture from cutting through the soft muscle. If a muscle tear is chronic and the gastrocnemius apparatus functionally lengthened, it may be easier and safer to shorten the gastrocnemius tendon with the hope that the musculotendinous junction will remain intact.

Strain injury of the tendinous portion is a more common injury in working and sporting dogs. The tendon and the tendon-bone junction may be involved. This site is more likely to sustain injury from repeated high-level loading because of its limited vasculature and healing capacity. Mild strain will cause lameness, particularly after heavy work. The tendon or area around the proximal calcaneus may be swollen and slightly painful to deep palpation. There will be no change in hock angle. From this point, the injury may heal if loading does not damage the repair tissue or other partially injured fibers. Even if healing proceeds as fast as possible, the area will often remain thickened for months as the tendon inflammation resolves and the early repair tissue is remodeled. Light physical therapy and heat may assist healing.

If the injured and healing tissues are overloaded, the percentage of damaged tendon increases. The eventual end result is complete disruption. Surgical intervention then becomes necessary. Techniques are similar to those described above for severance.[16]

Luxation of the Superficial Digital Flexor Tendon from the Calcaneus. The superficial digital flexor tendon meets the tendon of the gastrocnemius muscle on its deep surface and wraps around its lateral aspect to course over the top of the calcaneus before continuing to the foot. The tendon is held on the top of the calcaneus by a firm retinaculum that is continuous with the periosteum. A bursa is present between the tendon and the bone.

Luxation has been reported to occur in both medial and lateral directions,[17] but based on the anatomy of the region and the forces involved, lateral luxation is considered more likely. Reinke and Mughannam[18] describe a series of 12 cases, all of which involved

lateral displacement. Luxation occurs when the medial retinacular support tears. The tendon displaces the lateral aspect of the calcaneus. It is prevented from dropping completely by the lateral retinacular attachments. The injury usually occurs in association with vigorous activity. Affected dogs may be slightly dropped in the hock. They have mild lameness that worsens with exercise. On physical examination, the area around the calcaneus is thickened. Careful palpation is necessary to differentiate this situation from partial gastrocnemius tendon damage. The tendon may be felt in its abnormal location and can often be returned to the correct position if the process is not chronic. The area is not usually painful. Replacement of the tendon to its normal position and surgical repair of the torn retinaculum carry an excellent prognosis. Monofilament suture in a horizontal mattress or interrupted pattern is used. The repair is protected by a firm, soft, padded bandage that extends above the stifle for 2 to 3 weeks. A further 4 to 6 weeks of activity limitation is suggested to allow maturation of the healing tissue.

References

1. Vogel KG, Ordog A, Pogany G, Olah J: Proteoglycans in the compressed region of human tibialis posterior tendon and in ligaments. J Orthop Res 11:68–77, 1993.
2. Gelberman RH, Khabie V, Cahill CJ: The revascularization of healing flexor tendons in the digital sheath: A vascular injection study in dogs. J Bone Joint Surg 73-A:868–881, 1991.
3. Peacock EE, Van Winkle WV: Surgery and Biology of Wound Repair, 3rd ed. Philadelphia, WB Saunders Company, 1984.
4. Gelberman RH, Goldberg V, An KN, Banes A: Tendon. In Woo SL-Y, Buckwalter JA (eds): Injury And Repair of the Musculoskeletal Soft Tissues. Park Ridge, Ill, AAOS, 1988.
5. Tomlinson J, Moore R: Locking loop tendon suture use in repair of five calcaneal tendons. Vet Surg 3:105–109, 1982.
6. Berg RJ, Egger EL: In vitro comparison of the three loop pulley and locking loop suture patterns for repair of canine weightbearing tendons and collateral ligaments. Vet Surg 15:107–110, 1986.
7. Gelberman RH, Woo SL-Y, Lothringer K, et al: Effects of early intermittent passive mobilization on healing canine flexor tendons. J Hand Surg 7:170–175, 1983.
8. Lanyon LE: Mechanical function and bone remodeling. In Sumner-Smith G (ed): Bone in Clinical Orthopaedics. Philadelphia, WB Saunders Company, 1982, p 273.
9. Pettit GD: Studies on the pathophysiology of infraspinatus muscle contracture in the dog. Vet Surg 7:8–11, 1978.
10. Lincoln JD, Potter K: Tenosynovitis of the biceps brachii tendon in dogs. J Am Anim Hosp Assoc 20:385–392, 1984.
11. Stobie D, Wallace LJ, Lipowitz AL, et al: Chronic bicipital tenosynovitis in dogs: 29 cases (1985–1992). JAVMA 207:201–207, 1995.
12. Barthez PY, Morgan JP: Bicipital tenosynovitis in the dog—Evaluation with positive contrast arthrography. Vet Rad Ultrasound 34:325–330, 1993.
13. Goring RL, Parker RB, Dee L: Medial displacement of the tendon of origin of the biceps brachii muscle in the racing greyhound. J Am Anim Hosp Assoc 20:933–938, 1984.
14. Dee JF, Dee LG, Eaton-Wells RD: Injuries in high performance dogs. In Whittick WG (ed): Canine Orthopedics, 2nd ed. Philadelphia, Lea & Febiger, 1974.
15. Reinke JD, Kus SP, Owens JM: Traumatic avulsion of the lateral head of the gastrocnemius and superficial digital flexor muscles in the dog. J Am Anim Hosp Assoc 18:252–256, 1982.
16. Reinke JD, Mughannam AJ, Owens JM: Avulsion of the gastrocnemius tendon in 11 dogs. J Am Anim Hosp Assoc 29:410–418, 1993.
17. Milton JL, Henderson RA: Surgery of muscles and tendons. In Bojarb MJ (ed): Current Techniques In Small Animal Surgery, 2nd ed. Philadelphia, Lea & Febiger, 1983.
18. Reinke JD, Mughannam AJ: Lateral luxation of the superficial digital flexor tendon in 12 dogs. J Am Anim Hosp Assoc 29:303–309, 1993.

CHAPTER 17

CARPAL INJURIES

KENNETH A. JOHNSON

Anatomy. The carpus is a relatively complex, three-level hinge joint that is quite important in shock absorption. The seven major bones of the carpus are arranged in proximal (radial, ulnar, and accessory carpal bones) and distal (first to fourth carpal bones) rows[1, 2] (Fig. 17–1). The antebrachiocarpal joint is between the distal end of the radius and ulna and the proximal row of carpal bones. The middle carpal joint is between the proximal and distal rows of carpal bones. The carpometacarpal joint is between the distal row and the metacarpus. A thick palmar fibrocartilage attaches to the palmar aspect of the carpal bones and the metacarpal bones. Together with numerous individual ligaments, these structures provide significant support and stability for the carpus during weight bearing. Normally 70 per cent of carpal motion is at the antebrachiocarpal joint, 25 per cent is at the middle carpal joint, and 5 per cent is at the carpometacarpal joint.[3]

Injury. Diagnosis and surgical correction of carpal injuries can be demanding because of the relative complexity of this articulation. Types of injuries to the carpus include sprain, fracture, hyperextension, luxation, open fracture, and shearing injury. Each of these can potentially result in osteoarthritis, especially when they go undetected or untreated. Carpal injuries are common in racing greyhounds, and a serious carpal injury may be career ending. One survey of racing greyhounds in the United Kingdom found that 11 per cent of a total of 786 injuries occurred in the carpus.[4] The right carpus is more frequently injured than the left.[4, 5] In the survey by Prole,[4] 78 per cent of the carpal injuries were diagnosed as unspecified sprains and 14 per cent as accessory carpal bone fracture.

Palpation of the joint to detect swelling, sensitivity, crepitus, instability, and decreased range of motion, combined with routine and stressed radiographs, provides most of the information needed to make a diagnosis of carpal injury.[6] The following descriptions of sprains, luxations, and fractures deal with specific repair techniques for each injury. However, it must be appreciated when planning treatment that carpal fractures are frequently complicated by ligamentous injury and subluxation, which may affect prognosis adversely.

SPRAINS AND DISLOCATIONS

Ligament Injury

Carpal ligaments and the palmar fibrocartilage seem to be at relatively high risk for injury, as carpal ligament injuries are perhaps more common than carpal fractures and other injuries. Injury to a ligament is defined as a sprain. Sprain injury may either disrupt the midsubstance of the ligament fibers or disrupt its insertions into bone.[7]

An insertion of ligament into bone (enthesis) is a highly specialized junction, with four distinct zones: ligament, fibrocartilage, mineralized fibrocartilage, bone.[8, 9] Injuries at this junction can vary in severity from mild perturbations at the cellular and collagen matrix level to complete disruptions. A single excessive force (as in a sports injury) or chronic repetitive trauma to a ligament insertion, without gross disruption, causes a localized cycle of injury, inflammation, and repair.[10] One common outcome is that fibrocartilage at the insertion undergoes endochondral ossification, resulting in localized deposition of new bone at and around the ligament insertion.[10] This may be visible radiographically as a bone spur. Called enthesophytes[9] (Greek *enthesis* = insertion; Greek *phyte* = plant), these bony excrescences are different and distinct from osteophytes. Osteophytes are the chondro-osseous proliferations formed at the junction between articular cartilage and synovial membrane in osteoarthritis and other joint diseases. The radiological finding of enthesophytes in the vicinity of ligamentous insertions is generally indicative of chronic traumatic injury.

Complete disruption of insertions occurs most commonly at a site adjacent to the actual enthesis, either through the substance of the ligament or by avulsion fracture of a piece of bone containing the ligamentous insertion.[10] Radiographically these fracture fragments may appear to be inconsequential bone chips. In fact, they are frequently a sign of serious bone-ligament injury that may be accompanied by joint instability and subluxation.

Midsubstance ligamentous injuries have been arbitrarily graded into three degrees of severity.[7] Grade 1 (mild) sprain is overstretching of the tissue without disruption. Although the ligament is grossly intact, microscopically there is hemorrhage, and tearing and stretching of collagen fibers. Grade 2 (moderate) sprain is partial ligament rupture. Although ligament continuity is grossly maintained, strength is greatly reduced. Grade 3 (severe) sprain is complete disruption of all collagen fibers. A diagnosis of sprain injury is based on the finding of pain and inflammation in the region of the ligament, and perhaps palpable joint instability. Grades 1 and 2 sprains can be difficult to diagnose by physical examination because joint instability is minimal. However, magnetic resonance is a sensitive, noninvasive method for imaging these soft tissue injuries, and it is likely to become more widely used in diagnosis. Grade 3 injuries allow fairly obvious joint instability. In these cases, stressed radiology is usually successful in demonstrating subluxation, with increased width of joint space and an alteration in relationship of joint surfaces, relative to one another.[6]

Principles of Ligament Repair

Midsubstance ruptures of ligament heal by fibroplasia, remodeling, and maturation.[7] Healing ligaments are quite weak and regain only about 60 per cent of normal tensile strength after 1 year.[7] Also, gap formation between the ruptured ends results in considerable elongation of the healed ligament. With time, remodeling may return the ligament to normal length.[10] However, ruptured palmar carpal ligaments are under constant load during weight bearing, and there is potential for persistent elongation or further disruption, permitting chronic subluxation. Primary repair of ruptured palmar

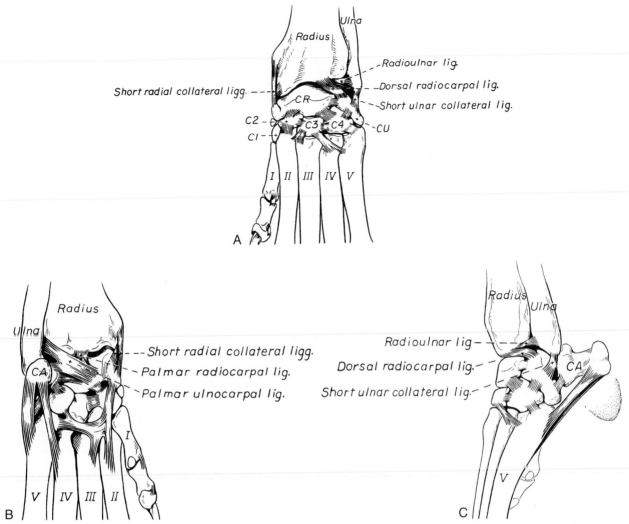

FIGURE 17–1. Dorsal (A), palmar (B), and lateral (C) aspects of canine left carpus illustrating bones and ligaments. CA = accessory carpal; CR = radial carpal; CU = ulnar carpal; C1 to C4 = first, second, third, and fourth carpals; I to V = metacarpals. (From Evans HE: Miller's Anatomy of the Dog. 3rd ed. Philadelphia, WB Saunders Company, 1993, pp 239–243.)

carpal ligaments with sutures is not feasible, as the palmar ligaments are small, numerous, and relatively inaccessible for surgery.

Collateral ligament disruptions are repaired by suturing with nylon in a modified locking loop or three-loop pulley suture pattern, or by autologous tissue grafting with fascia or tendon.[11–14] Sprain-avulsion fractures potentially have the best prognosis for healing, with complete functional restoration of ligament integrity. Provided that the fractured fragments are not multiply fragmented or too small, open reduction and internal fixation with small-diameter lag screws or pin and tension band wire are indicated. These fractures heal within 2 to 4 months, restoring ligament integrity.

Short Radial Collateral Ligament Sprain

The medial side of the antebrachiocarpal joint is stabilized by the short radial collateral ligament, which is composed of two parts[1] (Fig. 17–1). The straight part is orientated in an axial direction, and it runs from the tubercle that is proximal to the radial styloid process, distally to the most medial part of the radial carpal bone. It primarily provides stability while the joint is in extension. The oblique part of the ligament lies deep to the long part. It runs from the radial styloid process, obliquely to the palmaro-medial surface

of the radial carpal bone. The abductor pollicis longus tendon, which crosses the medial styloid process of the radius within a groove, passes between the two parts of the short radial collateral ligament.[1] A sesamoid bone within this tendon may be appreciated radiographically and should not be mistaken for a fracture.

Rupture of the short radial collateral ligament results in medial joint instability and later secondary osteoarthritis. Because the paw is normally in 5 to 10 degrees of valgus, weight bearing on the limb tends to open the medial side of the joint in case of ligament rupture.[11] Acute isolated ruptures of this ligament should be repaired with sutures, although the initial strength of the sutured ligament will be low. Therefore the repair is buttressed with an additional suture of nonabsorbable material placed in a figure-of-eight pattern, through three bone tunnels to replicate the action of the two parts of the ligament[11] (Fig. 17–2). Use of autologous tissue grafts derived from the abductor pollicis longus or flexor carpi radialis tendons, to replace the short radial collateral ligament, is reported to be successful.[12, 13] Tendon grafts are placed through body tunnels, similar to the suture technique.

In antebrachiocarpal luxation, the palmar carpal ligaments as well as the short radial collateral ligaments are likely to be disrupted. Primary repair of the short radial collateral ligament alone

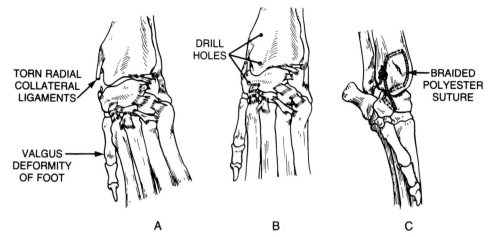

TORN RADIAL
COLLATERAL
LIGAMENTS

VALGUS
DEFORMITY
OF FOOT

DRILL
HOLES

BRAIDED
POLYESTER
SUTURE

A   B   C

FIGURE 17–2. Subluxation of the antebrachiocarpal joint resulting from tearing of the short radial collateral ligament. *A,* Valgus deformity of the foot develops from medial instability. *B* and *C,* Synthetic nonabsorbable suture is threaded through three bone tunnels placed in the radial carpal bone and radius to simulate both the straight and oblique parts of the short radial collateral ligament. An attempt also is made to suture the disrupted ligaments. (From Brinker WO, Piermattei DL, Flo GL: Handbook of Small Animal Orthopaedics and Fracture Treatment. 2nd ed. Philadelphia, WB Saunders Company, 1990.)

will not prevent antebrachiocarpal instability and hyperextension, and pancarpal arthrodesis is indicated. This procedure is described later in this chapter.

Enthesophytes formed on the craniomedial surface of the radius, proximal to the styloid process, are indicative of chronic sprain injury of the short radial collateral ligament (Fig. 17–3). These bony proliferations, at the proximal insertions of both parts of the ligament, accentuate the radiographic visibility of the groove in between containing the abductor pollicis longus tendon. These lesions may occasionally be bilateral and have accompanying radiographic signs of chronic joint instability and osteoarthritis. Some dogs have carpal pain and mild lameness, while other dogs are

apparently asymptomatic, and the full clinical significance of these abnormalities is not well understood. In young dogs these exostoses are considered by some to be a form of osteochondroma.[15]

Short Ulnar Collateral Ligament Sprain

Rupture of the short ulnar collateral ligament allows varus subluxation of the antebrachiocarpal joint when this joint is in slight flexion. In extension, the intact palmar ulnocarpal ligament prevents joint instability. One greyhound that had sustained this injury during a race also had rupture of the antebrachiocarpal joint capsule and the dorsal radiocarpal ligament.[14] Repair of the ruptured short ulnar collateral ligament was augmented with a strip of the dorsal one third of ulnaris lateralis tendon.[12] The distal insertion of the tendon graft was preserved, and the graft was passed transversely through a 2-mm drill hole in the ulnar styloid and sutured back upon itself distally. This procedure immediately restored joint stability, and the dog became sound but did not return to competitive racing.[14]

Radial Carpal Bone Luxation

Luxation of the radial carpal bone is a rare injury that is usually sustained as a result of jumping, falling from a height, or running on uneven terrain. Approximately half the reported cases have been in collie-type dogs, some of which were working or agility trial dogs.[16, 17] Immediately following the injury, the carpus is very painful, swollen, and relatively immobile in a straight extended position. Palpation may detect crepitus, medial instability, and a depression in the proximal row of the carpus, where the radial carpal bone is normally located.

The radial carpal bone is invariably luxated in a palmaro-medial direction (Fig. 17–4). It is rotated by 90 degrees around both the dorsopalmar and mediolateral axes, such that the proximal articular surface of the bone faces palmarly and medially.[16] In a study of four cases, it was found that the short radial collateral ligament and dorsal joint capsule were always ruptured as well.[16] However, the palmar ligament connecting the radial carpal bone to the second and third metacarpal bones was intact, and the bone had rotated around this ligament. In conjunction with the luxation, some cases also have a fracture of the ulnar styloid or ulnar carpal bone.

On the basis of a cadaveric study, Miller et al[16] found that radial

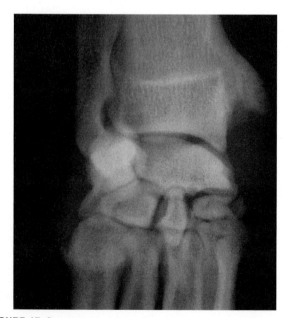

FIGURE 17–3. Enthesophytes on the radial styloid process and the medial tubercle just proximal to it. These enthesophytes are due to chronic sprain of the insertion of the short radial collateral ligament. There are also enthesophytes on the proximal end of metacarpal bone V and soft tissue swelling on the medial and lateral sides of the carpus.

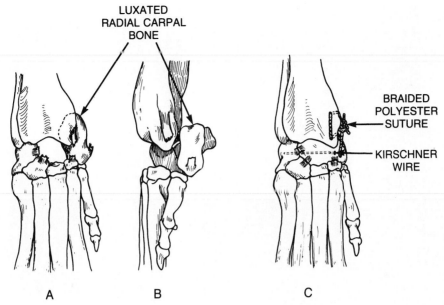

LUXATED
RADIAL CARPAL
BONE

BRAIDED
POLYESTER
SUTURE

KIRSCHNER
WIRE

A B C

FIGURE 17–4. *A* and *B,* Palmaro-medial luxation of the radial carpal bone. The bone is rotated 90 degrees medially and dorsopalmarly. *C,* The bone is reduced, and a Kirschner wire is driven through the bone into the ulnar carpal bone. The short radial collateral ligament is repaired, as described in Fig. 17–2. (From Brinker WO, Piermattei DL, Flo GL: Handbook of Small Animal Orthopaedics and Fracture Treatment. 2nd ed. Philadelphia, WB Saunders Company, 1990.)

carpal bone luxation could be induced only after transection of the short radial collateral ligament, the radioulnar intercarpal ligament, and the dorsal joint capsule. At this point, hyperextension of the carpus and pronation of the foot caused palmar rotation of the radial carpal bone, the proximodorsal edge of which engaged the palmar margin of the distal radial articular surface. Supination of the foot induced medial rotation of the radial carpal bone, such that its proximal surface faced palmaro-medially.

Closed reduction of very recent luxations may be possible.[11, 17] However, without repair of the short radial collateral ligament, the medial side of the joint remains unstable, and there is risk of reluxation and impaired function. For open reduction, a dorsal approach is made.[18] To achieve reduction, the bone is first rotated around a dorsopalmar axis, then a mediolateral axis.[11, 16] To facilitate reduction, Miller et al[16] have used a temporary transfixing pin, placed through the radial carpal bone from the medial side, as a handle. To stabilize the radioulnar intercarpal joint, a small Kirschner wire is inserted from the medial, nonarticular side of the radial carpal bone, transversely into the ulnar carpal bone[17] (Fig. 17–4). Remnants of the short radial collateral ligament are sutured if possible and then buttressed with a figure-of-eight suture, as described previously in this chapter. Finally the joint capsule is sutured. Fractures of the ulnar styloid are reduced and stabilized with a small lateral plate or tension banding wiring in the case of very distal fractures. Postoperatively the carpus is immobilized in slight flexion for 4 to 6 weeks, with gradual reduction in splint rigidity and increased extension of the carpus. Based on reports of a few cases, the prognosis for recovery is good following open reduction and stabilization of the luxated bone by this technique.[16, 19]

Pancarpal arthrodesis is indicated in luxations of greater than 3 weeks' duration because the radial carpal bone becomes irreducible. A modification to the standard arthrodesis procedure, as described later in this chapter, is to insert a corticocancellous bone graft taken from the iliac crest into the defect left by the luxated radial carpal bone. Immediate arthrodesis is also indicated if there has been concurrent fracturing of the ulnar carpal bone, unless such fractures

are amenable to anatomical reduction and stable fixation with lag screws.

Antebrachiocarpal Luxation and Subluxation

Complete luxation is accompanied by disruption of both the collateral ligaments, and the palmar ulnocarpal and radiocarpal ligaments (Fig. 17–5). Some cases also have fractures or luxation of the radial carpal, ulnar carpal, or accessory carpal bones. Although open reduction and reconstruction of the collateral ligaments are feasible, palmar instability persists, and in the long term this results in antebrachiocarpal hyperextension and osteoarthritis. Pancarpal arthrodesis produces acceptable restoration of limb function in these cases. Partial arthrodesis of the antebrachiocarpal joint alone is inadvisable, because of the subsequent development of osteoarthritis in the middle and carpometacarpal joints.[12]

Subluxation of the antebrachiocarpal joint occurs in conjunction with isolated injuries to the short radial or ulnar collateral ligaments, as described in the preceding sections, and also with sprain-avulsion fractures of the styloid processes. Another form of antebrachiocarpal subluxation, which we have seen in a greyhound and a coursing Afghan, was associated with a sprain-avulsion fracture of bone on the palmar margin of the distal radial articular surface, at the proximal insertion of the palmar radiocarpal ligament.[20, 21] The avulsion fracture could be visualized best on the mediolateral radiographic view. The greyhound also had a fracture of the distal ulnar styloid.[20] The Afghan had chronic pain and lameness, progressive osteoarthritis, and reduced range of motion in the carpus. Ultimately this was resolved by pancarpal arthrodesis.[21]

Middle Carpal and Carpometacarpal Luxation and Subluxation

Complete luxation of these joints is uncommon, and when present it results in gross instability and deviation of the paw. Reduction is usually possible if attempted within a few days of injury. However, treatment by coaptation is invariably followed by breakdown

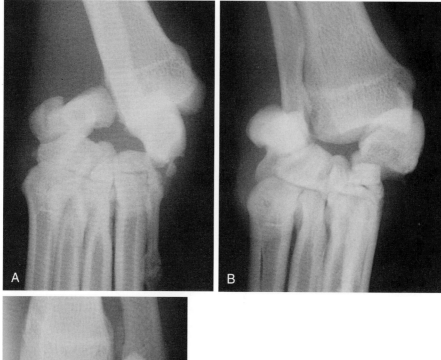

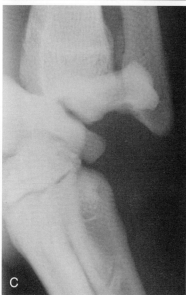

FIGURE 17–5. *A–C,* Complete luxation of the antebrachiocarpal joint in a 6-year-old Labrador. The ulnar carpal and radial carpal bones are also luxated, and both collateral ligaments are ruptured. This injury was treated by pancarpal arthrodesis (see Fig. 17–35).

at the joint, and so is not recommended. Partial carpal arthrodesis of both the middle carpal and carpometacarpal joints is necessary for long-term stability and limb function.

The majority of carpal hyperextension injuries result in subluxation at the middle carpal or carpometacarpal joints or both. Instability is considered to be primarily due to rupture of the palmar carpal ligaments and fibrocartilage. Weight bearing on the limb causes the carpus to become hyperextended, and the metacarpus assumes a palmar-grade stance. The extent of these injuries is best characterized with mediolateral radiographic views with the carpus stressed into a hyperextended position (Fig. 17–6). Specific alterations in the relationship of the carpal bones that are indicative of middle carpal or carpometacarpal hyperextension injury include the following: (1) angle between the dorsal face of the radial carpal bone or the distal row, and the metacarpus less than 180 degrees, (2) proximal tilting of the accessory carpal bone due to disruption of the two accessoro-metacarpal ligaments, (3) proximal elevation of the palmar part of the ulnar carpal bone, with widening of the

articulation between the distal articular surface of the ulnar carpal bone and the base of the fifth metacarpal bone, and (4) chip fractures along the dorsal margin of the distal row due to impingement of the carpal bones.

Subluxation of the medial part of the middle carpal joint occurs after disruption of the dorsal ligament from the radial carpal bone to the second carpal bone, or the ligament from the palmar process of the radial carpal bone to the second and third metacarpal bones. This injury allows valgus deviation of the paw. Isolated injuries are treated by a figure-of-eight wire from the palmar process of the radial carpal bone to the second metacarpal bone.[11] However, often this injury occurs in conjunction with palmar carpal ligament injury with carpal hyperextension.

Treatment of severe carpal hyperextension injuries by external coaptation with casts or splints invariably fails. Even though the palmar ligaments may heal, subsequent weight bearing on the limb causes elongation or breakdown of the repair tissue and return to palmar-grade stance. Partial arthrodesis of both the middle carpal

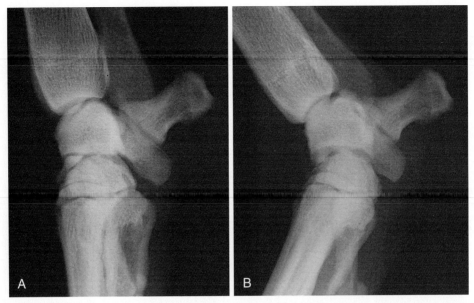

FIGURE 17–6. Carpal hyperextension injury of the middle carpal joint, with disruption of palmar ligaments and fibrocartilage. *A*, Proximal elevation of the ulnar carpal bone off metacarpal bone V with the carpus in a neutral position. *B*, Stressed in hyperextension, the middle carpal joint is subluxated, and the angle between the dorsal face of the radial carpal bone and the metacarpus is much less than the normal of 180 degrees. The injury was treated by partial arthrodesis (see Fig. 17–37).

and carpometacarpal joints is the recommended treatment for hyperextension injury, provided that the antebrachiocarpal joint is normal.[22] If it is not, pancarpal arthrodesis is indicated.[22, 23]

FRACTURES

Most carpal fractures in sporting dogs can be considered to be of two types: avulsion fractures in the vicinity of a tendon or ligament insertion and fractures due to compressive or shear forces on the bone. Most of the fractures in the latter group are intra-articular, while those in the former group may or may not be. Nevertheless, with nonsurgical management, most carpal fractures will unite only by fibrous tissue, not bone, and will cause varying degrees of osteoarthritis. This is because sprain-avulsion fractures allow subluxation, while intra-articular fractures cause damage to articular cartilage surfaces. Therefore, early diagnosis is essential if surgical treatment is to be considered so severity of secondary osteoarthritis can be minimized. While fractures of certain carpal bones like the accessory are common, involvement of others is rare. Because so few of these other fractures have been treated, very little can be said about prognosis, based on published case studies. Where possible, available data have been cited, although clearly more are needed.

Distal Radial Fractures

Radial Styloid Process. Fractures of the radial styloid process are most commonly a sprain-avulsion of bone at the proximal insertion of the straight or oblique parts of the short radial collateral ligament, or both (Fig. 17–7). Accurate anatomical alignment is essential if the fracture has extended into the main articular cartilage surface of the distal radius. As with rupture of the short radial collateral ligament, these fractures destabilize the medial side of the antebrachiocarpal joint. Small fracture fragments are fixed with fine Kirschner wires and a tension band, while lag screw fixation is preferable for larger fragments.[11]

Dorsal Radius. Fractures of the dorsal margin of the distal

articular surface of the radius in racing greyhounds are usually at the proximal insertion of the dorsal radiocarpal ligament that runs in a distolateral direction and inserts on the ulnar carpal bone.[24] Carpal swelling may be present, and there is pain on carpal flexion or direct palpation of the region. The fracture is seen best in a straight mediolateral radiographic view.[24] Fractured bone fragments may be multiply fragmented or quite large single pieces. One dog had a fragment 14 mm by 4 mm by 2 mm.[25] Despite the apparent

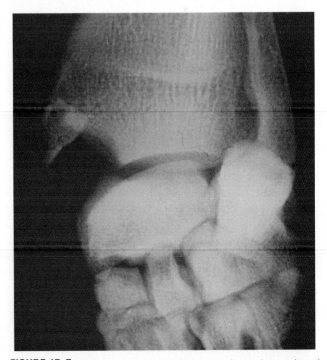

FIGURE 17–7. Fracture of the radial styloid process in a racing greyhound. (Courtesy of Jon F. Dee.)

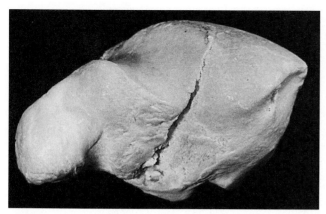

FIGURE 17–8. Incomplete fracture of right radial carpal bone viewed from the palmar aspect. (Courtesy of Jon F. Dee.)

potential for lag screw fixation, the most common treatment seems to be fragment excision to expedite return to racing. For excision of the fragment, a dorsal surgical approach and arthrotomy are carried out between the extensor carpi radialis and common digital extensor tendons. The fragment is excised from soft tissue attachments, and in chronic injuries fibrovascular tissue and bony callus on the radius are removed with rongeurs. With nonsurgical treatment these fractures do not heal, and racing time is lost.[24] However, it is not known if fragment removal and loss of insertion of the dorsal radiocarpal ligament have any significant deleterious effects on the joint in the long term. In 18 racing greyhounds with this injury (one bilateral), 17 had the bone fragment removed, 13 returned to trialing or racing, and 8 won races.[25]

Ulnar Styloid Process Fractures

The ulnar styloid articulates with both the ulnar carpal and accessory carpal bones. The distal end of this bone is crucial to stability of the carpus, because the short ulnar collateral, radioulnar, and palmar ulnocarpal ligaments insert upon it. Although there will be exceptions, fractures can be broadly divided into two types: transverse fractures 1 to 3 cm proximal to the end of the bone and sprain-avulsion fractures of a relatively small, distal fragment.

Proximal fractures may be accompanied by antebrachiocarpal

subluxation or luxation of the radial carpal bone (see these sections earlier in this chapter). Separation of the distal ulnar fragment from proximity to the radius implies that the distal radioulnar synovial articulation and the fibrocartilaginous articular disc have been disrupted. The latter structure provides the smooth transition between the distal ends of the radius and ulna and forms an integral part of that joint surface.[26] The ulnar fracture is repaired with a small, laterally positioned plate (veterinary cutable plate or 2.7 dynamic compression plate). Distal screws in the plate are kept short, within the ulna, to avoid interference with the distal radius and the distal radioulnar joint. However, planning of the fracture fixation and the expected prognosis must take into consideration any associated soft tissue injuries.

Fractures of the styloid with a small distal fragment destabilize the medial side of the antebrachiocarpal joint in a manner similar to ruptures of the short ulnar collateral ligament. Repair of these fractures is with small-diameter Kirschner wires and tension band wiring.[11]

Radial Carpal Bone Fractures

Body of Radial Carpal Bone. Fractures of this bone are rare and considered to be caused by compressive forces in dogs engaged in heavy work, such as field trialing and sled races.[11] In greyhounds, one type of fracture is oblique and intra-articular through the body of the bone. This type of fracture is more common in the right foreleg. The diagnosis may be delayed, and dogs have chronic lameness or the problem of drifting wide and slowing in the turns. On examination, there is reduced range of carpal flexion and pain. The fracture may not be radiographically apparent for several weeks until there has been some widening of the fracture gap due to bone resorption at the fracture or displacement of the fragments. The fracture is seen on the dorsopalmar view as a hairline fracture, beginning in the middle of the proximal articular surface and extending in a distomedial direction, to end above the second carpal bone (Figs. 17–8 and 17–9). Although some fractures are incomplete, and most are minimally displaced, best results are achieved by repair with lag screw fixation. A 2.7-mm cortical screw is introduced from the palmar process of the radial carpal bone and directed dorsolaterally, stopping short of the radioulnar intercarpal joint. The near fragment is overdrilled to allow interfragmentary compression, and the screw head is countersunk.[20] In six racing greyhounds with this fracture, three were treated by lag screw fixation, and of these, one was retired for breeding, one was

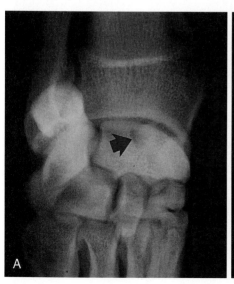 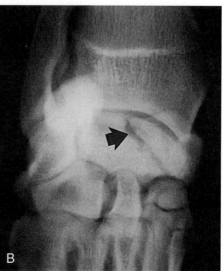

FIGURE 17–9. Early incomplete fracture (*arrow*) of the radial carpal bone (*A*). Three weeks later (*B*), the fracture line (*arrow*) extends completely through the bone. (Courtesy of Jon F. Dee.)

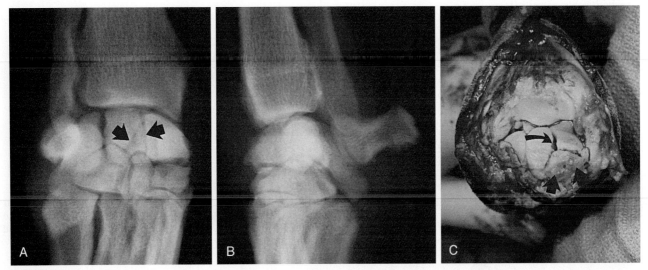

FIGURE 17–10. *A,* Chronic fracture of radial carpal bone *(arrows)* in a 6-year-old springer spaniel. *B,* Osteophytes on the distal end of the radius and dorsal margin of the radial carpal bone indicate secondary osteoarthritis. *C,* Fracture *(curved arrow),* fibrillated articular cartilage, and marginal osteophytes *(arrows)* seen intraoperatively during pancarpal arthrodesis.

lost to follow-up, and one returned to racing and won a race (Jon F. Dee, personal communication).

Because these fractures of the radial carpal bone are intra-articular and show little tendency to unite without internal fixation, delayed diagnosis leads to further resorption of the fragments, abrasion of articular cartilage of the apposing joint surfaces, and osteoarthritis. Chronic fractures with osteoarthritis are treated by pancarpal arthrodesis (Fig. 17–10).

Palmar Process. Avulsion fractures of the palmar process are a sprain-avulsion fracture of the proximal insertion of the palmar radial carpometacarpal ligament and are stabilized by lag screws or pin and tension band wire.[13, 27]

Dorsal Margin. Dorsal slab and chip fractures of the radial carpal bone probably result from compression and impingement by the distal radius during hyperextension of the joint. Fragments may be inapparent on mediolateral radiographic views, and several oblique views may be needed for diagnosis. Just as with other intra-articular fractures, the fragments may cause continued local irritation and pain and generally require surgical intervention. Most of these fracture fragments are too small or comminuted to permit

internal fixation, and these are excised. Large slab fractures are stabilized with 1.5-mm cortical lag screws if they are of sufficient size and the articular cartilage is normal in appearance. Screws are directed in a dorsopalmar direction and angled slightly proximally; screws must remain entirely within the bone. The screw is started quite distal on the dorsal margin of the radial carpal bone to avoid interference by the screw head with the articular cartilage or distal end of the radius. In one study of 15 racing greyhounds with dorsal fracture of the radial carpal bone, 12 were treated by a combination of fragment excision and various drugs, 6 returned to training, and 1 won a race.[25]

Ulnar Carpal Bone Fractures

Fractures of this bone are very rare. Both simple and comminuted fractures have been seen in conjunction with hyperextension injury, which in some cases was treated by pancarpal arthrodesis (Fig. 17–11). Also, fractures of this bone can occur in association with radial carpal bone luxation and antebrachiocarpal joint luxation.[16, 22]

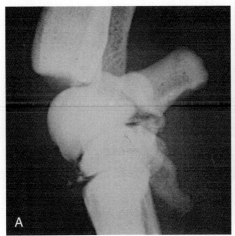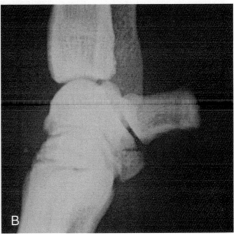

FIGURE 17–11. Flexed *(A)* and extended *(B)* mediolateral carpal radiographs of an Australian cattle dog that sustained a hyperextension injury. The palmar part of the ulnar carpal bone that articulates with the accessory carpal bone is fractured, and there are chip fractures dorsal to the numbered carpal bones.

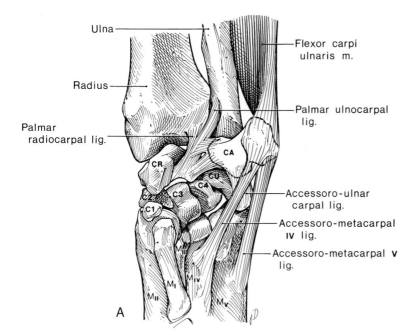

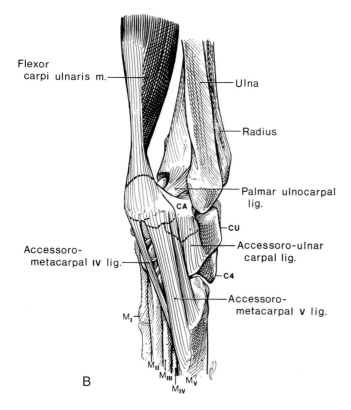

FIGURE 17–12. Ligaments of the accessory carpal bone are shown in palmaro-medial *(A)* and palmaro-lateral *(B)* views. CA = accessory carpal; CR = radial carpal; CU = ulnar carpal; C1 to C4 = first, second, third, and fourth carpals; MI to V = metacarpals. (From Johnson KA, et al: Characteristics of accessory carpal bone fractures in 50 racing greyhounds. Vet Comp Orthop Traumatol 2:104–107, 1988.)

Accessory Carpal Bone Fractures

Fracture of the accessory carpal bone is a common injury in greyhounds. This type of fracture is usually sustained while racing, and it is considered to be due to the stress of competitive performance, rather than an inherent breed susceptibility. Fractures of this bone are also occasionally seen in dogs of other breeds.

Anatomy. The accessory carpal bone is rod shaped, enlarged at each end, and positioned palmaro-lateral to the other carpal bones. The dorsal end is covered by hyaline cartilage, and it articulates primarily with the ulnar carpal bone and the ulnar styloid process to a lesser extent.[1] The accessoro-ulnar carpal joint is supported by both joint capsule and ligaments proximally, distally, and laterally. Also, two large accessoro-metacarpal ligaments extend from the palmar tip of the accessory carpal bone to the fourth and fifth metacarpal bones. The ligaments inserting on the accessory carpal bone support the accessoro-ulnar articulation, as well as stabilize the bone against the action of the flexor carpi ulnaris muscle that inserts upon it[5] (Fig. 17–12). The accessory carpal bone seems to be more prone to injury than the other carpal bones, perhaps because it acts as a fulcrum for the palmar carpal ligaments and flexor tendons, preventing hyperextension of the carpus during full weight bearing.

Etiopathogenesis. Most fractures in racing greyhounds occur while racing. Greyhounds race on circular or oval tracks in a counterclockwise direction, and it has been postulated that these fractures occur as the dog is rounding a bend, when all the body weight is taken on the right foreleg.[28] These injuries cause the dog to slow during the race or pull up lame afterward. With rest, the lameness may resolve, but lameness returns once racing resumes. Some dogs that subsequently sustain fractures are said to have low-grade pain in the region of the accessory carpal bone beforehand. Pain may be detectable by digital pressure applied laterally to the accessory carpal bone or a combination of this maneuver with carpal flexion.[5]

Fracture Classification

Bateman[29] was the first to describe a fracture involving the distal margin of the articular surface, and he originally proposed that the distracting pull of abductor digiti quinti muscle contributed to development of the fracture. However, it was later appreciated that the origin of this muscle was not in the vicinity of most fractures, and it was unlikely to be involved.[15, 30] It is currently believed that most accessory carpal bone fractures are avulsion fractures of ligamentous and tendinous insertions. On the basis of their radiological and pathological features, these fractures have been classified into five types[30] (Fig. 17–13). This classification was proposed as a basis for further study of incidence, treatment, and outcome of these fractures. The classification will undoubtedly require revision as more is learned. Diagnosis is made by detection of carpal swelling and pain on flexion. Fractures are usually most readily appreciated in mediolateral radiographic views with the carpus in flexion or extension.

Type I injury is an avulsion fracture of the distal articular margin of the articular surface in the region of the insertion of the ac-

Accessory Carpal Bone Fractures

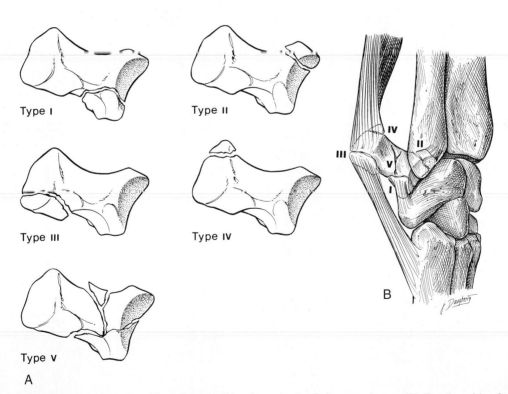

Type I

Type II

Type III

Type IV

Type V

A

B

FIGURE 17–13. Classification of accessory carpal bone fractures *(A)* and associated soft tissue attachments *(B)*. Type I: avulsion fracture of the distal margin of the articular surface at the origin of the accessoro-ulnar ligament. Type II: avulsion fracture of the proximal margin of the articular surface at the insertions of the palmar radiocarpal and ulnocarpal ligaments. Type III: avulsion fracture at proximal insertions of accessoro-metacarpal IV and V ligaments. Type IV: avulsion fracture at the insertion of flexor carpi ulnaris tendon. Type V: comminuted fracture. (From Johnson KA, et al: Characteristics of accessory carpal bone fractures in 50 racing greyhounds. Vet Comp Orthop Traumatol 2:104–107, 1988, and Johnson KA, Dee JF, Piermattei DL: Screw fixation of accessory carpal bone fractures in racing greyhounds: 12 cases (1981–1986). JAVMA 194:1618–1625, 1989.)

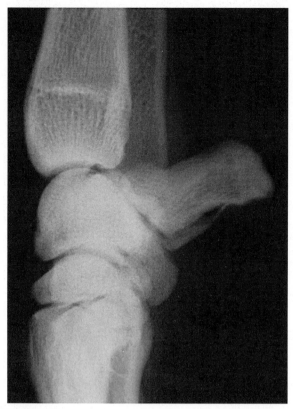

FIGURE 17–14. Type I avulsion slab fracture of the distal margin of the articular surface of the accessory carpal bone. (From Johnson KA: Accessory carpal bone fractures in the racing greyhound: classification and pathology. Vet Surg 17:60–64, 1987.)

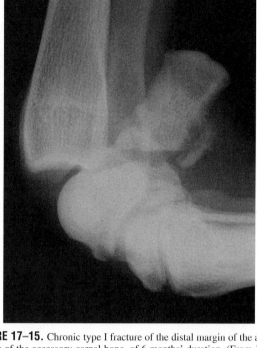

FIGURE 17–15. Chronic type I fracture of the distal margin of the articular surface of the accessory carpal bone, of 6 months' duration. (From Johnson KA: Accessory carpal bone fractures in the racing greyhound: classification and pathology. Vet Surg 17:60–64, 1987.)

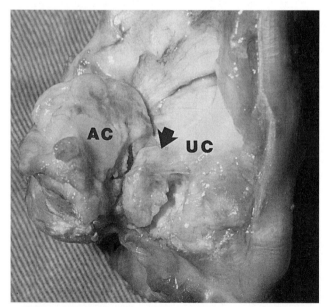

FIGURE 17–16. Chronic type I fracture of accessory carpal bone (AC) of six months' duration. The fractured bone fragment (*arrow*) is adhered to the articular surface of the ulnar carpal bone (UC) by fibrous tissue. (From Johnson KA: Accessory carpal bone fractures in the racing greyhound: classification and pathology. Vet Surg 17:60–64, 1987.)

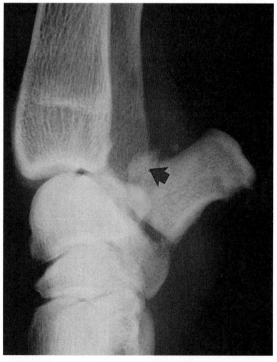

FIGURE 17–17. Type I and II (*arrow*) fractures at the distal and proximal margins of the articular surface of the accessory carpal bone. (From Johnson KA: Accessory carpal bone fractures in the racing greyhound: classification and pathology. Vet Surg 17:60–64, 1987.)

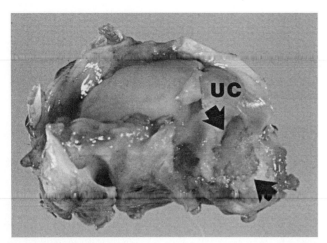

FIGURE 17–18. Ulceration of the articular cartilage *(arrows)* of the ulnar carpal bone (UC), 8 weeks after type I and II fractures of the accessory carpal bone, shown in Fig. 17–17. (From Johnson KA: Accessory carpal bone fractures in the racing greyhound: classification and pathology. Vet Surg 17:60–64, 1987.)

cessoro-ulnar ligament (Fig. 17–14). Fracture fragments may vary in size from single large slabs about 10 by 5 by 2 mm to multiple comminuted chips. Because these fractures are intra-articular and allow joint instability, they cause subluxation, articular cartilage abrasion, and secondary osteoarthritis (Fig. 17–15). Chronically the fractured bone fragments become surrounded by proliferative bone and fibrous tissue but do not usually proceed to bony union (Fig. 17–16).

A recently recognized variation to the typical type I injury is an avulsion fracture of the lateral articular prominence of the accessory carpal bone.[31] In some dogs the accessoro-ulnar ligament consists of two parts, one ventral and one lateral.[31] In one greyhound the avulsion fracture of the lateral prominence was at the proximal insertion of this lateral part of the accessoro-ulnar ligament. Unlike a type I fracture, the fragment could not be appreciated on the mediolateral radiographic view and could be visualized only on a dorsolateral palmaro-dorsal oblique view.[31]

Type II injury is an avulsion fracture of the proximal margin of the articular surface at the insertion of the palmar ulnocarpal and radiocarpal ligaments that connect to the caudo-medial surface of the distal ulna and the caudal surface of the distal radius (see Fig. 17–12). These types of fractures have been observed in conjunction with a type I injury. Similar to type I injuries, these fractures also allow subluxation and produce articular cartilage damage and secondary osteoarthritis. In the case in Figure 17–17 there was gross, deep fibrillation of articular cartilage on the ulnar carpal bone after 8 weeks (Fig. 17–18). The fracture fragments were surrounded by callus composed of woven bone and fibrocartilage (Fig. 17–19).

Type III injury is an avulsion fracture at the distal surface of the palmar end of the bone, at the origin of the two large accessoro-metacarpal ligaments that connect to the fourth and fifth metacarpal bones (Fig. 17–20). This disrupts the stay apparatus provided by these large ligaments, which normally counteracts the action of flexor carpi ulnaris muscle and acts to prevent carpal hyperextension during full weight bearing.

Type IV injury is a strain-avulsion fracture of bone from the proximal surface of the palmar end of the bone, at the tendon of insertion of the flexor carpi ulnaris muscle (Fig. 17–21). Bone fragments are distracted proximally by the flexor tendon. In immature animals, the fracture may be an epiphyseal avulsion from the accessory carpal bone[15] (Fig. 17–22). Radiological closure of the canine accessory carpal bone growth plate occurs between 10 weeks and 3 months of age, after which dogs are less susceptible to this type of injury.[32]

Type V injury includes all other fractures of the body of the bone, and these fractures may be comminuted or intra-articular (Figs. 17–23 and 17–24). Longitudinal fractures in a transverse plane that divide the bone roughly into two halves, and are intra-articular, have also been reported, and perhaps belong in this group.[15]

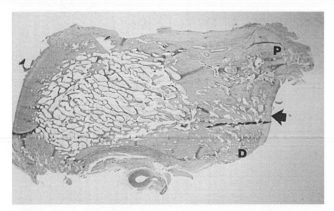

FIGURE 17–19. Histologic section of the accessory carpal bone in Fig. 17–17, showing location of the fractures of the proximal (P) and distal (D) margins of the articular surface *(arrow)*, 8 weeks later (H&E, × 3.6). (From Johnson KA: Accessory carpal bone fractures in the racing greyhound: classification and pathology. Vet Surg 17:60–64, 1987.)

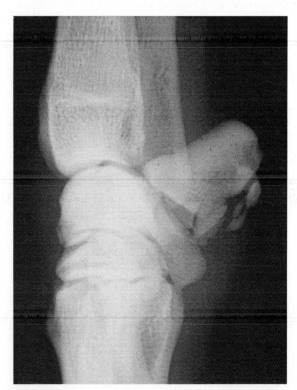

FIGURE 17–20. Type III fracture of the accessory carpal bone, at the insertion of the accessoro-metacarpal IV and V ligaments, in combination with a comminuted type I fracture. (From Johnson KA: Accessory carpal bone fractures in the racing greyhound: classification and pathology. Vet Surg 17:60–64, 1987.)

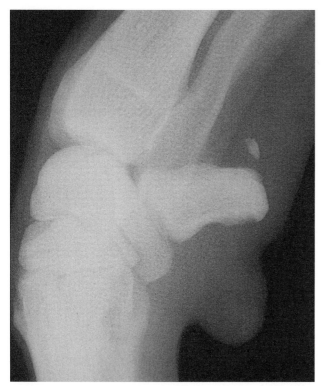

FIGURE 17–21. Type IV avulsion fracture from the proximal surface of the palmar end of the accessory carpal bone, from the insertion of flexor carpi ulnaris tendon. (From Johnson KA: Accessory carpal bone fractures in the racing greyhound: classification and pathology. Vet Surg 17:60–64, 1987.)

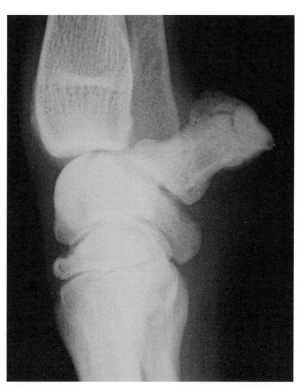

FIGURE 17–22. Epiphyseal avulsion fracture at the palmar end of the accessory carpal bone, healed in malunion in an 18-month-old greyhound.

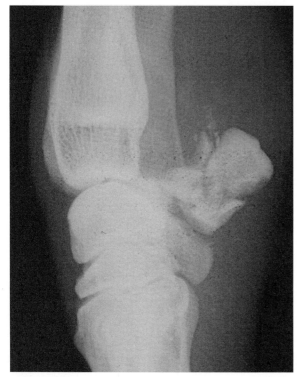

FIGURE 17–23. Type V comminuted fracture of the accessory carpal bone with fracture lines involving both the body and articular surface. (From Johnson KA: Accessory carpal bone fractures in the racing greyhound: classification and pathology. Vet Surg 17:60–64, 1987.)

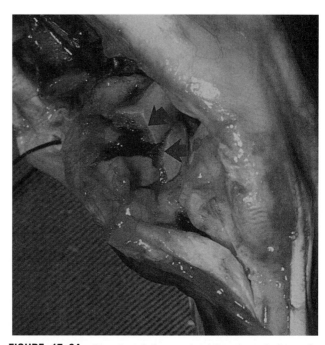

FIGURE 17–24. Comminuted fracture involving the articular surface *(arrows)* of the accessory carpal bone shown in Fig. 17–23. (From Johnson KA: Accessory carpal bone fractures in the racing greyhound: classification and pathology. Vet Surg 17:60–64, 1987.)

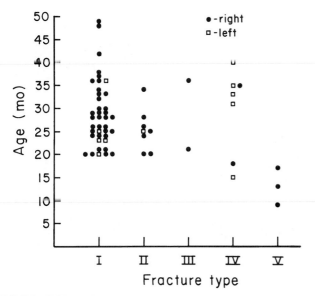

FIGURE 17–25. Age distribution in months of 50 greyhounds with accessory carpal bone fractures. The five fractures types are defined in Fig. 17–13. (From Johnson KA, et al: Characteristics of accessory carpal bone fractures in 50 racing greyhounds. Vet Comp Orthop Traumatol 2.104–107, 1988.)

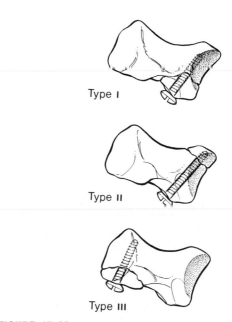

FIGURE 17–26. Screw fixation of fracture types I, II, and III. (From Johnson KA, Dee JF, Piermattei DL: Screw fixation of accessory carpal bone fractures in racing greyhounds: 12 cases (1981–1986). JAVMA 194:1618–1625, 1989.)

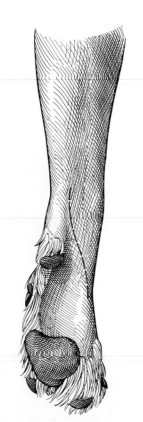

FIGURE 17–27. Surgical approach to accessory carpal bone fractures. A palmaro-lateral skin incision centered over the right carpus. (From Johnson KA, Dee JF, Piermattei DL: Screw fixation of accessory carpal bone fractures in racing greyhounds: 12 cases (1981–1986). JAVMA 194:1618–1625, 1989.)

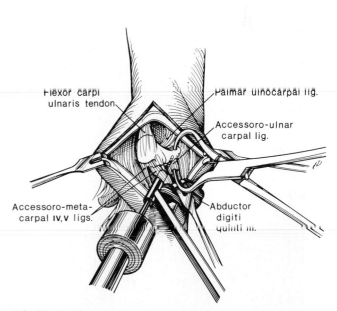

FIGURE 17–28. Reduction of a type I fracture with pointed reduction forceps and drilling a 1.1 hole for screw fixation. (From Johnson KA, Dee JF, Piermattei DL: Screw fixation of accessory carpal bone fractures in racing greyhounds: 12 cases (1981–1986). JAVMA 194:1618–1625, 1989.)

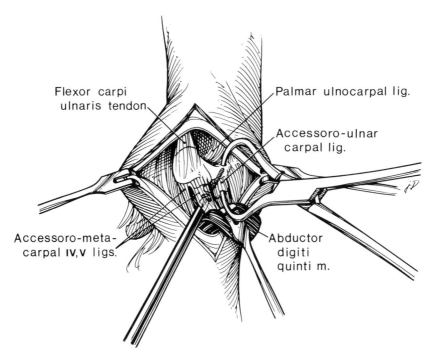

FIGURE 17–29. Fixation of a type I fracture with a 1.5-mm cortical screw. (From Johnson KA, Dee JF, Piermattei DL: Screw fixation of accessory carpal bone fractures in racing greyhounds: 12 cases (1981–1986). JAVMA 194:1618–1625, 1989.)

Distribution of Fractures

In racing greyhounds, 80 per cent of accessory carpal bone fractures overall occur in the right foreleg. This distribution is probably due to the stress of racing in a counterclockwise direction. One study of 50 greyhounds racing in New South Wales and Colorado found that the incidence of the five types of injury was influenced by age and limb[5] (Fig. 17–25). Sixty-seven per cent of fractures were type I injuries of the right carpus, and they were all sustained while racing. Unlike the other types of injury, type IV injuries tended to occur more in the left foreleg. Comminuted fractures occurred in young dogs being schooled or trained for racing. The male to female ratio of affected dogs was 1.8:1, which was similar to the sex ratio of greyhounds competing in races in

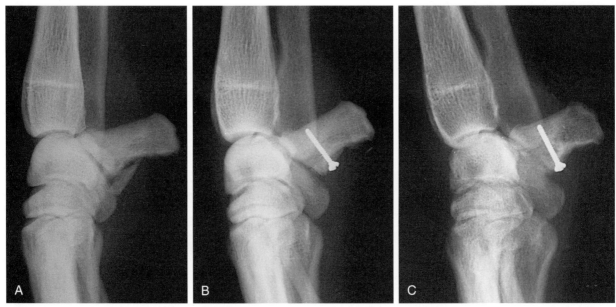

FIGURE 17–30. Type I fracture of the distal margin of the articular surface of the accessory carpal bone before (A), immediately after (B), and at 8 weeks (C) after repair by use of a 1.5-mm cortical screw. (From Johnson KA, Dee JF, Piermattei DL: Screw fixation of accessory carpal bone fractures in racing greyhounds: 12 cases (1981–1986). JAVMA 194:1618–1625, 1989.)

Colorado at that time.[5] Mean age of affected dogs was 27.9 months. This is relatively early in their racing career, which usually begins at age 18 to 20 months.

Treatment and Outcome

It is of historical interest that the first described treatment for accessory carpal bone fracture was transection of the abductor digiti quinti muscle, based on the erroneous belief that tension in this muscle contributed to the fracture.[29] Thereafter, fracture fragment excision was widely performed with little consideration given to restoration of ligamentous integrity.[28, 33, 34] More recently, open reduction of selected fractures and internal fixation with screws has been reported.[35] While it seems more logical to attempt fracture repair, this is a technically demanding operation, and some fracture fragments are simply too small to permit screw fixation, so excision becomes unavoidable.

Screw Fixation

Dogs with types I, II and III injuries, in which the avulsed bone fragment is relatively large and noncomminuted, may be candidates for repair with screw fixation[35] (Fig. 17–26). For the surgical operation, dogs are positioned in lateral recumbency with the affected limb uppermost.* A 5-cm longitudinal skin incision is made palmaro-lateral to the carpus to expose the palmar carpal retinacular fascia (Fig. 17–27). This fascia is incised to expose the accessory carpal bone and supporting ligaments. The abductor digiti quinti muscle is separated from the accessoro-metacarpal 4 and 5 ligaments and retracted medially. In dogs with types I and II injuries, lateral arthrotomy of the accessoro-ulnar joint is performed to allow inspection of the articular cartilage surface. This may facilitate

---

*Editors' comment: We find it technically expedient to have the patient in dorsal recumbency.

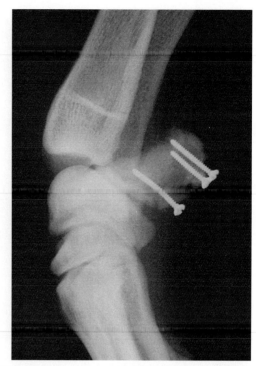

FIGURE 7–32. Incompletely healed type I and type III fractures, shown in Fig. 17–20, that were repaired with three 1.5-mm cortical screws, 7 weeks after surgery. The screw in the type I fracture is bent. (From Johnson KA, Dee JF, Piermattei DL: Screw fixation of accessory carpal bone fractures in racing greyhounds: 12 cases (1981–1986). JAVMA 194:1618–1625, 1989.)

precise anatomical reduction. Fracture reduction is maintained with small, pointed AO/ASIF reduction forceps (Figs. 17–27 and 17–28). Avoid damage to the ulnar nerve and palmar interosseous artery, which lie medial to the accessory carpal bone. Internal fixation is with 1.5- or 2.0-mm cortical screws inserted in lag fashion (Figs. 17–29 and 17–30). If there is concern about splitting the near fragment, overdrilling may be omitted, and the screw is inserted as a positional screw. Furthermore, countersinking of the bone for the screw head may also have to be omitted if the fragment is very thin. Prior to screw insertion, the hole is measured carefully and then tapped completely, to minimize friction between the screw and the bone during tightening. Breakage of 1.5-mm screws has been a problem in several cases (Fig. 17–31).

Following surgery, the carpus is protected with a palmar fiber glass slab splint and cast padding for 4 to 6 weeks. Initially the carpus is immobilized in about 40 degrees of flexion, but then with each splint change, the joint is progressively moved to a more extended weight-bearing position. Radiographs are obtained at 6 and 12 weeks postoperatively to monitor fracture healing (Fig. 17–32). Regular training may resume after 12 to 16 weeks postoperatively provided the dog is sound.

One study of 12 greyhounds with fractures treated by internal fixation found that 10 returned to racing and five of those won one or more races.[35] One greyhound with an avulsion fracture of the lateral articular prominence of the accessory carpal bone (a recently recognized variation on the type I injury), had returned to racing 11 weeks after screw fixation of the fracture.[25] While types I, II and III injuries are sprain-avulsion fractures causing accessoro-ulnar subluxation, it would be expected that types I and II would have a worse prognosis because they are intra-articular. Further outcome studies are needed.

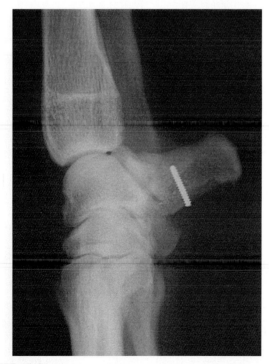

FIGURE 17–31. Healed type I fracture. Although the head broke off this 1.5-mm screw during insertion, fracture fixation was maintained, apparently because the screw was a positional screw. (Courtesy of Jon F. Dee.)

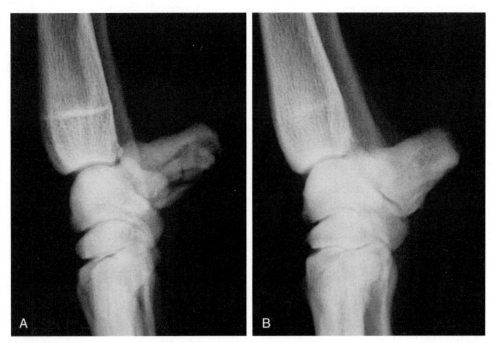

FIGURE 17–33. Comminuted intra-articular type V fracture in a 20-month-old racing greyhound *(A)* that was immobilized with external coaptation with the carpus in flexion. After 5 months *(B)* fractures are healed, but with malunion and articular incongruity; the dog subsequently raced and won. (Courtesy of Jon F. Dee.)

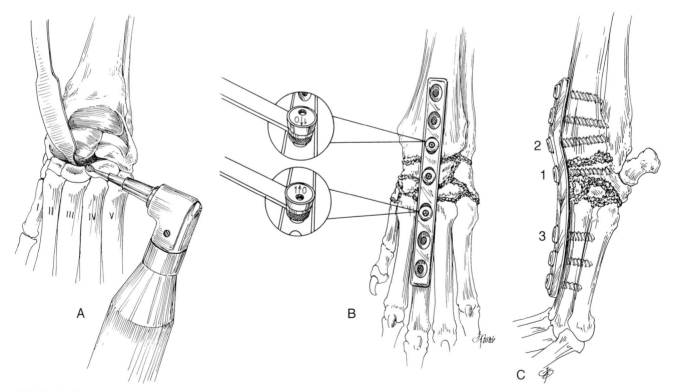

FIGURE 17–34. Pancarpal arthrodesis. *A,* Articular cartilage removal with an air-driven bur. A Hohmann retractor facilitates exposure of the joint compartments. *B,* Seven-hole 3.5-mm dynamic compression plate applied to the distal radius, radial carpal bone, and metacarpal bone III. The initial screw *(1)* is inserted into the radial carpal bone. Screws into the distal radius *(2)* and metacarpal bone III *(3)* are inserted in a load position to produce interfragmentary compression in the arthrodesis. *C,* Precontouring of the plate positions the carpus in approximately 10 degrees of extension. (From Johnson KA: Arthrodesis. *In* Olmstead ML (ed): Small Animal Orthopedics. St Louis, CV Mosby, 1995, pp 503–529.)

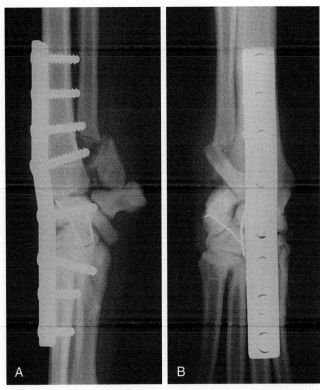

FIGURE 17–35. Luxation of antebrachiocarpal joint and the radial carpal and ulnar carpal bones (see Fig. 17–5), treated by pancarpal arthrodesis. *A* and *B,* The distal ulnar styloid process was caught behind the accessory carpal bone, and it was necessary to perform an ulnar osteotomy to reduce the luxation. After removal of articular cartilage, the radial carpal and ulnar carpal bones were held in reduction with Kirschner wires while the bone graft and plate were applied.

Fragment Removal

Removal of avulsed fracture fragments is apparently the most common treatment for accessory carpal bone fractures, especially type I fractures. The surgical approach for fragment removal is similar to that used for lag-screw fixation, except that it is more limited. A lateral approach is made to the ventral aspect of the bone and the joint capsule opened to allow visualization of fragments. Fragments are found attached to joint capsule and accessoro-ulnar ligament and are removed by sharp dissection with a no. 11 or no. 15 scalpel blade.

In removal of these fragments, it is recognized that no attempt is being made to suture the damaged ligament or stabilize the joint, and healing proceeds by fibroplasia. Since these are intra-articular fractures that do not naturally heal by bony union, and they are also associated with damage to the articular cartilage on the ulnar carpal bone, then fragment excision may perhaps be preferable to nonsurgical management. However, not much objective data are available on outcome of this commonly performed operation. A study in Scotland found that of 19 racing greyhounds that had type I fragments removed, 13 returned to race and 9 won races; of the other 6, 3 became sound but were unable to race, while the other 3 remained lame.[33]

External Coaptation

Immobilization of the carpus in flexion by means of a splint or cast is indicated for comminuted fractures that are not amenable to open reduction and internal fixation and for minimally displaced epiphyseal fractures in young dogs. Some malunion may be accept-

able, although fractures involving the articular surface would, in general, have a poorer prognosis (Fig. 17–33).

Numbered Carpal Bone Fractures

Chip and slab fractures of the dorsal margin of the third and fourth carpal bone occur in racing greyhounds. Initially the fracture may be detected by palpation, with pressure directly over the fragment causing pain. Fractured fragments off the third carpal bone are commonly about 5 mm by 3 mm by 2 mm.[25] Small chips are excised, while internal fixation of large slabs with 1.5-mm cortical lag screws has been recommended.[27] Prognosis for return to racing after fragment removal seems to be good. Of six racing greyhounds with dorsal fractures of the third carpal bone treated by fragment excision, one was lost to follow-up, five returned to training, and three of these won races.[25]

Multiple Carpal Bone Fractures

These fractures are the result of severe trauma, shearing injury, gunshot injury, carpal luxation, or hyperextension injury. Open reduction and internal fixation are often not feasible, and pancarpal arthrodesis may be indicated.[22]

ARTHRODESIS

Arthrodesis is a surgical procedure that results in complete bony fusion across an articulation.[22, 23] Although an arthrodesis precludes any further joint motion, it restores limb function by eliminating instability, osteoarthritis, and pain. Some of the indications for arthrodesis in sporting dogs are carpal luxation, hyperextension injury, irreparable fractures, gunshot injuries, and chronic osteoar-

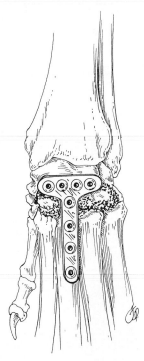

FIGURE 17–36. Partial carpal arthrodesis with a T plate applied to the proximal row of carpal bones and to metacarpal bone III. (From Johnson KA: Arthrodesis. *In* Small Animal Orthopedics. Olmstead ML (ed): St Louis, CV Mosby, 1995, pp 503–529.)

thritis. Fusion of the entire carpus is called pancarpal arthrodesis, whereas fusion that spares one or more normal joints of the carpus is called partial carpal arthrodesis. To achieve arthrodesis the joint cavities are opened by a dorsal approach.[18] The tendon of extensor carpi radialis is transected at its insertion on the third metacarpal bone III, and the digital extensor tendons are retracted laterally. For pancarpal arthrodesis, the distal end of the radius is also exposed to allow subsequent application of a plate. Articular cartilage is removed from all the joint surfaces with an air-driven bur until subchondral bone is exposed (Fig. 17–34). During removal of the cartilage, irrigation of the joints with saline prevents thermal damage to bone. Cancellous bone collected from the proximal metaphysis of the ipsilateral humerus is packed into the joint spaces to stimulate more rapid osseous union at the arthrodesis.[36, 37] Internal fixation of the carpus is required to stabilize the carpus in a slightly extended position. The internal fixation is protected with a splint until there is osseous union at the arthrodesis. This usually takes 8 to 12 weeks.[36, 37]

Pancarpal Arthrodesis

Pancarpal arthrodesis is indicated for injuries and abnormalities involving the antebrachiocarpal joint. If arthrodesis of the antebrachiocarpal joint is being planned, a pancarpal arthrodesis is performed, regardless of whether the middle carpal or carpometacarpal joints are normal. This is because there is normally very

little mobility at the two distal joints in the carpus, and attempts at partial arthrodesis of the antebrachiocarpal joints alone in a few cases subsequently resulted in secondary osteoarthritis of the joints that were spared. A pancarpal arthrodesis is usually stabilized with a plate on the radius, radial carpal bone, and third metacarpal bone. For medium- to large-sized dogs, a seven-hole 3.5-dynamic compression plate is of appropriate size. Outside this range, 2.7- and broad 3.5-dynamic compression plates are occasionally needed. In cases of open shearing injuries with infection or extensive tissue loss, stabilization is with a type II external fixator. Compared to arthrodesis of other joints, restoration of limb function and ambulation after carpal arthrodesis is generally good. In 45 dogs of various breeds, 74 per cent regained "normal" limb function after pancarpal arthrodesis with a plate.[38] It was not specified if any of these dogs were sporting animals. Nevertheless, the procedure can be recommended in severe carpal injuries in sporting breed dogs, if the goal is to use the animal subsequently for breeding or noncompetitive purposes (Fig. 17–35).

Partial Carpal Arthrodesis

Partial carpal arthrodesis is performed on the metacarpal and carpometacarpal joints, preserving the antebrachiocarpal joint when it is normal. The most common indication is carpal hyperextension injuries at these levels. Stabilization is achieved with a T plate from the radial carpal bone to the third metacarpal bone (Figs.

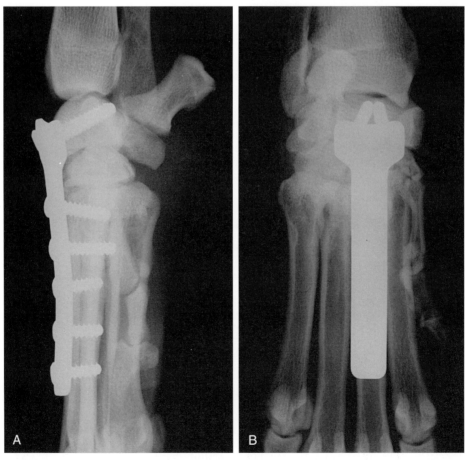

FIGURE 17–37. *A* and *B,* Partial carpal arthrodesis of the middle and carpometacarpal joints with an AO/ASIF small veterinary T plate, immediately after operation on a dog with middle carpal hyperextension injury (see Fig. 17–6).

8. Cooper RR, Misol S: Tendon and ligament insertion: A light and electron microscopic study. J Bone Joint Surg 52-A:1–20, 1970.
9. Resnick D, Niwayama G: Entheses and enthesopathy. Anatomical, pathological and radiological correlation. Radiology 146:1–9, 1983.
10. Woo S, Maynard J, Butler D, et al: Ligament, tendon, and joint capsule insertions to bone. *In* Woo SL-Y, Buckwalter JA (eds): Injury and repair of the musculoskeletal soft tissues. Park Ridge, Ill, American Academy of Orthopaedic Surgeons, 1987, pp 133–166.
11. Brinker WO, Piermattei DL, Flo GL: Handbook of Small Animal Orthopaedics and Fracture Treatment. 2nd ed. Philadelphia, WB Saunders Company, 1990.
12. Earley TD: Canine carpal ligamentous injuries. Vet Clin North Am 1978; 8:183–199.
13. Earley TD, Dee JF: Trauma to the carpus, tarsus, and phalanges of dogs and cats. Vet Clin North Am 10:717–747, 1980.
14. Roe SC, Dee JF: Lateral ligamentous injury to the carpus of a racing greyhound. JAVMA 189:453–454, 1986.
15. Vaughan LC: Disorders of the carpus in the dog I. Br Vet J 141:332–341, 1985.
16. Miller A, Carmichael S, Anderson TJ, Brown I: Luxation of the radial carpal bone in four dogs. J Small Anim Pract 31:148–154, 1990.
17. Vaughan LC: Disorders of the carpus in the dog. II. Br Vet J 141:435–446, 1985.
18. Piermattei DL: An atlas of surgical approaches to the bones and joints of the dog and cat, 3rd ed. Philadelphia, WB Saunders Company, 1993, pp 204–213.
19. Punzet G: Luxation of the os carpi radiale in the dog—pathogenesis, symptoms, and treatment. J Small Anim Pract 15:751–756, 1974.
20. Dee JF, Dee LG, Eaton-Wells RD: Injuries of high performance dogs. *In* Whittick WG (ed): Canine Orthopedics, 2nd ed. Philadelphia, Lea & Febiger, 1990, pp 519–570.
21. Johnson KA: Unpublished observations.
22. Johnson KA: Arthrodesis. *In* Olmstead ML (ed): Small Animal Orthopedics. St Louis, CV Mosby, 1995, pp 503–529.
23. Johnson KA: Carpal arthrodesis in dogs. Aust Vet J 56:565–573, 1980.
24. Ferguson RG: Chip fractures of the right distal radius involving the carpal joint in the racing greyhound. Aust Vet Pract 16:127–129, 1986.
25. Boemo CM: Chip fractures of the dorsal carpus in the racing greyhound: 38 cases. Aust Vet Practit 23:139–147, 1993.
26. Mikic ZDj, Ercegan G, Somer T: Detailed anatomy of the antebrachiocarpal joint in dogs. The Anatomical Record 233:329–334, 1992.
27. Dee JF: Fractures in racing greyhounds. *In* Bojrab MJ (ed): Disease Mechanisms in Small Animal Surgery, 2nd ed. Philadelphia, Lea & Febiger, 1993, pp 1060–1075.
28. Bateman JK: The racing greyhound. Vet Rec 72:893–897, 1960.
29. Bateman JK: Fracture of the accessory carpal (pisiform) bone in the racing greyhound and its repair. Vet Rec 62:154–155, 1950.
30. Johnson KA: Accessory carpal bone fractures in the racing greyhound: Classification and pathology. J Vet Surg 17:60–64, 1987.
31. Boemo CM: Fracture of the accessory carpal lateral articular prominence in a racing greyhound. Aust Vet Practit 24:70–73, 1994.
32. Sumner-Smith G: Observations on epiphyseal fusion of the canine appendicular skeleton. J Small Anim Pract 7:303–311, 1966.
33. Chico AC: Accessory carpal bone fracture in greyhounds: Assessment of prognostic indicators and outcome following surgical management by fragment removal. M Vet Med thesis. University of Glasgow, 1992.
34. Hickman J: Greyhound injuries. J Small Anim Pract 16:455–460, 1975.
35. Johnson KA, Dee JF, Piermattei DL: Screw fixation of accessory carpal bone fractures in racing greyhounds: 12 cases (1981–1986). JAVMA 194:1618–1625, 1989.
36. Johnson KA: A radiographic study of the effects of autologous cancellous bone grafts on bone healing after carpal arthrodesis in the dog. Vet Radiol 22:177–183, 1981.
37. Johnson KA, Bellenger CR: The effects of autologous bone grafting on bone healing after carpal arthrodesis in the dog. Vet Rec 107:126–132, 1980.
38. Parker RB, Brown SG, Wind AP: Pancarpal arthrodesis in the dog: A review of 45 cases. J Vet Surg 10:35–43, 1981.
39. Smith MM, Spagnola J: T-plate for middle carpal and carpometacarpal arthrodesis in a dog. JAVMA 199:230–232, 1991.
40. Willer RL, Johnson KA, Turner TM, Piermattei DL: Partial carpal arthrodesis for third degree carpal sprains. A review of 45 carpi. J Vet Surg 19:334–340, 1990.

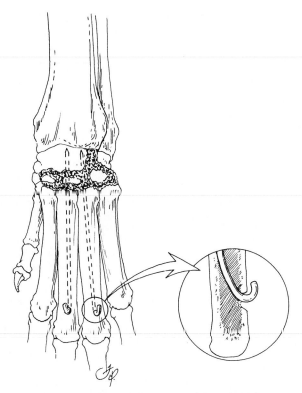

FIGURE 17–38. Partial carpal arthrodesis with pins. Articular cartilage is removed from the middle and carpometacarpal joints; autologous cancellous bone is packed into the joint cavities; and intramedullary pins inserted in slots made distally are driven up metacarpal bones III and IV, to be seated into the radial carpal bone. (From Johnson KA: Arthrodesis. *In* Small Animal Orthopedics. Olmstead ML (ed): St Louis, CV Mosby, 1995; pp 503–529.)

17–36 and 17–37) or small-diameter intramedullary pins driven from the third and fourth metacarpal bones (Fig. 17–38).[11, 39] In one study of 39 dogs of various breeds, 68 per cent regained good limb function[40]; 16 per cent of dogs subsequently developed osteoarthritis of the antebrachiocarpal joint, but none required further surgery. Although carpal mobility at the antebrachiocarpal joint is diminished by this procedure, some dogs have returned to heavy work. Further outcome studies are needed.

References

1. Evans HE: Miller's Anatomy of the Dog. Philadelphia, WB Saunders Company, 1993, pp 239–243.
2. Nickel R, Schummer A, Seiferle E, et al: Carpal joints. *In* Nickel R, Schummer A, Seiferle E (eds): Anatomy of the Domestic Animals. Berlin, Verlag Paul Parey, 1981, pp 184–188.
3. Yalden DW: The functional morphology of the carpal bones in carnivores. Acta Anat 77:481–500, 1970.
4. Prole JHB: A survey of racing injuries in the greyhound. J Small Anim Pract 17:207–218, 1976.
5. Johnson KA, Piermattei DL, Davis PE, Bellenger CR: Characteristics of accessory carpal bone fractures in 50 racing greyhounds. Vet Comp Orthop Traumatol 2:104–107, 1988.
6. Farrow CS: Stress radiography: Applications in small animal practice. JAVMA 181:777–784, 1982.
7. Woo SL-Y, An K-N, Arnoczky SP, et al: Anatomy, biology, and biomechanics of tendon, ligament and meniscus. *In* Simon SR (ed): Orthopaedic Basic Science. Park Ridge, Ill, American Academy of Orthopaedic Surgeons, 1994, pp 45–87.

CHAPTER 18

TARSAL INJURIES

JON F. DEE

ANATOMY

Bones

The *tarsus*, or *hock*, consists of seven tarsal bones. The term also applies collectively to the several joints between the tarsal bones, as well as the region between the crus and the metatarsus. The tarsus is arranged in two rows. The medially located talus and the laterally located calcaneus make up the proximal row. The distal row consists of four bones. Three small bones, the first, second, and third tarsal bones, are located side by side and are separated from the proximal row by the central tarsal bone. The distal row is completed laterally by the large fourth tarsal bone, which lies against the third and central tarsal bones[1] (Fig. 18–1A).

The talus articulates proximally with the tibia and fibula, distally with the central tarsal, and on the plantar side with the calcaneus. The surface of the trochlea of the talus articulates with the sagittal grooves and the intermediate ridge of the distal articular surface of the tibia. The sides of the trochlea articulate with the medial and lateral malleoli (Fig. 18–1B). The talus articulates with the calcaneus via three separate facets. The large concave proximal articular surface of the talus articulates with the convex dorsal articular facet of the calcaneus. The oval middle articular surface of the talus articulates with the concave medial articular facet of the calcaneus (Fig. 18–1C). The distal articular surface of the talus articulates with the distal articular facet of the calcaneus. This surface is confluent with a small articular facet for the central tarsal on the distal surface. Between the middle and distal articular surfaces of the calcaneus is the calcaneal sulcus, which concurs with a similar one on the talus to form the tarsal sinus.[1]

The calcaneus is the largest and longest bone of the tarsus. The tuber calcanei, or proximal half, is a sturdy traction process that serves as the insertion of the calcanean tendon. The distal half is wide transversely and possesses three facets and two processes; these mortise with the talus to form a stable articulation. A jutting shelf, the sustentaculum tali, leaves the medial side of the bone, over which the tendon of the flexor hallucis longus glides plantarly[1] (Fig. 18–1D).

The central tarsal bone lies medially between the proximal and distal rows of tarsal bones. It articulates with all of the other tarsal bones. The first, second, and third tarsal bones articulate with the central tarsal bone proximally and their respective metatarsals distally. The third tarsal bone also articulates with the fourth tarsal bone laterally. The fourth tarsal bone articulates proximally with the calcaneus and distally with metatarsals IV and V. It articulates with the central and third tarsal bones on its medial surface. The tuberosity of the fourth tarsal bone is a palpable landmark located on the midplantar aspect of the bone.[1]

Joints

The tarsal joints are composite articulations. The talocrural, or ankle joint, permits the greatest degree of movement. Some side movement is possible from the collective tarsal joints; however, the vertical joints between the individual bones (the intratarsal joints) are exceedingly rigid.[1] The talocrural joint is the articulation between the tibia and the talus. The talocalcaneal joint is the articulation between the talus and the calcaneus. The talocalcaneocentral joint is the joint between the talus, calcaneus, and central tarsal bones. The articulation between the calcaneus and the fourth tarsal bone forms the calcaneoquartal joint. The centrodistal joint is formed between the central tarsal bone and the first, second, and third tarsal bones. The tarsometatarsal joints are formed between the second, third, fourth, and fifth metatarsal bones and the second, third, and fourth tarsal bones.[2]

Ligaments

The tarsus is supported by a medial and lateral collateral ligament arising from the medial and lateral malleoli. Each ligament has a short and long component. The long, more superficial part of the tibial collateral inserts primarily to the first tarsal bone and strongly to the free surface of the central tarsal bone. The short part, originating craniodistal to the long part, divides as it passes under it. One part extends plantarly to attach on the talus, while the other longer part attaches primarily to the first tarsal and metatarsal bone. The long, more superficial part of the fibular collateral ligament inserts on the lateral aspect of the base of metatarsal V, attaching to the calcaneus and fourth tarsal bone along its course. The short part has one band that extends to the tuber calcanei; a second band goes to the more dorsally located talus (Fig. 18–2A).

The intraordinary ligament between the talus and calcaneus is referred to as the *talocalcaneal ligament.*[3]

On the plantar surface of the tarsus the special plantar ligaments are heavier than those on the dorsal side. Most of these fuse distally with the thickened part of the joint capsule at the tarsometatarsal junction. Several of these are distinct and are discussed under the section on plantar intertarsal subluxations. On the dorsal surface of the tarsus there are various short ligaments. One prominent ligament unites the talus with the third and fourth tarsals. A small band connects the second and third tarsals. Oblique bands exist between the central and second tarsals, as well as between the central and third tarsals. The distal row of tarsal bones are joined to the proximal ends of the metatarsal bones by small vertical ligaments on the dorsal surface (Fig. 18–2B).

INJURY

Fractures of the tarsus are common and frequently involve articular surfaces; therefore, to attain success, the tenets of joint surgery must be rigidly followed. In most cases, a thorough orthopedic examination of the tarsus in conjunction with the appropriate radiographic views utilizing detail cassettes and/or films will identify

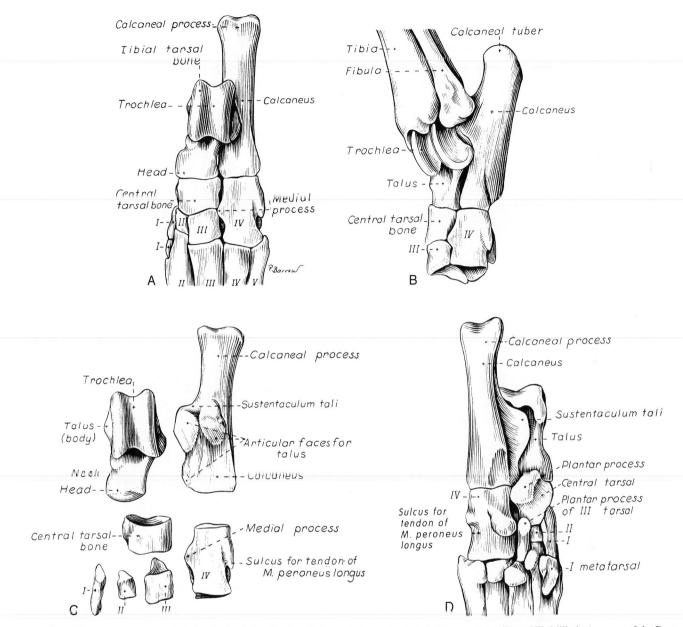

FIGURE 18–1. Dorsal *(A)*, lateral *(B)*, disarticulated dorsal *(C)*, and plantar *(D)* aspects of the left tarsus. (From Evans HE: Miller's Anatomy of the Dog, 3rd ed. Philadelphia, WB Saunders Company, 1993.)

the fractured bone. The tarsus should be palpated for localized areas of soft tissue swelling, point pain, deformity, instability, and crepitation. Doubts about the regional anatomy should be dispelled by radiography of the contralateral normal extremity. Radiographs should be hot-lighted and read with magnification to appreciate subtle lesions.

The principles of lag screw fixation or pin and figure-of-eight tension band wire will be utilized to manage most tarsal fractures that are technically repairable. Repairs that have potentially significant forces acting upon them will frequently be stress-protected by some form of coaptation. Chips that are too small to be stabilized are removed.

Subtle ligamentous (sprain) injuries of the tarsus are not always obvious on the routine examination of the tarsus. A typical scenario of a tarsal sprain is as follows: First, the tarsus was swollen and painful, therefore an inadequate examination was performed.

Second, no fractures were readily apparent on routine plain films; therefore, the owner was informed that nothing was broken and the tarsus was splinted and/or anti-inflammatories were given. The reasons for this mismanagement of sprains, as described by Farrow,[4] are a lack of appreciation of the pathology involved, ignorance of the specific anatomy, poor understanding of radiographic signs (especially of soft tissues), failure to correlate clinical and radiographic information, and lack of use of stress films.

The ideal scenario for the management of tarsal sprains is as follows:

1. Patients with painful extremities are given the appropriate analgesics.
2. Swollen extremities are placed in a modified Robert Jones padded splint to reduce swelling before a second examination in 12 to 72 hours.

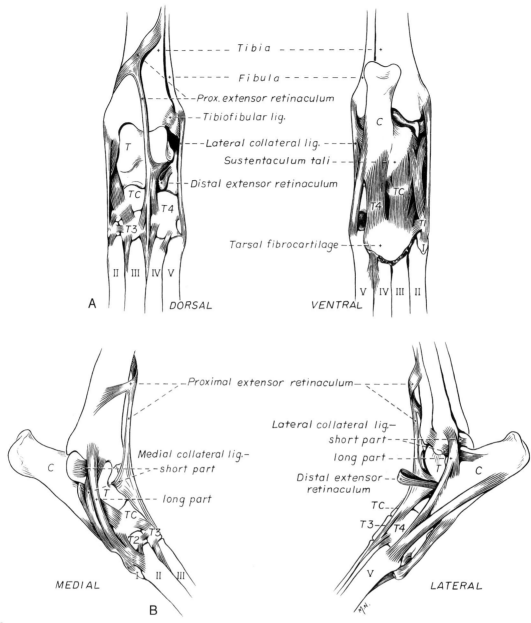

FIGURE 18–2. Medial and lateral collateral ligaments *(A),* dorsal and plantar ligaments *(B)* of the left tarsus. C = calcaneus, T = talus. T1, T2, T3, T4 = first, second, third, and fourth tarsals. TC = central tarsal. I to V = metatarsals. (From Evans HE: Miller's Anatomy of the Dog, 3rd ed. Philadelphia, WB Saunders Company, 1993.)

3. A complete examination of the tarsus is performed, with varus, valgus, flexion, extension, and rotational stability checked throughout the range of motion.
4. The appropriate stress radiographs are taken and, when there is doubt, compared with the opposite limb.
5. Definitive therapy is then undertaken.

Because tarsal sprains are seen by all veterinarians and occur in all breeds, it is imperative that an early, accurate diagnosis be made so that early reconstruction (when indicated) can be attempted. The improper management of sprains often yields persistent instability leading to secondary degenerative joint disease that usually requires arthrodesis for stabilization. To minimize the number of patients that end up as "comfortable cripples" via arthrodesis, these injuries should be detected and managed early.

FRACTURES

Malleolar Fractures

Malleolar fractures may be unilateral, bilateral, or "trimalleolar." Repair should always be with rigid internal fixation if a return to full function is to be achieved. Repair of medial or lateral malleolar fractures involves use of Kirschner wires and figure-of-eight tension band wire fixation to maintain reduction. The K-wires are seated in the distal tibial metaphyseal area (Fig. 18–3A,B).[5] "Third malleolar" fractures are axial fractures of the posterior triangle component of the distal tibia and are managed by countersunk leg screws. These fractures may be seen as isolated injuries or more commonly in conjunction with bimalleolar fractures[6] (Fig. 18–4).

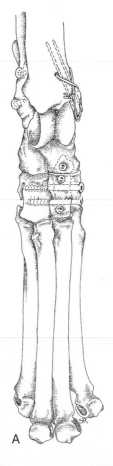
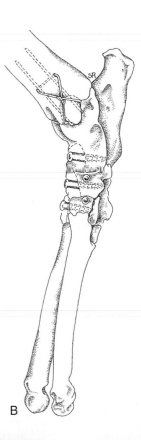

FIGURE 18–3. Dorsal *(A)* and medial *(B)* aspects of a right tarsus. The grade III sprain avulsion of the medial malleolus has been repaired with paired Kirschner wires and a figure-of-eight tension band wire. The spiral fracture of the lateral malleolus has been managed with small (1.5-mm–2.0-mm) cortical screws. The fractures of the talus, second, third, and central tarsal bone have all been managed with countersunk lag screws. All screws are left in situ. *C,* A/P preoperative view of the right tarsus of "L.A. Law," a racing greyhound. Note the type IV central tarsal fracture and an associated medial sagittal slab fracture of the head of the talus. *D,* A/P postoperative view. The central tarsal fracture has been repaired with a 4.0-mm cancellous screw and a 2.7-mm cortical screw. The talar component has been managed with a 1.5-mm cortical screw.

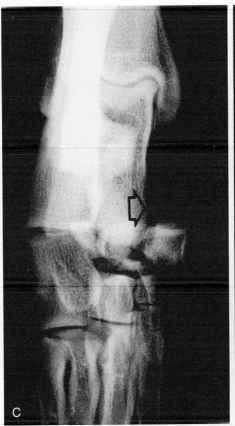
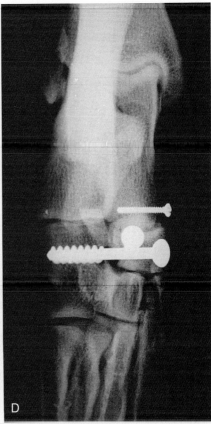

the screw is subjected to microshear forces in the tarsal sinus and is prone to failure.[8]

Damage to the articular surface of the head of the talus is a frequent finding in the more severe central tarsal bone fractures. Occasionally, a dorsal or medial slab fracture will be seen associated with a central tarsal bone fracture.[9] Repair is by countersinking and lagging a cortical bone screw (Fig. 18–3A–D).[8] Fractures of the talar head not amenable to reconstruction and stabilization may be treated by arthrodesis of the talocalcaneocentral joint.

Calcaneal Fractures

Calcaneal fractures may be solitary lesions; however, they are seen more commonly in conjunction with the more severe (type IV) central tarsal bone fractures. Chronologically, the central tarsal

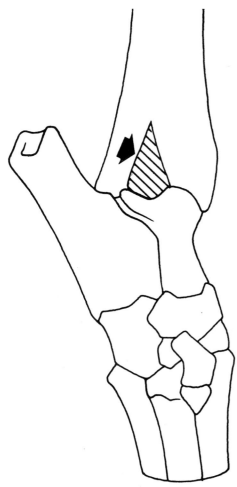

FIGURE 18–4. Medioplantar aspect of the left talocrural joint. Arrow indicates the area of the posterior distal tibial margin fracture in the racing greyhound. The fracture line incorporates the bony ridge located between tendinous sulci and has intra-articular extension. It is best appreciated radiographically on the medial lateral projection. (From Montavon PM, Dee JF, Weiss R: Distal tibial articular fractures in racing greyhounds: A review of six cases. Vet Compar Orthopaed Traumatol 6:147, 1993.

Rarely, a spiral fracture of the lateral malleolus is encountered and is repaired with multiple countersunk lag screws (Fig. 18–3A).[7]

Talar Fractures

The *talus* is the second largest tarsal bone, consisting of a body, neck, and head. The body is the enlarged proximal portion that articulates with the distal tibia and fibula via the condyles and trochlea.[1] Although quite rare, fractures of the body may involve one or both condyles and may be quite difficult to visualize radiographically. With suspected condylar fractures, stress radiographs should be taken. Dorsally located fractures may be exposed by the appropriate dorsomedial or dorsolateral approach. More proximally located and comminuted fractures require an osteotomy of the appropriate malleolus. Repair is by countersunk implants.[8]

Talar neck fractures are extra-articular fractures that may be reduced and stabilized with either a Kirschner wire or a lag screw that is started at the medial aspect of the head of the talus and seated in the lateral condyle. The placement of a screw (positional or lag) from the head of the talus to seat in the base of the calcaneus has been advocated.[8] No compression is obtained and

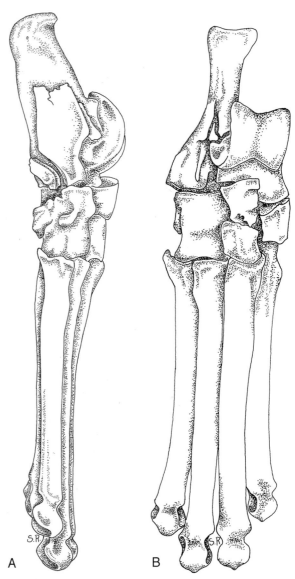

FIGURE 18–5. Dorsal *(A)* and medial *(B)* classical type IV central tarsal bone fracture. Although the fourth tarsal bone is intact, the calcaneus is fractured and subluxated laterally. The calcaneal fracture consists of a lateral sagittal slab fracture that extends into the proximal lateral articular facet dorsally and a smaller plantar lateral component. Concomitant dorsomedial axial slab fractures of the base may also be seen. The plantar support mechanism was intact.

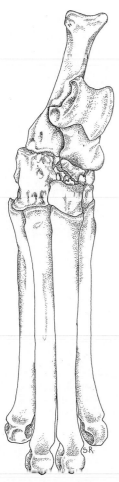

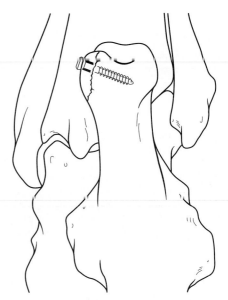

FIGURE 18–7. A plantar projection depicting an avulsion strain of the medial aspect of the insertion of the retinaculum of the superficial digital flexor tendon to the tuber calcanei. The fragment has been replaced with a small lagged cortical bone screw.

FIGURE 18–6. Dorsal plantar view of a right tarsus demonstrating a varus deformity subsequent to a comminuted central tarsal bone fracture. The major fragments of the central tarsal have been removed to aid in visualization of the deformity. Note the secondary compression fracture of the dorsal medial aspect of the fourth tarsal bone.

bone fails, extruding a large medial fragment and a smaller dorsal component, with a subsequent loss of craniomedial support. The integrity of the calcaneus is bound to the talus because of the intimate relationship of the medial, dorsal, and distal talar faces of the calcaneus to the talus.

As the head of the talus travels distally, the continued craniomedial tension applied by the Achilles tendon to the tuber calcanei allows the lowered talus to act as a fulcrum, over which the calcaneus fractures (Fig. 18–5A,B). If the calcaneus remains intact, as the central tarsal bone collapses, the brunt of the remaining compressive forces are placed on the fourth tarsal bone. Approximately 40 per cent of the severe central tarsal bone fractures have an associated compression fracture of the fourth tarsal bone[9] (Fig. 18–6).

The following types of calcaneal fractures are seen:

1. Avulsions of the medial or lateral attachment of the superficial digital flexor (SDF) tendon to the tuber calcis—managed by removal of small fragments, followed by soft tissue reconstruction. Larger strain avulsions are managed with internal fixation (Fig. 18–7).

2. Avulsions of the tuber calcis—primarily a problem of the skeletally immature tarsus. Repair is via figure-of-eight tension band wire and/or pin fixation (Fig. 18–8).

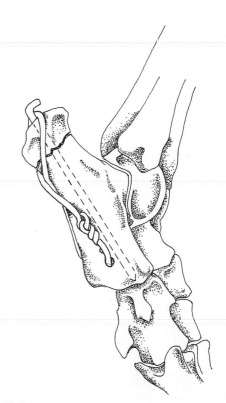

FIGURE 18–8. Lateral aspect of the calcaneus. An avulsion of the tuber calcis—primarily a problem of the skeletally immature—is managed with small Kirschner wires and coaptation or a pin and figure-of-eight tension band that is removed early in the course of healing.

3. Comminuted shaft fractures—require additional fixation in the form of lag screws and/or hemicerclage or cerclage wires (Fig. 18–5A,B and Figs. 18–9A–C and 18–10A–D).
4. Lateral sagittal slab fractures of the base and shaft of the calcaneus—use multiple lateral-to-medial lag screws (Fig. 18–11).
5. Large oblique plantar-distal chip fractures of the base of the calcaneus—repair with a pin and a figure-of-eight tension band wire placed in the calcaneus (Fig. 18–12).
6. Large oblique cranial-distal fractures of the base of the calcaneus—utilize a pin and figure-of-eight wire seated into the body of the fourth tarsal bone (Fig. 18–13).
7. Small oblique plantar-distal chip fractures of the base—manage as a plantar proximal intertarsal subluxation (PIS). Support the arthrodesis of the calcaneoquartal joint by a pin and figure-of-eight tension band wire into the fourth tarsal bone (Fig. 18–14).
8. Dorsomedial axial slab fractures of the base of the calcaneus

rarely go to non-union and can be managed by lag screw fixation or, more commonly, coaptation (Figs. 18–15 and 18–16A,B).

Calcaneal fracture management decisions include several options:

1. Size and number of pins (small vs. large, one vs. two).
2. Location of pins (medial and lateral placement vs. cranial and caudal).
3. Configuration of pins as related to wire placement (bent vs. countersunk and wire around pin or in a transosseous tunnel, respectively).
4. Significance of figure-of-eight tension band wire vs. pin in contributing to rotational stability. (Are pins required for rotational stability or does the tension band wire alone solve the problem in the calcaneal fracture?) The pin is definitely the weaker component, whereas the wire is the workhorse.
5. Plates vs. other methods of fixation—a calcaneal fracture that

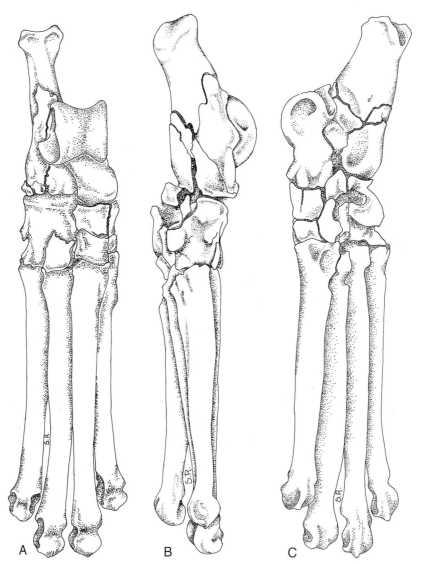

FIGURE 18–9. Dorsal *(A)*, plantar lateral oblique *(B)*, and plantar medial oblique *(C)* views of a right tarsus. A type IV central tarsal bone fracture, an unusual dorsal slab fracture of the base of T4 are all visualized on the dorsal projection *(A)*. The lateral sagittal slab fracture and the two plantar components of the fractured base of the calcaneus are best visualized from the plantar lateral oblique perspective. *B,* The extent of the damage to the sustentaculum tali is appreciated from the plantar medial oblique view *(C)*. Little wonder that some pristine central and calcaneal repair combinations may fare poorly after we see the extent of the trauma.

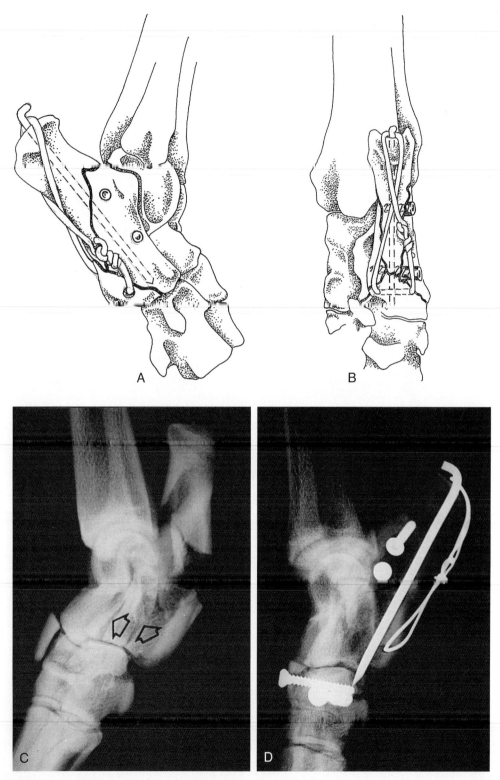

FIGURE 18–10. Lateral *(A)* and plantar *(B)* views of a comminuted calcaneal fracture of a right tarsus. A combination of lateral to medial countersunk lag screws and a pin and figure-of-eight tension band wire have been used to maintain anatomical reduction. Medial lateral preoperative *(C)* and medial lateral 3-week postoperative *(D)* views of the right tarsus of a comminuted calcaneal fracture seen in conjunction with a type IV central tarsal bone fracture in a racing greyhound. Repair was maintained with lag screws and a pin and tension wire band.

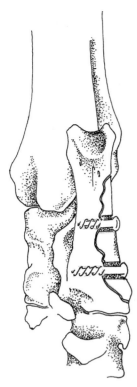

FIGURE 18–11. A plantar view of a right tarsus with an isolated lateral sagittal slab fracture of the base and shaft of the calcaneus repaired with lag screws.

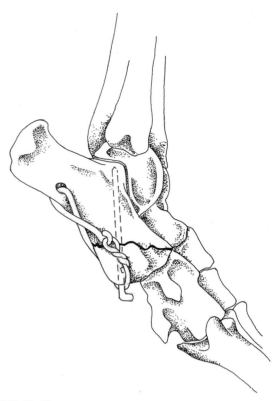

FIGURE 18–12. A lateral view of a right tarsus with an unusual and large oblique plantar to dorsal distal fracture of the base of the calcaneus. The plantar support mechanism was intact and the fracture was managed with a pin and figure-of-eight tension band.

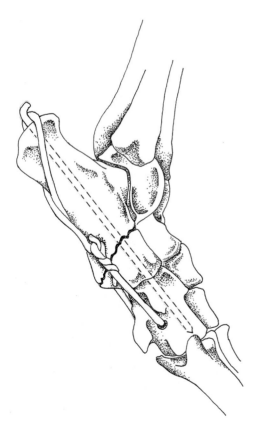

FIGURE 18–13. Lateral view of a right tarsus with an oblique cranial-distal fracture of the base of the calcaneus managed with a pin seated in the fourth tarsal bone and a figure-of-eight wire from the proximal end of the pin to engage in the body of the fourth tarsal bone in the area of the plantar process.

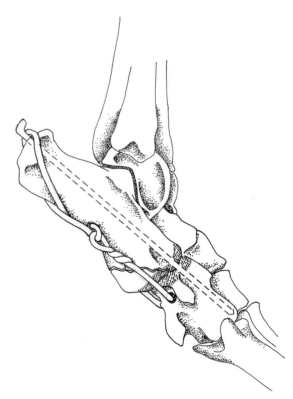

FIGURE 18–14. Lateral view of a right tarsus with a small oblique plantar distal chip that represent an avulsion of the origin of the middle plantar ligament. This is managed as a plantar intertarsal subluxation via a primary arthrodesis of the calcaneoquartal joint supported with a pin and figure-of-eight tension band wire.

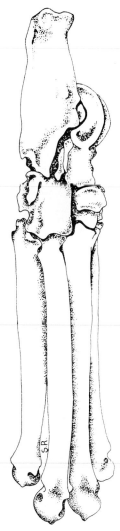

FIGURE 18–15. Dorsal lateral plantar medial oblique view of a right tarsus that has sustained a type IV central tarsal bone fracture. Additionally, an isolated dorsomedial axial slab fracture of the base of the calcaneus is seen. This fracture extends proximally to enter the proximal lateral articulation with the talus and plantarly to create a sagittal fracture of the sustentaculum tali. This is often not readily appreciated radiographically. T4 is intact.

may be plated may be managed via pin and wire at less cost, whereas the converse is not true.[7]

Central Fractures

The importance of the central tarsal bone to the integrity of the hock is appreciated when one recalls that it articulates with all of the other tarsal bones. Fractures of the central tarsal bone are most commonly seen in the large active, sporting, or working breeds. The most common injury to the central tarsal bone is a fracture that usually occurs in the right hock of a racing greyhound. Unlike many articular fractures, loss of joint motion does not appear to be a clinical problem, but loss of "bone space" or joint collapse leads to skeletal angular deformity (varus) and inevitable loss of limb function[10] (Fig. 18–6). These fractures are caused by an indirect force that is apparently greater on the outer rear or right rear limb, since greyhounds run the track counterclockwise. It is hypothesized that the lateral side of the hock is under tension and the medial

side under compression, forcing the central tarsal bone to act anatomically as a pivot or buttress for the other tarsal bones. This buttress effect causes the greatest force and consequently the highest incidence of fracture to occur in the central tarsal bone. The fractures frequently show radiographic evidence of compression, subluxation, and comminution but are rarely open.[10, 11] Fractures of the left central tarsal bone have been documented when the greyhound was moving in a clockwise direction or was off stride in a turn.[11]

Various short intertarsal ligaments bind the central tarsal bone to the other tarsal bones. A small oblique band connects the central and second tarsal bones. A larger oblique band connects the central and third tarsal bones. Another larger ligament leaves the plantar surface of the sustentaculum tali and passes under the long and short tibial collateral ligaments to attach on the dorsomedial surface of the central tarsal bone[1] (Fig. 18–2B). Fractures of the central tarsal bone commonly occur between the insertions of the latter two oblique ligaments. These ligaments lie just beneath the tendon of insertion of the tibialis cranialis muscle as it passes obliquely from laterally to medially over the central tarsal bone.[10]

Just as the short collaterals of the talocrural joint are under greatest tension during full flexion, it is supposed that this plantar ligament is under extreme tension during flexion. This plantar ligament tension, in conjunction with the compressive forces of the talus from above, contribute to the occurrence of central tarsal bone fractures. These have been classified into the following types according to their radiographic and surgical appearance (Fig. 18–17).[11]

- Type I—Dorsal slab fracture, nondisplaced.
- Type II—Dorsal slab fracture, displaced.
- Type III—Large displaced medial fragment without a dorsal slab fracture.
- Type IV—Dorsal slab fracture with a medial slab fracture.
- Type V—Comminuted fracture.

Types I and II fractures are suspected when point pain is produced over the central tarsal area by digital pressure. They are verified with detail radiography. Clinically, the patient does not bear full weight and has minimal soft tissue swelling. Historically, type I fractures have been overlooked by inexperienced observers.[12] Although rare, type III fractures are more readily apparent on physical and radiographic examination. The type IV fracture is classified by appearance as having two major displaced fragments, although it is common to have comminuted chips posteriorly. The limb has a varus deformity and plantigrade stance. Soft tissue swelling is profuse. Although uncommon, the type V fracture is a comminuted disaster that historically has been coapted or shored up with a "buttress" plate and a cancellous bone graft.

Five distinct types of fractures have been described. Of these, two main categories exist: those requiring one-screw fixation and those requiring two-screw fixation. Approximately one-fourth of the central tarsal bone fractures require one screw; the remainder require two-screw fixation. Fractures that can be repaired with one screw are either nondisplaced or displaced dorsal slab fractures or medial slab fractures without a dorsal component. Two screws are required to repair the combination of dorsal and medial slab fractures, which constitute approximately two-thirds of the cases.

Solitary dorsal slab fractures are replaced and repaired with a 2.7-mm screw that is overdrilled and countersunk. Because the dorsal fragment is often thin, excess compression may cause a fracture through the drill hole if one is not careful. The rare, solitary medial slab fracture is repaired with a 3.5-mm screw, which is overdrilled and countersunk. Dogs with these fractures have an excellent prognosis for returning to racing.

Central tarsal fractures that radiographically demonstrate two or more major fragments can usually be repaired with two screws.

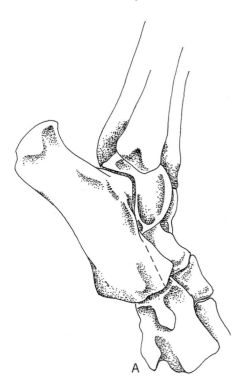
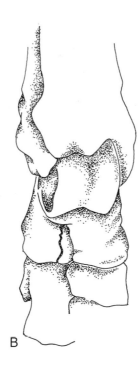

FIGURE 18–16. Lateral *(A)* and dorsal *(B)* aspect of a right tarsus depicting a dorsomedial axial slab fracture of the base of the calcaneus.

The first screw is a 4.0-mm cancellous bone screw placed medially to laterally to stabilize the medial fragment. The drill hole is placed as low as possible on the central tarsal bone without invading the distal joint space. This screw is countersunk and seated in the fourth tarsal bone. The second screw to be placed is a 2.7-mm cortical and is carefully overdrilled and countersunk in a dorsoplantar direction. It is placed just proximal to the mediolateral screw, neither hitting it nor entering the proximal joint space (Fig. 18–3*A,B*).[13]

First described some 20 years ago as a severely comminuted and displaced fracture, the type V (unreconstructable) central tarsal bone has remained unchanged in its radiographic and surgical description, which was based on the number and type of displaced fragments.[11] However, the surgical management, and subsequently the prognosis, of these fractures has changed and continues to do so.

As the surgeon's learning curve flattens and the technical expertise improves, the number of type V (unreconstructable) central tarsal bone fractures decreases. The combination of improved equipment availability and improved surgical expertise has allowed surgical reconstruction of many heretofore inoperable type V central tarsal bone fractures. Examples are as follows:

1. As many as four lag screws have been utilized to reconstruct a central tarsal bone fracture (Fig. 18–18*A,B*).
2. A single hole of a one-quarter tubular plate has been utilized (as a square washer) beneath the head of the medial to lateral lag screw in order to shore up or buttress the medial component of the fracture (Fig. 18–19*A,B*).
3. A medially placed bone plate has been utilized as a buttress to stress protect a tenuous repair.
4. "Flying Farley," belonging to prominent greyhound owner Dick Andrews, won grade A stakes elimination races after a type V central tarsal bone repair (Fig. 18–18*A,B*).

Those few that cannot be reconstructed by screw fixation are potential candidates for autogenous cortical cancellous bone grafts, synthetic replacement, or perhaps a central tarsal allograft. All of these techniques are in their infancy; further experience and additional numbers are needed before a firm recommendation can be made. These procedures require additional internal fixation for support.

Approximately two-thirds of the cases encountered in our practice have associated secondary fractures—most commonly, fractures of the fourth tarsal bone, fractures of the calcaneus, and

Types I & II 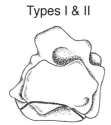   Type III 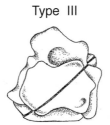   Type IV 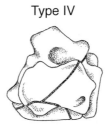   Type V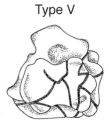

FIGURE 18–17. An interarticular view from above of a right central tarsal bone schematically depicting the five main types of central tarsal bone fracture. Types I and II are distinguished only by the amount of or lack of displacement of the dorsal slab component.

FIGURE 18–18. A/P view of the right tarsus of a racing greyhound that sustained a classical triad of the tarsus *(A)*. A highly comminuted (type V) fracture of the central tarsal bone was followed by a compression fracture of the fourth tarsal and an avulsion of the lateral aspect of the base of metatarsal varus. The nine-week postoperative A/P view illustrates healing via multiple lag screw fixation *(B)*.

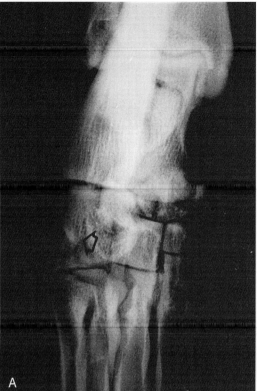
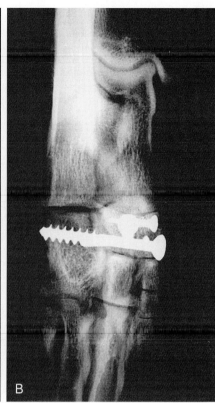

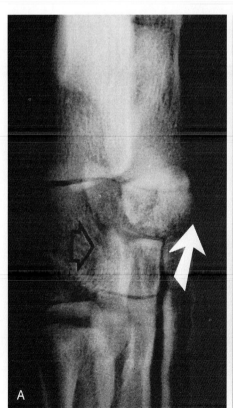
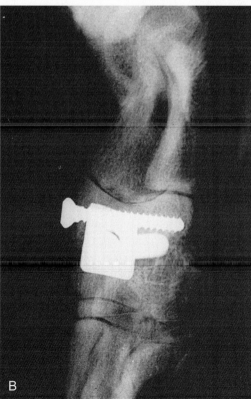

FIGURE 18–19. A/P preoperative *(A)* and medial-lateral one-month postoperative *(B)* view of the right tarsus of a racing greyhound. A highly comminuted (type V) central tarsal bone fracture in conjunction with a compression fracture of the fourth tarsal bone is appreciated on the preoperative A/P view. The medial to lateral 4.0-mm cancellous screw was passed through a single hole of a one-quarter tubular plate to act as a buttress to shore up the highly fragmented medial component as seen in this one-month postoperative medial view.

avulsion fractures of the lateral aspect of the base of metatarsal V.[9] Therefore, it is imperative that the total tarsus be examined, both physically and radiographically, lest subtle lesions go undetected.

All limbs are coapted in a soft roll and a double-thickness metasplint, prior to surgery and for 4 to 8 weeks postoperatively. We prefer to operate in the first 1 to 4 days but will operate up to two weeks after the injury. The earlier the surgery, the less need for a tourniquet. All screws are "lagged" and countersunk, and all are left in situ.

A survey was made of the records of greyhounds with central tarsal fractures for the period of 1975 to 1978 at the Hollywood Animal Hospital. Seventy-one per cent returned to winning after surgery. Given the benefit of time, experience, increased technical expertise, and improved equipment, we may realistically anticipate a 10 to 15 per cent improvement over the first series of 114 cases (i.e., an 80 to 85 per cent success rate). We have now operated on more than 300 animals.[7, 9, 13]

Fourth Tarsal Fracture

While we have seen a mere handful of compression fractures of the fourth tarsal bone in the pet population, we have seen more than 200 fourth tarsal bone fractures in the racing greyhound. These common fractures are seen in conjunction with approximately 40 per cent of the more severe types of central tarsal bone fractures. The sequence of events is as follows: as the craniomedial support of the central tarsal bone collapses under the compressive force of the calcaneus transmitted through the convex head of the talus, the brunt of the remaining compressive forces is placed on the fourth tarsal bone.[10] The fourth tarsal bone now assumes a trapezoidal shape as it shortens and subluxates laterally, frequently shearing off the lateral aspect of the base of metatarsal V (Figs. 18–3A and

18–18A). Repair of fourth tarsal bone fractures has been indirectly achieved by repairing the central tarsal bone and relying on the integrity of the central tarsal bone repair to provide support and maintenance of hock length and axial alignment. Additional shoring up of the fourth tarsal bone may be obtained by placing a second 4.0-mm cancellous screw medial to lateral from the second tarsal bone through the third tarsal bone and seated in the distal portion of the fourth tarsal bone (Fig. 18–3A,B). On occasion, the central and fourth tarsal bones are so badly comminuted as to make screw fixation impossible. Bone plates have been used to buttress the medial tarsus but the results have been better with screw fixation.[7]

Third Tarsal Fractures

Third tarsal bone fractures present as a solitary lesion, although on occasion there is an associated second tarsal bone subluxation/ fracture present (Figs. 18–3A,B and 18–20B). If the fracture is acute, slight soft tissue swelling is present and joint pain may be elicited directly over the fracture. If it is chronic, periosteal new bone formation is palpable to the astute clinician.[5, 14]

Radiographic changes may vary from the subtle to the obvious; they are determined by the amount of displacement of the solitary dorsal slab fracture. Experience has shown that whether the displacement is minimal or significant, the most predictable results with the least amount of degenerative joint disease are obtained by using a countersunk cortical bone screw in a lag manner. The extremity is coapted in slight extension for approximately six weeks.

Second Tarsal Fracture

Injuries to the second tarsal bone are rare. When seen, these uncommon injuries are nearly always associated with a severe

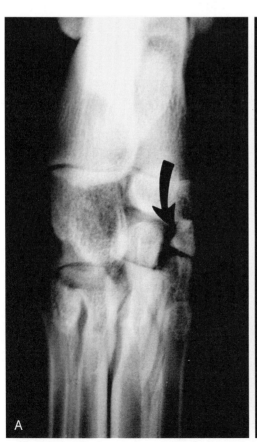
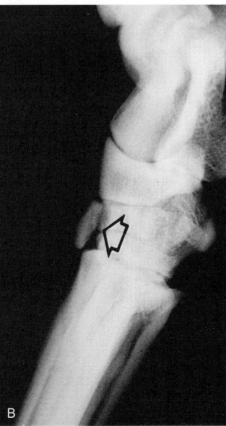

FIGURE 18–20. A/P preoperative *(A)* and medial lateral preoperative *(B)* view of a right tarsus that has sustained a subluxation of the second tarsal bone in conjunction with a dorsal slab fracture of the third tarsal bone, respectively.

fracture of the third tarsal bone (Figs. 18–3*A,B,* and 18–20*A*). Occasionally, one may see a subluxation of the second tarsal bone in association with a centrodistal instability or with a tarsometatarsal instability.[5, 15]

Radiographic signs are subtle and generally best appreciated on the P/A (A/P) view. An increase in the intratarsal joint space between T2 and T3 is seen. Fractures are extremely rare; subluxations are somewhat more common. Screw sizes as small as 1.5-mm cortical to as large as 4.0-mm cancellous have been successfully utilized. All screws are countersunk, seated in T4 and/or T3, and left in situ. Screws in T2 fractures are lagged. Screws in T2 subluxations may be lagged or positional. Most repairs require some form of postoperative coaptation.

Metatarsal Fractures

There exists a classical triad of fractures of the tarsus consisting of type IV central tarsal bone fracture, fourth tarsal fracture, and fracture of the lateral aspect of the base of metatarsal V.[10] Anatomically, the distal tendon of the peroneus (fibularis) brevis muscle crosses under the long fibular collateral ligament of the tarsus and then attaches to the proximal end of metatarsal V. The abductor digiti quinti muscle arises from the tuber calcanei, under the tendon of the superficial digital flexor, and courses distally to insert with the peroneus brevis on the base of the fifth metatarsal bone. A ligament from the body of the calcaneus is attached distally to the bases of metatarsals IV and V. Laterally, a conspicuous band leaves the caudolateral surface of the calcaneus and blends with the long fibular collateral ligament attached to the base of metatarsal V.[1]

When the craniomedial (compressive) side of the right hock collapses because of a central tarsal fracture, additional tensile forces are placed on some of the ligaments and tendons that have their insertions on the lateral base of metatarsal V, often resulting in an avulsion fracture (Figs. 18–3*A* and 18–18*A*). In addition, if the fourth tarsal bone is severely compressed, it will subluxate laterally and aid in shearing off the lateral portion of the base of metatarsal V.[10]

SPRAINS/SUBLUXATIONS AND STRAINS

Ligament Injury and Repair

The structure, function, mechanics, injury mechanisms, healing, and repair of many injuries of ligaments are well described in Chapter 17. Our comments center on the diagnosis and repair of comparable injuries of the tarsus.

Talocrural Subluxation/Luxation

Ligamentous injuries of the talocrural joint may be either partial or complete sprains, with or without an avulsion fracture component. Mild sprains may heal with support and rest. Complete sprains or avulsions are repaired by primary repair, if possible. Midsubstance tears may be sutured and supported. Tears at origins and insertions may be captured with suture material and reattached to the bone by way of transosseous tunnels.

Frequently, primary repair of the torn ligament is not possible and prosthetic replacement is required. The origin of the collateral ligaments is mimicked by the placement of a soft tissue "anchor" in the appropriate malleolus[16] or by the establishment of an anterior-posterior transosseous tunnel through the malleolus. The insertions of the long and short collateral ligaments are established by

the placement of two additional anchors in the talus medially or the calcaneus laterally, depending on whether you have a medial or lateral collateral instability. This technique of double prosthetic ligament replacement mimics the natural support of the long and short portions of the collateral ligaments.[17] These "reconstructed" ligaments are best protected with an external fixator initially and then decreasing amounts of support via splints, and finally soft roll bandages. Prognosis for return to athletics is poor.[7]

Talocrural Arthrodesis

Any unstable condition of the talocrural joint that cannot be reconstructed successfully is an indication for talocrural arthrodesis. Additional indications are degenerative joint disease that is not responsive to medical therapy, unrepairable calcaneal tendon injuries, and sciatic nerve palsy when combined with transposition of the long digital extensor tendon.[18]

Lag screw fixation of the talocrural joint is a commonly utilized method of arthrodesis.[19] The joint is approached by incising the origins of the medial collateral ligaments. Prior to insertion of an autogenous cancellous bone graft, all articular cartilage of the distal tibia and fibula is removed, as is the articular cartilage of the condyles of the talus. With the tarsus held in the functional position for the individual patient, a screw is lagged from the dorsal medial aspect of the distal tibia through the body of the talus to sit in the lateral plantar portion of the base of the calcaneus. An additional screw may be lagged from the dorsal lateral aspect of the distal tibia through the body of the talus to sit in the head of the talus. Some form of coaptation is required until fusion is achieved. Coaptation may be avoided and a more rigid form of protection may be achieved by the use of a transarticular external fixator[20] (Fig. 18–21). An alternate method of arthrodesis of the talocrural joint that has been useful is the application of DC plate on the dorsal aspect of the distal tibia, tarsus, and metatarsal III. The exposure is more extensive but provides for good fixation. The extremity is then coapted. Although both of these methods leave us with a "comfortable cripple" that cannot successfully return to competition, they allow salvage of the limb for pain-free ambulation.

Plantar Intertarsal Subluxations

This injury is caused by severe dorsiflexion, resulting in either tearing or avulsion of the plantar ligament that attaches proximally to the body of the calcaneus and distally to the fourth tarsal bone on its way to the base of the metatarsals IV and V. The plantar ligaments are much thicker and stronger that those on the dorsal side of the hock. Three distinct ligaments are noted, all of which are fused distally with the joint. Standard anatomical texts do not provide a specific nomenclature for the plantar ligaments. Therefore, the three plantar ligaments shall be referred to as the medial, middle, and lateral plantar ligaments.[3] One ligament (the medial) leaves the plantar surface of the sustentaculum tali and attaches to the central tarsal bone before ending at the tarsometatarsal joint capsule. Another (the lateral) leaves the caudolateral surface of the calcaneus and unites with the long fibular collateral ligament before attaching to the base of the fifth metatarsal bone. The third (the middle) and most commonly injured plantar ligament originates at the body of the calcaneus and attaches to the fourth tarsal bone before inserting at the base of the fourth and fifth metatarsals[1] (Fig. 18–2*B*).

The integrity of the plantar support apparatus is usually preserved in central or calcaneal fractures. Generally, the converse is also true. If the integrity of the plantar support apparatus is violated,

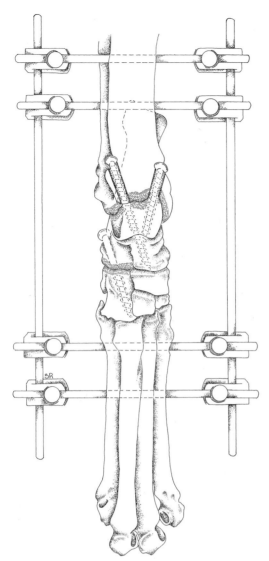

FIGURE 18–21. A dorsal view of a right tarsus showing the utilization of countersunk screws used in a lag manner across the talocrural joint and seated in the talus and calcaneus to facilitate, via compression, an arthrodesis of the joint. This is secondarily supported by a pre-bent (to the normal standing angle) external fixateur. In addition, an unrelated dorsal intertarsal subluxation with a primarily lateral instability has been stabilized by a arthrodesis of the calcaneoquartal joint via a lag screw. Fixator support is not required for this instability.

resulting in a plantar intertarsal subluxation, the patient exhibits a plantigrade walk, but the tarsal bones are usually free of fractures.[3]

Proximal intertarsal joint subluxations may involve either the dorsal or the plantar joint surfaces. Plantar subluxations are often associated with partial avulsions of the plantar ligament of the distal end of the calcaneus. The degree of involvement is best appreciated via stress radiography. Although locally swollen, the affected hock often is not particularly painful. Plantar subluxations are dorsiflexed; if weight bearing is attempted, the hock collapses and the patient has a plantigrade walk, like that of a rabbit.

For surgical repair, the patient is placed in sternal recumbency and the limb is extended posteriorly. A plantar incision is made beginning just proximal and lateral to the calcaneal tuber before extending distally to the base of metatarsal IV. The collateral

insertion of the superficial digital flexor on the lateral aspect of the tuber calcanei is incised, allowing the tendon to be reflected medially. A 2.0-mm hole is drilled from lateral to medial in the middle one-third of the fourth tarsal bone and a 1.0-mm cerclage wire is threaded through the drill hole. A hole is now drilled from the tuber calcanei distally down the medullary canal to emerge at the level of the joint (calcaneoquartal). The drill hole is filled with an appropriate-sized Steinmann pin. The articular cartilage of the calcaneoquartal joint is removed and replaced with a cancellous graft from the ipsilateral proximal humerus. With the tarsus in the normal position of function, the Steinmann pin is seated in the fourth tarsal bone. The cerclage wire is threaded in a figure-of-eight manner beneath the superficial digital flexor tendon and dorsal to the proximal bent end of the pin before being tightened (Fig. 18–14). The lateral portion of the superficial flexor is reattached. Any plantar ligament remnants are sutured prior to closure. The limb is then placed in a padded metasplint for 8 weeks. Fusion takes 8 to 12 weeks.[3, 5, 10, 21, 22]

An alternate method of repair is to countersink the pin and place the proximal loop of the wire through a hole drilled in the proximal one-fourth of the calcaneus. The advantage is no irritation to the flexor tendon from the pin—the disadvantage, the permanency of the pin[3, 5] (Fig. 18–22).

Dorsal Intertarsal Subluxation

This is a rare and subtle hyperextension injury of the limb. Soft tissue swelling is minimal and the patient is able to bear weight. Associated bone fragments are not present. This is a self-compress-

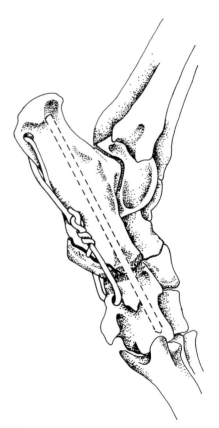

FIGURE 18–22. A lateral view of a tarsus with an arthrodesis of the calcaneoquartal joint to stabilize a plantar intertarsal subluxation via a countersunk pin and a tension band that is seated in the tuber calcis and the fourth tarsal bone.

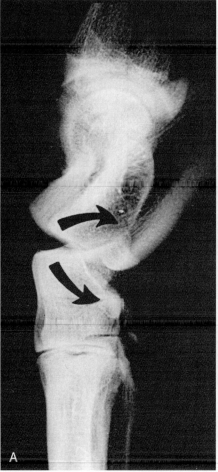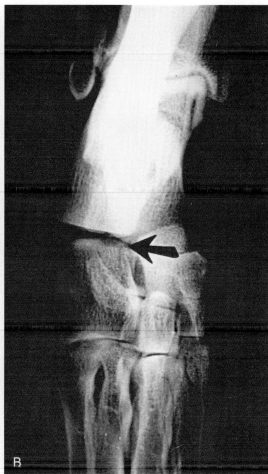

FIGURE 18–23. A medial *(A)* and a dorsal *(B)* view of a right tarsus. The dorsally stressed medial lateral view depicts a dorsal intertarsal subluxation. The laterally stressed A/P demonstrates some increased lateral instability of the calcaneoquartal joint. The plantar support mechanism is intact.

ing injury that becomes more stable with weight-bearing and less stable during the swing phase of the gait. In contrast, a plantar intertarsal subluxation becomes less stable during weight-bearing because the lesion is on the tension side of the tarsus rather than the compression side.

The tarsus can be hyperextended—opening the face or front of the joint space—allowing diagnosis by physical examination that is verified by medial-lateral stress radiography. As demonstrated by "stressed" dorsoplantar films, either the medial (talocalcaneoce-ntral, the joint primarily between the calcaneus and the talus and the central tarsal bone) or the lateral (calcaneoquartal, the joint between the calcaneus and the fourth tarsal bone) portion of the joint may be predominantly affected (Fig. 18–23A,B).

If the lesion is predominantly one sided, an arthrodesis is performed on that portion of the proximal intertarsal joint prior to screw compression. A bone screw is lagged through either the head of the talus into the fourth tarsal bone, or more commonly through the base of the calcaneus into the fourth tarsal bone[5, 8, 10, 21, 22] (Fig. 18–21).

Because this instability is inherently more stable with the limb loaded, an initial repair by coaptation alone may be considered before arthrodesis, especially in the individual with low functional requirements.

Plantar Tarsometatarsal Subluxation

Tarsometatarsal subluxations may be either plantar or dorsal. Plantar subluxations are more common despite thicker and stronger ligaments. Plantar tarsometatarsal joint subluxation is secondary to a severe sprain injury caused by excessive dorsiflexion damaging the plantar ligamentous support mechanism of the tarsometatarsal joint. Repair is by primary arthrodesis, utilizing a plantar approach that is simply a distal extension of the approach used for plantar intertarsal subluxations. An orthopedic wire is placed through a lateral to medial tunnel that has been drilled through the bases of the metatarsals, and an arthrodesis is performed. A Steinmann pin is placed from the tuber calcanei through a drill hole to seat in the base of metatarsal IV. The wire is placed under the superficial digital flexor and in front of the proximal portion of the pin prior to tightening in a figure-of-eight manner (Fig. 18–24A,B).[8] Some surgeons prefer a laterally placed DC plate for stabilization.

Dorsal Tarsometatarsal Subluxation

This is a rare and subtle hyperextension injury. Swelling is minimal and full weight bearing is possible. Physical examination and stress radiography are necessary for diagnosis. Bone fragments are rarely present. Although coaptation may be attempted, these injuries generally respond poorly to conservative management and are candidates for a primary arthrodesis via crossed pins.

Medial/Lateral Intertarsal Subluxation/Luxation

Intertarsal luxations involve the centrodistal (the joint between the central tarsal bone and the distal tarsal bones) joint and either the calcaneoquartal (the joint between the calcaneus and the fourth

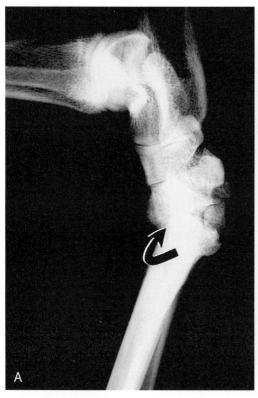
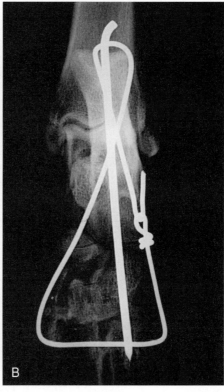

FIGURE 18–24. A preoperative medial *(A)* and a postoperative *(B)* view of a right tarsus. The plantarly stressed medial lateral views depicts a plantar tarsometatarsal subluxation. The nine-week P/A view shows early fusion of the tarsometatarsal arthrodesis site that has been stabilized and stress protected by a pin and figure-of-eight tension band wire.

tarsal bone) joint or the tarsometatarsal joint. Instability is present at one or more of these joint levels at the time of physical examination. The plantar support mechanism remains intact. Stressed radiographs demonstrate the amount of medial and/or lateral instability.

The most common instability involves the centrodistal joint and the calcaneoquartal joint. Repair is by arthrodesis. A seven-hole DC plate is placed laterally, incorporating three screws in the calcaneus. A two-hole plate is utilized medially with one screw in the central and one in the second tarsal bone that is seated in T3.[8]

Centrodistal tarsometatarsal subluxations involve the joint between the central tarsal bone and the distal tarsal bones and the joint between the fourth tarsal bone and the metatarsal bones.

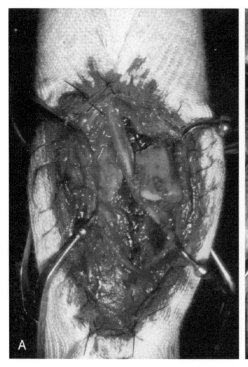
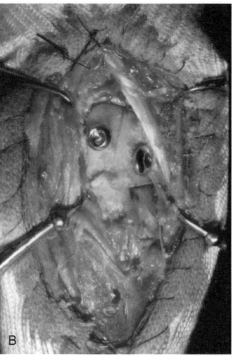

FIGURE 18–25. Repair of type IV central tarsal fracture. Both views, dorsal surface of right hock. *A,* Note the entrapment of the tibialis cranialis tendon between the dorsal and medial components of the fracture. Towel clamps are utilized as retractors. *B,* A 4.0-mm partially threaded cancellous screw has been lagged medial to lateral, through the medial fragment engaging the threads in the fourth tarsal bone. A 2.7-mm cortical screw has been lagged in a dorsoplantar direction through the dorsal slab component. Both are countersunk.

Arthrodesis may be achieved by utilizing two plates applied to the dorsal aspect of the central and fourth tarsal bones, and extending to incorporate the proximal portions of metatarsals III and IV.[8] If the instability is primarily one sided, that side of the tarsus may be plated.

Tendon Injury and Repair—Tibialis Cranialis

Many injuries of tendons are discussed in Chapter 16. An additional injury peculiar to the racing greyhound that is associated with the more severe central tarsal bone fractures (type IV and V) is the infrequent trauma to the tendon of insertion of the tibialis cranialis when it becomes entrapped between the fragments of a central tarsal bone fracture[7] (Fig. 18–25A,D). The tibialis cranialis muscle passes over the craniomedial surface of the crus, and near to its distal third becomes a thin, flat tendon. This tendon extends obliquely over the tarsus to the rudiment of metatarsal I, which is often fused with the first tarsal bone and to the proximal end of metatarsal II. The thread-like tendon of the muscle extensor hallucis longus encroaches closely upon the lateral edge of this tendon throughout its extent as far as the metatarsus, both turning toward the medial edge of the tarsus.[1]

One or both of these tendons may be injured at the time of fracture, while supported prior to repair, or during manipulation at the time of surgical reduction. The extension hallucis longus is too small to attempt reconstruction. The tibialis cranialis is managed via standard methodology.

References

1. Evans HE: Miller's Anatomy of the Dog. 3rd ed. Philadelphia, WB Saunders Company, 1993.
2. Shively MJ: Tarsal nomenclature. Veterinary Orthopedic Society. 6th Annual Conference. 1978.
3. Ost PC, Dee JF, Dee LG, Hohn RB. Fractures of the calcaneus in racing greyhounds. Vet Surg 16:53, 1987.
4. Farrow CS: Carpal sprain injury in the dog. J Am Vet Rad Soc 18:38–44, 1977.
5. Dee JF, Dee LG, Eaton-Wells RD: Injuries of high-performance dogs. In WG Whittick (ed): Canine Orthopedics II. Philadelphia, Lea and Febiger, 1990.
6. Montavon PM, Dee JF, and Weiss R: Distal tibial articular fractures in racing greyhounds: A review of six cases. Vet Comparat Orthopaed Traumatol 6:146–152, 1993.
7. Dee JF: Unpublished observations.
8. Dee JF, Dee LG, Earley T: Fractures of the carpus, tarsus, metacarpus, metatarsus, and phalanges. In Brinker WO, Hohn RB, Prieur WP (eds): Manual of Internal Fixation for Small Animals. Berlin, Springer-Verlag, 1984.
9. Boudrieau RJ, Dee JF, Dee LG: Central tarsal bone fractures in the racing greyhound: A review of 114 cases. J Am Vet Med Assoc 184:1486–1491, 1984.
10. Dee JF: Fractures in the Racing Greyhound. In Bojrab MJ (ed): Pathophysiology in Small Animal Surgery. Philadelphia, Lea and Febiger, 1981.
11. Dee JF, Dee J, Piermattei DL: Classification, management and repair of central tarsal fractures in the racing greyhound. JAAHA, 12:398–402, 1976.
12. Dee JF, Dee LG: Fractures and dislocations associated with the racing greyhound. In Nunamaker DM and Newton CD (eds): Textbook of Small Animal Orthopedics. Philadelphia, Lea and Febiger, 1985.
13. Boudrieau RJ, Dee JF, Dee LG: Treatment of central tarsal bone fractures in the racing greyhound. J Am Vet Med Assoc 184:1492–1500, 1984.
14. Dee JF: Third Tarsal Bone Fractures. In Refresher Course for Veterinarians. Proceedings No. 122, Greyhound Medicine and Surgery. University of Sydney, 1989.
15. Dee JF: Second Tarsal Bone Fracture. In Refresher Course for Veterinarians. Proceedings No. 122, Greyhound Medicine and Surgery. Sydney, University of Sydney, 1989.
16. Beale BS, Lewis DD: Clinical use of titanium anchors for treatment of trauma-induced joint instability in small animals. Veterinary Orthopedic Society, 23rd Annual Conference. Telluride, CO, 1996.
17. Aron DN: Prosthetic ligament replacement for severe tarsocrural joint instability. JAAHA 23:41, 1987.
18. Lesser A, Solimen SS: Experimental evaluation of tendon transfer for the treatment of sciatic nerve paralysis in the dog. Vet Surg 9:72, 1980.
19. Newton CD, Nunamaker DM: Arthrodesis of the tibiotarsal joint. In Brinker WO, Hohn RB, and Prieur WD (eds): Manual of Internal Fixation for Small Animals. Berlin, Springer-Verlag, 1984.
20. Ellison GW, Tarvin GB: The use of external fixators for selected juxta-articular injuries in the dog and cat. Presented at the 9th annual meeting, Veterinary Orthopedic Society, Park City, UT, 1982.
21. Dee JF: Injuries of the distal tibia and tarsus. Proceedings of the AAHA, 359, 1984.
22. Dee JF: Proximal Intertarsal Subluxation. In Refresher Course for Veterinarians. Proceedings No. 122, Greyhound Medicine and Surgery. Post-Graduate Committee in Veterinary Science. University of Sydney, 1989, pp 550–553.

CHAPTER 19

STIFLE INJURIES

LOIC M. DEJARDIN \ JEAN A. NEMZEK \ STEVEN PAUL ARNOCZKY

Stifle injuries comprise the majority of problems responsible for rear limb lameness in the adult dog, and the recognition and treatment of these conditions are an important part of any small animal practice. While lesions of the stifle can encompass a wide variety of traumatic and degenerative manifestations of bone, cartilage, and ligaments, this chapter examines the more commonly encountered injuries of this joint. This discussion includes epidemiology and mechanism of injury, treatment options, postoperative considerations, and prognosis.

FUNCTIONAL ANATOMY OF THE STIFLE

Successful treatment of any stifle injury centers around the ability to maintain or restore normal joint kinematics. Knowledge of the functional anatomy of the stifle is therefore a prerequisite to any discussion of stifle disorders.

Stifle Kinematics

The stifle joint represents the movable link between the femur and the tibia. In anatomical terms, the stifle is classified as a diarthrodial, condylar joint and is made of two functionally distinct articulations: the femorotibial joint and the femoropatellar joint. The femorotibial joint functions like a hinge about which the leg mainly extends and flexes. The femoropatellar joint consists of the patella which glides in the femoral trochlea and acts like a pulley. This joint can be seen as an enhancing feature that potentiates the extensor function of the quadriceps muscles. Because of its complex motion and the presence of various intra-articular structures (cruciate ligaments and menisci), the stifle joint is perhaps the most complex joint in the body.

In the most basic terms, the free movement of the femur relative to the tibia can be described by a set of three mutually orthogonal axes (x, y, z) (Fig. 19–1). The x axis passes through the femoral condyles parallel to the joint line in a medial-lateral direction. The y axis is parallel to the shaft of the tibia and passes through the medial tibial condyle just medial to the center of the tibial plateau. The z axis passes through the center of the joint space in a craniocaudal orientation.

Rotation about each axis, as well as translation (sliding) along each axis, results in six basic movements of the stifle joint (also termed the six degrees of freedom). While each motion (eg, flexion-extension, valgus-varus angulation, axial rotation, cranial-caudal translation) may be present to some extent in normal stifle motion, individual movements on or about a specific axis are limited by various ligamentous constraints:

x axis Rotation: normal flexion and extension of the stifle joint
        Translation: prohibited by cruciate and collateral ligaments
y axis Rotation: axial rotation of the tibia on the femur; prohibited by the collateral ligaments (extension: internal and external

rotation; flexion: external rotation) and limited by the cruciate ligaments (flexion: internal rotation)
        Translation: prohibited by cruciate and collateral ligaments in tension and by the articular cartilage and menisci in compression
z axis Rotation: varus and valgus angulation; prohibited by the collateral ligaments
        Translation: drawer movement; prohibited by cruciate ligaments

Thus, abnormal movement on or about a specific axis indicates damage to the specified constraints.

Normally, the stifle moves in two planes. Flexion-extension takes place about the x (or transverse) axis, while rotary movement of the tibia on the femur occurs about the y (or longitudinal) axis. In general, flexion-extension takes place between the femur and me-

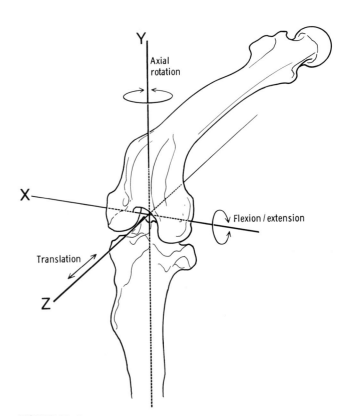

FIGURE 19–1. The stifle of the dog showing the three axes of motion (x, y, and z) and their orientation. (From Arnoczky SP: Cruciate ligament rupture and associated injuries. *In* Newton CD, Nunamaker DM (eds): Textbook of Small Animal Orthopaedics. Philadelphia, JB Lippincott, 1985.)

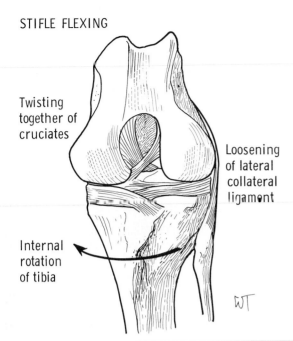

STIFLE FLEXING

Twisting together of cruciates

Loosening of lateral collateral ligament

Internal rotation of tibia

FIGURE 19–2. As the stifle is flexed the lateral collateral ligament loosens, allowing internal rotation of the tibia on the femur. The cruciate ligaments "twist" on each other to limit this internal rotation. (From Arnoczky SP, Torzilli PA, Marshall JL. Evaluation of anterior cruciate ligament repair in the dog: An analysis of the instant center of rotation. J Am Anim Hosp Assoc 13:553–558, 1977.)

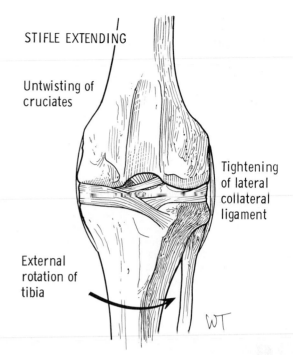

STIFLE EXTENDING

Untwisting of cruciates

Tightening of lateral collateral ligament

External rotation of tibia

FIGURE 19–3. As the stifle is extended, the lateral collateral ligament tightens and the tibia rotates externally. The cruciate ligaments "untwist" and thus have no effect on limiting external rotation. (From Arnoczky SP, Torzilli PA, Marshall JL. Evaluation of anterior cruciate ligament repair in the dog: An analysis of the instant center of rotation. J Am Anim Hosp Assoc 13:553–558, 1977.)

nisci while rotational movements occur between the tibia and menisci. The rotary motions are controlled by condylar geometry and ligamentous constraints. As the stifle is flexed (Fig. 19–2), the femoral and tibial attachments of the lateral collateral ligament move closer together and the ligament begins to relax. This allows caudal displacement of the smaller lateral femoral condyle on the tibial plateau (rotation about the y axis) and results in internal (medial) rotation of the tibia on the femur. Conversely, as the stifle is extended (Fig. 19–3), the lateral collateral ligament tightens, and the lateral femoral condyle moves cranially on the tibial plateau, causing external (lateral) rotation of the tibia on the femur. In humans, this motion has been classically termed the screw-home mechanism.

Because of their anatomical relationship and spatial orientation within the joint, the cruciate ligaments begin to "twist" about one another as the stifle is flexed and the tibia internally rotates on the femur. This twisting action limits the amount of normal internal rotation of the tibia. As the stifle is extended, the cruciate ligaments "untwist" and therefore have no individual effect in limiting external rotation of the tibia.

While the cruciate and collateral ligaments are considered the major static stabilizers of the stifle, the menisci also contribute to joint stability during the flexion-extension and rotary movements of the joint. As the stifle is flexed, the menisci slide caudally on the tibial plateau (Fig. 19–4). Because of its attachments to the medial collateral ligament and joint capsule, the medial meniscus displaces considerably less than the lateral meniscus. The caudal displacement of the lateral femoral condyle on the tibia during flexion makes the caudal displacement of the lateral meniscus even more pronounced, and in extreme movements of flexion, the meniscus may protrude over the edge of the tibial plateau. Conversely, as the stifle is extended, both menisci slide cranially on the tibial plateau.

Stifle Kinetics

Ground reaction forces (GRF) are forces exerted by the ground against a body in reaction to gravity. These external forces are transmitted through the bones and the joints and are counteracted by internal muscular forces that help maintain postures (state of

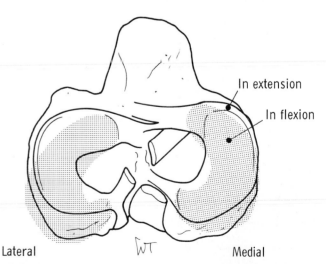

In extension
In flexion

Lateral   Medial

FIGURE 19–4. The dorsal aspect of the tibia illustrating the normal excursion of the menisci in extension and flexion (shaded). Note the limited movement of the medial meniscus. (From Arnoczky SP, Torzilli PA, Marshall JL. Evaluation of anterior cruciate ligament repair in the dog: An analysis of the instant center of rotation. J Am Anim Hosp Assoc 13:553–558, 1977.)

equilibrium) or generate motion (state of imbalance). Ground reaction forces can be divided into three basic components along mutually orthogonal axes (vertical, craniocaudal, mediolateral).

At rest in a standing position, about 60 to 65 per cent of the body weight is evenly borne by the front legs and 35 per cent of the body weight by the rear legs. During motion, the percentage of body weight carried by each leg increases because of kinetic energy. The higher the velocity, the more weight is placed on the limbs. In normal dogs moving forward at the trot (about 2 m/s), the vertical force corresponds to about 110 per cent of the body weight for each front leg and approximately 70 per cent of the body weight for each rear leg. Craniocaudal components of the GRF can be divided into a "braking" force followed by a "propulsive" force. The braking effect results from friction forces that tend to slow the animal each time a paw hits the ground. The propulsive effect follows as the animal propels itself to maintain its velocity. The braking force is greater for the front legs (16 per cent of the body weight at the trot) than for the rear legs (8 per cent of the body weight at the trot). The propulsive force is greater for the rear legs (10 per cent of body weight) than for the front legs (7 per cent). This force distribution pattern shows the importance of the rear legs in propulsion.

EPIDEMIOLOGY, CLINICAL SIGNS, AND DIAGNOSIS OF STIFLE INJURIES

Ligamentous Injuries

Cruciate Ligaments

Cranial cruciate ligament rupture is the most common injury to the stifle joint of dogs and is often the primary cause of degenerative arthritic changes diagnosed in that joint. Although associated with many breeds of dogs, rupture of the cranial cruciate ligament occurs with greatest frequency in large breeds of dogs, including rottweilers, Newfoundlands, and Staffordshire terriers. There is also a high prevalence in several sporting breeds, including Chesapeake Bay retrievers, Labrador retrievers, and German shorthair pointers. Rupture of the cranial cruciate ligament has been reported but with a lower incidence in golden retrievers, setters, spaniels, and greyhounds. The problem occurs most often in middle-aged and older dogs. Females have a higher incidence of cranial cruciate ligament rupture than males.

Acute traumatic rupture of the cranial cruciate ligament is diagnosed infrequently but is generally the cause of ruptures observed in young animals (<5 years old). The injury occurs as a result of specific, sudden stresses such as internal rotation and/or hyperextension of the limb.

In smaller breeds the majority of cranial cruciate ligament ruptures are associated with slow degeneration of the ligament. This process may result in partial tearing and minor instability that progresses over several months. The cause of degeneration is largely unknown, but several factors may contribute to the ultimate failure of the ligament. It is known that the strength of the ligament decreases as the dog ages, and chronic ruptures are diagnosed most frequently in older dogs. This decrease in strength is associated with changes in the microscopic structure of the ligament. The ligament may be further weakened by the repeated stresses produced by other conditions such as patellar luxation and abnormal conformation (straight legs, bowlegs, or knock-knees). Likewise, obesity can overload the stifle joint, creating additional stress on the cranial cruciate ligament. Because the initial degeneration and any contributing factors affect both rear legs, rupture of the cranial cruciate ligament can occur bilaterally in older dogs.

The clinical signs associated with cranial cruciate ligament rupture vary depending upon the cause of rupture. Dogs with traumatic ruptures will initially be non–weight-bearing. Over the course of several weeks, they begin to bear weight and may exhibit only a mild limp as fibrous tissue partially stabilizes the joint. Degenerative ruptures have an ill-defined course and may show episodic, mild to moderate lameness for several weeks to months. Lameness usually worsens with exercise. Dogs may also demonstrate difficulty in rising and shifting weight from one leg to the other, particularly if both stifles are affected. In all cases of untreated cranial cruciate ligament rupture, lameness is progressive as secondary arthritic degeneration develops. Dogs may become non–weight-bearing, usually a sign of secondary meniscal damage.

Diagnosis is made from the history of lameness and physical examination, which usually reveals some degree of rear limb lameness. Conformational abnormalities, obesity, and muscle atrophy of the affected leg may also be observed. Palpation of the joint usually does not elicit a pain response except in very acute cases. Gross enlargement of the joint due to thickening and fibrosis of the surrounding tissues, particularly on the medial aspect of the joint, is evident in chronic cases. Joint effusion is present in most cases and may be manifested by swelling of the joint with loss of palpable definition of the patellar tendon. Definitive diagnosis is made by demonstrating the cranial "drawer sign," in which the tibia slides forward with respect to the femur (Fig. 19–5). The drawer sign is generally present in dogs with acute, complete tears of the cruciate ligament. In dogs with chronic lameness and partial cruciate tears, the drawer sign may be minimal or absent. For large

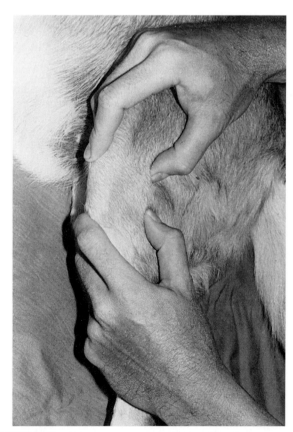

FIGURE 19–5. The drawer movement. With the stifle slightly flexed, the tibia is forced cranially and caudally while the femur is maintained in place. Forward motion of the tibia relative to the femur indicates a rupture of the cranial cruciate ligament. Backward motion reveals a rupture of the caudal cruciate ligament. (From Arnoczky SP, Tarvin GB. Physical examination of the musculoskeletal system. Vet Clin North Am Small Anim Pract 11:575–593, 1981.)

dogs, apprehensive dogs, and those with chronic fibrosis, sedation may be necessary to overcome any muscle rigidity that might suppress the drawer sign. Radiographs will detect joint effusion but will not detect the ruptured ligament except in rare cases involving avulsion of the ligament with a detectable bony fragment. Radiographs can also provide prognostic information by demonstrating the degree of arthritic change present.

Isolated rupture of the caudal cruciate ligament results when a cranial to caudal force is applied to the proximal tibia. Such trauma is rare, and therefore rupture of the caudal cruciate ligament alone is seldom diagnosed. Injury to the caudal cruciate is more often seen with severe trauma and disruption of multiple ligaments. In these cases, rupture of the caudal cruciate is often accompanied by trauma to the cranial cruciate ligament, one or both collateral ligaments, and the menisci. Dogs with caudal cruciate ligament rupture have non–weight-bearing lameness and joint swelling. Diagnosis is made by demonstrating the caudal drawer sign in which the tibia glides caudal with respect to the femur. The motion elicited in the unstable joint may be confused with the cranial drawer sign, and accurate diagnosis depends upon recognition of the normal position of the tibia with respect to the femur.

Collateral Ligaments

Rupture of a single collateral ligament, either medial or lateral, occurs rarely and produces only minor medial or lateral joint instability. Injury to the collateral ligaments is most commonly associated with severe trauma resulting in multiligamentous damage and severe joint instability.

Trauma to a collateral ligament may produce a complete tear of the ligament itself or create an avulsion of the ligament from the femur. Because multiple injuries are usually involved, dogs with collateral ligament rupture usually have non–weight-bearing lameness and diffuse swelling of the joint. The diagnosis is made by demonstrating medial or lateral joint instability by palpation and radiography of the stressed joint. Radiographs may also demonstrate fragments of bone avulsed with the ligament.

Meniscal Injury

Meniscal injury seldom occurs as an isolated event. Usually, meniscal injury is associated with joint instability caused by rupture of the cranial cruciate ligament. The medial meniscus is more susceptible to damage than the lateral because its ligamentous attachments make it relatively immobile. With rupture of the cranial cruciate ligament, there is increased internal rotation of the tibia on the femur and crushing of the stationary medial meniscus. Repeated abnormal wear can result in tearing of the meniscus (Fig. 19–6). In addition, the attachments of the caudal horn may be torn, allowing the meniscus to fold upon itself. Meniscal injury may also be associated with multiligamentous injury as previously described.

A tentative diagnosis of meniscal tear can be made by history and physical examination. A history of chronic lameness that suddenly worsens is a common finding with degenerative cruciate disease resulting in meniscal injury. During manipulation of the joint, a clicking sound may be elicited as the damaged portion of the meniscus snaps back and forth. This click is considered diagnostic for a meniscal tear; however, the absence of a click does not exclude the presence of meniscal injury. Meniscal damage and wedging of the meniscus between the femur and tibia may confound the diagnosis of a concurrent cranial cruciate ligament rupture by preventing the drawer sign. Definitive diagnosis of meniscal injury is made during exploratory arthrotomy.

Injury of the Extensor Apparatus

The extensor apparatus is composed of the quadriceps femoris, the patella, and the patellar tendon. From a cranial view the normal

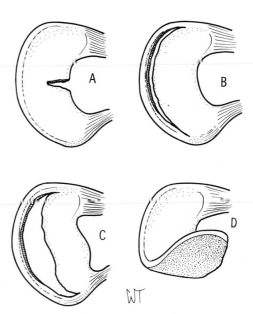

FIGURE 19–6. Common lesions of the medial meniscus showing: a transverse tear *(A),* a longitudinal tear *(B),* a bucket-handle tear *(C),* and a cranial horn tear with folding over the caudal horn *(D).* (From Arnoczky SP: Pathomechanics of cruciate ligament and meniscal injuries. *In* Bojrab MJ (ed): Disease Mechanisms in Small Animal Surgery. 2nd ed. Philadelphia, Lea & Febiger, 1993.)

extensor mechanism runs in a straight line from the subtrochanteric area to the tibial tuberosity. The patella glides within the femoral groove, which enhances the power of the quadriceps (pulley effect) and allows efficient extension of the leg.

Problems associated with the extensor mechanism occur less frequently than the ligamentous injuries described but are reported occasionally in sporting breeds of dogs. These abnormalities may be congenital (patellar luxations) or traumatic (fractures, tendon ruptures, some patellar luxations) in origin.

Patellar luxation in medium and large-breed dogs may be either medial or lateral. Lateral patellar luxation is diagnosed more often in large-breed than in small-breed dogs. Luxations are usually diagnosed in young dogs (<2 years of age). Several congenital and developmental abnormalities that allow malalignment of the extensor apparatus may be associated with patellar luxations, including a shallow trochlear groove, abnormal hip conformation, displacement of the quadriceps tendon, rotation of the distal femur, redundant joint capsule, and deviation of the proximal tibia. Clinically, patellar luxations are graded (from I to IV) according to severity. Mild cases may exhibit only occasional luxation of the patella (grade I). In these cases the dogs are lame only rarely, and patellar luxation may be an incidental finding during routine physical examination. The majority of patellar luxations are diagnosed as either grade II or grade III, in which displacement of the patella occurs more frequently and lameness is more persistent. Severe cases have permanent patellar luxation and severe skeletal abnormalities (grade IV). In extreme situations the patella becomes located caudal to the center of rotation of the stifle and thus transforms the quadriceps into a flexor muscle. Deprived of its major stifle extensor group, the animal is unable to stand or walk. Diagnosis is made by palpation of the lateral patellar luxation. Radiographs are useful to assess the degree of related skeletal abnormalities.

The remaining conditions associated with the extensor apparatus are the result of trauma; all of these conditions are diagnosed infrequently compared to ligamentous injuries. Patellar fractures are most often the result of a direct blow. Avulsion of the tibial tuberosity is diagnosed in young dogs. This lesion occurs when a traumatic incident results in hyperflexion of the stifle with concurrent contraction of the quadriceps muscle. Ruptures of the patellar tendon have been associated with direct laceration, but often the cause of rupture is unknown. With all of these conditions the affected dog exhibits sudden onset of non–weight-bearing lameness, painful swelling of the stifle joint, and inability to extend the leg. Palpation of the joint will localize the problem, and radiographs will provide the definitive diagnosis.

Miscellaneous Conditions

Other conditions of the stifle include osteochondritis dissecans, avulsion of the long digital extensor tendon, avulsion of the gastrocnemius, and avulsion of the popliteal tendon.

Osteochondritis dissecans occurs in the stifle joint of young large-breed dogs. Osteochondritis often results in a dissecting flap of articular cartilage with inflammatory joint changes. The cartilage flap may become fully detached from normal articular cartilage and stimulate synovitis until removed. Most often the lesion is seen in the lateral femoral condyle, but the medial condyle may be affected. The dogs have variable degrees of lameness, depending on the extent of the lesion. Diagnosis is made by history, physical examination, and radiographic signs. For additional information see Chapter 27.

The most commonly diagnosed strain in the stifle joint involves the tendon of origin of the long digital extensor muscle (LDE). The LDE originates from the extensor fossa of the lateral femoral condyle and inserts on the distal phalanges. Its functions are to extend the digits and flex the hock. Avulsion of the tendon of origin of the LDE is usually seen in young large-breed dogs and results in painful joint effusion with weight-bearing lameness. Diagnosis can be made by radiographic identification of an avulsed bone fragment or by exploratory arthrotomy.

Avulsion of the head(s) of the gastrocnemius muscle has been reported in working breeds such as the fox terrier, German shepherd, and Labrador retriever. The gastrocnemius muscle normally arises from the lateral and medial supracondylar tuberosities of the femur and inserts on the calcaneus. Dogs with avulsion of the head of the gastrocnemius will often have acute, non–weight-bearing lameness. Because the gastrocnemius muscle is a major extensor of hock, avulsion will result in hyperflexion of the hock during weight bearing. Radiographs may reveal displacement of the fabellae, which are contained within the tendons of origin of the gastrocnemius muscle.

Avulsion of the origin of the popliteal muscle also occurs in large-breed dogs. The popliteal muscle runs caudally from the lateral femoral condyle to the medial aspect of the proximal tibia and functions to flex the stifle and internally rotate the tibia. The tendon of the popliteal muscle includes a sesamoid bone that faces the caudolateral angle of the tibial plateau. Avulsion of the tendon of origin of the popliteal muscle results in weight-bearing lameness. Diagnosis is made by radiography, which reveals distal displacement of the sesamoid bone located within the tendon. After avulsion of the tendon, the sesamoid bone lies in a more distal and medial position.

TREATMENT AND PROGNOSIS OF STIFLE INJURIES

To assume its function as a weight-bearing joint and as a key structure in locomotion, the stifle joint must be stable, and the extensor mechanism must work efficiently. While the integrity of ligamentous constraints guarantees the stability of the joint, the effectiveness of the extensor mechanism depends on its proper alignment and on the adequate positioning of the patella in the femoral trochlea. The goal of treatment in stifle injuries is restoration of the stability and function of the joint to prevent or limit degenerative joint disease (DJD).

Nonoperative versus Operative

Several factors should be carefully considered prior to making an appropriate therapeutic decision. The nature of the stifle lesion is by itself a key factor. For instance, a patellar fracture is unlikely to improve without surgical attention, whereas a grade I luxated patella may benefit from physical therapy and controlled activity. As a general rule, small dogs may adequately function with nonoperative management of certain isolated ligamentous injuries such as rupture of the cranial cruciate ligament or collateral ligaments, while larger dogs show greater benefit with surgical intervention. For any size of dog, obesity may complicate surgical treatment and compromise its outcome by placing additional stress on the repair. Age and systemic pathology, such as Cushing's disease, may interfere with postoperative healing, making a medical/nonoperative approach more appropriate. In general, concurrent orthopedic conditions such as hip dysplasia or fracture justify surgical intervention over nonoperative management. Prior to consideration of surgery, it is always important to anticipate client and dog compliance to postoperative instructions. Finally, the client's expectation regarding the dog's future performance is crucial in determining the appropriate course of action.

Few stifle injuries, regardless of the mode of treatment, will recover fully and allow return to peak performance. However, in most instances, treatment will significantly improve the quality of life.

Nonoperative Management

Nonoperative treatment consists mainly of controlled activity for a period of 8 to 12 weeks. Rest during acute episodes of pain should alternate with moderate activity during remission periods. Short leash walks and non–weight-bearing activity such as swimming are recommended to improve muscular fitness. Passive range of motion, which helps in decreasing joint capsule adhesions, can also be implemented. Massages and heat are very beneficial in relieving muscle spasm and pain. A warm, water-soaked towel is applied around the joint for 10 minutes two or three times a day. However, in acute joint injuries, cold rather than heat is indicated to decrease pain, joint swelling, and hematoma formation. Body weight must be controlled during the postoperative period. Weight reduction in overweight animals will effectively contribute to clinical improvement of chronic lameness.

In addition, several anti-inflammatory drugs have been used to reduce local inflammation associated with loss of joint stability. Aspirin (buffered or not) is the most commonly used and one of the most potent anti-inflammatory drugs. Effective, readily available, inexpensive, and free from most side effects, aspirin is the first drug of choice in the treatment of osteoarthritis. Aspirin or buffered aspirin is recommended at a dose of 10 mg/kg two times a day. Feeding prior to aspirin administration helps prevent gastrointestinal upsets. Treatment should be suspended if vomiting persists. Other nonsteroidal anti-inflammatory drugs (ibuprofen, phenylbutazone, meclofenamic acid) have been used with varying success. Steroids administered orally or intra-articularly at anti-inflammatory doses may reduce cartilage erosion and osteophyte production. Although efficient, steroids have serious, undesirable systemic side effects and should be used only as a last resort. Hyaluronic acid injected intra-articularly significantly reduces cartilage damage by acting on the synovial membrane to decrease the inflammatory reaction. Glycosaminoglycan polysulfate reduces connective tissue breakdown and therefore DJD. Although of great potential, clinical use of hyaluronic acid and glycosaminoglycan should be postponed until conclusive results of clinical trials are available. It should be emphasized that most medications do not reverse DJD and should always be used cautiously, if needed, as determined by the animal's discomfort or decreased activity.

Specific Operative Management

This section examines some of the basic principles involved in the repair of various injuries of the stifle. While specific operative techniques will not be described in detail (these are available in numerous veterinary surgical texts), indications for repair, postoperative management, and prognosis are discussed.

Cranial Cruciate Ligament

Numerous procedures have been described to repair cranial cruciate ligament rupture. However, none is clearly superior to the others. All procedures are designed to improve joint stability either by reconstructing or replacing the ligament (intracapsular techniques) or by transposing or implanting periarticular structures or sutures (extracapsular techniques). Selection of a procedure is based on factors such as body weight, presence of DJD, and/or surgeon's preference. Although clinical improvement in lameness is observed postoperatively in most instances, the long-term success of a surgical procedure must be measured by its ability to slow the progression of DJD.

All surgical protocols start with exploratory arthrotomy. During arthrotomy the menisci are evaluated and medial meniscectomy is performed if necessary. The remnants of the cruciate ligament are debrided, and large osteophytes are removed. Then the surgeon can proceed with the chosen stabilization protocol.

Surgical Techniques

Primary Repair. Primary repair of midsubstance tears is technically difficult, if feasible at all, in dogs. Because the majority of cranial cruciate ligament ruptures in dogs are chronic, collagen degeneration and atrophy of ligament stumps will be present at time of surgery. Furthermore, the cranial cruciate ligament is thought to have limited healing ability.

Avulsion of the cranial cruciate ligament from the tibial plateau can theoretically be treated by direct reimplantation using a small lag screw or pins and tension band wire. The procedure is rarely successful because the small avulsed bone fragment is usually deprived of cancellous bone and heals poorly.

Intracapsular Techniques. Intra-articular procedures involve the use of a graft in the joint space. Although the grafts may be of different origin, the patellar tendon and/or the fascia lata are often chosen. The graft follows a direction that closely resembles that of the original cranial cruciate ligament and therefore mimics its natural function. These procedures are often preferred in large-breed dogs (greater than 15 kg) with little or no arthritic changes in the joint.

Since the introduction of two original procedures (Paatsama and "over-the-top"), several variations of each technique have been developed. In the Paatsama technique, a graft of fascia lata is introduced into the joint through a bony tunnel drilled in the lateral femoral condyle and the tibial plateau. In the over-the-top technique the graft is composed of a band of patellar tendon and a strip of fascia lata. The graft is routed into the intercondyloid fossa and exits the joint over the top of the lateral femoral condyle (Fig. 19–7).

Extracapsular Techniques. Extracapsular procedures rely on enhancement of periarticular fibrosis to provide long-term stability of the joint. Extracapsular procedures are easier to perform than intra-articular techniques. In general, they yield far better results in small-breed dogs (less than 15 kg) than in large-breed dogs. However, some techniques, such as fibular head transposition and retinacular imbrication, have shown very good results in large-breed dogs.

In fibular head transposition, internal rotation and forward translation of the tibia are prevented by moving the fibular head and the collateral ligament to a more cranial position. The major advantage of this procedure over imbrication methods, which require implantation of heavy suture, is that only autogenous structures are used. In retinacular imbrication techniques, joint stability is achieved by tightening large nonabsorbable sutures between the fabellae and the tibial crest (Fig. 19–8). The sutures mimic the function of the cranial cruciate ligament and induce local fibrosis. Ultimately, stability of the joint depends on secondary scar tissue deposition. The major complication associated with this procedure is a risk of implant failure and/or rejection.

Postoperative Regime

Ideally, passive range of motion should be implemented soon after surgery to prevent muscle atrophy, cartilage degeneration, and excessive intra-articular adhesions. However, as a result of low dog/owner compliance for postoperative physical therapy, it is often not possible. Practically, immobilization is recommended to protect the graft, facilitate its healing, and limit excessive joint motion. Typically a heavy padded bandage such as a Robert Jones is applied for 2 weeks, and activity is drastically reduced to leash-walks only for 6 to 8 weeks. Non–weight-bearing exercise, such as swimming, is the best physical therapy to improve joint motion, joint stability, and musculature, while respecting the implants. Progressive increase in activity level is permitted during the following 6 to 8 weeks. Before returning to competition or field trial activity, athletic dogs should be slowly rehabilitated. Their training should be gradually intensified over a 6-month period. Excessive weight should be controlled during and after the rehabilitation period.

Prognosis

Prognosis after surgical repair depends on several factors such as preexisting degenerative joint disease, meniscal damage, obesity, underlying systemic disease, concomitant orthopedic lesions, and compliance with the postoperative nursing care regimen. In an ideal situation, such as acute rupture of the cranial cruciate ligament in a well-conditioned and healthy dog, return to previous activity level is conceivable with appropriate joint stabilization. Peak performance is, however, unlikely to be reached. Hunting dogs should be able to perform adequately by the following season. In obese giant-breed dogs with preexisting DJD, prognosis is poor to guarded not only for functional recovery of the operated-on stifle but also for soundness of the opposite joint.

Caudal Cruciate Ligament

Surgical Techniques

Many surgeons believe that isolated rupture of the caudal cruciate ligament does not require surgical repair because, under load, the stifle tends to work against caudal displacement of the tibia, and the powerful quadriceps-patellar tendon unit seems to provide adequate joint stability. However, caudal cruciate ligament ruptures are rarely isolated injuries and most of the time necessitate surgical attention.

Retinacular imbrication techniques involve the use of suture material tightened outside of the joint. The medial imbrication suture runs between the patella and the caudal angle of the tibial plateau. A second suture is placed around the patella and the fibular head laterally. The major complication associated with this

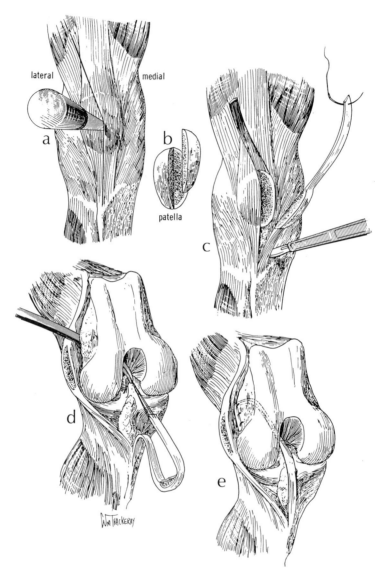

FIGURE 19–7. Over-the-top patellar tendon graft. Placement of osteotome to remove craniomedial wedge of patella (a). Extend of patellar osteotomy which respects the caudal articular surface of the patella (b). The graft includes joint capsule, patellar tendon, and fascia lata (c). Cranial view of flexed stifle showing tips of the hemostatic forceps emerging from over the top of the lateral femoral condyle, into the joint, and grasping the sutures placed in the free end of the graft (d). Cranial view of the stifle showing the graft passing through the joint and over the top of the lateral femoral condyle. The graft is then sutured to the soft tissues of the lateral femoral condyle (e). (From Arnoczky SP, et al: The over the top procedure. A technique for cranial cruciate ligament substitution in the dog. J Am Anim Hosp Assoc 15:283, 1979.)

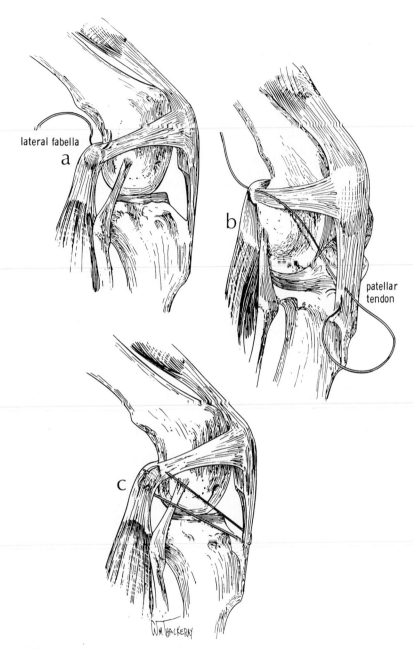

lateral fabella

a

b

patellar
tendon

c

WM HACKERY

FIGURE 19–8. Lateral retinacular imbrication. The imbrication suture is placed in the connective tissue surrounding the fabella (a), then into the lateral third of the patellar tendon just proximal to the tibial tuberosity (b). Alternatively, the suture can be directed through a hole drilled in the tibial crest. Finally, the imbrication suture is anchored into the connective tissue caudoventrally to the lateral fabella where it is tied with the limb in a functional position (c). In some instances, stability is improved by placing a similar suture on the medial side. A third suture may be pulled between the lateral fabella and the patella to enhance lateral retinacular fibrosis. (From Arnoczky SP: Surgery of the stifle: The cruciate ligaments. Comp Cont Ed 2:106, 1980.)

technique is secondary luxation of the patella due to asymmetrical tension applied to the sutures.

Ligament displacement techniques can also be used. Laterally the long digital extensor tendon is pulled caudally beyond the fibular head, then maintained in place and allowed to glide on a screw and a smooth washer anchored in the fibula. A similar procedure involving the medial collateral ligament is performed on the medial aspect of the joint. This procedure is technically challenging but provides better stability than the retinacular imbrication. There is a risk of collateral ligament or extensor tendon rupture due to premature wear.

Postoperative Regimen

Postoperative recommendations are identical to those previously described for cranial cruciate ligament rupture.

Prognosis

Isolated midsubstance rupture usually carries a fair prognosis even with nonoperative management. In many cases the prognosis must be guarded because multiple injuries, including rupture of the cranial cruciate and medial collateral ligaments, are involved. Although quality of life is greatly improved by surgery, dogs should be retired from strenuous activity and competition.

Collateral Ligaments

Surgical Techniques

Decision making in collateral ligament repair is based on location of the lesion, its extent, and its association with other ligamentous/meniscal injuries.

Avulsions are best treated by immediate reimplantation, provided that the bony fragment is large enough to accept either a lag screw and washer or a couple of pins and a tension band. Primary repair of midsubstance tears can be attempted using a locking loop suture pattern. To protect these tenuous repairs, screws and figure-of-eight wiring over the ligament should always be used to reinforce primary reconstruction.

Postoperative Regimen

Postoperative considerations are similar to those recommended after cranial cruciate ligament surgery.

Prognosis

In caudal cruciate ligament rupture, isolated lesions of collateral ligaments are rare and usually have a favorable prognosis when nonoperatively managed. Compound lesions are associated with a guarded prognosis, and retirement from competition is recommended.

Meniscus

Surgical Techniques

Because of the poor healing ability of the menisci, nonoperative management of meniscal injuries is not recommended. For the majority of surgeons, total meniscectomy is the treatment of choice because it is less technically challenging than partial meniscectomy. However, the meniscal regeneration that may occur after total meniscectomy offers little cartilage protection compared to the original structure, and usually fails to prevent degenerative joint disease. Because the deleterious effect of meniscectomy has been shown to be proportional to the amount of meniscus removed, partial meniscectomy should always be attempted.

Postoperative Regimen

No specific aftercare is required after meniscectomy. The postoperative regimen dictated by the repair of associated ligament is usually similar to the one that follows cranial cruciate ligament surgery.

Prognosis

Meniscal damage rarely occurs as a primary injury. Almost always, at least one stifle ligament is torn or stretched at time of injury. Meniscectomy will consistently worsen the prognosis associated with the specific ligamentous injury.

Extensor Mechanism

Treatments of extensor mechanism injuries are aimed at realigning and stabilizing the patella in the trochlear groove.

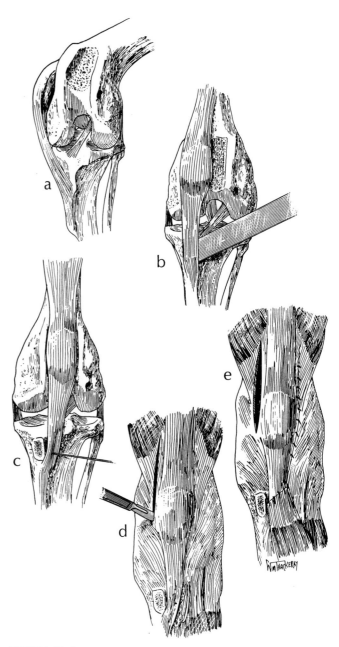

FIGURE 19–9. Surgical correction of a medial luxation of the patella. Regrooved femoral trochlea (a). Osteotomy of the tibial tuberosity (b). Lateral transplantation and fixation of the tibial tuberosity with a Kirschner wire (c). A medial releasing incision and/or a lateral imbrication of the joint capsule can be added if necessary (d and e). (From Arnoczky SP, Tarvin GB: Surgery of the stifle: The patella. Comp Cont Ed 2:200, 1980.)

Excessive internal rotation of the tibia, observed with a medially luxated patella, can be reduced by means of the same lateral imbrication suture used in repair of the cranial cruciate ligament rupture.

Finally, the redundant joint capsule opposite the side of the luxation may be imbricated or resected to tighten the retinaculum.

Patellar Fracture. These lesions are best treated by primary repair using various internal fixation devices (Fig. 19–11). In some instances, severe comminution makes reconstruction impossible, and then patellectomy must be performed. However, this procedure should be avoided if at all possible because of the importance of the patella to the mechanics of stifle extension.

Patellar Tendon Rupture/Avulsion. To restore normal extensor function, patellar tendon ruptures/avulsions must be surgically repaired. Primary repair of midsubstance tears can be performed

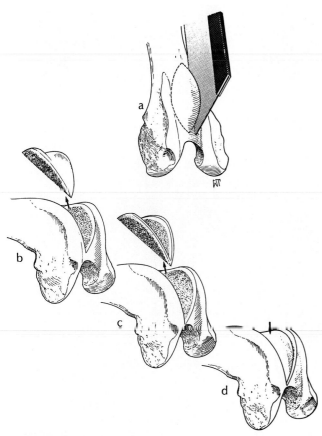

FIGURE 19–10. Trochlear wedge recession technique. Location of medial and lateral saw cuts (a). Removal of osteochondral wedge (b). Deepening of the trochlear bed by removal of a second wedge (c). Replacement of osteochondral wedge with original cartilage surface into the trochlear bed (d). (From Arnoczky SP, Tarvin GB: Surgical repair of patellar luxations and fractures. *In* Bojrab MJ (ed): Current Techniques in Small Animal Surgery. 3rd ed. Philadelphia, Lea & Febiger, 1990.)

Surgical Techniques

Luxated Patella. Nonoperative treatment as previously described is usually reserved for grade I luxated patella. As the severity of the luxation increases, surgical management is recommended. Several surgical procedures can be used either independently or in combination. The femoral trochleoplasty is a procedure used to deepen and widen the trochlear groove. In one technique the articular cartilage and the subchondral bone are removed using a high-speed bur or a rongeur. Once adequate depth is obtained, the groove is smoothed with a rasp. In immature dogs the cartilage covering the trochlea can be elevated and replaced after the remodeling of the trochlea. This minimizes development of DJD postoperatively. Unfortunately this technique is not applicable in adult dogs because the articular cartilage is too thin. To preserve articular cartilage in the adult dog, a wedge resection technique can be used. A V-shaped ostectomy of the trochlea is performed, and the articular wedge is then replaced in a deeper position (Fig. 19–9). The pressure generated by the patella on the wedge precludes the need for internal stabilization.

In more severe cases, deepening of the trochlear groove may be combined with one or more procedures to straighten the extensor apparatus. To realign the muscle/tendon unit, the insertion of the patellar tendon on the tibia may be displaced (Fig. 19–10). Following osteotomy, the tibial tuberosity is reimplanted medially or laterally to correct lateral or medial luxation, respectively.

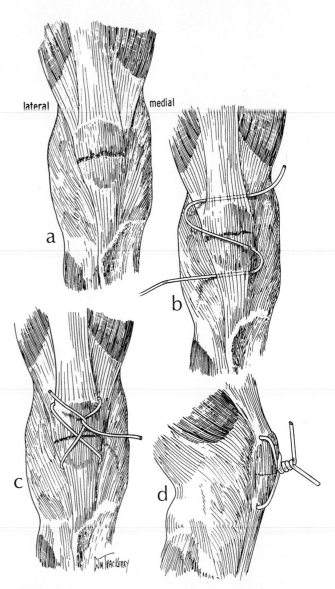

FIGURE 19–11. Surgical repair of an undisplaced transverse fracture of the patella (a). Wire is brought across the cranial surface of the patella and is reinserted into the patellar tendon (b). The wires are tightened while the joint is extended (c). Lateral view of a properly placed tension band (d). (From Arnoczky SP: Surgery of the stifle: The cruciate ligaments. Comp Cont Ed 2:106, 1980.)

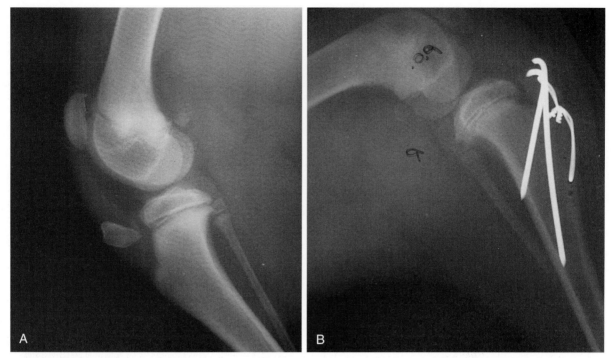

FIGURE 19–12. Lateral view of a stifle showing tibial tubercle avulsion in a young dog *(A)*. Avulsion can be repaired with pins and tension band wires *(B)*.

using a locking loop suture pattern. These repairs should always be protected by an internal splint to alleviate tension on the sutures and allow proper healing of the tendon. To this effect, a wire is placed from the patella to the tibial tuberosity. The wire often needs to be removed, as it eventually breaks and causes lameness. Pins and a tension band through the avulsed bony fragment are used for stabilization of patellar tendon avulsion. The same procedure is used to reduce and stabilize avulsed tibial tuberosity in young dogs (Fig. 19–12).

Postoperative Regimen

After extensor mechanism surgery, a well-padded Robert Jones bandage is applied for a week to help reduce joint effusion. Once it is removed, passive range of motion and massages are encouraged. Activity is limited to leash-walks for 4 to 6 weeks. Non–weight-bearing exercise such as swimming is highly recommended.

Prognosis

With moderate luxated patella (grade II and III), the prognosis for functional recovery is usually good providing that degenerative joint disease is not present at the time of surgery. Severe ligamentous and bony deformities are often present when the patella is permanently luxated (grade IV). For this reason the prognosis for functional recovery after treatment of severe (grade IV) patellar luxation is guarded. Because patellar fracture repair is associated with a high incidence of nonunion, the prognosis is fair at best. However, if proper healing occurs, normal activity level can be expected. Patellectomy is associated with a severely guarded prognosis. The functional prognosis for isolated patellar tendon rupture is usually very good once complete healing has occurred.

Miscellaneous

Only a brief overview of the following musculotendinous conditions is given here, as these specific injuries are addressed in separate chapters to which the reader is referred for more information. Osteochondritis dissecans lesions of the femoral condyle are addressed in more detail in a related chapter as well.

Osteochondritis Dissecans of the Femoral Condyle

Surgical Technique. Early surgical treatment is recommended to remove loose cartilage flaps and minimize degenerative joint disease. Once the cartilage flap has been excised, the edges of the defect are trimmed until healthy cartilage is reached (Fig. 19–13). Drilling of the defect may promote revascularization of the lesion. Meniscectomy is performed when the edges of the defect have damaged the underlying meniscus.

Postoperative Regimen. Postoperatively the dog is confined for 4 weeks followed by 4 weeks of gradual increase of activity.

Prognosis. The functional prognosis, poor at the best, depends on the extent of the lesion and meniscal involvement. While surgical treatment will limit further degeneration, affected dogs may not return to competitive levels.

Avulsion of the Long Digital Extensor Tendon

Surgical Technique. Whenever possible the avulsed long digital extensor (LDE) tendon should be reattached using a bone screw or pins. However, primary repair is rarely feasible because of the small size of the avulsed bone fragment. Suture of the tendon to the joint capsule or fixation to the proximal tibia with bone screw and spike washer is an effective alternative.

Postoperative Regimen. Postoperatively the repair should be protected for 2 weeks using a Robert Jones bandage or a full leg cast, the leg being kept under extension to alleviate the stress on the repair. Activity is restricted for 4 weeks after bandage removal, then gradually increased.

Prognosis. The functional prognosis is excellent. Return to pre-surgical activity level and performance can be expected, provided that repair and healing are adequate.

Avulsion of the Head(s) of the Gastrocnemius Muscle

Surgical Technique. Because the gastrocnemius is the most powerful extensor of the hock, the only acceptable treatment is surgical reimplantation of the avulsed tendon. Nonabsorbable suture material or cerclage wire can be used to secure the fabella to the femur.

Postoperative Regimen. Postoperative recommendations are similar to those after LDE tendon surgery, the leg being kept under slight flexion to protect the repair.

Prognosis. Prognosis for return to normal function is very good, provided that healing is uneventful. Return to peak performance however is unlikely.

Avulsion of the Origin of the Popliteal Muscle

Surgical Technique. Because the popliteal muscle participates in flexion of the stifle, its surgical repair is always recommended. As with LDE tendon avulsion, primary repair should be attempted when possible.

Postoperative Regimen. Postoperative recommendations are identical to those described for gastrocnemius and LDE tendon avulsion.

Prognosis. Functional prognosis depends on the quality of the repair. Although return to normal function can be expected, return to peak performance may not occur.

Salvage Procedures: Arthrodesis/Amputation

Surgical Technique. In rare instances, severe multiple injuries and/or DJD precludes surgical reconstruction. Arthrodesis of the stifle or amputation of the rear leg may then represent an alternative to improve quality of life.

Arthrodesis of the stifle joint is best performed using plate and screw fixation in large-breed dogs (Fig. 19–14). Alternatively, transfixation pins or screws are used in small dogs in whom plates are considered too large.

Amputation can be performed by disarticulation of the hip joint

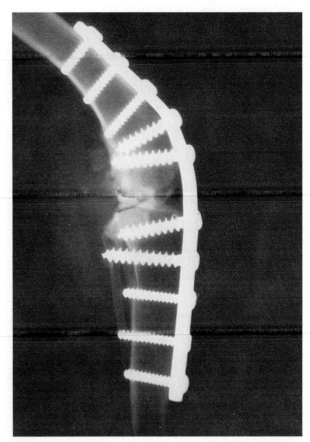

FIGURE 19–14. Lateral view of a stifle following arthrodesis. The plate is placed on the cranial aspect of the joint. The angle should be determined from the opposite leg (usually 130 to 150 degrees). Fusion of the joint markedly affects the function of the limb, especially at faster gaits.

or osteotomy of the proximal one third of the femur. Distal limb amputations (below the stifle) should be avoided because they are prone to skin ulceration because of lack of muscle padding and overuse of the stump by the dog.

Postoperative Regimen. Following arthrodesis, stifles must be placed into external fixation for 6 to 8 weeks. Ideally the bandage should include a hip spica so that the entire limb is immobilized. After bandage removal, activity is gradually increased over a four-week period.

Following amputation, assistance in standing and walking is provided to prevent bruising of the surgical site. Ambulation is expected within 3 to 5 days after surgery.

Prognosis. Arthrodesis provides a pain-free environment for the animal and an acceptable cosmetic result for the owner. However, as the joint is fused at a defined angle (140 degrees), the function of the limb is markedly affected, especially at faster gaits. For the same reason, bilateral stifle arthrodesis is not compatible with the most simple functions (rising, negotiating stairs, lying down) and therefore should not be performed. Amputation yields better overall functional results in most dogs provided that the opposite rear leg is sound. Owners should be aware that despite the cosmetic appearance, amputation of the rear leg may provide a better quality of life than arthrodesis.

Suggested Readings

Arnoczky SP, Marshall JL: The cruciate ligament of the canine stifle: An anatomical and functional analysis. Am J Vet Res 38:1807, 1977.

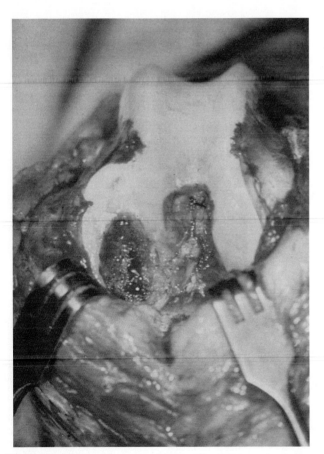

FIGURE 19–13. Osteochondritis dissecans of lateral femoral condyle. The cartilage flap has been excised and the edges of the defect have been debrided by curettage.

Arnoczky SP, et al: The over the top procedure. A technique for cranial cruciate ligament substitution in the dog. J Am Anim Hosp Assoc 15:283, 1979.

Arnoczky SP: Cruciate ligament rupture and associated injuries. *In* Newton CD, Nunamaker DM (eds): Textbook of Small Animal Orthopaedics. Philadelphia, JB Lippincott Co, 1985.

Arnoczky SP: Pathomechanics of cruciate ligament and meniscal injuries. *In* Bojrab MJ (ed): Disease Mechanisms in Small Animal Surgery, 2nd ed. Philadelphia, Lea & Febiger, 1993.

Brinker WO, Piermattei DL, Flo GL: Handbook of Small Animal Orthopedics and Fracture Treatment, 2nd ed. Philadelphia, WB Saunders Company, 1990, pp 377–435.

Flo GL: Modification of the lateral retinacular imbrication technique for stabilizing cruciate ligament injuries. J Am Anim Hosp Assoc 17:569, 1975.

Hayes AG, Boudrieau RJ, Hungerford LL: Frequency and distribution of medial and lateral patellar luxation in dogs: 124 cases (1982–1992). JAVMA 205:716–721, 1994.

Paatsama S: Ligamentous injury of the canine stifle joint. A clinical and experimental study. Helsinki, These, 1952.

Roush JK: Stifle surgery. Vet Clin North Am 23:4, 1993.

Vasseur PB: Stifle joint. *In* Slatter D (ed): Textbook of Small Animal Surgery, 2nd ed. Philadelphia, WB Saunders Company, 1993.

Whitehair JG, et al: Epidemiology of the cranial cruciate ligament rupture in dogs. JAVMA 203:1016–1020, 1993.

CHAPTER 20

Injuries of the Metacarpus and Metatarsus

CHRISTOPHER M. BOEMO

The metacarpal and metatarsal bones of the young greyhound sustain an inordinate degree of injury during the rearing, education, and early racing career relative to the other bones of the animal. These injuries are generally stress-related and reflect the bone's response to an increase in frequency, magnitude, and direction of forces acting on it. The type and severity of metacarpal or metatarsal bone injury is influenced by many factors, the most important of which is the rate at which corrective repair and remodeling occur relative to the rate of damage to the bone. The clinical signs of metacarpal injury vary with the severity of the damage, as do the treatments.

INCIDENCE

Injury to the metacarpal and metatarsal bones is most commonly observed when the greyhound begins pursuing the lure around turns on a trial track or racetrack during the breaking-in (initial education) process or during the early stages of the animal's racing career. Because of the variation in the ages at which greyhounds begin their training and racing, the incidence of metacarpal injury varies, with the earliest cases occurring at approximately 11 months of age, and with peak incidence at 16 to 22 months of age.[1] This represents the highest incidence of any bone injury in the young greyhound.[2] These injuries are seldom seen after 30 months of age.[1] The incidence of metacarpal injury is reported to vary from 2.8 to 32 per cent of stress fractures seen in racing greyhounds and that of metatarsals from 5 to 16.9 per cent.[2–4] In Australia the incidence of metacarpal injury is higher than that of metatarsal, whereas the reverse is the situation in the United States.[2, 4]

ETIOLOGY AND PATHOPHYSIOLOGY

Bone is a dynamic tissue, responding to forces applied to it. Under normal circumstances fatigue occurs, only to be repaired by secondary osteonal repair. An increase in the size, type, or rate of application of externally applied forces results in an increased extent and rate of damage to the bone matrix, which, if the integrity of the skeletal system is to be maintained, must be repaired and adaptively remodeled. If the increase in physical activity is high, the level of repair and adaptive remodeling is comparably high. Further increase in the rate and level of activity will result in more extensive damage to the bone matrix, and remodeling will occur with adaptive hypertrophy via the formation of periosteal and endosteal new bone and hypertrophy of the trabecular bone.[5, 6]

The initial process in the repair of damaged or fatigued cortical bone involves a destructive process with the osteoclastic resorption of damaged matrix[6]; hence, the removal of cores of load-bearing bone results in reduction of an already weakened cortex prior to the formation of the secondary osteons. It then follows that if the level of physical activity remains high while the reparative processes are occurring, the forces that were sufficient to cause cortical bone matrix injury initially will be applied to a consequentially weakened cortex and result in a greater strain per unit of applied force. Accumulation of cortical defects may follow. If, with an excessive rate of physical activity, the damage accumulates more rapidly than can be repaired by the biological repair processes, coalescence of the cortical defects will occur and may in turn lead to the development of fatigue (stress) fracture or total bone fracture.[1]

While metacarpal and metatarsal injuries in other domestic canines result from direct trauma,[7] injuries to these bones in the greyhound are more commonly truly stress-related injuries with only the occasional injury being due to direct trauma.

Greyhounds are designed to run primarily in straight lines with most of the forces being borne by the larger, stronger central metacarpal bones (MC-III, MC-IV).[8–10] Anticlockwise racing on circular tracks results in "body lean" and the transfer of weight to the lateral pair of metacarpal bones of the left forepaw (LMC-IV, LMC-V), and to the medial pair of metacarpal bones of the right

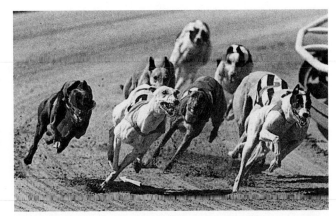

FIGURE 20–1. Body lean and weight transfer. Pursuit of the lure on circular racetracks of inadequate track banking results in body lean toward the inside of the track and transfer of weight from the central metacarpal bones to the railing side pairs (right medial and left lateral) of metacarpal bones *(arrow).* There is also transfer of weight to the left side of the animal with the metacarpals of the left forepaw experiencing greater forces than when the dog is running in a straight line. (With permission of Leader Newspapers.)

forepaw (RMC-II, RMC-III).[8–10] Leaning of the body also transfers weight to the left side of the animal, accounting for the bias observed in injury to LMC-V relative to the other metacarpal bones[1] (Fig. 20–1).

The metacarpus and metatarsus of the young greyhound are subjected to increased forces when it is placed into long galloping enclosures during rearing, and more so when it begins training. Such forces are manifested as an increased rate (the greyhound is run more often), altered direction (the animal is run in a circular manner instead of in a straight line), increased magnitude (the greyhound is run at higher speeds with body lean resulting in weight transfer to metacarpals closer to the inside of the track),

and increased duration (the animal is enticed to run farther and farther as it progresses through its training).

The metacarpus is subjected to compressive and bending forces with each stride of the galloping action as weight is borne by the foot and as the body passes over it (Fig. 20–2). Bones subjected to bending are subjected to high-compressive stresses on the concave side of the bone and tensile forces on the convex side, with the highest stresses centered on the surface of the bone.[5] The dorsal surface of each of the bones of the metacarpus experiences compressive stresses when the greyhound runs in a straight line. When the greyhound negotiates a bend, the leaning of the body results in these forces being exerted to a greater extent on the dorsolateral

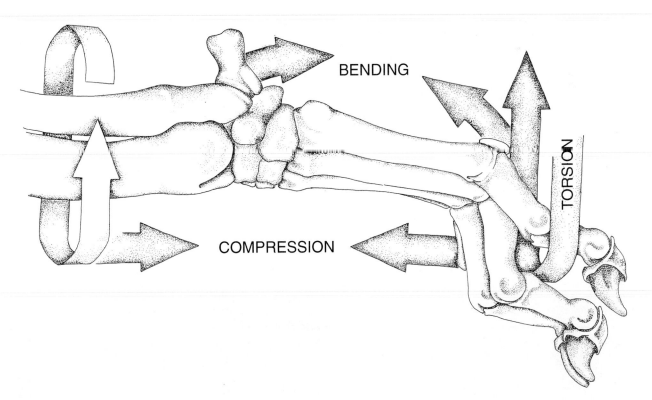

FIGURE 20–2. Forces acting on the metacarpal bones. With each stride the bones on the metacarpus and metatarsus are subjected to compressive and bending forces as each foot bears weight and as the body passes over it. Racing on circular tracks introduces torsional forces.

aspect of the left metacarpus (LMC-IV, LMV-V) and the dorsomedial aspect of the right metacarpus (RMC-II, RMC-III). The palmar aspect of the metacarpus experiences tensile stresses[1] (Fig. 20–3). Propulsive efforts of the hindlimbs subject the metatarsal bones to similar loadings. Pursuit of the lure on a circular track adds torsional forces to the bones. Torsional forces result in significant shear stresses axially and radially through the bone with their magnitudes greatest at the surface of the bone. Significant tensile stresses develop within the bone oriented in an oblique spiral around the bone's long axis (Fig. 20–4). Tensile forces of clinical significance are also observed to act on MC-II and MC-III at the insertion of the extensor carpi radialis tendon at the base of the bone, and at the origin of collateral ligaments[1] (Fig. 20–5). At these points, high tensile stresses develop within the cortical bone tissue along a plane perpendicular to the direction of the applied force.[5] The development of these stresses, either singly or in combination, results in the characteristic bone injury and fracture patterns seen in the metacarpals and metatarsals of the racing greyhound.

Poorly designed racetracks and inadequately maintained racing surfaces produce a higher incidence of metacarpal and metatarsal injury.[1, 11–13] Tight racetrack bends, inadequate camber (track banking), and loose surfaces, coupled with the field of greyhounds jostling for position, increase the magnitude of the forces experienced by each greyhound during a race.

Greyhounds that develop higher terminal velocities appear to be more prone to metacarpal and metatarsal injury. Faster animals experience greater centrifugal forces on turns and develop higher

momentum, making them more prone to metacarpal and metatarsal injuries.[1]

The changes observed clinically, radiographically, and grossly in cases of metacarpal and metatarsal bone injury are due to the osseous response to overload. To date there has been no scientific investigation in the dog of the physiological response of the bones of the metacarpus or metatarsus to repetitive compressive strain of the dorsal cortex. One report of experimental overload of the porcine radius describes hypertrophy of the periosteum, rapid proliferation of new bone on the periosteal surface, secondary osteonal remodeling of the existing cortex, and endosteal new bone production in response to ulnar osteotomy that resulted in compressive overload of the cranial aspect of the radius. With time the rate of new bone formation slowed, and with secondary osteonal remodeling the new bone tissue took on the appearance of normal circumferential lamellar bone.[6]

The changes observed in that report are similar to what is observed clinically in the greyhound metacarpal and metatarsal bones subjected to dorsal compressive overload. The periosteum becomes thickened, inflamed, and painful to touch, with proliferation of subperiosteal new bone over a period of 2 to 4 weeks. In older greyhounds in which adaptive remodeling has occurred, there is thickening of the dorsal cortex and narrowing of the medullary cavity as a result of endosteal remodeling[1] (Fig. 20–6).

The influence of genetics on the incidence of metacarpal injury is an issue of contention. Even though a familial incidence is noted in practice,[1] this may reflect poor nutrition and rearing rather than

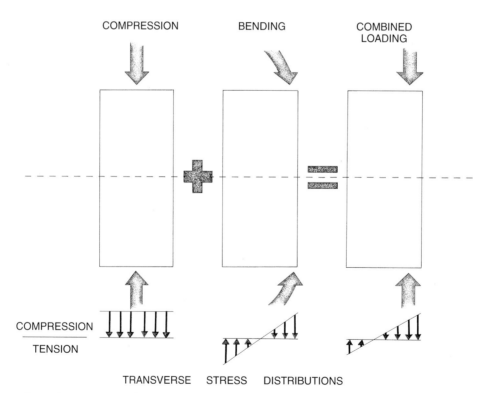

FIGURE 20–3. Stresses imposed on a transverse plane through a uniform bar that is subjected to a combination of compressive and bending loading. High compressive stresses are developed on the side subjected to concave strain, while the convex side experiences either a lower compressive stress or a tensile stress, depending on the relative magnitudes of each separate loading. Similar stress distributions occur in the metacarpal and metatarsal bones as weight is borne by the bone. The dorsal aspect is subjected to concave strain with the development of compressive stresses within the dorsal cortex. (Diagram reproduced from Carter DR, Spengler DM: Biomechanics of Fracture. *In* Summer-Smith G (ed): Bone in Clinical Orthopedics, Philadelphia, WB Saunders Company, 1982, p 311.)

palpated for the presence of edema, periosteal pain, periosteal callus, and, in the case of complete bone fracture, crepitus. Further clinical assessment of the bones is then made by having the patient place full weight on the foot and metacarpus (metatarsus) that is under examination by holding the contralateral limb off the ground. The entire length of each of the bones is then palpated, using the thumbnail to exert gentle pressure by drawing it over the surface of the bone from the head proximally to the base (Fig. 20–8). The presence of even minor periosteal pain will result in the dog's knuckling over on the foot and attempting to regain weight-bearing with the opposite foot.

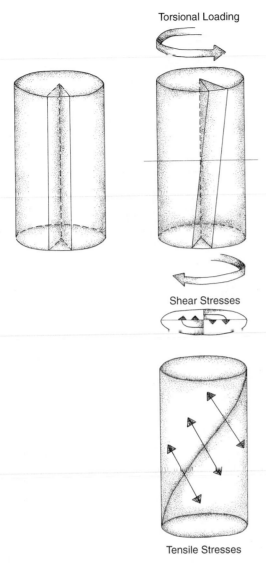

Torsional Loading

Shear Stresses

Tensile Stresses

FIGURE 20–4. Deformation and stress distribution in a cylindrical bar subject to torsional loading. Shear stresses are developed along the longitudinal and transverse planes while tensile and compressive stresses are imposed on planes that make an oblique spiral through the bar. When LMC-V is subjected to torsional forces that deform the bone beyond its yield strain it will fail along the lines of tensile stress, resulting in spiral fracture. (Diagram reproduced from Carter DR, Spengler DM: Biomechanics of Fracture. *In* Sumner-Smith G (ed): Bone in Clinical Orthopedics, Philadelphia, WB Saunders Company, 1982, p 312.)

genetic factors that result in reduced bone strength or reduced capacity of bone to respond to the increased forces experienced.

EXAMINATION OF THE METACARPUS AND METATARSUS

Physical examination of the metacarpus/metatarsus should be part of the clinical examination of the greyhound. Visual assessment and careful palpation of the dorsal and palmar/plantar aspects of the bones should be the minimum examination performed. Each foot should be lifted off the floor and palpated (Fig. 20–7). The entire length of all four metacarpal or metatarsal bones should be

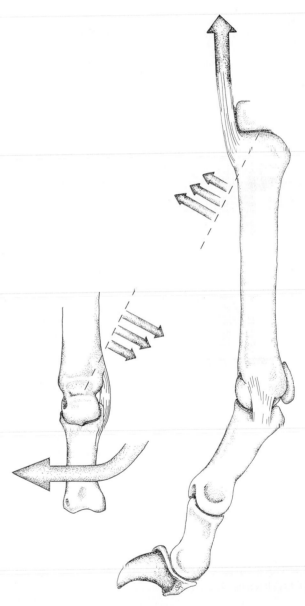

FIGURE 20–5. Tensile forces of significance in the metacarpus and metatarsus. The tensile force exerted by the tendon of insertion of the extensor carpi radialis muscle on the proximal cortex of RMC-II, and to a lesser extent RMC-III, results in tensile stresses along a plane perpendicular to the direction of the force. Fatigue of the bone matrix along that plane results in the failure of the bone observed in stress fracture of RMC-II. Collateral ligaments can also produce tensile stresses within the cortex (*insert*) and may result in avulsion fracture.

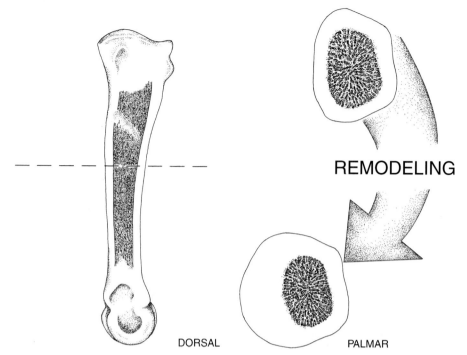

REMODELING

DORSAL   PALMAR

FIGURE 20–6. Response of metacarpal and metatarsal bones to overload. Dorsal compressive overload results in periosteal hypertrophy, proliferation of subperiosteal new bone, osteonal remodeling of the existing cortex, and adaptive hypertrophy of the endosteum. This reduces the strain experienced by the bone subjected to increased loads, resulting in a marked increase in the width of the dorsal cortex and a reduction in medullary canal diameter.

Radiography is used routinely as an aid to diagnosing the severity and the chronicity of metacarpal or metatarsal injury. Proper radiographic technique is essential if it is to assist in the diagnosis of subtle changes in the cortex or the periosteal region of the bone (Fig. 20–9). Because the metacarpal and metatarsal bones are arranged in an arch with their bases in close communication with their adjacent number, mach effects are commonly seen and may be misdiagnosed as a fracture. Subtle rotation of the metacarpus (metatarsus) will greatly reduce this effect on the bone under investigation.[1]

Thermography and bone scintigraphy are additional diagnostic procedures that may be utilized in the diagnosis of metacarpal and metatarsal injury. The advantages of thermography in the racing greyhound are that it provides a means of diagnosing injuries before they become radiographically apparent and may be used to justify resting the animal before the injury deteriorates further.[14] Bone scintigraphy, like thermography, has the advantage of being able to detect the presence of "hot spots" prior to their being detectable radiographically, and although it has been used on a small number of greyhound patients with metacarpal injuries,[15] the restrictions in relation to operating a nuclear medicine facility are disadvantageous to its acceptance as a routine diagnostic procedure.

CLINICAL SIGNS OF METACARPAL AND METATARSAL INJURY

Although it is common to define three principal categories of metacarpal or metatarsal injury (periostitis, stress fracture, and complete fracture), this demarcation is arbitrary, representing an empirical division of what is a continuum of bone change in response to cyclic injury. Clinical and radiographic signs will vary with the extent of bone injury, its rate of onset, and the time delay in presentation for examination.

Acute Metacarpal and Metatarsal Periostitis

Metacarpal periostitis is the earliest stage of injury to the metacarpus. Metacarpal edema may be present but is an inconsistent clinical sign. The animal usually has a history of a shortened stride and raising its head. The dog may lift and whirl its tail as it negotiates the turn. The greyhound runs awkwardly through the turn at a reduced speed or drifts wide. The affected foot may be lifted off the ground momentarily after the run or when the foot is being hosed down in the washing-down bay. Although the animal is not lame, as the condition worsens there may be shortening of gait as it attempts to reduce the time the affected foot spends bearing weight. Most commonly affected are left metacarpal V (LMC-V) and right metacarpal II (RMC-II) with LMC-IV, and RMC-III also frequently affected.[1, 16, 17]

Carpal flexion is resented, often leading to misdiagnosis of carpal sprain by the owner or trainer. Palpation of the dorsal aspect of the affected bone elicits a pain response (limb withdrawal, attempts at reduced weight bearing, or vocalization). Edema and periosteal hypertrophy may also be detected. Depending on the time delay between the last run and examination, no pain may be detectable on examination.

Metatarsal periostitis is more commonly observed during rearing when the pups are placed into long turnout pens. Affected animals frequently are reluctant to run up and down the enclosure. In my practice, metatarsal periostitis is more commonly observed to affect the more lateral bones (LMT-IV, LMT-V, RMT-IV, and RMT-V). The extent of the injury varies from periosteal pain and small amounts of periosteal new bone on the proximal dorsal aspect of the bone (commonly seen on MT-V) to extensive callus involving much of the bone surface and microfracture or complete bone fracture. Edema, periosteal pain, periosteal hypertrophy, and callus production are commonly observed during examination. Forced flexion of the tarsus may be met with resentment, and this must be differentiated from tarsal sprains and tarsal bone fractures.

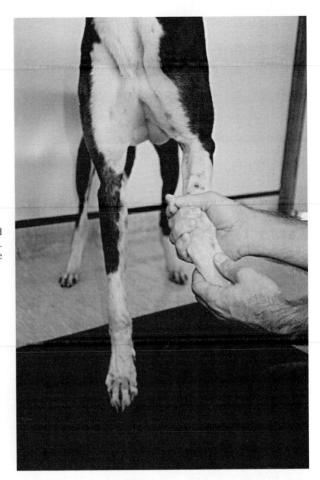

FIGURE 20–7. Palpation of the metacarpus. The foot under examination is held off the ground, and the dorsal aspect of the metacarpus is palpated with the thumb. The entire length of all four bones should be palpated with firm pressure for the presence of pain, periosteal hypertrophy, callus, or crepitus.

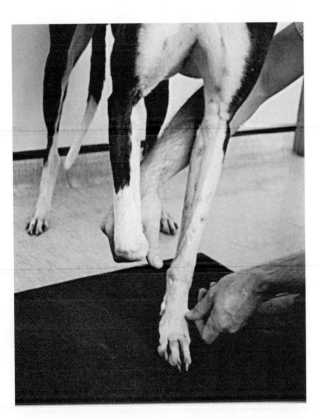

FIGURE 20–8. Examination of the metacarpus while weight bearing. While the contralateral limb is held off the ground, the dorsal aspect of each metacarpal of the foot under examination is palpated by drawing the thumbnail from the head proximally to exert gentle pressure on the bone's surface. The presence of even minor periosteal tenderness will result in the patient knuckling over on the foot, attempting to take weight off the affected bone, and placing the held paw onto the ground.

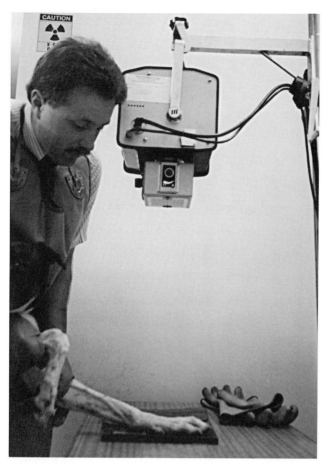

FIGURE 20–9. Radiographic positioning of the performance patient. A patient table height of approximately 450 mm is convenient for radiography of limb extremities. The distal limb may be elevated onto the radiographic cassette without discomfort to the patient. Direct dorsopalmar (plantarodorsal), rotated, and skyline views are often taken in the course of radiographic evaluation of metacarpal or metatarsal injury.

Chronic Metacarpal and Metatarsal Periostitis

Chronic metacarpal and metatarsal periostitis result from repeated injury and inadequate treatment and convalescence. Postperformance periosteal pain may be observed in some greyhounds despite diligent treatment and convalescence recommendations. Such animals usually have a history similar to that described for metacarpal periostitis, although the reduction in the animal's performance is usually more marked.[1]

With chronic periostitis, palpation reveals periosteal hypertrophy, pain, and often extensive periosteal callus. The ridges of periosteal new bone develop over 3 to 6 weeks, varying from irregular nodules of new bone to a thick ridge up to 4 mm occupying up to 70 per cent of the length of the bone.[1] Periosteal callus tends to be more extensive on LMC-V because of the greater forces acting on this bone commonly occupying the greater proportion of the dorsolateral surface. The development of periosteal callus on RMC-II, however, tends to be confined to the proximal third of the shaft of the bone. It is closely associated with the insertion of the extensor carpi radialis tendon (Fig. 20–10).

Greyhounds with clinical signs of extensive callus production are prone to repeated recurrences of reduced performance. Recurrences are due to the altered biomechanics associated with the presence of the callus on the surface of the bone.[1] When a bone with significant periosteal callus is subjected to the same degree of bending strain as the same bone before the production of the callus, the compressive stresses developed on the surface of the callus are far greater than those at the surface of the original cortex, resulting in greater injury to the new periosteal bone and a vicious circle of injury and response to injury ensues[1] (Fig. 20–11).

Palpation of periosteal callus per se is not pathognomonic for metacarpal or metatarsal periostitis; it merely represents a prior response to bone injury that may have fully resolved. The clinical findings of periosteal pain and radiographically detected active periosteal new bone in such cases are important.

Radiological changes in cases of early periostitis are negligible, although careful radiographic technique will reveal soft tissue swelling. Within 3 weeks, radiographic examination will reveal slight increases in radiodensity of the affected region of the bone.[1] Cortical width increases with subsequent reduction of the caliber of the medullary shadow, and there is an increase in radiodensity of the medullary shadow proportional to the amount of periosteal and endosteal new bone production (Figs. 20–12, 20–13A, and 20–13B). Although these radiographic changes are observed more commonly in the middle third of the diaphysis of LMC-V and the proximal third and base of RMC-II, they are not confined exclusively to these bones. When observed in other metacarpal bones, the changes are usually mid shaft and similar to those of LMC-V. Oblique (skyline) radiographs taken in cases of chronic periostitis show extensive periosteal new bone with the surface of the callus exhibiting active bone resorption and deposition, giving a feathery appearance to the surface (Fig. 20–14). Rotated dorsopalmar or plantarodorsal views of chronically affected bones reveal marked narrowing of the medullary canal shadow, thickening of the cortical shadow, marked sclerosis of the overall shaft of the bone indicative of increased bone deposition, and increased size of the trabecular network (Figs. 20–14 and 20–15).

Stress (Fatigue) Fractures of the Metacarpus and Metatarsus

Fatigue fracture results as the bone structure of the metacarpus or metatarsus deteriorates further after continued exposure to excessive levels of physical activity or inadequate convalescence. The greyhound's performance is poor, with the animal tending to drift wide markedly, shorten stride, and reduce its speed as it negotiates the turn. Lameness is present after racing or trials as a subtle or more obvious weight-bearing lameness that may persist for up to 3 days, although commonly the lameness persists for 12 to 36 hours. The more advanced the bone fatigue, the more prolonged the duration of post-run lameness. Mild transient episodes of lameness may have occurred and have been treated by the owner or trainer, and it is not until several episodes of lameness, increasingly severe lameness, or whole-bone fracture occur that the patient is presented for veterinary evaluation. There is obvious resentment to carpal flexion, and there may be a period of reduced weight bearing following carpal flexion. Palpation reveals signs referable to periostitis and usually some periosteal callus, although cases of acute-onset microfracture in which the animal has been subjected to a concentrated period of intense trialing or racing may not show any callus.

The radiological changes associated with fatigue fracture are variable, depending on the duration of time leading up to the development of the fracture and the extent of the fatigue. In cases in which the animal has been subjected to an intense workload in a short period early in its racing career, fatigue microfracture can ensue with minimal, if any, radiographically demonstrable lesion. More commonly, however, fatigue develops over some considerable time, usually many weeks, allowing radiographic signs of osseous damage together with attempts at repair and remodeling to become

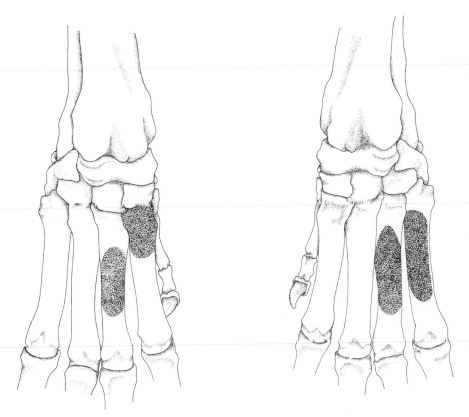

FIGURE 20–10. Callus production on the metacarpals. Periosteal new bone develops commonly in the dorsal mid-diaphyseal region of LMC-V and proximal third of the shaft of RMC-II. On other metacarpals the callus is usually apparent in the midshaft region.

evident radiographically. Increased cortical thickness, increased size and prominence of trabecular bone, reduced medullary canal diameter, reduced radiolucency through the fatigue area (even to the extent of the medullary shadow being obliterated), and variable degrees of periosteal and endosteal new bone production are commonly encountered. The periosteal new bone surface exhibits distinct areas of osteolysis and even distinct fissure fracture lines through the callus. The fissure fracture lines are sometimes observed to coalesce on skyline radiographs. The osteolysis and fissuring may extend even into the original cortical bone, as is often the case in fatigue failure of proximal RMC-II (Fig. 20–16, 20–17, 20–18C).

Complete Metacarpal and Metatarsal Fractures

Complete metacarpal and metatarsal bone fracture occurs as a result of either progressive weakening of the bone structure through fatigue or relatively normal bone being excessively loaded beyond its yield strain.[1, 5] The greyhound pulls up or fails to perform well, often trailing the field in the trial or race. The history is one of obvious lameness (severe weight-bearing or non–weight-bearing lameness) immediately post run. If the fracture occurs on the turn, the greyhound fails to negotiate the turn satisfactorily, slowing dramatically and drifting off the turn. Clinical signs of lameness and swelling are present. The degree of swelling observed depends on the severity of the fracture and any post-injury first-aid measures instituted by the owner or trainer. Palpation of the affected region is usually resented and often reveals crepitus. Usually only one metacarpal or metatarsal is affected, although when there is a history of collision with a stationary object, multiple bones may be involved. The swelling observed clinically (edema and hemorrhage)

is cool, doughy, pits on pressure, and often gravitates distally to cause digital swelling and even interdigital weeping of serosanguineous fluid. The principal differential diagnosis is that of cellulitis, but the history of exercise-precipitated lameness together with swelling and crepitus is diagnostic. Radiographs utilizing standard and rotated views reveal the number extent and type of fracture(s) present. In three reports[2, 16, 17] detailing a total of 174 metacarpal fractures, 79.3 per cent involved fractures of the left metacarpus, with 68 per cent of all metacarpal fractures involving LMC-V, and 82 per cent involving either LMC-V or RMC-II. The fracture patterns seen reflect the forces acting on the bone to cause the fracture[5] (Fig. 20–18A and 20–18B). LMC-V is subject to oblique, spiral, and comminuted fracture patterns with the most common being Y-shaped with a dorsal or dorsolateral fragment of variable size (Fig. 20–18A). Comminution is common and reflects the high-energy status of the bone at the point of failure. Compression, bending, and torsional forces act to varying degrees to produce the range of fracture patterns seen. Metacarpal and metatarsal fractures are rarely intra-articular,[1] and transverse fractures of metacarpals are uncommon, although they do occur.[1, 8, 17] The most common fracture of RMC-II (75 per cent of right metacarpal fractures in one study[16]) is a butterfly fragment of the dorsal aspect of the proximal shaft and is usually seen as a result of chronic fatigue of the bone.[18]

There are three common types of metatarsal fractures. The most common is a small avulsion from the plantar aspect of RMT-V that is usually detected on radiographs taken for other reasons (Fig. 20–19A). This represents an avulsion of the lateral plantar tarsometatarsal ligament and is of no clinical significance. The second is a transverse or short oblique fracture in the distal shaft just proximal to the metatarsophalangeal joint (Fig. 20–19B), and the

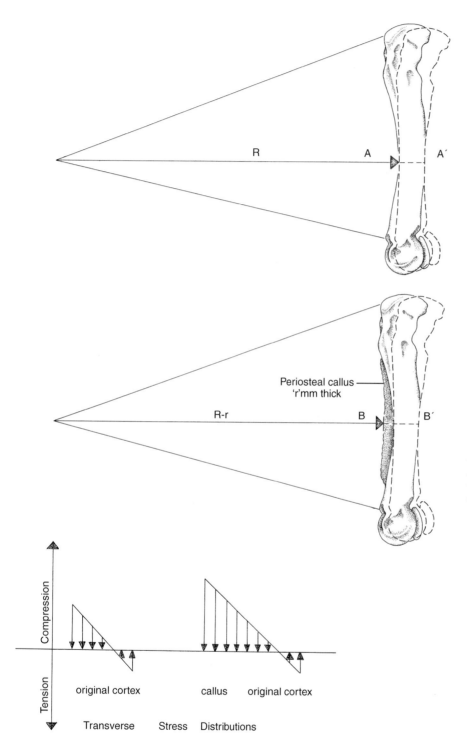

Periosteal callus —
'r'mm thick

R-r   B ►   B′

Compression

Tension

original cortex   callus   original cortex

Transverse   Stress   Distributions

FIGURE 20–11. Stresses developed in a transverse plane through a metacarpal subjected to compression and bending (a) prior to callus and (b) after callus production. Under combined compressive and bending load, the metacarpal bends through an arc of radius "R" and the plane A–A′ experiences compressive and tensile stresses. Bone matrix injury occurs, and there is periosteal callus production ("r" units thick) and secondary osteonal remodeling of the existing cortex. If the bone is then subjected to a force sufficient to strain the surface of the original cortex through an arc of the same radius, the magnitude of the compressive strain experienced along a transverse plane (B–B′) through the callus is greater than that which induced the bone matrix injury in the original cortex. A cycle of injury and response to injury ensues unless sufficient time is allowed for repair and adaptive remodeling to occur.

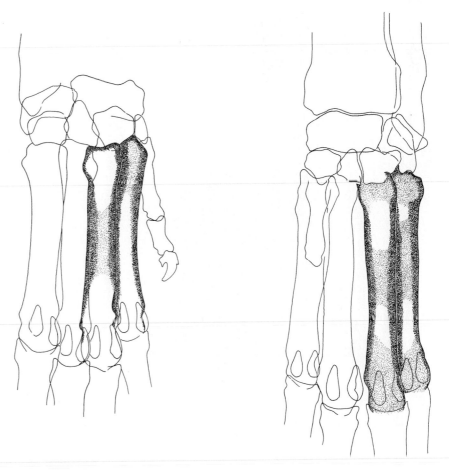

FIGURE 20–12. Representation of the radiological changes seen with metacarpal remodeling. There is increase in the cortical width, reduction in the medullary canal caliber, and increase in the radiodensity over the medullary canal shadow indicative of increased cortical thickness primarily apparent in the mid-diaphyseal region of LMC-V, and proximal third of RMC-II, and to a lesser extent in the midshaft region of LMC-IV and RMC-III. (Rotated dorsopalmar views redrawn from Boemo CM: Metacarpal Injury. In Proc Post-Grad Committee Vet Sci Uni Syd 122:272, 273, 1989.)

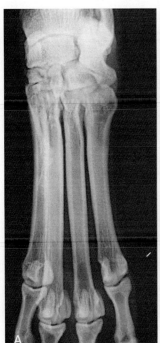
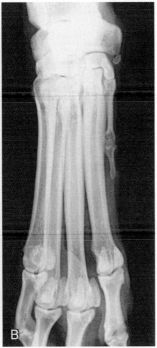

FIGURE 20–13. Periostitis. *A,* Rotated dorsopalmar radiograph of left metacarpus of a greyhound with periostitis. Note the increased radiodensity of the mid-diaphyseal region of both LMC-IV and LMC-V and to a lesser extent LMC-III. *B,* Dorsopalmar radiograph of the right metacarpus of the same greyhound showing more extensive osseous changes. There is increased cortical width and reduction of the diameter as well as increased sclerosis of the medullary canal shadow. The changes are proportional to the amount of periosteal and endosteal new bone produced in response to the increased stresses experienced by the metacarpal bones. Note how the rotated view in *A* provides clear separation of the metacarpal bones under investigation.

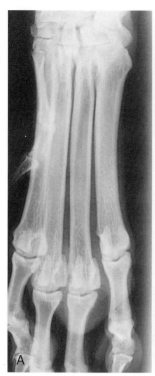
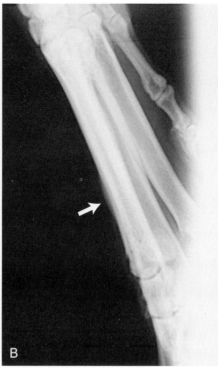

FIGURE 20–14. Chronic periostitis. *(A)* Rotated dorsopalmar and *(B)* rotated lateral radiographs of the metacarpus of a greyhound with chronic periostitis. There is an increase in the radiodensity of the junction of the middle and distal thirds of the diaphysis of LMC-V with an increase in the size and radiodensity of the trabecular bone. The skyline view demonstrates a distinct periosteal callus with a "feathery" surface *(arrow)* in response to cortical injury.

third is an explosive fracture of the mid shaft of RMT-III where, as a result of excessive propulsive force generated by the right hind, there is excessive bending strain of the metatarsal beyond its yield strain. The resultant fracture characteristically is a comminuted Y-shaped fracture with a dorsal butterfly fragment, and the proximal end of the distal fragment is displaced plantaro-proximally (Fig. 20–19*C*, 20–19*D*). Oblique and spiral fractures are observed also, but less frequently.

TREATMENT OF METACARPAL AND METATARSAL INJURIES

The principles in the treatment of metacarpal and metatarsal injuries are to return the dog to competitive racing.[1] Irrespective of the type of therapy, the correction of improper training regimens and time cannot be overly emphasized, although the greyhound practitioner is faced with the need to minimize the patient's downtime.

Periostitis

In cases of acute periostitis with no radiographic change evident, cryotherapy and the use of anti-inflammatories are indicated. Ice packs or cold water should be applied immediately (10 to 15 minutes four to six times a day) and continued for 3 or 4 days. Cryotherapy is most effective when performed within the first 24 to 72 hours of injury, reducing blood flow, tissue metabolic rate, and pain perception.[19, 20] Topical and systemic nonsteroidal anti-inflammatories are indicated. The use of subperiosteal short-acting corticosteroids has been described.[21] If present, dietary imbalances should be corrected.[1] The training program should be adjusted so that the frequency of circle-based trialing or racing is reduced to once every 12 to 14 days for 6 to 8 weeks,[1, 21] after which the frequency of such running may be gradually increased. The animal should be confined to the leash until edema and pain have subsided,

usually 7 to 10 days, after which time free galloping and straight runs are permitted.

Commonly, the greyhound has advanced periostitis. These cases are treated as discussed, with the addition of ultrasound and counterirritants.[1, 6, 21, 22] The regimen that has proved successful in my practice involves the use of ultrasound under water using settings of 1.5 to 1.7 watts/sq cm with continuous output for 5 to 7 minutes daily for 5 days then on alternate days for 5 to 10 sessions. A counterirritant liniment is applied twice daily for 5 days then twice daily on alternate days for a further 2 to 3 weeks. The affected region must be dried thoroughly before application of the liniment. The patient is confined to the leash or swimming or both for 10 to 21 days followed by free galloping and return to work in the manner as described previously. The interval between trials or races should be 12 to 14 days with gradual return to increased work as described above.

With chronic periostitis there may be recurrence of the injury upon return to work, causing practitioners some frustration. If the affected bone radiographically appears to be adequately remodeled and the periosteal callus exhibits a firm, sharp distinct edge to its surface, anti-inflammatory therapy is indicated. Short-acting corticosteroid may be injected subperiosteally and followed by topical and oral nonsteroidal anti-inflammatories for 5 to 7 days. The patient should be rested for at least 3 weeks. It is advantageous to wrap the affected region with two or three rounds of elastic adhesive tape for subsequent trials or races where permitted by racing regulations.

Chronic proliferative periostitis with inadequate remodeling, and active bone production may represent active periostitis or progressive degeneration of the bone with failing attempts at repair. Treatment should consist of anti-inflammatory therapy and 4 to 6 weeks of confinement and controlled exercise. Follow-up radiographs should be taken after approximately 4 weeks to assess improvement. With sufficient improvement, the animal may be permitted to return to light work, eg, free galloping for 2 to 3 weeks before any further increase in workload. These cases are often bordering on fatigue fracture, and lameness may not be apparent.

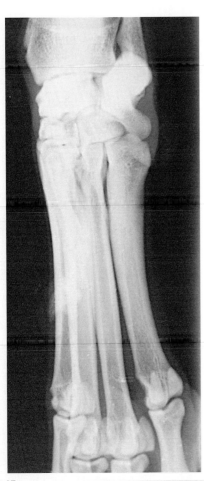

FIGURE 20–15. Chronic periostitis. Rotated lateral radiograph of a greyhound with chronic periostitis of LMC-V showing marked thickening of the cortical bone, loss of the medullary canal shadow in the proximal shaft, and extensive periosteal remodeling with prominence of the trabecular bone. These changes are indicative of longstanding and repeated exposure to excessive loads.

Stress Fracture

Fatigue (stress) fractures can be treated medically or surgically. Acute fatigue microfracture without extensive periosteal callus production and no radiographically demonstrable cortical fracture lines requires conservative treatment via the application of cold and anti-inflammatories together with kennel confinement for 7 to 10 days or until lameness has subsided, with the patient then being restricted to lead-controlled exercise for a period of 6 to 8 weeks. Counterirritant therapy is commonly instituted after the acute phase of the inflammation has subsided.

Follow-up radiographs and physical examination 4 to 5 weeks later usually reveal production of periosteal callus in response to superficial cortical fatigue. The greyhound is then gradually returned to work as previously described but should not be returned to circle work until there is radiographic and clinical evidence of subsidence of periosteal bone activity.

Fatigue fracture with extensive periosteal callus may be conservatively or surgically managed. Surgical therapy involves a dorsal approach to the affected area,[23] sharp incision, elevation and careful reflection of the hypertrophic periosteum, and removal of the periosteal bone. The periosteal callus is poor-quality bone and is readily removed, care being taken to minimize iatrogenic trauma to the

reflected periosteum during the procedure. The periosteum is then sutured with a 4/0 synthetic absorbable suture material. If the periosteum becomes excessively traumatized during the procedure, it is apposed and surrounding soft tissues are sutured. The foot is supported in a padded bandage for 14 days (changed at 5 to 6 days postoperatively). The patient may be given anabolic steroids for the purpose of enhancing collagen synthesis.[24] The animal is confined to its kennel while bandaged and restricted to lead exercise for 6 to 10 weeks before being allowed any free exercise.

Conservative treatment of such cases is met with less success (approximately 60 per cent satisfactory return to racing) than that achieved with surgical intervention (approximately 90 per cent).[1] Various treatment regimens to produce an acute inflammatory response on the surface of the bone have been described.[1, 8, 18, 21, 22] These patients are then given 2 to 3 months off all running, and I believe that it is not so much the type of treatment but the prolonged period of convalescence that allows the bone structure to repair and remodel without incurring further injury that is more important.

Complete Metacarpal and Metatarsal Fractures

Most commonly only one bone is fractured. The prognosis for return to racing reduces with the number of bones and the degree of comminution.[1] Fractures of LMC-V, RMC-II, RMT-III are the most common. The type of repair performed may be either conservative or surgical, depending on the fracture type, the degree of distraction of the fracture fragments, the performance potential of the animal, and the financial constraints of the owner or the trainer.

A nondisplaced long obliquely fractured metacarpal or metatarsal bone may be treated satisfactorily with coaptation for 3 to 4 weeks, followed by bandaging for 2 weeks. In cases of conservatively managed fractures there will be overriding and shortening. The adjacent bone is therefore subjected to an increased load and will sustain increased strain. This will result in a period of remodeling, evidenced by periostitis.

Surgery is indicated in the majority of metacarpal and metatarsal fractures. Cerclage, hemicerclage, and interfragmentary wiring, lag screw fixation, plating, and intramedullary pinnings using rush pins or K wires have been described as suitable methods of repair.[1, 9, 10, 17, 18, 21, 22, 25] Each fracture must be individually assessed to choose the most appropriate method of repair. Often more than one mode of repair is possible and the method chosen will be dictated by the surgeon's preference.

Some authors do not advocate cerclage as the sole mode of internal fixation.[26, 27] One survey of 120 cases of metacarpal fracture[16] showed this method achieved the highest percentage of successful return to racing. Cerclage wires are excellent for long oblique (Fig. 20–20A) and Y-shaped fractures with large butterfly fragments. Lag screws utilizing 1.5- or 2.0-mm diameter cortical screws can be used effectively in the repair of long oblique (Fig. 20–20B), spiral, and comminuted fractures as well as those fractures of proximal RMC-II with a dorsal butterfly fragment. Screws may be left in situ.[28, 29] Removal of screws extends convalescence by 8 to 10 weeks,[1] as the bone defects act as stress concentrators and the strength of the bone is significantly reduced.[5]

Bone plates are usually indicated in transverse or severely comminuted fractures. They may be used in conjunction with lag screw repair. Neutralization, compression, and buttressing techniques can be employed. Dynamic compression, semitubular, small-fragment, and miniplates are used routinely. The advent of the veterinary cutable plate with its low profile, slight concavity, and increased number of screw holes per unit length makes it ideally suited to metacarpal and metatarsal fractures.[25] Dorsal plating is the method of choice in the repair of the comminuted RMT-III fracture (Fig. 20–20C). It is customary to place the implants on the lateral or

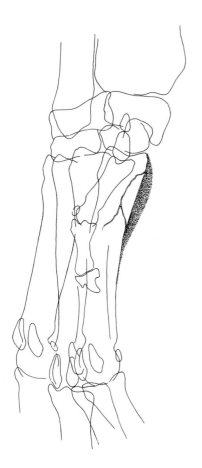
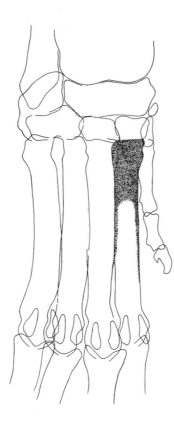

FIGURE 20–16. Representation of radiological changes seen with fatigue (stress) fracture of RMC-II. There is loss of the normal medullary canal shadow (now sclerotic) in the rotated dorsopalmar view. The rotated lateral (skyline) view can be exploited to highlight the dorsomedial aspect of the cortex. There is usually extensive periosteal new bone with a highly reactive surface, areas of osteolysis and maybe even fissure fractures extending into the dorsal cortex. Advancement of the fatigue fracture will result in the typical dorsal butterfly fragment with or without fracture of the palmar cortex. (Diagrams redrawn from Boemo CM: Metacarpal Injury. *In* Proc Post Grad 122: Committee Vet Sci Uni Syd p 274, 1989.)

FIGURE 20–17. Fatigue fracture. *(A)* Rotated dorsopalmar and *(B)* rotated lateral radiographs of the right metacarpus of a greyhound with fatigue fracture of RMC-II. Marked reduction of the medullary canal shadow diameter, increased radiodensity, and an increase in cortical width are evident in *(A)*, but the extent of the injury requires the skyline view *(B)* in which there is evidence of periosteal new bone, osteolysis, and fissuring of the callus *(black arrows)*. Active periosteal callus is also evident more distally on the dorsal aspect of RMC-II *(white arrow)*.

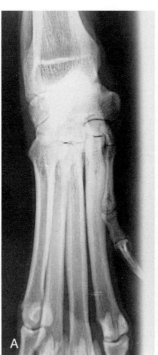
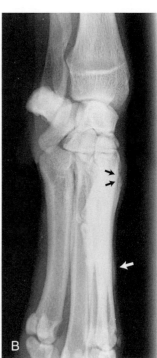

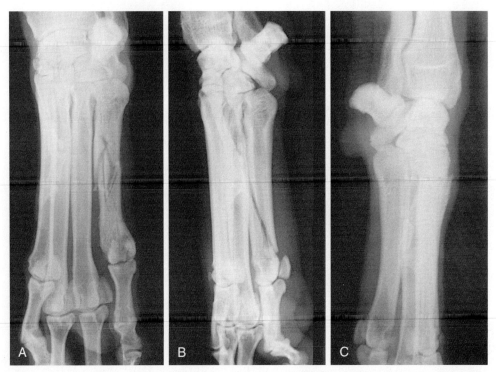

FIGURE 20–18. Complete metacarpal fracture. *A*, Rotated dorsopalmar radiograph of a comminuted fracture of LMC-V with multiple fissure fracture lines and dorsolateral butterfly fracture fragment. *B*, Rotated lateral radiograph of a long oblique fracture of LMC-V. *C*, Rotated lateral radiograph of RMC-II with fatigue fracture that has progressed to complete bone fracture with evidence of fissure lines extending into the dorsal callus.

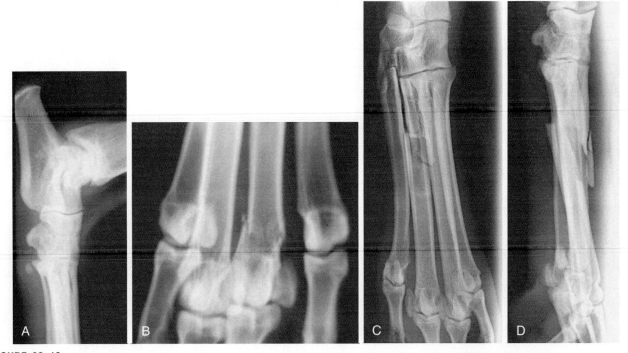

FIGURE 20–19. Complete metatarsal fracture. *A*, Lateral radiograph of right tarsus with medial trochlear ridge osteochondrosis dissecans lesion with evidence of avulsion of lateral plantar tarsometatarsal ligament from the base of RMT-V. *B*, Dorsoplantar view of distal metatarsal shaft fracture. *C*, Rotated plantarodorsal and *D*, lateral radiographs of a greyhound with the characteristic fracture of RMT-III. Excessive propulsive effort results in an explosive fracture with a dorsal butterfly fragment and plantaro-proximal displacement of the proximal end of the distal fracture fragment.

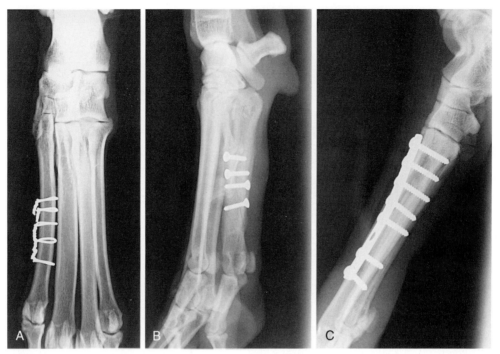

FIGURE 20–20. Metacarpal and metatarsal fracture repair. *A,* Rotated plantarodorsal postoperative radiograph of a greyhound with an oblique fracture of RMT-II required by cerclage wiring. Cerclage wiring is not recommended for the repair of short oblique fractures but is quite satisfactory for long oblique fractures. *B,* Rotated lateral postoperative radiograph of a greyhound with a long oblique fracture of LMC-V repaired with 2.0-mm lag screws. Note the periosteal new bone indicative of the osseous responses prior to bone failure. *C,* Lateral postoperative radiograph of the RMT-III fracture of Fig. 20–19 repaired with a dorsally placed 8-hole 2.7-mm DCP.

dorsolateral aspect of lateral metacarpal or metatarsal bones, and the dorsal or dorsomedial aspect of medial metacarpal or metatarsal bones. When metacarpal or metatarsal III or IV is involved, a dorsal approach is necessary.

Intramedullary pins inserted in the traditional normograde-retrograde manner[29] are not suitable for use in the performance animal, because their placement necessitates invasion of the metacarpo(tarso)phalangeal joint. Intramedullary pinning is indicated in transverse fractures in the region of the distal physeal plate, utilizing the rush pin technique, with the points of entry extra-articular on the lateral, dorsolateral, medial, dorsomedial, or dorsal aspects of the bone.

Postoperatively, animals in which adequate reduction and stability have been achieved are discharged to kennel confinement in a padded support bandage until suture removal. If the surgeon is not satisfied that rigid internal fixation has been achieved, or if there is reasonable concern that the animal will not remain quiet or is inclined to jump up or paw at the kennel wire, some form of molded external splinting should be applied for at least 3 weeks.

Early return to normal ambulation is imperative with the greyhound orthopedic patient.[1, 30] Prolonged disuse results in extensive muscle atrophy, reduced bone strength, and reduced intermetacarpal (tarsal) movement. Consideration must be given to ensure that premature return to work does not jeopardize the repair of the injury, but because of the limited racing life of the canine athlete, it is essential that this downtime be minimized. With adequate internal fixation, walking is begun at approximately 2 weeks postoperatively, and free running in a small enclosure might be encouraged from 4 to 6 weeks postoperatively. Follow-up radiographs should be taken at 4 to 5 weeks after surgery. Plates may be removed as soon as there is radiographical evidence of adequate healing. Bone plates should not be left in place as the bone is stress protected between the proximal and distal screws, resulting

in excessive stresses being exerted at the ends of the plate[31] with fracture of the bone through the distal or proximal screw holes a common side effect. When screws are removed the bone defects created act as stress concentrators,[5] and it is necessary to allow 8 to 10 weeks for these defects to be filled in and for the cortex to adapt to the increased stresses occurring with removal of the plate.

References

1. Boemo CM: Metacarpal Injury. *In* Proc Post-Grad Committee Vet Sci Uni Syd 122:257, 1989.
2. Gannon JR: Stress fractures in the greyhound. Aust Vet J 48:244, 1972.
3. Bloomberg MS: Incidence and characteristics of orthopedic injury of the racing greyhound between 1984–1990 at 6 racetracks in Florida, U.S.A. *In* Proc 7th Int Racing Greyhound Symp Eastern States Vet Conf Orlando, Florida, 1991, p 8.
4. Bloomberg MS: Racing greyhound injury survey update for 1990–1992. *In* Proc 9th Int Racing Greyhound Symp North Am Vet Conf Orlando, Florida, 1993, p 13.
5. Carter DR, Spengler DM: Biomechanics of fracture. *In* Sumner-Smith G (ed): Bone in Clinical Orthopedics, Philadelphia, WB Saunders Company, 1982, p 305.
6. Goodship AE, Lanyon LE, McFie H: Functional adaptation of bone to increased stress. J Bone Joint Surg Am 61:539, 1979.
7. Philips IR: A survey of bone fractures in the dog and cat. J Sm Anim Prac 20:661, 1979.
8. Kidd P: Forelimb injuries in the racing greyhound. *In* Proc Post-Grad Committee Vet Sci Uni Syd 34:286, 1977.
9. Kelman DA: Diagnosis, prevention and treatment of metacarpal injuries. Proc Ann Conf Aust Greyhound Vet Assoc Melbourne, 1984.
10. Kelman DA: Fractures in the hindlimb. *In* Proc Post-Grad Committee Vet Sci Uni Syd 64:366, 1983.
11. Hickman J: Greyhound injuries. J Sm Anim Pract 16:455, 1975.
12. Vines G: Science goes to the dogs. New Scientist p 44. 29/10/87.
13. Ireland BW: Greyhound racetrack design related to injury. *In* Proc Post-Grad Committee Vet Sci Uni Syd 122:355, 1989.

14. Bloomberg MS: Thermography: A new diagnostic aid for orthopedic injuries. *In* Proc 2nd Annual Mile High Kennel Club Greyhound Symp. Denver, Colorado, 1987, p 16.
15. Zuber RM: Personal communication. 1994
16. Homer DR: Metacarpal fractures in the racing greyhound. Vth Yr thesis (BVSc), University of Sydney, 1985.
17. Bellenger CR, Johnson KA, Davis PE, et al: Fixation of metacarpal and metatarsal fractures in greyhounds. Aust Vet J 57:205, 1981.
18. Cooper HL: Fracture of the medial metacarpal of the right front leg. *In* Proc Post-Grad Committee Vet Sci Uni Syd 64:547, 1983.
19. Taylor RA: Post-surgical physical therapy: The missing link. Comp Cont Ed 14:1583, 1992.
20. Whitney SL: Physical agents. Heat and cold modalities. *In* Scully RM, Barnes MR (eds): Physical Therapy. Philadelphia, JB Lippincott Co, 1989, p 849.
21. Gannon JR: Some aspects of greyhound practice. *In* Proc 41st Ann Meeting AAHA 1974, p 49.
22. Yore P: Practical treatments for orthopaedic problems in the forelimb. *In* Proc Post-Grad Committee Vet Sci Uni Syd 64:569, 1983.
23. Piermattei DL, Greeley RG (eds): An Atlas of Surgical Approaches to the Bones of the Dog and Cat, 2nd ed. Philadelphia, WB Saunders Company, 1979, p 120.
24. Pemberton PL: The use of anabolic steroids, vitamins and related substances in the racing greyhound. *In* Proc Post-Grad Committee Vet Sci Uni Syd 34:191, 1977.
25. Dee JF: Peak performance patients: Current surgical therapy, *In* Waltham Int Focus 1(2):2, 1991.
26. Brinker WO, Hohn RB, Prieur WD (eds): Manual of Internal Fixation in Small Animals. Berlin, Springer Verlag, 1984, p 57.
27. Kelman DA: Personal communication, 1992.
28. Eaton-Wells R: Personal communication, 1995.
29. Brinker WO, Piermattei DL, Flo GL (eds): Handbook of Small Animal Orthopedics and Fracture Treatment, Philadelphia, WB Saunders Company, 1983, p 175.
30. Eaton-Wells R: Prognosis for return to racing following surgical repair of musculo-skeletal injury. *In* Proc Post-Grad Committee Vet Sci Uni Syd 22:241, 1989.
31. Lanyon LE: Mechanical function and bone remodelling. *In* Sumner-Smith G (ed): Bone in Clinical Orthopedics, Philadelphia, WB Saunders Company, 1982, p 273.

CHAPTER 21

INJURIES OF THE DIGITS AND PADS

RICHARD D. EATON-WELLS

The digits of the forelimb are made up of the following joints: the metacarpophalangeal, the metacarposesamoid, the proximal phalangeal, or P1–2, and the distal phalangeal, or P2–3. The general anatomy of the area has been described,[1] as has the palmar sesamoids' anatomy.[2, 3] The anatomy of the interphalangeal joints in the racing greyhound has also been described in detail.[4] The digits and their respective metacarpal bones are numbered 1 through 5, starting on the medial side; digit 1 is also called the dewclaw. The anatomy of the equivalent area in the hind legs is similar. The problems associated with the sesamoids are covered in Chapter 29.

ANATOMY

Metacarpophalangeal Metatarsophalangeal Joints

The four weight-bearing metacarpophalangeal/metatarsophalangeal joints in either the fore or the hind limb are compound saddle joints, each involving the distal end of a metacarpal/metatarsal bone, the proximal end of the first phalanx, and two palmar/plantar sesamoids all supported by a complex arrangement of ligaments.[1]

The Proximal Interphalangeal Joint

The proximal interphalangeal articulation is a saddle joint involving the distal end of the first and the proximal end of the second phalanx. It is supported by a medial and lateral collateral ligament and the joint capsule, in conjunction with the common digital extensor tendon and its associated sesamoid dorsally and the insertion of the superficial digital flexor on the proximal palmar/plantar aspect of the second phalanx. Experimental studies have stressed the importance of the joint capsule in the joint's stability.[4] A small dorsal sesamoid is embedded in the joint capsule and supported by fibers from the common digital extensor tendon and the interosseous muscle anteriorly and a small ligament that extends distally to the dorsal surface of the middle phalanx.

The Distal Interphalangeal Joint

This joint involves the distal end of the second phalanx and the proximal end of the third. It is supported by the joint capsule and the medial and lateral collateral ligaments, each of which has a single origin but fans out to a diffuse attachment on the third phalanx. The tendons of insertion of the common digital extensor and the deep digital flexor cross the joint on the dorsal and palmar/plantar surfaces, respectively.

SURGERY OF THE EXTREMITIES

The phalangeal area is difficult to clip and prepare for aseptic surgery. A surgical scrub brush or toothbrush used on the digital and metacarpal pads, the toenails, and the nail bed during the initial preparation will help to remove any particulate matter. The area can then be prepared routinely for aseptic surgery. The use of a protective barrier wipe and sterile adhesive drape applied over the area from the metacarpus and metatarsus distally may help reduce the incidence of contamination. Prophylactic antibiotics should be given intravenously before surgery and repeated in 4 to 6 hours. All surgical approaches are made over the involved area and the structure concerned exposed by sharp dissection, as there is little or no subcutaneous tissue. Good hemostasis is essential, and blood vessels should be cauterized or ligated. A tourniquet, if used, will produce a relatively blood-free surgical field; however, there is the possibility of postoperative hemorrhage if hemostasis has been inadequate. The skin and subcutaneous tissues are closed routinely and a light dressing applied. The dressing is changed in 24 hours and then as necessary. The foot should be supported for 7 to 10 days and bandaged in such a way as to give maximum support to the injured structure. It is important to place sufficient padding between the digits to prevent pressure sores. As a general rule, the sooner the dog uses the foot after surgery the better the prognosis.

The prognosis for phalangeal collateral ligament injury has improved with careful dissection, debridement, and primary repair of the ligaments. The use of 4/0 polyglyconate sutures is desirable, as they have an initial breaking strength greater than both 4/0 nylon and polypropylene, measured in pounds per square inch to allow for the differences in suture diameter. They maintain approximately 40 per cent strength at 6 weeks postoperatively.[5]

METACARPOPHALANGEAL/ METATARSOPHALANGEAL LUXATION

Luxation occurs following injury to the collateral ligaments. It is more common in racing dogs but can occur in any breed. The injury usually occurs during exercise, and gross luxation may be evident (Fig. 21–1). The owner or trainer may have reduced the luxation before the dog's presentation to the veterinarian. The amount of swelling and pain is variable, and the dog may allow flexion and extension of the joint but resent rotation, as this causes the sesamoids to luxate over the sagittal crest; this luxation occurs

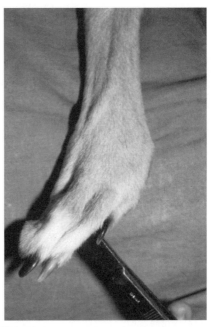

FIGURE 21–2. Multidigit metacarpophalangeal luxation.

with varying degrees of crepitus and is readily palpable. Once the joint has been reduced it should be stressed to ascertain which collateral ligament is injured. The injury usually affects either the medial or lateral digit; however, single luxations of the third or fourth digit may occur, or multiple digits may be involved (Fig. 21–2). Radiographs should be taken because of the high incidence of avulsion fractures associated with ligamentous injury (Fig. 21–3). Dissection of these joints after amputation will often reveal extensive articular cartilage erosion suggestive of a chronic injury. A complex injury involving more than one of the sesamoid liga-

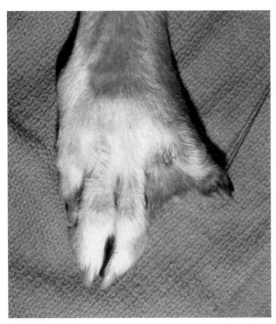

FIGURE 21–1. Gross luxation of the metacarpophalangeal joint.

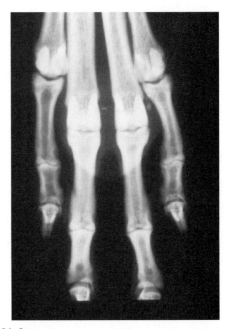

FIGURE 21–3. Radiograph of multidigit metacarpophalangeal luxation showing chips associated with the ligament injury.

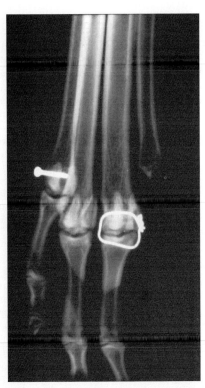

FIGURE 21–4. Insertion of 1.5-mm cortical screws to stabilize a metacarpophalangeal luxation.

ments results in a guarded prognosis for successful return to racing.[6]

Treatment

A simple padded dressing or light cast applied for 14 to 21 days will result in acceptable repair for those dogs that are to be retired from racing. The time-honored treatment of this injury in the racing greyhound has been amputation of the digit just proximal to the joint. This produces an acceptable result and the dog will return to the race track quickly; however, it can result in decreased performance. The ultimate aim for treatment of this injury in the racing dog should be primary surgical repair. However, there is no one technique that gives consistent results and therefore would avoid the loss of performance associated with some amputations. The involvement of multiple sesamoid ligaments and the presence of chronic sesamoid luxation even after surgical repair account for the poor to guarded prognosis given with these more complex injuries.[7] Chronic sesamoid luxation often results in the dog's failing to return to successful racing. Chronic luxation and degenerative joint disease do not always respond to sesamoid removal.

Surgical Repair of the Metacarpophalangeal Collateral Ligament

If the medial ligament on the second digit or the lateral ligament on the fifth digit is involved, the skin incision is made directly over the injury; approach to the ligaments between the metacarpals is more difficult. The ligament is repaired with one or two sutures of 4/0 polyglyconate. If primary repair is not possible, or the repair needs support, a 1.5-mm screw can be placed either at the site of the origin and/or insertion and a polyglyconate suture used to reattach or support it during the healing phase (Fig. 21–4).

INTRA-ARTICULAR FRACTURES OF THE DISTAL METACARPUS/METATARSUS AND PROXIMAL FIRST PHALANX

These fractures cause acute onset of lameness accompanied by swelling, pain, and crepitus on palpation. The diagnosis is confirmed radiographically. The fracture is repaired by open reduction and internal fixation using interfragmentary compression with either 1.5-mm or 2.0-mm screws (Fig. 21–5). The foot should be supported with a light dressing for 10 to 14 days.

SESAMOID FRACTURES

Acute sesamoid fractures in racing dogs may be slab, mid body, sagittal, or chip.[8] They are associated with acute onset of lameness and soft tissue swelling around the area concerned. There is reduction in range of motion with pain and crepitus on flexion and extension of the joint. The diagnosis is confirmed radiographically.

Treatment

Acute sesamoid fractures should be treated by surgical excision. The incision is made directly over the sesamoid involved; the superficial digital flexor tendon is identified, and the annular ligament incised on the affected side. Retraction of the superficial digital flexor and the annular ligament will reveal the sesamoid, which is carefully isolated from the tendon of the interosseous muscle by sharp dissection. The area is flushed and the annular ligament, subcutaneous tissue, and skin are then closed routinely. The foot should be supported with a light dressing for 5 to 7 days. The dog is confined to leash-walking for 2 weeks and is then allowed increasing amounts of free exercise. Small chips may be removed and the rest of the sesamoid left in situ. However, in fractures that involve large fragments, the whole sesamoid should be removed; in fact, both sesamoids may be removed with no obvious deleterious effects.

CHRONIC SESAMOID DISEASE

Chronic sesamoiditis has been recognized as both a cause of lameness and an incidental finding in the racing greyhound and

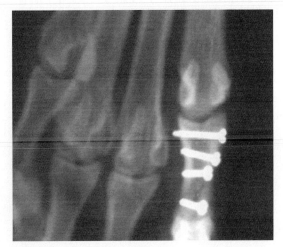

FIGURE 21–5. Postoperative radiograph of an intra-articular fracture of the metacarpophalangeal joint.

other breeds.[2] Using high-definition screens, radiographs of both forefeet should be taken for comparison. Congenital bipartite sesamoids may have minimally displaced fragments with rounded smooth edges (Fig. 21–6). The presence of these radiographic changes does not give any indication of the extent of the disease or the prognosis.[2]

Insofar as treatment and prognosis are concerned, sesamoid injuries can be divided into those that occur in the pet dog and those that occur in sporting, racing, and show dogs. The pet dog is rarely stressed to its maximum capacity, and conservative treatment is usually sufficient. However, a sporting dog needs to perform optimally over an extended time, a race dog must perform to its maximum for short periods, and a show dog needs to withstand the rigors of the show ring.

Once clinically significant degenerative joint disease has become established, sesamoid removal may not be beneficial. Treatment then consists of either rest and the use of nonsteroidal anti-inflammatory agents or amputation of the affected digit. If the degenerative joint disease is not clinically significant, no treatment is warranted.

The immune-mediated polyarthritis reported in young greyhounds often affects the metacarpophalangeal or the metatarsophalangeal joints first. This discussion is beyond the scope of this chapter.

THE PROXIMAL INTERPHALANGEAL JOINT

Soft tissue injuries to this area primarily involve the collateral ligaments, the joint capsule, and the dorsal sesamoid, resulting in sprains or luxations. Intra-articular fractures of the distal end of the first or the proximal end of the second phalanx may also occur. Injury to the joint capsule or the collateral ligaments may or may not result in lameness, and the clinical signs may vary. The joint should be fully flexed and extended; pain or inability to extend the joint may indicate palmar joint capsule sprain, partial avulsion of

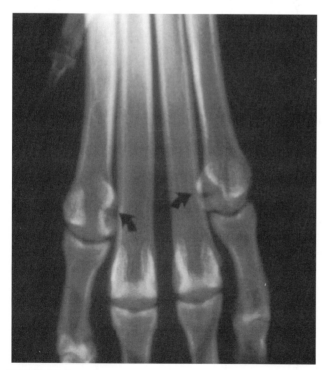

FIGURE 21–6. Radiograph showing multipartite sesamoid from clinically normal greyhound.

the superficial digital flexor tendon, chronic luxation, or degenerative joint disease. The interphalangeal collateral ligaments should always be tested with the toe in extension, as slight laxity in the neutral or flexed position is normal. Rupture of either the collateral ligament or the joint capsule alone does not produce marked joint instability. It is only when both occur simultaneously that the joint will luxate readily when stressed.[4] This may be accompanied by pain and/or crepitus. The position of the dorsal sesamoid should also be checked; minor instability is significant and indicates damage to its supporting structures. Occasionally, more than one joint may be involved on the same toe, the same foot, or another leg, or both medial and lateral collateral ligaments may be ruptured on the same digit.

Dogs that resent palpation of an injured digit should have a digital nerve block performed to enable a full examination. The block is performed by infiltration of approximately 0.25 ml of local anesthetic on the medial and lateral sides of the digit.

Surgical Approach

A 15-mm skin incision is made from the anterodistal end of the first phalanx to the proximopalmar aspect of the second. The soft tissues are retracted and the ligament remnants identified. The ligament ends are thickened in a chronic injury and may have to be dissected out of the surrounding fibrous tissue. The joint should be checked for small bone chips that will interfere with return of normal joint function. Two or three sutures of 4/0 polyglyconate placed in a "pulley" or near-far-far-near pattern are used to repair the collateral ligament. Total avulsion of the collateral ligament will necessitate anchoring the ligature in whatever subcutaneous tissue is available. This will provide sufficient stability if the toe is supported postoperatively. The use of synthetic "anchors" provides excellent stability, although the cost is high. The stability of the joint mediolaterally is tested and further sutures placed if the joint is still unstable. The stability of the dorsal sesamoid should also be checked and sutures placed to restore it if necessary. Once the joint is stable, it is important to check that it can be fully extended. Sutures that have been overtightened will prevent full extension of the joint and will result in chronic pain and reduced performance. The subcutaneous tissue and skin are closed routinely and the toenail cut short to reduce the mechanical leverage during the healing phase.

Severe instability may require placement of a wire suture through the distal end of the first and the proximal end of the second phalanx (Fig. 21–7). The placement of this suture is more technically demanding than primary ligament repair, but it will produce better stability. However, it often results in reduced range of motion. Arthrodesis of the interphalangeal joint may also be necessary. This may be performed by removal of the articular cartilage and application of a miniplate or with a pin and tension band wire (Fig. 21–8). The use of a cancellous bone graft will aid the arthrodesis. The joint should be fused in slight extension to decrease the incidence of postoperative complications. Provided that the joint has not been fused in flexion, the prognosis for return to racing after arthrodesis is good.

There is some controversy regarding toenail amputation when treating proximal interphalangeal ligament injuries. In my opinion if the second or fifth digit is involved it is preferable to amputate the toenail just proximal to the ungual crest. This reduces the stresses applied to the joint and hence the likelihood of recurrence. If the injury involves the central two digits the toenail should be cut short and hemorrhage controlled by bone wax or soap. Soap is preferable as it dissolves in the postoperative period and reduces the incidence of chronic problems.

Toenail amputation is accomplished by the use of an inverted Y-shaped incision around the nail. The soft tissues are carefully

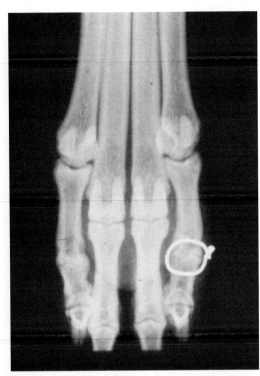

FIGURE 21–7. Wire suture placed to stabilize gross displacement of a P1–2 luxation.

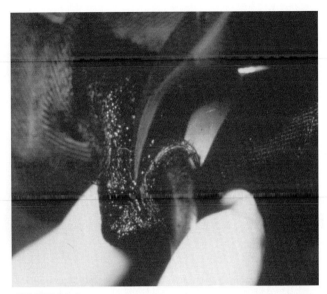

FIGURE 21–9. Placement of a curved rongeur for toenail amputation.

the toes, and a light dressing applied for 5 to 7 days. The dog may then be started on leash- or walking-machine exercise for 2 weeks and then allowed to free-gallop for another 2 weeks prior to being returned to race training.

Intra-articular Fractures

Simple fractures involving the proximal interphalangeal joint should be handled by either removal of small chips or replacement of large fragments. Lag screw fixation is achieved with either 1.5-mm or 2.0-mm screws. This is particularly important in the racing dog as accurate reduction and rigid internal fixation result in more rapid return to function and less degenerative joint disease. The subcutaneous tissue and skin are closed routinely. A light Robert Jones dressing is applied. This dressing is changed at 24 hours and

dissected back to the ungual crest and a pair of curved bone cutters is used to remove the nail (Fig. 21–9). It is essential to remove all the horny nail, or regrowth can occur, causing persistent lameness (Fig. 21–10). Skin closure is routine. Padding is placed between

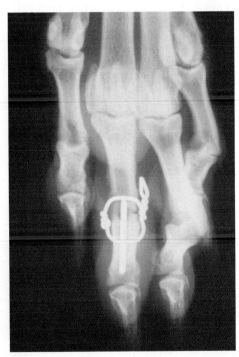

FIGURE 21–8. Pin and tension band used for P1–2 arthrodesis.

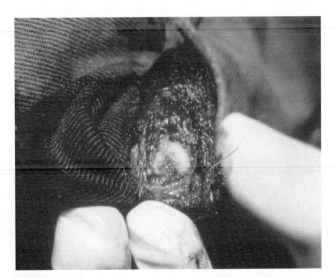

FIGURE 21–10. All of the corium layer is removed to prevent nail regrowth.

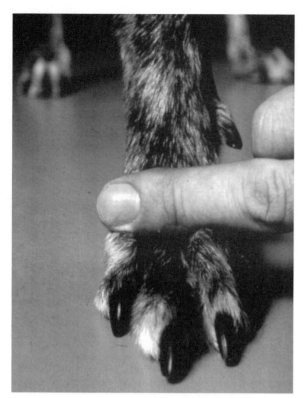

FIGURE 21–11. Dropped toe. Note that the proximal interphalangeal joint has collapsed.

then as necessary. The joint is supported for 10 to 14 days.* Comminuted fractures or ones that involve severe joint damage may require either arthrodesis or amputation.

AVULSION OF THE SUPERFICIAL DIGITAL FLEXOR TENDON

Avulsion of the superficial digital flexor tendon insertion off the first phalanx will result in loss of tension in that tendon and consequently a flat toe. This is called a dropped toe because of the flat appearance of the digit (Fig. 21–11). This injury is of little significance except in breeds in which the foot conformation is important for show purposes. The treatment, if necessary, is reattachment of the tendon with either a wire suture or a screw and washer. The wire suture technique requires two small holes to be drilled, from the anterior to the posterior surface, in the proximal end of the second phalanx. A suitable locking pattern suture, using multifilament wire, is placed in the tendon. The ends of the suture are then passed through the tunnels and tied on the dorsal aspect of the phalanx. Alternatively, a small spiked washer may be shaved with either a scalpel or a high-speed drill to decrease the "profile" of the washer. A screw is then used to reattach the avulsed tendon. The toes should be supported in flexion for 2 weeks, then in a weight-bearing position for another 2 weeks before the dog is allowed to bear weight normally. The prognosis for repair of this injury is excellent.

---

*Editor's note: Early joint manipulation and passive range of motion are important for complete recovery.

DISTAL INTERPHALANGEAL JOINT

The collateral ligaments of this joint should also be tested in extension because of the normal laxity in a neutral position. Injury to the collateral ligament may be accompanied by a small, profusely bleeding wound on the affected side of the joint (Fig. 21–12). In my experience, surgical repair of the ruptured ligament plus amputation of the nail will result in a faster return to function than if the third phalanx is amputated either at the joint or through the distal end of P2.

Two sutures of 4/0 polyglyconate are used to repair the ligament and stabilize the joint. The skin is closed routinely. A separate incision is then made around the nail and up the dorsal aspect of the second phalanx so that the toenail can be amputated proximal to the ungual crest. This reduces the mechanical leverage on the repair.[9] Postoperative care consists of administration of antibiotics for 5 days and use of a light dressing for 7 to 10 days with restricted exercise during this time. Progressively increasing amounts of leash-exercise are allowed for the next 2 weeks before allowing the dog free exercise.

Pain on forced extension and pain and swelling on palpation of the ventral aspect of the joint may indicate chronic synovitis of the deep digital flexor tendon. This may be treatable with a nonsteroidal anti-inflammatory agent and antibiotics; however, the amputation of the toe through the end of the second phalanx brings a more rapid return to racing. Rupture of the deep digital flexor tendon results in a "kicked-up" or "knocked-up" toe (Fig. 21–13). This is of little clinical importance. Some animals develop a painful "corn" on the affected pad that is treated by surgical excision or amputation of the digit through the end of the second phalanx. Avulsion fractures of the flexor process will appear similar clinically and may be treated by amputation of the third phalanx if clinically significant.

Intra-articular fractures involving the second phalanx may be amenable to open reduction and internal fixation. However, frac-

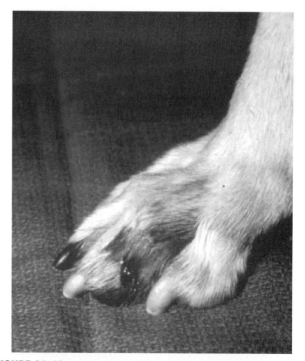

FIGURE 21–12. Distal phalangeal joint luxation showing bleeding from a small skin split.

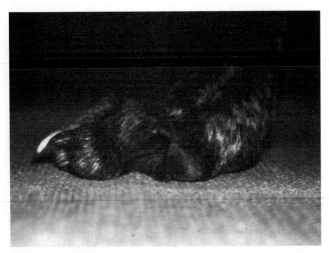

FIGURE 21–13. Rupture or avulsion of the deep digital flexor causing the toenail to be elevated.

tures of the third phalanx, severe degenerative joint disease, and chronic tenosynovitis due to penetrating pad wounds are best handled by amputation of the third phalanx through the distal end of the second phalanx. The joint may be disarticulated, but if so, the articular cartilage should be removed as it is prone to chondromalacia and degeneration (Fig. 21–14). This results in inflammation and chronic pain on palpation of the area. Close attention to hemostasis is essential to decrease the incidence of postoperative problems. The fibrocartilaginous pads that protect the deep digital flexor tendon as it crosses the palmar aspect of the joint may be excised or left in situ. The soft tissues and skin are closed routinely. It is important to preserve the digital pad regardless of the technique used.

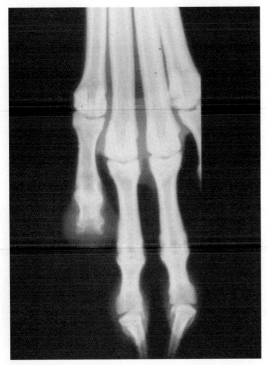

FIGURE 21–14. Chondromalacia of the distal P2 articular surface.

Acute cellulitis and septic arthritis cause sudden onset of lameness. The digit involved will have a discrete area of erythema, feel warmer than the others, and be acutely painful. The pain may be such that local anesthesia and radiographs may be necessary to rule out fractures. The dog should be treated with systemic antibiotics, a nonsteroidal anti-inflammatory agent, and hot compresses.

PAD INJURIES

The treatment of many pad injuries depends on the racing status of the dog. Breeding stock can often be treated conservatively, whereas racing dogs require aggressive treatment to reduce the likelihood of secondary problems and to ensure that they are returned to the track as soon as possible. The pads of racing dogs are subjected to many insults. Poorly maintained track surfaces may produce pad lacerations. In Australia, running dogs on grass or dry sand on hot days often results in blistering and then sloughing off of the cornified pad surface in a so-called burn. These superficial injuries are treated conservatively by application of products such as Friar's Balsam or Pad Paint and the cornified epithelium allowed to become reestablished. Pad lacerations should be sutured with a simple interrupted pattern to reappose the cut edges and a mattress suture to support the repair. Puncture wounds of the pad should always be radiographed to ensure that no foreign material is present. In countries where dogs are exercised outside the track area, the presence of glass and small stones is common. These should be removed under local anesthesia and the wound either closed primarily or the pad protected and allowed to heal by granulation. Systemic broad-spectrum antibiotics should be administered to reduce the likelihood of secondary infection and synovitis of the deep digital flexor tendon. Small fresh wounds may be treated by application of a small rubber patch applied with cyanoacrylate.

Nonrecognition or inappropriate treatment of a pad puncture wound may result in development of a corn (Fig. 21–15). Corns are cone-shaped hard fibrous masses that result from a puncture wound and cause chronic pain and discomfort to the dog. They should become immediately obvious during the physical examination. Treatment is by surgical excision and primary closure, and care should be exercised that the deep digital flexor tendon has not become involved in the corn base, as this will often result in a less than satisfactory outcome.

WEBBING INJURIES

The most common webbing injury involves lacerations between two toes. Small tears may be handled by primary closure, using 4/0 polyglyconate sutures, making sure that the thickened leading edge is carefully apposed. More extensive splits can be handled by creation of a permanent deficit in the webbing brought about by extending the split and suturing the dorsal and ventral surfaces together (Fig. 21–16). The foot should be supported with a light dressing for 5 to 7 days. After this, the use of a rubber band made of a bicycle tire or similar material will provide support while the wound is healing. This support needs to be used when the dog is exercised for approximately 1 month to allow the tissues to strengthen before the dog's return to full training.

The webbing, pad, and nailbed areas are also common sites for viral papillomas, or warts (Fig. 21–17). They are quite painful and occur more commonly in young dogs that have not developed an immune response to them. They are best managed by expression under local anesthesia; occasionally they are deep enough that the skin will need to be incised. Pressure will result in expulsion of

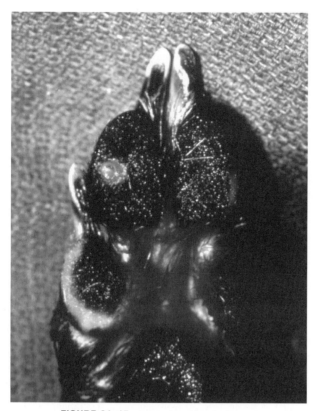

FIGURE 21–15. A corn is evident in this pad.

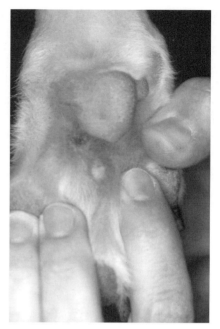

FIGURE 21–17. A viral papilloma is present.

the majority of the papilloma, which will leave a hole that bleeds excessively for a short period. A light dressing will control this.

"Sand ulcers" also occur on the under side of the webbing; these are usually heat related and may result when the dog is run in very hot conditions, especially on one of the artificial surfaces, although these lesions occur after exercise on any surface if the conditions are right (Fig. 21–18).

PARONYCHIA

Simple infection around the nailbed is a common cause of chronic inflammation and a debilitating paronychia. Most owners

and trainers have their own special treatment of this problem. However, use of a soft toothbrush for diligent removal of as much sand/track material as possible and application of dimethyl sulfoxide (DMSO) containing a broad-spectrum antibiotic will greatly aid in its control. In those countries that allow dogs to race with dressings in place, a small strip of adhesive tape applied to the nail will give some protection to the area (Fig. 21–19). Because of the loss of the protective hairs in the area once an infection has become established, this problem is rarely cured during the dog's racing life. Fungal infections and the immune-mediated disease pemphigus also occur.

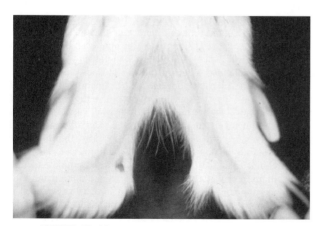

FIGURE 21–16. Split webbing with top-to-bottom repair.

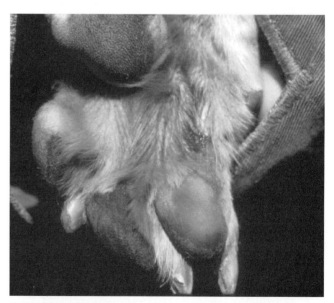

FIGURE 21–18. Sand ulcers are the result of environmental heat and poorly conditioned pads.

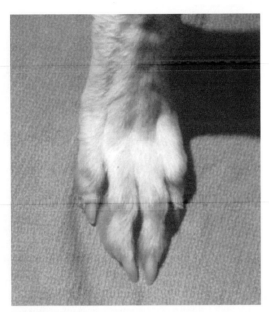

FIGURE 21–19. Nail bed is protected with adhesive strip.

TOENAIL INJURIES

As a result of the forces being placed on the digit during exercise, toenails are often split or torn off. If the keratinous horn is torn off, the "quick" can be protected by application of one of the epoxy cements, such as dental acrylic, while the new nail is growing. Alternatively, the quick can be cut off as short as necessary. If the nail has been stripped only partially, judicious use of one of the cyanoacrylate adhesives to reattach the nail and protect the exposed quick will decrease the amount of pain and allow the dog to be returned to the track earlier.

DIGITAL AMPUTATION

As our ability to repair greyhound injuries improves, so, it is hoped, will the incidence of toe amputation decrease. There are several levels at which a toe or whole digits may be amputated: If the entire digit is to be removed, the metacarpal or metatarsal bones should be amputated just above the joint, the sesamoids removed, and the bone smoothed and tapered. Care must be taken to ensure that sufficient metacarpal and tarsal bone is left so that the adjacent bone does not have to undergo major remodeling changes. Amputation may also be performed through the distal end of the second phalanx by "filleting" out the distal interphalangeal joint and third phalanx. The digital pad is retained to protect the second phalanx. The third level of amputation is just proximal to the corium of the nail. At this level the pad is retained. Closure for all of these procedures is routine, and the foot is supported in a padded bandage for 7 to 10 days. The dog is then started on walking exercise.

For pet or working dogs the prognosis for digital amputation is excellent. The prognosis for greyhounds returning to racing after full digital amputation is good, although it appears to be better if the second or fifth digit is involved rather than the third or fourth. There is also some variation in the outcome among dogs, depending on their keenness to chase. The prognosis for return to racing after distal second or third phalanx amputation is excellent.

References

1. Evans HE, Christensen GC. Miller's Anatomy of the Dog, 2nd ed. Philadelphia, WB Saunders Company, 1993.
2. Bennett D, Kelly DF: Sesamoid disease as a cause of lameness in the dog. J Small Anim Pract 26:567, 1985.
3. Robins GM, Read RA: Diseases of the sesamoid bones, *In* Borab MJ (ed): Disease Mechanism in Small Animal Surgery, 2nd ed. Philadelphia, Lea & Febiger, 1993, Ch 145.
4. Davis PE: Personal communication
5. Katz AR, Mukherjee DP, Kaganov AL, Gordon S: A new synthetic monofilament absorbable suture made from polytrimethylene carbonate. Surg Gynecol Obstet 161:213–222, 1985.
6. Dee JF, Dee LG, Eaton-Wells RD: Injuries of high performance dogs *In* Whittick WG (ed): Canine Orthopedics, 2nd ed. Philadelphia, Lea & Febiger, 1990.
7. Eaton-Wells RD: Prognosis for return to racing following surgical repair of musculoskeletal injury. *In* Greyhound Medicine and Surgery. Proceedings 122. University of Sydney Postgraduate Committee in Veterinary Science, 1989.
8. Davis PE, Bellenger CR, Turner DM: Fractures of the sesamoid bones in the greyhound. Aust Vet J 45:15, 1969.
9. Hickman J: Greyhound injuries. J Small Anim Pract 16:455, 1975.

CHAPTER 22

DISORDERS OF THE HIP JOINT IN THE CANINE ATHLETE

KIRK L. WENDELBURG

Disorders of the hip in a canine athlete can be categorized into injuries produced by severe external trauma, training-induced injuries, and hip dysplasia. Physical examination and patient management may vary depending on the signalment, history, and functional use of the patient. The most frequent cause of hip joint injuries in all types of dogs results from external trauma, such as a fall, a gunshot wound, or an automobile accident. Racing greyhounds can also develop a stress fracture of the hip joint resulting from the tremendous muscular and concussive forces transferred to the bones during training and racing. Fractures of this type are very similar to stress fractures reported in human athletes.[1] Hip dysplasia, an inherited developmental malformation, can also predispose the canine athlete to lameness. Hip dysplasia unfortunately continues to be recognized as a common cause of lameness in sporting dogs, despite efforts of breeders and veterinarians to reduce the prevalence of the disease by selective breeding.

ANATOMY

The hip joint or *coxofemoral* joint is an articulation of the femur onto the pelvis through a ball-and-socket design. The femoral head fits congruently into the horseshoe-shaped *lunate surface* of the acetabular socket. This ball-and-socket design provides the highest range of motion of all rear limb joints while maintaining stability.

To achieve normal function as a ball-and-socket joint, it is required to have 3 degrees of rotational freedom: Flexion-extension, abduction-adduction, and internal-external rotation. A fourth degree of freedom, lateral translation (hip joint laxity), in excess can lead to potential joint incongruency.[2] Functional joint congruity is imperative to the demands placed on the hip by canine athletes. Any degree of incongruity within the ball-and-socket joint will lead to abnormal mechanics, excessive cartilage wear, and eventual degenerative joint disease. Development joint of anatomical components of both the femur and the acetabulum are important for the normal function of the joint.

Fusion of the ilium, ischium, pubis, and acetabular bone during the 12th postnatal week creates the *acetabulum*.[3] The weight-bearing or articular cartilage surface of the acetabulum is called the *lunate surface*. The *acetabular angle* represents the angle formed by the tangent of the midlunate surface to a horizontal axis[4] (Fig. 22–1). Central to the lunate surface is the nonarticular, thin, depressed area called the *acetabular fossa*. Extending medially from the fossa is a notch, the *acetabular incisure*. The *transverse acetabular ligament* extends across the ventral aspect of the acetabular fossa. It serves to support the femoral head ventrally. It continues around the periphery of the acetabulum as a fibrocartilaginous structure called the *acetabular labrum*.

The proximal femur contributing to the hip joint includes the head, the neck, and the greater, lesser, and third trochanters. The

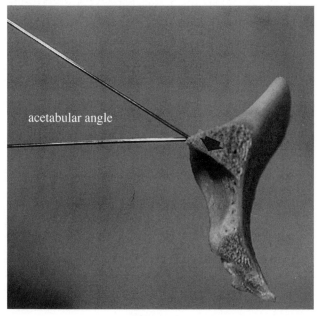
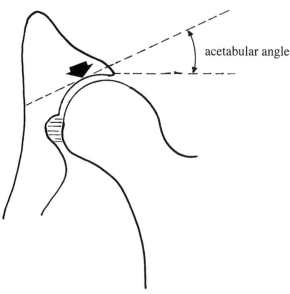

FIGURE 22–1. Tangent to the mid-lunate surface *(arrow)* forms the acetabular angle.

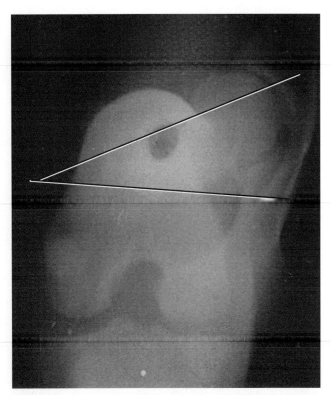

FIGURE 22–2. Axial view of the femur demonstrates normal femoral anteversion.

head is the hemispherical articular cap of the femoral neck originating from the epiphysis. Growth of the femoral head is through the endochondral ossification of its articular cartilage. Its surface is composed primarily of articular cartilage, except for a small depression on the caudomedial aspect, the *fovea capitis*. This small area serves as the attachment of the *ligament of the head of the femur* (round ligament).[3, 5] The ligament extends from the fovea to the acetabular fossa. The ligament of the head of the femur is important primarily as a constraint at the extremes of hip motion.[6]

The *neck* represents the most proximal aspect of the femoral diaphysis and unites the head to the trochanters and remaining body. The length of the femoral neck and the angles at which it leaves the proximal femur are important in maintaining the congruency and distribution of forces in the hip joint.[7–11] Neck length is controlled by endochondral growth from the *capital growth plate*. Premature closure of the growth plate or developmentally shortened neck length can lead to subluxation and incongruency of the hip joint.[8, 12, 13]

The angle between the plane of the femoral condyles and the axis of the femoral neck is called the *declination angle* or *femoral torsion*. A femoral neck projecting parallel to the plane of the femoral condyles is said to have 0 degrees of femoral torsion. If the axis of the femoral neck projects cranial to the condylar plane, the angle of torsion is positive and is called anteversion. The angle of torsion is negative and is called *retroversion* when the femoral neck axis projects caudally. Dogs normally have some degree of anteversion or positive femoral torsion. Normal angles of torsion have been reported to range from +12 to +40 degrees, with a mean of +27 degrees when measured by a direct radiographic technique (axial view), and from +18 to +47 degrees, with a mean of 31 degrees when measured by a method using trigonometry and biplanar radiography[14, 15] (Fig. 22–2).

The angle formed from intersection of the femoral neck axis and the femoral shaft axis is the *angle of inclination* or *cervicofemoral angle*. This angle as measured on the ventrodorsal radiographic view is influenced by technique of measurement, positioning, and the amount of femoral torsion present.[5, 16, 17] As the amount of anteversion increases, it falsely increases the apparent angle of inclination as measured on ventrodorsal radiographs.[14, 17] The angle of inclination has a reported range of 137 to 155 degrees, with a mean of 144.7 degrees when it is corrected for femoral torsion.[14]

The *joint capsule* completely encloses the hip joint. It is important in maintaining the femoral head within the acetabular socket. The capsule and a small amount of joint fluid produce a hydrostatic stability factor, preventing lateral translation of the femoral head.[6] As a distractive load is placed on the femoral head, the intra-articular pressure becomes negative, "sucking" the femoral head and joint capsule back into the acetabulum. The hydrostatic stability factor is lost with defects through the joint capsule or increases in the joint fluid volume. The mean joint fluid volume increases in dysplastic dogs to 2.52 ml as compared with 0.80 ml in dogs with normal hip conformation.[18] As fluid volume increases, lateral translation of the femoral head is limited by the tensile forces of the joint capsule and round ligament. The capsule may stretch in response to hip dysplasia as a result of misdirected lateral and upward forces in the hip joint.[2] It is still controversial whether these differences in joint fluid and joint capsule elongation are primary, or secondary to subluxation.[2]

Blood supply to the hip joint capsule and femoral head in the immature dog is from an extracapsular ring supplied by the *medial and lateral circumflex and caudal gluteal arteries*.[3, 19] Branches of these vessels, called *ascending cervical arteries* (retinacular arteries), travel within the joint capsule to ascend over the capital growth plate and enter the femoral head as *epiphyseal arteries*.[19, 20] The femoral head and capital growth plate are supplied primarily by the epiphyseal arteries with a very small portion of the epiphysis supplied by an artery in the ligament of the head of the femur.[19, 20] The femoral head of the immature dog depends totally on the ascending cervical arteries for its blood supply because of the physeal barrier and limited supply from the artery in the ligament of the head of the femur. Because of this limited vascular pattern, the femoral head and capital physis of the immature dog are highly susceptible to disruption by traumatic injury. Hip injuries in immature animals may produce disruption of the blood supply resulting in developmental changes in the hip joint.[19, 21, 22] The *nutrient artery of the femur* is a branch of the *medial circumflex femoral artery*, which enters the caudal surface of the femur at the junction of the proximal and middle thirds. The nutrient artery continues proximally as the *metaphyseal arteries*. The metaphyseal arteries do not cross the capital growth plate until the animal is mature and the growth plate closes. They will then penetrate the closed physis to anastomose with the epiphyseal arteries. Most of the intraosseous vascular supply to the acetabulum is derived from the nutrient artery of the ilium, a branch of the iliolumbar artery.[19] The medial and lateral circumflex femoral, cranial gluteal, and caudal gluteal arteries also contribute to the acetabular blood supply.

Muscles that provide function and support to the hip joint include flexors, extensors, external and internal rotators, adductors, and abductors. The flexors of the hip are responsible for the forward swing phase of the gait and include the iliospoas, the tensor fascia lata, articularis coxae, sartorious, and rectus femoris muscles.[3] Extensors are the largest muscles acting about the hip joint and produce the powerful propulsion phase of the gait. These muscles include the gluteals, biceps femoris, semimembranosus, semitendinosus, quadratus femoris, piriformis, gracilis, and adductor muscles.[3] The adductors (adductor longus and adductor magnus et brevis) along with the pectineus, and gracilis muscles adduct the femur. Gluteal muscles and the tensor fascia lata also act to produce internal rotation and abduction of the femur. External rotators of the hip are the internal obturator, external obturator, gemelli, quadratus femoris, and iliopsoas.

INJURIES RESULTING FROM EXTERNAL TRAUMA

External trauma necessary to produce a hip joint fracture or luxation is usually caused by automobile injuries. Severe falls, blunt trauma, gunshot wounds, and dog fights are other causes of injury to the hip. The degree of trauma necessary to cause fracture or dislocation of the hip is usually significant and often produces associated injuries. Therefore a thorough examination of the entire pelvis, rear limbs, and spine, along with the adjacent soft tissues and organs must be performed. Along with a complete physical examination, a complete blood count and serum chemistry should be performed. Thoracic and abdominal radiographs are taken if indicated.

Assessment of the urinary tract is necessary in all pelvic trauma patients. Any animal with hematuria, inability to urinate, or a bloody urethral discharge must be evaluated closely. Rupture of the bladder or ureteral avulsion occurs with similar frequencies in males and females, while urethral tears are more common in male dogs.[23, 24] A history of whether or not the dog urinated before or after the injury is important. Along with direct perforation from the fracture, compressive forces transmitted to a distended bladder are more likely to produce injury than when the bladder is empty. The ability to urinate normal volumes of clear urine following an accident does not preclude, but indicates an unlikelihood, that there is a serious injury to the urinary tract. Rising level of blood urea nitrogen (BUN) is highly indicative of an intra-abdominal urine leak. Suspicion of urinary tract trauma can be confirmed with

contrast radiography. An excretory urogram is used to evaluate the upper urinary tract while a urethrogram-cystogram is used to evaluate the urethra and bladder.

Pelvic fractures are commonly multiple because of the box-like configuration of the pelvis. Pelvic symmetry can be evaluated by comparative palpation of the iliac crest, tuber ischii, and greater trochanters. Inconsistency in distances between these structures is an indication of a pelvic fracture or luxation (coxofemoral or sacroiliac). A medially displaced greater trochanter that is difficult to palpate is often indicative of an acetabular fracture. Crepitus, pain, and decreased range of motion are also consistent findings of a fracture in the hip joint. A cranially and dorsally displaced greater trochanter along with decreased range of internal rotation is observed with craniodorsal hip luxations.

Trauma-induced injuries of the pelvis require a neurological evaluation of the femoral and sciatic nerves. Pain responses are appraised for both nerves. Absence of a pain response to the lateral digit is suggestive of an injury to the sciatic nerve. The lack of sensation to the medial digit or loss of patellar reflex may indicate an injury to the femoral nerve.

Radiographic examination of the pelvis may require sedation if the patient's condition is stable. Lateral and ventrodorsal views are necessary. A more detailed examination of the acetabulum or femoral head and neck may require a medial to lateral view of the hip joint. A slipped capital epiphysis in a young dog may become reduced and difficult to visualize on an extended ventrodorsal radiographic view. If this disorder is suspected, a ventrodorsal view with the hips and stifles flexed and abducted into a frog-leg position is also necessary (Fig. 22–3).

Acetabular Fractures. Fractures in the canine athlete involving any part of the acetabulum, or that produce hip joint instability (ilial fracture, sacroiliac luxations), are best repaired with open anatomical reduction and internal fixation. Surgical repair of reduc-

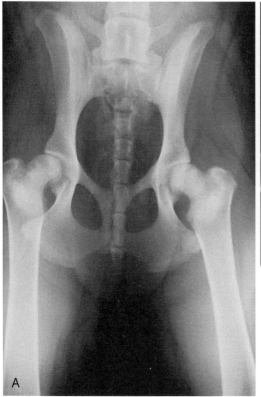
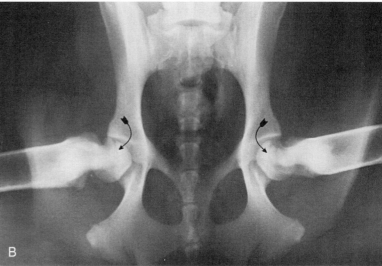

FIGURE 22–3. Extended *(A)* and frog-legged *(B)* ventrodorsal radiographs of bilateral capital physeal fractures. Note that the lesion is difficult to detect in the extended ventrodorsal view while clearly visible in the frog-leg view.

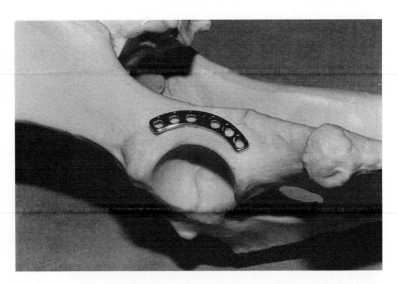

FIGURE 22–4. A semicircular acetabular plate is placed dorsal to the acetabulum for fracture stabilization.

ible acetabular fractures is reported to result in pain-free hip joints with minimal or no osteoarthrosis.[21, 25] Thirteen of 15 nonsurgically treated dogs with caudal third acetabular fractures had radiographic evidence of moderate to severe osteoarthrosis; 7 of these dogs were clinically lame, while 12 had a decreased range of motion or pain in the affected hip.[26] Another study, based on observations of lameness by owners, reported satisfactory results of conservative management in cases of minimally displaced caudal acetabular fractures in pet dogs.[27] Rigid, anatomical, surgical reduction is more likely to preserve function required in an athletic dog when fractures involve the lunate surface.

The prognosis for surgical management of acetabular fractures greatly depends on the ability to achieve a stable, anatomical repair. The repair is influenced by the amount of damage to the articular surface, the location, the amount of comminution, and the presence or absence of other pelvic fractures. Adequate exposure of the fracture site is essential to achieve reduction and stable fixation. Different approaches to the acetabulum can be used, but a dorsal approach via a trochanteric osteotomy provides the greatest exposure to the acetabulum and is usually preferred.[21, 25, 28–32] Reduction and fixation are best accomplished with bone plating through Association for the Study of Internal Fixation (ASIF) technique.[28, 29, 33] Mini- or small-fragment plating is used most commonly to stabilize the fractures. ASIF reconstruction plates are often useful for contouring over comminuted or multiple acetabular and ilial fractures. Lag screws are incorporated for interfragmentary compression, while multiple K-wires are sometimes necessary for positional stabilization of comminuted fragments. Since plate positioning is inevitably on the tension side of the bone, small finger plates or precontoured, lunate-shaped, acetabular plates (2.0 and 2.7 mm) will usually suffice (Fig. 22–4). Inaccurate contouring of a large plate may result in unsatisfactory functional results. It is essential for the repair to provide anatomical reduction of the cartilage surface. Secure joint capsule closure with an absorbable monofilament in a horizontal mattress or cruciate pattern helps prevent postoperative subluxation.

Strict activity limitations should be enforced for 6 weeks postoperatively. If comminution is present or positional stabilization with K-wires is required, a non–weight-bearing sling is placed on the dog for 2 to 3 weeks, unless injuries to the other legs make it impractical. Physical therapy with range-of-motion exercises is encouraged. Follow-up radiographic reevaluation is done at 4 to 6 weeks after surgery. A slow return to athletic function will follow radiographic union of the fractures. Athletic function can be expected to return with minimal degenerative joint disease (DJD) if

anatomical reduction is accomplished and maintained. Conservative medical management is recommended in dogs that develop DJD. Athletic function can be reestablished in those dogs with severe DJD by carrying out a total hip replacement after complete bony union.

Fractures of the Proximal Femur. Proximal femoral fractures that affect the hip joint can be divided into (1) capital epiphyseal (femoral head), (2) capital physeal (slipped capital epiphysis), (3) femoral neck, (4) trochanteric, (5) subtrochanteric, and (6) multiple.[13] All of these fractures can directly or indirectly affect coxofemoral joint congruency and function. Most of the fractures into the hip joint can be approached craniolaterally.[30] Exposure should be kept limited in the immature patient to prevent trauma to the highly vulnerable blood supply of the femoral head and physis. In mature animals, exposure can be facilitated by partial tenotomy of the deep gluteal and periosteal reflection of the vastus lateralis muscle origin. A dorsal approach to the coxofemoral joint by osteotomy of the greater trochanter provides a much increased exposure but is seldom required unless comminution is present.[30] A ventral approach to the coxofemoral joint is useful in surgical repair of small avulsion fractures of the femoral head[30] (Fig. 22–5). Trochanteric and subtrochanteric fractures of the femur are exposed by the lateral approach to the proximal femur.[30]

Capital Epiphyseal Fractures. Fractures of the femoral head are most commonly small avulsion fractures and are usually associated with coxofemoral luxations in immature animals. If the fragment is small and does not involve a significant weight-bearing area, it can be excised with the ligament of the head of the femur before reduction and repair of the coxofemoral luxation. Larger fractures involving the weight-bearing surface and subchondral bone are best repaired with internal fixation. Lag screw, multiple K-wire, or combination screw and pin techniques are most successful. Countersunk lag screw and/or K-wire placement through a ventral approach is accomplished from the insertion area of the ligament of the head of the femur (Fig. 22–5). Compression lag screw combined with K-wire repair resulted in excellent or good results in 4 of 5 cases.[34]

Capital Physeal Fractures (Slipped Capital Epiphysis). Capital physeal fracture is the most common proximal femur fracture in immature dogs.[35–37] Because the femoral physis is rather flat and prone to shear forces, trauma in this area most often results in a Salter-Harris type I fracture of the physis. It is important that a frog-legged, ventrodorsal radiographic view is taken when this fracture is suspected. An extended leg, ventrodorsal view will cause

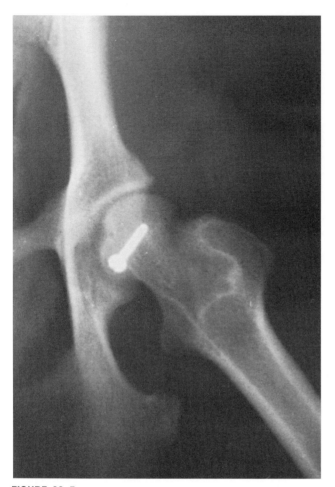

FIGURE 22–5. A 4-year postoperative radiograph of a lag screw repair done through a ventral approach for an epiphyseal avulsion fracture.

torsional tightening of the joint capsule that may result in reduction of the fracture, making it radiographically inapparent (Fig. 22–3).

Although avascular necrosis is always a concern with capital physeal fractures, most heal satisfactorily with early internal fixation.[35–38] It is expected to observe some degree of femoral neck resorption (apple core effect) on radiographic examinations 3 to 6 weeks after surgery.[36, 38] Although neck resorption does not usually cause a clinical failure, abnormal femoral head and neck development is likely, especially in animals less than 5 months of age with considerable growth potential remaining. Premature closure of the physis can result in shortening of the femoral neck, coxa vara, and overgrowth of the greater trochanter. These changes, if severe enough, will result in incongruency and early degenerative joint disease adversely affecting future athletic function. The prognosis depends on the severity of the soft tissue trauma (joint capsule and blood supply), the age of the animal, and early atraumatic and anatomical surgical repair.

Repair is best accomplished within the first 2 to 3 days of the injury. Remodeling and fibrosis can make repair of a chronic fracture difficult or unsuccessful. The most common method used to stabilize the femoral head involves multiple K-wires or pins[36, 39] (Fig. 22–6). Three K-wires are inserted at slightly converging angles into the femoral head and neck. Pins may be retrograded or normograded with the help of an ASIF C-guide. All pins are placed in the proximal femur and femoral neck with points flush at the level of the fracture. The femoral head is then reduced and the pins

are driven into the subchondral bone. The articular surface of the femoral head is visually inspected for pin penetration and checked for smooth, stable range of motion. An alternative repair can be accomplished with a compression lag screw and a pin. This technique may promote increased stabilization and revascularization but is also more likely to cause early physeal closure and growth deformities.

Femoral Neck Fractures. Femoral neck fractures occur primarily in the adult dog. The weaker physeal area usually becomes the location of a fracture in an immature patient. Although comminution is possible, most are simple fractures and occur near the base of the femoral neck (basilar). Compromise of the blood supply can vary depending on the displacement and the concurrent trauma to the joint capsule and adjacent femur.

A favorable prognosis for return to athletic function results from early surgical repair with a stable anatomical reduction. Stability and early bone healing are enhanced through accurate reduction and compression at the fracture site. An open reduction and internal fixation with a lag screw and K-wire combination are the strongest repair in the adult patient.[40] Although the three-pin configuration of fracture repair is almost as strong, it does not provide the compression at the fracture site. This method of femoral neck fracture repair is most appropriate in the immature animal with an open capital physis.

Postoperative patient management is important for successful repair and return to athletic function. The dog is placed in a non–weight-bearing or Ehmer sling for approximately 2 weeks. Activity is then restricted to short leash walks for 1 month or until clinical union is reached. Nonrepairable fractures of the femoral neck are treated by a salvage surgical procedure. Total hip replacement is preferable in the canine athlete if the fracture does not involve the more basilar area of the neck, which is required to support the femoral prosthesis. If a total hip replacement cannot be performed, a femoral head and neck excision is usually considered the second choice, because it is more likely to adversely affect demanding athletic functions.

Hip Dislocation. The coxofemoral joint is the most commonly luxated joint in the dog and may account for as many as 90 per cent of all luxations.[41] Most result from automobile accidents or falls and cause disruption to the joint capsule and ligament of the head of the femur.[42] The direction of luxation can be craniodorsal, cranioventral, caudodorsal, caudoventral, and medial (associated with acetabular fractures). Craniodorsal luxations are the most common type of hip luxation and account for approximately 90 per cent.[42]

Most patients will have a sudden onset of minimal to non–

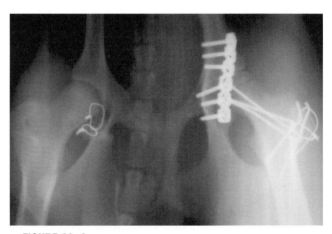

FIGURE 22–6. Multiple K-wire repair of a capital physeal fracture.

weight-bearing lameness. Craniodorsal luxation will cause the affected limb to appear externally rotated and slightly adducted. The much less common caudoventral luxation will produce an internally rotated and abducted limb.

In the standing animal, craniodorsal luxation will display medial and craniodorsal displacement of the greater trochanter. External rotation of the limb while firmly placing the examiner's thumb between the greater trochanter and ischial tuberosity will cause displacement of the thumb in a normal hip joint. Failure to displace the thumb from the depression is indicative of coxofemoral luxation (can also occur with femoral head and neck fractures). The anesthetized patient can be evaluated for differences in leg length. In craniodorsal luxations the affected limb is longer than the normal limb when in flexion, but it becomes shorter as the limbs are moved into extension. Diagnosis is confirmed with ventrodorsal and lateral radiographs. The radiographs are also necessary to evaluate the joint for the presence or absence of avulsion fractures of the femoral head, accompanying fractures of the pelvis or proximal femur, degenerative joint disease, and hip dysplasia.

Treatment options for coxofemoral luxations include both closed (nonsurgical) and open (surgical) reduction. Reduction should be performed as soon as possible to limit damage to the articular cartilage and to reduce the amount of fibrin filling of the acetabulum. The initial treatment method of choice is usually closed reduction if it can be performed within 5 to 7 days post trauma. Reported recurrence rates of closed reduction have been reported ranging from 15 to 71 per cent.[43-46] Open reduction is indicated if there are any associate fractures of the hip joint or if closed reduction is unsuccessful. Evidence of hip dysplasia or degenerative joint disease can dramatically affect success of an open or closed reduction. A salvage surgical procedure (total hip replacement or femoral head and neck excision) may be indicated in those patients.

Protection and maintenance of closed or open reduction is most commonly accomplished by the use of a figure-of-eight bandage or Ehmer sling. The bandage should remain in place for 10 to 14 days. A properly applied Ehmer sling will cause flexion, abduction, and internal rotation of the femur, giving the femoral head maximal acetabular coverage. Optimal positioning of the femur can be augmented by placing a cotton pad on the lateral surface of the stifle and incorporating it and the metatarsus in a body bandage. An Ehmer sling is not necessary after closed reduction of a caudoventral luxation.[42] Abduction should be prevented with the use of hobbles.

Alternative methods of maintaining closed or open reductions include DeVita pinning and a flexible external fixator.[47, 48] The primary advantage of these techniques is to allow early mobilization of the limb. This becomes extremely important in dogs having injuries in more than one limb. DeVita pinning is performed using a positive-profile threaded pin or Ellis pin through a stab incision just ventral to the ischiatic tuberosity. The pin is directed ventral to the ischiatic tuberosity, dorsal to the femoral neck, and embedded into the wing of the ilium.[47] The pin acts to augment the dorsal support of the femoral head and is left in place for 4 to 6 weeks.[49] Complications of DeVita pinning include damage to the sciatic nerve, pin migration, and reluxation.

A flexible external fixator maintains forces on the femoral head similar to an Ehmer sling yet allows early weight bearing and joint motion. Two threaded pins are connected by a 1-cm wide flexible, elastic rubber band, cut from a bicycle inner tube[48] (Fig. 22–7). The ilial pin is inserted perpendicular to the spine at the dorsal surface of the ilial body cranial to the acetabulum.[48] The trochanteric pin enters at the proximal, craniolateral aspect of the greater trochanter in a caudomedial direction, exiting distal to the lesser trochanter.[48] The elastic band can be held on the pins with a cyanoacrylate adhesive or an external fixator clamp. In an experi-

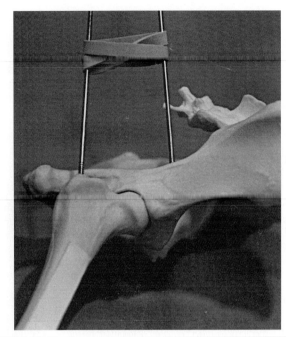

FIGURE 22–7. Flexible external fixator is used to maintain coxofemoral reduction, allowing early weight bearing and joint motion. Pins are placed into the ilial body, just cranial to the acetabulum, and the craniolateral aspect of the greater trochanter.

mental study, in none of the dogs with the flexible external fixator was the hip reluxated during or after the 14-day period of use.[48] Complications may include pin loosening, superficial pin tract infections, band deterioration, and enlargement of the stab incision over the greater trochanter.

Open reduction of a dislocated hip is indicated when closed reduction fails or if open examination of the joint is indicated as a result of a fracture. Techniques for open reduction include capsular repair (capsulorrhaphy), transposition of the greater trochanter, extracapsular suture stabilization, transarticular pinning, toggle pins, tissue anchors, purse string sutures, and the use of prosthetic or bone graft reinforcement of the acetabular rim.[8, 41, 50-62] The primary goal of open reduction is stable reconstruction of the joint capsule. A craniolateral approach is performed to assess trauma to the hip joint and joint capsule. If extensive damage exists to the joint capsule or acetabular labrum, osteotomy of the greater trochanter will be necessary for the additional required exposure. The torn remnants of the ligament of the head of the femur are excised, and the torn joint capsule is reconstructed. If stable reconstruction is possible, a capsulorrhaphy is the only method necessary.[44] When an osteotomy of the greater trochanter is used to achieve the necessary exposure, it can be relocated caudal and distal to its original position and held in place with a pin and tension band wire. The translocation of the greater trochanter results in increased tension of the gluteal musculature to produce internal rotation and abduction of the limb.

When the joint capsule, acetabular labrum, or gluteal musculature has been severely damaged from a traumatic luxation, an additional method of support is necessary to maintain reduction. A prosthetic joint capsule repair provides support of the femoral head within the acetabulum until the other natural support structures have healed.[63] Following a trochanteric osteotomy, two screws and washers are placed in the dorsal acetabular rim, cranial and caudal to the femoral head. Another screw and washer are placed in the trochanteric fossa. While the limb is held in slight abduction, a heavy, nonabsorbable suture material is placed in a figure-of-eight pattern from the femoral screw to each acetabular screw. Of 21 hip luxations greater than 7 days' duration or recurrent treated with this technique,[63] none of the hips reluxated and 65 per cent had excellent to good function on follow-up examination.[62] A salvage procedure (total hip replacement or femoral head and neck excision) is indicated in patients with recurrent luxations following open repair or with associated nonrepairable femoral head or acetabular fractures.

ACETABULAR FRACTURES IN RACING GREYHOUNDS

In general, an acetabular fracture in the small animal patient is produced by severe external trauma causing significant fracture displacement and is accompanied by a concurrent pelvic fracture or sacroiliac luxation. Racing greyhounds impose tremendous stresses on their musculoskeletal system, producing injuries not commonly seen in pet animals. Greyhounds sustain a unique stress-induced fracture of the acetabulum during racing or training.

Of more than 28 acetabular fractures reported, none was associated with concurrent pelvic fractures or dislocations, and there was no history of external trauma.[1, 64] All injured greyhounds were racing or training and did not fall, run into the rail, or clash with other dogs. Several of the dogs were injured while accelerating out of the starting boxes with an audible crack heard by the trainer followed by a slowing stride. The fractures resulted solely from tremendous stresses imposed on the caudodorsal rim of the acetabulum during running. The powerful gluteal, hamstring, and external rotator muscles produce tremendous tensile stresses concentrated dorsally over the caudal third of the acetabulum. Muscle forces are produced during the propulsion phase of the gait, while compressive forces of the femoral head within the acetabulum are greatest. A stress riser is generated from opposing force vectors pulling the ischium (lever arm) distally and compressing the femoral head (fulcrum) within the acetabulum (Fig. 22–8). Overstressed bones undergo plastic deformation which can eventually result in either adaptive hypertrophy or a stress fracture. In the racing greyhound, if intensity and duration of stress result in excessive bone resorption at sites of maximal stress (stress risers) and if recovery time is insufficient to permit bone remodeling and strengthening, a stress fracture may occur.[1]

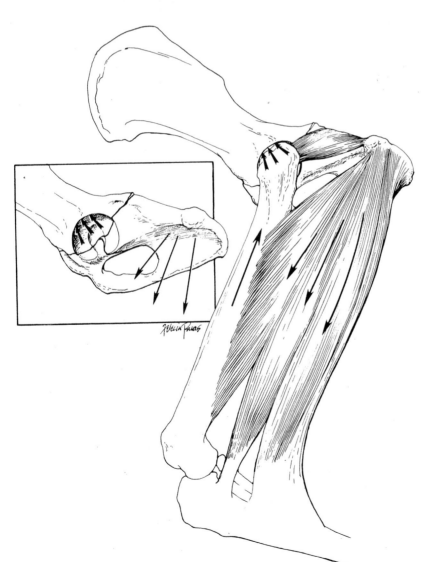

FIGURE 22–8. Muscular forces produce a stress riser in the caudal aspect of the acetabulum.

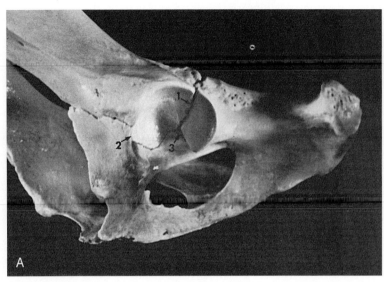

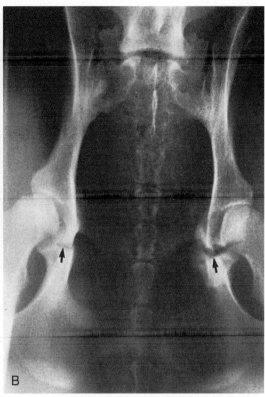

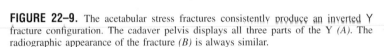

FIGURE 22–9. The acetabular stress fractures consistently produce an inverted Y fracture configuration. The cadaver pelvis displays all three parts of the Y *(A)*. The radiographic appearance of the fracture *(B)* is always similar.

Acetabular stress fractures are minimally displaced (<3 mm) and have a consistent configuration (x-ray). The inverted Y fracture configuration branches in three directions within the acetabular fossa. The fracture lines exit the lunate surface and acetabular rim in the caudal and cranial thirds[1] (Fig. 22–9). Unlike other stress fractures in racing greyhounds (metacarpal, metatarsal, tarsal), acetabular stress fractures occur with equal frequency on the right and left sides (unrelated to counterclockwise racing). The injury occurs in both male and female dogs from 16 to 36 months of age. Bilateral fractures have been observed in dogs that are rested for "obscure" hind limb lameness. When subsequently returned to the track, these dogs suffered an acute fracture in the opposite acetabulum.

Clinical signs range from subtle lameness to non–weight bearing on the affected leg. Dogs examined soon after the injury will have pain and swelling over the sacrotuberous ligament. Pain is also elicited by applying pressure over both greater trochanters and extension of the coxofemoral joint. Greyhounds with more chronic fractures have histories of poor performance, slow standing up after lying down, reluctance to load-up into the truck, and unwillingness to jump into the crate. These dogs will also have muscle atrophy and a decreased range of motion on extension in the affected hip.

Radiographic appearance is characterized by little or no displacement of the fracture. Ventrodorsal views show a fracture line in the caudal third of the acetabulum. An open leg mediolateral view of the affected hip best displays the fracture line as it exits the cranial acetabulum and extends through the caudoventral ilium (Fig. 22–10).

Conservative management of an acetabular stress fracture yields a nonbridging callus or unacceptable degree of DJD resulting in decreased range of motion, pain, and subsequent poor performance. Surgically treated dogs have returned to competitive racing as early as 5 months after the injury. The current recommendation based on small numbers of patients is to stabilize the caudodorsal acetabular fracture (tension side) with a dorsal acetabular compression plate. A dorsal approach without tenotomy or osteotomy is preferred. Although promising, the prognosis for a successful racing career after acetabular repair is still unknown because of the small number of cases that have been repaired surgically and the unproven racing abilities of most of the dogs before injury.[1]

CANINE HIP DYSPLASIA IN THE ATHLETIC DOG

Canine hip dysplasia is an inherited developmental disorder of the coxofemoral joint resulting in abnormal biomechanical stresses

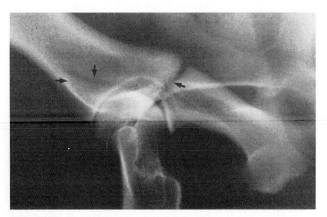

FIGURE 22–10. The fracture line exiting the cranioventral acetabulum and extending into the ilium is best visualized with an open-leg, mediolateral radiograph.

within the hip. The severity of involvement can range from subclin-ical structural changes in the joint to complete destruction of the hip with crippling of the dog. Although it has been diagnosed in almost all breeds of dogs, the incidence is highest in the medium, large, and giant breeds.[65-68] Unfortunately, many of the sporting breeds are overly represented. Both male and female dogs are affected with similar frequencies.

The development of the disease is multifactorial. The influence of dog size, growth rate, body type, muscle mass, and neuromuscular alterations—along with endocrine and vitamin imbalances—have been explored as potential causes. Although hip dysplasia has a genetic basis, the pattern of inheritance indicates that more than one gene is involved (polygenetic mode of inheritance).[69, 70] The architecture of a newborn hip is predetermined by a genetic blue-print that makes the coxofemoral articulation a ball-and-socket joint, determines muscle locations and size, establishes innervation, and forms all the bones of the hip joint.[4] As expected, breeding disease-free dogs is more likely to produce dogs with normal hips, while the progeny of dogs with hip dysplasia have an increased risk of developing the disease.[67, 71] Estimates of heritability index have ranged from 20 to 80 per cent.[65, 69, 70, 72-76]

While both genetic and environmental factors have been impli-cated, the phenotypic expression of the disease is determined by an interaction of genetic and environmental factors.[74] Three things have been identified that affect a growing hip's postnatal modeling activity:[4] (1) The basic genetic properties determine the original shape, size, anatomical relationships, musculature, and innervation of the coxofemoral joint; (2) the mechanical forces and motions put on the hip by daily activities influence its growth and modeling; and (3) how and where stiff bone replaces soft, more compliant cartilage affects the modeling of both.

Etiology and Pathogenesis. The common denominator in the pathogenesis of canine hip dysplasia is joint laxity or lateral transla-tion of the femoral head. Coxofemoral joints in puppies that later develop hip dysplasia are structurally and functionally normal at birth and are stable during the first 10 to 14 days of life.[77, 78] The most crucial period in the development of the hip joint is in the next 2 months.[79] Bones have not fully formed from cartilage models, the muscles and nerves have not fully developed, and the soft plastic tissues of the hip can be strained beyond their elastic limits.[80] Ensuing hip joint laxity will produce incongruency between the femoral head and acetabulum, resulting in modeling changes in endochondral ossification that constitute hip dysplasia. Once the cartilage model of the acetabulum and the femoral head lose con-gruency secondary to joint laxity, the resulting bone formation will be abnormal.

The pathogenesis of hip dysplasia depends primarily on how endochondral growth from articular cartilage in the acetabulum responds to abnormal mechanical loads. Biomechanical studies show the resultant of the normal hip's mechanical loads runs obliquely upward and medially, approximately through the middle of the acetabular articular cartilage.[4, 81] This mechanical load resul-tant is a sum of all forces (axial, vertical, medial, lateral) acting about the hip. In a normal hip, the mechanical load resultant is nearly perpendicular to the acetabular articular cartilage. The chon-dral growth force response curve suggests that both overloads and underloads on the cartilage will retard its growth but that overloads are much more likely to because of the curve's greater steepness to the right of its peak[4] (Fig. 22–11). A laterally translated mechani-cal load resultant or joint laxity will shift the hip load toward the dorsal acetabular rim. This in turn will retard downward growth laterally, while allowing the medial aspect of the articular cartilage continued outward growth, resulting in a progressively increased acetabular angle[4] (Fig. 22–12). Because endochondral ossification tends to follow the shape of the cartilage it replaces, radiographs of a chronically subluxated hip will show retarded development of

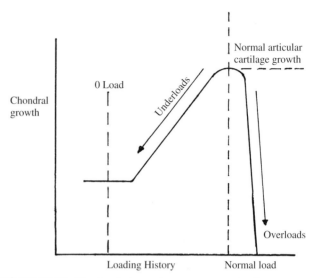

FIGURE 22–11. The chondral growth response curve. Cartilage growth is dramatically reduced with weight-bearing loads that exceed the load re-quired to produce normal articular cartilage growth.

the bony dorsal acetabular rim relative to the lateral growth of the socket's medial wall. This acetabular dysplasia is evident in dorsal acetabular rim (DAR) view x-rays as an increased acetabular slope and shallow socket[82-85] (Fig. 22–13).

The magnitude of medial directed force necessary to prevent subluxation is proportional to the acetabular angle where it contacts the femoral head. The normal hip with zero-degree acetabular angle requires a medial force of zero to maintain reduction regardless of the axial load applied.[82] As the acetabular angle increases, more medially directed force is required to maintain reduction. As a more shallow socket and increased acetabular angle produce lateral and upward sliding forces, medially directed forces may no longer maintain reduction, causing further stretching of the joint capsule and round ligament.

But what is the etiology of the hip joint laxity or lateral transla-tion of the femoral head? Biochemical, neuromuscular, and struc-tural factors have been studied. It appears that one or many of the causes could be responsible for the development of hip dysplasia, depending on the specific genotype of the dog. Breeds with a rapid rise in weight gain have been observed to have a high incidence of hip dysplasia.[86] Increased puppy weight will produce increased biomechanical stresses on the hip joint.[77] In a study involving 222 German shepherds, pups that weighed more than the mean at 60 days of age were almost twice as likely to have dysplastia at 1 year of age.[86] A high level of nutrition can be responsible for increased weight gains in pups. Environmental factors such as nutrition have been shown to have a secondary influence on the incidence, onset, progression, and severity of the disease.[87] Al-though studies have been conflicting, some researchers have shown that the incidence and severity of hip dysplasia in pups with a genotype for hip dysplasia are increased by feeding high-calorie diets and decreased by feeding low-calorie diets during their growth periods.[71, 72, 87] In a group of Labrador retrievers, the triradiate growth plates of the acetabula fused significantly earlier in pups with a high rate of growth compared to pups with restricted growth.[10] Early fusion of the triradiate bones of the acetabulum may lead to incongruency of the hip joint resulting in hip dysplasia. A restricted feeding program during the rapid growth phase has been suggested to lessen the possibility of an increased incidence of hip dysplasia and other skeletal diseases in fast-growing dogs.[88]

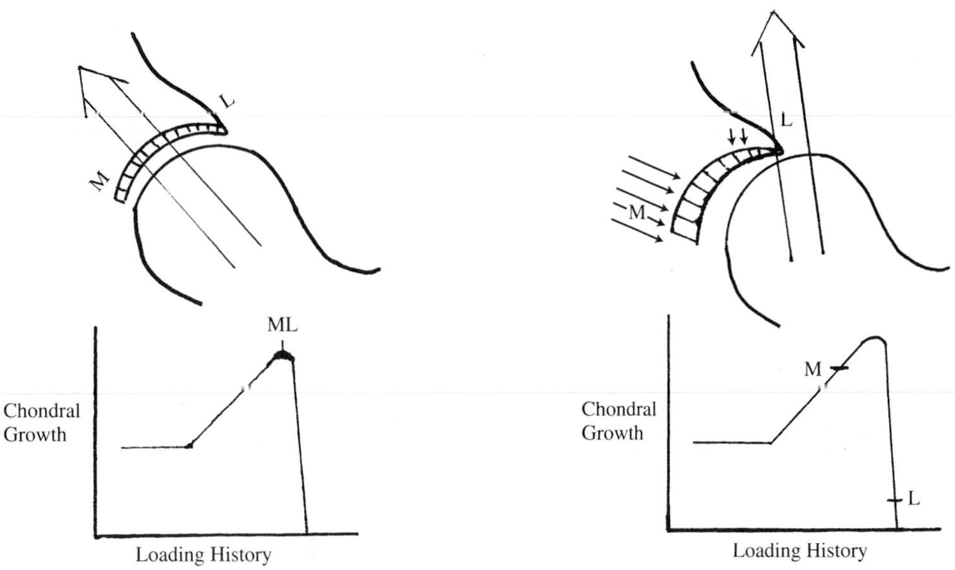

FIGURE 22–12. Endochondral bone growth of the acetabulum follows the chondral growth response curve. Note the lack of growth on the lateral (L) rim of the lunate surface while the medial (M) aspect continues to grow, resulting in progressive increase in the acetabular angle.

Chondral Growth

Loading History

Chondral Growth

Loading History

The role of ascorbic acid (vitamin C) in hip dysplasia has been studied and evaluated.[89] Most studies report no significant effects of oral vitamin C supplementation in preventing hip dysplasia, and its use cannot be supported.[89, 90]

The hormonal effects of estrogen, relaxin, insulin, growth hormone, and parathyroid hormone have been implicated as causal in hip dysplasia.[91] Experimentally, the administration of estrogens in young dogs has induced skeletal changes similar to hip dysplasia.[92] Increased urine concentrations of estrone and estradiol-17β have been documented with abnormal estrogen metabolism.[90] Dogs genotypic for hip dysplasia have reportedly greater urinary estradiol-17β concentrations than dogs with normal genotypes.[93] However, elevated levels of estrogen are likely to produce systemic effects, causing abnormalities in several joints. Estrogen levels in a normal biological range have not been shown to be related to the incidence of hip dysplasia.[77, 93, 94]

Hip dysplasia may be related to alterations in pelvic muscle mass and function. Biomechanical analysis has revealed how a balanced muscle support along with limb position, femoral neck angles, and subluxation are important factors in maintaining proper joint congruency.[7, 95] The correct balance between muscles of abduction and adduction helps to produce the medially directed forces necessary to prevent joint laxity. Abnormal muscle forces, whether neurological or myogenic in origin, could influence chondral modeling of the hip.

The role of the pectineus muscle, an adductor of the hip, in hip dysplasia has been controversial. Several studies have examined the mechanical, neuromuscular, histological, and biochemical properties of the pectineus muscle in normal and dysplastic dogs.[77, 96–101] A developmental myopathy with type II fiber hypotrophy of the pectineus muscle was identified in German shepherd pups.[99] Histologically the affected pectineal muscles showed features resembling neurogenic muscle disease. The myofiber composition of pectineus muscles from 2-month old German shepherd pups was evaluated.[100] The predysplastic dogs had smaller relative and absolute myofiber components, and larger non myofiber components, than dogs that subsequently had normal hips at 24 months. Another study reported an increased fibrous component in pectineus muscles of dysplastic dogs.[102] It is possible that if the relative growth of the pectineus muscle is not equal to the growth rate of the femur, abnormal upward and lateral force may be exerted on the femoral head. During the periods of rapid growth, this may produce lateral translation, hip joint laxity, and abnormal modeling of the acetabulum. Based on studies of pelvic muscle mass, pectineus muscle histology, and biomechanical influences of muscles, it is clear that hip dysplasia may develop as a sequel to neuronal-dysfunction-myofiber-dysfunction. A stable hip joint requires a balance between muscular forces and skeletal forces. Loss of the proper balance will influence the development of hip dysplasia.

The importance of the angle of inclination, the angle of femoral torsion, and the femoral neck length in the development of canine hip dysplasia remains controversial.[5, 7, 9, 16, 17, 78, 95, 103–106] Although no normal range for the angle of anteversion has been established, experimental osteotomies resulting in anteversion angles over 45 degrees are associated with osteoarthritic changes of the hip. The mechanical load resultant (femoral force vector) runs obliquely upward and into the acetabulum.[4] This force vector is a result of axial, vertical, and medial forces directed through the femoral head.[4, 82] The medially directed force results from the length of the moment arm (directly influenced by femoral neck length, femoral torsion, the angle of inclination) and muscular forces about the hip joint. The moment arm is a result of the perpendicular distances between (1) the abductor muscle force vectors and the center of the femoral head and (2) the axial directed force and the center of the femoral head (Fig. 22–14). Theoretically the femoral force

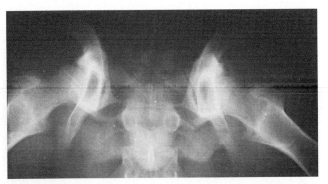

FIGURE 22–13. Dorsal acetabular view radiograph. The dorsal rim wear, increased acetabular slope, and shallow socket are due to laterally translated loading.

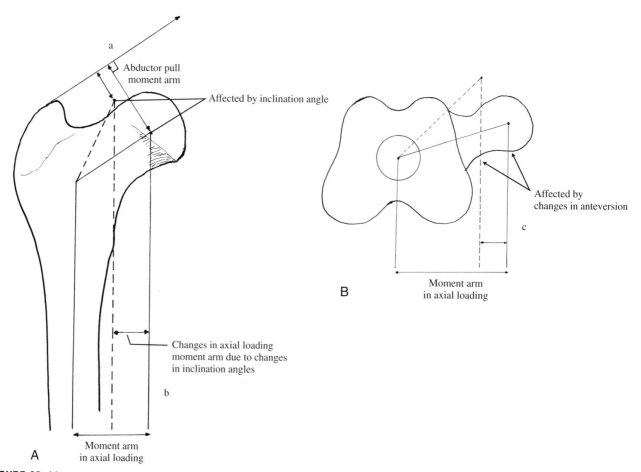

FIGURE 22–14. Angles of anteversion and inclination affect the moment arms producing medially directed forces. *A,* Moment arms for abductor muscle pull and axial loading of the femur. Note the decreases (a and b) due to an increased inclination angle. *B,* Moment arm in axial loading is decreased by increased anteversion (c).

vector or mechanical load resultant should be perpendicular to the acetabular angle to maintain reduction and congruency. Lateral deviations in the femoral force vector caused by increased angles of anteversion or inclination, decreased femoral neck length, or a decrease in abductor muscle forces will direct the hip load toward the socket's rim. The lateralization of hip load will produce incongruency or subluxation of the joint and greatly increase the forces transmitted through a small area on the dorsal acetabular rim.

Hip joint laxity and subluxation of the femoral heads were related to increased synovial fluid and round ligament volume in young dogs genetically predisposed to hip dysplasia.[18, 107] It is probable that joint laxity secondarily produces the early changes of synovitis, increased synovial effusion, and thickening of the round ligament and joint capsule.

History and Clinical Signs. Three clinically recognizable groups of dogs have hip dysplasia: (1) young and subclinical, (2) young and clinical, (3) adult and osteoarthritic. The first group are young dogs between 4 and 14 months of age that lack visible clinical signs and in whom diagnosis is made by orthopedic examination and radiography. If accurate early screening is not performed, these dogs will not be apparent until they become adults with clinical signs of osteoarthritis. The second group will develop visible clinical signs first observed generally between 4 and 14 months of age. The onset can be acute and may result from microfractures in the dorsal acetabular rim.[108] The clinical signs vary from mild discomfort to severe acute crippling pain affecting

one or both rear limbs. The owner may observe decreased exercise tolerance, reluctance or inability to jump up or to go up hills and stairs, difficulty in rising, a bunny-hop gait while running, lameness after periods of exercise, more aggressive or subdued behavior secondary to pain, and an audible click from one or both hips produced by subluxation as the dogs walk. If affected bilaterally, the dogs will stand with an arched back, shifting more weight to the front legs. The third group consists of the adult dogs with signs associated with osteoarthritis or DJD disease either unilaterally or bilaterally. These usually have more chronic lameness, although an acute exacerbation is possible if athletic activity of increased duration or intensity is performed. Owners will observe the same signs as those seen in younger dogs.

Physical Findings. Both orthopedic examination and radiography are required to gather the necessary information for the diagnosis, prognosis, and treatment recommendations. The diagnostic and treatment goals will depend on the group of dogs. Primary goals when evaluating the two younger groups of dogs are (1) early identification of the disease and (2) prevention of the progressive DJD and pain resulting from hip dysplasia. Adult dogs are evaluated primarily because of apparent pain or decreased ability to function athletically.

Diagnosis is accomplished through a combination of gait analysis, orthopedic manipulation, and radiographic examination. Prior to a hands-on examination, the dogs are observed standing and gaiting at fast and slow speeds. Often, subtle lameness is more easily detected after vigorous exercise. Along with evaluation for lameness, the range of motion of all joints should be closely observed. A dog with a painful hip may show a decreased range of extension in the hip prior to displaying lameness. After a complete physical examination, a thorough orthopedic examination and neurological examination of the pelvic limbs are performed. Disorders that can be clinically similar to hip dysplasia and that can occur concurrently in the same dog include injuries to the more distal part of the rear limb (cranial cruciate ligament and meniscal injuries), metabolic bone diseases (panosteitis, osteochondritis dissecans), immune-mediated arthropathies, neoplasia, and spinal diseases (lumbosacral compression, degenerative myelopathy, intervertebral disc disease). Other causes of lameness to the rear limbs must be ruled out before clinical signs are attributed solely to hip dysplasia.

Measurements of thigh circumference will detect unilateral muscle atrophy in dogs with chronic subtle lameness in one limb. Muscle atrophy can be detected in both rear legs in more severely affected dogs with bilateral hip dysplasia. Manipulation of the hips may produce mild to severe pain in clinically affected dogs. Forced extension is the most sensitive manipulation to produce pain. In younger dogs the range of motion may be restricted because of pain. Restricted range of motion in older dogs is also due to periarticular fibrosis and osteoarthritis. With severe DJD and capsular fibrosis, the range of motion in the anesthetized dog may be reduced from the normal of 110 degrees to as little as 45 degrees.[108] Crepitus can sometimes be detected early, as subluxation produces dorsal acetabular rim wear, but it is generally observed in hips with advanced degenerative osteoarthritis.

Early detection of canine hip dysplasia through orthopedic examination relies primarily on the detection of joint laxity by means of the trochanteric compression test, the Ortolani test, and the Barden test.[96, 109, 110] The presence of a positive Ortolani sign in a newborn infant has been used to accurately detect hip dysplasia in humans.[111] All dogs, especially young athletic dogs, with or without clinical signs should be palpated for the presence or absence of joint laxity.

The dog should be sedated or anesthetized for adequate performance of the Ortolani test (Fig. 22–15). The test can be performed in lateral or dorsal recumbency. The limb is held at the stifle and placed in a sagittal plane and perpendicular to the spine. Pressure is applied from the stifle, down the axis of the femur, toward the coxofemoral joint. This in theory simulates loading of the hip in neutral position. A normal coxofemoral joint will stay reduced while coxofemoral laxity will allow the femoral head to subluxate dorsally. As constant axial pressure is applied, the limb is slowly abducted, thereby progressively increasing medially directed forces. A positive Ortolani sign is felt and sometimes heard as a click when the subluxated femoral head suddenly drops back into the socket. The positive Ortolani can be variable in depth of reduction. As the acetabular angle increases and the socket becomes shallower, so does the intensity of the click as the femoral head reduces into the socket. The manipulation will produce crepitus in dogs that have significant dorsal acetabular rim cartilage wear. When the dorsal acetabular rim wear and central acetabular filling become severe, the subluxated femoral head can no longer reduce, and the positive Ortolani sign is lost. Adult dogs with osteoarthritis, or younger dogs with severely affected hips, usually do not have a positive Ortolani sign.

There is a close correlation between palpable joint laxity and the presence of radiographic signs of hip dysplasia in young dogs 3 months of age and older.[112] The Ortolani sign is less reliable at identifying pups at 8 weeks of age that eventually become dysplastic. Perhaps not all pups with tight hip joints at 8 weeks of age are going to continue to be normal. Some dogs over 3 months of age may not reveal any degree of subluxation on conventional ventrodorsal radiographs, but have a positive Ortolani sign. In most

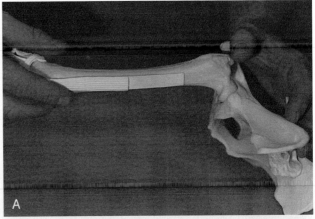
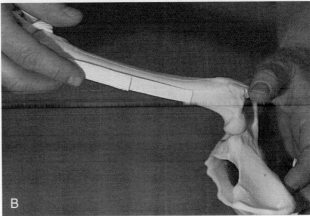
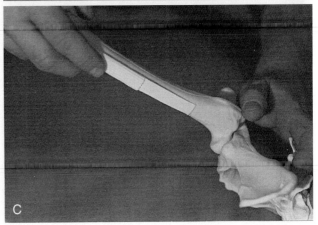

FIGURE 22–15. A positive Ortolani test. *A,* Axial loading of the femur producing subluxation. *B* and *C,* Slow abduction of the femur until it drops back into the acetabulum. The reduction of the femoral head can be palpated and sometimes heard by the examiner.

cases, if observed long enough, these dogs will develop radiographic signs consistent with hip dysplasia.

The Ortolani test is also necessary for prognosis and recommendations for treatment in young dogs with hip dysplasia. This is accomplished through measurements of angles of reduction and subluxation.[82–85] The amount of abduction necessary to cause reduction of the subluxated femoral head without assistance from muscular forces is measured as an angle from the sagittal plane to the point of reduction. The measurement is termed the angle of reduction. An increasing reduction angle is indirectly related to increasing joint laxity.

With the femoral head in the reduced position, the leg is slowly adducted toward the sagittal plane. As medially directed forces are reduced and axial loading is kept constant, the femoral head will slide laterally and dorsally as it subluxates. The angle measured from the sagittal plane to the point of subluxation is called the angle of subluxation. The angle of subluxation is directly related to the amount of dorsal acetabular rim wear and acetabular angle. The measured angle is the optimal rotation angle for a pelvic osteotomy, as it represents the angle of abduction at which medially directed muscle forces will be necessary to maintain hip congruency and stability. As the subluxation angle increases and approaches the angle of reduction, the prognosis for surgical correction with a pelvic osteotomy worsens. Hips with a 5-degree or less difference between the angle of reduction and angle of subluxation have a guarded prognosis with reconstructive surgery. No recommendation for surgery is given to dogs with reduction angles less than 20 degrees and subluxation angles near zero degrees. These dogs should be reevaluated monthly if less than 8 months of age and bimonthly if over 8 months of age.

The trochanteric compression test is performed on a heavily sedated or anesthetized animal in lateral recumbency. A medial directed force is applied to the greater trochanter. Medial movement of the greater trochanter is a positive test for a subluxated femoral head.[82, 85] No movement of the greater trochanter indicates that either the femoral head resides within the acetabulum or the hip is irreducible and cannot be relocated within the socket.[85] An irreducible femoral head associated with hip dysplasia indicates there is severe dorsal acetabular rim wear, central acetabular filling, and a significantly increased acetabular angle. Such a finding suggests that the hip probably will not benefit from pelvic osteotomy.[82, 85]

The Barden test is a method to estimate the distance of lateral translation of the femoral head out of the acetabulum.[96, 109] Whether or not the pup will become dysplastic can be predicted on the basis of the amount of laxity. Pups are best tested for hip joint laxity between 8 and 9 weeks of age. To perform the test, the animal is placed in lateral recumbency while under general anesthesia. The lower thigh is grasped with one hand while the index finger of the other hand is placed on the greater trochanter. While stabilizing the pelvis with the thumb and remaining fingers, the thigh is lifted laterally without abduction. The index finger lightly lying on the greater trochanter is used to estimate the amount of hip joint laxity. The test is positive if the amount of lateral laxity is more than ¼ inch.

Other studies have also found correlation between hip joint laxity in 8-week-old pups and radiographic evidence of hip dysplasia when the dog is a year old.[61, 98, 99, 113–116] Accuracy of over 80 per cent has been reported in predicting hip dysplasia in 4- to 8-week-old pups.[5, 6, 7, 61] Unfortunately the Bardens test is subjective and interpretation or results on the same pup can differ between clinicians. It should be used primarily as a screening test for detecting extreme laxity in the predysplastic dog. The manipulation becomes more difficult to accurately perform in pups over 12 weeks of age because of increased leg size. Other less subjective testing should be performed when the pup is older.

Radiographic Examination. While a thorough orthopedic examination is invaluable for evaluation of the coxofemoral joint, it requires experience and skill to produce consistently accurate results. The combination of palpation and radiography will greatly increase the sensitivity and accuracy of the diagnosis, prognosis, and treatment recommendations. Three radiographic views are used in the diagnosis of hip dysplasia: (1) the standard Orthopedic Foundation for Animals (OFA), extended leg, ventrodorsal view; (2) the dorsal acetabular rim view; (3) the distraction view.

The OFA was founded in 1966 as a nonprofit organization to serve as a diagnostic service and a registry for hip status for all breeds of dogs. The Foundation uses seven grades for the radiographic evaluation of canine hips. Three grades, excellent, good, and fair, are considered to be within normal radiographic limits for the breed and age. If a dog is given any of these grades and is at least 2 years of age at the time of radiography, it is eligible for a Foundation number. Four grades are given for dysplastic hips—borderline, mild, moderate, and severe dysplasia. Dogs with these grades are not eligible for Foundation numbers and are not recommended to be used as breeding animals.

A standard correctly positioned ventrodorsal view is required for accurate radiographic interpretation. The dog should be sedated or lightly anesthetized. A ventrodorsal radiograph of the pelvis (including the stifles) is obtained with the rear legs fully extended, the femurs parallel to each other, the patellae centered dorsally in the trochlear grooves, and the pelvis positioned symmetrically. In adult dogs with clinical lameness or pain, a lateral pelvic radiographic view is also obtained to evaluate for evidence of lumbosacral instability.

The first radiographic indication of hip dysplasia in the young animal is subluxation. It is visualized in the ventrodorsal radiographic view by (1) incongruency of the joint space between the cranial acetabular rim and the femoral head in the cranial one third of the joint (between the acetabular rim and fovea capitis); (2) shifting of the femoral head and neck position; (3) less than three fifths (60 per cent) of the femoral head covered by the acetabulum; and (4) a Norberg angle of less than 105 degrees (Fig. 22–16). As hip dysplasia progresses, radiographic signs of osteoarthritis will be apparent on the femoral head and neck and acetabulum.

The primary problem of the standard ventrodorsal radiographic view is that it is an insensitive test for early diagnosis of mild hip dysplasia. The reliability for detecting evidence of dysplasia in the German shepherd was 69.9 per cent at 12 months and 95.4 per cent at 24 months.[65] In the Vizsla, reliability was 32.4 per cent at 12 months and 92.5 per cent at 24 months.[117] As the legs are extended caudally, an unnatural strain is placed on the joint capsule, round ligament, and muscles, producing passive restraints on hip joint laxity at the extremes of hip motion. The spiral tensioning of the joint capsule acts to force the femoral head into the acetabular socket and masks the true coxofemoral joint laxity.[6] Therefore,

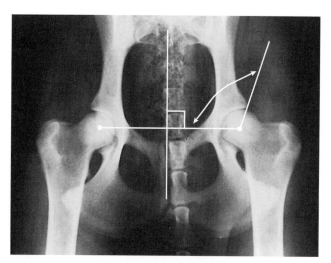

FIGURE 22–16. The Norberg angle is produced from a line perpendicular to the axis of the body going through the center of the femoral head, and from the center of the femoral head to cranial rim of the acetabulum. A normal acetabulum has a minimum Norberg angle of 105 degrees.

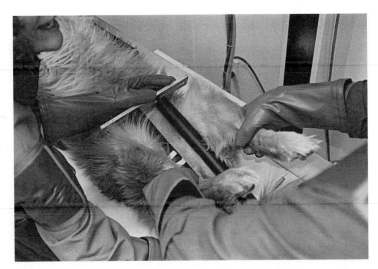

FIGURE 22–17. Positioning for distraction radiography.

some young dogs with palpable joint laxity may have hips that appear radiographically normal on the ventrodorsal view.

Early diagnosis of hip dysplasia is not only important for identifying the predysplastic pup but also for identifying pups as candidates for pelvic reconstruction. The distraction radiographic technique, using a fulcrum, was developed to improve the radiographic sensitivity for evaluation of hip joints in young dogs by revealing the presence of coxofemoral joint laxity in hip joints that appeared radiographically normal on the standard ventrodorsal view.[116, 118] The technique was later standardized and expressed as a distraction index.[6, 75, 119] Positioning for distraction radiography is performed under heavy sedation and with the dog in dorsal recumbency. An adjustable distracter device set at approximately the interacetabular distance is placed between the legs and held firmly down onto the pelvis. The hocks are grasped and the femurs positioned approximately 90 degrees to the pelvis and in the sagittal plane. This places the legs in a natural position, eliminating the spiraling tension of the joint capsule produced by extension. A medially directed force is then applied to the knees, causing the distracter device to act as a fulcrum, laterally distracting the femoral head from the acetabulum. Distraction is maintained for 1 to 2 seconds while the film is exposed (Fig. 22–17).

A unitless distraction index (DI) is used to quantitate the degree of laxity for direct dog-to-dog comparison regardless of the hip size, dog size, or breed-specific hip conformation.[6] The magnitude of femoral head distraction (lateral translation distance) is a direct measure of passive hip joint laxity. It is calculated by using circle gauges to determine the femoral head center and the acetabular center. The lateral translation distance (d) is the distance between the femoral head center and the acetabular center (Fig. 22–18). The DI is derived by dividing d by the measured radius of the femoral head,

$$r \ (DI = d/r)$$

(Fig. 22–18). A DI of zero indicates no joint laxity and absolute congruity while a DI of 1 indicates complete luxation.

In a study involving 142 dogs, a DI of less than 0.30 at 4 months showed that only 13 per cent went on to ultimately develop DJD.[75] None of the randomly selected hips with a DI less than 0.30 after 6 months of age had evidence of DJD when the dog was later evaluated at the age of 3 years. The biological variability between 4-month and 6-month evaluations indicates a need for follow-up examination on hips with a DI less than 0.30 at 4 months. All hips that ultimately developed DJD had DI values of 0.30 or greater. In

contrast, the rate of false-negative diagnoses in using the subjective OFA method (7-point scoring by a board certified radiologist) was 24 per cent from 4 to 24 months.

Although hips with a DI of 0.30 or greater have passive laxity and are considered to be genotypically predisposed to hip dysplasia, not all will develop DJD; 50 per cent of hips with a distraction index of 0.30 or greater at 6 months did not develop DJD at 3 years.[75] Some well-muscled breeds of dogs may have greater tolerance for passive laxity. Therefore, passive hip laxity measured by DI can be considered a risk factor, or possibly a genotypic carrier state, for hip dysplasia.

Conventional ventrodorsal, lateral, and distraction radiographic views of the pelvis do not permit clear visualization of the weight-bearing portion of the acetabulum. The dorsal acetabular rim (DAR) view radiographic technique was developed to evaluate the dorsal rim of the acetabulum for damage and secondary osteoarthritis, to correlate radiographs with palpation of joint capsule laxity and crepitation, to show acetabular filling, and to determine whether a hip was normal, dysplastic, or injured by trauma.[82] The DAR view is important for early diagnosis and as a method to help determine surgical recommendations for the young dog with hip dysplasia.

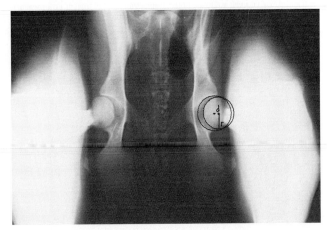

FIGURE 22–18. A distraction view radiograph is used to calculate a distraction index based on the lateral translation distance (d) between the center of the femoral head and the center of the acetabulum, and the radius of the femoral head (r).

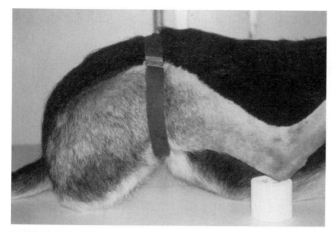

FIGURE 22–19. The proper positioning of a dog for a dorsal acetabular view x-ray.

For proper radiographic technique, the dog is placed in sternal recumbency while heavily sedated or under anesthesia. The hind limbs are pulled cranially and the femurs held close to the body by a restraining belt (Fig. 22–19). The tuber calcis of the hock is positioned 2 inches above the table with a roll of tape. This causes the pelvis to be aligned vertically so that the x-ray beam passes through the center of the ilial shaft with superimposition of the ilium, acetabulum, and tuber ischii (Fig. 22–20). The vertical alignment of the pelvis is recognizable on radiographs by visualizing the cross-section of the dorsal acetabular rim directly under the tuber ischii (Fig. 22–21).

In normal hips, the lateral aspect of the dorsal acetabular rim comes to a sharp point on the DAR radiograph. The acetabulum and femoral head fit congruently as evident by an even joint space. The normal acetabular slope (measured as a tangent to the acetabulum at the point of lateral femoral head contact) is zero degrees to less than 10 degrees (Fig. 22–22). Dogs with a combined right and left acetabular angle of less than 15 degrees have positive correlation with hips judged as OFA normal.[82, 85] As a dysplastic hip worsens, there becomes progressively more rounding of the lateral aspect of the dorsal rim, sclerosis, filling of the acetabular fossa, and osteophyte formation above the dorsal rim. Acetabular slope will gradually increase as the hip dysplasia worsens. A combined acetabular slope of right and left hips over 15 degrees has positive correlation with hips judged dysplastic by OFA.[82, 85]

Other radiographic views are used in the evaluation of predysplastic and dysplastic dogs. A lateral radiograph is useful for evaluation of the joint space and the lumbosacral abnormalities. Although femoral moment arm length can be accessed from an extended leg, ventrodorsal view, the degree of coxa valga (inclination angle) and anteversion angles are difficult to assess accurately from this view alone. If the femoral moment arm is determined to be abnormally short, the anteversion and inclination angles should be evaluated. An axial view of the femoral shaft is used for direct measurement of anteversion. The biplanar calculation of anteversion and inclination angles requires an additional sagittal (mediolateral) view of the femur.[14, 17] Anteversion angles exceeding 45 degrees are associated with osteoarthritic changes of the hip.[9, 14, 103, 104]

Treatment of Hip Dysplasia

Canine hip dysplasia can be recognized in hips with varying degrees of joint laxity and mild or no degenerative changes or in the postosteoarthritis state. Treatment is aimed at preventing the inevitable osteoarthritis associated with the disease or at relieving the pain and discomfort with a return to normal function. Maintenance of normal athletic function is an important aspect of treatment when recommendations are made for a sporting or working

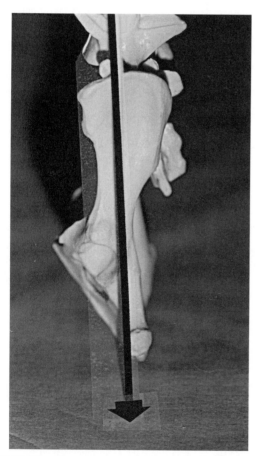

FIGURE 22–20. The pelvis is positioned to allow the vertical path of the x-ray beam to align the dorsal acetabular rim just below the tuber ischii on the x-ray film.

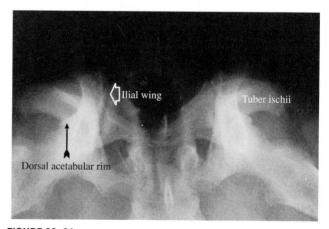

FIGURE 22–21. A normal DAR view radiograph with the dorsal acetabular rim just below the tuber ischii. Under-rotation will be viewed as an increased distance between the rim and tuber ischii causing the caudal acetabular rim to be visualized. Over-rotation will produce superimposition of the tuber ischii and dorsal acetabular rim.

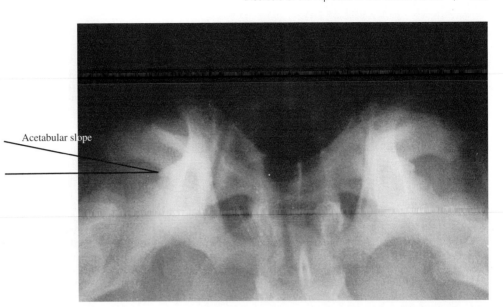

Acetabular slope

FIGURE 22–22. A normal DAR view radiograph. The acetabular slope is approximately 5 degrees.

dog. Prevention of debilitating osteoarthritis, through hip stability, is the primary objective when joint laxity or early hip dysplasia is diagnosed in a young dog. To stabilize the hip joint and prevent or reduce further osteoarthritic changes, reconstructive surgical procedures are recommended rather than conservative medical management. Age alone is not the determining factor for reconstructive procedures designed at prevention. Important considerations for surgery are the condition of the articular surfaces and the amount of abnormal modeling changes that have occurred. The amount of subluxation, femoral dysplasia, and acetabular dysplasia must be evaluated to make surgical recommendations. Dogs with significant osteoarthritis do not have an acceptable prognosis with reconstructive, preventive surgical procedures. Those dogs become candidates for conservative medical management or salvage surgical procedures.

Conservative and Medical Management. In spite of advanced degenerative joint disease, some dogs with hip dysplasia may live a comfortable life with conservative management.[120] The primary goals in the sporting dog are to alleviate pain of osteoarthritis and maintain athletic function. Both environmental influences and medical management must be addressed to accomplish these objectives. Although analgesics may help alleviate pain, they do not alter the degenerative changes that take place with hip dysplasia. Obese dogs should lose weight to decrease the load placed on the hip joints. Sporting dogs should be rested if pain is apparent. Repetitive and traumatic activities such as long runs and jumping are discouraged in pet dogs but unfortunately are often required activities in a canine athlete. Swimming is an excellent nonconcussive exercise to help maintain muscle mass and joint motion. Passive range-of-motion exercises may aid in cartilage nutrition.[121]

Nonsurgical treatment of early hip dysplasia has been recommended in 6- to 16-week-old pups with excessive joint laxity.[122] The treatment involves daily repetitive abduction manipulations to force the femoral heads deep into the acetabulum. Although reported to be successful, there were no data to correlate clinical findings with joint laxity or radiographic evidence of hip dysplasia.

Nonsteroidal anti-inflammatory drugs (NSAIDs) are the most widely recommended drugs for the treatment of hip dysplasia. A buffered aspirin (acetylsalicylic acid) product has been the most commonly administered NSAID in treating osteoarthritis (10 to 25 mg/kg orally every 12 hours). Other oral NSAIDs have been used successfully, including phenylbutazone (40 mg/kg divided three times daily, not to exceed 800 mg/day), meclofenamic acid (1.1 mg/kg divided two times daily), ibuprofen (15 mg/kg divided three times daily), ketoprofen (1 mg/kg orally every 24 hours) and piroxicam (0.3 mg/kg orally every other day).[121, 123] Because of the potential severe side effects and toxicity, the most commonly recommended NSAIDs in this group are aspirin and phenylbutazone. Carprofen (Rimadyl), a member of the propionic acid class of NSAIDs, has been recently approved for use in dogs (2.2 mg/kg orally twice daily). This drug is a reversible inhibitor of cyclooxygenase and a moderately potent inhibitor of phospholipase A_2. It may have some actions similar to corticosteroids, but without the side effects of steroid use. Minimal side effects have been reported. The gastrointestinal toxicity appears to be limited, and the negative effects observed with other NSAIDs on glycosaminoglycan synthesis in cartilage may be minimal.[124, 125] NSAIDs have been associated with gastrointestinal irritation and should be administered with food. If any gastrointestinal problems (vomiting, inappetence, or diarrhea) occur, the drug is discontinued until the dog is normal. If the drug is to be continued, it should be administered at a lower dose.

Corticosteroids are potent inhibitors of inflammation. Although corticosteroids suppress periarticular inflammation, the systemic side effects of long-term use can be potentially severe. Corticosteroids can also stimulate proteoglycan loss in normal or osteoarthritic cartilage after a relatively short period of administration.[126-131] Destruction of cartilage can be an end result of corticosteroid use; therefore it can be recommended only as a drug of last resort.

Polysulfated glycosaminoglycans (PSGAG; Adequan) is a semisynthetic compound derived from bovine trachea and lung and is chemically similar to the mucopolysaccharides that make up joint cartilaginous tissue. PSGAG has chondroprotective effects when used either prophylactically or therapeutically.[132, 133] These effects are produced through the ability to inhibit the function and release of specific enzymes (cathespin and hyaluronidase) implicated in the pathogenesis of DJD.[134]

Similar serum and joint concentrations of PSGAG are present with intramuscular and intra-articular injections.[135] It binds strongly to noncollagenous protein and proteoglycans of the extracellular cartilaginous matrix, resulting in high concentrations in articular cartilage, menisci, and the annulus of intervertebral discs.[134, 136] Concentrations of PSGAG in pathological cartilage can exceed concentrations found in normal cartilage.[136]

A variety of anecdotal doses of PSGAG have been used. After intramuscular injection, effective concentrations of PSGAG persisted in articular cartilage for up to 96 hours.[135] Therefore, recommended dosing of PSGAG is 5 mg/kg intramuscularly every 3 to 5 days for 5 to 10 injections.[134] No studies have reported any toxic effects systemically or in the joints. However, PSGAG does potentiate antithrombin III activity, resulting in prolongation of activated partial thromboplastin time, prothrombin time, and activated coagulation time.[137, 138] This inhibition of coagulation is dose dependent.[137]

Studies on clinical efficacy appear to have mixed results. PSGAG was successfully used for prevention of DJD in puppies susceptible to hip dysplasia and for treatment of naturally occurring DJD in humans.[135] Another study reported no significant clinical effects from PSGAG in the treatment of adult dogs with clinical signs of severe hip dysplasia.[135]

Reconstructive Surgery. Reconstructive operations are designed to restore stability and congruency to the hip joint. A functionally normal joint can develop if the abnormal biomechanical forces acting on the hip are corrected early. Stability and congruency of the joint are required to prevent progression of DJD. Subluxation and early acetabular dysplasia are best corrected by reorientation of the acetabulum with a *pelvic osteotomy* procedure to provide better coverage of the femoral head and prevent joint laxity.[84, 139–141]

Femoral dysplasia, although less frequent, is surgically corrected by procedures that increase the length of the femoral moment arm. A shortened femoral neck, increased angle of inclination, and excessive anteversion will individually or in combination cause shortening of the moment arm. Procedures designed to increase the moment arm include *intertrochanteric osteotomy* and *femoral neck lengthening*.[12, 142–145]

Pelvic Osteotomy. The basic principle of pelvic osteotomy (triple pelvic osteotomy) is to biomechanically stabilize the hip joint by improving dorsal coverage of the femoral head through axial rotation of a free acetabular bone segment. The degree of acetabular rotation is specific for an individual hip and is determined by orthopedic examination (angle of reduction and subluxation) and DAR view radiographs. Earlier methods for stabilization of the rotated acetabulum included orthopedic wire, a single screw, and a torqued bone plate. Recent modifications in technique have produced pre-angled plates (Slocum Canine Pelvic Osteotomy Plates) available at 20-, 30-, and 40-degree rotation angles (Fig. 22–23). The canine pelvic osteotomy plate lateralizes the acetabular segment and provides additional plate width to help stabilize torsional forces.[85]

Good candidates for pelvic osteotomy are young dogs with a reduction angle under 30 degrees and a subluxation angle below 10 degrees.[85] DAR view radiographs show a mild acetabular slope of 10 to 15 degrees or less, and slight rounding of the dorsal

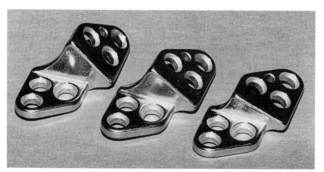

FIGURE 22–23. Slocum Canine Pelvic Osteotomy Plates. Available in 20, 30, and 40 degrees.

acetabular rim. These dogs may or may not be clinically lame and will not have evidence of DJD on the ventrodorsal radiographic view. A pelvic osteotomy candidate with moderate dysplasia will have a good to fair prognosis for full athletic function, depending on the amount of damage to the acetabular cartilage. These dogs have clinical lameness. Hips have a subluxation angle that is at least 10 degrees less than the reduction angle. The reduction angles are usually 35 degrees or less (25 to 35 degrees). DAR view radiographs show increased rounding of the dorsal acetabular rim, incongruency, and an acetabular slope of 15 to 20 degrees. Both DAR and ventrodorsal radiographs may show the presence of osteophytes. Dogs that have subluxation angles within 5 degrees of the reduction angle (usually over 30 degrees) have a guarded to poor prognosis for full athletic function.[82, 85] Although the function may improve, normal activity will not be restored. DAR view radiographs will show an acetabular slope of more than 20 degrees, incongruency, acetabular filling, severe deformation and wear of the rim, and dorsal acetabular osteophytes. These dogs are not candidates for pelvic osteotomy and are generally treated by a salvage surgical procedure.

The surgical procedure involves three osteotomies of the hemipelvis.[82, 83, 85] The free acetabular segment is then rotated and stabilized with a predetermined pelvic osteotomy plate. Intraoperative Ortolani testing is performed after plate stabilization. If subluxation is detected, the next larger angle pelvic osteotomy should be applied. Pelvic osteotomy can be performed unilaterally or bilaterally (Fig. 22–24).

Significant osteoarthritis (dorsal acetabular rim wear, acetabular filling, and femoral neck osteophytes) of the hip are contraindications to pelvic osteotomy. Also, medially directed pelvic muscle force is required to keep the femoral head in the acetabulum. A permanent neurological deficit involving pelvic muscles will contribute to failure of pelvic osteotomy and is reason to exclude a potential candidate.[82, 83, 85] Femoral anteversion over 45 degrees will not respond to pelvic osteotomy alone and will require the addition of a corrective femoral osteotomy.[83]

Intertrochanteric Osteotomy. The purpose of intertrochanteric osteotomy is to improve the congruency and biomechanical function of the hip joint.[143–146] It does so by increasing the moment arm of the femoral neck. The intertrochanteric osteotomy changes the femur's position to the acetabulum in three planes. Inclination of the femoral neck is changed to a more varus position.[146] The degree of anteversion is reduced toward normoversion, while the femoral head is shifted more medially in relation to the femoral shaft.[9, 146]

The intertrochanteric osteotomy is best indicated on hips with abnormally elevated anteversion and inclination angles. Since modeling of the hip is greatest early in life, the procedure ideally should be performed prior to abnormal modeling changes.[146] The presence of acetabular dysplasia will significantly worsen the prognosis for long-term success with an intertrochanteric osteotomy. Unfortunately, early correction by this procedure is limited by the complication of closure to the greater trochanteric physis. Although degenerative changes within the coxofemoral joint continue, the benefit gained from the procedure is relief of pain for an average of 5 to 6 years.[146]

Femoral Neck Lengthening. Femoral neck lengthening is a procedure designed for early correction of femoral dysplasia. Some dogs such as Akitas and chows have a high incidence of shortened femoral neck.[85] If this is diagnosed early, before damage to the acetabular rim has occurred, the procedure may be curative.[85] The primary advantage over intertrochanteric osteotomy is the ability to perform the procedure at an early age, prior to acetabular remodeling, and without physeal interference. In addition, femoral neck lengthening will decrease the amount of acetabular rotation necessary in pelvic osteotomy.[85]

The procedure involves osteotomy of the proximal femoral shaft

Total Hip Replacement. Total hip replacement (THR) is the recommended salvage procedure of the hip for medium- and large-breed dogs[147–150] (Fig. 22–25). Improvements in the implant design and materials, surgical technique, and prevention of surgical wound infection have made THR a common and highly successful surgical procedure in the dog. A study evaluating 146 dogs with Richard's Canine type II THRs reported a 95.2 per cent success rate (full clinical range of motion with no pain, increased muscle mass, and no limping).[151] Thousands of THRs have since been performed in dogs. Many veterinary surgical centers currently report success rates over 95 per cent.

Both cemented and cementless (press fit, bone ingrowth) prostheses are successfully used in THR. Currently the most commonly used prosthesis is the cemented Canine Modular Total Hip System. The system provides five high-density polyethylene acetabular cup sizes, four cobalt chrome femoral stem sizes, and three neck lengths through the use of a Morris taper neck design and three variable-depth cobalt chrome heads. Compatibility of the components allows full-size versatility between acetabular and femoral prostheses. The components are cemented in place with polymethylmethacrylate (PMMA) bone cement.

Recently, a porous-coated anatomical total hip system (PCA Canine Total Hip System) was developed for cementless implantation in dogs. The porous coating allows for bony and fibrous tissue ingrowth to stabilize the implant.[119, 160, 161] Initial short-term results

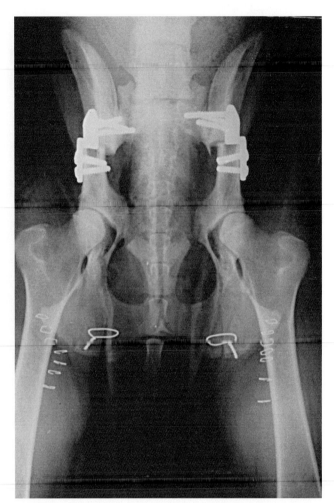

FIGURE 22–24. Postoperative radiograph of a dog with a bilateral TPO. Notice the excellent dorsal acetabular rim coverage. This dog would be expected to have normal performance in the hip joints.

in the sagittal plane. Preformed polyacetyl resin wedges are driven into the osteotomy to split the femoral head and neck in a medial direction. Stabilization is accomplished with pins and circlage wires.[12]

Pectineal Myectomy. The purpose of pectineal myectomy is to release its adductor muscle forces on the hip and increase the range of abduction in the hip. This in turn will decrease the stresses on the joint capsule and allow for better congruency. Because stability of the hip joint is not corrected, degenerative changes will continue to progress. The procedure does provide some dogs with temporary relief of pain. The procedure is usually reserved as a semiconservative method of pain relief for those dogs with acetabular changes too severe for pelvic osteotomy yet too young for total hip replacement.

Salvage Surgical Procedures. Salvage surgical procedures for dogs with hip dysplasia include *total hip replacement* and *femoral head and neck excision*. A salvage surgical procedure for hip dysplasia in the canine athlete is reserved for dogs with osteoarthritis exhibiting clinical pain and associated loss in function. Other indications are chronic hip luxation, irreparable fractures of the coxofemoral joint, avascular necrosis of the femoral head, or osteoarthritis of the hip unrelated to hip dysplasia. If a dog is clinically sound, a salvage procedure is not indicated, regardless of the radiographic evidence of DJD.

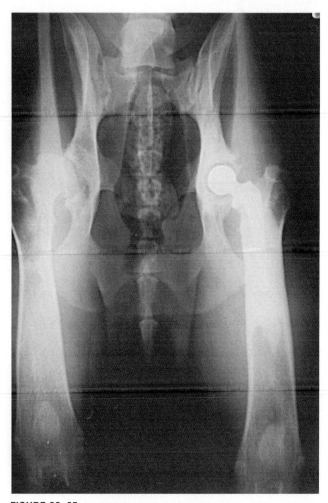

FIGURE 22–25. Ventrodorsal radiograph of a dog with a total hip replacement.

have been comparable to cemented implants.[152, 155] A reported potential benefit of a cementless system is the lack of aseptic implant loosening or "cement disease," resulting from a response to PMMA or polyethylene debris, which produces enzymatic erosion of the bone.[156, 157] However, this same type of osteolysis is also observed in cementless implants and is produced from polyethylene acetabular cup debris that can track between the implant and the bone.[28, 55] It is now known that wear debris—whether metal, polyethylene, or cement—is responsible for the initiation of osteolysis and eventual fixation failure.[156, 157] Cement fixation achieves a more reliable bone-implant interlock initially, and the mechanisms that may result in the loss of this interlock apply no more and perhaps less in cemented fixation.[157] The absence of a cement mantle in the cementless total hip arthroplasty necessitates precise bone preparation to result in an initial press fit stability that will allow bone ingrowth.

To be a candidate for THR, a sporting dog must have pain isolated to the hip, resulting in lameness, reluctance to perform intended activities, deficiencies in the athletic functions, or exercise intolerance. If hip dysplasia is bilateral, the clinically more severe hip is operated on first. The second THR can be performed 2 months later in the opposite hip if it exhibits continued clinical pain and functional deficiencies on repeat evaluation. Most bilaterally affected dogs require THR on only one side because the increased weight bearing provides relief to the nonoperated hip. The earliest a cemented THR can be performed is when the proximal femoral physis is closed (approximately 10 months of age). The upper age limit is governed by the general health of the patient. Prosthesis size limits implantation to dogs that are generally over 15 kg. Although a failed femoral head and neck excision is an indication for THR, bone resorption and remodeling may preclude femoral prosthesis implantation.

Contraindications to THR include accompanying neurological disease (most commonly lumbosacral disease, but also degenerative myelopathy, intervertebral disc disease, infection, and spinal tumors), systemic disease, and skin or other organ system infection. Lumbosacral (LS) disease producing nerve root compression or inflammation will have similar clinical findings as hip dysplasia. Dogs with this disease will have a history and clinical findings similar to those observed from hip dysplasia. It is not unusual for dogs to be clinically affected by both diseases. Like hip dysplasia, LS disease will produce pain on hip extension. Unlike hip dysplasia, it will also typically produce pain on palpation of the dorsal and ventral nerve roots at the lumbosacral junction or by extreme lifting of the tail. The indication for THR can be reevaluated if the neurological problem is resolved.

Systemic disease or infection must be treated and controlled before THR can be performed. Other orthopedic causes for rearlimb lameness must be ruled out or successfully treated prior to THR.

Surgical techniques for cemented and cementless THRs have been described.[2, 152, 158–165] As with any technically involved surgical procedure, there is a learning curve. The risk of complication is significantly reduced with thorough understanding of the biomechanics, the instrumentation and implants, and the principles of their application. Potential complications of THR include dislocations of the prosthesis, infection, aseptic loosening of the acetabular or femoral component, neuropraxia, and fractures.[166, 167] A reported 6.3 per cent complication rate was observed in dogs implanted with a cemented Richard's Canine II Total Hip Replacement.[151] Approximately half of these complications were successfully resolved.

Femoral Head and Neck Excision. In the past, the most frequent surgical treatment for osteoarthritis associated with hip dysplasia was a femoral head and neck excision or excision arthroplasty. A smooth excision of the femoral head and neck is crucial in creating a fibrous, pain-free false joint. The success with this procedure is limited by the size of the dog and the desired athletic function.[16, 147, 148, 150, 168–173] Most reports describe some long-term functional impairment ranging from mild lameness to intermittent non-weight bearing.[147, 148, 168, 172, 174] Reduced hip extension, limb shortening, and muscle atrophy can be expected. Smaller dogs and cats not expected to perform athletically are more likely to have adequate functional results with a pain-free false joint.

Although the use of a biceps muscle sling has been advocated, subjective owner evaluations show only about 50 per cent of the dogs functioned without lameness or gait abnormality.[172] Objective evaluations of a biceps muscle sling in normal hips reported no benefit over conventional head and neck excision.[175, 176] Because of the lack of beneficial effects, and the increased morbidity with the procedure, it cannot be recommended.

Control of Hip Dysplasia. Control of an inherited disease is possible only through eliminating the disease within the gene pool. Because of the polygenetic nature of canine hip dysplasia, environmental influences, and the lack of regulatory control, it is unrealistic to expect to eliminate the disease. However, the frequency of the disease can be reduced through selective breeding of normal dogs to normal bitches.[66, 177] Currently, the OFA serves as a voluntary all-breed hip dysplasia registry for dogs 24 months of age or older. Dogs are phenotypically graded, based on radiographic evaluation from three randomly selected board-certified radiologists. A breed registry number is issued only to dogs interpreted as phenotypically normal.

Although the frequency of hip dysplasia is slightly reduced in the population of dogs submitted to the OFA, it unfortunately continues to be a common orthopedic disease in dogs.[66] The phenotype of a quantitative trait, such as hip dysplasia, reflects the genotype of the dog as influenced by superimposed environmental factors.[75] For screening purposes it is important to select a method of phenotypic measurement that is the least influenced by environmental factors. The subjective phenotypic grading of the extended leg–ventrodorsal view used by the OFA on dogs over 2 years of age can be influenced by environmental factors. It is possible that because of environmental influences and the quantitative nature of the disease, dogs graded normal by the OFA method transmit a susceptible hip dysplasia genotype to their offspring.

Functional hip joint laxity, producing lateral translation during weight bearing, is an important pathogenic factor in the development of osteoarthritis observed with hip dysplasia. Passive laxity is a prerequisite for functional laxity, although not all dogs with passive laxity develop functional laxity. Distraction radiography is an effective method for early diagnosis and quantification of passive hip joint laxity.[6, 75] None of the randomly selected dogs over 6 months of age with a DI less than 0.30 developed DJD at 3 years of age.[75] All hips in that study that ultimately developed radiographic signs of DJD had DI values > 0.29, but not all dogs with DI > 0.29 developed DJD within 3 years. Passive laxity is therefore necessary for the development of DJD and may indicate a genetic carrier state for hip dysplasia but is not necessarily causal by itself. When selecting breeding stock, perhaps the high ability to accurately predict which dogs are not susceptible to hip dysplasia is more important than the low (50%) ability to predict which dogs will eventually get DJD.

Distraction radiography may become useful as a selection criterion to reduce the prevalence of hip dysplasia. Although superior to the OFA method, the heritability of passive hip laxity for each breed is not clear at this time. PennHIP (International Canine Genetics, Inc.) is currently compiling a data base as it relates to age, breed, sex, and expression of DJD. More studies need to be performed before using this method for clinical selection of breeding stock.

References

1. Wendelburg K, Dee J, Kaderly R, et al: Stress fractures of the acetabulum in 26 greyhounds. Vet Surg 17:128, 1988.
2. Manley P: The hip joint. In Vasseur P, Slatter D (eds): Textbook of Small Animal Surgery, 2nd ed. Philadelphia, WB Saunders Company, 1993, Vol 2, p 1786.
3. Evans H, Christensen G (eds): Miller's Anatomy of the Dog. Philadelphia, WB Saunders Company, 1979.
4. Frost H: Pathogenesis of congenital hip dysplasia (CDH). A proposal. Vet Compara Orthopaed Traumatol 1:1, 1989.
5. Hauptman J, Cardinet G, Morgan J, et al: Angles of inclination and anteversion in hip dysplasia in the dog. Am J Vet Res 46:2033, 1985.
6. Smith G, Biery D, Gregor T: New concepts of coxofemoral joint stability and the development of a clinical stress-radiographic method for quantitating hip joint laxity in the dog. JAVMA 196:59, 1990.
7. Arnoczky S, Torzilli P: Biomechanical analysis of forces acting about the canine hip. Am J Vet Res 42:1581, 1981.
8. Bennett D, Duff S: Transarticular pinning as a treatment for hip luxation in the dog and cat. J Small Anim Pract 21:373, 1980.
9. Dueland D: Femoral torsion and its possible relationship to canine dysplasia (abstract). Vet Surg 9:48, 1980.
10. Lust G, Rendano V, Summers B: Canine hip dysplasia: Concepts and diagnosis. JAVMA 187:638, 1985.
11. Rendano V, Ryan G: Canine hip dysplasia evaluation: A positioning and labeling guide for radiographs to be submitted to the Orthopedic Foundation for Animals. Vet Radiol 26:170, 1985.
12. Slocum B: Femoral neck lengthening. In The Cutting Edge in Veterinary Orthopedics. Eugene, Ore, Slocum Enterprises, 1988, pp 1–4.
13. Milton J: Fractures of the femur. In Slatter (ed): Textbook of Small Animal Surgery, 2nd ed. Philadelphia, WB Saunders Company, 1993, vol 2, p 1805.
14. Montavon P, Hohn R, Olmstead M, et al: Inclination and anteversion angles of the femoral head and neck in the dog. Vet Surg 14:277, 1985.
15. Nunamaker D: Femoral neck anteversion in the dog: Its radiographic measurement. J Am Vet Radiol Soc 14:45, 1973.
16. Hauptman J: The Hip Joint. In Slatter DH (ed): Textbook of Small Animal Surgery, Philadelphia, WB Saunders Company, 1985, p 2153.
17. Hauptman J, Prieur W, Butler H, et al: The angle of the canine femoral head and neck. Vet Surg 8:74, 1979.
18. Lust G, Beilman W, Dueland D, et al: Intra-articular volume and hip joint instability in dogs with hip dysplasia. J Bone Joint Surg Am 62-A:576, 1980.
19. Kaderly R, et al: Intracapsular and intraosseous vascular supply to the mature dog's coxofemoral joint. Am J Vet Res 44:1805, 1983.
20. Rivera L, et al: Arterial supply to the canine hip joint. J Vet Orthop 1:20, 1979.
21. Hulse D, Root C: Management of acetabular fractures: Long term evaluation. Comp Cont Educ 2:189, 1980.
22. Schoenecker P, et al: A dynamic canine model of experimental hip dysplasia. J Bone Joint Surg Am 66A:1281, 1984.
23. Selcer B: Urinary tract trauma associated with pelvic trauma. JAVMA 18:785, 1982.
24. Wingfield W: Lower urinary tract injuries associated with pelvic trauma. Canine Pract 25, 1974.
25. Hulse D: Acetabular fractures. In Bojrab M (ed): Current Techniques in Small Animal Surgery, 2nd ed. Philadelphia, Lea & Febiger, 1983.
26. Boudrieau R, Kleine L: Nonsurgically managed caudal acetabular fractures in the dog: 15 cases (1979–1984). JAVMA 193:701, 1988.
27. Butterworth S, Gribben S, Skerry T, et al: Conservative and surgical treatment of canine acetabular fractures: A review of 34 cases. J Sm Anim Pract 35:139, 1994.
28. Betts C: Pelvic Fractures. In Vasseur P, Slatter D (eds): Textbook of Small Animal Surgery, 2nd ed. Philadelphia, WB Saunders Company, 1993, Vol 2, p 1769.
29. Brinker WO: The pelvis. In Bojrab MJ (ed): Current Techniques in Small Animal Surgery. Philadelphia, Lea & Febiger, 1975.
30. Piermattei D, Greely R: An Atlas of Approaches to the Bones of the Dog and Cat, 2nd ed. Philadelphia, WB Saunders Company, 1979.
31. Slocum B, Hohn R: A surgical approach to the caudal aspect of the acetabulum and the body of the ischium in the dog. JAVMA 167:65, 1975.
32. Wheaton L, et al: Surgical treatment of acetabular fractures in the dog. JAVMA 162:385, 1973.
33. Brinker W, Braden T: Fractures of the pelvis. In Brinker W, Hohn R, Prieur W (eds): Manual of Internal Fixation in Small Animals. New York, Springer-Verlag, 1984, p 152.
34. Vernon F, Olmstead M: Femoral head fractures resulting in epiphyseal fragmentation: Results of repair in five dogs. Vet Surg 12:123, 1983.
35. Daly W: Femoral head and neck fractures in the dog and cat: A review of 115 cases. Vet Surg 7:29, 1978.
36. DeCamp C, et al: Internal fixation of femoral capital physeal injuries in dogs: 40 cases (1979–1987). JAVMA 194:1750, 1989.
37. Nunamaker D: Repair of femoral head and neck fractures by interfragmentary compression. JAVMA 163:569, 1973.
38. Hulse D, et al: Revascularization of femoral capital physeal fractures following surgical fixation. J Vet Orthop 2:50, 1981.
39. Anderson W, et al: Method for treatment of fractures of the femoral neck in the dog: An experimental study. JAVMA 122:158, 1953.
40. Lambrechts N, Verstraete F, Sumner-Smith G, et al: Internal fixation of femoral neck fractures in the dog—an in vitro study. Vet Compara Orthopaed Traumatol 6:188, 1993.
41. Fry P: Observations on the surgical treatment of hip dislocation in the dog and cat. J Small Anim Pract 15:661, 1974.
42. Thacher C, Schrader S: Caudal ventral hip luxation in the dog: A review of 14 cases. J Am Anim Hosp Assoc 6:645, 1984.
43. Basher A, Walter M, Newton C: Coxofemoral luxation in the dog and cat. Vet Surg 15:356, 1986.
44. Bone D, Walker M, Cantwell H: Traumatic coxofemoral luxation in dogs. Results of repair. Vet Surg 13:263, 1984.
45. Dobbelaar M: Dislocation of the hip in dogs. J Small Anim Pract 4:101, 1963.
46. Greene J, Hoerlein B, Hayes H, et al: Orthopedic surgery. North Am Vet 34:50, 1953.
47. DeVita J: A method of pinning for chronic dislocation of the hip joint. Proc 89th Annu Meet Am V MA 191, 1952.
48. McLaughlin R, Tillson D: Flexible external fixation for craniodorsal coxofemoral luxations in dogs. Vet Surg 23:21, 1994.
49. Pettit G: Coxofemoral luxations. Vet Clin North Am 1:503, 1971.
50. DeAngelis M, Prata R: Surgical repair of coxofemoral luxation in the dog. J Am Anim Hosp Assoc 9:175, 1973.
51. Denny H, Minter H: Recurrent coxofemoral luxation in the dog. Vet Ann 14:220, 1973.
52. Durr J: The use of Kirschner wires in maintaining reduction of dislocation of the hip joint. JAVMA 130:78, 1957.
53. Fuller W: Reduction and fixation of chronic coxofemoral luxations with the threaded point of a Steinman pin. Vet Med Small Anim Clin 67:406, 1972.
54. Gendreau C, Rouse G: Surgical management of the hip. J Am Anim Hosp Assoc 1:393, 1975.
55. Hammer D: Recurrent coxofemoral luxations in fifteen dogs and one cat. JAVMA 177:1018, 1980.
56. Helper L, Schiller A: Repair of coxofemoral luxations in the dog and cat by extension of the acetabular rim. JAVMA 143:709, 1963.
57. Horne R: Trochanteric pinning procedure for reduction of coxofemoral luxations. Vet Med Small Anim Clin 66:331, 1971.
58. Knowles A, Knowles J, Knowles R: An operation to preserve the continuity of the hip joint. JAVMA 123:508, 1953.
59. Marvich J: Use of bone screw in repair of traumatic coxofemoral luxations. Vet Med Sm Anim Clin 67:302, 1972.
60. Thompson R: A purse-string technique for retention of coxofemoral luxations. Iowa State Univ Vet 30:4, 1968.
61. Vincent Z: The use of Steinman stainless steel pin in recurrent coxofemoral luxation in the dog and cat. S Afr Vet Med J 32:423, 1961.
62. Edwards M, Taylor R, Franceschi R: Clinical case applications of Mitek tissue anchors in veterinary orthopaedics. Vet Compara Orthopaed Traumatol 6:20, 1993.
63. Johnson M, Braden T: A retrospective study of prosthetic capsule technique for the treatment of problem cases of dislocated hips. J Vet Surg 16:346, 1987.
64. Dee J: Fractures in racing greyhound. In Bojrab M (ed): Disease Mechanisms in Small Animal Surgery, 2nd ed. Philadelphia, Lea & Febiger, 1993, p 1060.
65. Corley E: Hip dysplasia: A report from the Orthopedic Foundation for Animals. Semin Vet Med Surg (Small Anim) 2:141, 1987.
66. Corley E: Role of the orthopedic foundation for animals in the control of canine hip dysplasia. Vet Clin North Am: Small Anim Pract 2:597, 1992.

67. Corley E, Hogan P: Trends in hip dysplasia control: Analysis of radiographs submitted to the Orthopedic Foundation for Animals, 1974–1984. JAVMA 187:8, 1985.

68. Priester W, Mulvihill J: Canine hip dysplasia: Relative risk by sex, size, and breed, and comparative aspects. JAVMA 160:735, 1972.

69. Hutt F: Genetic selection to reduce the incidence of hip dysplasia in dogs. JAVMA 151:1041, 1967.

70. Jessen C, Spurrell F: Heritability of canine hip dysplasia. In Proceedings Canine Hip Dysplasia Symposium and Workshop. St. Louis, Orthopedic Foundation for Animals, 1972, p 53.

71. Lust G, Geary J, Sheffy B: Development of hip dysplasia in dogs. Am J Vet Res 34:87, 1973.

72. Hedhammar A, Wu F, Krook L, et al: Overnutrition and skeletal disease. An experimental study in growing Great Dane dogs. Cornell Vet (supp5) 64:1, 1975.

73. Lust G: Other orthopedic disease: Hip dysplasia in dogs. In Slatter D (ed): Textbook of Small Animal Surgery, 2nd ed. p 1938. Philadelphia, WB Saunders Company, 1993, vol 2.

74. Lust G, Farrell P: Hip dysplasia in dogs; the interplay of genotype and environment. Cornell Vet 67:447, 1977.

75. Smith G, Gregor T, Rhodes H, et al: Coxofemoral joint laxity from distraction radiography and its contemporaneous and prospective correlation with laxity, subjective score, and evidence of degenerative joint disease from conventional hip-extended radiography in dogs. Am J Vet Res 54:1021, 1993.

76. Willis M: Hip dysplasia. In Genetics of the Dog, New York, Howell Book Company, 1989, p 144.

77. Riser W: The dog as model for the study of hip dysplasia. Vet Pathol 12:229, 1975.

78. Riser W, Shirer J: Hip dysplasia: Coxofemoral abnormalities in neonatal German Shepherd dogs. J Small Anim Pract 7:7, 1966.

79. Morgan J, Stephens M: Pathogenesis of dysplasia. In Radiographic Diagnosis and Control of Canine Hip Dysplasia. Ames, Iowa, Iowa State University Press, 1985.

80. Alexander J: The pathogenesis of canine hip dysplasia. Vet Clin North Am: Small Anim Pract 12:503, 1992.

81. Maistrelli G, Gerundini M, Bombelli R: The inclination of the weight bearing surface in the hip joint. The clinical significance of abnormal force. Orthop Rev 5:271, 1986.

82. Slocum B, Devine T: Pelvic Osteotomy. In Whittick W (ed): Canine Orthopedics, Philadelphia, Lea & Febiger, 1990, p 471.

83. Slocum B, Devine T: Pelvic osteotomy in the dog as treatment for hip dysplasia. Semin Vet Med Surg 2:107, 1987.

84. Slocum B, Devine T: Pelvic osteotomy technique for axial rotation of the acetabular segment in dogs. J Am Anim Hosp Assoc 22:331, 1986.

85. Slocum B, Slocum T: Pelvic osteotomy for axial rotation of the acetabular segment in dogs with hip dysplasia. Vet Clin North Am Small Anim Pract 22:645, 1992.

86. Riser W, Cohen D, Lindquist S, et al: Influence of early rapid growth and weight gain on hip dysplasia in the German shepherd dog. JAVMA 145:661, 1964.

87. Kasstrom H: Nutrition, weight gain, and development of hip dysplasia. An experimental investigation in growing dogs with special reference to the effect of feeding intensity. Acta Radiol Suppl 344:135, 1974.

88. Olson S: Canine hip dysplasia. In Kirk R (ed): Current Veterinary Therapy VII. Philadelphia, WB Saunders Company, 1980, p 802.

89. Bennett D: Hip dysplasia and ascorbate therapy: Fact or fancy? Semin Vet Med Surg Small Animal 2:152, 1987.

90. Rettenmaier J, Constantinescu G: Canine hip dysplasia. Compend Contin Educ Pract Vet 13:643, 1991.

91. Paatsama S: Somatotropin, thyrotropin and corticotropin hormone induced changes in the cartilage and bones of young dogs. J Small Anim Pract 12:603, 1971.

92. Gustaffson P: Estradiol induced skeletal changes. Acta Radiol Suppl 344:53, 1975.

93. Pierce K, Bridges C: The role of estrogens in the pathogenesis of canine hip dysplasia. Metabolism of exogenous estrogens. Small Anim Pract 8:383, 1967.

94. Riser W, Rhodes D, Newton C: Hip dysplasia. In Newton C, Nunamaker D (eds): Textbook of Small Animal Orthopedics. Philadelphia, JB Lippincott Co, 1985, p 953.

95. Prieur W: Coxarthritis in the dog. I: Normal and abnormal biomechanics of the hip joint. Vet Surg 9:145, 1980.

96. Bardens J, Hardwick H: New observations on the diagnosis and cause of hip dysplasia. Vet Med Small Anim Clin 63:238, 1968.

97. Bowen J: Electromyographic analysis of reflex and spastic activities of canine pectineus muscles in the presence and absence of hip dysplasia. Am J Vet Res 35:661, 1974.

98. Cardinet G, Fedde M, Tunell G: Correlates of histochemical and physiological properties in normal and hypotrophic pectineus muscles of the dog. Lab Invest 27:32, 1972.

99. Cardinet G, Wallace L, Fedde M, et al: Developmental myopathy in the canine. Arch Neurol 21:620, 1969.

100. Ihemelandu EC, Cardinet G, Guffy M, et al: Canine hip dysplasia: Differences in pectineal muscles of healthy and dysplastic German shepherd dogs when two months old. Am J Vet Res 44:411, 1983.

101. Riser W, Shirer J: Correlation between canine hip dysplasia and pelvic muscle mass: A study of 95 dogs. Am J Vet Res 124:769, 1967.

102. Lust G, Kindlon C: Biochemical studies on hip dysplasia in dogs. In Proceedings of the 19th Gaines Veterinary Symposium. Lafayette, Ind, Purdue University Press, 1969, p 16.

103. Bardet J: Femoral torsion and experimental midshaft femoral osteotomies in dog (thesis). Columbus, Ohio State University, 1981.

104. Forsyth H, Paschall H: A study of congenital hip dysplasia in dogs. J Bone Joint Surg 45:1781, 1963.

105. Schneider M: The effect of growth on femoral torsion. J Bone Joint Surg 45:1439, 1963.

106. Smith W, Coleman C, Olix M, et al: Etiology of congenital dislocation of the hip. J Bone Joint Surg 45:491, 1963.

107. Lust G, Beilman W, Rendano V: A relationship between degree of laxity and synovial fluid volume in coxofemoral joints of dogs predisposed for hip dysplasia. Am J Vet Res 41:55, 1980.

108. Riser W, Newton C: Canine hip dysplasia as a disease. In Bojrab M (ed): Pathophysiology in Small Animal Surgery. Philadelphia, Lea & Febiger, 1981, p 618.

109. Bardens J: Palpation for the detection of joint laxity. In Proceedings Canine Hip Dysplasia Symposium and Workshop. St. Louis, Orthopedic Foundation for Animals, 1972:105.

110. Chalman J, Butler H: Coxofemoral joint laxity and the Ortolani sign. J Small Anim Hosp Assoc 21:671, 1985.

111. Ortolani M: The classic: Congenital hip dysplasia in the light of early and very early diagnosis. Clin Orthop 119:6, 1976.

112. Samuelson M: Correlation of palpation with radiography in diagnosis and prognosis of canine hip dysplasia. In Proceedings Canine Hip Dysplasia Symposium and Workshop. St Louis, Orthopedic Foundation for Animals, 1972, p 110.

113. Giardina J, MacCarthy A, Jr: Hip palpation: Evaluation of a technique for early determination of predysplastic dogs. Vet Med Small Anim Clin 63:878, 1971.

114. Lust G, Craig P, Geary J, et al: Changes in pelvic muscle tissues associated with hip dysplasia. Am J Vet Res 33:1097, 1972.

115. Lust G, Craig P, Ross G, et al: Studies on pectineus muscles in canine hip dysplasia. Cornell Vet 62:628, 1972.

116. Bardens J: Palpation for the detection of dysplasia and wedge technique for pelvic radiography. Proceedings of the 39th Annual Meeting of the American Animal Hospital Association. Denver, American Animal Hospital Association, 1972, pp 468–471.

117. Jessen C, Spurrell F: Radiograph detection of canine hip dysplasia in known age groups. In Proceedings Canine Hip Dysplasia Symposium and Workshop. St. Louis, Orthopedic Foundation for Animals, 1972, p 93.

118. Henry J, Jr, Park R: Wedge technique for demonstration of coxofemoral joint laxity in the canine. Proceedings Canine Hip Dysplasia Symposium and Workshop. St. Louis, Orthopedic Foundation for Animals, 1972, p 93.

119. Heyman S, Smith G, Cofone M: Biomechanical study of the effect of coxofemoral positioning on passive hip joint laxity in dogs. Am J Vet Res 54:210, 1993.

120. Barr A, et al: Clinical hip dysplasia in growing dogs: The long term results of conservative management. J Small Anim Pract 28:243, 1987.

121. Wallace L: Canine Hip Dysplasia. Semin Vet Med Surg Small Anim 2:92, 1987.

122. Candlin F: The diagnosis and treatment of hip dysplasia: One point of view. J Am Anim Hosp Assoc 8:323, 1972.

123. Bloomberg M: Canine hip dysplasia: What's old, what's new, what's true. Vet Tech 11:303, 1990.

124. Vasseur P, Johnson A, Budsberg S, et al: Randomized, controlled trial of the efficacy of carprofen, a non-steroidal antiinflammatory drug, in the treatment of osteoarthritis in dogs. JAVMA 206:807, 1995.
125. Benton H, Vasseur P, Broderick-Villa G, et al: Effect of carprofen on sulfated glycosaminoglycan metabolism, protein synthesis, and prostaglandin release by cultured osteoarthritic canine chondrocytes. J Vet Res 58(3):286, 1997.
126. Clark D: Current concepts in the treatment of degenerative joint disease. Comp Contin Educ Pract Vet 13:1439, 1991.
127. Behrens F, Shepard N, Mitchell N: Alteration of rabbit articular cartilage by intra-articular injections of glucocorticoids. J Bone Joint Surg 57(A):70, 1975.
128. Chunekamrai S, Krook L, Lust G, et al: Changes in articular cartilage after intra-articular injections of methylprednisolone acetate in horses. Am J Vet Res 50:1733, 1989.
129. Glade M, Krook L, Schryver H: Morphologic and biochemical changes in cartilage in foals treated with dexamethasone. Cornell Vet 73:170, 1983.
130. Silberberg M, Silberberg R, Hasler M: Fine structure of articular cartilage in mice receiving cortisone acetate. Arch Pathol 87:569, 1986.
131. Mclaughlin D: Veterinary Pharmaceuticals and Biologicals, 6th ed. Lenexa, Kan, Veterinary Medicine Publishing Co, 1988, p 697.
132. Altman R, Dean D, Muniz O, et al: Prophylactic treatment of canine osteoarthritis with glycosaminoglycan polysulfuric acid ester. Arthritis Rheum 32:759, 1989.
133. Hannan N, Ghosh P, Bellenger C, et al: Systemic administration of glycosaminoglycan polysulfate (arteparon) provides partial protection of articular cartilage from damage produced by meniscectomy in the canine. J Orthop Res 4(8):16, 1987.
134. Huber M, Bill R: The use of polysulfated glycosaminoglycan in dogs. Compendium 16:501, 1994.
135. DeHaan J, Goring R, Beale B: Evaluation of polysulfated glycosaminoglycan for the treatment of hip dysplasia in dogs. Vet Surg 23:177, 1994.
136. Burkhardt D, Ghosh P: Laboratory evaluation of antiarthritic drugs as potential chondroprotective agents. Semin Arthritis Rheum 17:3, 1987.
137. Beale B, Goring R, Clemmons R, et al: The effect of semisynthetic polysulfated glycosaminoglycans on the hemostatic mechanism in the dog. Vet Surg 19:57, 1990.
138. Bianchini P: Therapeutic potential of non-heparin glycosaminoglycans of natural origin. Semin Thromb Hemost 15:365, 1989.
139. Hohn R, Janes J: Pelvic osteotomy in the treatment of canine hip dysplasia. Clin Orthop 62:976, 1972.
140. Schrader S: Triple osteotomy of the pelvis as a treatment for canine hip dysplasia. JAVMA 178:39, 1981.
141. Schrader S: Triple osteotomy of the pelvis and trochanteric osteotomy as a treatment for hip dysplasia in the immature dog: The surgical technique and results of 77 consecutive operations. JAVMA 189:659, 1986.
142. Nunamaker D: Surgical correction of large femoral anteversion angles in the dog. JAVMA 165:1061, 1974.
143. Prieur W: Intertrochanteric osteotomy in the dog: Theoretical consideration and operative technique. J Small Anim Pract 28:3, 1987.
144. Prieur W: Intertrochanteric osteotomy. In Bojrab M (ed): Current Techniques in Small Animal Surgery. Philadelphia, Lea & Febiger, 1990, p 667.
145. Walker T, Prieur W: Intertrochanteric femoral osteotomy. Semin Vet Med Surg Small Anim 2:117, 1987.
146. Braden T, Prieur D: Three-plane intertrochanter osteotomy for treatment of early stage hip dysplasia. In Alexander J (ed): Vet Clin North Am Small Anim Pract 22:623, 1992.
147. Duff R, Campbell J: Long term results of excision arthroplasty of the canine hip. Vet Rec 101:181, 1977.
148. Gendreau C, Cawley A: Excision of the femoral head and neck: The long-term results of 35 operations. J Am Anim Hosp Assoc 13:603, 1977.
149. Montgomery R, Milton J, Pernell R, et al: Total hip arthroplasty for treatment of canine hip dysplasia. Vet Clin North Am 22:703, 1992.
150. Vasseur P: Femoral head and neck ostectomy. In Bojrab M (ed): Current Techniques in Small Animal Surgery. Philadelphia, Lea & Febiger, 1990, p 674.
151. Olmstead M: Total hip replacement in the dog. Semin Vet Med Surg 2:131, 1987.
152. DeYoung D, DeYoung B, Aberman H, et al: Implantation of an uncemented total hip prosthesis; technique and initial results of 100 arthroplasties. Vet Surg 21(3):168, 1992.
153. DeYoung D, Schiller R: Radiographic criteria for evaluation of uncemented total hip replacement in dogs. Vet Surg 21:88, 1992.
154. Schiller T, DeYoung D, Schiller R, et al: Quantitative ingrowth analysis of a porous-coated acetabular component in a canine model. Vet Surg 22:276, 1993.
155. Rothman R, Cohn J: Cemented versus cementless total hip arthroplasty. Clin Orthop Rel Res 254:153, 1990.
156. Callaghan J: Total hip arthroplasty. Clin Orthop 276:33, 1992.
157. Freeman M, Tennant R: The scientific basis of cement versus cementless fixation. Clin Orthop Rel Res 276:19, 1992.
158. Josefsson G, Lindberg L, Wiklander B: Systemic antibiotics and antibiotic-containing bone cement in the prophylaxis of postoperative infections in total hip arthroplasty. Clin Orthop Rel Res 159:194, 1981.
159. Murray W: Use of antibiotic-containing bone cement. Clin Orthop Rel Res 190:89, 1984.
160. Olmstead M, Hohn R, Turner T: Technique for canine total hip replacement. Vet Surg 10(1):4, 1981.
161. Paul H, Bargar W: A modified technique for canine total hip replacement. J Am Anim Hosp Assoc 23:13, 1987.
162. Petty W, Spanier S, Shuster J: Prevention of infection after total joint replacement. J Bone Joint Surg 70:536, 1990.
163. Richardson D, Aucoin D, DeYoung D, et al: Pharmacokinetic disposition of cefazolin in serum and tissue during canine total hip replacement. Vet Surg 21:1, 1992.
164. Sorensen T, Anderson M, Glenthoj J, et al: Pharmacokinetics of topical gentamicin in total hip arthroplasty. Acta Orthop Scand 55:156, 1984.
165. Soto-Hall R, Saenz S, Tavernetti R, et al: Tobramycin in bone cement. Clin Orthop Rel Res 175:60, 1983.
166. Olmstead M: Pathomechanics and complications of total hip prostheses. In Bojrab M (ed): Disease Mechanisms in Small Animal Surgery, 2nd ed. Philadelphia, Lea & Febiger, 1993, p 1129.
167. Olmstead M, Hohn R, Turner T: A five-year study of 221 total hip replacements in the dog. JAVMA 183:191, 1983.
168. Berzon J, Howard P, Covell S, et al: A retrospective study of the efficacy of femoral head and neck excisions in 94 dogs and cats. Vet Surg 9:88, 1980.
169. Bjorling D, Chambers J: The biceps femoris flap and femoral head and neck excision in dogs. Compend Contin Educ Pract Vet 8:359, 1986.
170. Dueland R, Bartel D, Antonson E: Force plate technique for gait analysis of the total hip and excision arthroplasty. J Am Anim Hosp Assoc 13:547, 1977.
171. Lippincott C: Femoral head and neck excision in the management of canine hip dysplasia. Vet Clin North Am Small Anim Pract 22:721, 1992.
172. Lippincott C: Excision arthroplasty of the femoral head and neck. Vet Clin North Am Small Anim Pract 17:857, 1987.
173. Tarvin G, Lippincott C: Excision arthroplasty for the treatment of canine hip dysplasia using the biceps femoris muscle sling: An evaluation of 92 cases. Semin Vet Med Surg (Small Anim) 2:158, 1987.
174. Montgomery R, Milton J, Horne R, et al: A retrospective comparison of three techniques for femoral head and neck excision in dogs. Vet Surg 16:423, 1987.
175. Lewis D, Bellah J, McGavin M, et al: Postoperative examination of the biceps femoris muscle sling used in excision of the femoral head and neck in dogs. Vet Surg 17(5):269, 1988.
176. Mann F, Tangner C, Wagner-Mann C, et al: A comparison of standard femoral head and neck excision using a biceps femoris muscle flap in the dog. Vet Surg 16(3):223, 1987.
177. Hedhammar A, Olsson S, Anderson S, et al: Canine hip dysplasia: study of 401 litters of German shepherd dogs. JAVMA 174:1012, 1979.

CHAPTER 23

LUMBOSACRAL STENOSIS IN THE SPORTING DOG

KIRK L. WENDELBURG

Diseases of the cauda equina or lumbosacral spine continue to be recognized more frequently because of improved diagnostic techniques and veterinary awareness. Several terms used to describe the disease include *cauda equina syndrome, lumbosacral disease, lumbosacral nerve root compression, lumbosacral instability,* and *lumbosacral stenosis.* Both congenital and acquired diseases of the lumbosacral spine are observed in dogs. Acquired lumbosacral nerve root compression is most often observed in middle-aged German shepherds, but is also seen frequently in other working breeds and a number of sporting breeds.[1] Although trauma, infection, and neoplasia can produce lumbosacral nerve root disease, the more common underlying cause of compression in athletic dogs is lumbosacral instability with associated degenerative lumbosacral arthritis and/or intervertebral disc protrusion. Acquired diseases result in compression and impingement of the nerve roots in the lumbosacral canal or intervertebral foramen, producing clinical signs of sensory and/or motor nerve dysfunction.

I will confine my discussion to the acquired disorders that frequently affect the canine athlete. These disorders, which result from the excessive stress, instability, and motion in the lumbosacral spine, include idiopathic lumbosacral stenosis and degenerative lumbosacral stenosis with intervertebral disc protrusion.

ANATOMY

Differential growth of the neural and skeletal systems results in the termination of the spinal cord or *conus medullaris* to occur between caudal L4 vertebral body (giant-breed dog) and L6 vertebral body (small-breed dog).[2, 3] The *cauda equina* represents the terminal group of nerve roots descending from the conus medullaris within the spinal canal, lateral recesses, and intervertebral foramen. The cranial extent of the cauda equina can vary, depending on the size of the dog, but includes L6, L7, S1–3, and coccygeal nerve roots. These nerve roots leave their spinal cord segments and travel caudally within the spinal canal until exiting the intervertebral foramen, caudal to their respective vertebral body (Fig. 23–1).

The sciatic nerve performs many of the sensory and motor functions of the rear legs and is formed from the L6, L7, and S1 nerve roots. These nerve roots exit the L6–7, L7–S1, and S1–2 intervertebral foramen respectively. The S1 and S2 nerve roots contribute to both the pudendal and pelvic nerves. The pudendal nerve innervates the external anal sphincter and perineum. The pelvic nerve provides the autonomic innervation that controls urinary and fecal continence. The coccygeal nerves supply motor and sensory innervation to the tail.

The *spinal canal* formed by adjoining vertebrae supports and protects the spinal cord and cauda equina. The canal space is oval, becoming more flattened dorsoventrally at the level of the lumbosacral junction. At the intervertebral spaces, the cauda equina are bordered dorsally by the dorsal vertebral lamina, interarcuate ligament, and articular facets and joint capsule and ventrally by the vertebral bodies, dorsal longitudinal ligament, and annulus fibrosus.

Just prior to a nerve root exiting an intervertebral foramen, it courses through a depression called the *lateral recess,* bordered laterally by the caudal pedicle of its respective vertebra. The L7 nerve root then exits through the intervertebral foramen cranial to the L7–S1 intervertebral disc and S1 pedicle. The S1, S2, S3, and coccygeal nerve roots course over the L7–S1 disc. Paired venous sinuses travel over the vertebral bodies, diverging laterally as they approach the disc spaces, while exiting nerve roots are accompanied by a radicular artery and vein.

PATHOPHYSIOLOGY

Compression of one or more nerve roots of the cauda equina or its vasculature is the common factor in the pathogenesis of pain or neurological dysfunction associated with cauda equina syndrome. Flexion and extension forces produced from the rear limbs and pelvis during the gait are transmitted directly into the sacrum. Since the L7–S1 intervertebral junction is the first area of the spine that absorbs these forces, it becomes the area of greatest stress in the lower spine. Diseases that produce decreased extension of the hip joint (eg, canine hip dysplasia) may cause the other joints of the rear limb and the lower lumbar or lumbosacral spine to hyperextend during the propulsion phase of the gait. This additional stress resulting from compensatory lumbosacral hyperextension may secondarily cause dogs with osteoarthritis of the hip joints to be more prone to stenosis of the lumbosacral spine (unpublished personal observation).

A number of changes can take place when excessive stress produces abnormal motion and instability at the lumbosacral junction. Extension of the area (produced in the propulsion phase of the gait) is limited primarily by the ventral longitudinal ligament, ventral annulus, and joint capsules of the articular facets. Flexion is limited by the supraspinous, interspinous, interarcuate, and dorsal longitudinal ligaments, as well as the joint capsule of the articular facets.[4] Excessive forces producing abnormal motion at the lumbosacral junction are responded to by hypertrophy of the structures involved. Instability in extension produces cranial and ventral sliding of the dorsal lamina of S1, bulging of the interarcuate ligament, joint capsules, dorsal longitudinal ligament, and annulus. This results in a narrowed spinal canal and intervertebral foramen. Excessive flexion at the lumbosacral junction could also result in stretching of the nerve roots causing associated clinical signs.[5]

Vessels of the cauda equina dilate in response to exercise to provide the necessary metabolic demands of the nerves.[6–9] Vascular impingement prevents dilatation of blood vessels, which can produce intermittent nerve root ischemia during exercise. The vascular phenomena producing an intermittent ischemic neuropathy is referred to as *neurogenic intermittent claudication.*[3, 9] Transient ischemic neuropathy results in nerve root pain and referred pain to the back, rear limbs, tail, and perineum.[3] In humans, symptoms of neurogenic ischemia can be exacerbated in extension and alleviated

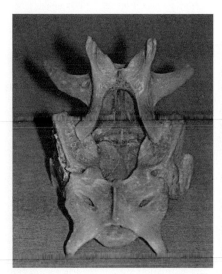
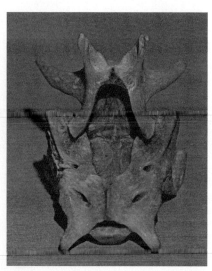
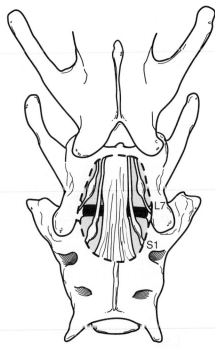

FIGURE 23–1. Dorsoventral view of lumbosacral canal. Nerve roots exit their respective foramen. The L7 nerve root exits the intervertebral foramen just cranial to the lumbosacral disc while the S1 nerve root courses dorsally over the disc to exit the S1 foramen.

by flexion of the lumbosacral spine.[5, 8] Neurogenic claudication may be difficult to elicit on examination but is an important part of the clinical history of a dog with cauda equina syndrome.

Degenerative Lumbosacral Stenosis

Degenerative lumbosacral stenosis is the most common cause of lumbosacral nerve compression in the canine athlete and nonathlete.[4, 10, 11] The degenerative changes are the result of long-term mechanical stresses acting upon the lumbosacral junction. Stenosis results from multiple changes that occur in the lumbosacral anatomy, but is usually associated with a Hansen type II intervertebral disc degeneration.[12] The disc degeneration may produce bulging of the annulus or extrusion of the nucleus pulposus and annular material causing ventral nerve root compression. When the nucleus

pulposus is extruded, an inflammatory reaction commonly produces significant adhesions around the nerve roots.

Instability at the lumbosacral articulation causes the S1 facet to slide cranially and ventrally below the L7 caudal facets.[1, 11] Collapse of the facets will produce dorsal attenuation from the infolded interarcuate ligament and downward displacement of the S1 dorsal lamina. The intervertebral foramen is also reduced in size because of the collapsing pedicles. Degenerative osteoarthritis of the facets produces periarticular osteophytes and hypertrophied joint capsules, attenuating dorsolaterally and within the intervertebral foramen. Abnormal stresses on the vertebral body end plates at the attachment sites of the annulus and dorsal and ventral longitudinal ligaments eventually produce the commonly observed ventral spondylosis, and occasionally the more clinically significant dorsal and lateral spondylosis (Fig. 23–2).

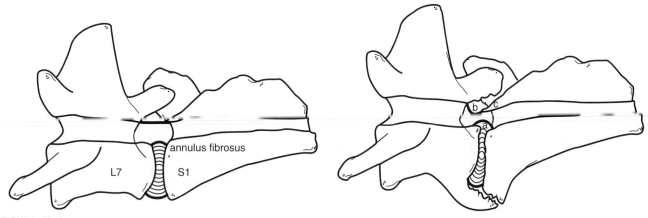

FIGURE 23–2. *Left,* Normal lumbosacral junction. *Right,* Instability of the lumbosacral junction. Collapse of the facets and disc space produces dorsal bulging of the annulus fibrosus and dorsal longitudinal ligament (a), infolding of the interarcuate ligament (b), and downward displacement of the S1 dorsal lamina (c). Results are narrowed canal and intervertebral foramen.

Idiopathic Lumbosacral Stenosis

Congenital stenosis, characterized by shortening of the pedicles, thickened lamina and articular processes, hypertrophy and infolding of the interarcuate ligament, and sclerotic, bulbous articular facets, has been clinically documented in humans.[7, 9, 13–15] These changes in neural arch development are thought to decrease the spinal canal and intervertebral foramen diameters independent of any disc degeneration.[3, 16] Since lumbosacral stenosis is very rarely reported in dogs less than 1 year of age, it is unlikely that the developmental abnormalities alone are responsible for the clinical signs. While the entity is viewed as congenital stenosis in dogs, objective spinal canal measurements could not document stenosis in one report of 15 dogs.[16] A congenitally compromised canal in a dog may be more prone to instability or minor changes in the joint capsule and interarcuate ligament, resulting in dynamic idiopathic stenosis. It is quite possible that idiopathic lumbosacral stenosis is just a more subtle presentation of acquired degenerative stenosis.

The clinical onset for idiopathic lumbosacral stenosis is usually not until middle or old age.[3, 16] The pathophysiology of the disease is similar to degenerative lumbosacral stenosis except that the anatomical changes do not have to be as pronounced or result from a degenerative disc. The resulting stenosis not only produces direct compression on the cauda equina, but results in neurogenic intermittent claudication. Pain and lameness may be observed primarily when the dog is exercised. As a protective response, the dog will maintain the caudal spine in a flexed position to increase the spinal canal diameter. Increased activity, producing further neurogenic claudication, will enhance this "tucked-up" appearance (Fig. 23–3).

German Shepherd Lumbosacral Stenosis

Lumbosacral stenosis in German shepherd dogs may also be associated with other causative factors. It has been associated with both degenerative disc disease and transitional vertebral segments.[17] Radiographic and pathological abnormalities compatible with osteochondrosis of the sacral end plate was associated with 30 per cent (21 of 65) of German shepherd dogs with clinical signs of cauda equina compression.[18] Male dogs were more often affected than females. Osteochondrosis lesions of the sacral end plate were also found in clinically normal growing and young adult dogs. The dogs in this study with clinical signs of lumbosacral stenosis also had severe degenerative disc disease with protrusion of the lumbosacral disc and compression of the cauda equina, suggesting

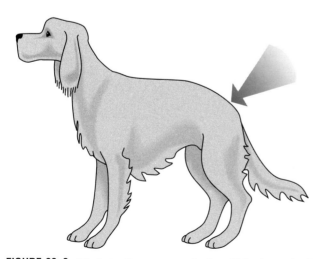

FIGURE 23–3. "Tucked-up" appearance of a dog with lumbosacral pain.

that clinical signs are more likely directly related to degenerative lumbosacral stenosis and disc protrusion than to the osteochondrosis. Because these dogs were, on average, 2 years younger than dogs with cauda equina compression and without sacral osteochondrosis, it suggests the sacral osteochondrosis may predispose them to early degenerative disc disease and lumbosacral stenosis.

CLINICAL FINDINGS AND NEUROLOGICAL ASSESSMENT

The most common clinical sign associated with lumbosacral stenosis is pain. The pain may occur as back pain, unilateral or bilateral lameness (nerve root signature), or tail pain. The dogs commonly have a history of difficulty rising but may tend to warm out of the initial stiffness. Owners may report an unwillingness to run, jump, or climb that is exacerbated with increased activity. The dogs often have a stilted gait in the rear or appear tucked-up (Fig. 23–3). Root signature lameness or referred pain in the rear legs is the result of L7 and/or S1 nerve root (sciatic nerve) compression or ischemia. The pain may be acute or chronic, intermittent or persistent, or exercise induced.

Further neurological signs develop as attenuation and ischemia of entrapped nerve roots progress. These include muscle atrophy and progressive weakness in the sciatic distribution, tail weakness, paresthesias producing self-mutilation, overflow urinary incontinence (S2 and S3 pelvic nerve attenuation), and, uncommonly, fecal incontinence. The external anal sphincter may become hypotonic or atonic. As coccygeal nerves become further compressed, weakness and pain may progress to an anesthesia and paralysis of the tail.

Physical Examination

Observation of the gait is the first element in examining for rear limb pain or weakness. The patient should be observed at the walk and jog, and if possible, ascending and descending a hill or stairs. The most common gait observation will be the tucked-up appearance in the rear, with the dog failing to extend at the hips. This gait is very similar to that of a dog with hip dysplasia and has often been mistakenly attributed to that disease. Gait abnormalities, although typically bilateral, can be unilateral. Unilateral L7 or S1 nerve root impingement may cause the dog to limit hip extension on the affected side while quickly advancing the opposite leg.

After a general physical examination (including a rectal examination), the orthopedic and neurological systems should be evaluated. The standing dog is first observed for postural reactions (conscious proprioception, hopping, hemiwalking) and then for hyperesthesia. Abnormalities in postural reactions may or may not be observed with diseases of the cauda equina, but when present, are indicators of neurological disease. Palpation for hyperesthesia is initiated by gentle dorsal pressure over the lower lumbar and lumbosacral spine. If there is no response, the pressure is increased while the tail is lifted. The most sensitive palpation test for lumbosacral pain is done by the examiner applying dorsal pressure over the lumbosacral junction with the thumbs while using the fingers to apply medially directed pressure just ventral to the iliac body and wings (Fig. 23–4). All tests for hyperesthesia can be exacerbated by extending the hips of the dog, thereby producing lordosis and additional nerve root compression. Unfortunately, some dogs with disease of the lumbosacral spine also have hip dysplasia. Because osteoarthritis of the hip joints can produce a severe pain response with hip extension, this test is unreliable in patients with hip dysplasia.

In lateral recumbency the spinal reflexes are evaluated along with a complete orthopedic examination. Atrophy of the gluteal and hamstring muscles may be apparent. The pelvic limb spinal

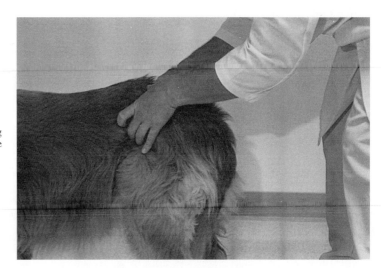

FIGURE 23–4. Lumbosacral hyperpathia is detected by applying downward pressure dorsally over the lumbosacral junction while medial pressure is directed just ventral to the ilium.

reflexes are usually normal but may be hypoactive to sciatic innervation (cranial tibial, sciatic, and peroneal) because of L6, L7, or S1 impingement. Although the patellar reflex is usually normal, it can occasionally appear brisk because of the decreased antagonistic hamstring tone. An anal reflex is usually present, even though rectal examination will often reveal decreased anal tone.

Lumbosacral spinal hyperpathia is again assessed with the dog in lateral recumbency. Medially directed pressure is applied just ventral to the ilium while downward pressure is applied dorsal to the lumbosacral junction. Rear limb extension will concurrently produce extension forces on the lumbosacral junction and will intensify a pain response. If hip dysplasia is also present, slowly extend the dog's hips, stopping just before the angle of a pain response, then apply pressure over the lumbosacral spine and ventral to the ilium (Fig. 23–5). This palpation sequence may help differentiate between neurogenic and orthopedic pain.

Radiographic Examination

Survey radiography is required to evaluate the lower spine for osseous changes and to evaluate for coxofemoral joint disease. Lumbosacral spondylosis alone is not diagnostic of lumbosacral stenosis, although when combined with compatible clinical signs, it becomes very suggestive evidence of lumbosacral stenosis. A narrowed disc space, end plate sclerosis, and the presence of calcified material (osteophytes or disc) in the ventral canal are also very suggestive of lumbosacral stenosis when accompanied by compatible clinical signs (Fig. 23–6).

Because nerve root compression is usually the result of soft tissue impingement, contrast radiography is the primary means of definitive diagnosis in the dog. Myelography, although required to rule out compressive diseases cranial to L6, is usually inadequate for examination of the lumbosacral junction. Combined epidurography and myelography is the preferred method of radiographic evaluation for lower lumbar compression and/or lumbosacral stenosis in the dog. Epidurography best demonstrates compressive lesions at the L6–L7 or L7–S1 intervertebral disc spaces and has been shown to strongly correlate with findings at surgery[19] (Fig. 23–7).

The procedure is performed under anesthesia using 0.2 to 0.4 ml/kg of iohexol or iopamidol as the contrast agent. Injection into the spinal canal can be performed cranial or caudal to the lumbosacral junction. An epidurogram from the caudal injection is obtained at any of the dorsal intervertebral spaces between S3 and Cd3. The cranial injection is performed with the larger dose at the dorsal

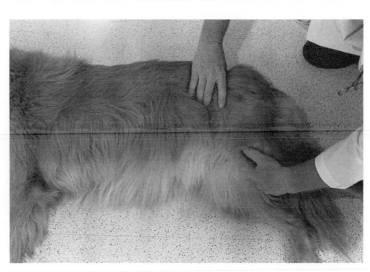

FIGURE 23–5. Both hip dysplasia and lumbosacral stenosis may be present in the same dog. Extension of the rear limb can produce pain from the affected hip or lumbosacral stenosis. Extension is stopped just prior to a pain response, then digital pressure is applied over the lumbosacral spine and ventral to the ilium.

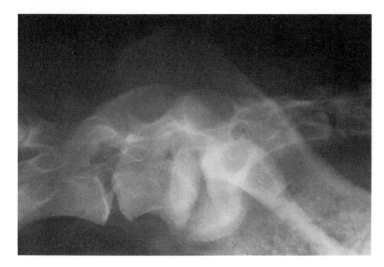

FIGURE 23–6. Survey radiographs may demonstrate spondylosis or a collapsed disc space.

intervertebral space of L5–L6 or L6–L7. If combined myelography and epidurography is done, the L5–L6 injection is made with half the dose first injected into the subarachnoid space, then the remainder injected epidurally by advancing the needle to the floor of the canal and rotating the bevel to face in the caudal direction. The injection should be performed with the spine in flexion to allow flow of the contrast agent over the compressed lumbosacral junction. Lateral radiographs are obtained in flexion, neutral, and extension. Ventrodorsal views are also taken but are often difficult to interpret.

Epidurograms are considered abnormal if there is obstruction to contrast flow or dorsal deviation of the ventral epidural space at the lumbosacral junction or L6–L7. One study evaluating caudally injected epidurography showed a 96 per cent correlation between compressive lesions at surgery, and epidurogram findings of a 50 per cent elevation of the epidural space or total contrast obstruction.[19]

Advanced Imaging Techniques

Contrast computerized tomography (CT) and magnetic resonance imaging (MRI) have revolutionized the diagnosis of lumbosacral stenosis in humans and recently has become available in veterinary referral centers. Magnetic resonance imaging has become particularly useful because of its extremely sensitive ability to visualize soft or bony tissue compression on nerve roots (Fig. 23–8).[20–22] MRI is also preferred, since it is noninvasive (does not require radiographic contrast media) and does not subject the patient or technical staff to radiation. The main disadvantages of MRI are the cost and limited availability.

TREATMENT OF LUMBOSACRAL STENOSIS

Treatment of lumbosacral stenosis can be categorized as conservative (nonsurgical) or surgical. The recommendation for the type of treatment depends on the severity and duration of clinical signs, the expected athletic function, and in some cases, the response to previous medical treatments. Conservative management is recommended only in dogs with an initial episode of mild pain. Along with anti-inflammatory medication, strict rest is recommended for 6 to 8 weeks. Dogs are generally much more responsive to steroidal than to nonsteroidal anti-inflammatory drugs. Prednisone is given at a tapering dose over a 3-week period. Methocarbamol is adminis-

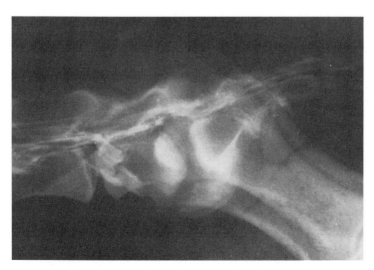

FIGURE 23–7. Combined myelography and epidurography demonstrate dorsal deviation of the ventral epidural space and attenuation of the contrast in the lumbosacral area.

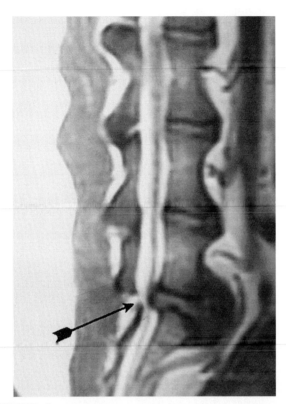

FIGURE 23–8. Magnetic resonance imaging demonstrates both soft tissue and bony stenosis of the lumbosacral canal *(arrow).*

tered at 10 mg/pound three times a day for 1 week if muscle spasms are observed.

Conservative management with strict rest and steroidal anti-inflammatory medication gives an athletic dog a guarded prognosis at best for return to its original athletic function.[1, 4, 16, 23] Pain may be temporarily relieved while the dog is rested but will usually return once athletic activity is resumed. A delay in surgical treatment may lessen the prognosis for return to athletic function or produce increased morbidity associated with the disease and the surgery.[1, 4]

Surgical Management

Early surgical management should be recommended if initial conservative management is unsuccessful, if pain is severe, or if lower motor neuron signs are apparent. The two basic techniques for surgical management of lumbosacral stenosis are fusion and decompression. Fusion is aimed at stabilization of the abnormal motion, thereby preventing subluxation, disc herniation, and hyperplastic degeneration.[11] Decompression through a dorsal laminectomy removes soft tissue and bony impingement from the nerve roots.

Since the majority of dogs with lumbosacral stenosis have discrete type II disc lesions, and motion is pathological only to the degree of encouraging further hyperplastic changes, the recommended surgical treatment in dogs is decompression alone. Fusion is generally not necessary and has a high risk of complications such as nonunion, bony overproduction with recurrent stenosis, pin failure, pin migration, and facet or spinous process fracture.[1, 3, 4, 24–26] Laminectomy allows direct examination of the cauda equina and removal of compressive tissues.

Dorsal laminectomy is performed in the area of visible nerve

root compression on the epidurogram or MRI. This generally includes L7–S1 but may also involve L5 or L6. A partial facetectomy is performed, preserving the dorsal and lateral aspects of the pedicles. The partial preservation of the pedicles and facets retains stability. Preservation is accomplished by performing the laminectomy and foramenotomy with upcutting Kerrison or Schlesinger rongeurs, thereby removing only the bone necessary to achieve complete decompression. After removal of the dorsal lamina and medial aspects of the pedicles, the annular ligament and redundant joint capsule are excised and removed. All nerve roots are followed through the spinal canal, lateral recesses, and intervertebral foramen, examining for evidence of tension or impingement.

The intervertebral disc is visible by gentle lateral retraction of the cauda equina. A bulging intervertebral disc is not always apparent in surgery since the surgical positioning (flexion) can act to smooth out the dynamic bulging effect of the disc visible in extension radiography. If the annulus is ruptured, and nucleus pulposus is extruded into the spinal canal, a severe inflammatory response results in formation of perineuronal adhesions. These adhesions must be gently "teased" apart to remove the offending disc material. After sharp excision through the annulus, the dorsal annulus and nucleus are removed with rongeurs. Any remaining soft tissue or bony compression is removed with rongeurs or curettes. An autologous free fat graft is then placed in the laminectomy site before routine closure.[3, 27, 28] Neither instability nor laminectomy scarring is a complicating problem.

Postoperatively, the dogs receive a 2-week tapering course of prednisone. This may lessen formation of perineuronal adhesions. The dogs are limited to only short walks for a period of 2 months, and then gradually returned to full athletic activity. Although alleviation of pain is usually within a few days of surgery, it may take several weeks. Improvement in preexisting urinary incontinence can take weeks to months, and the incontinence may not fully resolve.[4]

Surgical management of lumbosacral stenosis in athletic dogs is generally rewarding and often curative, allowing full return to athletic function. The most important prognostic indicators for return to athletic function are the duration and severity of neurological signs and the presence or absence of a ruptured nucleus pulposus. The perineuronal adhesions resulting from the ruptured disc material may continue to "tether" nerve roots, producing varying degrees of postoperative pain. Residual pain occasionally occurring as stiffness after heavy exercise is usually managed easily with steroidal anti-inflammatory medication.

References

1. Chambers J: Degenerative lumbosacral stenosis in dogs. Vet Med Rep 1:166, 1989.
2. Evans H, Christensen G: Miller's Anatomy of the Dog. Philadelphia, WB Saunders Company, 1979.
3. Prata R: Diseases of the lumbosacral spine. *In* Bojrab M (ed): Disease Mechanisms in Small Animal Surgery, 2nd ed. Philadelphia, Lea & Febiger, p 987, 1993.
4. Chambers J, Selcer B, Oliver J: Results of treatment of degenerative lumbosacral stenosis in dogs by exploration and excision. Vet Compar Orthop Trauma 3:130, 1988.
5. Lenehan T: Canine cauda equina syndrome. Compend Cont Educ Pract Vet 5:941, 1983.
6. Naylor A: Factors in the development of the spinal stenosis syndrome. J Bone Joint Surg 61(B):306, 1979.
7. Paine K: Clinical features of lumbar spinal stenosis. Orthop Clin 115:77, 1976.
8. Snyder E, Mulfinger G, Lambert R: Claudication caused by compression of the cauda equina. Am J Surg 130:172, 1975.
9. Wilson C, Enhig G, Grollmus J: Neurogenic intermittent claudication. Clin Neurosurg. 18:62, 1971.
10. Palmer R, Chambers J: Canine lumbosacral diseases: I. Anatomy,

pathophysiology, and clinical presentation. Compend Cont Educ Pract Vet 13:61, 1991.
11. Slocum B, Devine T: L7-S1 fixation-fusion for treatment of cauda equina compression in the dog. JAVMA 188:31, 1986.
12. Hoerlein B: Intervertebral disk disease. *In* Oliver J, Hoerlein B, Mayhew I (eds): Veterinary Neurology. Philadelphia, WB Saunders Company, 1987, p 321.
13. Kirkaldy-Willis W, McIvors G: Lumbar spinal stenosis. Clin Orthop 115:2, 1976.
14. Lee C, Hansen H, Weiss A: Developmental lumbar spinal stenosis. Spine 3:246, 1978.
15. Verbiest H: A radicular syndrome from developmental narrowing of the lumbar vertebral canal. J Bone Joint Surg 36B:230, 1954.
16. Tarvin G, Prata R: Lumbosacral stenosis in dogs. JAVMA 177:154, 1980.
17. Morgan J, Bahr A, Franti C, et al: Lumbosacral transitional vertebrae as a predisposing cause of cauda equina syndrome in German shepherd dogs: 161 cases (1987–1990). JAVMA 202:1877, 1993.
18. Lang J, Hani H, Schawalder P: A sacral lesion resembling osteochondrosis in the German shepherd dog. Vet Radiol Ultrasound 33:69, 1993.
19. Selcer B, Chambers J, Schwensen K, et al: Epidurography as a diagnostic aid in canine lumbosacral compressive disease. Vet Compar Orthop Trauma 2:97, 1988.
20. de Haan J, Shelton S, Ackerman N: Magnetic resonance imaging in the diagnosis of degenerative lumbosacral stenosis in four dogs. Vet Surg 22:1, 1993.
21. Forristal R, Marsh H, Pay N: Magnetic resonance imaging and contrast CT of the lumbar spine. Spine 13:1049, 1988.
22. Schneiderman G, Flannigan B, Kingston S, et al: Magnetic resonance imaging in the diagnosis of disc degeneration: Correlation with discography. Spine 12:276, 1987.
23. Oliver J, Selcer R, Simpson S: Cauda equina compression from lumbosacral malformation and malarticulation. JAVMA 173:207, 1978.
24. Brodsky A: Post laminectomy and post fusion stenosis of the lumbar spine. Clin Orthop 115:130, 1976.
25. Rothman R, Simeone F: Lumbar disc disease. *In* Rothman R (ed): The Spine. Philadelphia, WB Saunders Company, 1975, p 447.
26. Shelby D: When to operate and what to operate upon. Orthop Clin N Am 14:577, 1983.
27. Gill G, Sakovich L, Thomson E: Pedicle fat grafts for prevention of scar formation after laminectomy: An experimental study in dogs. Spine 4:176, 1979.
28. Langenskild A, Kiviluoto O: Prevention of epidural scar formation after operations on the lumbar spine by means of free fat transplants: A preliminary report. Clin Orthop 115:92, 1976.
29. Trevor P, Martin R, Saunders G, et al: Healing characteristics of free and pedicle fat grafts after dorsal laminectomy and durotomy in dogs. Vet Surg 20:282, 1991.

CHAPTER 24

LONG-BONE FRACTURES IN THE RACING GREYHOUND

RICHARD D. EATON-WELLS \ JON F. DEE

The veterinarian managing long-bone fractures in the racing greyhound is faced with many difficult decisions. Our goal always should be to return a dog to winning form. However, there are numerous reasons why this may not be feasible. The dog may be too old, destined for retirement and/or breeding, or it may not be fast enough to warrant an expensive repair. In each case, the treatment regimen may be different.

Greyhound fractures are rarely caused by vehicular trauma. They are usually due to a collision with a stationary object or another dog or are a result of excessive intrinsic forces that produce failure of the skeletal system. High-energy fractures occur in the femur and tibia and are typically severely comminuted. Radius and ulnar fractures are characteristically transverse with a small comminuted fragment, and they may be open. Fractures of the humerus are usually spiral or comminuted with a single butterfly segment. The quality and worth of the dog, the bone involved, type of fracture, method of repair, implant used, timing of implant removal, and the postoperative rehabilitation must all be considered part of the fracture management.

Internal or external fixation of long-bone fractures is essential if the dog is to be returned to the race track in the shortest time possible. Open anatomical reduction and interfragmentary compression techniques with plates and screws provide excellent stability and result in rapid bone union and subsequent return to racing.[1] The use of a cancellous bone graft will decrease the healing time

in the more severely comminuted fractures. Rigid stability improves patient comfort and allows greater postoperative patient mobility, thereby maintaining muscle mass. However, implant removal is difficult and more disruptive.

Open or closed application of an external fixation device is less likely to result in anatomical fracture alignment, the repair is not as rigid, and there is more soft tissue irritation. However, the fracture can be progressively destabilized, and implant removal is not as difficult or traumatic to the dog. External fixation is the method of choice for the fixation of severely comminuted radius and ulna or tibial fractures.

FRACTURES OF THE SCAPULA

Scapular fractures are usually caused by collision with a stationary object or another greyhound. They are more common on rearing or spelling establishments. Fractures of the scapular spine or body with minimal fragment displacement can be managed with kennel rest with or without a body dressing. Those involving the scapular neck or scapular body fractures with marked displacement require open reduction and internal fixation if the dog is to be returned to racing. An appropriate length of veterinary cuttable plate, which may be applied "upside down," is fixed to the base of the spine (Fig. 24–1). The cortical bone of the scapula is very thin, and great

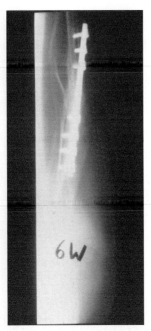

FIGURE 24-1. Comminuted scapular fracture repaired with a veterinary cuttable plate applied close to the junction of the scapular spine.

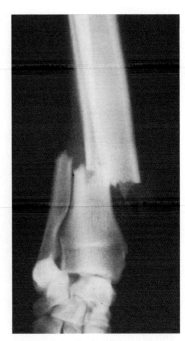

FIGURE 24-2. Characteristic distal radial and ulnar fracture in a mature racing dog.

care is necessary to ensure that the screw threads are not stripped. In our opinion these plates do not need to be removed.

The prognosis for return to racing in dogs with a nondisplaced fracture of the scapular spine is excellent. Conservatively treated, minimally displaced fractures of the scapular body have a good to excellent prognosis. Surgically repaired scapular body fractures carry a fair prognosis for eventual return to the track. Avulsion fractures of the supraglenoid tubercle carry a poor prognosis for successful return to racing.

FRACTURES OF THE HUMERUS

Humeral fractures can occur secondarily to a fall or collision and are more common in young, as opposed to racing, animals. We prefer to repair humeral fractures by open reduction and internal fixation using a plate and screws. Healing is usually uneventful. However, in young dogs, excessive callus production may occur because of the tendency of the thick periosteum to "strip" off the bone. This excessive callus formation may affect racing performance. Intramedullary (IM) pinning with or without cerclage wires or an external fixator for rotational stability will result in satisfactory fracture repair but lacks accurate anatomical reduction and hence adversely affects racing performance. The implants are removed as soon as radiographic evidence of union is evident.

FRACTURES OF THE RADIUS AND ULNA

Fractures of the radius and ulna that occur during racing classically involve the distal third of the diaphysis (Fig. 24-2). In younger dogs on rearing farms, the fracture is usually mid shaft. It can be repaired by application of a dynamic compression plate to the radius and a neutralization plate to the ulna. The anatomical reduction of the ulna prevents distraction of the styloid process and subsequent reduced flexion of the carpus. The application of plates to both bones means that smaller implants may be used.

In distal fractures the radial plate should be applied to the medial aspect of the bone to minimize soft tissue disruption. Plating the

dorsal aspect of the radius may cause apparent shortening of the extensor muscles and subsequent loss of carpal flexion. In addition, disuse of the extensor tendons may lead to disuse atrophy and adhesions to the radius. Historically, radial and ulnar fractures were repaired with a medially applied 4.5-mm radial plate and a laterally applied 2.7-mm ulnar plate.[3] It is now recommended that a 2.7-mm plate be applied medially to the radial fracture and a suitable small plate applied laterally to the ulna (Fig. 24-3).

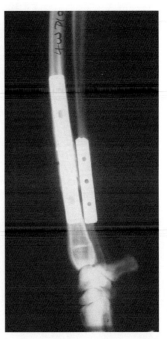

FIGURE 24-3. Radius and ulna fracture repaired with a 2.7-mm dynamic compression plate on the medial aspect of the radius and a veterinary cuttable plate on the lateral side of the ulna.

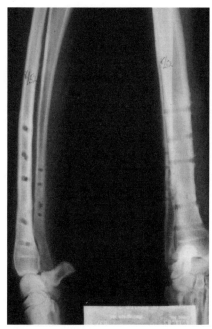

FIGURE 24–4. Plate removal at 8 weeks post surgery.

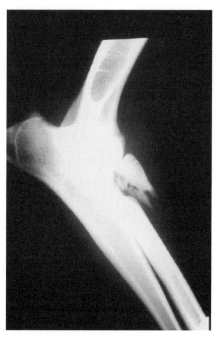

FIGURE 24–5. Intra-articular proximal radial fracture.

In proximal or mid-shaft fractures the plate should be applied to the dorsal aspect of the radius as the natural curve of the bone in the mid-shaft area results in distraction of the fracture when compression is applied to the medial side. The radial fracture alone may be repaired in those dogs that are to be retired from racing.

A modified Robert Jones dressing is applied to the limb for 5 to 7 days postoperatively* and the dog confined to leash exercise for the first 3 weeks. Thereafter, exercise in a small galloping yard is allowed. Radiographs of the fracture should be taken at 3-week intervals and the implants removed as soon as cortical continuity has become reestablished, usually between 6 and 8 weeks† (Fig. 24–4). After implant removal the leg is again supported with a padded dressing and a similar postoperative regimen is followed. If no problems are evident radiographically at 3 weeks the dog is allowed exercise in a small galloping yard for 3 more weeks. At that time, additional radiographs are taken. If healing is progressing well, free activity is allowed for 6 to 8 weeks before the dog is placed back into training. Thus, a layoff time of 4.5 to 5.5 months is anticipated prior to the dog's returning to competitive racing.

The use of external fixation devices by those skilled in their application will result in a satisfactory outcome. However, initial stability is less, and soft tissue irritation is greater, with this type of repair when compared to plate fixation. Areas of reduced tissue morbidity have been described.[4] Intra-articular fractures of the proximal radius can occur as a result of a fall. These fractures must be repaired by internal fixation and interfragmentary compression if the dog is to be returned to racing (Figs. 24–5 and 24–6). Fractures in dogs that are to be retired can be treated in a manner

that suits the veterinary surgeon, always bearing in mind the exuberant nature of the greyhound, its thin skin, and the often poor outcome if the limb is immobilized in a cast.

Stress fractures of the radius or ulna can be difficult to diagnose; the history and clinical signs are vague, and the area involved is small and located in an area not routinely palpated. They are treated by rest plus some form of physiotherapy. In our opinion, laser acupuncture appears to decrease the healing time.

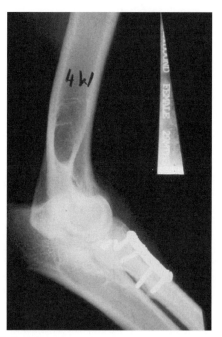

FIGURE 24–6. Four-week postoperative radiograph of fracture shown in Figure 24–5.

---

*Editor's note: With adequate internal fixation, bandage immobilization may not be warranted. Absence of a bandage facilitates early physical therapy efforts.

†Editor's note: Timing of implant removal is based on radiographic evidence of fracture repair, normal use of the leg, and clinical judgment. In general, early implant removal is favored in Australia with good results. Implant removal required general anesthesia, some surgical morbidity, and additional costs. In many cases the dog is transported to another location, making follow-up and implant removal more challenging.

FRACTURES OF THE FEMUR

In the young dog, femoral fractures are usually spiral with or without a butterfly fragment. They may be repaired by open reduction and stabilized with an IM pin and multiple cerclage wires. However, because of the boisterous nature of these pups, additional support with a half-Kirschner will reduce the likelihood of failure from overuse. The external fixator should be removed after 2 to 3 weeks and the fracture monitored radiographically so that the IM pin can be removed as soon as possible. Because of the irritation of the large muscle mass by the external fixator and the IM pins, exercise should be restricted until these pins have been removed. Open anatomical reduction and the application of a plate to these fractures will result in excellent repair. However, the morbidity associated with implant removal is significant.

The high-energy femoral fractures that occur in racing dogs are usually highly comminuted (Fig. 24–7). Open reduction and fixation with the use of lag screws and the application of a neutralization plate are necessary (Fig. 24–8). Severely comminuted fractures in which anatomical reduction is not possible may be repaired by the application of a buttress plate after the limb has been stretched to length (Figs. 24–9 and 24–10). A suction drain, placed adjacent to the femur, in the immediate postoperative period aids in removing excess tissue fluid. Since a large amount of hardware is placed during the repair of these fractures, implant removal is essential if the dog is to be returned to competitive racing. The fracture is evaluated radiographically every 3 weeks and the implant removed as soon as cortical continuity is reestablished. Decreased bone density due to late plate removal may require application of an external fixator apparatus to provide support in the immediate postoperative period. This device should be removed 10 to 14 days later. The prognosis for racing following repair of a spiral fracture in a young dog or an anatomically reduced comminuted fracture is fair. However, the results following the repair of comminuted fractures that were not anatomically reduced has been poor. Compression fractures of the distal femur should be treated by an appropriate technique to realign the articular surfaces (Figs. 24–11 and 24–12).

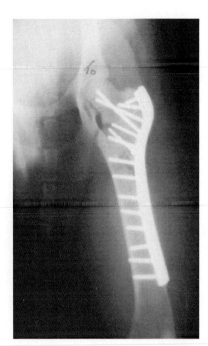

FIGURE 24–8. Postoperative repair showing anatomical reduction and interfragmentary compression plus a neutralization plate.

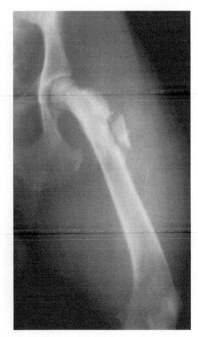

FIGURE 24–7. High-energy comminuted femoral fracture sustained while racing.

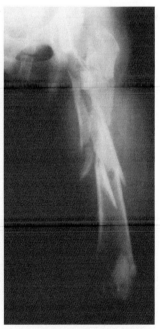

FIGURE 24–9. High-energy femoral fracture with too many pieces for anatomical reduction.

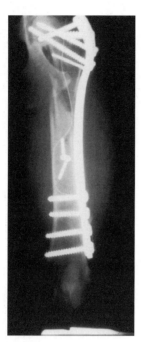

FIGURE 24–10. Postoperative radiograph showing leg distracted to length and buttress plate applied.

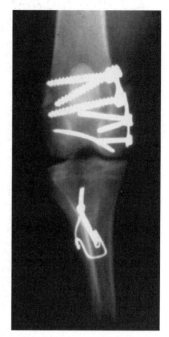

FIGURE 24–12. Postoperative radiograph showing tuberosity osteotomy, for exposure, and application of a multifragment (serpentine) plate as a buttress to maintain alignment.

TIBIAL FRACTURES

Tibial fractures may be divided into those occurring in immature dogs and those occurring in racing dogs.

Tibial Fractures in Immature Dogs. Tibial fractures in immature dogs include (1) malunion fractures resulting from early puppy trauma and (2) physeal injuries. Malunions are amenable to corrective osteotomy and stabilization with a type 1 external fixation device. Proximal tibial physeal injuries may involve a Salter type I fracture of the tibial tuberosity or Salter type II fracture of the proximal tibial plateau. Salter type I and II fractures of the distal tibial physis also occur.

Tibial tuberosity avulsions are replaced and maintained with two K-wires placed across the physis (Figs. 24–13 and 24–14). One of the pins should be removed at 10 days and the other at 3 weeks postoperatively in an attempt to reduce the incidence of premature

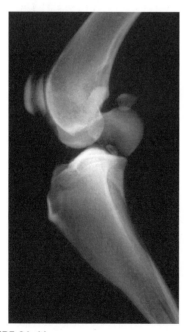

FIGURE 24–11. Distal femoral intra-articular fracture.

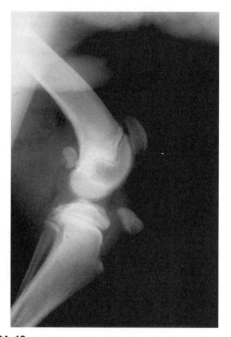

FIGURE 24–13. Avulsion of the tibial tuberosity due to the traction of the quadriceps.

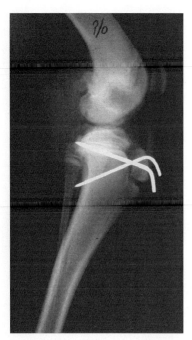

FIGURE 24-14. Postoperative radiograph showing reduction of avulsed tibial tuberosity with two K-wires.

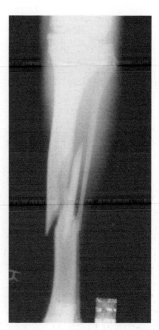

FIGURE 24-16. High-energy tibial shaft fracture in a racing dog.

closure of the physis and subsequent deformity of the proximal tibia (Fig. 24-15). Occasionally, premature closure of the physis will still occur. Lag screw or tension band techniques should be avoided. However, if the temptation to apply a compressive device cannot be resisted, it should be removed at 10 days. Long-standing avulsions of the tibial tuberosity require debridement of any accu-

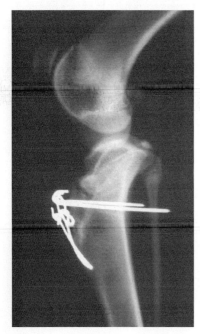

FIGURE 24-15. Premature closure of the tibial tuberosity due to compression of the growth plate by the repair. (Courtesy of Dr. Ken Johnson.)

mulated fibrous tissue filling the deficit prior to stabilizing the tubercle and stabilizing as before.

Proximal tibial plateau fractures may occur in combination with a tibial crest avulsion; they are usually displaced caudally and laterally. The fracture may include a piece of the proximal caudal metaphysis and is hence classified as a Salter type II. They are treated by open reduction and maintained by the placement of small K-wires in the medial and lateral condyles and the tibial tuberosity.

Fractures of the distal tibial and fibular physis should be managed by careful reduction and placement of small K-wires, then supported by a modified Robert Jones dressing. The distal tibial physis apparently is less prone to premature closure than the proximal physis, and the pins are often left in place. Occasionally, isolated injuries to the distal fibula growth plate may occur. Initial evaluation following acute injury may reveal some soft tissue swelling. Radiographs are not unusual at this time. As growth continues, lateral bowing of the distal limb may appear. The bowing is secondary to premature closure of the distal fibular growth plate and asynchronous growth of the tibia and fibula. The deformity often regresses spontaneously and the limb appears normal. However, the dog will usually have chronic problems with the lateral aspect of the stifle when training starts. This is thought to be due to distraction of the fibula head distally to accommodate the shortened fibula.

Tibial Shaft Fractures in Racing Dogs. The majority of tibial shaft fractures occur in older racing dogs and are usually comminuted. They are best managed by closed-reduction stabilization, using an external fixation (Figs. 24-16 and 24-17). Lag screws may be used in conjunction with an external device (Figs. 24-18 and 24-19) or with a neutralization plate (Figs. 24-20 and 24-21) to stabilize large fragments. Plates and screws are removed as soon as radiographic union is apparent. Early destabilization of the external device helps reduce the incidence of "stress protection" in the fractured bone. Safe corridors for insertion of external fixator pins at various levels have been described.[5]

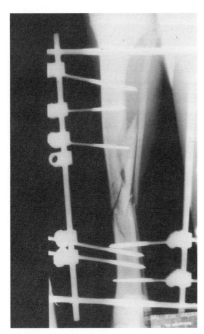

FIGURE 24–17. Postoperative radiograph showing closed reduction and application of an external fixation device.

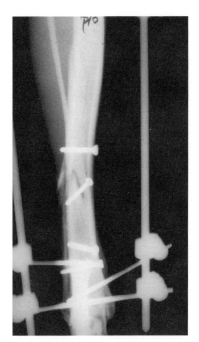

FIGURE 24–19. Postoperative radiograph of repair of a tibial fracture with external fixation and interfragmentary compression.

FRACTURES OF THE FIBULA

Two distinct types of fracture occur in the fibula. The first type is a proximal third fracture, under the belly of the anterior tibialis muscle (Fig. 24–22), associated with direct trauma, usually the result of the dog slipping on the kennel floor. Clinically the dog has a discrete area of pain directly over the injury. The diagnosis is confirmed radiographically. The dog is managed with cage rest and restricted exercise. The second type is a stress fracture of the distal third of the shaft, usually in the region of the saphenous vein (Fig. 24–23). These fractures respond well to cage rest; however, they may progress to delayed union or nonunion. If this nonunion is pain free it is not treated. Fractures that have progressed to painful nonunion may be treated by packing the fracture site with

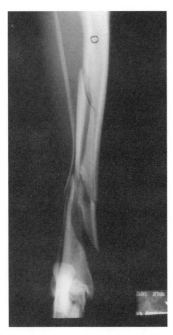

FIGURE 24–18. Tibial fracture with larger fragments suitable for repair by interfragmentary compression and an external fixator.

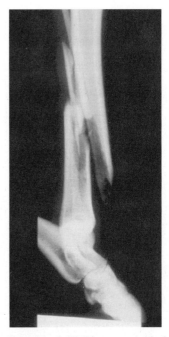

FIGURE 24–20. Comminuted tibial fracture suitable for application of a neutralization plate.

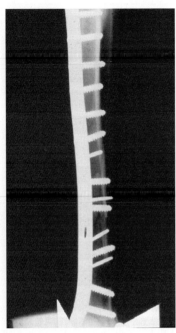

FIGURE 24–21. Use of a neutralization plate in a comminuted tibial fracture.

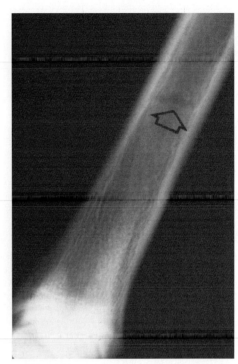

FIGURE 24–23. Stress fracture of distal fibula.

a cancellous bone graft.[6] They may also be treated by ostectomy of the nonunion site with a small pair of bone rongeurs. The prognosis for the return to racing of dogs with tibial or fibula fracture is excellent.

The overall prognosis for return to racing following long-bone fractures in the racing greyhound is improving. A few years ago few dogs that fractured a major long bone were returned to the track. Currently, dogs with fractures of the scapula, radius, and ulna and tibia are commonly returned to the track with an excellent prognosis for return to winning. Even some dogs with femoral fractures may return or progress to racing.

References

1. Eaton-Wells RD: Surgical management of long bone fractures and their prognosis for return to racing. Proc Aust Greyhound Vet Assoc 1990, pp 1–4.
2. Piermattei D: An Atlas of Surgical Approaches to the Bones and Joints of the Dog and Cat, 3rd ed. Philadelphia, WB Saunders Company, 1993.
3. Eaton-Wells RD: The specialized treatment of radius and ulna fractures in the racing greyhound utilizing interfragmentary and axial compression. Aust Vet Pract 13(4):175, 1983.
4. Marti JM, Miller A: Delimitation of safe corridors for the insertion of external fixator pins in the dog. II: Forelimb. J Small Anim Pract 35:78–85, 1994.
5. Marti JM, Miller A: Delimitation of safe corridors for the insertion of external fixator pins in the dog. I: Hindlimb. J. Small Anim Pract 35:16–23, 1994.
6. Boemo CM: Proc Aust Greyhound Vet Assoc 1992.

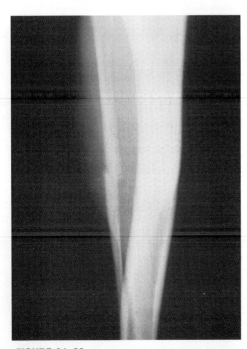

FIGURE 24–22. Traumatic proximal fibula fracture.

CHAPTER 25

ARTHROPATHIES

BRIAN S. BEALE

THE NORMAL JOINT

Anatomy

Diarthrodial joints are composed of two oscillating surfaces covered with hyaline cartilage and bathed in synovial fluid contained within a joint capsule. The joint capsule is composed of two layers, an outer fibrous layer and an inner synovial membrane (synovium). The outer fibrous layer is composed predominantly of collagen. It has a poor blood supply but contains numerous nerve endings associated with proprioception and pain sensation.[1] The synovial membrane is highly vascular and is composed of delicate areolar tissue covered by one or two layers of synoviocytes.[1] Two types of synoviocytes are recognized. Type A synoviocytes function as phagocytes in the joint.[1] Type B synoviocytes produce hyaluronic acid.[1] Synovial fluid is an ultrafiltrate of plasma to which has been added hyaluronic acid.[1] Synovial fluid is the primary source of nutrition for articular cartilage and the route by which metabolic by-products are eliminated from the joint. Synovial fluid also plays an important role in lubrication of synovial membrane tissues. Hyaluronic acid is thought to have both structural and regulatory functions.[2, 3] Proper viscosity of synovial fluid, which is important for joint lubrication, depends on the molecular weight and concentration of hyaluronic acid.[1] Hyaluronic acid also affects synovial fluid content by modifying the ultrafiltration of plasma at the level of the synovial endothelial cell. In addition, it may regulate synthesis of proteoglycans in articular cartilage.[2] The synovial fluid cell count is usually low (20 to 60 cells/μl) with small and large mononuclear cells predominating.[1]

Articular surfaces are covered with hyaline cartilage, which functions to provide nearly friction-free movement.[4] Hyaline cartilage is composed of an extracellular matrix within which are embedded proportionately few chondrocytes.[1, 4] Mature cartilage is 70 to 80 per cent water by weight.[1] Extracellular matrix is composed of two major components, type II collagen and proteoglycans, both of which impart viscoelastic properties, important for proper joint movement and lubrication. The function of chondrocytes is synthesis of collagen and proteoglycans, which compose the ground substance (matrix) of articular cartilage.[4] Chondrocyte death and destruction of hyaline cartilage lead to clinical signs of degenerative joint disease.

Physiology

Articular cartilage lives in relative isolation from other tissues, owing to its avascular, alymphatic, and aneural state.[4] As a result of its avascularity, cartilage alone cannot initiate an inflammatory response to injury. Because healing of vascularized tissues occurs in the presence of an inflammatory response, partial-thickness wounds of cartilage do not readily heal.[1, 4] On the other hand, full-thickness wounds heal by invasion of subchondral blood vessels with eventual formation of fibrocartilaginous repair tissue.[1, 4] Fibro-cartilage is composed of type I collagen, in contrast to type II found in hyaline cartilage, resulting in replacement tissue that does not tolerate stress and structural deformation as well as normal hyaline cartilage.[4] Mature chondrocytes have limited ability to undergo mitosis, and so are relatively ineffective in assisting healing of cartilage wounds.[4] On the other hand, immature chondrocytes in superficial and deep zones are capable of mitosis and may assist healing.[1, 4]

Because of the avascularity of cartilage in mature animals, it is almost exclusively dependent on synovial fluid for nutrition and removal of metabolic waste products.[1, 4] Nutrition of articular cartilage depends on nutrient content of synovial fluid and pumping action associated with joint motion.[1] Health of articular cartilage also depends on maintenance of proper lubrication. Joint lubrication can be divided into two components: lubrication of opposing surfaces of articular cartilage and lubrication of synovial membrane as it glides over non–weight-bearing articular cartilage.[5]

DISEASE OF THE JOINT

Joint disease in both the cat and dog can be divided into two general categories, inflammatory and noninflammatory. Noninflammatory joint disease includes degenerative joint disease. Degenerative joint disease is in fact associated with periods of mild inflammation, characterized by increased mononuclear cells within synovial fluid. Inflammatory joint disease includes infective and noninfective forms, both of which are characterized by a purulent synovial effusion. Noninfective inflammatory joint disease includes immune-mediated arthropathies, which are in turn divided into erosive and nonerosive forms.

NONINFLAMMATORY JOINT DISEASE

Degenerative Joint Disease

Pathophysiology

Degenerative joint disease (DJD) is best described as a progressive, self-perpetuating destructive process commonly affecting weight-bearing diarthrodial (synovial) joints. Characteristic pathological changes associated with this syndrome include progressive damage to articular cartilage and subchondral bone, joint capsular thickening, and production of periarticular new bone (osteophytosis). Two broad classes of DJD are primary (idiopathic) and secondary. Primary DJD is often referred to as *wear-and-tear joint disease,* owing to its insidious onset, which is thought to be due to long-term use combined with aging. Primary DJD is not associated with an identifiable predisposing cause; however, this may be due only to our inability to detect subtle abnormalities. Secondary DJD, identified more commonly, results from an initiating cause such as joint instability, trauma, osteochondral defects, or joint incongruity.

Any condition that directly or indirectly affects the normal homeostasis of the joint may result in secondary DJD, depending on the severity and duration of the insult.

Degenerative joint disease is characterized by changes in the structural components of articular cartilage. The initial change involves the loss of proteoglycans from the extracellular matrix because of increased destruction and decreased production.[6, 7] Proteoglycan content can be restored if catabolic processes cease and anabolic processes are stimulated. The breakdown and loss of collagen and chondrocytes occur as disease progresses, leading to irreversible change.

Although DJD is usually categorized as a noninflammatory joint disease, low-grade inflammation plays an important role in its pathogenesis.[8] Inflammation of the synovial membrane leads to extravasation of inflammatory cells, primarily mononuclear cells, from synovial capillaries to synovial fluid. Leukocytes and synoviocytes release a variety of inflammatory mediators, including prostaglandins, leukotrienes, neutral metalloproteinases, serine proteases, oxygen-derived free radicals, lysosomal enzymes (proteases, glycosidases, and collagenases), oncoproteins, interleukins, tumor necrosis factor, and other cytokines. Prostaglandins and leukotrienes cause pain, increased vascular permeability, and vasodilation and are chemotactic.[9] Interleukin-1 and tumor necrosis factor function as cytokines to increase production of prostaglandins and neutral metalloproteinases (stromelysin and collagenase).[18, 19] Oncoproteins, c-Fos and c-Myc, are produced after induction by cytokines; oncoproteins appear necessary for maximal stimulation of cells to produce neutral metalloproteinases such as stromelysin.[19] The neutral metalloproteinase stromelysin is thought to be the primary factor responsible for proteoglycan degradation in degenerative cartilage.[6, 7, 13, 16, 18, 20–23] Collagenase also plays a role in the long-term destruction of cartilage in DJD.[7, 10, 17, 21, 23, 24] Stromelysin and collagenase are secreted in a latent state by synoviocytes and chondrocytes and are subsequently activated by serine proteases and metalloproteinases.[6, 8, 17, 18, 25–27] Prostaglandins, oxygen-derived free radicals, interleukins, and tumor necrosis factor also lower the proteoglycan content of cartilage by decreasing proteoglycan synthesis and increasing proteoglycan degradation.[7, 8, 11, 14, 27, 28] Viscosity of synovial fluid decreases because of breakdown and dilution of hyaluronic acid by hyaluronidase, oxygen-derived free radicals, and influx of plasma components.[28, 29]

Treatment

There are several basic tenets of treatment that apply to both idiopathic and secondary DJD: Relieve pain and discomfort, improve joint function and minimize progression of disease. Treatment may include weight loss, exercise restriction, pharmacological therapy, or surgery (Fig. 25–1). In cases of secondary DJD the underlying cause must be identified in an attempt to minimize the long-term effects. This may imply removal of an osteochondral fragment or stabilization of a stifle after rupture of a cranial cruciate ligament.

Weight loss, when indicated, will lessen clinical signs of DJD as a result of decreased forces being placed on abnormal joint surfaces. Weight reduction before surgery will reduce postoperative

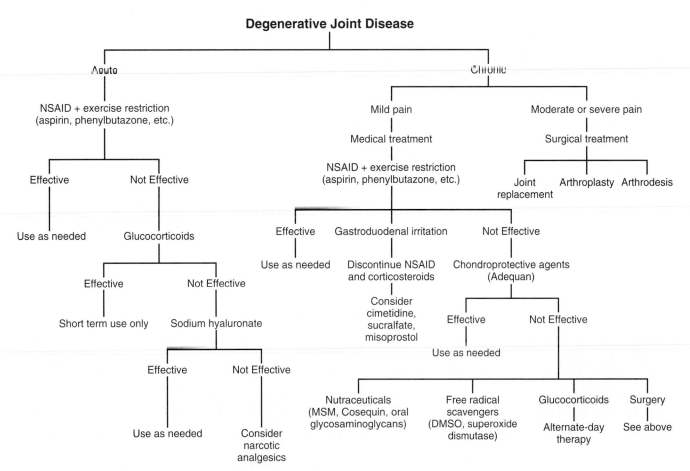

FIGURE 25–1. Treatment of degenerative joint disease.

Table 25–1. Treatment of Degenerative Joint Disease in Dogs

Drug	Dose	Frequency	Side Effects
NSAIDs			
Aspirin	10–25 mg/kg, PO	q 12 hr	Gastric irritation, platelet inhibition
Phenylbutazone	3.0–7.0 mg/kg, PO	q 8 hr	Gastric irritation, platelet inhibition
Carprofen	2.2 mg/kg, PO	q 12 hr	Idiosyncratic hepatotoxicity
Chondroprotectants			
Glycosaminoglycan polysulfate (Adequan)	4.4 mg/kg, IM	q 4–5 days, 8 treatments	Inhibition of hemostasis, neutrophils and complement
Pentosan polysulfate (Cartrophen)	3.0 mg/kg, IM or SQ	q 7 days, 4 treatments	Inhibition of hemostasis
Sodium hyaluronate	7.0 mg, IA	q 7 days	None known
Free radical scavengers			
DMSO	topical, prn	q 12 hr	Garlic odor
Superoxide dismutase	5.0 mg, SC	q 24 hr for 6 days then q 48 hr for 8 days	None known
Nutraceuticals			
Glucosamine (Cosequin)	See manufacturer recommendation, PO	q 24 hr	None known
Glycosaminoglycans	See manufacturer recommendation, PO	q 24 hr	None known
Methyl 1-sulfonyl-methane (MSM)	See manufacturer recommendation, PO	q 24 hr	None known

stress placed on the surgical repair. Enforced rest and restricted activity provide an opportunity for transient episodes of inflammation to resolve, in addition to decreasing stress placed on the repair.

Pharmacological management of DJD includes a wide variety of pharmaceuticals, most of which have gained popularity based on use in humans (Table 25–1). The objectives of phamacological therapy are to reduce inflammation when present, alleviate pain, and improve function. Consideration should be given to drugs that inhibit the release or activity of prostaglandins, leukotrienes, neutral metalloproteases (stromelysin, collagenase), serine proteases, oncoproteins, interleukins, and tumor necrosis factor. Nonsteroidal anti-inflammatory drugs and glucocorticoid drugs are common examples. Other drugs, such as the chondroprotective agents, not only inhibit mediators of inflammation within the joint, but also may stimulate metabolic activity of synoviocytes and chondrocytes.[30] Examples of these drugs include glycosaminoglycan polysulfate ester, pentosan polysulfate, and hyaluronic acid. Nutritional supplements have also been proposed as an aid to treatment of DJD.

Nonsteroidal Anti-inflammatory Drugs. Nonsteroidal anti-inflammatory drugs (NSAIDs) are widely used as a means of reducing prostaglandin synthesis (primarily PGE_2) through inhibition of cyclooxygenase. Aspirin and phenylbutazone are the most commonly used agents in dogs. In dogs, aspirin is ideally administered with food at a dose of 25 mg/kg body weight every 8 hours.[31] Phenylbutazone can be given at a dosage of 10 to 22 mg/kg body weight divided three times a day in dogs.[32, 33] When the higher dose is selected it is decreased after 48 hours to the lowest effective level, not to exceed a total daily dosage of 800 mg regardless of patient body weight.[34] Although NSAIDs are used effectively to control pain and inflammation that may accompany DJD, some of these drugs have been shown to promote progressive degeneration of cartilage by inhibiting proteoglycan synthesis.[8, 34–36] Because of the potential for gastric ulceration, NSAIDs should be used cautiously in dogs with orthopedic problems.[37] Although many references have suggested dosages for naproxen, piroxicam, flunixin meglumine, and ibuprofen,[38–40] they appear to have increased ulcerogenic potential as compared with aspirin; therefore, their use is discouraged. Carprofen is a recently developed NSAID that has been found to relieve clinical signs of DJD in dogs, while causing less gastrointestinal side effects.[41] Carprofen is given at a dose of 2.2 mg/kg, orally, every 12 hours. A reversible, idiosyncratic, hepatotoxic reaction has been reported in Labrador retriever dogs

given carprofen, but this side effect is considered to be rare. Acetaminophen has analgesic and antipyretic properties, but little anti-inflammatory effect.[42] Its use for treatment of DJD in the dog is underwhelming because of its decreased anti-inflammatory properties. In addition, acetaminophen can be toxic in the dog, leading to cyanosis, anemia, hemoglobinuria, icterus, and hepatic necrosis.[43]

Glucocorticoids. Glucocorticoids have been traditionally used to treat DJD only when other more conventional means of therapy have been ineffective. Glucocorticoids effectively reduce inflammation by inhibiting chemotaxis of neutrophils, decreasing microvasculature permeability, inhibiting cyclooxygenase and thereby decreasing prostaglandin production, inhibiting lipoxygenase and thereby decreasing leukotriene production, inhibition of interleukin-1 release, inhibition of oxygen-free radical generation, inhibition of metalloproteinases, and stabilization of lysosomal membranes.[8, 12, 31, 44–47] Glucocorticoids have been shown to prevent the formation of osteophytes and cartilage lesions in models of DJD.[48] The use of glucocorticoids for treatment of DJD would appear to be ideal because of their generalized inhibition of inflammatory mediators and cytokines; however, long-term use of these drugs has been found to delay healing and initiate damage to articular cartilage.[48] Prednisone is given orally at an initial dose of 1 to 2 mg/kg once daily in dogs and 4 mg/kg once daily in cats.[32] The potential systemic side effects of glucocorticoids are well documented[49]; therefore, low-dose (0.5 to 2.0 mg/kg in dogs and 2 to 4 mg/kg in cats) alternate-day therapy is the goal if long-term therapy is instituted.[32] Intra-articular injection of 5 mg triamcinolone hexacetonide in dogs suggested a protective effect not only under prophylactic but also under therapeutic conditions in an experimental DJD model.[19] The sparing effect on cartilage appeared to be due to decreased production of stromelysin, interleukin-1, and oncoproteins.[19] At best, treatment of DJD with corticosteroids is controversial. This class of drugs may become more routinely used in the future if protocols can be developed that take advantage of their chondroprotective effects, while eliminating their systemic catabolic effects.

Free-Radical Scavengers. Another class of drugs effective in reducing inflammation are the free radical scavengers such as dimethyl sulfoxide (DMSO) and superoxide dismutase. Oxygen-derived free radicals (superoxide, hydrogen peroxide, hydroxyl radical) are thought to play a role in the progression of DJD through their ability to damage cells by oxidative injury. Oxidative injury leads to depolymerization of hyaluronic acid, destruction of collagen, and decreased production of proteoglycans.[9, 29, 31]

DMSO, which is used as a topical agent when treating musculoskeletal problems, has the ability to penetrate most tissues, including skin.[9, 31] Topical application of 20 ml/day of a medical grade DMSO (70 to 90 per cent solution) every 6 to 8 hours for up to 14 days has been recommended to treat local inflammation.[50] Side effects with topical use are minimal, but impart a garlic odor to the breath.[31]

Superoxide dismutase is an endogenous antioxidant present in mammalian cells that inhibits production of oxygen free radicals. This enzyme acts to stabilize phagocyte cell membranes and lysosomes, and reduce superoxide radical levels in tissues, with a resultant decrease in free radical generation.[9, 29, 31] The efficacy of exogenous superoxide dismutase is unknown. One author recommends giving 5 mg subcutaneously daily for 6 days in the dog, followed by alternate-day therapy for 8 days.[9] The manufacturer recommends giving 2.5 mg/kg subcutaneously five times a week for 2 weeks for treatment of spondylitis or disc disease.

Chondroprotective Agents. These agents are emerging as a new class of drugs used to slow progression of and treat chronic DJD. These drugs not only should be anti-inflammatory but also should support anabolic (repair) processes in cartilage, bone, and synovium essential for normalization of joint function.[30] This class of drugs includes the glycosaminoglycans. Examples of these drugs are glycosaminoglycan polysulfate ester, pentosan polysulfate, and sodium hyaluronate.

A drug (Adequan) that is gaining popularity for use in dogs is a glycosaminoglycan polysulfate ester (GAGPS). It is purported to be both chondroprotective and chondrostimulatory. Chondroprotec-

tion is achieved because of the inhibition of various destructive enzymes and prostaglandins associated with synovitis and DJD (Fig. 25–2). GAGPS has been found to inhibit neutral metalloproteinases (stromelysin, collagenase, elastase), serine proteases, hyaluronidase, and a variety of lysosomal enzymes.[8, 23, 30, 51–53] The drug has also been found to inhibit PGE$_2$ synthesis, generation of oxygen-derived free radicals, and the complement cascade.[53–56] Protection of articular cartilage has also been seen on gross and histological examination in numerous experimental studies.[23, 57–59] GAGPS has been found to stimulate anabolic activity in synoviocytes and chondrocytes. Chondrostimulatory effects are characterized by increased synoviocyte secretion of hyaluronate and enhanced proteoglycan, hyaluronate, and collagen production by articular chondrocytes.[43, 52, 60–65] GAGPS also has anticoagulant and fibrinolytic properties that facilitate clearing of thrombotic emboli deposited in the subchondral and synovial blood vessels.[30] While the majority of experimental and clinical studies support the premise that GAGPS possesses properties of chondroprotection and chondrostimulation, some studies have found GAGPS either to have no beneficial effect or to actually have a detrimental effect on cartilage metabolism.[23, 66]

A recent clinical study in hip dysplastic dogs found the greatest improvement in orthopedic scores at a dose of 4.4 mg/kg (2 mg/pound) given intramuscularly every 3 to 5 days for 8 injections.[67] The improvement in orthopedic score was not statistically significant, however. Another study found twice weekly intramuscular administration of 5 mg/kg GAGPS from 6 weeks to 8 months of age in growing pups that were susceptible to hip dysplasia resulted in less coxofemoral subluxation.[68] The longevity of relief provided by GAGPS is unknown. Most studies have evaluated its effect in

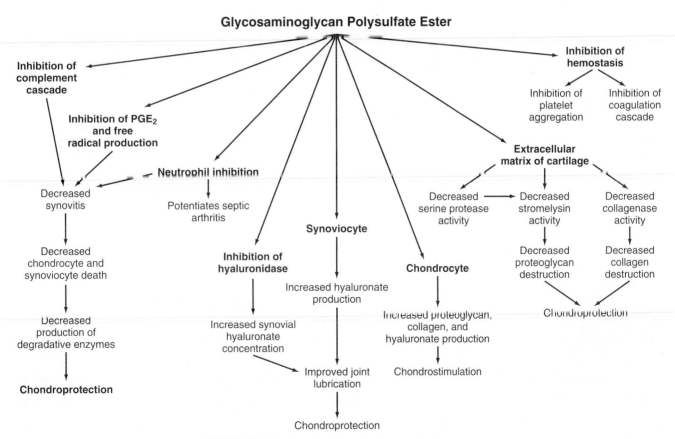

FIGURE 25–2. Actions of glycosaminoglycan polysulfate ester.

the short term only. Anecdotal reports of duration of amelioration of clinical signs range from days to months. It is also not known whether the complete series of injections are needed once clinical signs return or whether a shorter regimen would suffice.

Side effects of GAGPS in dogs include short-term inhibition of the intrinsic coagulation cascade as well as inhibition of platelet aggregation when given 5 mg/kg or 25 mg/kg intramuscularly.[69] Also, GAGPS has been found to inhibit neutrophils and complement, which may predispose to infections, especially when injected intra-articularly under contaminated conditions.[55] GAGPS has been reported to cause sensitization reactions in humans, but this has not been reported in the dog.[70, 71]

Pentosan polysulfate (SP54, Cartrophen-Vet) is a polysaccharide sulfate ester (mean molecular weight of 6000 daltons) prepared semisynthetically from beech hemicellulose.[8, 31] The drug is approved for use in dogs and horses in Australia and is used in a similar manner to GAGPS for relieving clinical symptoms of DJD.[31] Pentosan polysulfate can be given intra-articularly, intramuscularly, subcutaneously, or orally. The recommended dosage for intra-articular use is 5 to 10 mg per joint weekly, as necessary.[31] The intramuscular or subcutaneous dosage in dogs is 3 mg/kg once weekly for 4 weeks; this regimen can be repeated as necessary.[31, 72] A relatively recent double-blind study evaluating the efficacy of this product for treatment of DJD in the dog found this dose to be ideal.[72] An oral preparation of pentosan polysulfate is available and appears to have some anecdotal success.[73]

Sodium hyaluronate has been touted to promote joint lubrication, increase endogenous production of hyaluronate, decrease prostaglandin production, scavenge free radicals, inhibit migration of inflammatory cells, decrease synovial membrane permeability, protect and promote healing of articular cartilage, and reduce joint stiffness and adhesion formation between tendon and tendon sheaths.[74, 75] The molecule lines the synovial membrane and acts like a sieve, excluding bacteria and inflammatory cells from reaching the synovial compartment by steric hindrance.[28, 74] The actions of exogenous and endogenous hyaluronate appear to be similar.[75] As of this writing, sodium hyaluronate is generally recommended for mild to moderate synovitis and capsulitis, rather than DJD.[75] The drug appears to have a chondroprotective effect, but it is unclear whether this is a direct effect or as a result of its effect on the articular soft tissues.[69, 75, 76] Sodium hyaluronate is administered intra-articularly or intravenously. Hyaluronate was used in experimental dogs at a dose of 7 mg per joint, intra-articularly, once weekly with success in slowing DJD.[1, 52]

Nutraceuticals. A new class of "oral drugs" that is claimed to be effective in treating DJD has flooded the market. These preparations are actually promoted as nutritional supplements, rather than pharmaceuticals. Manufacturers have labeled these products as nutraceuticals. The obvious advantage to this is the ability to avoid expensive toxicity and efficacy studies required by the FDA for approval of pharmaceuticals. Unfortunately, most of these products have little controlled experimental or clinical research in dogs to substantiate manufacturer claims. As additional studies are performed in the future, some of these products may warrant classification as chondroprotective compounds.

Oral glycosaminoglycan products are currently being marketed, including Ultraflex and Pet Flex. These products reportedly contain purified chondroitin sulfates. Anecdotal success with these products has been purported; however, no controlled studies have been performed in the dog to substantiate these claims. Likewise, data are not available describing the absorption and activity following absorption of these products in dogs. Up to 40 per cent absorption of dietary chondroitin sulfates has been reported in mice. Dosages vary between products; therefore manufacturer recommendations should be followed.

Glyco-Flex is a food supplement containing a mixture of proteins, glycosaminoglycans, amino acids, minerals, enzymes, and vitamins. The source of this product is the *Perna canilicus* mussel, alfalfa, and brewers' yeast. The product is promoted for use in small animals for management of DJD and is available only through veterinarians.

Another product (Cosequin) is marketed as a glycosaminoglycan enhancer, capable of providing raw materials needed for the synthesis of endogenous synovial fluid and extracellular matrix of cartilage. Cosequin contains glucosamine, which has been described as the building-block of the matrix of articular cartilage.[77] It also has been described as a preferential substrate and stimulant of proteoglycan biosynthesis, including hyaluronic acid and chondroitin sulfate.[77, 78] Cosequin also contains chondroitin sulfate, mixed glycosaminoglycans, and manganese ascorbate for the purpose of promoting glycosaminoglycan production.[79] Orally administered glucosamine sulfate has been associated with relief of clinical signs of DJD and chondroprotection in clinical and experimental studies in man.[77, 80-82] Although glucosamine has a slower onset of relief of clinical signs associated with DJD as compared to ibuprofen, two clinical trials found it to have equal long-term efficacy.[83, 84] The product is available with recommended doses in capsules for small animals and powder for horses. Glucosamine has been found to be 95 per cent absorbable and to have 30 per cent long-term retention in musculoskeletal tissues when given orally.[85, 86] Numerous experimental and clinical studies are in progress to assess this product's efficacy in the dog.

Methyl-sulfonyl-methane (MSM) is a white, crystalline, water-soluble, odorless, and tasteless compound that is a derivative of DMSO.[87, 88] MSM is reported to supply bioavailable sulfur, a macronutrient required by animals and plants for a variety of uses, including hair, skin, connective tissue, enzymes, hormones, and immunoglobulins.[87] MSM has been suggested as an agent for management of pain and inflammation and as an antioxidant. Radiolabeled sulfur from MSM has been found in amino acids (methionine and cysteine) of proteins in guinea pigs following experimental oral administration.[87] The rationale behind its use, according to the manufacturer and others, is the possibility of a dietary sulfur deficiency.[87, 88] The product (MSM, Flex-A-Gan 2) is available with recommended doses in capsules and powder form for use in small and large animals. Similar to most other nutraceuticals, there are no controlled experimental or clinical studies available to support the use of this product for management of DJD in dogs.

INFLAMMATORY JOINT DISEASE

Inflammatory joint diseases can be categorized into noninfectious and infectious types. Noninfectious types are generally associated with polyarthritis, occurring as a result of an immune-mediated process not directly attributable to a local infectious agent. Infectious arthritis, on the other hand, is associated with an infectious agent that localizes in the joint, causing inflammation.

Noninfectious (Immune-Mediated) Arthritis

Immune-mediated arthritis is commonly divided into nonerosive and erosive forms. Nonerosive immune-mediated arthropathies include idiopathic polyarthritis, systemic lupus erythematosus (SLE, lupus polyarthritis), polyarthritis associated with chronic disease (chronic infectious, neoplastic, or enteropathic disease), polyarthritis-polymyositis syndrome, polyarthritis-meningitis syndrome, polyarteritis nodosa, familial renal amyloidosis in Chinese Shar Pei dogs, lymphocytic-plasmacytic synovitis, villonodular synovitis, and juvenile-onset polyarthritis of Akitas. Erosive immune-mediated arthropathies include rheumatoid arthritis (RA) and erosive polyarthritis of greyhounds (EPG).

Nonerosive Arthritides

These diseases are often cyclic and may appear to respond to antibiotic therapy when in actuality the disease may be spontaneously undergoing remission. Radiographic changes typical of this group of diseases include periarticular swelling, joint effusions, and occasional periosteal reaction. Unlike erosive arthritides, articular cartilage destruction is extremely uncommon with nonerosive forms.

Idiopathic Polyarthritis

Pathophysiology. Idiopathic polyarthritis is the most common form of immune-mediated, nonerosive polyarthritis in the dog.[39] The disease affects both large and small breeds but is more common in the former. Breeds that appear to be overrepresented include German shepherds, Doberman pinschers, retrievers, spaniels, pointers, toy poodles, Lhasa apsos, Yorkshire terriers, and Chihuahuas.[3] Clinical signs include lameness affecting one or more limbs, swelling of joints, fever, lethargy, anorexia, and stiffness. This condition can affect all joints but is most commonly seen in the carpus and tarsus. When the disease is monoarticular, it most frequently affects the elbow.[3] Radiographic changes are limited to joint capsular distention and occasionally osteophytosis in prolonged or recurrent cases. A diagnosis is usually made based on clinical signs, synovial fluid analysis, and exclusion of other diseases causing polyarthritis. Synovial fluid cell counts are 5000 to 100,000/μl with the predominant cell being the neutrophil.[3] Synovial fluid cultures are negative for bacteria, *Mycoplasma,* and *Chlamydia.* Rickettsial titers (*Ehrlichia, Borellia, Rickettsia*) should not be indicative of active infection. The patient should also have a negative antinuclear antibody and rheumatoid factor titer.

The cause of the disease is unknown, but it is associated with deposition of immune complexes in the synovial membrane resulting in synovitis. Synovial hypertrophy and hyperplasia are associated with a mononuclear cell infiltrate. Neutrophils are also seen in the synovial tissues as they migrate from synovial capillaries to the synovial fluid.

Treatment. Glucocorticoids are usually used for the initial treatment of idiopathic polyarthritis. If response is poor, combination chemotherapy using glucocorticoids and cytotoxic drugs is started. Complete remission is usually achieved; however, a recurrence rate of 30 to 50 per cent can be expected once therapy is discontinued.[3] Glucocorticoid therapy is usually initiated with prednisone at 1.5 to 2.0 mg/kg orally, twice daily for 10 to 14 days (dexamethasone can be substituted at one-fifth this daily dosage).[3] If synovial fluid cell counts return below 4000/μl and mononuclear cells predominate, the dose of prednisone can be slowly tapered over several weeks to 1.0 mg/kg orally, every other day.[3] If clinical signs persist or synovial fluid analysis is abnormal, cytotoxic drugs should be started with prednisone. If clinical signs do not recur with alternate-day glucocorticoid therapy for 2 to 3 months, the drug can be discontinued.[3]

Combination chemotherapy is used if initial glucocorticoid therapy is unsuccessful. Cytotoxic drugs are used in combination with glucocorticoids because of their synergistic effect.[3] The most commonly used cytotoxic drugs include cyclophosphamide and the thiopurines, azathioprine and 6-mercaptopurine. Cyclophosphamide is given at 2.5 mg/kg for dogs less than 10 kg, 2.0 mg/kg for dogs between 10 and 25 kg, and 1.75 mg/kg for dogs heavier than 50 kg.[3] This dosage is given orally, once daily for 4 consecutive days of each week. Prednisone is also given as described above, although some clinicians reduce the total daily dose by half.[3] If either azathioprine or 6-mercaptopurine is used, it is given at 2.0 mg/kg

orally for 14 to 21 days, then every other day. Prednisone is given as with cyclophosphamide; however, it is given on alternating days with the thiopurine.[3] Combination chemotherapy will usually induce remission within 2 to 16 weeks.[3] Cytotoxic drugs are discontinued 1 to 3 months after remission is achieved; this is determined by resolution of clinical signs and confirmation of a normal synovial fluid analysis.[3] Alternate-day glucocorticoid therapy (prednisone, 1.0 mg/kg orally) is generally successful in maintaining remission. If clinical signs or synovial neutrophilia recurs, long-term cytotoxic drug therapy may be necessary.[3] If clinical signs do not recur while the patient is receiving alternate-day glucocorticoid therapy for 2 to 3 months, the drug can be discontinued. If clinical signs recur when glucocorticoids are discontinued, treatment should be extended; if remission does not ensue, long-term cytotoxic drug therapy may be necessary.

Long-term administration of glucocorticoids can lead to iatrogenic hyperadrenocorticism-like disease or iatrogenic secondary hypoadrenocorticism. To reduce the chance of developing these side effects, glucocorticoids should be given every other day or discontinued if possible. It is also prudent to slowly reduce the dose over several weeks if therapy has been prolonged (over 2 weeks). Administration of cytotoxic drugs frequently induces bone marrow suppression. Complete blood counts should be monitored for reductions in the leukocyte count to below 6000/μl and platelet count to below 125,000/μl. If this occurs the dose of the cytotoxic drug should be reduced by one-fourth.[3] If the leukocyte count falls below 4000/μl and platelet count below 100,000/μl, cytotoxic drugs should be discontinued for 1 week, then reinstituted at three-fourths the normal dose when the leukocyte and platelet counts return to normal.[3] The thiopurines (2 to 6 weeks) generally cause bone marrow suppression earlier than cyclophosphamide (several months).[3] Use of cyclophosphamide should be limited to less than 4 months because of the possibility of developing sterile hemorrhagic cystitis, which results in hematuria and dysuria.[3] If these symptoms occur, the drug should be discontinued immediately. One of the thiopurine drugs can be substituted for cyclophosphamide if therapy is required for greater than 4 months or if cystitis occurs.[3]

Systemic Lupus Erythematosus

Pathophysiology. Canine systemic lupus erythematosus (SLE) affects many organ systems, including the hematopoietic, renal, articular, neuromuscular, and the integumentary.[3] Articular and dermal manifestations of SLE are seen most commonly in the dog.[3] Classic hematological abnormalities such as thrombocytopenia and hematolytic anemia are seen in only 10 to 20 per cent of all cases of SLE.[3] A thorough discussion of the pathophysiology of SLE can be found elsewhere.[3, 4]

The age of onset of canine SLE ranges from 2 months to 12 years.[4] In contrast to RA, SLE has a tendency to affect larger-breed dogs. Breeds reported more often include collies, German shepherds, poodles, beagles, and Shetland sheepdogs.[4] Unlike human SLE, for which a familial tendency is recognized, no hereditary component has been observed in canine SLE.[4] Early in the course of the disease, dogs typically have nonspecific signs such as lethargy, anorexia, and occasionally pyrexia. These bouts of malaise tend to last several days, until they spontaneously regress. Clinical signs, however, may recur several weeks to months later.[4] As the disease progresses, characteristic clinical signs of SLE appear. Polyarthritis, which is found in 60 per cent of canine cases, is characterized by multiple joint effusions, periarticular fibrosis, and decreased range of motion. In advanced states if the disease goes untreated, joint instability may ensue, leading to DJD.

Typical radiographic changes include joint capsular effusion, periarticular soft tissue swelling, and periosteal bone production; DJD ensues in the later course of the disease, associated with apparent joint instability and chronic synovitis.[4]

Specific criteria have been established for diagnosis of both human and canine SLE. Both serological and clinical evidence of SLE must be present.[4] Serological abnormalities include either a positive LE preparation or a positive antinuclear antibody (ANA) test.

Findings of synovial fluid analysis of canine SLE patients do not consistently differ from those of other immune-mediated arthropathies. Synovial leukocyte counts vary widely depending on the stage of disease. Canine synovial leukocyte counts have been reported to range from 6000 to 371,000/μl (mean 74,500/μl).[89] The predominant cell type is usually the neutrophil, but small and large mononuclear cells may represent the major cell type in the early or recovery phase.

The pathological changes that may be seen with canine SLE include polyarthritis, dermatitis, myositis, glomerulonephritis, thickening of serosal membranes, and occasionally hypoplastic bone marrow.[2] Pathological lesions associated with these tissues are typical of immune complex disease. The antigen stimulating the formation of immune complexes is nucleic acid.[3] Nearly 80 per cent of dogs affected with SLE show synovial tissue changes characterized by synoviocytic proliferation and fibrous villous synovitis.[2] The subsynoviocytic tissues become infiltrated with plasma cells, monocytes, and neutrophils.[2] Perivascular cuffing or inflammatory cells may also been seen in deeper regions of subsynoviocytic tissues.[2] In contrast to RA, pannus and erosion of articular cartilage usually do not occur except in later stages of uncontrolled SLE. Articular erosion associated with chronic SLE is probably a result of chronic joint instability rather than immune complex disease, as in RA arthritis. It is beyond the scope of this chapter to discuss pathological findings in other organs affected by canine SLE, but these changes are well described in other reports.[1, 2, 5]

Treatment. The treatment of choice of canine SLE is initially immunosuppressive treatment with prednisone or prednisolone. Patients that do not respond to prednisolone treatment alone should be switched to a combined chemotherapy protocol utilizing cytotoxic drugs such as cyclophosphamide or azathioprine. Treatment protocols are similar to that described under treatment of idiopathic polyarthritis. Many cases of canine SLE respond favorably, resulting in remission for periods of weeks to months without any maintenance therapy. Unfortunately, recurrence of the disease usually leads eventually to organ failure and death.

Polyarthritis Associated with Chronic Disease

Pathophysiology. Polyarthritis associated with chronic infectious, gastrointestinal, or neoplastic disease has been recognized in both human and canines. This syndrome is sometimes referred to as reactive arthritis or postinfectious arthritis in human medicine. Polyarthritis in canine patients has been associated with the presence of concurrent gastrointestinal disease, neoplasia, urinary tract infection, periodontitis, bacterial endocarditis, heartworm disease, pyometra, chronic otitis media or externa, fungal infections, and chronic actinomyces infections.[1, 4]

No specific breed, age, or sex predilection has been observed in canines.[2] Clinical signs consist of those associated with the primary disease process plus pain and lameness in one or more joints. Typically, dogs become anorectic, depressed, and pyrexic during bouts of polyarthritis. Joint swelling and pain occur most frequently in distal joints of the extremities, especially tarsal and carpal joints.[3] Episodes of lameness may spontaneously regress, only to recur days to weeks later if the primary disease is not resolved. Radiographic changes are indistinguishable from those of SLE and other nonerosive immune-mediated arthropathies. Soft tissue changes such as joint capsular distention secondary to synovial effusion and periarticular swelling are typically the only radiographic changes. In chronic cases, degenerative joint disease and osteophytosis may ensue.

Clinicopathological changes are variable, depending on the primary disease. Changes in the hemogram are consistent with a nonspecific inflammatory reaction, including neutrophilia and hyperfibrinogenemia. Synovial fluid findings are identical to those of other nonerosive immune-mediated arthropathies. The synovial leukocyte count is elevated (5000 to 150,000/μl), with the predominant cell type being the neutrophil.[3] Neutrophils appear nontoxic and have morphologically normal cytoplasmic granules.[3] Joint-associated pathological changes are similar to those of canine SLE. Synovial hypertrophy and hyperplasia are associated with a mononuclear inflammatory cell infiltrate.[3] Neutrophils can be seen throughout the synovial tissue, especially in the subsynoviocytic tissues; these cells are probably in the process of marginating into the synovial fluid toward various chemotactic factors.

Numerous hypotheses have been proposed to describe the pathogenesis by which chronic infectious disease induces polyarthritis. In canine patients the pathogenic mechanism is thought to occur primarily because of immune complex disease.[1–3] Either viable bacteria or bacterial cell products are thought to act as a foreign antigen or hapten, which subsequently induces an immune response. The production of circulating antibodies against this antigen allows the formation of circulating immune complexes, which localize in synovial tissue. The presence of immune complexes in synovial tissue leads to a type III hypersensitivity reaction, attracting and activating inflammatory cells (neutrophils primarily).

Treatment. Treatment is usually unnecessary if the primary disease can be eliminated. Symptomatic therapy with NSAIDs or glucocorticoids can be used to alleviate joint pain during treatment of the primary disease.

Drug-Induced Arthritis

Pathophysiology. Polyarthritis can occur secondarily to a hypersensitivity reaction involving the deposition of drug-antibody complexes in blood vessels of the synovium.[3] Other body systems can also be involved, leading to fever, lymphadenopathy, and skin disease.[3] Antibiotics of the following classes have been suspected of initiating this syndrome: sulfas, cephalosporins, lincomycin, erythromycin, and penicillins.[3] Doberman pinschers appear to have an increased sensitivity to developing polyarthritis secondary to administration of sulfa drugs.[90] Synovial fluid analysis is consistent with sterile, inflammatory arthritis having a predominance of polymorphonuclear cells. Clinical signs are generally not seen until after completion of 10 to 21 days of treatment.[3, 90] Subsequent exposure to the offending drug leads to acute exacerbation of polyarthritis.

Treatment. Treatment usually is unnecessary if the offending drug is discontinued. Clinical signs generally resolve in 2 to 3 days. If necessary, symptomatic therapy with NSAIDs or corticosteroids can be used while awaiting spontaneous resolution of clinical signs.

Polyarthritis-Polymyositis Syndrome

Pathophysiology. Polyarthritis-polymyositis syndrome (PPS) is an immune-mediated, nonerosive, symmetrical polyarthritis occuring in young dogs. Five of six dogs in one report were spaniels.[91] Clinical signs include stiffness, swelling and pain of multiple joints, muscle atrophy, muscle pain and contracture, and pyrexia.[91] Clinicopathological changes include mild, systemic neutrophilia, elevated synovial fluid cell counts associated with a dramatic increase in neutrophils, and increased creatine phosphokinase.[91] Serum titers for ANA and rheumatoid factor are normal. Radiographic changes are identical to the other nonerosive, immune-mediated polyarthropathies. Evaluation of muscle biopsies reveal muscle necrosis without inflammation in some areas, while other areas are characterized by active inflammation.[91] Synovial histopathological changes include synovial hypertrophy and hyperplasia associated with chronic-active inflammation.[91]

Treatment. Combination chemotherapy using cyclophosphamide and prednisolone is usually tried initially in an attempt to induce remission of clinical signs.[91] Some dogs respond poorly; others may require maintenance levels of glucocorticoids and some dogs recover completely, allowing discontinuation of therapy.[91]

Polyarthritis-Meningitis Syndrome

Pathophysiology. Clinical signs of pyrexia, stiffness, neck pain, neurological signs, lameness, joint swelling, and pain have been reported in the Weimaraner, German shorthair pointer, Boxer, Bernese mountain dog, and Japanese Akita.[39] The arthritis is typically nonerosive and involves multiple joints. Diagnosis is made by synovial and cerebrospinal fluid analysis and synovial histopathology and exclusion of other infectious and immune-mediated inflammatory arthropathies.[39] Synovial fluid analysis and synovial histopathology are typical for nonerosive immune-mediated arthropathies (see idiopathic polyarthritis). Cerebrospinal fluid shows increased protein, white blood cells, and creatine phosphokinase.[39]

Treatment. Dogs usually respond to treatment with corticosteroids.[39] Treatment should be initiated using the same protocol as with idiopathic polyarthritis.

Polyarteritis Nodosa

Pathophysiology. This condition is considered rare and has similarities to polyarthritis-meningitis syndrome and juvenile-onset polyarthritis of Akitas. All three of these syndromes can be associated with clinical signs and clinicopathological changes consistent with polyarthritis and meningitis. Clinical signs of polyarteritis nodosa include cyclical pyrexia, depression, stiffness, neck pain, lameness, joint swelling, and pain.[39] Diagnosis is made by correlation of clinical signs, clinicopathological changes, and histopathological identification of arteritis; the arteritis typically affects small arteries and may be granulomatous.[39]

Treatment. Some of these cases may spontaneously resolve, while other dogs require treatment with corticosteroids.[39] Treatment should be initiated using the same protocol as with idiopathic polyarthritis.

Familial Renal Amyloidosis in Shar Pei Dogs

Pathophysiology. Amyloidosis and synovitis are prominent features of a syndrome affecting young Shar Pei dogs. Clinical signs initially include episodes of fever and swelling of the hocks and occasionally other joints; the period between attacks can vary, but is often 4 to 6 weeks.[39] Later in the course of the disease, signs of renal failure, including vomiting, anorexia, lethargy, polydipsia, polyuria, edema, ascites, and dehydration are seen.[39] Synovial fluid analysis shows an inflammatory synovia, with an increased cell count and increased numbers of neutrophils.[39] Amyloid eventually deposits within many organs, but particularly in the kidneys.[39] Urinalysis shows isosthenuria and proteinuria. Amyloid deposits can be seen in the renal medulla and glomeruli of renal biopsies.[39]

Treatment. Dogs recover spontaneously from episodes of arthritis within a few days.[39] Amyloidosis of the kidneys will eventually lead to renal failure between 1.5 and 6 years of age.[39] Prognosis for treatment is poor as no effective treatment is known. Colchicine has been suggested as a possible treatment, but its efficacy is unproven.[39]

Plasmacytic-Lymphocytic Synovitis

Pathophysiology. This condition is most commonly seen in the stifles of small and medium breeds of dogs and is thought to be a variant of rheumatoid arthritis.[3] This disease can be confused with rupture of the anterior cruciate ligament because of its predilection for the stifle and associated severe joint instability that results.[3] Clinical signs are often limited to hindlimb lameness only. The cause of plasmacytic-lymphocytic synovitis is unknown. Typical pathological findings include a thickened, edematous synovium with a reddish-yellowish tint and a cloudy synovial fluid with increased numbers of lymphocytes (about 60 to 90%) and neutrophils (about 10 to 40%).[3] Synovial histopathology shows a diffuse lymphocytic plasmocytic infiltrate and hypertrophy. Cartilage erosion is mild or absent.[3]

Treatment. Immunosuppressive therapy is often successful in treating this condition. Treatment is similar to that described for idiopathic polyarthritis. Glucocorticoids are administered alone or in combination with cytotoxic drugs such as azathioprine or cyclophosphamide.[39] If cytotoxic drugs are used, animals should be monitored for bone marrow suppression with frequent complete blood counts. Long-term maintenance therapy may be necessary if clinical signs recur after discontinuation of therapy.

Juvenile-Onset Polyarthritis of Akitas

A clinical syndrome has been seen in Akita dogs less than 1 year of age that is characterized by marked pyrexia, polyarthritis, generalized myalgia, lymphadenopathy, and meningitis.[92] Although the etiology is unknown, the disease is believed to be heritable and immune mediated.[92] Anemia and leukocytosis are commonly seen.[39] Antinuclear antibody testing is normal. Microbiological and serological evaluation have failed to identify an infectious etiological agent.[92] Affected dogs may not respond to immunosuppressive therapy.[92] Some clinical improvement has been observed following aggressive anti-inflammatory or immunomodulatory therapy.[92]

Erosive Arthritides

Erosive arthritides include RA and EPG, both of which have similar radiographic and gross pathological changes. Typical radiographic changes include the apparent loss of joint space, due to destruction of articular cartilage and subchondral bone, decreased trabecular bone density, periarticular osteophytosis, and subluxation or luxation during the later course of the disease. Characteristic changes may not be evident during early stages, when synovitis predominates. Early erosive arthritis may radiographically mimic the nonerosive arthritides, having only subtle changes such as periarticular soft tissue and joint capsule swelling. Typical radiographic findings of the erosive arthritides correlate well with gross pathological changes. Erosion of articular cartilage, which typically begins marginally, can be seen in many joints; the most severe changes usually involve carpal and tarsal joints. Other common gross pathological changes include synovial hypertrophy, periarticular osteophytosis, intra-articular-articular fibrin deposition, joint instability, subluxation or luxation, and occasional fibrous or bony ankylosis

Rheumatoid Arthritis

Pathophysiology. Rheumatoid arthritis (RA) is an uncommon disease in dogs but typically affects toy- or small-breed dogs ranging in age from 8 months to 9 years.[1-5] A thorough discussion of its pathophysiology can be found elsewhere.[1-5] The disease is severely debilitating and has clinical, serological, radiographic, and pathological changes remarkably similar to those of human RA.[1,93] A predisposition for females has been reported in humans; however, this has not been substantiated in dogs.[94,95] As in humans, the cause of RA in dogs remains unknown. Diagnosis of canine RA depends on correlating a typical clinical presentation with characteristic radiographic, serological, and pathological changes. Diagnosis of human RA is based on diagnostic criteria established by the American Rheumatism Association.[5]

Multiple joints—especially carpal, tarsal, and phalangeal joints—are persistently swollen and may exhibit instability or deformity associated with periarticular soft tissue weakening and cartilage-subchondral bone destruction. Characteristic histopathological lesions of RA are observed primarily in diathroidal joints.[2,3]

Villous synovial hypertrophy, a dense, plasmacytic, lymphocytic inflammatory infiltrate, and erosion of articular cartilage are seen.[2, 4]

Treatment. Treatment of RA in humans begins in the early stages with NSAIDs. As the disease becomes refractory, therapy is expanded to combination chemotherapy, including glucocorticoids, cytotoxics, and gold salts (chrysotherapy). Use of NSAIDs to treat canine RA has been unrewarding. Most authors recommend a combination of chemotherapy with glucocorticoids and cytotoxic drugs, such as cyclophosphamide, azathioprine, and methotrexate.[2-5] Weekly injections of 1.0 mg/kg sodium aurothiomalate (chrysotherapy) have also been successful in alleviating symptoms of RA.[5] Chrysotherapy is contraindicated in dogs with intercurrent renal disease, owing to possible nephrotoxic effects of gold compounds. Although resolution of RA has been reported in the dog, remission of the disease within 3 to 6 months of initiation of treatment should be considered a therapeutic goal. Once the disease is in remission, treatment may be either discontinued or modified by administering lower doses of induction agents or changing to alternate-day glucocorticoid therapy.[5]

Erosive Polyarthritis of Greyhounds

Pathophysiology. An erosive polyarthritis of greyhounds (EPG) has been described that does not fulfill RA diagnostic criteria. The disease affects primarily young greyhounds: the reported age of onset ranges from 3 to 30 months. The disease was initially reported in 1976 in Australia; however, affected dogs have recently been identified in the United States as well.[96-98] No familial predisposition has been observed.[96] Clinical presentation varies from an insidious onset to acute illness. Some dogs have only swelling of affected joints, while others display signs of systemic illness such as anorexia, weight loss, depression, and pyrexia. Typically, joints are extremely painful and animals are very reluctant to walk.

Extensive efforts have been made to identify an agent. Blood, synovial fluid, synovial membrane, and articular cartilage have been evaluated for the presence of aerobic bacteria, anaerobic bacteria, mycoplasmas, chlamydia, and viruses. To date, an infective agent has not been consistently isolated. One report isolated *Mycoplasma spumans* in a single case.[96] Serological tests, including titers for *Ehrlichia, Brucella, Borrelia* (Lyme disease), *Rickettsia* (Rocky Mountain spotted fever), and *Chlamydia* have been normal. Antinuclear antibody tests, rheumatoid factor tests, and LE cell preparations have also been normal.[96, 97]

Radiographic changes of EPG include synovial effusion, periarticular swelling, and apparent collapse of the joint space with progression of the disease. Gross pathological examination of affected joints reveals mild to moderate synovial hypertrophy and articular cartilage erosion, often in the stifle, elbow, carpus, and hock. Systemic changes of diffuse pneumonia in two dogs and diarrhea in two others have been identified in the United States.[97] Histologically, full-thickness necrosis of articular cartilage was observed in all joints of the appendicular skeleton.[97] A prominent feature was necrosis of deeper hyaline cartilage zones with relative sparing of surface regions. Necrosis extended beneath the tidemark, to the level of mineralized cartilage; however, underlying subchondral bone was not affected. Synovial hypertrophy associated with a lymphocytic inflammatory infiltrate was typically present.[96, 97] Other components of the infiltrate included plasma cells, macrophages, neutrophils, fibroblasts, and hemosiderin pigment. Pannus formation was present in many joints but was not extensive.[96] Severe cartilage degeneration in the absence of pannus formation was very common over most affected articular surfaces.[96] The pathogenesis of this disease is unknown. The presence of a dense lymphocytic inflammatory infiltrate and neutrophilic synovial effusion is highly suggestive of an immune-mediated mechanism; however, the possibility of an infective agent cannot be ruled out. Deposition of immunoglobulins (IgG, IgM) has been found around chondrocytes

and within the extracellular matrix of articular cartilage in affected joints.[99] Documented cases are few, and our ability to observe these dogs over time is limited.

Treatment. Treatment of EPG has proved to be extremely unrewarding. Immunosuppressive drugs have not produced the improvement that would be anticipated in immune-mediated arthritis. Various antibiotics, NSAIDs, glucocorticoids, cytotoxic drugs, and a semisynthetic polysulfated glycosaminoglycan (Adequan) have all failed to induce remission. The prognosis for racing these young greyhounds is grave, owing to the widespread erosion of articular cartilage, resultant joint dysfunction, and inability to halt the disease process. Although disabled, some dogs can function as pets with long-term medical (NSAIDs, chondroprotectants, corticosteroids) and surgical (arthrodesis, joint replacement, arthroplasty) therapy.

Infectious Arthritis

A vast array of infectious organisms can lead to debilitating arthritis in dogs. This chapter discusses some of the most common and newer causes of infectious arthritis in dogs. Etiological agents implicated include bacterial, spirochetal, mycoplasmal, fungal, rickettsial, protozoal, and viral organisms. We limit our discussion to the effect these agents have on diathrodial joints; a thorough discussion of the systemic effects can be found in other sources.

Bacterial Arthritis

Pathophysiology. Bacterial arthritis, often referred to as septic arthritis, can result from hematogenous routes, extension of a local infection from an adjacent site, and local inoculation from penetrating or open wounds. The most commonly isolated bacterial organisms from septic joints are beta-hemolytic streptococci (Lancefield group G), staphylococci, hemolytic *Escherichia coli, Pasteurella,* and *Erysipelothrix*[39]; however, any bacterial organism has the potential to cause infection in a suitable environment. Bacterial arthritis can occur in dogs of any age but appears to be more common in young dogs. Large-breed dogs are more commonly affected, and the male/female ratio has been reported to be 2:1.[100, 101] Most commonly, one joint is involved, but multiple joint involvement is also seen. Septic arthritis is seen most commonly in the carpus, tarsus, stifle, elbow, shoulder, and hip.

Clinical signs include single or multiple limb lameness, pyrexia, joint inflammation, lethargy, and anorexia. Early radiographic signs include joint capsular distention and occasionally apparent widening of the joint space due to increased intra-articular pressure associated with synovial effusion. Joint space collapse and subchondral destruction are seen in cases with chronic or highly virulent infections; this is indicative of cartilage erosion. Synovial fluid analysis yields an increased cell count ($>$ than $5000/\mu l$) with a predominance of neutrophils that commonly have degenerative changes. Decreased viscosity of synovial fluid is also present. Positive bacterial culture of the synovial fluid or synovial membrane is diagnostic of bacterial arthritis; however, false-negative results have been reported to be as high as 50 per cent.[102] Incubation of synovial fluid in a special blood culture medium prior to culturing may improve the chance of obtaining a positive culture.[102]

Intra-articular bacterial infection causes marked inflammation of the synovial membrane. Synovial capillaries become permeable to fibrin, complement, and clotting factors; intense chemoattraction and migration of inflammatory cells also occurs.[100] Cartilage erosion is due to the catabolic effects of destructive enzymes released by inflammatory cells and bacteria. Collagenase, stromelysin, and a variety of lysosomal enzymes are produced, leading to chondrocyte necrosis and breakdown of collagen and proteoglycans within the extracellular matrix of articular cartilage.[103, 104]

Treatment. If clinical signs and synovial fluid analysis are consistent with bacterial arthritis, treatment should be started immediately using appropriate antibiotics. An attempt should be made to isolate the causative agent by culture and sensitivity testing. Specimens for culture should be obtained prior to initial antibiotic therapy. While culture results are awaited, therapy should begin using a broad-spectrum, bactericidal antibiotic. A penicillinase-resistant synthetic penicillin or cephalosporin is often selected since greater than 50 per cent of bacterial arthritides are caused by *Staphylococcus aureus.*[100] Ampicillin, clavulanate-potentiated amoxicillin, and cephalexin are commonly used. Antibiotic therapy should be adjusted according to culture and sensitivity results. Antibiotics are given for a minimum of 4 weeks. It is unnecessary to administer antibiotics intra-articularly as therapeutic concentrations of drug reach the joint quickly with parenteral or enteral administration.[100] It may be wise to continue therapy for 2 to 3 weeks after resolution of clinical signs.

If clinical signs do not improve within 2 to 3 days of starting appropriate antibiotics, surgical drainage and lavage should be considered. Surgical intervention should also be considered in severely inflamed joints or if cartilage erosion is suspected. Surgical debridement of necrotic synovium and cartilage and removal of fibrinous debris should be carried out. If indwelling drains are left in place, they should be protected with sterile bandages that should be changed once or twice daily to reduce the chance of developing a nosocomial infection. Indwelling drains can be used to drain passively or actively with continuous suction. An ingress-egress drainage system can also be placed to allow daily mechanical debridement by copiously lavaging the joint. Drains are rarely needed for longer than 1 week.

In cases of open intra-articular wounds, daily sterile lavage with 0.9 per cent saline solution and bandage changes should be performed until a healthy granulation tissue bed either covers the joint surface or allows delayed primary closure.

Spirochetal Arthritis (Lyme disease)

Pathophysiology. *Borrelia burgdorferi* is a spirochete implicated as the cause of the systemic illness Lyme disease. The disease is transmitted primarily by ticks of the *Ixodes* genus.[39] Clinical signs of polyarthritis are seen along with pyrexia, anorexia, and lymphadenopathy. If left untreated, chronic Lyme disease can be associated with glomerulonephritis, meningitis, and myocarditis.[105] Diagnosis is made based on criteria that include a history of possible exposure in an endemic area, clinical signs consistent with Lyme disease, positive serum antibody, and response to treatment.[39, 105] Changes seen in synovial fluid include an increased cell count (> than 5000/μl) with a predominance of neutrophils. Serological testing is helpful, but false positives can occur because of cross-reactivity with other spirochetes and bacteria.[20] Direct visualization or culture of *Borrelia* from tissues or body fluids, although diagnostic, is difficult and rarely achieved.

Treatment. Treatment with appropriate antibiotics will usually lead to resolution of clinical signs within 7 days, although treatment should be continued for 2 weeks.[39, 105, 106] Tetracycline (22 mg/kg three times a day orally), doxycycline (2.5 mg/kg twice a day orally), ampicillin (22 to 66 mg/kg three times a day orally), amoxicillin (22 mg/kg twice a day orally), or cephalexin (22 mg/kg three times a day orally) are most often used. Tetracycline is the treatment of choice.[106] Treatment is most successful in earlier stages of the disease. To avoid reinfection, preventive control of tick infestation should be carried out.

Mycoplasmal Arthritis

Pathophysiology. Mycoplasmal arthritis is uncommon in healthy dogs, but is occasionally seen in immunocompromised or debilitated animals. The mucous membranes of the respiratory, urogenital, and alimentary tracts may act as sources of hematogenous spread to joints.[39] Synovial fluid analysis is similar to other nonerosive arthritides; cell counts are greater than 5000/μl with a predom-

inance of nondegenerate neutrophils. Definitive diagnosis is made by correlation of clinical signs, synovial neutrophilia, and isolation of mycoplasmal organisms in special culture media. *Mycoplasma spumans* has been isolated in a greyhound with erosive polyarthritis, but it is uncertain if a cause-and-effect relationship exists.[98] Attempts at isolating mycoplasma from numerous other suspected cases of this disease has failed.

Treatment. Mycoplasmal arthritis can be treated with tylosin, gentamicin, or erythromycin.[39] Treatment should generally be continued for at least 2 weeks following resolution of clinical signs. For this reason, gentamicin is not the best choice for treatment because of its tendency to cause renal compromise with prolonged treatment.

Fungal Arthritis

Pathophysiology. Fungal arthritis is rarely seen; when seen it is usually associated with adjacent fungal osteomyelitis. Organisms reported to cause fungal arthritis include *Coccidiodes immitis, Blastomyces dermatitidis, Cryptococcus neoformans, Sporothrix schenckii,* and *Aspergillus terreus.*[39] Clinical signs include lameness of affected limbs, pain and swelling over affected bones and joints, pyrexia, lethargy, and anorexia. Other organ systems, including the nervous, respiratory, and ophthalmologic, should be evaluated carefully for concurrent systemic infection. Fungal arthritis can occur by hematogenous routes or by extension from adjacent infection or local inoculation. Diagnosis is made by serological testing, fungal cultures, synovial histopathology, and synovial cytology. Occasionally, fungal organisms may be seen on synovial fluid smears along with an increased cell count with increased numbers of neutrophils. Histopathology will generally show granulomatous synovitis in cases of chronic fungal arthritis.[39]

Treatment. Because of the infrequent occurrence of fungal arthritis, a lack of data exists describing efficacy in treating this condition. Use of systemic fungicides including ketoconazole, itraconazole, and amphotericin B can be attempted. If only one joint is affected, topical therapy administered through an intra-articular ingress-egress drainage system using agents such as povidone-iodine, clotrimazole, and enilconazole could be considered. Fungal infections usually require prolonged treatment, typically 2 to 4 months. Successful treatment of sporothrix arthritis in a dog has been reported with ketoconazole following 14 weeks of therapy.[107] Kidney and liver function should be monitored carefully because of the possibility of adverse side effects associated with prolonged treatment with fungicides.

Rickettsial Arthritis

Pathophysiology. Neutrophilic, nonerosive polyarthritis has been associated with infections caused by *Rickettsia rickettsii,* the causative agent of Rocky Mountain spotted fever (RMSF), and *Ehrlichia canis,* the causative agent of ehrlichiosis. Both pathogens are transmitted by ticks. *R. rickettsii* is spread by the American dog tick, *Dermacentor variabilis,* in the eastern United States, and the wood tick, *Dermacentor andersoni,* in the central and western United States.[105] *E. canis* is spread by the brown dog tick, *Rhipicephalus sanguineus.*[105] In addition to arthritis, both diseases usually cause systemic illness.

Clinical signs associated with RMSF include edema of extremities and scrotum, petechial hemorrhaging of mucous membranes, fever, lethargy, anorexia, abdominal pain, vomiting, diarrhea, lymphadenopathy, splenomegaly, seizures, stupor, ataxia, dyspnea, coughing, uveitis, retinal hemorrhage, and muscle or joint pain.[39] The disease is usually seen in the spring and summer during periods of increased tick activity. The organism causes widespread vasculitis, endothelial cell necrosis, increased vascular permeability, vasoconstriction of capillaries, arterioles, arteries, and some venules.[39] These changes lead to edema, hemorrhage, hypotension, and shock.[106] Abnormalities seen on a complete blood count include early leukopenia followed by progressive leukocytosis, mono-cytosis, eosinopenia, lymphopenia, mild anemia, and mild thrombo-cytopenia.[108] Biochemical abnormalities include mild elevation of ALT and SAP, hypoproteinemia, hypoalbuminemia, azotemia, hy-ponatremia, and hypocalcemia.[108] Synovial and cerebrospinal fluids may have increased cell counts with a predominance of neutro-phils.[108] Definitive diagnosis is made by serological testing or direct immunofluorescent testing of tissue samples.[108] A four-fold rise between acute and convalescent sera titer is diagnostic.[108]

Clinical signs associated with ehrlichiosis during the acute phase of disease include depression, anorexia, pyrexia, weight loss, edema of extremities and scrotum, lymphadenopathy, ocular and nasal discharge, epistaxis, and muscle or joint pain.[108] Central nervous system signs can occasionally be seen due to meningeal hemor-rhage and inflammation.[108] The clinical signs associated with acute ehrlichiosis are often similar to those of RMSF and distemper.[108] Chronic infection often leads to clinical signs associated with thrombocytopenia-induced hemorrhage, anemia, abdominal pain, meningoencephalitis, debilitation, uveitis, and retinal hemor-rhage.[108] After initial infection with *E. canis*, the organism multi-plies in mononuclear cells within the circulatory system, liver, spleen, and lymph nodes.[108] Infected cells adhere to endothelial cells causing vasculitis. The organism initially results in a hypercel-lular response in the bone marrow, but as the disease becomes chronic a hypocellular bone marrow response is seen. Thrombocy-topenia is most commonly seen, but pancytopenia is present in approximately 25 per cent of cases.[108] Monoclonal or polyclonal hyperglobulinemia is seen in about 50 per cent of affected dogs.[108] Synovial fluid analysis generally has a high cell count (30,000 to 50,000/μl) of which 60 to 80 per cent are neutrophils.[105] Definitive diagnosis is made by finding *E. canis* morula in neutrophils, eosino-phils or monocytes in synovial fluid, peripheral blood, or buffy-coat smears or by serological testing using the indirect fluorescent antibody technique.[105, 108] A positive titer is generally diagnostic for active infection because dogs generally become seronegative within 3 to 9 months following resolution of disease.[108]

Treatment. Tetracycline (22 mg/kg three times a day orally) is the treatment of choice for both RMSF and ehrlichiosis.[108] Chlor-amphenicol and enrofloxacin are also effective.[108] Doxycycline (10 mg/kg every day orally) is also effective for treatment of ehr-lichiosis. Treatment of both diseases is generally continued for 14 days. Prolonged treatment may be required for several months in cases of chronic ehrlichiosis.

Protozoal Arthritis

Pathophysiology. Polyarthritis can occur from infection caused by the protozoal organism, *Leishmania donovani*.[105] The organism is endemic in parts of Asia, the Middle East, the Mediterranean basin, Africa, Central America, and South America; it is rare in the United States, but is endemic in parts of Texas and Okla-homa.[105] The organism is transmitted by the bite of sandflies (eg, *Phlebotomus* spp., *Lutzomyia* spp.).[105] Dogs act as a reservoir host in endemic areas.[105] Leishmaniasis is a zoonotic disease. In addition to clinical signs of polyarthritis (lameness, joint swelling, and pain), the visceral form of this disease is associated with weight loss, pyrexia, lymphadenopathy, and hepatosplenomegaly.[105] Hematolog-ical changes include nonregenerative anemia, monocytosis, hypo-globulinemia, and hypoalbuminemia.[105] Synovial fluid analysis may be normal, but occasionally the organism may be seen in macro-phages within the synovial fluid.[105] Diagnosis is made by identifi-cation of the organism on impression smears or histopathological sections of liver, lymph node, bone marrow, or synovial mem-brane.[105] Proliferative synovitis associated with an inflammatory infiltrate containing plasma cells and macrophages is seen.[105]

Treatment. A variety of agents can be used for treatment of leishmaniasis. These include meglumine antimonate (200 to 300 mg/kg intravenously every other day, for 15 to 20 treatments or 50 mg/kg subcutaneously every day for 2 days followed by 100 mg/kg subcutaneously every day for 10 days and repeated in 2 weeks), sodium stibogluconate (20 mg/kg intramuscularly daily for 8 days, repeated after an 8-day rest), pentamidine (4 mg/kg intramuscularly every other day, for 15 days), metronidazole (10 to 15 mg/kg orally twice a day for 15 days), ketaconazole (15 to 30 mg/kg orally every day for 60 or more days).[105]

Viral Arthritis

Arthritides of dogs caused by viral infections have rarely been identified. Transient, sometimes protracted, sterile polyarthritis is seen following vaccinations of puppies and kittens.[39] These animals display clinical signs of polyarthritis, including, lameness, joint pain, and swelling. Several viruses, including feline syncitium-forming virus, feline leukemia virus, feline immunodeficiency vi-rus, feline infectious peritonitis virus, and feline calicivirus have been implicated in a variety of arthritides in cats.[39, 105]

References

1. Pedersen NC, et al: Noninfectious canine arthritis: Rheumatoid arthri-tis. JAVMA 169:295, 1976.
2. Lipowitz AJ: Immune-mediated arthropathies. *In* Newton CD, Nuna-maker DM (eds): Textbook of Small Animal Orthopaedics. Philadel-phia, JB Lippincott Co., 1985, pp 1055–1078.
3. Pedersen NC, Wind A, Morgan JP, et al: Joint diseases of dogs and cats: *In* Ettinger SJ (ed): Textbook of Veterinary Internal Medicine, 3rd ed. Philadelphia, WB Saunders Company 1989, vol. 2, pp 2329–2377.
4. Lipowitz AJ: Immune-mediated articular disease. *In* Slatter DH (ed): Textbook of Small Animal Surgery. Philadelphia, WB Saunders Com-pany 1985, vol 2, pp 2302–2311.
5. Halliwell REW, and Gorman NT: Immune-mediated joint diseases. *In* Halliwell REW, Gorman NT (eds): Veterinary Clinical Immunology, Philadelphia, WB Saunders Company, 1989, pp 337–358.
6. Martel-Pelletier J, Pelletier JP, Cloutier JM, et al: (1984): Neutral proteases capable of proteoglycan digesting activity in osteoarthritic and normal human articular cartilage: Arthritis Rheum 27:305–312, 1984.
7. Tyler JA, Bolis S, Dingle JT, et al: Mediators of matrix catabolism. *In* Kuettner K, et al (eds): Articular Cartilage and Osteoarthritis. New York, Raven Press, Ltd., 1992, pp 251–264.
8. Burkhardt D, Ghosh P: Laboratory evaluation of antiarthritic drugs as potential chondroprotective agents. Semin Arthritis Rheum 17(2): 3–34, 1987.
9. Conlon PD: Nonsteroidal drugs used in the treatment of inflammation. Vet Clin North Am 18:1115–1129, 1988.
10. Bayne EK, Hutchinson NI, Walakovits LA, et al: Production, purifica-tion and characterization of canine prostromelysin. Matrix 12:173–184, 1992.
11. Dayer JM, Beutler B, Cerami A: Cachectin/tumor necrosis factor stimulates collagenase and prostaglandin E$_2$ production by human synovial cells and dermal fibroblasts: J Exp Med 162:2163–2168, 1985.
12. Frisch SM, Ruley HE: Transcription from stromelysin promoter is induced by interleukin-1 and repressed dexamethasone. J Biol Chem 262:16300–16304, 1987.
13. Hasty KA, Reife RA, Kang AH, et al: The role of stromelysin in the cartilage destruction that accompanies inflammatory arthritis. Arthritis Rheum 33:388–397, 1990.
14. Lefebvre V, Peeters-Joris C, Vaes G: Modulation by interleukin 1 and tumor necrosis factor alpha of production of collagenase, tissue inhibi-tor of metalloproteinases and collagen types in differentiated and dedifferentiated articular chondrocytes. Biochim Biophys Acta 1990;1052:366–378.
15. McDonnell J, Hoermer LA, Lark MW, et al: Recombinant human interleukin-1 beta-induced increase in levels of proteoglycans, stromel-ysin, and leukocytes in rabbit synovial fluid. Arthritis Rheum 35:799–805, 1992.
16. Mort AS, Dodge GR, Roughly PJ, et al: Direct evidence for active metalloproteinases mediating matrix degradation in interleukin 1-stim-ulated human articular cartilage. Matrix 13:95–102, 1993.

17. Ogata Y, Enghid JJ, Nagase H: Matrix metalloproteinase 3 (stromelysin) activates the precursor for the human matrix metalloproteinase 9. J Biochem Chem 267:3581–3584, 1992.

18. Wu JJ, Lark MW, Chun LE, et al: Sites of stromelysin cleavage in collagen types II, IX, X, and XI of cartilage. J Biol Chem 266:5625–5628, 1991.

19. Pelletier JP, DiBattista JA, Raynauld JP, et al: The *in vivo* effects of intraarticular corticosteroid injections on cartilage lesions, stromelysin, interleukin-1, and oncogene protein synthesis in experimental osteoarthritis. Lab Invest 72:578–586, 1995.

20. Hutchinson NI, Lark MW, MacNaul KL, et al: In vivo expression of stromelysin in synovium and cartilage of rabbits injected intraarticularly with interleukin-1 beta. Arthritis Rheum 35:1227–1233, 1992.

21. Lohmander LS, Hoermer LA, Lark MW: Metalloproteinases, tissue inhibitor, and proteoglycan fragments in knee synovial fluid in human osteoarthritis. Arthritis Rheum 36:181–189, 1993.

22. Okada Y., Shinmei M., Tanaka O., et al: Localization of matrix metalloproteinase 3 (stromelysin) in osteoarthritic cartilage and synovium: Lab Invest 66:680–690, 1992.

23. Todhunter RJ, Lust G: Polysulfated glycosaminoglycan in the treatment of osteoarthritis. JAVMA 204:1245–1251, 1994.

24. Howell DS, Carreno MR, Pelletier JP, et al: Articular cartilage breakdown in a lapine model of osteoarthritis. Clin Orthop 213:69–76, 1986.

25. Docherty AJ, Murphy G: The tissue metalloproteinase family and the inhibitor TIMP: A study using cDNAs and recombinant proteins. Ann Rheum Dis 49:469–479, 1990.

26. Murphy G, Cockett MI, Stephens PE, et al: Stromelysin is an activator of procollagenase. Biochem J 248:265–268, 1987.

27. Simon SR: Oxidants, metalloproteases and serine proteases in inflammation. *In* Proteases, Protease Inhibitors and Protease-Derived Peptides. Basel, Birkhauser Verlag, 1993, pp 27–37.

28. McIlwraith CW: Diseases of joints, tendons, ligaments and related structures. *In* Stayshak TS (ed): Adam's Lameness In Horses, Philadelphia, Lea & Febiger, 1987, pp 339–369.

29. Auer DE, NG JC, Seawright AA: Effect of palosein (superoxide dismutase) and catalase upon oxygen derived free radical induced degradation of equine synovial fluid. Equine Vet J 22:13–17, 1990.

30. Ghosh P, Smith M, Wells C: Second-line agents in osteoarthritis. *In* Dixon JS, Furst DE (eds): Second-Line Agents in the Treatment of Rheumatic Diseases. New York, Marcel Dekker, Inc, 1993, pp 363–427.

31. Johnson KA, Davis PE: Drug therapy in surgical musculoskeletal disease. *In* Bojrab MJ (ed): Disease Mechanisms in Small Animal Surgery, Philadelphia, Lea & Febiger, 1993, pp 1105–1110.

32. Johnson R: Table of common drugs: Approximate doses. *In* Kirk RW (ed): Current Veterinary Therapy X. Small Animal Practice. Philadelphia, WB Saunders Company, 1989, pp 1370–1380.

33. Rubin SI, Papich MG: Nonsteroidal anti-inflammatory drugs. *In* Kirk RW (ed): Current Veterinary Therapy X. Small Animal Practice. Philadelphia, WB Saunders Company, 1989, pp 47–54.

34. Kalbhen DA: Chemical model of osteoarthritis—a pharmacological evaluation. J Rheumatol 14(suppl):130–131, 1987.

35. Brandt KD: Effects of nonsteroidal antiinflammatory drugs on chondrocyte metabolism in vitro and in vivo. Am J Med 83(suppl. 5A):29–34, 1987.

36. Brandt KD, Slowman-Kovacs S: Nonsteroidal antiinflammatory drugs in treatment of osteoarthritis. Clin Orthop 213:84, 1986.

37. Wallace MS, Zawie DA, Garvey M: Gastric ulceration in the dog secondary to the use of nonsteroidal antiinflammatory drugs. J Am Anim Hosp Assoc 26:467–472, 1990.

38. Beale BS, Goring RL: Degenerative joint disease. *In* Bojrab MJ (ed): Disease Mechanisms in Small Animal Surgery, Philadelphia, Lea & Febiger, 1993, pp 727–736.

39. Bennett D, May C: Joint diseases of dogs and cats. *In* Ettinger SJ, Feldman EC (eds): Textbook of Veterinary Internal Medicine, 4th ed. Philadelphia, WB Saunders Company, 1995, vol 2, pp 2032–2076.

40. Manley PA: Treatment of degenerative joint disease. *In* Current Vet Therapy XII. Small Animal Practice, Philadelphia, WB Saunders Company, 1995, pp 1196–1199.

41. Holtsinger RH, Parker RB, Beale BS, et al: The therapeutic efficacy of carprofen (Rimadyl-V) in 209 clinical cases of canine degenerative joint disease. Vet Compar Orthop Trauma 5:140–144, 1992.

42. Weissman G: Pathogenesis of inflammation. Effects of the pharmacological manipulation of arachidonic acid metabolism on the cytological response to inflammatory stimuli. Drugs 33(suppl 1), 28–37, 1987.

43. Adam M, Krabcova M, Musilova J, et al: Contribution to the mode of action of glycosaminoglycan polysulfate (GAGPS) upon human osteoarthritic cartilage. Arzneimittelforschung 30:1730–1732, 1980.

44. Clark SD, Kobayashi DK, Welgus HG: Regulation of the expression of tissue inhibitor of metalloproteinases and collagenases by retinoids and glucocorticoids in human fibroblasts. J Clin Invest 80:1280–1288, 1987.

45. Fubini SL, Boatwright CE, Todhunter RJ, et al: Effect of intramuscularly administered polysulfated glycosaminoglycan on articular cartilage from equine joints injected with methylprednisolone acetate. Am J Vet Res 54:1359–1365, 1993.

46. Lipowitz AJ, Newton CD: Degenerative joint disease and traumatic arthritis. *In* Newton CD, Nunamaker DM (eds): Textbook of Small Animal Orthopedics. Philadelphia, JB Lippincott Co, 1985, pp 1029–1046.

47. Yang-Yen HF, Chambard JC, Sun YL, et al: Transcriptional interference between c-Jun and the glucocorticoid receptor: Mutual inhibition of DNA binding to direct protein–protein interaction. Cell 62:1205–1215, 1990.

48. Pelletier JP, Pelletier JM: Protective effects of corticosteroids on cartilage lesions and osteophyte formation in the pond-nuki dog model of osteoarthritis. Arthritis Rheum 32:181–193, 1989.

49. Papich MG, Davis LE: Glucocorticoid therapy: *In* Kirk RW (ed): Current Veterinary Therapy X. Small Animal Practice, Philadelphia, WB Saunders Company, 1989, pp 54–62.

50. Booth NH: Topical agents: *In* Booth NH, McDonald LE (eds): Veterinary Pharmacology and Therapeutics, Ames, Iowa State Press, 1982, pp 657–675.

51. Altman RD, Dean DD, Muniz OE, et al: Prophylactic treatment of canine osteoarthritis with glycosaminoglycan polysulfuric acid ester. Arthritis Rheum 32:759–766, 1989.

52. May SA, Hooke RE, Lees P: The effect of various drugs used in the treatment of equine joint disease on equine stromelysin (proteoglycanase). Br J Pharmacol 93:281, 1988.

53. Milkulikova D, Trnavsky K: Influence of a glycosaminoglycan polysulfate on lysosomal enzyme release from human polymorphonuclear leukocytes. Z Rheumatol 41:50–53, 1982.

54. Egg D: Effects of glycosaminoglycan polysulfate and two nonsteroidal anti-inflammatory drugs on prostaglandin E2 synthesis in Chinese hamster ovary cell cultures. Pharmacol Res Commun 15:709–717, 1983.

55. Rashmir-Raven AM, Coyne CP, Fenwick BW, et al: Inhibition of equine complement activity by polysulfated glycosaminoglycans. Am J Vet Res 53:87–90, 1992.

56. Tsuboi I, Matsuura T, Shichijo, et al: Effects of glycosaminoglycan polysulfate on human neutrophil function. Jpn J Inflamm 8:131–135, 1988.

57. Altman RD, Dean DD, Muniz OE, et al: Therapeutic treatment of canine osteoarthritis with glycosaminoglycan polysulfuric acid ester. Arthritis Rheum 32:1300–1307, 1989.

58. Carreno MR, Muniz OE, Howell DS: The effect of glycosaminoglycan polysulfuric acid ester on articular cartilage in experimental osteoarthritis: Effects on morphological variables of disease severity. J Rheumatol 13:490–497, 1986.

59. Hannen N, Ghosh P, Bellenger C, et al: Systemic administration of glycosaminoglycan polysulphate provides partial protection of articular cartilage from damage produced by meniscectomy in the canine. Ortho Res 5:47–59, 1987.

60. Glade M: Polysulfated glycosaminoglycan accelerates net synthesis of collagen and proteoglycans by arthritic equine cartilage tissues and chondrocytes. Am J Vet Res 51:779–785, 1990.

61. Nishikawa H, Mori I, Umemoto J: Influences of sulfated glycosaminoglycans on hyaluronic acid in rabbit knee synovia. Arch Biochem Biophys 240:146–148, 1985.

62. Smith MM, Ghosh P: The effect of polysulfated polysaccharides on hyaluronate (HA) synthesis by human synovial fibroblasts. Agents Actions 18:55–62, 1986.

63. Verbruggen G, Veys EM: The effect of sulfated glycosaminoglycan on the proteoglycan metabolism of synovial lining cells. Acta Rheumatol Belg 1:75–92, 1971.

64. Verbruggen G, Veys EM: Proteoglycan metabolism of connective tissue cells. An in vitro technique and its relevance to in vivo condi-

tions. *In* Degenerative Joints, Test Tubes, Tissues, Models, and Man, Amsterdam, Excerpta Medica, 1982, pp 113–126.

65. von der Mark K: Collagen synthesis in cultures of chondrocytes as effected by arteparon. *In* IX Europ Cong Rheumatol. Euler, Basil, 1980, pp 39–50.

66. Vance BA, Kowalski CG, Brinckerhoff CE: Heat shock of rabbit synovial fibroblasts increases expression of mRNAs for two metalloproteinases, collagenases and stromelysin. J Cell Biol 108:2037–2043, 1989.

67. de Haan JJ, Goring RL, Beale BS: Evaluation of polysulfated glycosaminoglycan for the treatment of hip dysplasia in dogs. Vet Surg 23:177–181, 1994.

68. Lust G, Williams AJ, Burton-Wurster N, et al: Effects of intramuscular administration of glycosaminoglycan polysulfates on signs of incipient hip dysplasia in growing pups. Am J Vet Res 53:1836–1843, 1992.

69. Abatangelo G, Botti P, Del Bue M, et al: Intraarticular sodium hyaluronate injections in the pond-nuki experimental model of osteoarthritis in dogs. I: biochemical results. Clin Orthop 241:278–285, 1989.

70. Dettmer N, Nowack H, Raake W: Platelet aggregation by heparin and arteparon. Munch Med Wschr 125:540–542, 1983.

71. Verbruggen G, Veys EM: Treatment of chronic degenerative joint disorders with a glycosaminoglycan polysulfate. *In* IX Europ Cong Rheumatol. Euler, Basil, 1980, pp 51–69.

72. Read R, Cullis-Hill D: The systemic use of the chondroprotective agent pentosan polysulfate in the treatment of osteoarthritis-results of a double-blind clinical trial in dogs. Proceedings Annual Mtg Vet Orthop Society. Lake Louise, Canada, 1993, p 32.

73. Read R: Personal communication, 1994.

74. Ghosh P, Smith M, Wells C: Second-line agents in osteoarthritis. *In* Dixon JS, Furst DE (eds): Second-Line Agents in the Treatment of Rheumatic Diseases, New York, Marcel Dekker Inc, 1993, pp 363–427.

75. Howard RD, Mcllwraith CW: Sodium hyaluronate in the treatment of equine joint disease. Compend Cont Educ 15:473–481, 1993.

76. Schiavinato A, Lini E, Guidolin D, et al: Intraarticular sodium hyaluronate injections in the pond-nuki experimental model of osteoartritis in dogs: II. Morphological findings. Clin Orthop 241:286–299, 1989.

77. D'Ambrosio E, Casa B, Bompani R, et al: Glucosamine sulphate: A controlled clinical investigation in arthrosis. Pharmatherapeutica 2:504–508, 1981.

78. Vidal y Plana RR, Bizzarri D, Rovati AL: Articular cartilage pharmacology: I. In vitro studies on glucosamine and non steroidal antiinflammatory drugs. Pharmacol Res Commun 10:557–569, 1978.

79. Leach RM: Role of manganese in mucopolysaccharide metabolism. Fed Proc 30:991–994, 1971.

80. Drovanti A, Bignamini AA, Rovati AL: Therapeutic activity of oral glucosamine sulfate in osteoarthrosis: A placebo-controlled double-blind investigation. Clin Ther 3:260–272, 1980.

81. Eichler J, Noh E: Therapy of arthrosis deformans by influencing the metabolism of cartilages. Orthop Praxis 9:225, 1970.

82. Pujalte JM, Liavore EP, Ylescupidez FR: Double-blind clinical evaluation of oral glucosamine sulphate in the basic treatment of osteoarthrosis. Curr Med Res Opin 7:110–114, 1980.

83. Vaz AL: Double-blind clinical evaluation of the relative efficacy of ibuprofen and glucosamine sulphate in the management of osteoarthrosis of the knee in out patients. Curr Med Res Opin 8:145–149, 1982.

84. Muller-Fabender H, Bach GL, Haase W, et al: Glucosamine sulfate compared to ibuprofen in osteoarthritis of the knee. Osteoarthritis Cartilage 2:61–69, 1994.

85. Setnikar I, Giachetti C, Zanolo G: Absorption, distribution and excretion of radioactivity after a single intravenous or oral administration of [^{14}C] glucosamine to the rat. Pharmatherapeutica 3:538–550, 1984.

86. Setnikar I, Giachetti C, Zanolo G: Pharmakinetics of glucosamine in the dog and in man. Arzneimittelforschung 36:729–736, 1986.

87. Herschler RJ: MSM: A nutrient for the horse. Equine Vet Data 7:268–269, 1987.

88. Jones WE: MSM reviewed. J Equine Vet Sci 7:2, 1987.

89. Maeda M, Cooke TDV: Destruction of rabbit knee hyaline cartilage associated with surface antigen-antibody interaction during the arthus reaction of antigen-induced arthritis. Clin Orthop 190:287, 1984.

90. Giger U, et al: Sulfadiazine-induced allergy in six doberman pinschers. JAVMA 186:479, 1985.

91. Bennett D, Kelly F: Immune-based non-erosive inflammatory joint disease of the dog: 2. Polyarthritis/polymyositis syndrome. J Small Anim Pract 28:891, 1987.

92. Doughery SA, et al: Juvenile-onset polyarthritis syndrome in akitas. JAVMA 198:849, 1991.

93. Newton CD: Canine rheumatoid arthritis. *In* Bojrab MJ (ed): Pathophysiology in Small Animal Surgery, Philadelphia, Lea & Febiger, 1981, pp 584–587.

94. Newton CD, et al: Rheumatoid arthritis in dogs. JAVMA 168:113, 1976.

95. Alexander RJW, et al: Rheumatoid arthritis in the dog; clinical diagnosis and management. J Am Anim Hosp Assoc 12:727, 1976.

96. Huxtable CR, Davis PE: The pathology of polyarthritis in young greyhounds. J Comp Pathol 86:11, 1976.

97. Woodard JC, et al: Erosive polyarthritis in two greyhounds. JAVMA 198:873, 1991.

98. Barton MD, et al: Isolation of *Mycoplasma spumans* from polyarthritis in a greyhound. Austr Vet J 62:206, 1985.

99. Beale, BS: Unpublished data.

100. Bennett D, Taylor DJ: Bacterial infective arthritis in the dog. J Small Anim Pract 29:207, 1988.

101. Kaderly RE: Infectious arthritis. *In* Bojrab MJ (ed): Disease Mechanisms in Small Animal Surgery. Philadelphia, Lea & Febiger, 1993, pp 737–741.

102. Montgomery RD, et al: Comparison of aerobic culturette, synovial membrane biopsy, and blood culture medium in detection of canine bacterial arthritis. Vet Surg 18:300, 1989.

103. Curtiss PH: The pathophysiology of joint infections. Clin Orthop 96:129, 1973.

104. Weissman G: Lysosomal mechanisms of tissue injury in arthritis. N Engl J Med 286:141, 1972.

105. Lau RE, Hay WH: Other infectious arthritides of the dog and cat. *In* Bojrab MJ (ed): Disease Mechanisms in Small Animal Surgery. Philadelphia, Lea & Febiger, 1993, pp 758–763.

106. Breitschwerdt EB: Borreliosis in small animals. *In* Proceedings of the North American Veterinary Conference, Orlando, Fla, 8:301–303, 1994.

107. Goad DL, Goad MEP: Osteoarticular sporotrichosis in a dog. JAVMA 189:1326, 1986.

108. Breitschwerdt EB: Ehrlichiosis and Rocky Mountain spotted fever. *In* Proceedings of the North American Veterinary Conference, Orlando, Fla, 8:297–300, 1994.

CHAPTER 26

PHYSEAL INJURIES

ROBERT B. PARKER

GENERAL COMMENTS

The physis is a complex anatomical structure composed of cartilage, bone, and fibrous components and is responsible for the majority of long-bone growth. The physis, which is also known as the metaphyseal growth plate, the epiphyseal plate, and the epiphyseal cartilage, is physically situated between the metaphysis and the epiphysis in immature animals.

During embryological development, mesenchymal cells form into bony precursors and are differentiated into cartilage forms. These forms are surrounded by a connective tissue perichondrium. This layer allows the cartilage model to circumferentially grow in size, and it differentiates later into the early periosteum. Following provisional mineralization, the primary ossification center develops in the center of the core, followed by chondrocyte death and vascular invasion. This process begins at the center of the bone and spreads proximally and distally to begin formation of the physis. Secondary centers of ossification typically develop in the proximal and distal ends of the cartilage model. As in the primary center, early mineralization, cell death, and vascular invasion occur. Endochondral ossification proceeds and expands centrifugally. The centrifugal expansion eventually reaches the physis at the metaphysis and also leaves behind a layer of cartilage that will remain as the articular cartilage.

The physis and surrounding tissues can be divided into three anatomical portions according to the type of tissue present. A cartilaginous component is divided into characteristic histological zones, a bony section represented by the metaphysis and a fibrous component that surrounds the periphery. Each anatomical portion in this area has a distinct blood supply. The epiphyseal artery penetrates the epiphysis, and small arterial vessels eventually branch perpendicularly to the main artery and penetrate through small cartilage canals in the reserve zone and terminate at the top of the cell columns in the proliferative zone. Four to ten cell columns are supplied by each small arterial branch. It is important to realize that the epiphyseal vessels supply the reserve zone of cells of the physis, and the origin of these vessels is from the epiphysis. The nutrient artery predominates in the metaphysis and is supplemented by specific metaphyseal vessels. Terminal branches from these vessels pass toward the bone-cartilage junction and end in vascular loops just below the last intact transverse septum at the base of the cartilage plate. These vessels do not pass into the hypertrophic zone. Of the actual cartilaginous physis, only the proliferative zone is primarily vascularized by vessels of epiphyseal origin.

The cartilaginous component of the physis can be divided into various morphological or functional zones. The *reserve zone* lies adjacent to the secondary growth center and contains cells that are actively storing lipids and other materials required for future development. The cells in this zone are somewhat disorganized and are separated from each other by more extracellular matrix than any other layer of the physeal cartilage. This zone can be classified as a germinal layer containing the so-called mother cells. In the *proliferative zone* the spherical cells in the reserve zone transform to flattened chondrocytes aligned perpendicular to the bone axis. These are the only cells that actually divide in the physeal cartilage. The top cell in the proliferative zone is the true mother for that column, and the longitudinal physeal growth is equal to the rate of new chondrocyte production multiplied by the maximum chondrocyte dimensions at the bottom of the proliferative zone. The major function of the proliferative zone is matrix production and cellular proliferation. In the *hypertrophic zone* the flattened chondrocytes in the proliferative zone become spherical and greatly enlarge. The average chondrocyte enlarges by approximately five times. This cellular enlargement is at the expense of the matrix, which is responsible for the strength of the physis. In the proliferative zone the chondrocytes begin to accumulate calcium within their mitochondria, and by the time the cells are in the top half of the hypertrophic zone, they are loaded with calcium. As the cells reach the bottom of the physis the intracellular calcium is depleted and is involved in cartilage calcification. Initial calcification takes place within or on matrix vesicles present on the longitudinal septa of the matrix. With hydroxyapatite crystal growth, the longitudinal septa become calcified in the bottom portion of the hypertrophic zone, which is referred to as the zone of provisional calcification. The significance of cartilage mineralization is threefold. First, by guiding vessel ingrowth into individual cell columns, it provides a template for vascular invasion; second, it protects delicate vascular structures from damage; and third, the mineralized septa act as a scaffold for bone deposition and serve as the core for the primary spongiosa. The invading vessels carry osteoprogenitor cells that can differentiate into osteoblasts that ultimately are responsible for osteoid deposition. Remodeling ultimately occurs, and the woven primary spongiosa is replaced by lamellar bone.

PHYSEAL FRACTURES

Physeal fractures are relatively common in skeletally immature animals. The cartilaginous physis is the "weak link" in the composite formed by adjacent soft tissue supporting structures and the bone. Histologically the weakest area of the physis exists at the hypertrophic zone, as this is the area where the chondrocytes have increased in size at the expense of the stronger, supportive matrix. At the secondary ossification centers located at the proximal and distal ends of long bones, it is also clinically important to realize that the germinal cells are present on the epiphyseal segment. Either direct or indirect trauma to this area results in arrest of the normal cascade of cellular maturation and produces premature physeal closure. This trauma can be initiated by the force of the fracture or by surgical manipulation. Careless handling of epiphyseal fragments can lead to premature closure.

Compression across a physeal plate can also lead to premature closure. The method of fracture fixation is therefore important so as not to cause iatrogenic damage. As a general rule, small K-wires placed parallel to the maturing cartilage rows cause the least damage; however, this type of fixation may not be sufficient in many veterinary applications. Orthopedic appliances that apply compression across a physis such as plates, external fixators, and Rush pins should also, theoretically, be avoided.

Physeal fractures in humans were initially classified by Salter and Harris in 1963. This system has been used extensively in the veterinary literature to describe similar fractures. A retrospective study evaluated the histological changes from excised physeal fractures. It found that the histological description did not coincide with the classic Salter-Harris radiographic scheme. The important point from this study is that, although the classic Salter-Harris system is helpful in preoperatively describing many fractures, it may not be used to predict the potential for continued growth. Following is the Salter-Harris classification of physeal fractures.

Type I

With a Salter-Harris I fracture, the fracture line begins and ends directly through the hypertrophic cartilage cells in a transverse manner (Fig. 26–1). Many times these fractures occur as a result of transverse shear or avulsion-type forces. Depending on the histological damage (which is impossible to ascertain on a radiograph) and the blood supply to the proliferating cells, the prognosis for continued physeal growth is theoretically good with adequate alignment and fixation. The aforementioned study of 13 naturally occurring unrepaired canine physeal fractures illustrated that many type I and II fractures had histological extensions into the proliferating cartilage zone, which more than likely would have caused premature physeal arrest (type V).

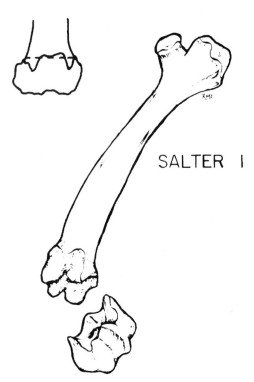

FIGURE 26–1. Diagram of a Salter-Harris I fracture.

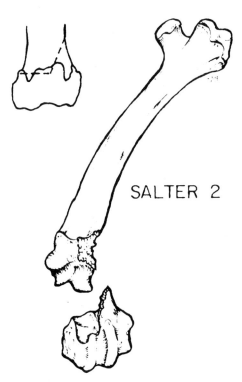

FIGURE 26–2. Diagram of a Salter-Harris II fracture.

Type II

A Salter-Harris type II physeal fracture classically begins transversely through the hypertrophic zone; however, at a variable distance across, the fracture line diverges to exit through the metaphysis (Fig. 26–2). Type II fractures are a relatively common form of physeal fracture, and the remaining metaphyseal piece of bone attached to the epiphysis has been termed the *Thurston-Holland sign* in human orthopedics. Because a corner of the metaphysis is usually involved and the fragment extension frequently resembles a sailboat sail, it also is termed the *corner* or *sail sign*. Classically, these fractures had a good prognosis for continued physeal growth with adequate surgical technique and stabilization; however, the aforementioned study casts doubt on continued growth with naturally occurring fractures.

Type III

With Salter-Harris type III injuries the fracture begins at the hypertrophic zone of the physis; however, in contrast to the type II, the fracture diverges into the joint space of the adjacent joint (Fig. 26–3). This particular fracture configuration, although relatively rare, is serious. As with all intra-articular fractures, the final clinical result depends on accurate anatomical alignment and rigid internal fixation. The prognosis for continued growth is probably guarded, and the final clinical outcome depends on the status of the intra-articular repair.

Type IV

This fracture begins at the metaphysis, passes across the physis, and terminates in the joint space (Fig. 26–4). With this relatively common fracture, the major surgical concern again is restoration

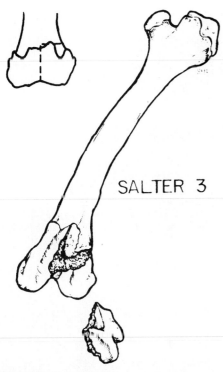

SALTER 3

FIGURE 26–3. Diagram of a Salter-Harris III fracture.

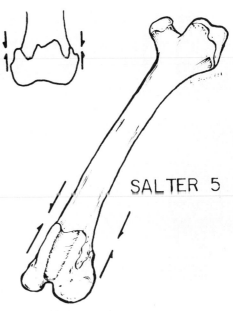

SALTER 5

FIGURE 26–5. Diagram of a Salter-Harris V fracture.

Type V

This is a crushing, compressive injury to all or part of the physis and implies that either the germinal cells are damaged or the epiphyseal blood vessels are compromised (Fig. 26–5). Because no true fracture results from the trauma, radiographic evaluation is difficult. It is important to advise all owners of traumatized immature animals that, although a bony injury is not apparent, premature closure could be a sequela. Follow-up radiographs are recommended to monitor continued physeal growth.

SPECIFIC PHYSEAL FRACTURES

Supraglenoid Tuberosity

The supraglenoid tuberosity arises as a separate center of ossification from the remainder of the scapular glenoid and normally fuses to the remaining scapula at a mean of 6 months. The tuberosity is the point of origin for the biceps brachii muscle and is subsequently subjected to traction forces. Because a significant portion of the glenoid surface is involved with this fracture, open reduction, precise alignment, and rigid internal fixation are necessary. Surgical exposure is difficult. For maximum visualization a cranial approach—including osteotomy of the greater tubercle—is usually employed. The cranial piece with the attached biceps muscle is gently levered into place and initially fixed with a single K-wire. Depending on the size of the fragment, additional K-wires and a tension band or the use of a lag screw is necessary to apply compression at the fracture site (Fig. 26–6). This is one area in which rigid fixation takes precedence over potential physeal growth. The prognosis depends primarily on the accuracy of the alignment and the rigidity of the fixation.

Proximal Humerus

The proximal humerus is composed of the proximal physis, which is primarily responsible for longitudinal growth, and a sec-

of the articular surface. The prognosis for continued growth from the physis is guarded; however, clinical signs related to symmetrical premature arrest are uncommon. When this type of fracture is being repaired, two fracture facets occur: the intra-articular component and the metaphyseal surface. It is important that both facets are perfectly aligned during reduction.

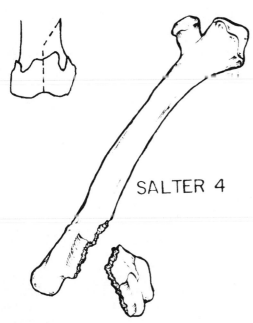

SALTER 4

FIGURE 26–4. Diagram of a Salter-Harris IV fracture.

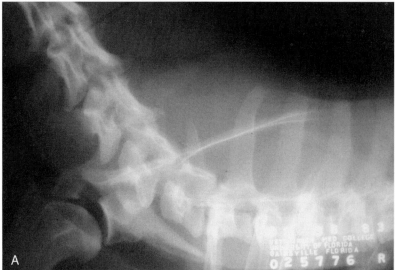
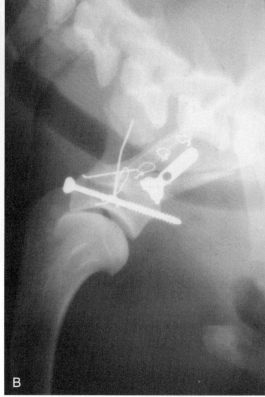

FIGURE 26–6. Pre *(A)* and postoperative *(B)* views of a supraglenoid tuberosity avulsion.

ondary center (apophysis) responsible for formation of the greater tubercle. Fortunately, most physeal fractures that occur in this area are Salter-Harris type I, with the epiphysis and the greater tubercle contained as a single bone fragment. Surgical exposure consists of a cranial approach to the area of the greater tubercle. The fragments are levered into place, reduction is verified along the cranial margins, and the fracture is usually stabilized with divergent pins or K-wires introduced through the greater tubercle (Fig. 26–7).

Distal Humerus

In the normal humeral condyle two centers of ossification develop. The lateral center develops into the capitulum (lateral condyle) and the medial side develops into the trochlea (medial condyle). These two ossification centers, separated by a cartilage plate, usually unite into a single growth center by 70 ± 14 days after birth. Cocker spaniels have been shown to have a propensity for incomplete ossification between these two centers, which predisposes this breed to various fractures in this area. Interestingly, most fractures in this breed occur in middle-aged males, without a history of major trauma.

The most common fracture in the immature dog is a Salter-Harris IV fracture involving the capitulum (lateral condyle). These fractures result from shearing forces that develop following a fall on an extended forelimb. The forces are transmitted through the radial head, fracture the lateral portion of the condyle, and continue across the supratrochlear foramen and exit through the lateral portion of the lateral epicondylar crest. This creates the usual lateral metaphyseal fragment (Fig. 26–8). If the fracture travels across both supracondylar crests, a bicondylar (T or Y) fracture can occur.

Because these are intra-articular fractures, precise anatomical alignment and fixation are necessary. Salter-Harris IV fractures involving the lateral aspect of the condyle have been treated by both open and closed methods. Some surgeons report on the use of closed manipulation, reduction with a condyle clamp, and percutaneous transcondylar screw placement. Although this form of treatment has been successful for some, most surgeons would recommend open reduction and internal fixation. The condyle is approached with either a lateral or a craniolateral approach, and the fracture site is identified, cleaned, and irrigated. I usually initiate the glide hole for the transcondylar lag screw at the lateral fracture facet after externally rotating the fracture fragment. After location of the center of the fracture surface, the over-drill is directed laterally and parallel to the joint and exits just distal and cranial to the lateral epicondyle. The use of a centering drill sleeve in the lateral fragment will provide a "handle" to facilitate manipulation and reduction. After reduction of both the intra-articular and metaphyseal fracture lines, the condyles are stabilized with pointed reduction clamps, and a single K-wire is driven in a transcondylar manner. The thread hole for the lag screw is drilled into the medial part using the centering drill guide. After the lag screw is tightened, a small K-wire is driven across the metaphyseal fracture, along the lateral epicondylar crest.

Although bicondylar fractures are seen more frequently in mature animals, a bicondylar physeal fracture can occur. Olecranon osteotomy or triceps tenotomy provides excellent exposure to the posterior, distal aspect of the joint. With bicondylar fractures the two aspects of the condyle are initially lagged together, and then the repaired condyle is secured to the distal humerus with either intramedullary pins alone or with external fixator augmentation, Rush pins, or plates and screws. The combination of medial and lateral plates provides secure fixation with bicondylar fractures in large sporting and hunting breeds. Alternatively, one aspect of the condyle can be secured to the shaft initially, followed by lag screw fixation of the lateral portion. Both types of fractures require early range of motion and vigorous physical therapy for a successful result.

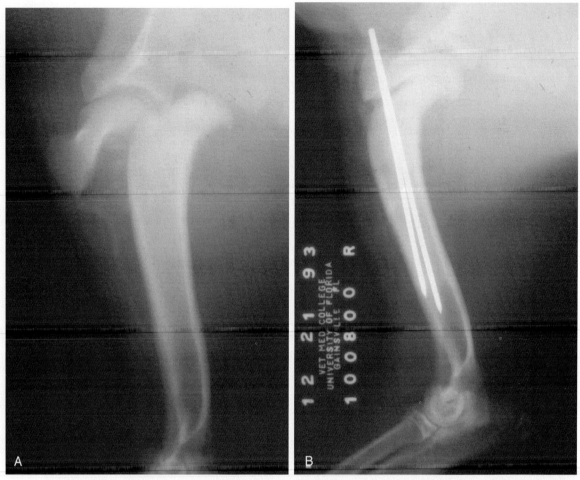

FIGURE 26–7. Pre (A) and postoperative (B) views of a Salter-Harris type I proximal humeral physeal fracture.

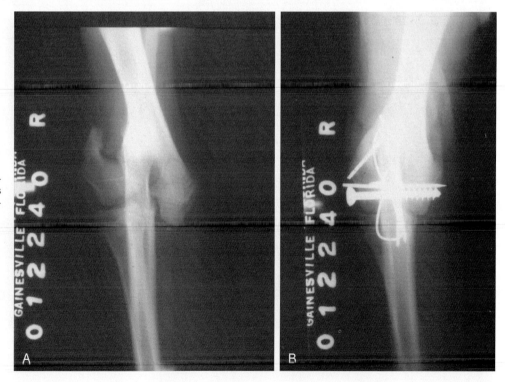

FIGURE 26–8. Pre (A) and postoperative (B) views of a Salter-Harris type IV distal humeral physeal fracture.

Proximal Radius

Actual fractures of the proximal radial physis are rare; however, cases with proximal radial growth arrest and radiohumeral subluxation secondary to Salter-Harris V injuries are not uncommon. Restoration of elbow congruency is preferable in performance animals. Remarkably, some smaller pet breed animals show minimal lameness with this abnormality.

Restoration of joint congruency is performed by means of high-radial osteotomy and reduction of the radiohumeral joint space (Fig. 26–9). Either a transverse or sliding-step osteotomy is performed, and the fixation is held with screws, plate, or external fixator. Although not yet described, the use of a ring fixator with distraction osteogenesis according to the principles of Illizarov would be applicable in this situation.

Proximal Ulna

The proximal ulnar growth plate contributes approximately 15 per cent of the total ulnar growth and is infrequently fractured. Iatrogenic fracture may occur during an attempt at olecranon osteotomy to provide posterior exposure of the elbow joint in an immature animal.

The proximal ulna is approached posteriorly, and the fracture site is visualized. Because of proximal traction provided by the triceps on the olecranon, the epiphysis is displaced proximally. Placing the elbow in extension will facilitate reduction. Stabilization is usually carried out with a pin and tension band. Although the tension band is dynamic and provides compression at the fracture site, complications related to premature physeal closure have not been reported.

Distal Ulna

Because the distal ulnar growth plate provides 85 per cent of the total length of the ulna (100 per cent of growth distal to the elbow) and the ulna is paired with the radius to form the antebrachium, injury to this growth plate has significant results. The anatomical conical shape of the physis predisposes it to Salter-Harris V injury when excessive axial or shear forces are applied. The radiographic appearance of a Salter-Harris V injury is usually normal at the time of injury; subsequently it is important to warn owners of acutely injured animals that unrecognized compressive injury may lead to clinically relevant consequences.

If premature closure of the ulna occurs, the ulna acts as a bowstring or tether to the radius and prevents longitudinal growth of the antebrachium. Because it can no longer grow longitudinally, the radius deviates and grows around the ulna. The radius bows cranially and medially and begins to externally rotate. This produces the valgus and externally rotated appearance of the paw typical of the radius curvis syndrome (Fig. 26–10). Subluxation of the antebrachial carpal joint occurs, and degenerative changes will progress if the condition is not corrected. Equally important is the humeroulnar subluxation that can occur at the elbow joint. Posterior subluxation of the trochlear notch and "fracture" of the anconeal process can occur.

The goal in reconstruction of angular limb deformities is to relieve the tethering effect of the ulna and to provide parallel and congruent joints. Limb length discrepancies may not be a clinical factor; however, this could also be factored into the reconstruction plan utilizing distraction osteogenesis according to the principles of Illizarov.

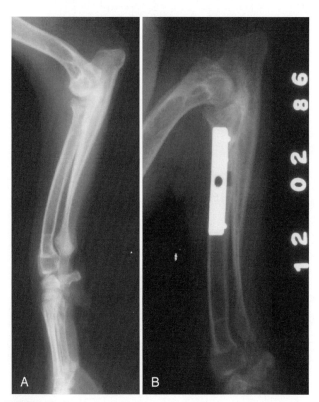

FIGURE 26–9. Pre *(A)* and postoperative *(B)* views of a premature proximal radial physeal closure.

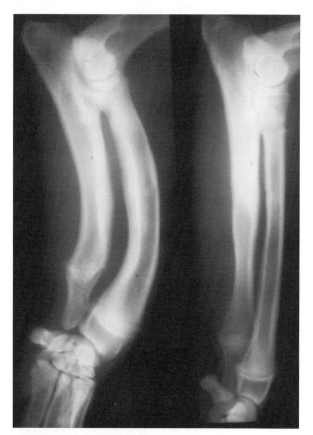

FIGURE 26–10. Premature distal ulnar physeal closure *(left)* with the normal antebrachium *(right)* for comparison.

Preoperative planning is essential for a successful result. In young animals, measures to remove the tether of the ulna require aggressive ulnar ostectomies, careful stripping of periosteum from the ostectomy site, and implantation of an interpositional material to retard healing and recurrence of a similar effect. The ulna is approached laterally, and the periosteum is incised over the distal one third of the ulna. After periosteal elevation, ostectomy of the distal one third of the physis and metaphysis is performed. After careful removal of the periosteum from the defect, autogenous fat harvested from the gluteal area is interposed, and the sutured muscular fascia is used to hold it in place. Humeroulnar subluxations may reduce themselves after the tether is relieved and dynamic traction is applied by the triceps tendon. Depending on the animal's age, some spontaneous radial correction may occur after the ulna is excised. The surgeon can wait until skeletal maturity to perform a definitive radial correction; however, many radial deformities can progress, which makes correction at a later date more difficult. If the ostectomy is performed early, a second correction may be necessary. An oblique radial osteotomy is usually performed at the area of maximum deformity; angular correction and parallel joints are achieved, and the limb is immobilized in a modified type II external skeletal fixation device. With more clinical experience, fine-wire ring fixators with hinges and motors may be recommended for complex deformities, especially with limb length discrepancies.

Distal Radius

The distal radial growth plate contributes approximately 60 per cent of longitudinal growth to that bone. Although a large review of physeal injuries in the dog indicated that Salter II fractures were the most common, other authors and clinical experience indicate that type II and V injuries are most common. Distal radial physeal fractures are commonly associated with distal ulnar physeal injuries; therefore, it is prudent to radiographically monitor the healing and growth of both bones following a distal radial physeal fracture. Many minimally displaced and stable distal radial physeal fractures can be treated with reduction and stabilized with external coaptation. If closed reduction is not possible, open reduction and stabilization with crossed pins or K-wires is necessary.

Premature closure of the entire distal radial physis (symmetrical epiphysiodesis) results in a clinical picture similar to proximal radial closure. The radius is straighter than normal or it is slightly curved posteriorly (Fig. 26–11). Subluxation of the antebrachial carpal joint may be present. Correction usually involves a transverse or stair-step osteotomy, distraction, and fixation with screws, plate, or external fixator. This is another location where the Illizarov apparatus can be useful.

Proximal Femur

Proximal femoral physeal (capital physeal) fractures are relatively common in immature animals sustaining injury to the hindlimbs. The lateral and medial circumflex femoral arteries send branches that ultimately give rise to the superior and inferior cervical arteries that supply the capital epiphysis. Salter-Harris I fractures occur most commonly, although Salter-Harris type II fractures have been reported (Fig. 26–12A). Although not directly related to success, early surgical repair is advised. A craniolateral or dorsal approach by either trochanteric osteotomy or partial tenotomy of the deep gluteal tendon provides adequate exposure without compromising revascularization. A number of fixation techniques have been described; however, I prefer the three-divergent K-wire technique (Fig. 26–12B). Three K-wires are normograded, beginning laterally in the area of the third trochanter, and progress across the neck to penetrate the metaphyseal side of the

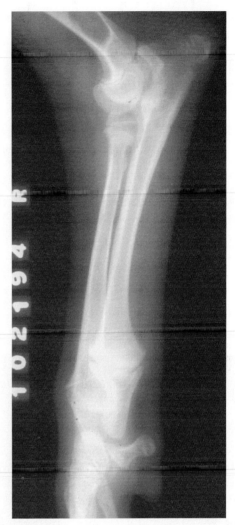

FIGURE 26–11. Premature distal radial physeal closure.

fracture site. Proper pin placement is facilitated by starting the pins slightly more distal than one would intuitively imagine. Proper orientation of the fracture fragments is sometimes confusing through a limited exposure; however, this can be facilitated by knowing that the epiphyseal fragment usually has an inverted L surface, with the long portion of the L directed superiorly. After reduction, the K-wires are driven into the capital epiphysis, care being taken not to penetrate the articular cartilage. Range of motion is checked, and with application of traction on the greater trochanter, the joint is subluxated to visualize the articular surface for inadvertent pin penetration.

Prognosis depends on a number of factors. A study revealed the incidence of degenerative joint disease increased when animals were younger (4 months or less) and when they had associated ipsilateral acetabular fracture, ipsilateral coxofemoral luxation, or ipsilateral coxofemoral subluxation after surgery. This is obviously of clinical importance in performance animals. Alternative salvage procedures include excision or total hip arthroplasty.

Distal Femur

The distal femoral physis was the most frequently fractured in a large review of physeal injuries in the dog. The distal femoral physis provides approximately 60 per cent of the ultimate long-bone growth of the femur. Although all forms of physeal fractures are possible, Salter-Harris II fractures are the most common. The normal physis has a W appearance when viewed on a lateral radiograph and physically has four metaphyseal projections or pegs and four corresponding epiphyseal sockets or depressions. With a Salter-Harris II physeal fracture, at least one of the metaphyseal pegs remains with the epiphysis. Because of the pull of the gastrocnemius muscle, the distal epiphyseal fragment displaces caudally (Fig. 26–13A).

Open and closed repair have been described. With a minimally displaced acute fracture, reduction can be attempted with the stifle flexed and the hock extended to relieve the gastrocnemius tension. After reduction, the joint would be placed in a modified Ehmer or 90-90 sling for 2 to 3 weeks. The "sockets and pegs" on either side of the fracture will add to the stability; however, the closed technique does not allow for early range of motion and is subject to patient and owner compliance. Early range of motion is helpful in preventing stiff stifle syndrome and quadriceps contracture. Open techniques are generally required for a successful result, and a

number of forms of fixation have been described, including single or modified intramedullary pins with or without cross-pin rotational support, Rush and Rush-like pin fixation, multiple pin fixation (Fig. 26–13B), and crossed-pin fixation. With all of these techniques it is important to anatomically or slightly overreduce the epiphyseal fragment. This enables maximum pin purchase in the epiphysis and allows the quadriceps muscle group to locate slightly off the healing bone. This and early range of motion may help prevent quadriceps tie-down. The choice of technique must depend on the surgeon's preference and experience.

Proximal Tibia and Tibial Tuberosity

The proximal tibial epiphysis is relatively flat and somewhat triangular. The tibial tuberosity is the proximo-cranial projection of the tibia and acts as an insertion point for the patellar tendon. These two epiphyses are joined together in the immature dog by cartilage, which eventually fuses both epiphyses together. Three fracture configurations are possible: the proximal tibial physis can fracture alone, the tibial tuberosity can fracture alone, or a com-

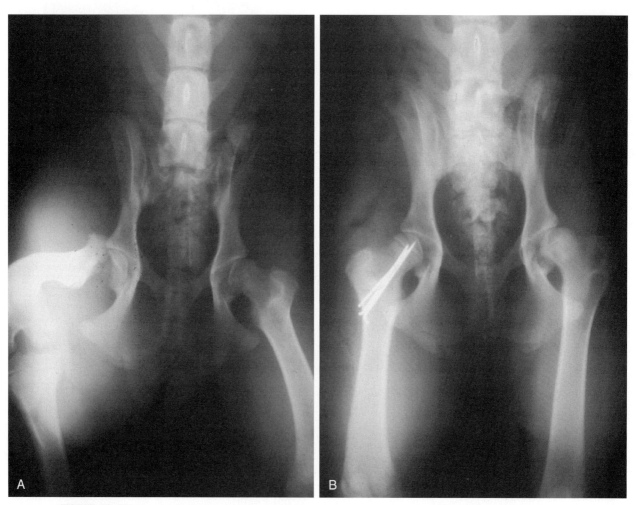

FIGURE 26–12. Pre *(A)* and postoperative *(B)* views of a Salter-Harris type I proximal femoral (capital) physeal fracture.

bined fracture can occur when the cartilage bridge remains intact (Fig. 26–14A, B).

When the proximal tibial physis is involved, Salter-Harris II fractures are the most common. Closed reduction and external fixation may be possible with minimally displaced fractures. Open reduction and internal fixation usually involve alignment of the fracture fragments and fixation with laterally and medially placed K-wires. The epiphyseal fragment is small, and care must be taken to prevent the pins from entering the stifle joint. When the tibial tuberosity remains attached to the proximal tibial epiphysis (as is frequently the case), additional K-wires can be placed through the tibial tuberosity for further stability (Fig. 26–14C, D).

The racing greyhound may have a predisposition to Salter-Harris I or II tibial tuberosity avulsion fractures. Cases have been reported in young dogs and in dogs as old as 21 months of age, thus the variability in growth plate closure time between breeds and even between closely related dogs. Some greyhounds have a history of chronic lameness and radiographic evidence of chronic fracture. Conservative treatment using a cast has been recommended for dogs with minimal displacement. Surgical treatment has usually involved the use of a pin and tension band; however, some signifi-

cant complications have occurred, especially in the greyhound. Most notably this breed has an unexplained tendency to develop distal translocation of the tibial tuberosity following pin and tension band repair (Fig. 26–15). In addition, some racing greyhounds develop an abnormality of the tibial plateau that is thought to be due to an unrecognized Salter-Harris V injury to the proximal tibial physis at the time of initial injury. My current recommendation for this fracture in the greyhound is stabilization of an acute, displaced fracture with crossed K-wires with external coaptation support for 3 to 4 weeks.

Distal Tibia

Fractures of the distal tibial physis are rare. Salter-Harris types I and II are the most common and usually also include a Salter-Harris I fracture of the distal fibula (malleolus). Open reduction is usually necessary for displaced fractures. Fixation is usually achieved with small crossed K-wires started in the lateral and medial malleoli. Fixation may be tenuous, and external support is advised (Fig. 26–16).

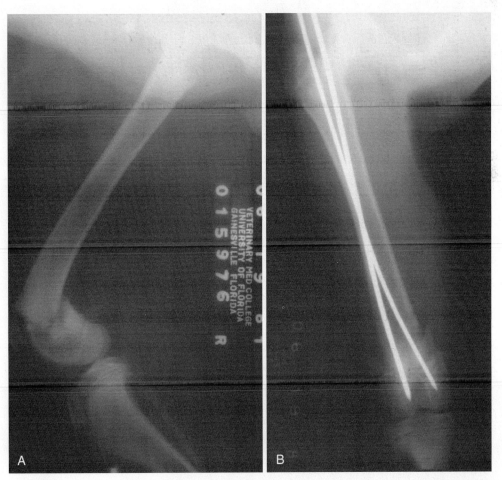

FIGURE 26–13. Pre (A) and postoperative (B) views of a Salter-Harris type II distal femoral physeal fracture.

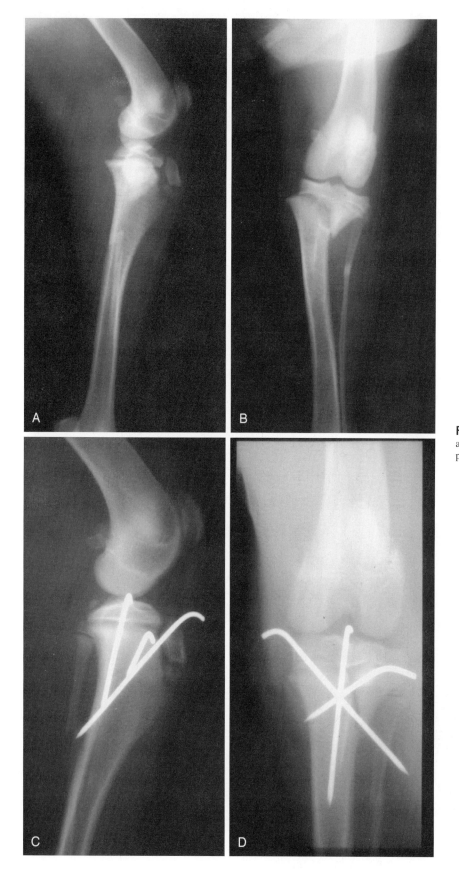

FIGURE 26–14. Pre *(A* and *B)* and postoperative *(C* and *D)* views of a Salter-Harris type II proximal tibial physeal fracture.

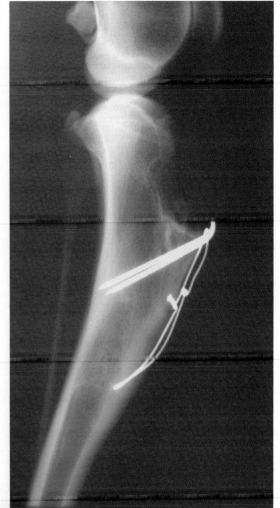

FIGURE 26–15. Lateral view of a 3-month follow-up of a Salter-Harris type I tibial tuberosity fracture in a 13-month greyhound repaired with a pin and tension band apparatus. Distal migration of the tibial tuberosity is evident.

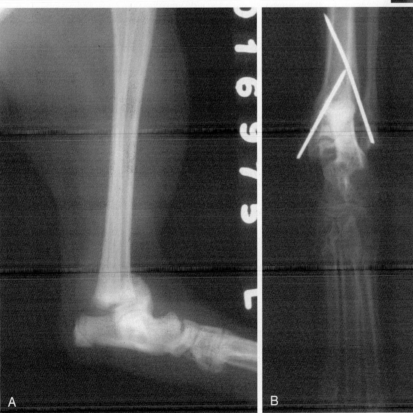

FIGURE 26–16. Pre *(A)* and postoperative *(B)* views of a Salter-Harris type II distal tibial fracture.

References

1. Braden TB: Histopathology of the growth plate and growth plate injuries. *In* Bojrab MJ (ed): Disease Mechanisms in Small Animal Surgery. Philadelphia, Lea and Febiger, 1993.
2. Salter RB and Harris WR: Injuries involving the epiphyseal plate. J Bone Joint Surg 45A:587, 1996.
3. Johnson JM, Johnson AL, and Eurell JC: Histological appearance of naturally occurring canine physeal fractures. Vet Surg 23:81, 1994.
4. Manley PA, Henry WB, and Wilson JW: Disease of the epiphyses. *In* Whittick WG: Canine Orthopedics. Philadelphia, Lea and Febiger, 1990.
5. Marcellin-Little DJ, DeYoung DJ, Ferris KK, et al: Incomplete ossification of the humeral condyle in spaniels. Vet Surg 23:475, 1994.
6. Marretta SM, Schrader SC: Physeal injuries in the dog: A review of 135 cases. J Am Vet Med Assoc 182:708, 1983.
7. DeCamp CE, Probst CW, Thomas MW: Internal fixation of femoral capital physeal injuries in dogs: 40 cases (1979–1987). J Am Vet Med Assoc 194:1750, 1989.
8. Shires PK, Hulse DA: Internal fixation of physeal fractures using the distal femur as an example. Compen Cont Ed 11:854, 1980.
9. Goldsmid S, Johnson KA: Complications of canine tibial tuberosity avulsion fractures. Vet Comp Ortho Trauma 4:51, 1991.

CHAPTER 27

OSTEOCHONDROSIS OF SPORTING AND WORKING DOGS

MARK S. BLOOMBERG \ DANIEL D. LEWIS

Osteochondrosis, a developmental orthopedic condition characterized by a disturbance in the normal process of endochondral ossification,[1–3] is one of the most common causes of secondary osteoarthrosis in domestic animals. It primarily affects the diarthrodial joints in dogs, including the shoulder, elbow, stifle, and tarsal joints. This chapter concentrates on the aspects of osteochondrosis that affect the canine athlete. The etiology, pathogenesis, incidence, treatment, and prognosis of various manifestations of osteochondrosis with respect to athletic performance are described.

Endochondral ossification is the process responsible for long-bone growth and involves the orderly formation of bone from cartilage.[1, 2, 4] In the pathogenesis of osteochondrosis, the normal process of cartilage resorption and subsequent calcification process is disrupted and affected articular or physeal cartilage becomes grossly thickened. Articular cartilage, which is avascular, depends on diffusion of synovial fluid for its metabolic needs. Chondrocytes in the deeper zones of abnormally thickened cartilage are deprived of nutritional support because of the increased distance synovial fluid must diffuse. The result is abnormal chondrocyte metabolism and dysfunction. Cartilage in these deeper layers may become necrotic and develop cracks and fissures. If a crack or fissure extends to the surface of the cartilage, synovial fluid dissects beneath the cartilage flap, and debris and inflammatory mediators are released from the necrotic cartilage, resulting in inflammation of the synovial tissues. When a cartilage flap or osteochondral fragment is present, the condition is more appropriately described as osteochondritis dissecans.[1–5]

An articular cartilage flap is the classic lesion of osteochondritis dissecans.[1, 5, 6] Articular cartilage flaps have been described as type I lesions and typically develop at or near the center of a convex joint surface.[1] At some locations, such as the trochlear ridges of the talus, lesions often exist as osteochondral fragments rather than cartilage flaps.[1, 7] These have been described as type II lesions that typically develop in the periphery of a joint surface in contact with the joint capsule and supporting ligamentous structures.[1] The

inflammation associated with osteochondritis dissecans lesions produces observable clinical signs such as pain and lameness.[3–5] As the cartilage flap or osteochondral fragment continues to separate from the subchondral bone, several sequelae can develop. Cartilage flaps may remain attached, causing lameness and osteoarthrosis. Cartilage flaps and osteochondral fragments often give rise to a superficial erosive (kissing) lesion of the apposing articular surface. Cartilage flaps may detach and be resorbed or develop into an attached or free-floating "joint mouse." The remaining articular cartilage defect will eventually fill in with fibrous repair tissue resembling fibrocartilage.[1–5]

ETIOLOGY

Osteochondrosis is thought to have many causes.[1, 2, 5, 6] Genetic factors that affect weight gain and growth, behavior, sexual development, and conformation undoubtedly are involved in the etiology of osteochondrosis.[1, 3, 7–10] Osteochondrosis occurs primarily in medium-, large-, and giant-breed dogs.[1, 3, 4, 7, 11–15] Rapidly growing representatives of these breeds seem to be predisposed. The genetic capacity for rapid growth and overfeeding may be influential during the dog's period of rapid growth. This is an important aspect in athletic dogs, as often it is the largest, most rapidly growing dog that is desired. In addition, the selective breeding of performance animals may be based on performance data, conformation, and other desired qualities without knowledge of subclinical articular disease or affected litter mates.

Biomechanical forces are another important etiological factor in the development of osteochondrosis.[2, 5, 16–18] Osteochondrosis lesions develop in areas of articular cartilage that are subject to increased loads.[16, 18, 19] Normal joint stresses and focal trauma likely are inciting and perpetuating factors involved in the pathogenesis of this condition.[2, 3, 18] The strenuous activity often imposed on performance dogs at very young ages may partially account for the high incidence of osteochondrosis in many breeds of working and racing dogs.

Overnutrition in the form of excessive amounts of food and/or nutritional supplements has been incriminated as another important etiological factor.[1, 2, 8, 20] This is evidenced by higher caloric intake in rapidly growing animals resulting in greater incidence of osteochondrosis.[8, 20, 21] Excessive calcium supplementation has been shown to increase the development of osteochondrosis.[22–24] Hormonal disturbances have also been incriminated through experimental production of osteochondrotic lesions following the administration of thyrotropin, growth hormone, estrogens, and androgens.[5, 25, 26] All of the aforementioned etiological factors may enter into the development of osteochondrosis as breeders, trainers, and owners search for the combination of the biggest, fastest, best-looking representatives of a breed, not infrequently placing the individual dog or breed at risk.

INCIDENCE

Osteochondrosis is usually seen in medium-, large-, and giant-breed dogs.[1, 14, 27, 28] The clinical manifestations of the disease typically occur between 4 and 9 months of age.[4, 5, 7, 29] It is interesting to note, however, that in a review of 626 dogs with osteochondrosis of the humeral head, 36 per cent were greater than 1 year of age at the time of diagnosis.[15] Osteochondrosis is usually seen more frequently in males than in females.[3, 7, 13, 29] The exception to this trend is osteochondrosis of the hock, which has been reported slightly more frequently in female dogs.[1, 30–32]

In dogs, osteochondrosis most commonly develops on the articular surfaces of the humeral head, humeral condyle, femoral condyles, and the trochlear ridges of the talus.[2, 3, 6, 7, 29] Less frequently reported sites of osteochondrosis include the femoral head, patella, distal end of the radius, articular facets of the spine, and glenoid surface of the scapula.[1, 2, 33–35] Multiple joint involvement is not uncommon.[1, 4, 7] A thorough physical and radiographic examination is necessary for early detection of this disease and to avoid giving an overly optimistic prognosis for return to athletic performance.

In the dog, many developmental orthopedic conditions affecting physeal and articular cartilage have been lumped under the general category of osteochondrosis. Definitions of osteochondrosis vary among some investigators, and the classification of certain developmental orthopedic conditions occurring in dogs as osteochondrosis is a contentious issue. Fragmented coronoid process and united anconeal process are two examples of developmental orthopedic conditions that have been purported to be osteochondroses,[1, 9, 36, 37] but likely have different causes.[18, 27, 38, 39]

OSTEOCHONDROSIS OF THE HUMERAL HEAD

The humeral head is the most frequently reported location for osteochondrosis in dogs.[6, 7, 40] The lesion most commonly involves the caudocentral aspect of the humeral head (Fig. 27-1).[2, 3, 4, 41] Although giant-breed dogs, such as mastiffs, Newfoundlands, Great Pyrenees, Saint Bernards, Bernese mountain dogs, and Irish wolfhounds, seem to be at particular high risk of developing osteochondrosis of the humeral head, the condition is also very common in many of the more popular large-breed working and sporting dogs, such as retrievers, setters, shepherds, and rottweilers.[3, 14, 15, 17, 28, 42] There are several reports of osteochondrosis of the humeral head in the racing greyhound.[43–49] Zuber reports finding three dogs with osteochondritis dissecans of the humeral head in a series of 50 racing greyhounds with forelimb lameness.[47] Milton et al reported

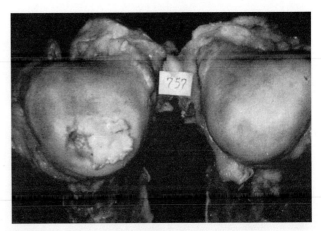

FIGURE 27–1. Gross specimen of the humeral heads of a Great Dane with a unilateral osteochondritis dissecans lesion. (From Lenehan TM, Van Sickle DC: Canine osteochondrosis. *In* Newton CD, Nunamaker CM: Textbook of Small Animal Orthopaedics. Philadelphia, JB Lippincott, 1985, pp. 981–997.)

on two clinical cases of osteochondritis dissecans in greyhounds, but found only one osteochondrosis lesion upon examining the humeral heads of 218 greyhound cadavers.[43] In contrast, a 5 per cent incidence of osteochondrosis of the humeral head was found in racing greyhounds presented to the University of Florida's Veterinary Medical Teaching Hospital (UF-VMTH) for euthanasia.[44] One litter of greyhounds presented to UF-VMTH had five dogs with osteochondritis dissecans of the humeral head; three were male, and two of the males were affected bilaterally.

Although most dogs with osteochondritis dissecans of the humeral head typically do not display clinical abnormalities before 6 months of age, some dogs develop lameness as early as 4 months of age.[14, 41, 42] Lameness may not become apparent in some greyhounds until the dogs are 11 to 15 months of age and begin breaking in for racing.[50] Dogs may initially have a mild, intermittent weight-bearing forelimb lameness that is insidious in onset.[4, 5, 42] The condition can progress to a profound weight-bearing or intermittent non–weight-bearing lameness.[4, 7, 42, 5, 51] Atrophy of the regional musculature is obvious in severely affected dogs.[4, 6, 42] Flexion and extension of the scapulohumeral joint elicit a marked pain response.[3, 5, 15, 41, 50]

The diagnosis of osteochondrosis is confirmed by the presence of a subchondral bone defect of the caudal aspect of the humeral head, most evident on a lateral-view radiograph of the scapulohumeral joint (Fig. 27-2).[7, 40] Supplemental lateral-view radiographs made with the humerus positioned in internal and external rotation may occasionally be necessary to tangentially outline lesions that are atypically medially or laterally positioned.[2, 40] Radiographic evidence of osteochondrosis of the humeral head has been reported to be bilateral in 43 to 65 per cent of affected dogs, but less than half of these dogs exhibit bilateral lameness.[14, 41, 52, 53]

Positive-contrast arthrography has prognostic value in evaluating the contralateral shoulder in dogs with unilateral lameness but bilateral radiographic lesions.[40, 52, 54, 55] The only means of distinguishing osteochondrosis from osteochondritis dissecans radiographically (unless the cartilage flap has mineralized) is to perform contrast arthrography, because cartilage has the same radiographic density as synovial fluid and cannot be visualized on plain radiographs. Contrast arthrography allows evaluation of the integrity of the cartilage overlying a defect in the subchondral bone. The presence of intact thickened cartilage over the subchondral bone defect is a favorable prognostic sign (Fig. 27-3).[52, 53] If, however,

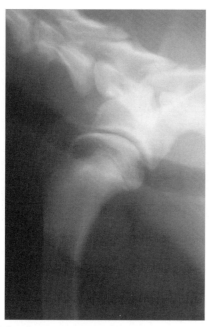

FIGURE 27–2. Lateral view radiograph of an 8-month-old greyhound with an osteochondritis dissecans lesion of the humeral head. Note the subchondral bone defect on the caudal aspect of the humeral head.

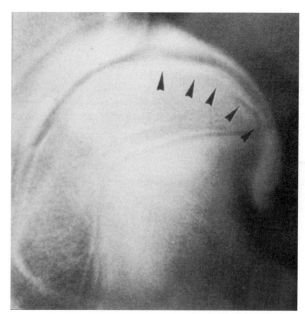

FIGURE 27–4. Positive contrast arthrogram of the scapulohumeral joint of a dog with an osteochondritis dissecans lesion of the humeral head. Note that the contrast agent dissects beneath the surface of the articular cartilage overlying the subchondral bone defect *(arrowheads)*. (From van Bree H: Comparison of the diagnostic accuracy of positive-contrast arthrography and arthrotomy in evaluation of osteochondrosis lesions in the scapulohumeral joint in dogs. JAVMA 203:84–88, 1993.)

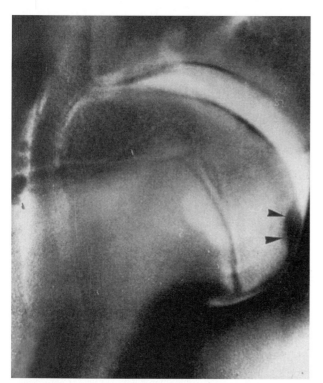

FIGURE 27–3. Positive contrast arthrogram of the scapulohumeral joint of a dog with an osteochondrosis lesion of the humeral head. The thickened cartilage overlying the subchondral defect on the caudal aspect of the humeral head is intact *(arrowheads)*. (From van Bree H: Comparison of the diagnostic accuracy of positive-contrast arthrography and arthrotomy in evaluation of osteochondrosis lesions in the scapulohumeral joint in dogs. JAVMA 203:84–88, 1993.)

contrast medium dissects under the thickened cartilage overlying a subchondral bone defect (substantiating the presence of a cartilage flap) (Fig. 27–4), there is a 50 per cent chance that arthrotomy will be required to remove the flap.[52] In working dogs or racing greyhounds that are being schooled, we have also found positive-contrast arthrography to be useful in dogs with a history of a subtle intermittent forelimb lameness associated with strenuous activity. These dogs are typically between 14 and 20 months of age and have equivocal pain associated with manipulation of the scapulohumeral joint. Although these dogs have a subchondral bone defect of the caudal aspect of the humeral head, the absence of a definitive corroborating pain response on flexion or extension of the scapulohumeral joint makes a diagnosis of osteochondritis dissecans somewhat questionable. Contrast arthrography and cytological examination of the synovial fluid obtained just prior to arthrography are useful in establishing a definitive diagnosis in such dogs.

In some dogs the cartilage flap may detach. A detached flap that adheres to the synovium of the caudal joint pouch is unlikely to cause lameness[52] (Fig. 27–5); however, greater than 50 per cent of dogs with a detached flap floating loose in the joint space have or develop substantial lameness.[52] Flaps that lodge in the bicipital tendon sheath also are associated with chronic lameness (Fig. 27–6).[52, 55] Contrast arthrography again is necessary to identify a detached flap radiographically unless the flap has mineralized.[52, 55]

At the initial onset of lameness, young animals may be treated conservatively with the idea that normal activity may dislodge the cartilage flap, causing it to adhere to the synovium of the caudal joint pouch, and lameness will resolve.[1] Although surgical excision and curettage of osteochondritis dissecans lesions is associated with a much higher rate of resolution of lameness, lameness will resolve in some dogs without surgical intervention.[50, 51] This therapeutic approach is supported somewhat by the fact that although approximately 50 per cent of dogs have bilateral radiographic lesions, less than half of these dogs develop bilateral lameness.[14, 52, 53] Many of

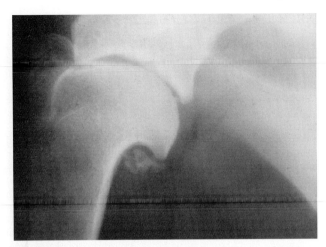

FIGURE 27–5. Lateral radiograph of the scapulohumeral joint of a 6-year-old Labrador retriever with a detached osteochondritis dissecans flap that has adhered to synovium of the caudal joint pouch and mineralized. There are degenerative changes of the scapulohumeral joint, but the dog had no associated lameness.

the dogs that do not develop lameness, however, probably have osteochondrosis and not osteochondritis dissecans lesions in the limb that does not develop lameness. Dogs with mild lameness that responds to conservative nonsurgical therapy will generally respond rapidly and will be sound on the affected limb in 2 to 3 months.[53] Dogs with more severe lameness that is not treated surgically may require a year or longer before becoming sound on the affected

limb and stop exhibiting lameness after vigorous exercise.[2] The probability for resolution of lameness in greyhounds that develop lameness during breaking in is reported to be 60 to 80 per cent.[50] Resolution of lameness in younger greyhounds with osteochondritis dissecans of the shoulder is stated to be even higher, since these dogs are not undergoing rigorous training.[50] These percentages seem exceptionally high, and we suggest that many of these dogs had lameness due to other causes. Intra-articular sodium hyaluronate and intramuscular polysulfated glycosaminoglycan therapy has been recommended for dogs that are managed without surgery.[50]

Surgical excision of the cartilage flap (Fig. 27–7) and curettage of the subjacent bed is indicated for dogs with chronic or severe lameness.[2–4, 41] Several surgical approaches have been described for this procedure.[3, 56–61] The craniolateral approach to the scapulohumeral joint, which requires tenotomy of the tendon of insertion of the infraspinatus muscle and if necessary the teres minor muscle, allows the humeral head to be subluxated and affords the surgeon the greatest exposure of the articular surface of the humeral head.[60, 62] Caudolateral and caudal approaches to the scapulohumeral joint have been described that do not require tenotomy or subluxation of the scapulohumeral joint.[56, 57, 58] While the craniolateral approach allows maximal exposure of the articular surface of the humeral head, slightly greater morbidity is associated with this approach.[56, 57, 62] A relatively recent study compared the morbidity of the craniolateral and caudolateral approach to the scapulohumeral joint in normal dogs using force plate analysis, lameness evaluation, and

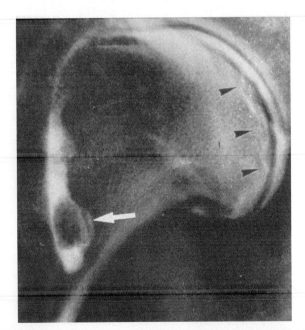

FIGURE 27–6. Positive contrast arthrogram of the scapulohumeral joint of a dog with a detached osteochondritis dissecans flap that has lodged in the bicipital tendon sheath *(white arrow)*. Contrast material has penetrated the articular surface at multiple sites *(black arrowheads)* suggesting that there is fragmentation of the articular cartilage. (From van Bree H: Comparison of the diagnostic accuracy of positive-contrast arthrography and arthrotomy in evaluation of osteochondrosis lesions in the scapulohumeral joint in dogs. JAVMA 203:84–88, 1993.)

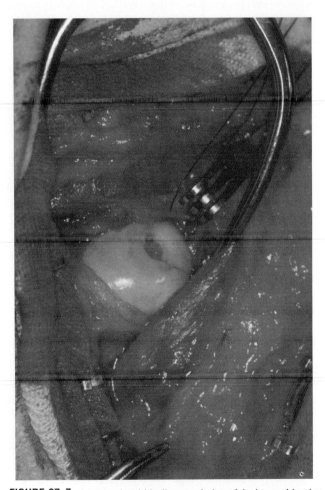

FIGURE 27–7. An osteochondritis dissecans lesion of the humeral head at arthrotomy.

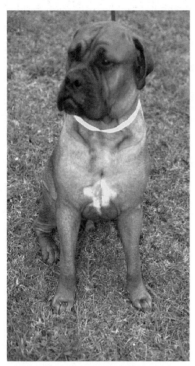

FIGURE 27–8. Eight-month-old mastiff with bilateral fragmented coronoid processes and an osteochondritis dissecans lesion of the left humeral condyle. Note the characteristics of the forelimb stance with the elbows abducted and the carpi held in a supinated position.

goniometry for 5 weeks following surgery. Dogs had a more rapid and complete return to function following the caudolateral approach, although significant differences were no longer present at 35 days.[62] Thus, while the craniolateral approach to the scapulohumeral joint may be acceptable for nonworking or nonracing dogs, a caudolateral or caudal approach should be used in performance animals. The caudal approach is also preferable if exploration of the caudal joint pouch is indicated.[56, 57]

Postoperative care consists of kennel confinement and leash exercise for 10 to 14 days followed by gradual return to normal activity over the subsequent 2 weeks. Seroma formation is a frequent complication following surgery and has been ascribed to vigorous activity in the early convalescent period.[4, 58, 63, 64] We have found seroma formation to be an uncommon problem with the caudal and caudolateral approaches. Seroma formation is probably also related to excessive dissection and poor closure techniques. The prognosis for return to previous performance levels following surgery is excellent.[4, 5, 14, 15]

OSTEOCHONDROSIS OF THE ELBOW

Three developmental conditions, osteochondrosis of the humeral condyle, ununited anconeal process (UAP), and fragmented coronoid process (FCP), can affect the elbow of many large and giant breeds of dogs.[1, 29, 39, 65] Although ununited anconeal process and fragmented coronoid process may not be true osteochondroses,[18, 27, 39, 66] all three conditions share many clinical similarities and will be discussed here. It should be noted that these lesions are often bilateral. Most commonly, osteochondrosis dissecans of the humeral condyle and fragmented coronoid process are recognized concurrently.[1, 67–70]

The history, signalment, and clinical signs are similar with all three conditions.[7, 29, 65, 71] Clinical abnormalities result from acute joint inflammation and progressive degenerative joint disease of the elbow. Affected animals may exhibit lameness as early as 4 months of age.[4, 7, 29] The lameness is intermittent and may be exacerbated by exercise or when the dog first ambulates following prolonged rest.[1, 72] Affected dogs may stand or sit with the carpus held in a "valgus" or supinated position and with the elbow abducted (Fig. 27–8).[7, 27, 39] The dog may circumduct the antebrachium during the swing phase of the stride.[7, 27] Full extension and flexion of the elbow may elicit a pain response. In dogs with ununited anconeal process it has been stated that a pain response also can be elicited by applying direct pressure to the anconeal process through the anconeus muscle as the dog's elbow is held in flexion.[68] Crepitus, joint capsule thickening, and decreased range of motion are present in advanced cases. Although synovial effusion is considered a classic sign of ununited anconeal process, synovial effusion can also be present with osteochondrosis of the humeral condyle and fragmented coronoid process (Fig. 27–9).[7]

These conditions can be differentiated by high-quality craniocaudal and lateral radiographic views of the elbow joint.[27, 70–73] Additional oblique and flexed lateral views of the elbow may also be warranted.[27, 29, 74] In all three conditions the prognosis for return to working or athletic performance, irrespective of whether or not surgical intervention has been carried out, is guarded. This guarded prognosis is based on the progression of degenerative joint disease with all three of these conditions regardless of whether or not surgery is performed. In addition, an arthrotomy is not a benign procedure, especially if a desmotomy or an osteotomy is performed. Although the apparent recovery following surgery is rapid, some morbidity should be expected. Also, elbow function depends on a normal anatomical relationship of the radioulnar, humeroulnar, and radiohumeral articulations, and abnormal elbow conformation is believed to be an integral component in the pathogenesis of these diseases.[1, 38, 39]

The heritability of fragmented coronoid process and osteochondrosis of the humeral condyle are well established, and a heritable basis is also suspected in ununited anconeal process.[7, 11–13, 66, 75] Thus, affected animals should be neutered and eliminated from breeding programs.

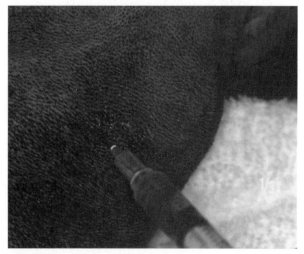

FIGURE 27–9. Arthrocentesis of the elbow joint of a 7-month-old rottweiler with a fragmented coronoid process and synovial effusion.

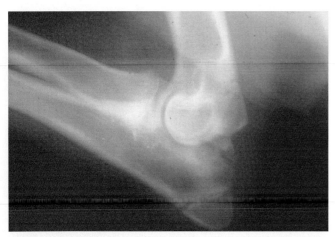

FIGURE 27–10. Flexed lateral view radiograph of the elbow of a 6-month-old German shepherd with an ununited anconeal process.

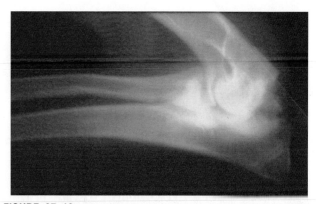

FIGURE 27–12. Flexed lateral view radiograph of the elbow of an 8-month-old Irish wolfhound with an ununited anconeal process and proximal humeroradial subluxation.

UNUNITED ANCONEAL PROCESS

Ununited anconeal process occurs primarily in large- and giant-breed dogs, most notably German shepherds.[29, 38, 76, 77] The condition is also recognized in chondrodystrophic breeds such as bassett hounds and bulldogs, because of retarded ulnar growth resulting in elbow incongruency.[66, 78] Male dogs are affected approximately twice as frequently as female dogs.[66, 79, 80] The condition is bilateral in 11 to 30 per cent of affected dogs.[76, 79, 80]

Diagnosis of ununited anconeal process is confirmed by a flexed lateral radiograph of the elbow (Fig. 27–10).[29, 65] In breeds that are predisposed to ununited anconeal process, the anconeal process develops as a distinct center of ossification separate from the ulna.[81] In German shepherd dogs, the anconeal process begins to mineralize at approximately 12 weeks of age and fuses with the ulna at 16 to 24 weeks of age (Fig. 27–11).[81] A definitive diagnosis

of ununited anconeal process thus should not be made before 24 weeks of age.[66] Congruency of the elbow must be assessed, as many chondrodystrophic and nonchondrodystrophic dogs with ununited anconeal process have humeroulnar subluxation (Fig. 27–12).[29, 76–79] Secondary degenerative changes of the elbow may be present.[7, 65, 80] Dogs with ununited anconeal process typically develop an intermittent, subtle-to-severe lameness of gradual onset between 5 and 9 months of age.[2, 66, 80] It should be noted, however, that ununited anconeal process can be a serendipitous radiographic finding in mature, middle-aged dogs with no prior history of fore-limb lameness, or it can be a cause of acute forelimb lameness in mature or middle-aged dogs that may not have had any previous history of lameness.[23, 80]

Excision of the ununited anconeal process is still the most widely accepted treatment for this condition.[29, 78, 82] If the anconeal process is to be excised, it is removed via a caudolateral approach to the

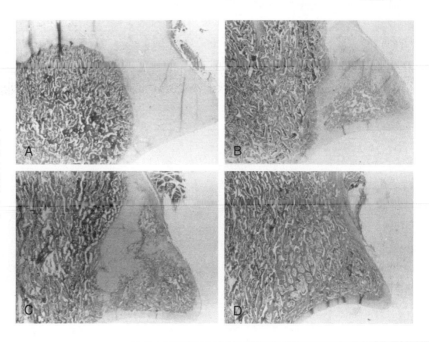

FIGURE 27–11. Developmental histology of the anconeal process. These sections were made from German shepherds euthanatized at *(A)* 10, *(B)* 12, *(C)* 16, and *(D)* 20 weeks of age. (From Lenehan TM, Van Sickle DC: Ununited anconeal process, ununited medial coronoid process, ununited medial epicondyle, patella cubiti, and sesamoidal fragments of the elbow. *In* Newton CD, Nanamaker CM: Textbook of Small Animal Orthopaedics. Philadelphia, JB Lippincott, 1985, pp 999–1012.)

elbow.[78]* The anconeal process is generally not freely movable because of numerous fibrous adhesions. These adhesions must be broken down with a periosteal elevator to remove the anconeal process (Fig. 27–13). Following surgery the limb is placed in a soft padded bandage for several days to limit swelling. Exercise is restricted for 21 days; however, passive flexion and extension of the elbow should be performed during this time.

Although the prognosis for working and athletic dogs with ununited anconeal process is guarded, many dogs obtain surprisingly good limb function following process excision. A recent retrospective study evaluated the long-term (mean follow-up 65 months following surgery) clinical results in six dogs that had ununited anconeal processes (one bilateral) excised between 5 and 12 months of age. Although degenerative joint disease progressed and range of motion was decreased in all affected elbows, limb function was considered good to excellent in six of the seven affected limbs.[82] Others have reported similar results,[76, 80] and we have had dogs with ununited anconeal process return to hunting, obedience, and field trial work after process excision. Some lameness after vigorous exercise, however, should be expected.

Stabilization of the ununited anconeal process utilizing lag screw fixation has been suggested; however, this procedure has met with technical difficulties and complications, and long-term results establishing the efficacy of lag screw fixation are lacking.[29, 66, 83–85] A recent report described radiographic union of six of ten ununited anconeal processes stabilized by lag screw fixation (Fig. 27–14). Detailed information describing limb function in these dogs, unfortunately, was not available.[86]

Some reports describe union of the ununited anconeal process with the olecranon following proximal diaphyseal ulnar osteotomy in young dogs with humeroulnar subluxation.[1, 77] The proximal diaphyseal ulnar osteotomy is performed to improve elbow joint congruency and relieve pressure on the anconeal process. The anconeal process fuses to the ulna in a slightly abnormal position (Fig. 27–15).[1, 77] The long-term functional results associated with proximal diaphyseal ulnar osteotomy appear to be superior to process excision.[77] The value of performing osteotomies to improve

---

*Editor's comment: In the uncommon event that a dog has a fragmented coronoid process and/or osteochondrosis of the medial humeral condyle with an associated ununited anconeal process, all may be removed via the medial incision if desired.

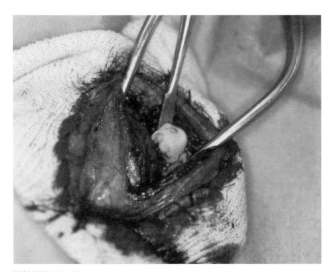

FIGURE 27–13. Surgical excision of an ununited anconeal process via caudolateral elbow arthrotomy.

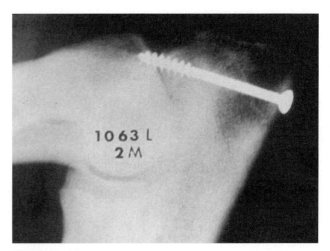

FIGURE 27–14. Two-month postoperative radiograph confirming fusion of an ununited anconeal process with the ulna following stabilization with a partially threaded 4.0-mm cancellous bone screw placed in lag fashion. (From Fox SM, et al.: Ununited anconeal process: Lag screw fixation. J Am Anim Hosp Assoc 32:52–56, 1996.)

joint congruency at the time of anconeal process excision in older dogs with humeroulnar subluxation has not been established. Empirically it would seem advantageous to restore normal joint congruency, particularly in dogs with marked subluxation; however, it is not known whether improving joint congruency results in improved limb function any more than fragment excision alone.

OSTEOCHONDROSIS OF THE HUMERAL CONDYLE

In our practice we recognize osteochondrosis of the humeral condyle infrequently in comparison to fragmented coronoid process and ununited anconeal process. Reports from Europe suggest that osteochondrosis of the humeral condyle occurs more frequently in Europe than in the United States.[1, 18, 67, 68, 70] This may reflect genetic differences in the populations. While osteochondrosis of the humeral condyle occurs in many large and giant breeds of dogs, golden and Labrador retrievers seem particularly prone to develop this condition.[12, 29, 70, 87, 88]

Osteochondrosis of the humeral condyle can be observed on the craniocaudal view radiograph of the elbow as a subchondral bone defect that affects the trochlea (the medial portion) of the humeral condyle. These lesions can be subtle and may not be identified unless the radiographs are of good quality and evaluated carefully. The pronated oblique craniocaudal view (Fig. 27–16) is often of value in identifying lesions that may not be apparent on non-oblique craniocaudal view radiographs.[4, 40, 87] If the lesion is large, an irregular subchondral bone defect or flattening of the articular surface of the trochlea may be visible on the lateral-view radiograph.[4, 40] Secondary degenerative changes are usually present in dogs 7 months of age and older. As previously stated, osteochondrosis of the humeral condyle often occurs concurrently with fragmented coronoid process. True osteochondrosis lesions of the humeral condyle can sometimes be difficult to distinguish radiographically from erosive lesions of the trochlea of the humeral condyle induced by fragmented coronoid process, particularly in older dogs with advanced degenerative changes.

Treatment involves excision of the cartilage flap and curettage of the subjacent subchondral bed. Several methods have been described for approaching the medial compartment of the elbow.[27.]

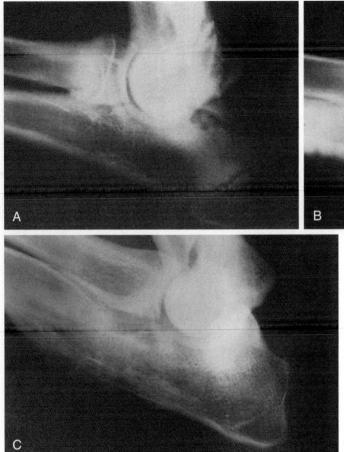

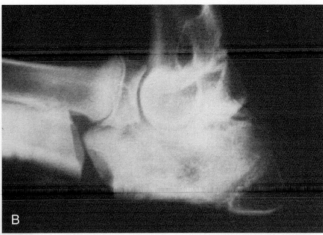

FIGURE 27–15. *A,* Preoperative radiograph of the elbow of a dog with an ununited anconeal process and humeroulnar subluxation. *B,* Eleven-day postoperative radiograph following proximal diaphyseal ulnar osteotomy. Note that the gap between the anconeal process and the ulna has narrowed. *C,* Thirty-one-month follow-up radiograph confirming union of the anconeal process with the ulna. Note that there are negligible degenerative changes in the elbow. (From Sjöström L, Kasström H, Källberg M: United anconeal process in the dog. Pathogenesis and treatment by osteotomy of the ulna. Vet Compar Ortho Trauma 8:170–176, 1995.)

[69, 73, 87, 89, 90] A recent study using cadaver limbs evaluated articular cartilage exposure and immediate postoperative stability afforded by three described approaches to the medial compartment of the elbow: osteotomy of the medial epicondyle, longitudinal myotomy of the flexor carpi radialis muscle, and desmotomy of the medial collateral ligament, which included tenotomy of the pronator teres muscle. The approach using an osteotomy of the medial epicondyle provided significantly greater exposures of the humeral articular cartilage (22 per cent) than either of the other two approaches, and the approach using desmotomy of the medial collateral ligament provided significantly greater exposure of the humeral articular cartilage (16.5 per cent) than the approach using longitudinal myotomy of the flexor carpi radialis muscle (6.6 per cent). The immediate postoperative stability of the approach using an osteotomy of the medial epicondyle and the approach using longitudinal myotomy of the flexor carpi radialis muscle was significantly greater than that of the approach using desmotomy of the medial collateral ligament. It must be noted, however, that testing of the limb was performed with both the elbow and carpus in 90 degrees of flexion to accentuate the soft tissue contributions to valgus stability of the elbow. At lesser angles of elbow flexion, interlocking of the anconeal process in the trochlea and olecranon fossa provided the valgus stability of the elbow.[91] This locking mechanism of the anconeal process in the trochlea and olecranon fossa probably negates much of the morbidity of any surgical approach to the medial compartment of the elbow and accounts for the lack of reported complications associated with the use of medial desmotomies in clinical cases.

We and others have experienced implant complications in clinical cases in which we used osteotomy of the medial epicondyle to approach the medial compartment of the elbow.[27, 92] We believe that exposure of the trochlea of the humeral condyle is sufficient to excise cartilage flaps and curette the lesion's bed using a muscle-separating approach between the flexor carpi radialis muscle and the pronator teres muscle. In some instances, exposure is sufficient by retracting the medial collateral ligament, but in many instances medial desmotomy is required to excise and curette an osteochondritis dissecans lesion of the humeral condyle. Myotenotomy of the pronator teres muscle can be performed if additional exposure is required; however, this is seldom necessary and should be avoided in performance dogs.

Osteochondritis dessicans lesions of the humeral condyle may not be as obvious as osteochondritis dissecans lesions of the humeral head. If a lesion is suspected based on the preoperative radiographs and is not readily apparent at arthrotomy, the articular surface of the trochlea of the humeral condyle should be probed with a Freer periosteal elevator (Fig. 27–17). In these instances the malacic cartilage will readily separate from the adjacent unaffected cartilage. All diseased cartilage should be excised and the subchondral bed curetted. Osteochondritis dissecans lesions of the humeral condyle should be differentiated from erosive or kissing lesions of the trochlea of the humeral condyle that frequently occur in response to fragmented coronoid process (Fig. 27–18).

Postoperatively the limb is placed in a soft padded bandage for several days following surgery to limit swelling, and exercise is restricted for 3 to 4 weeks. The prognosis for return to function is

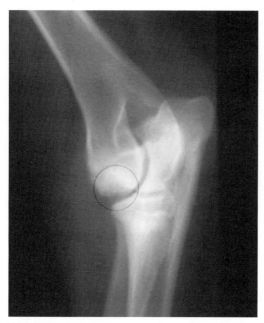

FIGURE 27–16. Pronated oblique, craniocaudal view radiograph of the elbow of a dog with an osteochondritis dissecans lesion of the humeral condyle *(circle).*

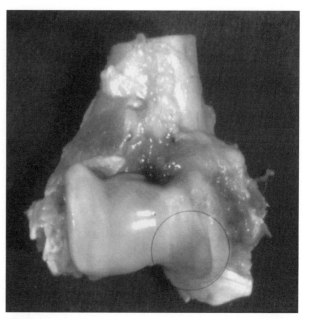

FIGURE 27–18. Erosive or "kissing" lesion *(circle)* of the trochlea of the humeral condyle that is the result of a fragmented coronoid process. (From Lewis DD, et al: Fragmented medial coronoid process of the canine elbow. Compend Contin Educ Pract Vet [Small Anim] 11:703–715, 1989.)

again somewhat guarded for dogs with osteochondrosis of the humeral condyle.[68, 90] The prognosis seems somewhat to depend on the size of the lesion and the extent of degenerative joint disease present at the time of surgery. Young dogs with small lesions and minimal degenerative joint disease appear to have a more favorable prognosis than older dogs with larger lesions and more advanced degenerative joint disease.[4] Although degenerative joint disease progresses irrespective of surgical intervention, some dogs may have acceptable limb function to return to hunting and other working activities on a limited basis.[68, 90]

FRAGMENTED CORONOID PROCESS

Fragmented coronoid process is the third developmental condition that affects the elbows of large- and giant-breed dogs, particularly retrievers, rottweilers, Bernese mountain dogs, and German shepherd dogs.[27, 39, 66, 71, 93] The etiopathogenesis of this condition is controversial. Fragmented coronoid process was initially believed to be a manifestation of the osteochondrosis complex[9, 37, 36, 71]; however, pathoanatomic studies have not fully supported this contention.[18, 38, 94] Fissures or fragmentation may result from abnormal stresses placed on the developing coronoid process secondary to conformational abnormalities of the elbow.[38, 94, 95] The medial coronoid process is most often involved.[38, 67, 69, 73, 96] The disease is more common in male dogs and is often bilateral.[38, 68, 69, 73, 97] Traumatic fracture of the medial coronoid process has also been reported in a racing greyhound.[98] Injury to the distal radial physis in skeletally immature dogs may also result in distal radiohumeral subluxation as the ulna continues to grow, with subsequent fragmentation of the coronoid process.[89, 99, 100]

Clinical signs are rarely noted before 5 months of age. Subtle weight-bearing lameness, exacerbated by prolonged rest or exercise, is typical.[27, 68, 71] The onset of lameness is insidious.[27, 71, 97] As lameness persists, it may increase in severity. Affected dogs often place the carpus in an exaggerated "valgus" or supinated position when sitting or standing and circumduct the antebrachium during the swing phase of the stride.[27, 39] A pain response is usually not elicited until the elbow is fully extended.[7] Some investigators suggest that the carpus should be placed in a flexed, externally rotated position while the elbow is extended.[66] Joint effusion may be detected as a fluctuant swelling beneath the lateral epicondyle of the humerus.

The fragmented coronoid process is rarely identified radiographically because of superimposition of the medial coronoid process and the head of the radius.[27, 29, 71] The mediolateral (extended and supinated) view made with the elbow maximally extended and supinated 15 degrees reportedly is a superior radiographic projec-

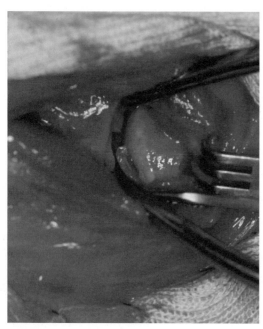

FIGURE 27–17. Osteochondritis dissecans lesions of the humeral condyle as seen via a medial elbow arthrotomy.

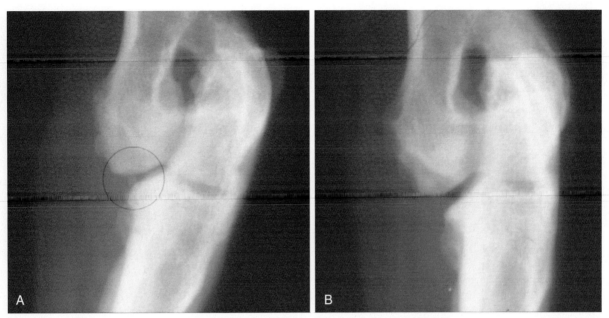

FIGURE 27–19. Preoperative *(A)* and postoperative *(B)* oblique pronated craniocaudal view radiographs of the elbow of a dog with fragmented coronoid process. Note that the fragment that can be visualized in the joint space overlying the medial coronoid process on the preoperative radiograph *(circle)* is no longer present on the postoperative radiograph following excision. Extensive degenerative joint disease is also present along the medial compartment of the elbow.

tion for demonstrating pathology of the medial coronoid process[74]; however, we have not found this view to be useful for specific identification of coronoid pathology. We have found the pronated oblique, craniocaudal view (Fig. 27–19) to be more useful for specific identification of medial coronoid pathology, but the percentage of dogs in which a specific fragment can be identified is still limited.

When fragmentation of the coronoid process cannot be identified radiographically, a clinical diagnosis of fragmented coronoid process is supported by the presence of degenerative changes in the elbow in the absence of an ununited anconeal process or osteochondrosis of the humeral condyle.[27, 71, 72, 74, 97] Osteophyte development on the anconeal process and increased density of the ulna subjacent to the coronoid process and the trochlear notch are early radiographic degenerative changes associated with fragmented coronoid process (Fig. 27–20).[27, 70, 71, 101] Degenerative changes are usually not radiographically evident before 7 months of age.[27, 72, 95] Distal humeroradial subluxation, a purported etiologic factor in fragmentation of the coronoid process, may be apparent in some dogs before degenerative changes become apparent.[27, 39, 95]

Definitive diagnosis of fragmented medial coronoid process is made at exploratory arthrotomy. The medial coronoid process is exposed via the previously described muscle-separating approach. Experience and adequate lighting facilitate definition of the pathology. In some dogs an isolated well-defined free fragment exists (Fig. 27–21) and is readily identified and removed. In other dogs, only fissuring of the articular cartilage is present (Fig. 27–22). These fissures can extend variable depths into the subchondral bone.[1, 38, 94] These lesions can be difficult to recognize and confusing. Probing the articular surface of the medial coronoid process with a Freer periosteal elevator can help identify fissures that are not readily apparent. Although optimal treatment of these fissures has not been determined, we generally excise the affected region as if it were a fragment.

Postoperative care is similar to that described in the section of osteochondrosis of the humeral condyle. The prognosis for dogs

with fragmented coronoid process is again guarded. The benefits and efficacy of surgery for dogs with fragmented coronoid process is a contentious issue. Although degenerative joint disease progresses irrespective of whether or not surgical intervention takes place,[67, 73, 90] most dogs will eventually become sound with a slightly stiff stilted gait.[86, 90, 102, 103] Although studies disagree regarding the benefits of surgery,[67, 73, 90, 92, 102–104] we believe that surgical

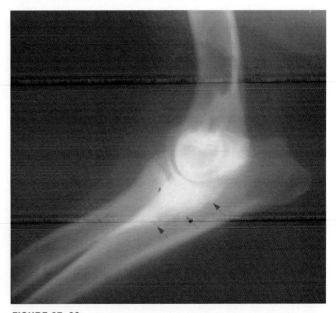

FIGURE 27–20. Lateral radiograph of the elbow of a 7-month-old rottweiler with fragmented coronoid process. The increased density of the ulna subjacent to the coronoid process and the trochlear notch *(arrows)* is the only degenerative change present.

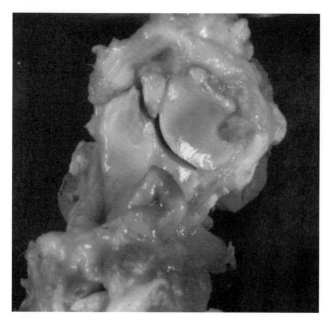

FIGURE 27–21. Proximal-to-distal view of a necropsy specimen of the proximal radius and ulna of a dog with an obvious fragmented coronoid process. A large fragment such as this should be easily identified at surgery. (From Lewis DD, et al.: Fragmented medial coronoid process of the canine elbow. Compend Contin Educ Pract Vet [Small Anim] 11:703–715, 1989.)

excision of fragmented coronoid process results in more rapid resolution of lameness in most dogs, particularly in dogs younger than 18 months of age. Many of these dogs can return to hunting, obedience, and field trial work; however, some lameness should be expected with vigorous activity.

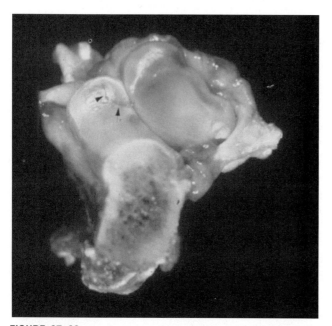

FIGURE 27–22. Proximal-to-distal view of a necropsy specimen of the proximal radius and ulna of a 9-month-old rottweiler with fragmented coronoid process. The ulna has been cut through the trochlear notch. This lesion (arrows) would be better characterized as a fissure and could be difficult to identify at surgery.

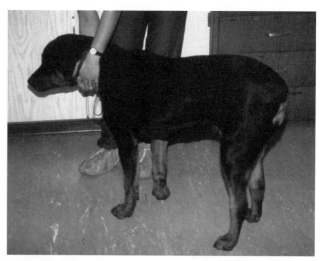

FIGURE 27–23. An 8-month-old rottweiler with osteochondritis dissecans lesions affecting both hocks. Note that both hocks are held in a hyperextended position.

OSTEOCHONDROSIS OF THE HOCK

Although osteochondrosis of the hock may affect any large-breed dog, rottweilers, Labrador retrievers, and Australian cattle dogs are particularly at risk.[30, 31, 32, 105–107] There may be a predisposition for female rather than male dogs to develop osteochondrosis of the hock.[30–32] Bilateral lesions occur in approximately 50 per cent of affected dogs, although clinical lameness is rarely symmetrical.[4, 30, 32, 107] Affected dogs often develop clinical lameness by 4 or 5 months of age.[30, 32] Most dogs have consistent weight-bearing lameness; however, this often progresses to intermittent non–weight-bearing lameness.[30, 31] The affected hock is often held in hyperextension (Fig. 27–23).[4, 105, 106] Muscle atrophy of the limb is often present.[7] Palpation of the hock demonstrates synovial effusion, which is detected as a fluctuant swelling most easily palpated immediately caudodistal to the malleoli.[4, 105, 106] In more chronic cases, the joint capsule becomes thickened, and range of motion is decreased, especially in flexion.[4, 106] Full flexion or extension of the hock may evoke a pain response.[7, 104] Crepitus may be elicited as the affected joint is moved through the range of motion.[4]

The radiographic appearance of osteochondrosis of the hock is variable and depends on the chronicity of the process and the location and extent of the lesion. Lesions vary from subchondral bony defects with associated subchondral sclerosis to mineralized flaps or osteochondral fragments.[30, 31, 32, 105, 106, 107, 108] Osteochondral fragments can comprise a substantial portion of the involved trochlear ridge.[7, 107, 108] Degenerative changes, including subchondral sclerosis of the articulating surfaces of the tibia and osteophyte formation, are frequently present (Fig. 27–24). The medial trochlear ridge of the talus is affected most often[30, 31, 105, 109, 110]; however, lesions affecting the lateral trochlear ridge are being recognized with increasing frequency.[30, 107] The primary lesion may occur anywhere along the arc of the trochlear ridges. Subchondral defects may not be visible on standard radiographic views. Oblique projection radiographs may be necessary to define some lesions, particularly those that involve the lateral trochlear ridge.[7, 30, 32, 107, 109] The dorsal 45 degree lateral–plantaromedial oblique projection has been reported to be the most useful view in identifying lesions of

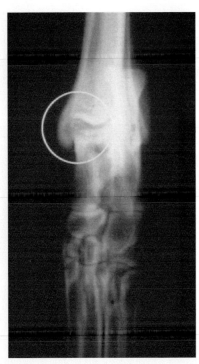

FIGURE 27–24. Dorsoplantar view radiograph of the hock of an Australian cattle dog with an osteochondritis dissecans lesion affecting the plantar aspect of the medial trochlear ridge of the talus (*circle*).

the lateral trochlear ridge.[107] The flexed dorsoplantar ("skyline") projection (Fig. 27–25) is useful in defining lesions involving the proximal aspect of either trochlear ridge.[109, 110]

There is some disagreement regarding appropriate treatment of osteochondritis dissecans of the hock. One study comparing the clinical results (mean follow-up 34 months) of dogs with osteochondritis dissecans of the hock managed with and without surgery found little difference in limb function and the radiographic progression of degenerative joint disease between the two treatment groups.[32] In our experience, however, nonsurgical management is frequently unrewarding and does not address the cause of the arthritic degeneration. Large osteochondral fragments have been successfully stabilized.[108, 111] Advocates of this approach cite maintenance of joint stability as the primary advantage, but adequate exposure may require an aggressive surgical approach via malleolar osteotomy, and the percentage of viable candidates for this approach is low.[108, 111]

Most surgeons advocate removal of osteochondral fragments and curettage of the lesion's bed.[4, 30, 105] Approaches (dorsomedial, plantaromedial, dorsolateral, and plantarolateral) that do not utilize a desmotomy or osteotomy are preferable.[98, 112, 113] Use of these approaches requires specific identification of the lesions prior to surgery and is associated with minimal morbidity. Fragment excision probably does not significantly reduce hock stability, and removal of the loose articular cartilage eliminates a source of intra-articular inflammation. A soft padded bandage is applied for 3 to 5 days following surgery, and the dog is restricted to kennel confinement and leash exercise for 2 to 3 weeks.

Although degenerative changes continue to progress irrespective of surgical treatment, substantial improvement in limb function is to be expected following surgical excision.[30, 31] The prognosis for return to athletic performance is guarded. It would be unreasonable to expect a dog to return to racing following surgery. Some working dogs, however, become sound enough on the affected limb follow-

ing surgery to return to hunting, field trial, or obedience competition, but some residual lameness should be expected.

OSTEOCHONDROSIS OF THE STIFLE

Osteochondrosis of the stifle occurs infrequently.[4, 6, 7, 114, 115] The signalment of affected dogs is similar to that of dogs affected with osteochondrosis at other locations; 76 per cent of reported cases have involved male dogs.[116] The condition is bilateral in 72 per cent of affected dogs.[113] Irish wolfhounds, German shepherd dogs, and Great Danes appear to be predisposed to develop the condition.[68, 116, 117]

The onset of lameness is usually insidious and may occur as early as 3 months of age.[6, 70, 118] While it is likely that most performance dogs would be evaluated for lameness at a young age, it is not uncommon for nonworking dogs to be several years of age when they are eventually presented to a veterinarian because of lameness. Lameness is exacerbated by exercise. Lameness is often asymmetrical in dogs that are bilaterally affected.[113] Range of motion, especially extension, is decreased, and manipulation of the stifle elicits a pain response. Crepitus may be palpated during joint manipulation, and effusion is a consistent finding.[4, 7, 113]

The most common radiographic abnormality associated with osteochondrosis or osteochondritis dissecans of the stifle is a flattening or subchondral bony defect that involves the medial aspect of the lateral femoral condyle (Fig. 27–26).[4, 7, 113] This abnormality should not be confused with the fossa of the long digital extensor tendon or an aberrant attachment of the cranial cruciate ligament.[119, 120] Although lesions are usually more obvious on the craniocaudal view, lesions can sometimes be identified more readily on the lateral view (Fig. 27–27). Oblique projections may be helpful in

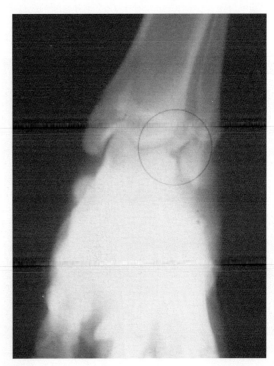

FIGURE 27–25. Flexed dorsoplantar ("skyline") view radiograph of the hock of a dog with an osteochondritis dissecans lesion affecting the dorsal aspect of the lateral trochlear ridge of the talus (*circle*).

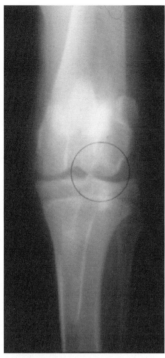

FIGURE 27–26. Craniocaudal view radiograph of the stifle of a 2-year-old Boxer with an osteochondritis dissecans lesion of the medial aspect of the lateral trochlear ridge of the talus *(circle).*

identifying lesions in some dogs. Lesions that affect the medial condyle have been reported in only 4 per cent of affected stifles.[113] In our experience this figure under-represents the true incidence of lesions in this location. Detached mineralized cartilage flaps, synovial effusion, osteophyte formation, and other degenerative changes may be observed on the radiographs.[7]

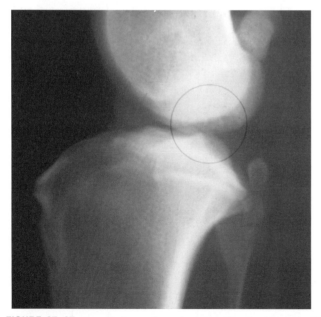

FIGURE 27–27. Lateral view radiograph of the stifle of a 16-month-old Great Dane with an osteochondritis dissecans lesion of the medial aspect of the lateral femoral condyle *(circle).*

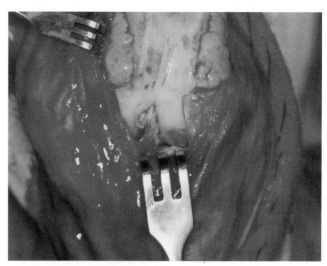

FIGURE 27–28. Osteochondrosis dissecans lesion of the lateral femoral condyle as seen at arthrotomy in a 4-year-old Akita. Despite the extensive degenerative joint disease, the dog had only a recent history of lameness.

Treatment of osteochondritis dissecans of the femoral condyle consists of removal of pathological cartilage and curettage of the underlying bed. Lesions can be variable in appearance. Some dogs may have large osteochondral fragments. Most dogs have cartilage flaps. Distinct cartilage flaps may not be present in some dogs, but rather there is often a depressed area on the articular surface in which the diseased cartilage has a granular mosaic appearance. Curettage is traditionally accomplished via standard parapatellar stifle arthrotomy (Fig. 27–28).[4, 68] Dogs with large lesions typically have substantial postoperative lameness that may persist for weeks to months following arthrotomy and curettage.[68] A limited arthrotomy has been described for the treatment of osteochondritis dissecans of the femoral condyle that is associated with less postoperative morbidity.[121]

We[122] and others[123] have managed osteochondritis dissecans lesions of the stifle with arthroscopic curettage and have obtained encouraging results. The technique can be performed rapidly and allows good visualization of the lesion (Fig. 27–29) as well as other intra-articular structures. With practice, arthroscopic curettage is simple to perform and greatly reduces postoperative morbidity. The long-term results, however, seem to be similar to those obtained following arthrotomy. The prognosis for performance dogs must be guarded, and some lameness should be expected with vigorous activity.[122, 123]

Osteochondrosis affecting the patella has been reported in four dogs.[35, 124] Three dogs were littermates. All four dogs were female greyhounds that developed a mild weight-bearing lameness between 2 and 3 months of age. Two dogs were affected bilaterally. The clinical presentation was similar to that in dogs with osteochondritis dissecans of the femoral condyle. The most striking clinical feature in each dog was a firm, prominent enlargement of the lateral aspect of the patella (Fig. 27–30). Radiographic examination, including a cranioproximal-craniodistal oblique (skyline) projection, revealed fragmentation of the lateral border of the patella (Fig. 27–31) in all dogs. Surgical excision of the osteochondral fragments was performed in three dogs. One dog was euthanatized and necropsy performed. Histological examination of specimens from each dog supported the diagnosis of osteochondrosis. All three dogs eventually had satisfactory limb function following surgery, although mild lameness persisted for 4 to 8 weeks following surgery. All three dogs eventually raced.[35, 124]

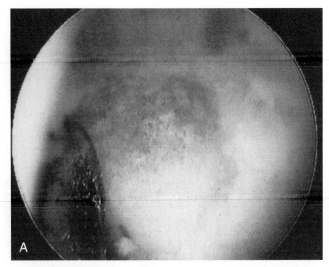
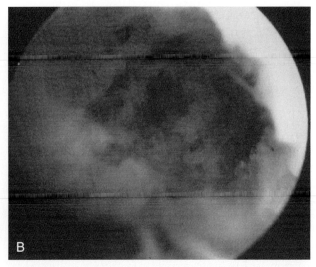

FIGURE 27–29. Arthroscopic view of an osteochondritis dissecans lesion of the lateral femoral condyle (*A*) before and (*B*) after curettage.

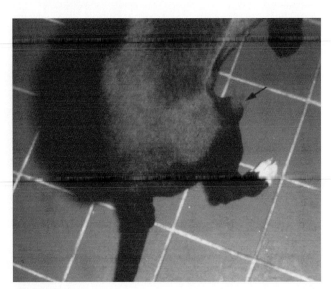
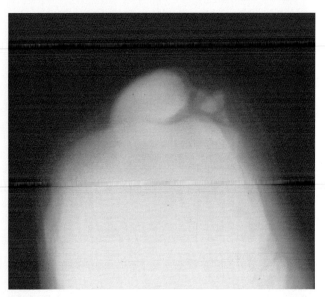

FIGURE 27–30. Right hindlimb of a greyhound with osteochondrosis of the patella. Note the prominent enlargement of the lateral aspect of the patella (*arrow*). (From Shealy PM, et al.: Osteochondral fragmentation [osteochondrosis] of the canine patella. Vet Compar Ortho Trauma 5:114–121, 1992.)

FIGURE 27–31. Cranioproximal-craniodistal oblique ("skyline") view radiograph of a greyhound with osteochondrosis of the patella. Note the osteochondral fragmentation of the lateral border of the stifle. (From Brizze-Buxton BL, et al.: What's your diagnosis? Osteochondral fragmentation of the patella. JAVMA 205:1537–1538, 1994.)

References

1. Olsson S-E: Pathophysiology, morphology and clinical signs associated with osteochondrosis in the dog. *In* Bojrab MJ (ed): Disease Mechanisms in Small Animal Surgery, ed 3. Philadelphia, Lea & Febiger, 1993, pp 777–796.
2. Lenehan TM, van Sickle DC: Canine osteochondrosis. *In* Newton CD, Nunamaker CM. Textbook of Small Animal Orthopaedics. Philadelphia, JB Lippincott Co, 1985, pp 981–997.
3. Milton JL: Osteochondritis dissecans in the dog. Vet Clin North Am Small Anim Pract 13:117–134, 1983.
4. Probst CW, Johnston SA: Osteochondrosis. *In* Slatter DH (ed): Textbook of Small Animal Surgery, 2nd ed. Philadelphia, WB Saunders Company, 1993, vol 2, pp 1944–1966.
5. Robbins GM: Osteochondritis dissecans in the dog. Aust Vet J 54:272–279, 1978.
6. Alexander JW, Richardson DC, Selcer BA: Osteochondritis dissecans of the elbow, stifle, and hock—a review. J Am Anim Hosp Assoc 17:51–56, 1981.
7. Lewis DD, McCarthy RJ, Pechman RD: Diagnosis of common development orthopedic conditions in canine pediatric patients. Compend Contin Educ Pract Vet (Small Anim) 14:287–301, 1992.
8. Grondalen T, Vangen O: Osteochondrosis and arthrosis in pigs: V. A comparison of the incidence in 3 different lines of the Norwegian land race breed. Acta Vet Scand 15:61–79, 1974.
9. Olsson S-E: Osteochondrosis—a growing problem to dog breeders. Gaines Progress 1–11, 1976.
10. Rejno S, Stromberg B: Osteochondrosis in the horse: II. Pathology reprint. Acta Radiol 1–28, 1976.
11. Grondalen J, Lingaas F: Arthrosis in the elbow joint of young, rapidly growing dogs: A genetic investigation. J Small Anim Pract 32:460–464, 1991.
12. Studdert VP, Lavelle RB, Beilharz RG, et al: Clinical features and heritability of osteochondrosis of the elbow in Labrador retrievers. J Small Anim Pract 32:557–563, 1991.
13. Hayes HM, Selby LA, Wilson GP, et al: Epidemiologic observations of canine elbow disease (emphasis on dysplasia). J Am Anim Hosp Assoc 15:449–453, 1979.

14. Smith CW, Stowater JL: Osteochondritis dissecans of the canine shoulder joint: A review of 35 cases. J Am Anim Hosp Assoc 11:658–662, 1975.
15. Rudd RG, Whitehair JG, Margolis JH: Results of management of osteochondritis dissecans of the humeral head in dogs: 44 cases (1982 to 1987). J Am Anim Hosp Assoc 26:173–178, 1990.
16. Scherrer PK, Hillberry BM, Van Sickle DC: Determining the in vivo areas of contact in the canine shoulder. J Biomech Eng 101:271–278, 1979.
17. Craig PH, Riser WH: Osteochondritis dissecans in the proximal humerus of the dog. J Am Vet Rad Soc 6:40–49, 1965.
18. Guthrie S, Plummer JM, Vaughan LC. Etiopathogenesis of canine elbow osteochondrosis: A study of loose fragments removed at arthrotomy. Res Vet Sci 52:284–291, 1992.
19. Kinzel GL, Van Sickle DC, Hillberry BM, et al: Preliminary study of the in vivo motion in the canine shoulder. Am J Vet Res 37:1505–1510, 1976.
20. Carlson CS, Hilley HD, Meuten DJ, et al: Effect of reduced growth rate on the prevalence and severity of osteochondrosis in gilts. Am J Vet Res 49:396–402, 1988.
21. Relland S: Osteochondrosis in the pig. Acta Radiol 1–118, 1975.
22. Hazewinkel HAW: Nutrition in relation to skeletal growth deformities. J Small Anim Pract 30:625–630, 1989.
23. Hazewinkel HAW, Goedegebuure SA, Poulos PW, et al: Influences of chronic calcium excess on the skeletal development of growing Great Danes. J Am Anim Hosp Assoc 21:337–391, 1985.
24. Hedhammer A, Wu FM, Knook L, et al: Overnutrition and skeletal disease. An experimental study in growing Great Dane dogs. Cornell Vet 64(suppl 5):1–160, 1974.
25. Paatsama S, Rokkanen P, Jussila J, et al: Somatotropin, thyrotropin and corticotropin hormone induced changes in the cartilage and bones of the shoulder and knee joint in dogs. J Small Anim Pract 12:595–601, 1971.
26. Paatsama S: Aetiological factors in osteochondritis dissecans. Acta Orthop Scand 46:906–918, 1975.
27. Lewis DD, Parker RB, Hager DA: Fragmented medial coronoid process of the canine elbow. Compend Contin Educ Pract Vet (Small Anim) 11:703–715, 1989.
28. Slater MR, Scarlett JM, Kaderly RE, et al: Breed, gender, and age as risk factors for canine osteochondritis dissecans. Vet Compar Orthop Trauma 4:100–106, 1991.
29. Read RA: Arthrosis in young dogs: Incidence, diagnosis and management. Waltham Intern Focus 3(2):2–10, 1993.
30. Beale BS, Goring RL, Herrington J, et al: A prospective evaluation of four surgical approaches to the talus of the dog used in the treatment of osteochondritis dissecans. J Am Anim Hosp Assoc 27:221–229, 1991.
31. Breur GJ, Spaulding KA, Braden TD: Osteochondritis dissecans of the medial trochlear ridge of the talus in the dog. Vet Compar Orthop Trauma 4:168–176, 1989.
32. Smith MM, Vasseur PB, Morgan JP: Clinical evaluation of dogs after surgical and nonsurgical management of osteochondritis dissecans of the talus. JAVMA 187:31–35, 1985.
33. Johnson AL, Pijanowski GJ, Stein LE: Osteochondritis dissecans of the femoral head of a Pekingese. JAVMA 187:623–625, 1985.
34. Butler HC, Wallace LJ, Ladds PW: Osteochondritis dissecans of the distal end of the radius in a dog. J Am Anim Hosp Assoc 7:81–86, 1971.
35. Shealy PM, Milton JL, Kincaid SA, et al: Osteochondral fragmentation (osteochondrosis) of the canine patella. Vet Compar Orthop Trauma 5:114–121, 1992.
36. Olsson S-E: Lameness in the dog: A review of lesions causing osteoarthrosis of the shoulder, elbow, hip, stifle and hock joints. J Am Anim Hosp Assoc 1:363, 1975.
37. Olsson S-E: Osteochondrosis in the dog. In Kirk RW (ed): Current Veterinary Therapy VI. Philadelphia, WB Saunders Company, 1977, pp 880–886.
38. Grondalen J, Grondalen T: Arthrosis in the elbow joint of young rapidly growing dogs: V. A pathoanatomical investigation. Nord Vet Med 33:1–16, 1981.
39. Wind AP: Elbow dysplasia. In Slatter D (ed): Textbook of Small Animal Surgery. Philadelphia, WB Saunders Company, 1993, pp 1966–1977.
40. Poulos PW: Canine osteochondrosis. Vet Clin North Am Small Anim Pract 12:313–328, 1982.
41. Whitehair JG, Rudd RG: Osteochondritis dissecans of the humeral head in dogs. Compend Contin Educ Pract Vet (Small Anim) 12:195–204, 1990.
42. Vaughan LC, Jones DGC. Osteochondritis dissecans of the head of the humerus in dogs. J Small Anim Pract 9:283–294, 1968.
43. Milton JL, Rumph PF, Reed AD: Osteochondritis dissecans of the shoulder in the racing greyhound: A report of two cases and a survey of 109 greyhound anatomy specimens. J Am Anim Hosp Assoc 17:617–622, 1981.
44. Riser WH, Woodard JC, Bloomberg MS, et al: Shoulder lesions in the greyhound with special reference to osteochondritis dissecans and chondrocalcinosis. J Am Anim Hosp Assoc 29:449–454, 1993.
45. Milton JL: Osteochondrosis in the greyhound. Proceedings of the 21st Annual American College of Veterinary Surgeons Forum, San Francisco, 1993, pp 513–515.
46. Needham DH: OCD in the greyhound. Racing Greyhound 3:65–70, 1981.
47. Zuber RM: Osteochondritis of the canine shoulder. Proceedings #64, Greyhound Medicine and Surgery. TG Hungerford Refresher Course for Veterinarians, Sydney, Australia, 1983, pp 21–26.
48. Eaton-Wells R: OCD of the shoulder, hock and stifle. Proceedings #122, Greyhound Medicine and Surgery. TG Hungerford Refresher Course for Veterinarians, Sydney, Australia, 1989, pp 231–237.
49. Hoskins RTS, Garnworthy PG, Daniel B: OCD of the proximal humerus in the racing greyhound. Racing Greyhound 3:71–74, 1981.
50. Blythe LL, Gannon IR, Craig AM: Care of the Racing Greyhound. A Guide to Trainers, Breeders and Veterinarians. Portland, Ore, American Greyhound Council, Inc., 1994, pp 223–224.
51. Birkeland R: Osteochondritis dissecans in the humeral head of the dog. Nord Vet Med 19:294–306, 1967.
52. van Bree H: Evaluation of the prognostic value of positive-contrast shoulder arthrography for bilateral osteochondrosis lesions in dogs. Am J Vet Res 51:1121–1125, 1990.
53. Griffiths RC: Osteochondritis dissecans of the canine shoulder. JAVMA 153:1733–1735, 1968.
54. van Bree H, Van Ryssen B, Desmidt M: Osteochondrosis lesions of the canine shoulder: Correlation of positive contrast arthrography and arthroscopy. Vet Radiol Ultrasound 33:342–347, 1992.
55. LaHue TR, Brown SG, Roush JC, et al: Entrapment of joint mice in the bicipital tendon sheath as a sequela to osteochondritis dissecans of the proximal humerus in dogs: A report of six cases. J Am Anim Hosp Assoc 24:99–105, 1988.
56. Tomlinson J, Constantinescu G, McClure R, et al: Caudal approach to the shoulder joint in the dog. Vet Surg 15:294–299, 1986.
57. Gahring DR: A modified caudal approach to the canine shoulder joint. J Am Anim Hosp Assoc 21:613–618, 1985.
58. Probst CW, Flo GL: Comparison of two caudolateral approaches to the scapulohumeral joint for treatment of osteochondritis dissecans in dogs. JAVMA 191:1101–1104, 1987.
59. Schulman AJ, Lusk R, Ettinger SJ, et al: Longitudinal myotomy of the acromial head of the deltoid: A modified approach for the surgical treatment of osteochondritis dissecans in the dog. J Am Anim Hosp Assoc 22:475–479, 1986.
60. Howard PE: Luxation of the canine shoulder joint to maximize exposure for treatment of osteochondritis dissecans. Vet Surg 13:15–17, 1984.
61. Dee JF: A simplified approach to the canine shoulder for the treatment of osteochondritis dissecans. J Am Anim Hosp Assoc 8:111–114, 1972.
62. McLaughlin RM, Roush JK: A comparison of two surgical approaches to the scapulohumeral joint in dogs. Vet Surg 24:207–214, 1994.
63. Jones DGC, Vaughan LC: The surgical treatment of osteochondritis dissecans of the humeral head in dogs. J Small Anim Pract 11:803–812, 1970.
64. Cechner PE, Knecht CD: Approach to the canine shoulder without myotomy, osteotomy, or tenotomy. J Am Anim Hosp Assoc 15:753–754, 1979.
65. Fox SM, Bloomberg MS, Bright RM: Developmental anomalies of the canine elbow. J Am Anim Hosp Assoc 19:605–614, 1983.
66. Lenehan TM, Van Sickle DC: Ununited anconeal process, ununited medial coronoid process, ununited medial epicondyle, patella cubiti,

and sesamoidal fragments of the elbow. *In* Newton CD, Nunamaker CM: Textbook of Small Animal Orthopaedics. Philadelphia, JB Lippincott Co, 1985, pp 999–1012.

67. Bennett D, Duff SRI, Kene RO, et al: Osteochondritis dissecans and fragmentation of the coronoid process in the elbow joint of the dog. Vet Rec 109:329–336, 1981.

68. Denny HR, Gibbs C: The surgical treatment of osteochondritis dissecans and ununited coronoid process in the canine elbow joint. J Small Anim Pract 21:595–608, 1980.

69. Berzon JL, Quick CB: Fragmented coronoid process: Anatomical, clinical and radiographic considerations with case analysis. J Am Anim Hosp Assoc 16:241–251, 1980.

70. Guthrie S: Use of radiographic scoring technique for the assessment of dogs with elbow osteochondrosis. J Small Anim Pract 30:639–644, 1989.

71. Houlton JEF: Osteochondrosis of the shoulder and elbow joints in dogs. J Small Anim Pract 25:399–413, 1984.

72. Olsson S-E: The early diagnosis of fragmented coronoid process and osteochondritis dissecans of the canine elbow. J Am Anim Hosp Assoc 19:616–626, 1983.

73. Henry WB: Radiographic diagnosis and surgical management of fragmented medial coronoid process in dogs. J Am Vet Med Assoc 184:799–805, 1984.

74. Voorhout G, Hazewinkle HAW: Radiographic evaluation of the canine elbow joint with specific reference to the medial humeral condyle and the medial coronoid process. Vet Radiol 28:158–165, 1987.

75. Guthrie S, Pidduck HG: Heritability of elbow osteochondrosis within a closed population of dogs. J Small Anim Pract 31:93–96, 1990.

76. Guthrie S: Some radiographic and clinical aspects of ununited anconeal process. Vet Rec 124:662–663, 1989.

77. Sjöström L, Kasström H, Källberg M: Ununited anconeal process in the dog. Pathogenesis and treatment by osteotomy of the ulna. Vet Compar Orthop Trauma 8:170–176, 1995.

78. Thacher C: Ununited anconeal process. *In* Slatter DH (ed): Textbook of Small Animal Surgery, 2nd ed, Philadelphia, WB Saunders Company, 1993, vol 2, pp 1977–1981. 1993.

79. Cawley AJ, Archibald J: Ununited anconeal process of the dog. JAVMA 134:454–458, 1959.

80. Sinibaldi KR, Arnoczky SP: Surgical removal of the ununited anconeal process in the dog. J Am Anim Hosp Assoc 11:192–198, 1975.

81. Van Sickle DC: The relationship of ossification to canine elbow dysplasia. J Am Anim Hosp Assoc 2:24–31, 1966.

82. Roy RG, Wallace LJ, Johnston GR: A retrospective long-term evaluation of ununited anconeal process excision on the canine elbow. Vet Compar Orthop Trauma 7:94–97, 1994.

83. Pritchard DL: Anconeal process pseudoarthrosis: Treated by lag-screw fixation. Canine Pract 18–23, 1976.

84. Brinker WO, Piermattei DL, Flo GL: Handbook of Small Animal Orthopedics and Fracture Repair, 2nd ed. Philadelphia, WB Saunders Company, 1990, pp 502–505.

85. Herron MR: Ununited anconeal process—a new approach to surgical repair. Mod Vet Pract 51:30–34, 1970.

86. Fox SM, Burbidge HM, Bray JC, et al: Ununited anconeal process: Lag screw fixation. J Am Anim Hosp Assoc 32:52–56, 1996.

87. Boudrieau RJ, Hohn RB, Bardet JF: Osteochondritis dissecans of the elbow in the dog. J Am Anim Hosp Assoc 19:627–635, 1983.

88. Wissler J, Sumner-Smith G: Osteochondrosis in the elbow joint in the dog. J Am Anim Hosp Assoc 13:349–354, 1977.

89. Macpherson GC, Lewis DD, Johnson KA, et al: Fragmented coronoid process associated with premature distal radial physeal closure in four dogs. Vet Compar Orthop Trauma 5:93–99, 1992.

90. Grondalen J: Arthrosis with special reference to the elbow joint of rapidly growing dogs: III. Ununited medial coronoid process of the ulna and osteochondritis dissecans of the humeral condyle. Surgical procedure for correction and postoperative investigation. Nord Vet Med 31:520–527, 1979.

91. Suess RP, Trotter EJ, Konieczynski D, et al: Exposure and postoperative stability of three medial surgical approaches to the canine elbow. Vet Surg 23:87–93, 1994.

92. Tobias TA, Miyabayashi T, Olmstead ML, et al: Surgical removal of fragmented medial coronoid process in the dog: Comparative effects of surgical approach and age at time of surgery. J Am Anim Hosp Assoc 30:360–368, 1994.

93. Grondalen J: Arthrosis in the elbow joint of young rapidly growing dogs: II. Occurrence in the rottweiler breed. Nord Vet Med 34:76–82, 1982.

94. Wind AP: Elbow incongruity and developmental elbow diseases in the dog: I. J Am Anim Hosp Assoc 22:711–724, 1986.

95. Wind AP: Incidence and radiographic appearance of fragmented coronoid process. Calif Vet 6:19–25, 1982.

96. Tirgari M: Clinical, radiographical and pathological aspects of ununited medial coronoid process of the elbow joint in dogs. J Small Anim Pract 21:595–608, 1980.

97. Grondalen J: Arthrosis with special reference to the elbow joint of rapidly growing dogs: II. Occurrence, clinical and radiographic findings. Nord Vet Med 31:69–75, 1979.

98. Goring RL, Beale BS: Fractured medial coronoid process in a racing greyhound. J Am Anim Hosp Assoc 26:157–160, 1990.

99. Olsson NC, Brinker WO, Carrig CB, et al: Asynchronous growth of the canine radius and ulna: Surgical correction following experimental premature closure of the distal radial physis. Vet Surg 10:125–131, 1981.

100. Vandewater A, Olmstead ML: Premature closure of the distal radial physis in the dog. A review of eleven cases. Vet Surg 12:7–12, 1983.

101. Mason T, Lavelle R, Skipper S, et al: Osteochondrosis of the elbow joint in young dogs. J Small Anim Pract 21:641–656, 1980.

102. Read RA, Armstrong SJ, O'Keefe JD, et al: Fragmentation of the medial coronoid process of the ulna in dogs: A study of 109 cases. J Small Anim Pract 31:330–334, 1990.

103. Bouck GR, Miller CW, Taves CL: A comparison of surgical and medical treatment of fragmented coronoid process and osteochondritis dissecans of the canine elbow. Vet Compar Orthop Trauma 8:177–183, 1995.

104. Huibregtse BA, Johnson AL, Muhlbauer MC, et al: The effect of treatment of fragmented coronoid process on the development of osteoarthritis of the elbow. J Am Anim Hosp Assoc 30:190–195, 1994.

105. Johnson KA, Howlett CR, Pettit GD: Osteochondrosis in the hock joints in dogs. J Am Anim Hosp Assoc 16:103–113, 1980.

106. Rosenblum GP, Robins GM, Carlisle CH: Osteochondritis dissecans of the tibiotarsal joint in the dog. J Small Anim Pract 19:759–767, 1978.

107. Wisner ER, Berry CR, Morgan JP, et al: Osteochondrosis of the lateral trochlear ridge of the talus in seven rottweiler dogs. Vet Surg 19:435–439, 1990.

108. Aron DN, Mahaffey MB, Rowland GN: Free chondral fragment involving the lateral trochlear ridge of the talus in a dog. JAVMA 186:1095–1096, 1985.

109. Carlisle CH, Robins GM, Reynolds KM: Radiographic signs of osteochondritis dissecans of the lateral ridge of the trochlea tali in the dog. J Small Anim Pract 31:280–286, 1990.

110. Miyabayashi T, Biller DS, Manley PA, et al: Use of a flexed dorsoplantar radiographic view of the talocrural joint to evaluate lameness in two dogs. JAVMA 199:598–600, 1991.

111. Aron DN, Gorse MJ: Clinical use of N-butyl 2-cyanoacrylate for stabilization of osteochondral fragments: Preliminary report. J Am Anim Hosp Assoc 27:203–210, 1991.

112. Beale BS, Goring RL: Exposure of the medial and lateral trochlear ridges of the talus in the dog: I. Dorsomedial and plantaromedial surgical approaches to the medial trochlear ridge. J Am Anim Hosp Assoc 26:13–24, 1990.

113. Goring RL, Beale BS: Exposure of the medial and lateral trochlear ridges of the talus in the dog: II. Dorsolateral and plantarolateral surgical approaches to the lateral trochlear ridge. J Am Anim Hosp Assoc 26:19–24, 1990.

114. Montgomery RD, Milton JL, Henderson RA, et al: Osteochondritis dissecans of the canine stifle. Compend Contin Educ Pract Vet (Small Anim) 11:1199–1205, 1989.

115. Denny HR, Gibbs C: Osteochondritis dissecans of the canine stifle joint. J Small Anim Pract 21:317–322, 1980.

116. Arbesser E. Osteochondrosis dissecans der Femor-kondylen beim Hund. Wien Tierarztl Monatschr 61:303–313, 1974.

117. Ponzet G, Walde I, Arbesser E. Zur osteochondrosis dissecans genu des Hundes. Kleintier-Praxis 20:88–98, 1975.

118. Knecht CD, Van Sickle DC, Blevins WE, et al: Osteochondrosis of the shoulder and stifle in 3 of 5 Border Collie littermates. JAVMA 170:58–60, 1977.

119. Losonsky JM, Kneller SK: Misdiagnosis in normal radiographic anat-

omy: Eight structural configurations simulating disease entities in dogs and cats. JAVMA 191:109–114, 1987.

120. Dueland RT, Sisson D, Evans HE: Aberrant origin of the cranial cruciate ligament mimicking an osteochondral lesion radiographically. Vet Radiol 23:175–177, 1982.

121. Shealy PM, Milton JL: Limited arthrotomy of the canine stifle for osteochondritis dissecans. Vet Compar Orthop Trauma 4:134–139, 1991.

122. Bertrand SG, Madison JB: Arthroscopic examination and treatment of

stifle osteochondritis dissecans in four dogs. Proceedings 22nd Annual Meeting of the Veterinary Orthopedic Society, Whistler/Blackcomb, Canada, 1995, pp 22.

123. McLaughlin RM, Hurtig MB, Fries CL: Operative arthroscopy in the treatment of bilateral stifle osteochondritis dissecans in a dog. Vet Compar Orthop Trauma 4:158–161, 1989.

124. Brizzee-Buxton BL, Lewis DD, Pechman RD, et al: What's your diagnosis? Osteochondral fragmentation of the patella. JAVMA 205:1537–1538, 1994.

CHAPTER 28

DIAGNOSTIC AND SURGICAL ARTHROSCOPY IN SMALL ANIMALS

BERNADETTE VAN RYSSEN \ HENRI VAN BREE

Arthroscopy is a frequently used technique for diagnosis and treatment of joint diseases in humans[1, 2] and horses.[3–5] In the dog, arthroscopy was first performed in the late 1970s.[6, 7] Siemering[7] and, a few years later, Kivumbi[8] described a technique for diagnostic arthroscopy of the knee. Several reports concerning arthroscopy of the knee joint followed,[9–14] with increasing interest in and rapid development of the procedure. This evolution was possible after development of an arthroscope with a small diameter. Techniques for arthroscopy of the shoulder,[15–17] elbow,[18] hip,[19] and hock joint[20] have been described. Arthroscopic surgery in small animals has only recently been developed. A few reports exist on arthroscopic reconstruction of the cranial cruciate ligament[21] and treatment of osteochondritis dissecans (OCD) in the shoulder[22] and stifle.[23] For a few years, we routinely have applied arthroscopy for the diagnosis and treatment of shoulder,[17, 24] elbow,[18, 25] stifle, and hock osteochondrosis.

Arthroscopy has some important advantages for the patient as well as for the surgeon. It allows detailed intra-articular inspection and provides valuable information, which cannot be obtained by a clinical and radiographic examination, the most frequently used diagnostic methods in veterinary medicine. Arthrosis can be diagnosed earlier by arthroscopy than by radiography. Because arthroscopy allows a "quick look" into the joint, it can provide additional information about certain joint diseases, it allows better understanding of the pathological changes, it permits detailed inspection of the synovial villi in their natural environment, and it provides important information after acute joint trauma. Arthroscopy also permits repeated examinations because of little tissue trauma, which allows more rapid return to function and a better cosmetic result. With increasing experience, the shorter surgery time allows treatment of bilateral lesions during the same surgical period.[5, 8, 13, 16, 24, 26, 27] Some surgical interventions that were not beneficial when performed through an arthrotomy are now justified when performed arthroscopically, because of the minimal invasive character. Arthroscopy is also suitable for semisurgical interventions such as joint lavage, lysis of adhesions, and taking biopsies. Disadvantages of arthroscopic surgery include the relatively high cost of the equipment, the intensive training required to perform the technique,[28] and the need for a trained assistant.

MATERIAL AND EQUIPMENT

Small arthroscopes are used to perform arthroscopy in small animals. Most examinations can be performed using a 2.7-mm, 25-degree foreoblique arthroscope in a 4-mm outside diameter trocar sleeve. In smaller animals (weighing less than 15 kg) and in fibrotic joints, a 2.4- or 1.9-mm scope is more convenient. A 25-degree viewing angle is helpful in increasing the field of vision by simply rotating the arthroscope. Viewing angles larger than 25–30 degrees can cause problems related to orientation and manipulation of instruments as the operator is no longer looking at the surgical field in front of the longitudinal axis of the arthroscope.

For inspection directly through the arthroscope, a fiberoptic light source of 150 watt (W) is sufficient. The use of a video system requires a 400 W light source, especially for examination of larger joints. Some of the more expensive light sources are equipped with an automatic light intensity controller, which regulates the light intensity according to the video signal. We perform the examinations using a 400 W automatic light source. For photographic documentation, we use a 150 W light source with an electronic flash generator. With this light source, photographic documentation can be obtained using a single-lens reflex camera with a 105-mm lens, a 200 ASA film, and an exposure time of 1/60 or 1/30 seconds. To display the procedure on a monitor, a camera is attached to the arthroscope. Advantages of a video system, although expensive, include a more comfortable position and better coordination during arthroscopic surgery, less chance for contamination, a higher education value for students and assistants, and capability to record and review the procedure.[22]

During the arthroscopic procedure the joint is continuously irrigated and distended with pressurized fluid. Pressure can be obtained with a sleeve around a fluid bag (1 or 3 L), the sleeve being inflated manually with a bulb or automatically with a rapid intravenous infuser. Fluid inflow is maintained via a sterile infusion set connected to the stopcock of the trocar sleeve. Although it is stated that lactated or acetated Ringer's solution is less harmful to the chondrocytes than saline,[29] we observed no difference in clinical situations. Alternatively, gas (air, CO_2, N_2O) can be used to distend the joint.[30] It provides a wider field of view, which can be advantageous in small joints. Discrete irregularities of the articular cartilage can be more easily discerned in gas.

Most arthroscopic surgical interventions can be performed using hand-held small instruments, including grasping and basket forceps, curettes, and cutting instruments. They can be introduced directly into the joint or through a drainage cannula (3 or 4 mm diameter) to avoid fluid accumulation and tissue trauma. An instrument cannula is very useful, especially in the shoulder and the elbow. Motor-driven rotating burs and cutting instruments can be helpful for the removal of loose cartilage fragments and for synovectomy in chronically inflamed joints to improve visualization. Disadvantages include the high cost and extensive bleeding. As space is limited in small animal joints, care must be taken in using these instruments because the opposite joint surface can be easily damaged.

Sterilization of the instruments can be performed in an autoclave or gas sterilizer or by immersion in an antiseptic solution, ie, cold sterilization. Autoclaving considerably reduces the life of the optical instruments. At present we use cold sterilization, and after more than 800 arthroscopies we have not had one case of infection.

GENERAL PRINCIPLES

All interventions are performed under general anesthesia. The involved area is clipped, disinfected, and draped with a self-adherent impermeable sheet. The joint is punctured with a 1.5-inch, 19-gauge needle, which can afterward serve as an egress cannula. Synovial fluid (when present) is withdrawn to ensure intra-articular placement. The joint is distended with irrigation solution. With a second needle the correct direction for the arthroscope is determined. A stab incision is made where the needle entered the skin. The joint capsule is penetrated using the sharp trocar locked in the arthroscopic sleeve. Outflow of irrigation fluid through the sleeve confirms the intra-articular position. Replacement of the sharp trocar with a blunt obturator allows further manipulation of the arthroscopic sleeve within the joint. The blunt obturator is replaced by the arthroscope, and the light cable is connected. The fluid inflow line is attached to the trocar sleeve. Joint inspection can then be started.

For insertion of an instrumental cannula, the joint is again first punctured with a needle. The right location and direction are confirmed when the needle can be visualized through the arthroscope. A stab incision is made where the needle entered the skin. A drainage cannula is inserted using a sharp trocar in the previously determined direction into the joint under arthroscopic control. After the cannula has entered the joint, instruments can be introduced into the joint. In some cases, instruments are inserted into the joint without a cannula. After the procedure the skin incisions are closed with staples or simple sutures. Antibiotics are not administered.

INDICATIONS FOR ARTHROSCOPY

In every situation in which the joint cartilage, synovial membrane, and intra-articular ligaments (structures not visible on plain film) have to be examined, arthroscopy is indicated as a less invasive alternative of exploratory arthrotomy. Thorough clinical and radiographic examinations always have to precede the arthroscopic procedure. Arthroscopy does not replace these examinations, but provides additional information. During the arthroscopic examination, guided biopsies of the different joint structures can be taken. Evaluation of synovial inflammation, judged by the aspect and pattern of the synovial villi, correlates well with histological findings.[31] Cartilage lesions can be detected in an early stage, which is especially important in the elbow joint. It is an excellent and reliable technique for early detection of osteochondrosis (OCD) lesions of the medial condyle and fragmented coronoid process [FCP]) before the development of degenerative joint disease.[32]

Arthroscopic surgery is indicated for the treatment of osteochondrosis lesions in the shoulder (OCD), elbow (OCD, FCP), stifle (OCD), and hock (OCD) joints, which we now routinely perform.

ARTHROSCOPY OF THE SHOULDER JOINT

Each arthroscopic procedure is performed with the dog in lateral recumbency, the affected limb uppermost. The joint is held in a neutral position, ie, the scapula and humerus in a 160-degree angle. Palpable landmarks to locate the joint space include the acromion, the greater tubercle, and the infraspinatus tendon (Fig. 28–1). A first puncture is performed with a 1.5-inch, 19-gauge needle cranio-lateral between the acromion and the caudal part of the greater tubercle in a caudomedial direction. The joint is distended with about 10 ml of irrigation fluid. The correct direction for the arthroscopic sleeve is determined with a second needle, 1 cm distal to the acromion. The joint capsule is penetrated using the sharp trocar locked in the arthroscopic sleeve. The trocar is replaced by the arthroscope (2.7 mm), and the light cable is connected. The fluid inflow line is attached to the trocar sleeve.

Examination of the entire joint, including the origin of the biceps brachii tendon sheath, the cartilage, and synovial membrane of the cranial and medial compartment, and caudal joint pouch, is completed before any surgical treatment is attempted. For insertion of the caudal instrumental portal, the joint is punctured with a 2-inch, 23-gauge needle 2 to 4 cm caudal and 1 cm distal to the arthroscopic portal. The right location and direction are confirmed when the needle can be visualized through the arthroscope. There are two methods to treat an OCD lesion: When the cartilage flap is small or almost completely detached, the flap is dislodged and removed completely with a large grasping forceps. Another method

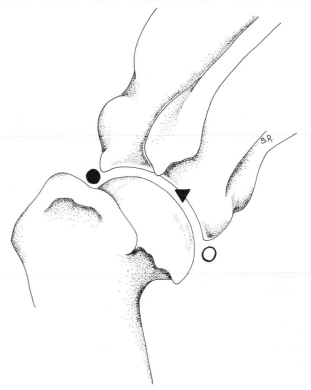

FIGURE 28–1. Lateral view of shoulder joint.

is to remove the flap piece by piece with a smaller forceps. This method is preferable, because treatment can be performed with more control, and the floating away of large flaps is avoided. In some cases a cranial instrumental portal is created when the flap is very large or to remove fragments that have migrated into the cranial joint compartment. This second instrumental cannula is inserted at the location of the first needle. After removal of the loose cartilage, the edges of the defect are probed and trimmed with a curette. The procedure is completed by thorough irrigation of the joint to remove small detached fragments and debris. At the end of the procedure, swelling of the shoulder region is possible because of leakage of irrigation fluid from the joint into the muscles and subcutaneous tissue. This swelling is absorbed within 24 hours. After the arthroscopic treatment, restricted exercise is advised for 6 weeks.

The most important indication for diagnostic and surgical arthroscopy of the shoulder joint is osteochondrosis. Although in the dog positive-contrast arthrography is useful in evaluation of the status of the articular cartilage,[35] arthroscopy is a complementary examination in painful joints when arthrography fails to demonstrate rupture of the articular cartilage.[31] However, arthrography remains the technique of choice to demonstrate joint mice within the bicipital tendon sheath.[31]

ARTHROSCOPY OF THE ELBOW JOINT

The anesthetized dog is positioned in lateral recumbency with the affected limb on the table and with the upper limb retracted caudally. The medial side of the elbow joint is prepared for aseptic surgery. The elbow is placed over the edge of the table to enable abduction. The puncture site is located proximally between the medial humeral condyle and the most proximal part of the olecranon. Irrigation fluid (8 to 10 ml) is injected to check for the exact location, which is confirmed by distention of the joint capsule and backflow through the needle. To enlarge the joint space, the limb is rotated internally and abducted. The arthroscopic sleeve is inserted into the joint, using the sharp trocar, 1 cm distal and 1 cm caudal to the medial epicondyle of the humerus (Fig. 28–2). Systematic examination of the elbow joint is performed with a 1.9- or 2.4- or 2.7-mm arthroscope. During elbow arthroscopy a large part of the joint can be examined: the medial coronoid process, the medial humeral condyle, the radial head, the lateral coronoid process, the proximal part of the ulna with the anconeal process, and a part of the lateral humeral condyle. Arthroscopically, different types of lesions in the area of the coronoid process can be differentiated including chondromalacia-like lesions, fissures of the articular cartilage, and nondisplaced and displaced fragments containing subchondral bone. In the area of the medial humeral condyle, kissing lesions and OCD lesions can be visualized. Inflammation of the synovial membrane and arthrotic changes can also be evaluated.

The instrumental portal is created 1 cm cranial to the arthroscope, just behind the medial collateral ligament. First, a needle is inserted under arthroscopic control, 1 to 2 cm cranial to the arthroscope, but still caudal to the medial collateral ligament. At this point, a stab incision (scalpel blade no. 11) is made. A cannula (3 mm) is introduced into the joint with the sharp trocar, under arthroscopic guidance. Through the cannula, instruments have access to the lesions. For treatment of large OCD lesions, a second instrumental entry can be created between the arthroscope and first instrumental portal. After a skin incision, a sharp trocar is inserted through the joint capsule to create an opening. Instruments are inserted into the joint without an instrumental cannula.

The FCP fragments or OCD flaps are detached completely or in small pieces, made with a banana-shaped knife or with a curette. In case of a coronoid fragment, the ligamentous connections, when

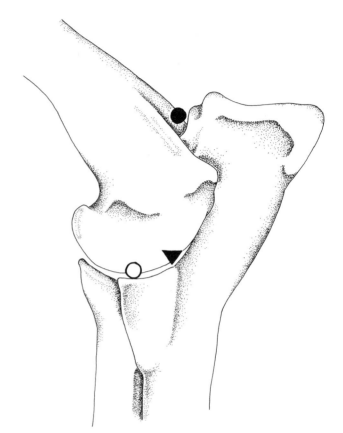

FIGURE 28–2. Lateral view of elbow joint.

present, are severed with a retrograde or Smiley knife or cut with a small biopsy forceps. Small fragments and flaps are retrieved from the joint with a small grasping forceps (2 mm) through the cannula. Larger fragments and flaps are grasped (2-mm or 2.7-mm forceps) and removed together with the cannula. To retrieve very large fragments, a large grasping forceps (3 mm) is introduced into the joint without a cannula. After removal of the fragment or flap, the edges of the defect and the subchondral bone are refreshed with a curette or shaver. Nondisplaced fragments can also be treated with a shaver: The fragment is destroyed and the particles are flushed out of the joint. In chondromalacia-like lesions, the soft and fibrillated cartilage is removed. Deep kissing lesions of the medial humeral condyle are treated by curettage. Superficial cartilage lesions are left untreated. The procedure is completed after thorough lavage of the joint.

Indication for elbow arthroscopy is present in every dog in which persistent foreleg lameness has been clinically localized within the elbow joint. Even in cases of negative radiography and computed tomography, arthroscopy can demonstrate early lesions before radiographic evidence of arthrosis, or discrete lesions not visible on CT.[32] If lesions (OCD, FCP) are present, diagnostic and surgical arthroscopy can be combined.

ARTHROSCOPY OF THE STIFLE JOINT

The dog is positioned in dorsal recumbency. The stifle region is prepared for aseptic surgery. The use of a legholder allows limited valgus and varus and more accurate inspection of the menisci. With a 20-gauge needle, the joint is punctured in the suprapatellar recess or medial/lateral to the straight patellar ligament. Synovial fluid is

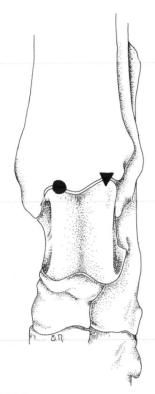

FIGURE 28–3. Anterior-posterior view of tarsal joint.

aspirated when possible and irrigation fluid injected. A skin incision of 5 mm is made medial or lateral to the straight patellar ligament halfway between the tibial crest and patella. The trocar assembly (trocar sheath plus sharp trocar) is inserted into the flexed stifle. Relocation of the arthroscopic sheath is carried out with the blunt obturator.

A systematic inspection of the joint is performed, starting with the suprapatellar pouch, and followed by the femoropatellar joint, the trochlear ridges, down to the medial compartment (medial femoral condyle, medial femorotibial joint line, medial meniscus). After inspection of the intercondylar area including the cruciate ligaments, the lateral compartment (lateral femorotibial joint line, the lateral meniscus) and the tendon of the long digital extensor muscle are examined. During the procedure, flexion, extension, varus, valgus, endorotation and exorotation are performed to enlarge the field of view and to visualize the different structures.

Although the arthroscopic technique for the knee joint is relatively simple, interpretation of the images can be very difficult. View obstruction due to the disrupted cranial cruciate ligament and/or excessive synovial villi is one of the major problems in chronic cases, making evaluation of the menisci difficult or even impossible. Evaluation of the cartilage, synovial membrane, and cruciate ligaments is relatively simple.

Indications for knee joint arthroscopy include lameness clinically located in a radiographic normal knee of a young dog, traumatic lesions, and synovial disease. OCD lesions can be treated arthroscopically.

ARTHROSCOPY OF THE TARSAL JOINT

Arthroscopic examination of the tarsocrural joint can be performed through three different portals: dorsolateral, dorsomedial, and plantarolateral.

Depending on the radiographic location, a suitable portal is used to evaluate the joint.

1. Dorsomedial portal (Fig. 28–3). The dog is fixed in dorsal recumbency. The dorsal region is prepared for aseptic surgery. The joint is punctured lateral to the extensor tendon (extensor digitorum longus muscle). Injection of irrigation fluid causes distention of the joint capsule. The arthroscopic sleeve is inserted medial to the extensor tendon, where joint distention is most pronounced. The instrumental cannula is inserted lateral to the extensor tendon after the needle is withdrawn.
2. Dorsolateral portal (Fig. 28–3). A similar technique is used as described for the dorsomedial portal. The arthroscope is inserted lateral to the extensor tendon, the instrumental cannula medial.
3. Plantarolateral portal (Fig. 28–4). The dog is positioned in lateral recumbency with the joint to be examined in the uppermost position. The lateral region is prepared for aseptic surgery. The joint is punctured dorsolaterally. A small incision is made plantarolateral, just behind the lateral malleolus, partially incising the joint capsule. The trocar sleeve is inserted using the sharp trocar or blunt obturator. An instrumental cannula can be introduced caudal to the arthroscope.

An instrumental portal for arthroscopic surgery is easily created in the dorsal part of the canine tarsocrural joint. Through this portal, surgical instruments can be introduced into the joint to treat osteochondrosis lesions of the dorsal part of the lateral trochlear ridge. In the plantar part of the joint, it is more difficult to insert an instrumental cannula. The plantar joint space is limited, certainly when (chronic) synovitis is present. Therefore, a small arthroscope (1.9- or 2.4-mm) is preferable, because it allows the additional insertion of an instrument cannula. Small OCD fragments can be removed arthroscopically. This is possible only with small instruments inserted through the instrument cannula. Arthroscopic surgery fails when the fragment is too large or has an unfavorable

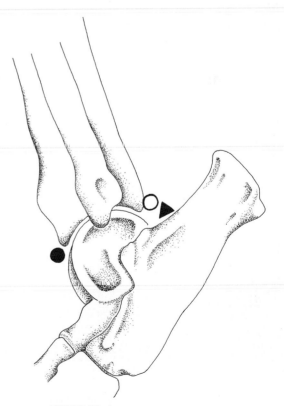

FIGURE 28–4. Lateral view of tarsal joint.

position (lateral ridge, covered by tibia). However, because the exact location can be determined by the arthroscopic examination, the fragment can easily be removed by a mini-arthrotomy, thus avoiding disruption of the medial collateral ligament complex, which can create postsurgical instability.

Similar to the elbow, cartilage lesions (OCD) within the tarsal joint can be demonstrated earlier by arthroscopy than with radiographs. Arthroscopy is indicated in young dogs in which lameness is clinically located in the tarsal joint, even without showing radiographic changes. The diagnosis can be made in an early stage in which no secondary arthrosis has developed, and treatment is performed using minimally invasive techniques (arthroscopy or mini-arthrotomy).

PROBLEMS AND COMPLICATIONS OF ARTHROSCOPY

Problems during the procedure are: difficulties with the insertion of the arthroscope or instruments, disadvantageous position of the arthroscope causing limited mobility and decreased field of vision, difficulties with the triangulation technique (localizing and manipulating the instrument), joint collapse due to periarticular fluid accumulation, dislodging the arthroscope out of the joint, instrument breakage,[33] view obstruction caused by synovial villi or the fat pad (knee), and incorrect interpretation of the arthroscopic findings. Other reported complications in humans include infection, neurovascular damage, and iatrogenic damage of joint structures.[33,34]

CONCLUSIONS

In the dog, as in humans and in horses, arthroscopy will have an important place in joint disease. In the shoulder and stifle joint, surgical arthroscopy can and will replace the classic surgical methods to treat OCD lesions. In elbow and tarsocrural joint disorders, the diagnostic potentials of arthroscopy are evident. With the established techniques, not only can the lesions be diagnosed with accuracy but they can also be treated within the same procedure, making arthroscopy the technique of choice to deal with OCD lesions.

References

1. Ogilvie-Harris DJ, Wiley AM: Arthroscopic surgery of the shoulder. J Bone and Joint Surg 68-B: 201–207, 1986.
2. Rockwood CA: Editorial: Shoulder Arthroscopy. J Bone and Joint Surg 70-A: 639–640, 1988.
3. Bertone AL, McIlwraith CW: Arthroscopic surgical approaches and intra-articular anatomy of the equine shoulder joint. Vet Surg 16:312–317, 1987.
4. Bertone AL, McIlwraith CW, Powers BE, et al: Arthroscopic surgery for the treatment of osteochondrosis in the equine shoulder joint. Vet Surg 16:303–311, 1987.
5. Nixon AJ: Diagnostic and surgical arthroscopy of the equine shoulder joint. Vet Surg 16:44–52, 1987.
6. Knezevics PF, Wruhs O: Arthroscopy in the horse, ox, pig and dog. Vet Med Rev 1:53–63, 1977.
7. Siemering GB: Arthroscopy of dogs. JAVMA 172:575–577, 1978.
8. Kivumbi CW, Bennett D: Arthroscopy of the canine stifle joint. Vet Rec 109:241–249, 1981.
9. Van Gestel MA: Arthroscopy of the canine stifle joint. Vet Q 7:237–239, 1985.
10. Van Gestel MA: Diagnostic accuracy of stifle arthroscopy in the dog. J Am Anim Hosp Assoc 21:757–763, 1985.
11. Person MW: A procedure for arthroscopic examination of the canine stifle joint. J Am Anim Hosp Assoc 21:179–186, 1985.
12. Miller CW, Presnell KR: Examination of the canine stifle: Arthroscopy versus arthrotomy. J Am Anim Hosp Assoc 21:623–629, 1985.
13. Lewis DD, Goring RL, Parker RB, et al: A comparison of diagnostic methods used in the evaluation of early degenerative joint disease in the dog. J Am Anim Hosp Assoc 23:305–315, 1987.
14. Siemering GB, Eilert RE: Arthroscopic study of cranial cruciate ligament and medial meniscal lesions in the dog. Vet Surg 15:265–269, 1986.
15. Person MW: Arthroscopy of the canine shoulder joint. Comp Cont Ed 8:537–548, 1986.
16. Goring RL, Price C: Arthroscopical examination of the canine scapulohumeral joint. J Am Anim Hosp Assoc 23:551–555, 1987.
17. Van Ryssen B, Van Bree H, Vyt P: Arthroscopy of the shoulder joint in the dog. J Am Anim Hosp Assoc 29:101–105, 1993.
18. Van Ryssen B, Van Bree H, Simoens P: Elbow arthroscopy in the clinically normal dog. Am J Vet Res 54:191–198, 1993.
19. Person MW: Arthroscopy of the canine coxofemoral joint. Comp Cont Ed 11:930–935, 1989.
20. Van Ryssen B, Van Bree H: Arthroscopic evaluation of osteochondrosis lesions in the canine hock joint. J Am Anim Hosp Assoc 28:295–299, 1992.
21. Person MW: Prosthetic replacement of the cranial cruciate ligament under arthroscopic guidance. A pilot project. Vet Surg 16:37–43, 1987.
22. Person MW: Arthroscopic treatment of osteochondritis dissecans in the canine shoulder. Vet Surg 18:175–189, 1989.
23. McLaughlin RM, Hurtig RM, Fries CL: Operative arthroscopy in the treatment of bilateral stifle osteochondritis dissecans in a dog. Vet Compar Orthop Trauma 4:158–161, 1989.
24. Van Ryssen B, Van Bree H, Missinne S: Successful arthroscopic treatment of shoulder osteochondrosis in the dog. J Small Anim Pract 34:521–528, 1993.
25. Van Ryssen B, Van Bree, H: Arthroscopic treatment of fragmented coronoid process in the dog. In preparation.
26. Patel D, Fahmy N, Sakayan A: Isokinetic and functional evaluation of the knee following arthroscopic surgery. Clin Orthop Rel Res 167:84–91, 1992.
27. Zarins B, Boyle J, Harris BA: Knee rehabilitation following arthroscopic meniscectomy. Clin Orthop Rel Res 198:36–42, 1985.
28. Van Ryssen B, Van Bree H: The use of the arthroscope in small animal practice: A review of the literature. Vlaams Diergeneesk Tijdschr 58:184–189, 1989.
29. Reagan BF, McInery VK: Irrigation solutions for arthroscopy. J Bone Joint Surg 65A:629–631, 1983.
30. Van Ryssen B, Van Bree H: A comparison of arthroscopy in a gas and a fluid medium. In preparation.
31. Van Bree H, Van Ryssen B, Desmidt M: Osteochondrosis lesions of the canine shoulder: Correlation of positive contrast arthrography and arthroscopy. Vet Radiol Ultrasound 33:342–347, 1992.
32. Van Bree H, Van Ryssen B, Simoens P: Correlation between Radiographic and Arthroscopic Findings in Dogs with Elbow Arthrosis. Proc 1st Annual Conf EVRA, 1992, p 1.
33. Kieser CH: A review of the complications of arthroscopic knee surgery. J Arthrosc Rel Surg 8:79–83, 1992.
34. Sherman OH, Fox JM, Snyder SJ, et al: Arthroscopy—"No problem surgery." J Bone Joint Surg 68A:256–265, 1986.
35. Van Bree H: Comparison of diagnostic accuracy of positive-contrast arthrography and arthrotomy in evaluation of osteochondrosis lesions in scapulohumeral joints in dogs. JAVMA 203, 84–88, 1993.

CHAPTER 29

Diseases of the Sesamoid Bones

GEOFFREY M. ROBINS \ RICHARD A. READ

In general terms, sesamoid bones are small rounded bodies located within tendons or joint capsules near freely moving joints, but they may develop in ligamentous tissue over which tendons pass. Occasionally they develop in response to friction, but usually they are present prenatally. Sesamoid bones serve three important functions: (1) to protect tendons as they pass over bony protuberances, (2) to increase the surface area of tendons over certain joints, and (3) to redirect the pull of tendons so that they can apply a more effective force to the part being moved.[1]

No sesamoid bones are present in the shoulder joint. In the elbow a sesamoid may be present within the sesamoid cartilage of the origin of the supinator muscle, articulating with the craniolateral aspect of the head of the radius. The incidence of this sesamoid has been studied and varies from about 10 to 30 per cent.[2] In the carpus there is a small sesamoid within the tendon of insertion of the abductor pollicis longus muscle, located on the medial side of the proximal end of the first metacarpal. Two small flat sesamoids may be present on the palmar surface of the carpus, located between the two rows of carpal bones.[1]

There are a number of prominent sesamoids in the metacarpophalangeal joints. In the four major digits there is a single small dorsal sesamoid in the extensor tendon, whereas on the palmar surface paired sesamoids are present, which cradle the flexor tendon complex. In the first digit there is a single palmar sesamoid. Cartilaginous nodules, which may be referred to as *sesamoids*, are found within the dorsal and palmar sides of the distal interphalangeal joints.[1]

There are no sesamoids in the hip joint. In the stifle the patella or knee cap is the largest sesamoid in the body. Contained within the tendon of the quadriceps femoris muscle, the patella articulates with the trochlea of the femur. There are three smaller sesamoids caudal to the stifle called the *fabellae*. Two are contained within the tendon of origin of the lateral and medial heads of the gastrocnemius muscle and articulate with the caudal surface of the corresponding condyles of the femur. The third fabella is located within the tendon of insertion of the popliteal muscle and articulates with the lateral tibial condyle.[1] In the hock there may be up to two sesamoids that are located within the thick tarsometatarsal fibrocartilage lying on the plantar surface of the distal part of the tarsus and proximal part of the metatarsus. It has been proposed that the prominent lateral sesamoid, present in 50 per cent of hocks in one study, be called the lateral plantar tarsometatarsal sesamoid and the smaller medial bone, detected in only 27 per cent of hocks, be named the intra-articular tarsometatarsal sesamoid bone.[3] The sesamoids in the metatarsophalangeal joints are the same as in the metacarpophalangeal joints of the forelimb.

Clinically, sesamoid problems are limited to the palmar and plantar sesamoids of the metacarpophalangeal/metatarsophalangeal joints and to the sesamoid bones in the stifle joint.

METACARPOPHALANGEAL/ METATARSOPHALANGEAL JOINT DISORDERS

Traumatic conditions of the sesamoid bones, such as fractures and dislocations, have been recognized in the racing greyhound in both the United Kingdom[4] and Australia[5, 6] for more than 30 years. More recently, attention has been focused on degeneration of the sesamoid bones, so-called *sesamoid disease*,[7] as a cause of lameness, especially in the larger breeds of domestic dogs, in the United States,[8] United Kingdom,[7, 9] Europe,[10–12] Australia,[13, 14] and Canada.[15] One survey in the United Kingdom revealed a 44 per cent incidence of sesamoid lesions in a consecutive series of 50 rottweilers with a variety of orthopedic problems, but the authors concluded that in no case was the lameness caused by the sesamoid abnormality.[9] However, a prospective study of 55 young rottweiler pups revealed a 22 per cent incidence of lameness attributable to sesamoid disease and a 73 per cent incidence of radiographic changes in the sesamoid bones. It was concluded that sesamoid disease will cause clinical lameness, but subclinical disease is common.[16] Other authors[7, 8, 11–13] have reported clinical lameness associated with sesamoid pathology, and rapid improvement has occurred once the affected sesamoid was removed. Read and colleagues[16] suggested that in more than 50 per cent of cases the lameness resolved without surgery, but in those dogs that were lame and in pain for more than 6 weeks, surgical excision of the affected sesamoid bones gave a satisfactory outcome. Sesamoid fractures[8] and degenerative disease[7] of the sesamoids are probably part of the same clinical problem. A discussion of the pathogenesis of sesamoid disease and suggested etiology has been published elsewhere.[14]

Anatomy

There are five metacarpophalangeal joints in the canine foot, one associated with each of the five digits. They are numbered from 1 to 5 in a medial to lateral direction.

Each metacarpophalangeal joint is made up of the distal end of the metacarpal bones and the proximal end of the first phalanx. The distal end of each of the third and fourth metacarpals has two symmetrical condyles separated by a sharp-edged sagittal crest, whereas the abaxial condyle of the second and fifth metacarpals is less well defined. In the four main digits (2 to 5) there is a pair of sesamoid bones on the palmar surface of each of the metacarpophalangeal joints and a single sesamoid on the dorsal surface. A single sesamoid bone exists on the palmar surface of the first digit. The palmar sesamoids of the main digits are numbered from 1 through 8 in a medial to lateral direction starting with the second digit.[1]

The shape of the palmar sesamoids varies. When viewed from behind, 1 and 8 are shorter, with a wider base than 3, 4, 5, and 6, while 2 and 7 are also shorter and almost pear shaped (Fig. 29–1). In cross section, all the sesamoids are roughly triangular, with the base of the bone articulating with the metacarpals (Figs. 29–2 and 29–3).

In each metacarpophalangeal joint, a joint capsule envelops the four bones that make up the joint, and collateral ligaments unite the metacarpal bone to the first phalanx.

The palmar sesamoid bones are supported by a complex arrangement of ligaments. There are no proximal sesamoidean ligaments; instead, the proximal ends of the sesamoid bones are embedded in the interosseous muscles of the second to the fifth digits. The middle sesamoidean ligaments consist of the lateral and medial collateral sesamoidean ligaments and a short cartilaginous transverse palmar ligament, or intersesamoidean ligament, that joins the two bones of each pair together. Each collateral is divided into two parts, with short flat bands of tissue extending from the sesamoid to attach to a corresponding area on the distal end of the metacarpal bone and the proximal end of the first phalanx. These sesamoidean collateral ligaments insert behind the attachment of the main metacarpophalangeal collaterals. The distal sesamoidean ligament consists of a broad flat band that unites the distal end of each sesamoid bone to the palmar surface of the proximal end of the first phalanx. Underneath this ligament and running diagonally from the base of each sesamoid bone extends a pair of cruciate ligaments that cross and attach to the tuberosity on the opposite side of the first phalanx.[17]

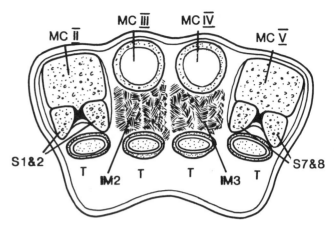

FIGURE 29–2. Cross section through paw at the level of first, second, seventh, and eighth sesamoid bones. MC = Metacarpal bones. T = Flexor tendon unit. IM = Interosseous muscle. (From Robins GM, Read RA: Diseases of the sesamoid bones. *In* Bojrab MJ [ed]: Disease Mechanisms in Small Animal Surgery. Philadelphia, Lea & Febiger, 1993, p 1094.)

Thus the sesamoids and their supporting soft tissues form a groove or pulley on the palmar surface of the foot over which run the digital flexor tendons. At this level, the deep flexor tendon passes through a sheath (manica flexoris) formed by the superficial flexor tendon.[1] These tendons are held against the sesamoids by a transverse annular ligament (Figs. 29–2 and 29–3).

The metacarpal bones do not lie parallel with the transverse axis of the limb. When viewed from above, they curve with the two central digits, being positioned more cranial than the others (Figs. 29–2 and 29–3), and when viewed from behind, they diverge distally (see Fig. 29–1). The digital flexor tendons have a similar orientation to the metacarpal bones, diverging as they divide at the level of the carpus with one bundle supplying each of the four main digits. As a consequence of this diverging pattern, the flexor tendons of digits 3 and 4 lie centrally in the groove between the palmar sesamoids, whereas the tendon is eccentrically located in the intersesamoidean groove of digits 2 and 5, lying predominantly

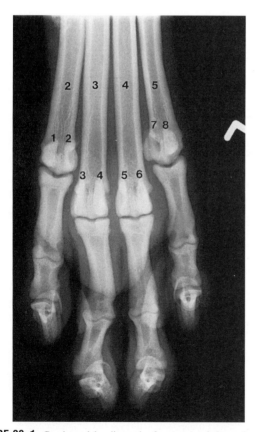

FIGURE 29–1. Craniocaudal radiograph of metacarpophalangeal region of an adult dog. The upper numbers identify the metacarpal bones, and the lower numbers the sesamoid bones. (From Robins GM, Read RA: Diseases of the sesamoid bones. *In* Bojrab MJ [ed]: Disease Mechanisms in Small Animal Surgery. Philadelphia, Lea & Febiger, 1993, p 1094.)

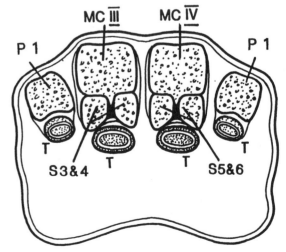

FIGURE 29–3. Cross section of paw at the level of sesamoids 3–6. (Modified from Robins GM, Read RA: Diseases of the sesamoid bones. *In* Bojrab MJ [ed]: Disease Mechanisms in Small Animal Surgery. Philadelphia, Lea & Febiger, 1993, p 1094.)

over and in contact with the second and seventh sesamoids[5] (see Figs. 29–2 and 29–3).

The anatomical features of the metatarsophalangeal joints and the plantar sesamoid bones are essentially the same as those described above.

Clinical Signs

The clinical signs of sesamoid fracture and sesamoid degeneration are similar, especially in chronic cases, and they will therefore be considered together. In the acute case there may be marked lameness with reluctance to bear weight, and in chronic cases the foot may be lifted from the ground immediately after the cessation of exercise.[8] The affected joint may be thickened, especially in chronic cases, and the joint capsule may be distended with an increased volume of synovial fluid. Palpation and manipulation of the joint are usually resented, but this can be difficult to interpret because some normal dogs resent manipulation of their toes. Both flexion and extension of the affected metacarpophalangeal joint will elicit pain and sometimes crepitus. Ventral flexion of the joint, which should normally be to about 90 per cent, is often markedly reduced. Direct palpation over the affected sesamoid is usually resented, especially in acute cases. Infiltration of local anesthetic around the affected sesamoid may relieve the lameness.[15] Occasionally in racing greyhounds an acute injury to the metacarpophalangeal joint will cause disruption of the collateral ligaments resulting in axial or abaxial displacement of the digital flexor tendons and associated sesamoids.[18] Affected animals have pain and swelling of the joint, and the affected joint may rotate in a longitudinal plane as the animal bears weight. Palpation and manipulation of the joint will confirm the extent of the soft tissue damage. Dissection of one acutely injured toe, which was removed surgically, revealed not only damage to the collateral support of both the sesamoid and the metacarpophalangeal joint but also chronic erosive changes of the articular surface of the sesamoids and the adjacent sagittal ridge of the metacarpal bone. This seemed to indicate that chronic subluxation of the sesamoids had been present before disruption of the collaterals.

In a survey of 25 cases of sesamoid degeneration,[13] clinical and radiographic signs were detected in 21 rottweilers, two greyhounds, one Labrador retriever, and one Queensland cattle dog. Fifteen of the cases were in males and 10 in females. The average age at presentation was 20 months with a range of 7 months to 7½ years. Nineteen of the patients were 18 months or younger. The right forefoot had a higher incidence of involvement than the left (30 sesamoids versus 19). Both forefeet were involved in 8 cases, and in 16 cases more than one sesamoid was involved. In the right foot, the second sesamoid was affected in 14 cases and the seventh in 12 cases. The third, fourth, fifth, and sixth sesamoids were each involved once. In the left forefoot the second sesamoid was involved in nine cases, the seventh in eight cases, and the sixth and eighth in one case each. The hind feet were involved in three cases. These findings agree with those of other surveys.[7, 8, 9, 12, 16]

The high incidence in rottweilers in this survey may reflect a predilection for sesamoid problems in this breed,[7, 9, 15] but it may also reflect a bias toward the breed, because many of the rottweilers were presented for other orthopedic problems, such as fragmentation of the medial coronoid process of the ulna (FCP) and hip dysplasia.

Synovial fluid analysis has been reported as being consistent with degenerative osteoarthritis. The fluid volume may be increased with a moderate increase of white cells (2.5 to 3.4 $\times$ 10^9/L) and a differential count revealing mostly mononuclear cells, particularly lymphocytes and macrophages.[7]

Radiography

Craniocaudal and oblique lateral projections using high definition x-ray film are an important part of the clinical assessment. The radiographic features vary according to the cause and chronicity of the problem. In acute cases of sesamoid fracture the bone may be divided into two or more fragments with sharp, well-defined irregular borders, but the fragments may not be displaced. A divided sesamoid bone with smooth, regular margins may be a congenitally malformed or bipartite sesamoid.[19] The radiographic features of sesamoid degeneration are quite varied and at times hard to distinguish from sesamoid fractures.

In many respects the changes are consistent with the general changes seen in degenerative joint disease, with one major difference being the presence of periarticular calcified bodies (Fig. 29–4). The size, number, and location of these calcifications vary considerably, ranging from single, rounded bodies to linear masses in the surrounding soft tissues (Fig. 29–5).

In some cases the outline of the affected sesamoid bone disappears, being replaced by numerous large calcified bodies.[7, 9, 13] Dorsal or axial displacement of the affected sesamoid has been noted in several cases (Fig. 29–6). Serial radiographs in one case revealed a gradual increase in the size of the calcified bodies, and in another, union of the small fragments[14] (Fig. 29–7A and B). The distal end of the adjacent metacarpal bone and proximal end of the first phalanges may be enlarged because of the presence of periarticular osteophytes (Fig. 29–6).

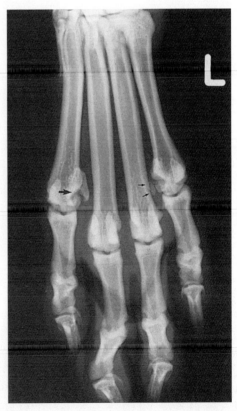

FIGURE 29–4. Craniocaudal radiograph of the forepaw of a 2.5-year-old rottweiler. The large arrow indicates a fracture in the second sesamoid bone with dorsal displacement of the larger fragment. The small arrows indicate a calcified body adjacent to the seventh sesamoid. (From Robins GM, Read RA: Diseases of the sesamoid bones. *In* Bojrab MJ [ed]: Disease Mechanisms in Small Animal Surgery. Philadelphia, Lea & Febiger, 1993, p 1094.)

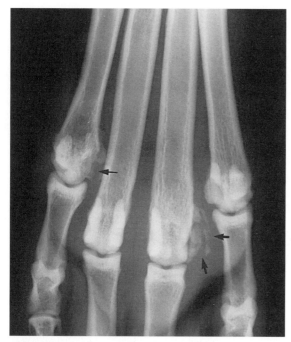

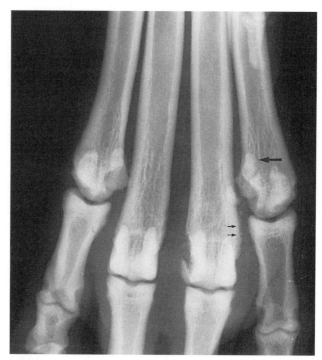

FIGURE 29–5. Craniocaudal radiograph of the forepaw of a 9-month-old rottweiler. The pair of arrows indicates multiple linear calcifications in the soft tissues adjacent to the third sesamoid. Note that this sesamoid appears totally disrupted. The single arrow indicates degeneration of the seventh sesamoid. (From Robins GM, Read RA: Diseases of the sesamoid bones. *In* Bojrab MJ [ed]: Disease Mechanisms in Small Animal Surgery. Philadelphia, Lea & Febiger, 1993, p 1094.)

FIGURE 29–6. Craniocaudal radiograph of the forepaw of an adult rottweiler. The large arrow indicates dorsal displacement of the second sesamoid. Calcified bodies are evident in the soft tissues near the base of the sesamoid. The small arrows indicate periosteal new bone formation on the medial side of metacarpal 3; the lateral side is also affected. (From Robins GM, Read RA: Diseases of the sesamoid bones. *In* Bojrab MJ [ed]: Disease Mechanisms in Small Animal Surgery. Philadelphia, Lea & Febiger, 1993, p 1094.)

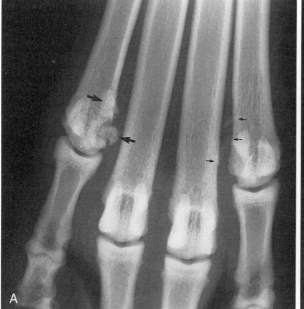

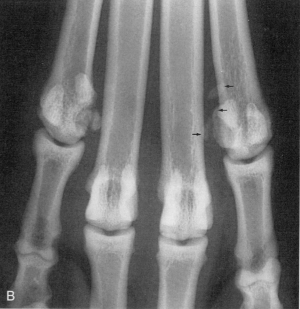

FIGURE 29–7. *A*, Craniocaudal radiograph of the forepaw of a rottweiler taken at 8 months of age. The small arrows indicate soft tissue calcification adjacent to the second sesamoid. The large arrows indicate dorsal displacement and disruption of the seventh sesamoid. *B*, Radiograph of the same forepaw of the dog in *A*, but taken 2 months later. Note that in this time the calcifications adjacent to the second sesamoid have grown and the sesamoid appears to have enlarged. (From Robins GM, Read RA: Diseases of the sesamoid bones. *In* Bojrab MJ [ed]: Disease Mechanisms in Small Animal Surgery. Philadelphia, Lea & Febiger, 1993, p 1094.)

Pathology and Pathogenesis

The pathogenesis of sesamoid fractures and degeneration remains unresolved. There does appear to be agreement among some authors[4, 5, 8, 11, 12, 19] that repeated stress on the palmar surface of sesamoids by the digital flexor tendons during overextension of the metacarpophalangeal joints may result in fatigue fractures and/or degeneration of the underlying bone and surrounding soft tissues. The high incidence of involvement of sesamoids 2 and 7 can be explained by the slight anatomical variation that exists in the relationship between the digital flexor tendons and the sesamoids in the second and fifth digits. In the central two digits the pressure of the flexor tendons during active extension is spread evenly across the sesamoids and the intersesamoidean ligaments. However, in the second and fifth digits the flexor tendon pressure is borne solely by the flat surface of the inner (axial) sesamoids, numbers 2 and 7. This uneven distribution of forces may also be due to the divergence of the metacarpals and flexor tendons of digits two and five (see Anatomy). The asymmetry of the distal end of metacarpals 2 and 5 also suggests that the axial condyle bears more load.

The high incidence of sesamoid problems in young large-breed dogs and the coexistence in many cases of other orthopedic problems associated with osteochondrosis has led some authors to postulate a similar etiology for sesamoid degeneration,[10, 20] but these claims have been rejected on the histopathological evidence of a limited number of cases.[7, 11, 12] A congenital disorder of ossification, or a bipartite sesamoid bone, has been cited as the possible underlying cause.[9, 12] Some other authors consider this to be rare,[10, 11] while another considers it to be common.[21] Direct trauma remains a possible cause, particularly when sesamoids other than 2 and 7 are involved.[8] Foot conformation has also been cited by one author, as some affected dogs have a flatfooted appearance.[13]

The possibility of vascular compromise has been suggested because of the similarities to a sesamoid condition seen in horses.[12, 22] We have examined the histopathological appearance of 18 affected sesamoids from 11 dogs (10 rottweilers and 1 greyhound) and 20 normal sesamoids from 3 normal dogs. All the grossly normal sesamoid bones were not unusual histologically. Mild infiltration of mononuclear cells was seen in the synovial membrane of affected joints. Affected sesamoid bones showed one or more fracture lines at various stages of attempted repair. In all the affected sesamoids there were areas of necrotic bone with empty osteocyte lacunae and no viable cells in the marrow. The extent of this bone necrosis was inversely correlated with the stage of fracture repair. In six of the sesamoids the entire bone was necrotic, with a marked distinction between the viable, apparently healthy chondrocytes of the articular cartilage and the underlying necrotic bone. In these cases, evidence of attempted fracture repair was restricted to fibrous proliferation in the fibromuscular attachments on the nonarticular surface and early signs of cell division in the articular cartilage overlying the fracture (Fig. 29–8). This histological picture was associated with a history of acute lameness spanning less than 3 weeks. In bones in which the fracture site was undergoing attempted repair, large amounts of fibrous callus with some areas of cartilage proliferation were present in the fracture site, surrounded by areas of active bone remodeling with osteoclasis of the adjacent necrotic bone (Fig. 29–9). This type of lesion was associated more with chronic lameness over several months. Most of the fracture lines were situated toward the apex of the bone, but in some cases the architecture was so disrupted that it was difficult to define the location of the fractures within the bone.

The extent of bone necrosis seen in this series of affected sesamoid bones supports the hypothesis that vascular compromise is important in the pathogenesis of this condition. In some sections examined, an artery could be seen penetrating the caudal (nonarticular) cortex in the proximal one third of the bone. Whether trauma

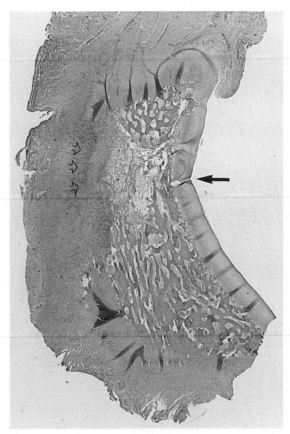

FIGURE 29–8. Low-power (12×) view of a midsagittal section through the seventh sesamoid from a young rottweiler with a history of acute foreleg lameness. The large arrow indicates the site of the fracture, with folding of the articular cartilage. The bone above and below the fracture is necrotic. An early fibrous reaction is beginning to invade the fracture site *(small arrows)*, but as yet there is no evidence of osteoclasis. (From Robins GM, Read RA: Diseases of the sesamoid bones. *In* Bojrab MJ [ed]: Disease Mechanisms in Small Animal Surgery. Philadelphia, Lea & Febiger, 1993, p 1094.)

to or occlusion of the nutrient artery causes necrosis of the bone and subsequent fracture, or conversely, whether the fracture traumatizes the vessel leading to necrosis, remains unclear and must await further investigation. A study of the microvasculature of the sesamoid complex of the human great toe led the authors to suggest that injury to the proximal or plantar aspects of the sesamoid bones could disrupt the vascular supply to these bones.[23] A similar study of the palmar metacarpal sesamoid bones of the dog has revealed an abundant blood supply, which presumably resists disruption.[24]

The finding of large areas of proliferating fibrous tissue and cartilage in a cleft in the bone associated with focal proliferation of articular cartilage is probably the basis for the hypothesis that sesamoid disease is associated with osteochondrosis. However, the evidence presented here suggests that these histological changes are simply a stage of fracture healing.

It would appear that bony union is rarely achieved in affected sesamoids, possibly because of the continual distracting forces on the fragments during weight bearing. Failure to achieve bony union does not, however, preclude resolution of the lameness.[14] Fragmented palmar sesamoids are a common incidental finding on radiographs of normal (sound) dogs, particularly rottweilers[9, 16] and greyhounds.[18]

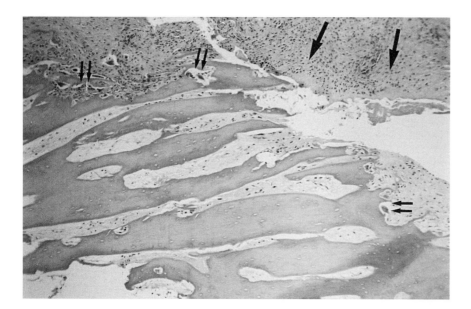

FIGURE 29–9. High-power (110×) view of a midsagittal section through the seventh sesamoid from a young rottweiler with a history of lameness spanning 2 months. A marked fibrous callous reaction is invading the fracture site *(large arrow)*, with active osteoclasis of adjacent bone *(double arrows)*. All osteocytic lacunae are empty, indicating death of the bone. The marrow spaces contain a sparse population of cells with stellate nuclei that appear similar to the cells in the fibrous callus. (From Robins GM, Read RA: Diseases of the sesamoid bones. *In* Bojrab MJ [ed]: Disease Mechanisms in Small Animal Surgery. Philadelphia, Lea & Febiger, 1993, p 1094.)

Treatment

Surgical treatment of sesamoid injuries remains controversial. It is well recognized that many dogs have advanced sesamoid disease but are never lame.[9, 13, 16, 18] However, numerous reports document patients with chronic lameness and pain that resolve once the affected sesamoid bone is removed.[7, 8, 12, 16] One author recommends removing the sesamoid only if the fragments have become displaced.[6] Conservative therapy by splinting the foot has been recommended in acute cases of sesamoid fracture.[8] Pain and lameness may resolve after a prolonged period of restricted exercise.[13, 16]

The surgical approach to removing the sesamoid involves making an incision directly over the affected bone. Fortunately, in most cases this involves sesamoids 2 and 7 and does not require incising through the metacarpal pad. A tourniquet or Esmarch's bandage may assist in keeping the operative field free of blood.

The superficial flexor tendon is located and the annular ligament that holds both it and the deep flexor to the sesamoids is incised on the side nearest the affected bone, and the flexor tendons are displaced away from the affected bone.[7, 25]

Alternatively, the superficial flexor tendon can be divided longitudinally and the deep flexor tendon located and retracted sideways.[12] The affected bone is carefully dissected free from the surrounding soft tissues. The joint is closed in layers and the foot supported in a padded bandage for 7 days. Exercise is then restricted for 7 more days. The results of surgery are usually very good, the lameness in most cases resolving within 4 weeks of surgery.

Long-term follow-up (mean 3.8 years) was obtained by one of the authors (RR) from 17 rottweilers that had undergone excision of one or more palmar metacarpal sesamoids for sesamoid disease. Of 46 radiographically affected sesamoids involving 21 limbs, 31 had been surgically removed, with 26 of these involving sesamoids 2 and 7. Mean duration of lameness immediately after surgery was 2.7 weeks. Seventeen (86%) of the surgically treated limbs were sound at long-term follow-up, and four dogs had mild residual lameness. Surgically treated joints were thickened and had reduced range of movement, but the animals were pain free on manipulation. Radiographs of surgically treated metacarpophalangeal joints revealed minimal osteoarthritis (Fig. 29–10).

Conclusions

There is some debate over the importance of sesamoid disease as a cause of lameness in dogs. When a lame dog exhibits marked pain on pressure and manipulation of a metacarpophalangeal joint and radiographs and physical examination fail to reveal any other causes of lameness in that limb, the diagnosis of lameness due to sesamoid disease can be made with confidence. However, problems arise because of the high incidence of other orthopedic problems in dogs with sesamoid disease. This is particularly true in rottwei-

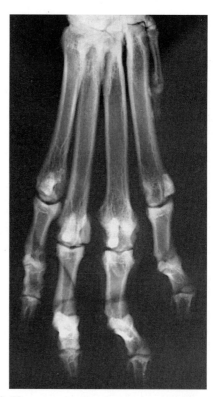

FIGURE 29–10. Craniocaudal radiograph of the forepaw of a mature rottweiler, 5 years following excision of the second, third, and seventh sesamoids. The dog is sound, although there is a restricted range of pain-free motion of the affected metacarpophalangeal joints. There is minimal evidence of degenerative joint disease in the second and fifth metacarpophalangeal joints, but in the third there is evidence of chronic changes.

lers, in which there is a high incidence of elbow lameness due to FCP.[26] A decision to surgically remove an affected sesamoid should be made only when a definite pain response is elicited from the affected joint and lameness has been evident for more than six weeks. Thickening and restricted movement of the metacarpophalangeal joint without a significant pain response suggests that an alternative cause of the lameness should be sought.

The prognosis for return to soundness is good, although one report suggests that chronic cases carry a less favorable prognosis.[12] This may be associated with the development of osteoarthritic changes in the affected metacarpophalangeal joints in more chronic cases. However, long-term follow-up of the 17 dogs referred to above showed minimal radiographic evidence of osteoarthritis.

The apparent high incidence of sesamoid disease in rottweilers suggests a genetic component in the pathogenesis, but to date this aspect has not been investigated.

PATELLAR LUXATION

Although luxation of the patella is a common cause of lameness—particularly in the toy and miniature breeds—it is an infrequent occurrence in working and racing dogs. It can occur unilaterally or bilaterally and in a medial or a lateral direction. It is usually the result of a congenital deformity, but it can be due to trauma. Medial luxation occurs five times more frequently than lateral luxation, although the latter form is observed more frequently in large breeds. Traumatic luxation can occur in any breed and at any age, whereas congenital luxation usually becomes evident before 4 to 6 months of age, although minor deformities may not lead to luxation until later in life.

Medial Patellar Luxation

It has been estimated that 95 per cent of dogs with patellar luxation have some form of related structural deformity. Although the clinical expression of patellar luxation is displacement of the quadriceps muscle with its associated sesamoid bone, the underlying cause of this displacement may be in the hip joint. A detailed but unpublished study of the condition revealed that a decrease in the angle of inclination of the femoral head (coxa vara) and a decrease in the femoral neck anteversion angle result in a series of structural changes in the whole limb.[27]

In an attempt to resolve some contradictory statements regarding the changes in the hip joint with patellar luxation, the radiographs of 40 cases were studied in detail.[26] Parameters measured were (1) the hip anteversion angles determined by the direct fluoroscopic method and/or the biplanar method, (2) inclination angles of the femoral head and neck, and (3) the transcondylar axis of the distal femur (Fig. 29–11, Table 29–1).

The results revealed that dogs with medial patellar luxation have a reduced anteversion angle that is most pronounced in the more severe grades of luxation. The inclination angle did not differ significantly from normal. The transcondylar axis was significantly altered.

Reduction of the anteversion angle may be a reflection of lateral torsion of the femur. The conformational changes in the femur and tibia seen in dogs with patellar luxation are probably caused by the abnormal loads being applied across the growth plates and epiphyses by the displaced patella and the quadriceps muscle. Whether changes in the hip joint or dysplasia of the quadriceps causes the initial displacement of the patella remains to be resolved.[28]

A detailed examination of dogs with medial patellar luxation may reveal a wide range of pathological changes related to the severity of the condition and the age of the animal. Untreated congenital luxation in a young pup is likely to result in progressive

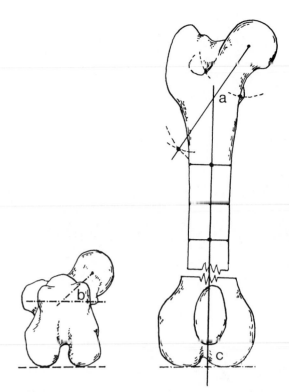

FIGURE 29–11. *a,* Inclination angle of the femoral head and neck relative to the midshaft of the femur. *b,* Anteversion angle of the femoral head and neck relative to the transcondylar axis. *c,* Transcondylar axis of the distal femur relative to the midshaft of the femur.

deformity. However, recent experience with a greyhound pup with a severe congenital (grade 4) medial patellar luxation revealed that the degree of the deformity improved (to grade 3) in the 6-week period between birth and surgical correction.

Because of the wide range of deformities associated with patellar luxation, it is helpful to categorize patellar luxations into four grades:[27]

Grade 1. Intermittent luxation that occasionally results in the dog carrying the leg. The patella can be manually luxated with the joint in full extension, but when released it returns to the trochlea immediately. There is no evidence of crepitus. Rotation of the tibia and displacement of the tibial tuberosity are minimal. When the joint is extended and flexed it moves in a straight line, with no abduction of the hock.

Grade 2. Frequent luxation, which may last for long periods, causing the dog to carry the limb. Some weight bearing may occur

TABLE 29–1. Radiographic Findings in 40 Cases of Medial Patellar Luxation

	Anteversion		Inclination		Transcondylar
	Direct Mean	Biplanar Mean	Direct Mean	Corrected	Mean
Medial (Gd ½)	23	22	146	142	75
Medial (Gd ¾)	14	21	145	144	67
Lateral	37	28	135	130	86
Normal	25	30	145	142	82
Published normal	31	31	149	145	87

with the limb in a flexed position. The patella can be replaced either manually or by extension of the joint and derotation of the tibia, but reluxates easily when the tension is released. Pain and crepitus may be apparent during relocation and reluxation because of focal erosion of the articular cartilage from the underside of the patella and the medial ridge of the femoral trochlear. The tibia is rotated and the tibial tuberosity is displaced medially up to 30 degrees from the midline. Mild angular and torsional changes may be present in the femur and tibia.

Grade 3. Permanent luxation with rotation of the tibia and tibial tuberosity from 30 to 60 degrees. Repositioning of the patella is possible with extension of the joint and derotation of the tibia, but reluxation occurs immediately. Although the luxation is permanent, many dogs use the limb in a semiflexed position. Flexion and extension of the stifle cause abduction or adduction of the hock. Distortion of the femoral and tibial articular surfaces is present with angulation and torsion of the femur and tibia. The trochlea is shallow or flat.

Grade 4. Permanent luxation with rotation of the tibia and the tibial tuberosity from 60 to 90 degrees. Repositioning of the patella is impossible, and extension of the stifle is limited by muscular contraction. The limb is carried or, if affected bilaterally, the animal moves in a crouched position with the limbs semiflexed. The trochlea is flat or convex, and articular surfaces are severely angulated. Angular and torsional changes are present in the tibia and femur. Despite severe rotation of the proximal tibia, there may be concurrent outward torsion of the tibial shaft to such a degree that the distal tibia and the foot are in approximately normal alignment.[29]

Although the relative incidence of each grade has not been determined in a large unbiased survey, it appears to be greater in grades 1 to 3 than in grade 4.

Subluxation of the patella onto the medial trochlear ridge has been identified recently by one of the authors (RR) in Australian cattle dogs and other working breeds. There is minimal bony deformity, and the dogs often have non–weight-bearing lameness associated with full-thickness erosion of the articular cartilage of the patellar and trochlear ridge, resulting in bone-on-bone contact.

Clinical Signs

As indicated in the grading system, the clinical signs of medial patellar luxation vary according to the degree of deformity, the duration of the condition, and whether the condition is present in one or both stifles.

A thorough clinical examination of the stifle should include observation of the animal's gait and posture and palpation of both the weight-bearing and non–weight-bearing limbs. Further information may be obtained by palpation after the animal has been anesthetized. Radiographs of the limb are not essential to confirm the diagnosis but may help in assessment of a grade 4 luxation.

Preoperative Assessment

After completion of a clinical examination, the following facts relevant to the choice of operation and to the prognosis should be established:

1. Direction of luxation
2. Duration of luxation (permanent or intermittent)
3. Presence of crepitus
4. Stability of reduction
5. Alignment of the tibial tuberosity to the trochlear groove with the patella reduced and the limb weight bearing
6. Depth of trochlear groove

7. Overall conformation and joint mobility
8. Presence of lameness

Treatment

Each case should be treated individually; there is no place for a stereotyped approach to the problem. The appropriate procedure(s) are selected after careful preoperative assessment and on decisions made during surgery. As a rule, surgical intervention should not be delayed, especially with young animals with grade 3 or 4 luxation. Realignment of the quadriceps apparatus during active growth may prevent some of the severe deformities from occurring.[30]

Surgical intervention should aim to:

I. Reinforce the patella in the trochlea by
   A. Lateral femoropatellar fascial tightening
   B. Medial femoropatellar fascial release
   C. Femoral trochlear deepening
   D. Fascial transplantation
II. Realign the quadriceps muscle by
   A. Tibial derotation with sutures
   B. Tibial tuberosity transplantation
   C. Femoral osteotomy
   D. Rectus femoris transplantation
III. Correct severe conformational defects by
   A. Femoral osteotomy
   B. Tibial osteotomy
IV. Pain relief by patellectomy

In most cases a number of these procedures are combined at one operation. Failures are more often related to undertreatment and are invariably associated with inadequate preoperative assessment.[31]

PATELLAR FRACTURES

Fractures of the patella are uncommon and are usually associated with direct trauma. Transverse fractures are ideally suited to fixation with a tension band wire so that the distracting forces generated by the quadriceps muscle can be converted into a compressive force. More stable fixation can be achieved if one or more K-wires are inserted in addition to the tension band wire. It is advisable to predrill the hole for the pin as the bone in the patella is very hard.[30] It is imperative to ensure accurate alignment of the intraarticular fracture surfaces to reduce the possibility of degenerative joint disease, but this can prove quite difficult. Approaching the fracture by performing an osteotomy of the insertion of the patellar ligament onto the tibial crest may facilitate reduction and fixation of the fracture. Fractures near the proximal or distal pole can be treated effectively by excision of the small fragments.

Comminuted fractures that cannot be accurately reduced may be better handled by excision of the fragments and reinforcement of the patellar ligament with a supporting figure-8 wire from the quadriceps tendon to the tibial crest. Alternatively, patellectomy has been shown to result in satisfactory long-term limb function in dogs.[31]

Some greyhound pups with tibial crest avulsion may also have a fracture of the distal pole of the patella, and it is advisable to remove the fragment when surgery is performed to repair the avulsed tibial crest.[32]

PATELLAR OSTEOCHONDROSIS

Osteochondral fragmentation of the lateral aspect of the patella has been reported in three 4-month-old female greyhound pups.[33] One was affected unilaterally, while the other two had bilateral

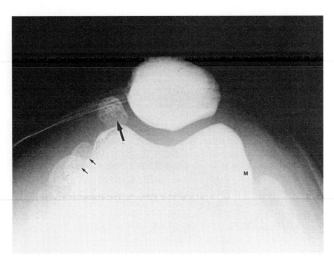

FIGURE 29–12. A skyline projection of the distal femoral trochlear and patella of a young greyhound with an osteochondral fragment adjacent to the lateral aspect of the patella (*single arrow*) and two additional fragments in the lateral aspect of the joint (*double arrows*). M = medial aspect.

lesions. Mild weight-bearing lameness was present with slight reduction in the range of joint motion, mild synovial effusion, and obvious prominence of the patella. Radiographs, particularly the skyline projection (Fig. 29–12), revealed the presence of osteochondral fragments and defects within the patella. Surgical exploration confirmed the presence of the lesions. In two cases the fragments were removed, and the lateral fascia reattached to the patella. In one case there was a transverse fracture in the patella that had all the characteristics of a congenitally deformed bipartite patella. In the other two cases the defect was a full-length sagittal lesion on the lateral aspect.

FABELLAR LESIONS

Fractures of the lateral fabella have been recorded as an uncommon cause of lameness in dogs.[34] In most cases there is no history of direct trauma, and it is postulated that the fracture occurs when there is an imbalance between the forces generated by the gastrocnemius and the quadriceps muscles, particularly when the stifle is extended and inward rotation of the tibia is largely restrained by the lateral collateral ligament. Clinical signs include weight-bearing lameness with a limited range of stifle movement during walking. The lameness was more apparent with exercise and after rest. Palpation of the stifle reveals pain localized over the lateral fabella with no evidence of instability or reduced passive range of motion. Chronic cases involve some atrophy of the quadriceps and gluteal muscles. Radiographs demonstrate fragmentation of the lateral fabella with the small pieces of bone having sharply defined borders in the acute cases and rounded borders in the chronic cases.

As with palmar sesamoid fractures, conservative treatment with restricted exercise and nonsteroidal anti-inflammatory drugs will usually produce a satisfactory outcome after about 10 weeks. Surgical excision may result in more rapid resolution of the lameness.[34] Fragmentation of the fabellae may be identified as an incidental observation on radiographs of the stifle.

Although displacement of the fabellae has been noted as a normal anatomical variation in the dog,[35] displacement of the medial fabella has been observed as part of a condition called *deformity of the proximal tibial plateau*.[36] In this condition, which is usually bilateral, there is abnormal cranial bowing of the tibia resulting in an exaggerated caudal slope to the tibial plateau. This results in inability of the dog to fully extend the stifle joint and subsequently leads to degenerative joint disease and failure of the cranial cruciate ligament. Displacement of the medial fabella may reflect the abnormal loads placed on the gastrocnemius muscle as a result of the abnormal gait and position of the stifle joint.

The lateral and medial fabellae may also become displaced as a result of traumatic avulsion of the respective heads of the gastrocnemius muscle. This is an uncommon cause of dysfunction of the common calcaneal tendon, and affected animals will have hyperextension of the stifle, hyperflexion of the hock, and a painful firm swelling over the affected fabella. Radiographs will confirm the displaced fabella and the presence of soft tissue swelling. Reattachment of the fabella and the head of the gastrocnemius muscle to the distal femur with nonabsorbable sutures is recommended.[31]

Avulsion of the tendon of origin of the popliteal muscle with its associated fabella from the lateral aspect of the femoral condyle is another uncommon cause of lameness in the dog. In an acute case the stifle will be swollen and painful. Radiographs reveal displacement of the popliteal sesamoid in a caudal and distal direction. Reattachment of the tendon to its origin with a screw and spiked washer is recommended in acute cases. In chronic cases this may be impossible, so the tendon is anchored with sutures to surrounding tissues.[31]

References

1. Evans HE, Christensen CG: Miller's Anatomy of the Dog, 2nd ed. Philadelphia, WB Saunders Company, 1979.
2. Wood AKW, McCarthy PH, Howlett CR: Anatomic and radiographic appearance of a sesamoid in the tendon of the origin of the supinator muscle of dogs. Am J Vet Res 46:2043, 1985.
3. Wood AKW, McCarthy PH: Radiologic and anatomic observations of plantar sesamoid bones at the tarsometatarsal articulations of greyhounds. Am J Vet Res 45:2158, 1984.
4. Bateman JK: Fractured sesamoids in the greyhound. Vet Rec 71:101, 1959.
5. Davis PE, Bellenger CR, Turner DM: Fractures of the sesamoid bones in the greyhound. Aust Vet J 45:15, 1969.
6. Gannon JR: Stress fractures in the greyhound. Aust Vet J 48:244, 1972.
7. Bennet D, Kelly DF: Sesamoid disease as a cause of lameness in young dogs. J Small Anim Pract 26:567, 1985.
8. Berg JA: Fractures of the palmar and plantar sesamoid bones as a cause of lameness in the dog. JAVMA 163:968, 1973.
9. Vaughan LC, France C: Abnormalities of the volar and plantar sesamoid bones in rottweilers. J Small Anim Pract 27:551, 1986.
10. Von Arbesser E: Division of sesamoids as a cause of lameness in the dog. Wien Tierarztl Mschr 61:144, 1974.
11. Punzet G, Grundschober F, Mayrhofer E: The aetiology and treatment of sesamoid injuries in the dog. Kleintierpraxis 1979; 24:303.
12. Krooshof Y, Hazewinkel HAW: Examination and treatment of fractures of sesamoid bones in the feet of dogs. Tijdschr Diergeneeskd 111:1167, 1986.
13. Robins GM: Sesamoid disease and metatarsal rotation. Aust Vet Pract 16:200, 1986.
14. Robins GM, Read RA: Diseases of the sesamoid bones. In Bojrab, MJ (ed): Disease Mechanisms in Small Animal Surgery, 2nd ed. Philadelphia, Lea & Febiger, 1993, p 1094.
15. Atilola M: A developmental abnormality of the fore-sesamoids in rottweilers—An introduction. Vet Comp Orthop Traumatol 3:129, 1989.
16. Read RA, Black AP, Armstrong SJ, et al: Incidence and clinical significance of sesamoid disease in rottweilers. Vet Rec 130:533, 1992.
17. Nichel R, Schummer A, Seiferle E: The Anatomy of Domestic Animals—The Locomotory System of Domestic Mammals. Berlin, Verlag Paul Parey, 1986.
18. Eaton-Wells R: Prognosis for return to racing following surgical repair of musculo-skeletal injury. In Greyhound Medicine and Surgery. Pro-

ceedings 122, University of Sydney Post-graduate Committee in Veterinary Science, 1989, p 245.

19. Dee JF: Fractures in the racing greyhound. *In* Bojrab MJ (ed): Pathophysiology in Small Animal Surgery. Philadelphia, Lea & Febiger, 1981.

20. Pobisch R: The diagnosis of acute lameness in the dog. Kleintierpraxis 14:37, 1969.

21. Morgan JP: Radiology in Veterinary Orthopaedics. Philadelphia, Lea & Febiger, 1972, p 392.

22. Nemeth F: The pathology of sesamoiditis. Tijdschr Diergeneeskd 98:1003, 1973.

23. Sobel M, Hashimoto J, Arnoczky S, et al: The microvasculature of the sesamoid complex: Its clinical significance. Foot and Ankle 13:359, 1992.

24. Cake MA, Read RA: The blood supply to the canine palmar metacarpal sesamoid bones. Vet Comp Orthop Traumatol 8:76, 1995.

25. Piermattei DL: An Atlas of Surgical Approaches to the Bones and Joints of the Dog and Cat, 3rd ed. Philadelphia, WB Saunders Company, 1993.

26. Read RA, Armstrong SJ, O'Keefe JD, et al: Fragmentation of the medial coronoid process of the ulna in dogs: A study of 109 cases. J Small Anim Pract 31:330, 1990.

27. Putman RW: Patellar luxation in the dog. Master's Thesis, University of Guelph, 1968.

28. Robins GM: Hip anterversion and inclination angles in dogs with patellar luxation. Aust Vet Pract 20:168, 1990.

29. Rudy RL: Stifle Joint. *In* Archibald J (ed): Canine Surgery, 2nd ed. Santa Barbara, American Veterinary Publications, 1974.

30. Brinker WO, Piermattei DL, Flo GL: Handbook of Small Animal Orthopaedics and Fracture Treatment, 2nd ed. Philadelphia, WB Saunders Company, 1990.

31. Robins GM: The Canine Stifle Joint. *In* Whittick (ed): Canine Orthopaedics, 2nd edition. Philadelphia, Lea & Febiger, 1990, p 693.

32. Eaton-Wells RD: Injuries of Traction Growth Plates. *In* Bojrab, MJ (ed): Disease Mechanisms in Small Animal Surgery, 2nd ed. Philadelphia, Lea & Febiger, 1993, p 1042.

33. Shealy PM, Miller JL, Kincaid SA, et al: Osteochondral fragmentation (osteochondrosis) of the canine patella: Clinical, radiographic, tomographic and pathological findings and surgical treatment. 19th Veterinary Orthopedic Society Conference Proceedings 1992, p 42.

34. Houlten JEF, Ness MG: Lateral fabellar fractures in the dog: A review of eight cases. J Small Anim Pract 34:373, 1993.

35. Rendano VT, Dueland R: Variation in location of gastrocnemius sesamoid bones (fabellae) in a dog. JAVMA 173:200, 1978.

36. Read RA, Robins GM: Deformity of the proximal tibia in dogs. Vet Rec 111:295, 1982.

SECTION VI

TREATMENT METHODOLOGIES

CHAPTER 30

PHYSICAL THERAPY IN CANINE SPORTING BREEDS

ROBERT A. TAYLOR \ MERRY LESTER \ JAMES R. GANNON

Physical therapy was once thought to consist of treatment of disease or trauma by the use of cold or heat, by massage, and by therapeutic exercise.[1] However, physical therapy has evolved into a dynamic field. Gone are the days of performing surgery or putting on a cast and then discharging the patient without follow-up care.[2] Research on the effects of immobilization on muscular atrophy[3] and variations in the nutrition of the intervertebral disc induced by motion,[4] the work of Salter and colleagues on the healing of articular cartilage,[5] and the study of Gelberman et al on effects of early intermittent passive mobilization on healing canine tendons have changed the postinjury and postoperative follow-up of small animals.[6]

What is physical therapy? In the human model, physical therapy started during World War I, when reconstruction aides worked to assist in the rehabilitation of wounded veterans. Physical therapy throughout the past 80 years has continued to grow. The U.S. Department of Labor statistics indicate that physical therapy is a highly sought health care profession and projects demand to exceed supply through the turn of the century.[7] Physical therapy for human patients is directly accessible in most states. Human and veterinary orthopedists acknowledge that all patients, regardless of age or athletic status, benefit psychologically and physiologically from postsurgical physical therapy.[8] Postoperative attention and "hands-on" therapy benefit the animal, while owners' participation helps them understand the animal's progress. They can play a vital role in functional return through their participation. Physiological benefits of physical therapy include reduction of muscle atrophy, earlier resolution of inflammation, improved joint hemostasis and biomechanics, promotion of wound healing, and earlier functional return.

Physical therapy can reduce muscle contracture by utilizing forms of passive range of motion, modalities such as ultrasound, active exercise, cold applications, and splinting. Without adequate physical therapy there will be increased swelling in the tissues and increased collagen formation that will create stiffer muscles and

tendons after injury. Stiffer joints, muscles, and tendons increase the risk for future injury.[9, 10]

It is known that as soon as surgery is attempted or an injury has occurred to a joint, the type II muscle fibers (fast-twitch glycolytic muscle fibers) in and around the area start to atrophy chemically. This chemical atrophy results in loss of control of the joint and increases forces along the surgical area or along the injured area. Booth has documented in animals the time course of muscle atrophy during immobilization and that muscle atrophy occurs almost immediately following immobilization.[3] Physical therapy can help decrease atrophy by utilizing modalities such as electrical stimulation, ultrasound, and massage.

Restricted joint motion causes rapid cartilage atrophy and reduced chondrocyte nutrition.[11] Early movement throughout the range of motion maintains synovial fluid in the joint and helps maintain cartilage nutrition and hence decrease degenerative changes.[5] By improving biomechanics in the joint and by increasing early weight bearing, there is less stress to the other limbs and functional training can begin earlier, with faster return of the animal to its sporting activity. It is interesting to note that in dogs subjected to operative repair of cranial cruciate ligament rupture as many as 37 per cent[12] suffer contralateral cranial cruciate ligament rupture within a year. Perhaps with appropriate physical therapy following repair the frequency of this problem might be diminished.[13]

Physical therapy, when properly applied, can promote wound healing. Physical therapy may be utilized initially over the first 72 hours to promote fibroblastic activity and increase formation of collagen. Ultrasound, massage, and microcurrent have all been shown to increase fibroblastic activity.[14, 15] Early physical therapy using ice with compression will decrease swelling[13] and hasten faster return to activity.[13] Early activity and passive range of motion decreases sarcomere atrophy,[6] and early weight bearing will enhance strengthening of the muscle. Appropriate physical therapy will also control the loads to joints and build stronger tissue by applying a slow low-load to the bone, muscle, or tendons to promote healing.[10]

A discussion of tissue–specific physical therapy would be incomplete without discussion of wound healing. Wolff's law (1892) states that bone is continually undergoing change and that compression will form stronger and harder bones. Therefore, to get it to heal, one needs to apply controlled forces to the bone. Internal fixation of fractures can limit loading of a fracture site to stimulate fracture repair. Physical therapy as well as early weight bearing can help to apply slow low-load forces in a correct direction to the bone to promote healing.[10]

Physiologically, as tendons heal, one can control the loads that in turn enhance healing times. During the early phase of tendon healing, swelling may interfere with proliferation of fibroblasts. By reducing the swelling, fibroblastic proliferation and deposition of orderly collagen bundles can be enhanced. From day 5 to 21 during tendon healing, there is early remodeling with fibroblasts producing type 3 collagen. Tendon injuries are usually immobilized for 3 to 4 weeks. This period of relative immobilization allows for myofibril tightening around the scar, and the collagen remains very stiff.[16] The scar can go beyond the tendon and adhere to muscle as well. A repaired tendon or injured tendon will reach maturation between 60 and 80 days. During this period, tension and compression are very important to promote healing. Both should be applied in low loads with high repetitions. The literature indicates that it will take a full 50 weeks for a ruptured tendon to reach full maturation in humans, and we possibly need to consider the load demands of the animal, whether racing, coursing, or hunting, to be sure we protect the tendon for the full year it needs to be protected.

Mild muscle injuries heal in about 21 to 30 days, provided that both effusion and force to the muscle are controlled. With use of ice and compression during the early phase immediately following the muscle injury, the animal can be returned to activity significantly earlier. Injured tendons are usually immobilized for 3 to 4 weeks. Muscle ruptures such as those that occur in the racing greyhound can be treated surgically. Following a period of immobilization, a functional training program can hasten the recovery. It is important to load muscle as it is healing but not load it more than 80 per cent of its maximum strength,[4] as overloading will cause reinjury. The muscular tendon junction heals poorly, and it will never be as strong as it was before injury. While this is a rare injury in the dog, the prognosis for functional return is guarded.

MODALITIES AND PROCEDURES

Modalities and procedures may be used in rehabilitating an animal. In this chapter, different modalities and procedures are discussed, including application of cold and heat and the use of electrical stimulation, ultrasound, electromagnetic therapy, cold laser, massage, and exercise.

Cold and Heat

The use of cold, cryotherapy, in therapeutic settings has become the most common treatment in human sports medicine. The physiological effects of cryotherapy are poorly understood; however, research has shown that cryotherapy along with compression significantly lowers the temperature in a joint,[13] constricts and then dilates blood vessels, produces an analgesic effect, and decreases swelling. In a study by Merrick et al, it was shown that ice application combined with compression can lower the skin temperature by 27 degrees centigrade. At 2 cm below the surface the temperature drops by 10 degrees Celsius (Fig. 30–1). Ice may be applied directly to a postoperative site, or ice packs that conform readily to the body area may be used. Intermittent use of ice with compression or an elastic bandage over the top of the ice pack causes reduction of the temperature deep within the tissue. Remem-

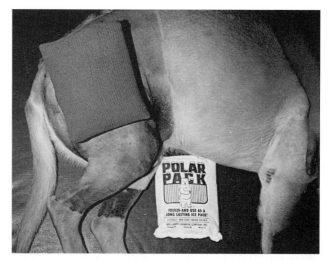

FIGURE 30–1. Cold application can be done with padded ice packs, refrigerated blankets, or ice in cups.

bering also that ice creates an analgesic effect, one may "ice" the painful area for 10 to 15 minutes before exercise. Following the exercise session the area is re-iced, allowing earlier mobilization of a painful joint.

Heat is perhaps one of the oldest methods of physical therapy; however, heat should not be used for at least the first week following injury or surgery. Heat may be applied through moist hot packs such as Hydrocollator packs or by means of a dry heating pack. Therapy tubs with warm water (101F/38.3C) may be used to apply heat, but caution should be used to avoid overheating.

Electrical Stimulation

Electrical stimulation is used for several different reasons: to enhance muscle reeducation, promote healing, reduce pain, and reduce swelling.[9, 10, 17] Unfortunately there is not a single machine on the market that produces all these effects. When an electrical stimulation machine is being chosen to use in a clinic or at a track, it is necessary to know the capabilities of each individual machine and its intended uses (Fig. 30–2).

The biphasic waveform of electrical stimulation is used most commonly in veterinary medicine. This waveform is ideal for muscle reeducation[18] (Fig. 30–2). Biphasic waveforms are sine waves, and a minimum of 10,000 cycles per second is necessary for electrical stimulation to get through the skin. An ideal setting of 50 pulses per second and a frequency of 175 macroseconds will help for maximum contraction. Research by Currier et al shows that electrical stimulation can actually cause a muscle to create 15 to 50 per cent of its maximum isometric contraction.[19] Bickford and associates[20] reported 50 per cent of the patient's maximum isometric contraction was possible utilizing electrical stimulation.[20] When utilizing electrical stimulation for muscle reeducation, one should strive for maximum contraction if the goal is to decrease muscle atrophy or to increase muscle strength. The optimal cycle of muscle contraction is 10 seconds on and 50 seconds off.[19] Ten maximum contractions of a muscle should be performed.

Transcutaneous electrical neuromuscular stimulation (TENS) should not be used for muscle reeducation. The waveform is different and is a very uncomfortable contraction, and the animal may protest if this form of battery stimulation is used. TENS currently has little use in veterinary physical therapy in the United States.

Electrical stimulation also can be used to reduce swelling. This is especially effective after a muscle injury. To reduce swelling

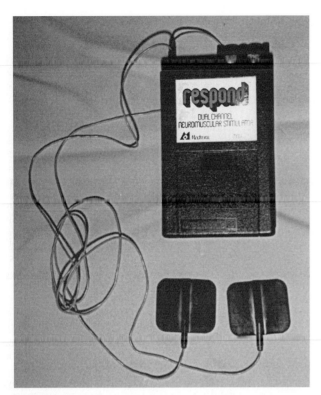

FIGURE 30–2. This neuromuscular electrical stimulation unit requires four AA batteries.

ideally, an electrical stimulation unit that is primarily monophasic in nature is desirable. Negative current is the most likely to cause decreased edema. The unit should be applied to threshold, the machine turned up until there is a mild muscle fasciculation. An ideal setting would be 5 to 20 pulses per second to decrease swelling. Electrical stimulation is very effective if used simultaneously with both compression and ice application to enhance all three of their individual effects.

Reduction of pain is another benefit of electrical stimulation. Either a monophasic or biphasic waveform device can be used. The unit should be set on a subthreshold application or where the stimulation is not felt. In cases of a monophasic waveform to reduce pain, a positive waveform consisting of fast pulses of 75 to 120 pulses per second should be used.

Electrical stimulation to promote healing should be used early after initial injury and is most effective in athletic animals as opposed to sedentary animals.[17] Microcurrent is most commonly used to enhance healing. There are several theories of how it functions, including enhancing calcium transport or exciting the mitochondria,[21] but at this point its method of operation is still being evaluated. Microcurrent, in either a biphasic or monophasic waveform, is applied to the subthreshold level. In human athletes when microcurrent is utilized immediately following an activity there is less pain and earlier return of activity.[22]

Ultrasound

Ultrasound has been used widely in physical therapy for many years. During this period, ultrasound has been utilized to promote healing,[23, 24] to remove exudate,[25] and to increase the strength of tendons[26] (Fig. 30–3).

Ultrasound utilizes the piezoelectric effect as voltage is pushed across a crystal. The crystal expands and contracts, producing a

nonaudible sound wave that will pass into the skin via a conductant and then create cavitations of the cells below the sound head. Ultrasound therapy units come with several different-sized sound heads. The frequency of the ultrasound heads may be 3 MHz or 1 MHz. The depth of penetration of ultrasound depends on the frequency of the sound wave from the head, not the intensity itself. A 3-MHz head penetrates at a superficial level only. This works much better in a bony area or in an area with little soft tissue coverage. The 1-MHz head is the most common and most widely used in humans. It penetrates from 3 to 5 cm, depending on the tissue below the surface of the skin. Some ultrasound units have interchangeable heads, possibly making them effective on both large and small animals.

Ultrasound units themselves come with both a pulsed and a continuous method of application. A pulsed application may use a 20- or a 50-per cent duty cycle. For example, the pulses are generated for 50 per cent of the time the machine is on. Continuous ultrasound may cause unstable cavitation, and unstable cavitation in the animal model is destructive to tissue. Scar tissue may be stretched or expanded by unstable cavitation. However, to enhance healing or remove swelling from an area, research shows that pulsed ultrasound at a 20-per cent duty cycle is enough to treat most areas.

Until recently it was believed that ultrasound via the piezoelectric effect of vibration produced heat in tissue as its primary effect. However, the effect of heat in muscle tissue itself was disproved by Enwemeka et al,[27] who showed that the muscle itself has adequate circulation, and all heat created by the sound wave application is recirculated through the circulation of the tissue. This fact also had been proven by Lehmann et al in 1967.[28] Lehmann et al[28] and Enwemeka et al[27] have shown that the muscle circulatory perfusion is capable of dissipating ultrasound heat as it occurs.

Differences in tissue density influence how muscle ultrasound energy is absorbed. Intense ultrasound energy at the periosteum bone interface may produce burns due to ultrasound absorption. If ultrasound is passed over a bony area repetitively, periosteal burns and pain can be created. Ultrasound is best suited for muscle injuries since muscle allows 76 per cent of available sound waves to pass through it. Fat and bone are poor conductors of ultrasound energy.

Ultrasound itself will increase fibroblastic activity and hasten wound healing, and increased acoustic streaming will enhance

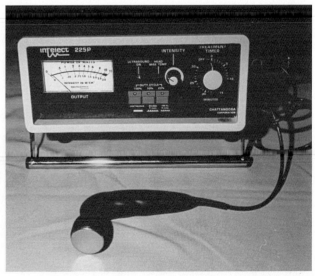

FIGURE 30–3. Ultrasound therapy can aid in rehabilitation.

cell metabolism.[14] Utilization of ultrasound in the first 48 hours immediately following tendon or muscle injury can decrease the inflammatory process. Ultrasound itself also can be used to increase circulation. Dyson reported a 66-per cent decrease in the size of indolent ulcers with the use of ultrasound as opposed to only a 10-per cent decrease in a control group that received sham ultrasound.[24] Enwemeka also showed significant increase in tendon healing using low-intensity ultrasound.[29] Ultrasound is applied in a watt/cm[2] dosage. Dyson reported that 0.6 watts/cm[2] is significant for enhancing wound healing. It is reported that 0.5 watts/cm[2] is important for removal of exudate and promotion of healing. Circulation has been shown to increase with a dosage of 1 watt/cm[2], and 1.0 to 1.8 watt/cm[2] has been shown to be very useful in reducing joint contractures, and it may be very useful for an animal who may have developed quadriceps contracture from a Salter IV fracture.[30]

Timing is very important in application of ultrasound in acute injuries. It should be applied between 48 and 72 hours after injury for ultimate results in healing. There has been no hard research on the optimal length of one treatment session. Lehmann originally used 5 minutes per 5-cm area, and that figure is still used. Treatment may be given daily, for a maximum of 10 to 12 treatments, unless benefit is still being derived after the 12 treatments.

Ultrasound should not be used directly over metal implants, malignant tumors, a gravid uterus, or the eye.

Electromagnetic Therapy

Electromagnetic therapy is not commonly used in the United States, but has widespread use in Australia. The three forms used in Australia are infrared therapy, microwave, and diathermy.

Infrared. The apparatus emits invisible light waves with wave lengths from 7500 to 100,000 Angstroms. Two types of apparatus are currently in use.

Nonluminous type. An electrically heated core embedded in a ceramic base and protected by an iron plate. No visible rays are emitted, and a reflector concentrates the rays upon the patient. Penetration from such sources is only slight; the maximum is 1 to 2 mm.

Incandescent type. A 50- to 100-watt gas-filled tungsten filament lamp mounted in an aluminum reflector. The rays from this source penetrate a maximum of 1 cm into the body, thus having an effect on blood, lymph, and nerve endings in the subcutaneous tissues.

Indications are

(1) to relieve pain and muscle tension and muscle spasm. These are quite marked.
(2) to relieve bruising, myositis, and localized infection. The increased vasodilation results in improved local circulation and phagocytosis.

A danger is that: The application of heat beyond physiological limits produces pain and tissue damage that may vary from hyperemia to actual sloughing of the skin and subcutaneous tissue.

Microwave. Has very limited application as the apparatus is expensive and not generally available for animal use. Microwave penetration is only a little deeper than infrared (1 to 2 cm). This form of therapy falls between infrared and diathermy and appears to have no distinct advantage over either. The disadvantages of microwaves are that the eyes must be protected to prevent cataracts, and the waves must be accurately directed to the area undergoing treatment.

Diathermy. This form of physical therapy generates heat in the deeper tissues of the body because of their resistence to high-frequency alternating current. With diathermy the deeper structures in the body can be heated without heating the skin or subcutaneous tissues, ie, conversive heating is used rather than conductive heating (conductive heating is the application of heat to the body surface and its transfer to deeper structures). Shortwave diathermy is usually employed for 10 to 15 minutes once daily for 3 to 7 days, depending on the severity of the injury.

The Diathermy Unity Method. This is basically a transformer producing a high-frequency electric current greater than 10,000 cycles/second, which flows from one electrode to another using the body of the patient as a conductor. The electrodes are composed of flexible pieces of metal vulcanized between two layers of rubber and connected to the transformer by insulated flexible leads. These electrodes come in various sizes and are usually rectangular.

Dry toweling or cloth must be interposed between the electrode and the skin to avoid accumulation of fluid skin secretions in this area. Such fluids act as zones of high electrical conductivity and may produce superficial burns on the patient.

Indications are contusions (to aid resorption of inflammatory exudate and to reduce muscular induration and pain) and myositis and similar athletic injuries. It is better than ultrasound as the deeper tissues are affected by the deeper penetration of the high-frequency current.

Diathermy is of value in tendon injury but skilled hands are necessary for its use. Potential hazards include (1) burning of the skin resulting from insufficient covering of the pads, pads too close to the skin, or undue pressure on the pads. (2) Excessive exposure time may lead to fat necrosis. (3) Crossing the leads may lead to short circuit—leads must be kept parallel.

Faradism

Faradism is widely used in Australia but not in the United States. Faradic current is derived from the secondary wiring of an induction coil. Two electrodes are used, and the current, at a surge frequency of 6 to 8 per minute, is passed through the tissues. The therapeutic effect is produced not by heat but by stimulation of rhythmic contractions of muscle that disperse inflammatory fluids, break down adhesions, increase circulation, and have a general "toning-up" effect on muscles.

The current is adjusted so that the strongest contractions that do not cause discomfort are produced. The muscle contractor enables production of local exercise to specific muscles without the need to exercise all muscles and is ideal in situations in which strengthening or building up of withered muscle groups is desirable.

The use of electrical muscle stimulation is regarded by some as an effective way of locating areas of muscle soreness. This is attributed to the fact that injured muscles are much more sensitive to the current than are normal muscles, but considerable skill is required to distinguish between superficial nerve stimulation and increased sensitivity of injured tissues.

Use of Faradic Machine. This is quick, clean, and effective therapy for muscle soreness. The following precautions are necessary:

The muscle being treated must be fully relaxed, preferably with the patient lying on its side, or with the limb being treated while held off the ground.

A good electrical coupling must be ensured, using a commercially prepared gel or a mixture of 1 L of water containing 1½ teaspoonfuls of ordinary table salt plus 1½ teaspoonfuls of any household detergent.

The "gain" (power) control is slowly turned up until a full contraction of the muscle—not just a twitch—is achieved.

The "rate" (frequency) control is turned up to give full relaxation between each contraction.

A minimum of 15 contractions (preferably 30) is given on each muscle being treated.

The sore muscle and each muscle that contacts the sore one on either side are treated. Each muscle receives the full 15 to 30 contractions.

Treatments can be given at intervals of 4 hours in urgent situations, but usually once or twice daily is sufficient.

Recovery from muscle soreness requires time as well as treatment—usually 1 to 4 days.

Magnetic Field Therapy

With this therapy, pulsating electromagnetic fields of extremely low frequency (ELF) are used for therapeutic purposes. It has been shown experimentally that magnetic fields with impulse frequencies in excess of 10 Hz cause active widening of blood vessel diameters. It is worth noting that the large blood vessels in the body dilate as do the nutritive arterioles of the periphery. As a consequence, there is improved diffusion of oxygen into peripheral tissue such as muscle. In experiments with 58 test subjects, an average increase in oxygen concentration in tissues of about 200 per cent was reached.[31] Also under the influence of pulsating magnetic fields, the flow rate of blood in capillaries within tissues is increased. Thus the higher the capillary flow rate, the higher the quantity of oxygen transported.

When the whole body or single areas of the body are exposed to magnetic fields, the magnetic field lines permeate these completely. In doing so, the field lines meet sodium and potassium necessary for the functioning of the cells. Ions are electrically charged carriers and are influenced by magnetic fields; hence the electrical potential difference on the marginal surface of the cell is changed, and the dynamics of the ions (exchange of ions between interior and exterior of the cell wall) is increased. The oxygen utilization of the cell is improved. A change in the voltage across the cell membrane can be found with most illnesses. This contributes to the slowing down of cellular metabolism, with subsequent reduction in oxygen efficiency. The aim of magnetic field therapy is to help to restore the affected cells to their normal operating voltage and hence to reestablish the cell's normal metabolism.[32]

As a result, the pulsating high–frequency magnetic fields are able to reduce pain sensations that are caused by acute or chronic oxygen deficiency due to compromised blood flow and accumulation of metabolites. Conversely, applying frequencies of around 5 Hz to soft tissues will slightly constrict the blood circulation to the affected area and reduce inflammation and edema associated with acute conditions such as torn muscles or joint ligament sprains.

Magnetic field therapy may be used alone as a primary treatment for sporting injuries or as supplementary therapy following application of ultrasound or faradism. As a general guide, severe injury associated with bleeding, swelling, or edema responds best to settings in the order of 5 to 15 gauss and 50 Hz. This has a vasoconstrictive, anti-inflammatory effect and consequently is applied for 10 to 20 minutes once or twice daily for 1 to 7 days following the initial trauma. Once swelling recedes or for less severe bruising or sprain, when repair processes are to be stimulated by a vasodilatory effect, the higher settings of 85 to 100 gauss and 55 to 65 Hz are used for 10 to 20 minutes, once or twice daily for up to 14 days.

Laser

Therapeutic laser is usually a cold or low-level laser (Fig. 30–4). These class II lasers have a 2-mw tube and emit no more than 1 mw from the tip of the fiberoptic cable, and visible light with a wavelength of 632.8 nm is emitted. They come in two different forms: gallium arsenide, which penetrates 5 mm, and helium, which penetrates 0.8 mm to 15 mm.

Low–level laser treatment has been reported to increase collagen synthesis.[33] This has been used to treat muscle injuries, provide pain relief, and stimulate trigger points.

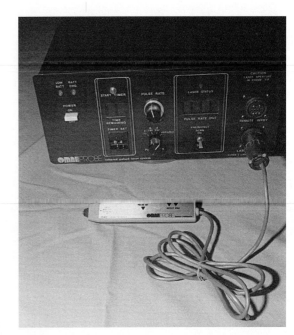

FIGURE 30–4. This soft laser is being used to increase collagen deposition.

Massage

Historically, massage was discussed as early as 1000 BC in the Chinese literature.[15] Recent studies indicate that massage will enhance spinal motor neuron excitability.[34] No one can question the psychological or physiological effects of massage. Massage can also remove exudate from an area, increase circulation, and stretch collagen matrix. Massage also can increase muscle relaxation. Cross-friction massage (CFM) can be used occasionally to create ischemia. As ischemia is created, and the deep pressure is then released, blood flow to an area will be increased.[35]

Massage can take several different forms. Initially there is a deep large milking stroke of an effleurage movement along the grain of the muscle toward the heart. Massage performed away from the heart may disrupt the venous integrity and damage the valve within the vein itself, so it is important that massage be performed along the grain of the muscle toward the heart. Massage is effective in decreasing swelling in an area. Pétrissage concentrates more on one muscle area and utilizes smaller strokes. The belly of the muscle is picked up and let go, during movement along or across the muscle fiber itself. Pétrissage is deeper than effleurage and will enhance circulation in the deeper tissue areas.[36]

Cross-fiber massage is deep massage along the scar tissue or crosswise to the muscle fiber itself. Deep-tissue or cross-fiber massage is designed to break down abnormal scar tissue to promote healing.[35] Cross-fiber massage should always be followed by effleurage massage to enhance circulation in and around the area. Massage not only gives physiological results but also can be very useful in calming an anxious animal following an injury or surgery. Massage can also help initiate contact with the animal before a more painful technique, such as passive range of motion, is carried out. Massage can be initiated on the day of surgery and continued throughout the physical therapy period. One important aim of massage is to decrease adhesions that occur underneath the scar and to allow the scar to be mobile, allowing maintenance of full range of motion of the joint.

Manipulation

Joint manipulation is described by Paris as a skilled passive movement to the joint.[11] All joints possess a classic range of motion

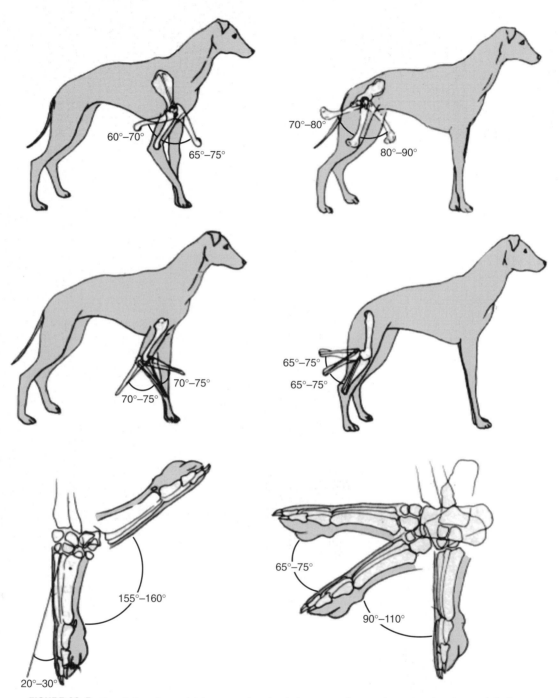

FIGURE 30–5. Knowledge of normal joint range of motion is important when passive range-of-motion work is done.

that is the actual motion that the muscles can allow the joint to move through. Along with this classic motion, all joints also possess what is called accessory motion or joint play that is movement within the joint that allows that joint to glide, roll, spin, and glide. When injury to a joint occurs, very often accessory motion and joint play are lost as well as classic movement. Full range of motion is then lost. If full classic range of motion and accessory motion are not returned, the joint involved will certainly be susceptible to future injury. Manipulation is basically taking a joint through its range of motion. Following manipulation both accessory movement and classic movements should return to normal. Manipulation in the spine and extremity joints will fire the type 3 mechanoreceptor that will inhibit muscle guarding and promote more full free range of motion.[37] Firing of type 3 mechanoreceptors also will decrease the pain so the animal is then able to accomplish more activity. Whenever a joint is stretched and there is more motion, one needs to be cognizant of the fact that the muscles must be strengthened in the new range of motion, so they are able to move the joint through that range.

Exercise

Exercise takes several different forms. Passive range of motion is started initially, progressing to more active range of motion in which the muscles themselves are taking the joint through its range, and followed by gentle resistive exercises. Progression through the exercise program depends on the aim for the animal. The goal of physical therapy is functional return, and to that end exercises should be based upon enhancing the activities the animal has to perform.

Passive Range of Motion

Passive range of motion (PROM) is similar to manipulation in that it moves a joint through and beyond its normal range of motion. Some of the important aspects of PROM are that a muscle needs to be relaxed, and movement must be performed slowly (see Fig. 30–5). Moving through the normal range of motion prevents formation of contractions. Research shows that it is possible to increase the number of sarcomeres by doing a slow low–load passive stretch.[10] This stretch would need to be taken into end range and held gently for at least 5 minutes. Splinting sometimes can be a form of PROM to actually increase the length of muscles. By performing PROM, an animal's owner can get involved with the animal's home care as well. Ideally, range of motion should be initiated the day of surgery and continued for 2 to 3 weeks. The goal certainly is to maintain or increase range of motion.

When performing PROM, the range should be performed slowly to the point of resistance and then a hold at the point of resistance slowing moving into new range. For a young animal, range-of-motion exercises may be scary and need to be done quite slowly. One would perform 10 to 15 repetitions three times per day. A goniometer should be used to measure the range of motion in a joint and compare it to the uninvolved side to see what normal range of motion is for the dog. PROM has been shown not to be age dependent; however, loss of range usually is related to injury and nonuse. Animals with loss of motion should have a slow progressive passive range-of-motion program to reduce all of the physical signs of restrictions. Certainly, contraindications for PROM would be unstable fracture sites, luxations, or hypermobile joints. Caution should be exercised when working around bone tumors or in cases of recent skin grafts.[2]

Active exercise is not as easy for animals to perform as it is for humans. To perform an active range of motion (AROM) basically we ask to see the muscle move the joint through its range of motion. Ways found to work with dogs on AROM would include

sit/stands or assuming a "play" position in which the upper extremity is fully flexed. Other ways to enhance AROM would be utilizing a pool or hydrotherapy (Fig. 30–6). Swim therapy can work well in reducing the amount of weight on an animal so that it can move more freely through a range of motion. In any animal that may have neurological conditions, hydrotherapy also will help prevent urine scalding and decrease the chance of ulcers associated with paralysis.[2] When hydrotherapy is used as an AROM form, it should be remembered that the animal may have very poor endurance and swimming is a vigorous exercise. Initially it should be limited to 3 to 5 minutes and then slowly increased to 15 minutes when possible. Animal hydrotherapy pools are specially designed to create a current of resistance against which the animal may swim. This may improve circulation and improve return to full activity.

Resistive exercise can help return an animal to its sport. Resistive exercise comes in two different forms—open kinetic chain or closed kinetic chain. Open kinetic chain activity is one in which the distal aspect of the limb is not attached to the ground or touching anything. It is quite difficult to perform open kinetic chain activities with animals because it generally involves a nonphysiological movement. In the human example, patients are asked to tighten a quadriceps muscle and then lift up the leg, keeping it straight. Certainly this is quite difficult in our canine counterparts. Open kinetic chain activities are very difficult to achieve in domestic animals and is rarely attempted.[2] Closed kinetic chain activities, however, are activities in which the distal aspect of the limb is closed or is striking the ground. Different aspects of closed kinetic chain activities include walking, trotting, the stance phase of running, and resistive exercises applied by a human through the use of straps or manual contacts. These resistive exercises can come in several forms. Swimming against a jet spray becomes a closed chain activity if the limb is encountering the resistance of water. Weight-bearing activities are a closed kinetic chain of activities.

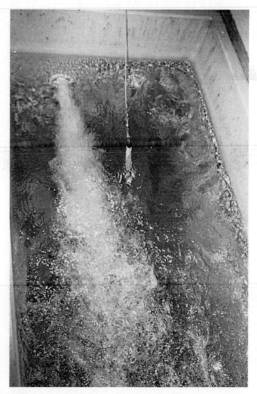

FIGURE 30–6. This therapy pool has a water pump that can be used to create resistance for swimming.

NAME: _____ Week Post-Op: _____
Procedure and Date: _____ Doctor: _____
Neurological Status: Pre-op _____ Technician: _____
             Post-op _____
Status: In hospital _____ Day Patient _____

	MONDAY	TUESDAY	WEDNESDAY	THURSDAY	FRIDAY
WEIGHT BEARING					
WEIGHT SHIFTING					
MASSAGE- # OF MIN					
SIT/STAND- # TIMES					
NEUROSTIM # MIN & MUSCLE GROUP					
RANGE OF MOTION # OF MIN					
TOWEL/TAIL WALKING: HOW FAR					
SWIMMING: # MIN					
STAIRS: # FLIGHTS & TIMES PER DAY					

PLAN—PROGRESS	INITIALS	LIMB MEASUREMENT
MONDAY: _____		MUSCLE GIRTH:
TUESDAY: _____		
WEDNESDAY: _____		JOINT SIZE:
THURSDAY: _____		
FRIDAY: _____		RANGE OF MOTION:

FIGURE 30–7. A therapeutic plan and periodic documentation are recorded on this form.

The animal is placed in proper standing position and pressure is applied to the forelimbs or hindlimbs. This is approximation and is very useful to increase proprioception as well as getting the muscles starting to work in a normal stance position. After standing, weight bearing, approximation, and weight shifting, the animal is then progressed to a walking program. Initially, start out walking on the straights, both slow and fast. Then progress to walking in a snake position with both right and left circles and then progress to walking in figure-of-eights or circles. When trying to increase weight bearing on the limb, the dog walks in circles to the injured side. As the animal is turning toward the inner side, it will be putting increased weight on the inner leg. A progression when working with coursing dogs would be to have the animal walk with harness weights, pulling chains behind it that will help increase the ability of the muscles to perform lateral movements with resistance and will actually increase proprioception in the joint. Next is progression to running in a straight line followed by cutting via snake figures and figure-of-eights. Walking, to running, to cutting would be sound progression. Before cutting is initiated, one may want the dog to walk on hills or stairs, which is a good way for the animal to pull its body weight against gravity. One then increases work and increases strength to the muscles. Stairs should be attempted very slowly. The animal should not be allowed to lean on the human walking it or to lean into the wall as it goes up the stairs. It should go up the stairs very slowly, using the legs one at a time. Climbing stairs can be a very useful resistive exercise.

FUNCTIONAL RETURN

Once the animal has gone through initial stages following surgery or injury, work should begin on PROM followed by slow AROM. The patient should be returned to both walking and some resistive activity. Then it is time to start to return to functional

TABLE 30–1. Suggested Physical Therapy Protocol After Surgical Repair of Type IV (Two-Screw) Central Tarsal Fracture

Week	Therapy
1–3	In general, a splint or cast is applied to the tarsal region following open reduction and stabilization of the tarsal fracture.
	1. Neuromuscular stimulation of the cranial tibial muscle and the gastrocnemius muscle
	2. PROM of the hip and stifle
4	Document: limb circumference, ROM, gait, weight-bearing status
	Reassess with radiographs
	ROM exercise of the tarsocrural joint, intertarsal joints, tarsometatarsal joint
	Short leash walks—on sand if possible; bandage support to the distal extremity
5, 6	Continued leash walks 10–15 min alone in a short turnout pen
End of week 6. The fracture should be reassessed by physical examination and radiographs. If there is sufficient healing, the dog can be worked at a trot behind a three-wheeler or whirlygig.	
7, 8	Progression to more walking, trotting actively to ensure muscle strength and joint ROM
9, 10	Short hand-slips on the straight portions of the track

activities. Depending on the animal, functional return should be based on the dog's activity. We recommend that in returning an animal to coursing, a leash should be used to control cutting activities and quick moves. With greyhounds, use hand-slipping at the track, starting with very short distances and slowly progressing. Aerobic and anaerobic training of animals and how to return them to full activity is beyond the scope of this chapter. However, we caution against too-soon rapid return of an animal to its activity. If the dog has increased swelling or is limping, the activity may be too difficult and may need to be decreased.

For the return of bird dogs to service, start them first in areas where there is no risk of reinjury. It is beneficial for them to work off a beach prior to their return to more difficult activities. Deconditioning initially starts 56 hours after the last exercise session, and the animal needs to be trained to return to competition. One may want to return a greyhound to one-half controlled work and have it run with some slower animals. A pond dog may be worked on short distances. Coursing animals should be worked in an open field prior to working in any type of thick brush. The animal should be progressed to 75 per cent work load. The animal may return to function when it can fully bear weight and 75 per cent work loads are done without difficulty.

DOCUMENTATION

Documentation is important to establish objectively if the animal is progressing and to know if it is returning to normal (Fig. 30–7). Means of documentation include girth measurements, goniometric measurements, amount of weight bearing, and observation. Documented findings and outcome can show the owner the animal's progress. Also, one will know when the animal is not progressing adequately on a home program and may require more formal physical therapy.

Normal measurements need to be known when documenting. Measure the uninvolved side of the animal to see what is normal. For measurement of girth, there should be weight on the animal's

limb, and landmarks should be used so that measurements are accurate. Always measure the unaffected area before the area being treated. For goniometric measurements, both proximal and distal landmarks should be utilized, the limb should be relaxed, and the joint should be taken through its full range of motion. For example, when measuring a stifle, one would line up the proximal end of the goniometer with the greater trochanter, and the distal end with the lateral malleolus; the center of the axis is directly through the stifle joint. If muscles are tight, it is difficult to get an accurate measurement.

One method of measuring the force the animal is putting on the limb is by using a force plate; however, force plates are not accessible to many veterinarians. An alternative is to utilize a rolled-up blood pressure cuff having a certain amount of mercury in it, eg, a tare weight of 40 mm Hg. Have the animal unweighted on the right and measure the weight on the left. Then switch and measure the difference. These measurements help identify when a dog is actually walking only on three legs.

Certainly observation is one of the best ways to detect deviations in an animal's gait. Nunamaker stated that locomotion of the dog requires proper functioning of every organ system in the body and up to 99 per cent of the skeletal muscles.[21] Always walking with its head down may indicate an injury in the rear end of a dog because lifting the head would put increased weight on its rear legs. Walking primarily with its head up may indicate a forelimb injury. Observation of how an animal runs, chases after a bird, or races also plays an important role. Observation can help decide at what point the dog starts to fatigue. Documentation of observations is very important to determine if the animal has improved.

PROTOCOLS

Tables 30–1 to 30–3 provide protocols for administration of physical therapy techniques for a central tarsal fracture, anterior cruciate ligament repair, and a Salter type II fracture in which the possibility of "quadriceps tie-down" is present.[30] None of these

TABLE 30–2. Suggested Physical Therapy Protocol After Intracapsular Repair of Anterior Cruciate Injury

Week	Therapy
1	Document preoperatively: Limb circumference, ROM, gait, weight bearing status
	Postsurgical: PROM (sets of 10—3 to 4 times daily), ice packs to peri-incision area (10–15 min three to four times daily), short leash walks
2	Suture removal, + ice packs, short leash walks, neuromuscular stimulation
3	Redocument circumference, ROM, gait, weight-bearing status, neuromuscular stimulation
	Extend leash walks; begin sit/stays, figure-of-eights
4–5	Continue leash walks 30–45 minutes at least three times weekly; begin gentle incline work (walk up and down gradual incline); NO STAIRS; continue with sit/stays
6	Document: limb circumference, ROM, gait, weight-bearing status
	Leash walks/trots; 1 hour plus stairs—8–10 flights three times daily; swimming (begin with dog standing in water); work on proprioception—try to unbalance leg while dog is walking.

At this juncture many dogs have a normal gait while walking. If further rehabilitation is needed for working dogs the protocol can be continued. During weeks 7, 8, 9 active forms of exercise are included and are directed at the semimembranosus, semitendinosus, quadriceps, biceps femoris, and sartorius. These forms of exercise may include swimming, trotting, specific neuromuscular stimulation to affected muscle groups, and resistive pulling.

TABLE 30–3. Suggested Protocol for Rehabilitation After Repair of a Salter II Fracture of the Distal Femur

Week	Therapy
1	PROM, ice packs
2	PROM, stimulation, massage of hamstrings/quads
3	Start leash walks, stimulation, reassessment
4	Continued work to ensure full ROM and muscle strengthening

protocols is designed to be followed exactly, but each should be used as a guide to help utilize physical therapy more effectively.

Many books and articles discuss physical therapy in depth. If resources are limited, ice cups and ice bags are the most important items for reducing both pain and edema. An ultrasound machine has many possibilities. There are inexpensive electrical stimulators on the market; in a battery-operated machine, the battery should be replaced about every 3 weeks.

Physical therapy, used appropriately, will help animals return faster to full function.

References

1. Tangner CH: Physical therapy in small animal patients: Basic principles and application. Compend Continuing Education 6:933–936, 1984.
2. Taylor RA: Physical therapy and rehabilitation. ACVS Veterinary Symposium, October 1993.
3. Booth FW: Time course of muscular atrophy during immobilization of hindlimbs in rats. J Appl Physiol 43:656, 1977.
4. Holm S: Variations in the nutrition of the canine intervertebral disc induced by motion. Spine 4:866–874, 1983.
5. Salter RB, et al: The biological effect of continuous passive motion on the healing of full thickness deficits in articular cartilage. J Bone Joint Surg 62A:1232–1251, 1980.
6. Gelberman RH, et al: Effects of early intermittent passive mobilization on healing canine flexor tendons. J Hand Surg 7:170, 1982.
7. US Department of Labor: US Department of Labor Report from the Bureau of Labor Statistics, 1992–1993.
8. Taylor RA: Postsurgical physical therapy: The missing link. Compend Continuing Education 14:1583, 1992.
9. Chipman R: Microcurrent Bio-therapy Treatment Protocol. Unpublished article, 1989.
10. Currier DP, et al: Dynamics of Human Biological Tissues. Philadelphia, F A Davis Co., 1992.
11. Paris SV: Introduction to spinal evaluation and manipulation. St. Augustine, Fla, Patris Press, 1991.
12. Doverspike M: Contralateral cranial cruciate ligament rupture: Incidence in 114 dogs. J Am Anim Hosp Assoc 29:167–169, 1993.
13. Merrick MA, et al: The effects of ice and compression wraps on intramuscular temperatures at various depths. J Athlet Train 28:236–245, 1993.
14. Edmond PD, et al: Protein synthesis by neuroblastoma cells enhanced by exposure to burst-mode ultrasound. Ultrasound Med Biol 14:219–223, 1988.
15. Basmajian JV, et al: Manipulation, traction and massage. Baltimore, Williams & Wilkins, 1985.
16. Cummings GS: Soft tissue changes in health and disease. Seminar Presentation, Denver, Colo, 1986.
17. Stanish WD, et al: The use of electricity in ligament and tendon repair. Physician Sports Med 13:109–116, 1985.
18. Greathouse DG, et al: Effects of short term electrical stimulation on the ultrastructure of rat skeletal muscles. Phys Ther 66:946–953, 1986.
19. Currier DP, et al: Effects of electrical and electromagnetic stimulation after ACL reconstruction. J Orthop Sports Phys Ther 17: 1993.
20. Bickford RG, et al: Magnetic stimulation of human peripheral nerve and brain: Response enhancement by combined magnetoelectrical techniques. Neurosurgery 20:110–116, 1987.
21. Nunamaker D: Normal and abnormal gait. In Newton CD, Nunamaker D (eds): Textbook of Small Animal Orthopedics. Philadelphia, JB Lippincott Co, 1985, pp 735–744.
22. Wallace L: Introduction to micro-amp electrical stimulation (M.E.N.S.) Seminar Presentation, Denver, Colo, 1990.
23. Young SR, Dyson M: The effect of therapeutic ultrasound on angiogenesis. Ultrasound Med Biol 16:261–269, 1990.
24. Dyson M, et al: Stimulation of tissue repair by therapeutic ultrasound. Infect Surg 37–44, 1982.
25. Fyte MC, et al: The effect of ultrasound on experimental oedema in rats. Ultrasound Med Biol 6:107–111, 1980.
26. Enwemeka CS, et al: The effect of therapeutic ultrasound on tendon healing: A biomechanical study. Am J Phys Med Rehab 68:283–287, 1989.
27. Enwemeka CS, et al: Non-thermal effects of ultrasound: Poster presentation. APTA Annual Conference Denver, Colo, 1992.
28. Lehmann JF, et al: Healing produced by ultrasound in bone and soft tissues. Arch Phys Med Rehabil 48:397–401, 1967.
29. Enwemeka CS, et al: The biomechanical effects of low-intensity ultrasound on healing tendons. Ultrasound Med Biol 19:801, 1990.
30. Shires PK, et al: Effect of localized trauma and temporary splinting on immature skeletal muscle and mobility of femorotibial joint in the dog. Am J Vet Res 43(3):454–460, 1982.
31. Warnke U: Biophysics and medicine proceedings. International Congress on Magnetic Medicine, Rome, 1980.
32. Hansen KM: Some observation of magnetic field upon the human organism. Acta Med Scand 97:339–364, 1938.
33. Michlovitz SL: Thermal Agents in Rehabilitation. Philadelphia, F A Davis Co, 1990, Ch. 9.
34. Sullivan SJ, et al: Effects of massage on alpha motoneuron excitability. Phys Ther 71:555, 1991.
35. Cryiax J: Treatment by manipulation, massage and injection. New York, Paul B. Hoeber, Inc. 1984.
36. Wood EC: Beard's Massage Principles and Techniques. Philadelphia, W B Saunders Company, 1974.
37. Wyke B: Articular neurology—a review. Physiotherapy 58(3):94–99, 1972.

CHAPTER 31

RACING PERFORMANCE IN GREYHOUNDS: MANIPULATION, TRACTION, TISSUE MOBILIZATION, AND SUSTAINED STRETCH EXERCISES

PHILLIP E. DAVIS

Physiotherapy is the physical treatment of injury. Massage and chiropractic manipulation are the traditional bases for both spinal diagnosis and treatment. Manipulation in humans as a form of healing predates most medical and surgical procedures. Both Hippocrates (*c*460–370 BC) and Galen (AD *c*130–202) described techniques of manipulation to treat spinal abnormalities.[1,2] Boje[3] in 1958 described veterinary therapy based on manipulation, and in 1963 Moltzen[4] described his techniques for manipulation in mixed-breed dogs. Davis[5] in 1989 and Hauler[6] in 1990 described manipulation as it applies to the racing greyhound. To enhance these methods, modern technology provides sophisticated equipment for treatment of tissue injury. In greyhounds, enhancement of racing performance through manipulation and massage is such a common training practice that a group of paraveterinary individuals skilled in these techniques, or "muscle men," flourishes among Australian greyhound trainers. This chapter details the procedure for chiropractic manipulation of the greyhound with particular focus on the spine, shoulder, and hip joints. Chiropractic theory is outside the scope of this chapter. Physiotherapy for specific injuries is presented.

GENERAL TECHNIQUES

The primary indication for chiropractic spinal manipulation is a reversible mechanical derangement of an intervertebral joint that produces a barrier to normal motion. Manipulation adjusts the position of individual vertebrae. Manipulation cannot be considered to have only a local effect. Interventions can initiate skeletal reactions some considerable distance from the site at which the force is applied. Lee et al[7] showed that clinically significant vertebral displacements occurred distant to the vertebra under manipulation. Two main types of manipulative forces are applied to vertebral and extravertebral articulations: (1) indirect adjustment, in which a high-velocity force is exerted on a point of the body some distance from the area where it is expected to have its beneficial effect, and (2) direct specific adjustment, in which a high-velocity thrust is directed at a particular joint.[8] Conditions that may respond to chiropractic are the spinal subluxation complex, reflex effects following nerve irritation, nerve compression, joint fixations, spinal muscle hypertonicity, muscle spasms, articular adhesions, ligamentous shortening, disc displacement, joint hypomobility, and any reversible mechanical derangement of joints. Vertebral disc prolapses may be modified by traction in so far as manipulation corrects vertebral displacement and diminishes pressure on the spinal nerves. Disc prolapse with neurological deficit should be referred to a neurosurgeon.

In humans, manipulation for neck pain may result in loss of pain, general relaxation, sleepiness, and sometimes slight euphoria.

On the assumption that the human response is not psychosomatic, similar relief may be anticipated and is seen in animals.

Joint fixation, joint locking, or joint blockage can be determined clinically by mobility palpation and stress radiography. Motion palpation is used to detect relative movement between palpable bony landmarks. An increase or decrease in the interspinous spaces, the intercostal spaces, or the spaces between the dorsal cranial iliac spines and the second sacral tubercle may be palpated. Increased resistance to joint movement can also be determined by "springing" or "tractioning" the joint. Tractioning a joint along its long axis is commonly used to determine movement restriction in extremity joints. Springing a spinal joint to test for end-feel can be done by pushing the spinous process through the three planes of motion.[8]

MASSAGE

Massage is the therapeutic use of friction, stroking, and kneading of the body tissue. There may be variation in the intensity of the pressure exerted, the surface area treated, and the frequency of application.[8] Effects of massage include removal of dry skin and opening of sebaceous glands, mechanical assistance to blood and lymph flow to increase circulation and reduce edema, maintenance of muscle flexibility and viability, breaking up of scar tissue, adhesions and fibrosis, sedation or stimulation, treatment of myofascial pain, and mobilization of lung secretions.

Types of Massage

Effleurage. Strokes should parallel the direction of the muscle fibers and should be heavier in the centripetal direction, ie, toward the heart. Massage should begin with light pressure, progress to heavier pressure as tolerated, and terminate with light pressure.

Petrissage. The muscles are stroked with a kneading or rolling motion either in a centripetal direction or transversely to the muscle fibers.

Rolfing. This is a system of deep massage that strives to separate the fascia between muscles.

Friction Massage. With the fingers placed on one spot on the skin, small circular or linear strokes are used to loosen the tissue beneath the skin. No lotion is used.

Transverse Friction Massage. Friction massage is performed perpendicular to the tendon sheath. The tendon is separated from the tendon sheath and may slide through it more easily.

Tapotement. Tapping, slapping, cupping, and hacking motions increase circulation and drainage of abnormal secretions from the lungs.

Pneumatic Massage. A machine provides intermittent air pressure and is useful for the reduction of extremity edema.[8]

Relief of Muscle Spasm by Massage

Prior to mobilization and manipulation of the spine, massage is used to relieve reflex spasm in the epaxial musculature. Two massage techniques are commonly used. The first is the application of deep sustained pressure over the belly of the affected muscles. To avoid stimulation of the spastic muscle the pressure is gradually increased to the limit of the greyhound's tolerance and is then maintained for about 1 minute. The pressure is then gradually released. With severe pain and muscle spasm the application of heat may be required. The second major method of relaxing spastic muscles is muscular kneading. Stretch is applied to the contracted muscle and transverse or circular kneading pressure is then applied across the belly of the muscle in a rhythmical fashion. The clinician's fingers do not rub across the dog's skin, but rather the skin becomes an extension of the clinician's fingers. Application of heat may be required.[6]

When heat is required, shortwave diathermy (SWD) and midwave diathermy (MVD) are convenient to use and provide heat in the deeper tissues and muscles without heating the skin. SWD is used at 25 to 40 percent power for 5 to 10 minutes, up to a maximum of 20 minutes for greyhound muscular spasm. Greyhounds have a much lower fat content in their tissues than do humans, and this should be taken into consideration when comparing recommendations for physiotherapy dosages between species. Hauler[6] recommended low-power SWD for 20 to 25 minutes using an automatic field, adjusting SWD to relax spastic musculature associated with spinal mobility faults in greyhounds. It is easy to produce subcutaneous burns as diathermy has the ability to heat subcutaneous tissue with little sensation to the animal. Veterinarians should be wary of exposing patients to shortwave and microwave radiation.[8]

MOBILIZATION

Mobilization is the process of returning a joint with a mobility fault to full movement. This is achieved by gentle movement that stretches the joint to the end point of its elasticity. Each vertebral joint has varying freedom of movement in flexion, extension, rotation, and sidebending. When a restriction exists in a vertebral joint, mobilization is achieved by gentle, smooth, rhythmical, and gradual stretching of the contracted musculature that acts upon the joint. There should be no forced, wrenching, or thrusting movements.[8] Treatment by massage and mobilization prepares for manipulation.

MANIPULATION

The primary indication for spinal manipulation is the presence of a reversible structural barrier to normal joint mobility. Three physical events in manipulation differentiate it from mobilization: (1) as the elastic barrier of the joint is passed, the articular surfaces separate suddenly; (2) a cracking noise is heard; and (3) a radiolucent space appears within the joint. Manipulation consists of forcing the joint beyond the end-feel elastic barrier. Gatterman[8] stated that the cracking noise heard as the articular surfaces move apart is the result of sudden cavitation of dissolved synovial gases. Remanipulation during an approximately 20-minute refractory period will not produce the familiar crack and is not recommended.

Indirect specific manipulation of vertebrae is possible only if some spinal joints are immobilized or locked and then used as a rigid lever to transmit force onto other joints. Rotation, sidebending, and flexion govern the level to which a joint or series of joints can be locked.[6] The vertebrae are positioned with the facet joints locked on one side and in ligamentous tension on the other. The unlocked joints are then moved through their full range by a direct thrust.

Greyhounds often receive a combination of mobilization and manipulation during physiotherapy. Manipulation should not separate the joint surfaces beyond their limit of anatomical integrity. In the greyhound, because of the difficulties with positioning and patient cooperation during positioning, direct specific manipulation is used only in the cervicothoracic junction area, the thoracic spine, and the thoracolumbar area.

SPINAL TRACTION

As early as 400 BC Hippocrates[1] recorded the therapeutic use of traction. Traction is used to stretch soft tissues, to separate articular surfaces, and to treat soft tissue injuries, joint fixations, nerve root compression, and degenerative and herniated disc disease. Traction may be useful for the relief of pain in both humans[9] and dogs[10] as a palliative alternative to surgery. Traction has also been used as a diagnostic aid in myelographic procedures. Distraction with the spine in flexion is achieved in humans using a specialized table. Manual and positional traction utilizing the weight of the patient and gravity is sometimes employed in humans. Traction may be static or intermittent, with static traction being used for minutes to hours.

MUSCLE INJURY

Dogs fed and trained for athletic performance and kenneled in a stress- and parasite-free environment have a lowered incidence of muscle injury. Racetrack design and surface are major correlates to muscle injury. Injuries may be common between racetracks, but individual tracks produce their own pattern of injury. Muscle strain accounts for 90 per cent of clinical muscular injury.[6]

Racing injury myositis may be mild when due to strain, or it may be severe in muscle fiber and connective tissue sheath rupture. Strain is the less serious but most common injury and responds to therapy without interfering with the racing program. Strain injury can be successfully treated the day before the race. With muscle fiber and sheath rupture the animal must be withdrawn from training. Continued galloping aggravates this type of injury.

Strain lesions result in palpable muscle spasm or hypertonicity and subsequent progressive athletic atrophy. There is a reduced range of active movement of the strained muscle.[6] Chronic athletic atrophy can be managed with sustained stretch physiotherapy. Injury is common in the medial gluteal, vastus, and semimembranosus muscles.[6]

Pain and Muscular Injury

Muscles respond to injury by self-immobilization. This complex mechanism is partly mediated by a pain reflex spasm. Pain is perceived by the individual greyhound in the context of its tolerance to pain. Performance with injury will depend on both structural and psychological criteria. Chronic inflammation or structural pain may reduce the active range of muscular movement, which, with further forced exercise, initiates a vicious cycle of inflammation, pain, and spasm. Muscles may be self-immobilized because of the phenomenon of referred pain. For example, cervical injury may produce pain in the triceps brachii muscle. It is important that this dual source of muscular pain be kept in mind when treatment of muscular injury is considered.[6] Chiropractic manipulation of the spine may relieve severe muscle pain in the limbs.

Functional Compensation for Muscle Pain

Hauler[6] observed that existing muscle pain leads to functional muscular compensation and predisposes to further injury. Greyhounds protect and reduce the use of injured muscles by distributing the work load to other portions of the body. With chronic right-sided strain of gluteal or groin areas, there is often subsequent sprain or rupture of the right long head of the triceps brachii muscle or severe ligamentous damage to the right carpus. In compensation, Hauler[6] correctly concluded that greyhounds can race with muscular fibrillar tearing but not with muscle tearing or rupture. If these greyhounds are further raced, gross tearing of the triceps muscle is often observed.

Treatment of Muscle Injury

Physiotherapy with cold, pressure, massage, mobilization, manipulation, heat (ultrasound, microwave, inductothermy, transcutaneous electrical stimulation, laser), and acupuncture has been used successfully in the greyhound to optimize healing and minimize inflammatory response and associated pain.

Treatment of muscle strains with a short-acting anti-inflammatory glucocorticosteroid, diluted in isotonic phosphorus solution and injected into the affected muscle, allows a greyhound to be galloped within a day of treatment. Medication aims at achieving a local physiological effect within the injured muscle rather than a systemic therapeutic effect. Local anesthetic may be injected into the strained muscle to relax local spasm. This method of treatment is termed *needling*.

Muscle rupture may be palpated as an area of discontinuity in the muscle fibers or muscle sheaths. This form of injury always leads to a "lay-off" period in the greyhound's training program. Medical treatment involves:

1. Application of cold packs and laser immediately after the injury and for the next 24 to 48 hours. Laser can be continued daily
2. Pressure bandaging if required to prevent further hemorrhage
3. Injections of cortisone
4. Concurrent administration of nonsteroidal anti-inflammatory drugs (NSAIDs). These significantly decrease the extent of scarification in the healing muscle[11] and are essential in the treatment of all muscle tears. The ideal time to undertake surgical correction following anti-inflammatory therapy is 4 to 5 days after injury occurred.

Passive extension exercise (PEE) and active extension exercise (AEE) together with deep friction massage assist return of function. PEE involves gradual extension of the injured muscle to its full range of passive movement. Initially 2 or 3 days of mobilization may be required to achieve this, followed by 10 to 15 passive extensions applied daily to the muscle for 3 weeks. PEE limits adhesion formation and scar tissue restriction of mobility in the injured muscle.

AEE involves walking the greyhound in water to a depth that requires it to propel its legs through the water rather than lift its feet out of the water. AEEs are initiated 20 to 30 days after anti-inflammatory therapy. The greyhound is water-walked every third day, beginning with 30 to 40 meters and increasing to a maximum of 60 to 70 meters. After 4 weeks the greyhound is allowed to frolic in a confined area, and at 6 to 8 weeks it is allowed free galloping and is returned to the race track 12 weeks after injury. Dogs with less severe, medically treated injuries usually return to the race track about 8 weeks post injury.

CLINICAL EXAMINATION AND TREATMENT
Visual Examination

The temperament, body condition, coat luster, eyes, mucous membranes, and stance of the dog are noted. Carriage of the head and neck, the levels of the shoulder joints, the scapular levels, the levels of the iliac wings, the gluteal muscles, and the position of the stifles and hocks give an indication of postural abnormality.[6] However, lameness or stiffness from muscle strain is rarely evident. Thoracic lordosis and exaggerated lumbar kyphosis predispose to spinal mechanical faults and muscle injury. Sacroiliac and low lumbar mobility faults are often associated with an exaggerated straight hindleg posture and exaggerated lumbar kyphosis. The lateral placement of the hindfeet may indicate a low lumbar mobility fault.

Physical Examination

The greyhound is examined standing on the floor. Greyhounds become tense when made to stand on an examination table, making it difficult for the clinician to assess muscle tone. The clinician will need to kneel or squat beside the dog as the limb musculature is examined.

Palpation

Palpation is essential for detecting musculoskeletal abnormalities in the greyhound. Detection of pain by palpation largely depends on the pain tolerance and tissue tenderness of the individual dog. The greater the pressure applied, the deeper the palpatory examination. Concurrent bilateral palpation allows simultaneous comparison of the pain thresholds of both sides of the body. Significant variation is often detected. The groin of a greyhound is a tender area. Discomfort on palpation is not diagnostic, whereas detection of muscular spasm during palpation is diagnostic. The spine is palpated to detect hypersensitivity of the spinal musculature, spasm, and reduced vertebral mobility. In the presence of spinal mechanical fault, forced movement results in muscular spasm and pain. To detect referred pain it is necessary to concentrate on the shape and reaction to palpation of the muscle in question. Exaggerated spasm on palpation rather than spasm per se is diagnostic of referred pain.

Tissue Tension

Tissue tension is detected by palpation. The clinician must become familiar with the "feel" of a fit greyhound's muscles. Myositis and muscle spasm limit joint movement, and this can be detected through abnormal muscle tissue tension.

Anatomy

The topographical anatomy of the greyhound is the starting point of greyhound manipulation. It is essential to be able to palpate commonly injured muscles such as the gluteus medius, tensor fasciae latae, vastus lateralis (origin), semitendinosus (insertion), gracilis, the lateral head of the deep digital flexor, teres major (insertion), and latissimus dorsi.

Spinal Cord Segments and Muscle Innervation

The thoracic limbs are innervated by the ventral branches of spinal nerves C6 to T2. These branches form the brachial plexus from which the specific peripheral nerves to the forelimbs emanate. Chiropractic adjustments to vertebrae C4 to T2 will affect the peripheral innervation to the muscles of the greyhound forelimb, eg, specific adjustment of vertebra T2 can eliminate triceps brachii hypersensitivity in some greyhounds. Figure 31–1 shows the importance of correction of spinal mechanical faults in the lower cervical and upper thoracic area for the normal function of the forelimb musculature. Following C5–7 and T1–2 vertebrae adjustments, it

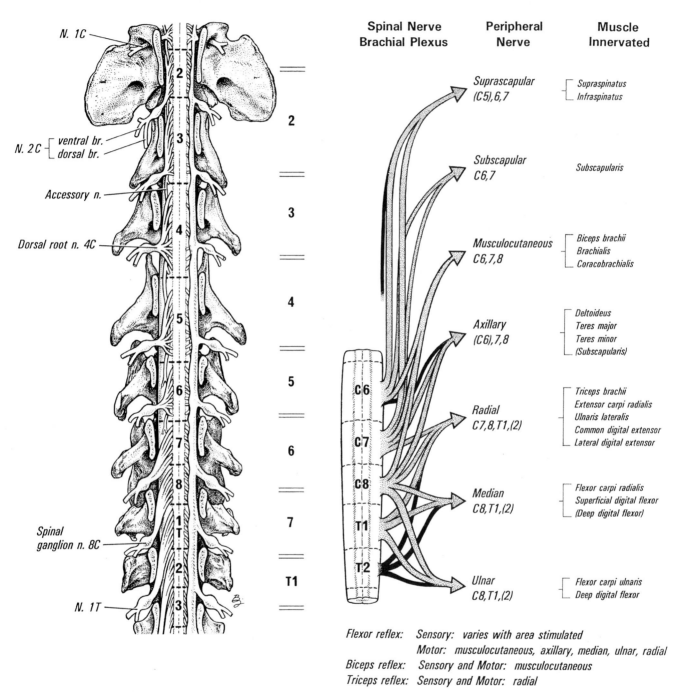

FIGURE 31–1. The cervical spinal cord segments, their relationships to the vertebrae, and the distribution of the spinal nerves to the muscles of the forelimb. In the greyhound the vertebral column shows maximum rotation in the area of C1–C2, maximum sidebending in the area C3–C5, and combined rotation and sidebending in the area of C6–C7. (Modified from Fletcher TF, Kitchell RI: Anatomical studies on the spinal cord segments of the dog. Am J Vet Res 27:1759, 1966; and DeLahunta A: Veterinary Neuroanatomy and Clinical Neurology, 2nd ed. Philadelphia, WB Saunders Company, 1983, p 62.)

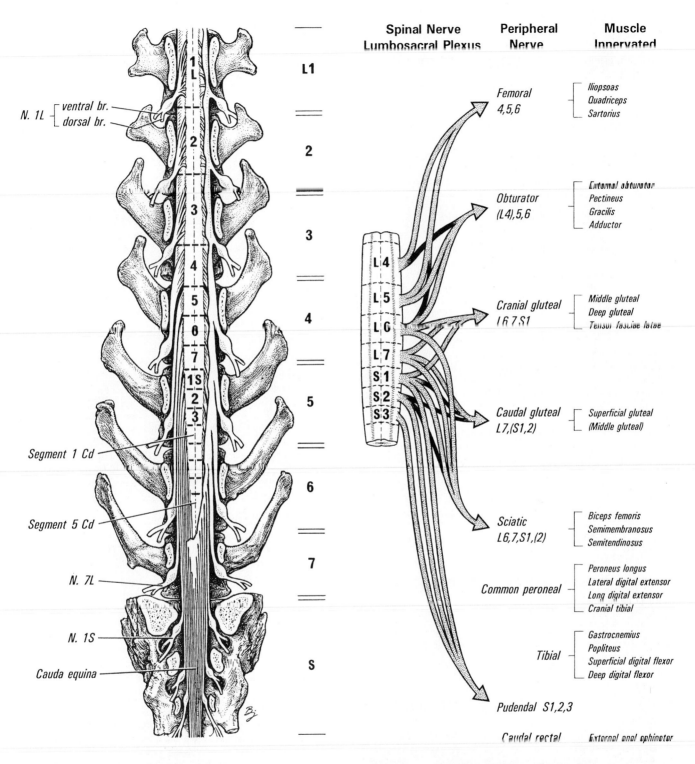

Spinal Nerve Lumbosacral Plexus	Peripheral Nerve	Muscle Innervated
	Femoral 4,5,6	Iliopsoas / Quadriceps / Sartorius
	Obturator (L4),5,6	External obturator / Pectineus / Gracilis / Adductor
	Cranial gluteal L6,7,S1	Middle gluteal / Deep gluteal / Tensor fasciae latae
	Caudal gluteal L7,(S1,2)	Superficial gluteal / (Middle gluteal)
	Sciatic L6,7,S1,(2)	Biceps femoris / Semimembranosus / Semitendinosus
	Common peroneal	Peroneus longus / Lateral digital extensor / Long digital extensor / Cranial tibial
	Tibial	Gastrocnemius / Popliteus / Superficial digital flexor / Deep digital flexor
	Pudendal S1,2,3	
	Caudal rectal	External anal sphincter

Flexor reflex: Sensory and Motor: Sciatic nerve
Patellar reflex: Sensory and Motor: Femoral nerve
Perineal reflex: Sensory and Motor: Pudendal nerve

FIGURE 31–2. Lumbar, sacral, and caudal spinal cord segments, their relationships to the vertebrae, and distribution of the spinal nerves to the muscles of the hindlimb. (Modified from Fletcher TF, Kitchell RI: Anatomical studies on the spinal cord segments of the dog. Am J Vet Res 27:1759, 1966; and DeLahunta A: Veterinary Neuroanatomy and Clinical Neurology, 2nd ed. Philadelphia, WB Saunders Company, 1983, p 63.)

is necessary to reassess the initial injury to determine if further physiotherapy is necessary.

With the pelvic limbs, spinal segments beginning as far forward as L1, but mainly involving L4 to S3, are involved with the lumbosacral plexus. L1 is involved with muscles that flex the hip[6, 12] (Fig. 31–2). Injuries to vertebrae in the thoracolumbar, lumbar, lumbosacral, and sacroiliac areas commonly affect racing performance. These areas must be free to flex, and any restriction hinders the greyhound's performance, especially its ability to leave the starting boxes. Spinal mobility injuries in the lumbar area such as lumbar rotation can lead to muscle cramping in the hindquarters or dysuria. Both conditions are common in the racing greyhound. Adjustments of the lumbar vertebral bodies may correct greyhound dysuria and should be considered prior to medical therapy for the condition.

Normal Spinal Movement

Mobility tests may be specific to a particular joint or may test the movement of an area. In examination of an individual joint it is necessary to locate the movement of the joint so that both joint-specific mobility tests and adjustive forces are directed to the joint.[6] Two major means available to test the mobility of an area are articular facet locking and ligamentous tension locking.

In greyhounds, mobility tests for the head and neck include extension, flexion, rotation, and sidebending. Trunk movements are limited because of the stability of the vertebral column, and faults are detected by palpation. With the spine, it needs to be appreciated that under compression joint surfaces become the pivot for movement through another plane. In the greyhound spine, except for the neck, only a few degrees of movement are possible in any plane before the articular facets come into contact with each other. With neck movement, if the full extent of joint movement in one plane is manipulated, eg, extension, further movement can be achieved only in a second plane (flexion/extension, sidebending, rotation). If a fully extended neck is sidebent to the point where the articular facets lock into apposition, further movement can still be achieved in the extended, sidebent neck by rotation. With sidebending, in the neck and thorax (T1 to T10), ipsilateral rotation occurs. In the thoracolumbar transitional zone and the lumbar spine, contralateral rotation occurs.[6] Sidebending of the neck produces contralateral

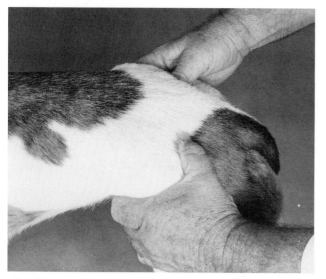

FIGURE 31–3. Mobility test of the sacroiliac joints. Direct palpation of the ilium with the patient standing.

articular facet lock. Vertebral rotation produces ipsilateral joint gapping (separation) and ligamentous tension lock. The rotation and sidebending locking effect is found to travel caudally in the cervical spine. Consequently the level of cervical treatment may be determined by the degree of sidebending and rotation.

Extension of the neck bilaterally locks the articular facets, allowing testing and manipulation of the caudally located cervico-thoracic junction. Ligamentous tension locking is the limit of articular surface separation available under normal ligament tension. Joint-snap is often a palpable rather than an audible sensation and is a good indicator that restoration of full joint mobility has been achieved. Clinically, articular facet locking and ligamentous tension locking can be used in two ways:[6] (1) Direct adjustment to an articulation. A shearing force is then applied directly to a facet-locked joint to free the restricted mobility of the joint. Greyhounds resent the positioning necessary for this technique, and it is most useful in the thoracic and cervical spine. (2) Indirect adjustment to an articulation. The spine is used to lever ligamentous tension-locked joints rather than application of direct force. During positioning for this procedure the movements are slower and produce a gapping effect upon the joints. This technique is used to treat the upper cervical, lumbar spinal, and sacroiliac regions.[6]

SACROILIAC JOINTS

Sacroiliac Pain

The pelvic ring complex includes the sacroiliac joints, coxofemoral joints, and pubic symphysis. Pain-free function is important in the racing greyhound, which must rapidly clear the starting boxes and maintain balance and drive when running. Both sacroiliac fixation and sacral rotation will produce asymmetry of the iliac crests. The clinical feature of sacroiliac joint fault is pain on palpation over the sacroiliac joint and elicited with lateral pressure to the wings of the ilium. Manipulation alleviates pain, and the greyhound will support full weight over the hindquarters.

Mobility of the Sacroiliac Joints

The articular surfaces of the sacroiliac joint are a rough interlocking series of projections and depressions that commonly become "hitched" or luxated in greyhounds.

Mobility Tests for the Sacroiliac Joints

Direct Palpation. Direct palpation of the sacroiliac joints is readily accomplished in the standing patient and is side specific[6] (Fig. 31–3).

Manipulation of the Sacroiliac Joints

Direct Manipulation of the Sacroiliac Joint. The greyhound is treated in a standing position. An assistant stands over the greyhound and uses both legs to grasp the animal firmly in the shoulder area while the head and neck are extended vertically in a comfortable position[6] (Fig. 31–4). With large powerful greyhounds of 40 kg or more, the assistant should face away from the veterinarian to better control the greyhound.

The veterinarian places the right forearm under both stifles so that the dog is elevated off the ground and resting comfortably on the forearm (Fig. 31–5). The right hand is rotated forward and the greyhound's stifle grasped so that the dog's lower spine is gently rotated. The palm of the left hand is placed on the dorsal wing of the ilium and is used to carry out the manipulation.

The range of rotation and flexion is increased to the point at

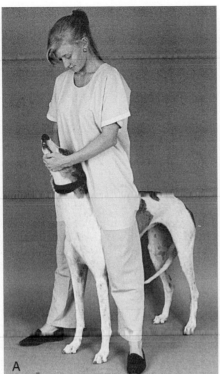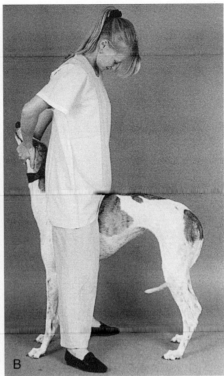

FIGURE 31–4. Position of greyhound and handler for manipulation of the sacroiliac joint. *A*, Manipulation of the sacroiliac joint with the handler facing away from the veterinarian. *B*, Manipulation of the sacroiliac joint with the handler facing the veterinarian.

which there is strong tension in the lumbar spine. Maximum lumbar flexion is necessary to effect the more caudal manipulation. The palm of the hand on the ilium is used to carry out the manipulation by directing a small-amplitude powerful thrust through the plane of the sacroiliac joint[6] (Fig. 31–6).

It is important not to pull on the hand holding the stifle as this could injure the dog by exerting excessive leverage. Manipulation of a sacral rotation is accompanied by a large movement (approximately 1 cm) and a distinct "clunk." This is different from the normal joint-snapping sound heard with other spinal manipulations.

It is important to remember that the manipulation should be gentle, forces applied should be of small amplitude, firm, powerful, and quick, with a minimum amount of pain to the animal. The manipulation is carried out in both directions and often has the desired effect of relaxing the greyhound, which is then more amenable to further handling. Poorly performing greyhounds have been observed to improve up to 10 lengths following diagnosis and manipulation for sacroiliac mobility fault.

LUMBOSACRAL JOINT

Lumbosacral Pain

Lumbosacral weakness and hypersensitivity are common in the greyhound. The dog lacking drive will be slow breaking from the starting box, the gait may be unbalanced, and muscle strain develops in the hindquarters. Sacral injuries mainly occur during jumping from the starting boxes or when the dog is run into from behind at the end of a race. This injury may be severely debilitating with acute pain and sidebending or elevation of the tail on palpation. Palpation between the spinous process of vertebrae L7 and S1 will elicit pain and may lead to total collapse of the hindquarters. Certain breed lines appear to be more susceptible to weakness

in this area. This injury, if left uncorrected, will lead to strain of the deep pectoral muscles and further loss of speed. Manipulative correction gives instantaneous relief. Greyhounds lose all pain from the area, are more relaxed, and sleep better, and bitches are able to squat fully to urinate.

LUMBAR SPINE

Mobility of the Lumbar Spine

The characteristic movement of the lumbar spine is rotation to the contralateral side during sidebending. This is crucial to the practice of manipulation. During sidebending to the right, rotation of the vertebral bodies will occur toward the left. In effect, the right articular facets approach apposition while the left articular facets approach ligamentous tension. This is the opposite to that found in the neck, and consequently indirect vertebral manipulation is directed to the convex side of the sidebending curve.[6]

When sidebending is induced in the lumbar spine, there is the opposite relationship of articular facet behavior to that occurring cranial to joint T10–11. A state of articular facet lock is approached on the concave side of the sidebending curve and a ligamentous tension lock on the convex side of the sidebending curve. Sidebending increases from L2–3 through to and including the lumbosacral joint. Rotation increases from L2–3 through to the lumbosacral joint where there is a sharp reduction in rotational ability. Extension increases to lumbar joint L6–7 and then markedly increases at the lumbosacral joint. The lumbosacral joint is frequently observed to show mobility faults.

Mobility Tests for the Lumbar Spine

Palpation of the Standing Patient. The clinician stands over the greyhound and either uses both thumbs to concurrently apply

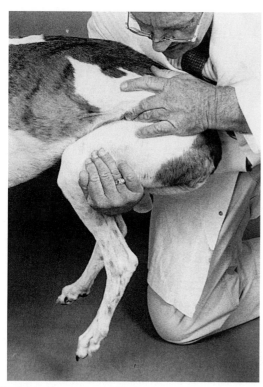

FIGURE 31–5. Manipulation of the sacroiliac joint showing the dog resting comfortably on the veterinarian's forearm.

bilateral pressure or unilaterally applies pressure over the area of the articular processes of each lumbar vertebra. Discomfort indicates mobility fault. With the greyhound either lying or standing, the finger of one hand is used to stabilize the spinous process of each lower lumbar vertebra while the adjacent cranial spinous process is subjected to rotational force.[6]

Manipulation of the Lumbar Spine

The greyhound is positioned for indirect vertebral manipulation as described under Sacroiliac Joints. To manipulate the cranial

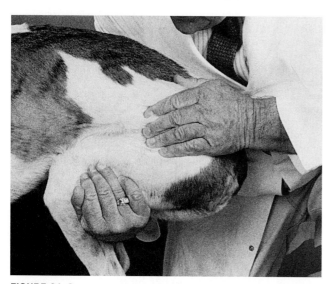

FIGURE 31–6. Manipulation of the sacroiliac joint. The palm of the hand is used to direct a small-amplitude powerful thrust through the plane of the sacroiliac joint.

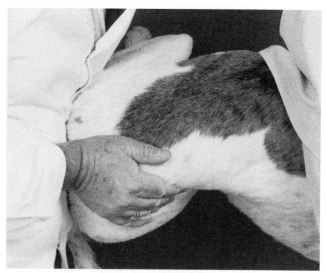

FIGURE 31–7. Manipulation of the lumbosacral and lumbar joints. The joints are in full flexion with rotatory tension.

lumbar spine the spine is extended and then increasingly flexed to manipulate the more caudal vertebrae.

Lumbar joints L6–7 and L7–S1 are manipulated with the joints in flexion. The joint capsules and the facet joints at these two lumbar levels are extensive, allowing relatively large ranges of movement in flexion, extension, rotation, and sidebending. To obtain sufficient ligamentous tension during manipulation, the L6–7 and L7–S1 joints must be brought into full flexion before application of rotatory tension and the final manipulative thrust (Fig. 31–7).

Spinal joints L5–6, L6–7, and L7–S1 routinely demonstrate a configuration of mobility fault that is defined as extension lock. The overextended joints are subsequently unable to be freely flexed. The manipulation technique employs direct manipulation to the extended joints and involves application of a cranial thrust to the vertebral joint.[6]

Direct Vertebral Manipulation of the Lumbar Spine. With the greyhound in lateral recumbency, and the spine either flexed or extended, a thrusting force is applied directly through the axis of each spinous process.[6]

THORACOLUMBAR JUNCTION

Thoracolumbar Pain

Greyhounds with thoracolumbar pain show a lordotic (sway-backed) or kyphotic (hump-backed) stance, stiff gait, reluctance to shake through the full length of their spine or to jump, hindlimb lameness, and, in severe cases, ataxia. Track performance may be decreased by 10 lengths. Greyhounds show hypersensitivity on bilateral horizontal palpation of the thoracic or lumbar spine. Palpation may detect strained and sore muscles and in a few cases localized myositis. There is always pronounced soreness with passive movements of the spine. Hammer-percussion may locate the vertebra in question.[4]

Mobility of the Thoracolumbar Junction. Mobility in the thoracic spine predominantly allows flexion and extension. There is limited sidebending with ipsilateral rotation. Contralateral rotation occurs caudal to joint T10–11 with sidebending. The lumbar mode of spinal movement is increasingly represented in the articulations caudal to T12–13, ie, rotation occurs after the first few degrees of sidebending movement, and the vertebral bodies rotate to the opposite side of the sidebending movement.

Thoracic joint T10–11 is ellipsoid with considerable freedom of flexion and rotation but limited extension. In sidebending, rotation may occur in either direction. Mobility of this joint is constrained by the rib cage. T10–11 is representative of the transitional region between the mobility characteristics of the thoracic and lumbar spinal segments and may be likened to the universal joint of an automobile, linking thoracic and lumbar movement. It is a joint subjected to stress and injury in the racing greyhound.

The anatomical limitations that allow for the graded introduction of lumbar movement modes beyond T10–11 are: (1) The accessory process. These effectively limit the degree of observed rotation and sidebending. (2) The shape of the facet articulations. At T11–12 sidebending is promoted while rotation is restricted. The facet articulations below T11–12 increasingly show the capacity for sidebending and rotation and do so in accordance with the lumbar movement modes. The spine between T10–11 and L1–2 demonstrates an extensor tone in the resting greyhound, while both the thoracic and lumbar spine demonstrate flexor tone. In states of mobility fault, the true thoracic spine will generally demonstrate lordosis, whereas the lumbar spine demonstrates kyphosis.[6]

Mobility Tests for the Thoracolumbar Transitional Zone

Springing Test. See the description of this test in Mobility Tests for the Thoracic Spine.

Direct Palpation. Palpable rotational movement is minimal as the short spinous processes do not impart the sensation of movement. Extensor tone further limits the detection of movement.[6]

Manipulation of the Thoracolumbar Junction

The most significant feature of this area is that T10–11 has a universal joint action and is prone to mobility faults.[6]

Indirect Vertebral Manipulation. With the greyhound standing, the veterinarian grasps the hindquarters and induces extension in the lumbar spine that acts as a rod to induce rotation and sidebending of the thoracolumbar area. When the lumbar spine is brought into extension, bilateral articular facet apposition occurs. With the thoracolumbar area in articular facet lock and ligamentous tension, a thrust is delivered via the lumbar spine. This fully mobilizes the thoracolumbar joints in the induced direction.[6]

Direct Vertebral Manipulation. A thrusting force is applied in flexion or extension. The spine of the laterally recumbent dog is brought into flexion, and a thrusting force is applied directly through the axis of the spinous processes. The same procedure is then applied in extension (Fig. 31–8).

Thrusting Force in Flexion. With the greyhound standing, the hindquarters are elevated with one hand under the cranial thigh to the region of the veterinarian's waist (Fig. 31–9). The palm of the opposite hand is placed over the dorsal spinous process and manipulates it by moving in a down and forward short arc thrust. Moltzen[4] described thoracolumbar manipulation for dogs with spinal pain, gait abnormalities, and paresis.

THORAX

Mobility of the Thoracic Spine

The thoracic spine has both a cranial and caudal transitional zone. The cranial transitional zone extends from C6 to T3. The caudal transitional zone begins at T10 and extends to L1. The direction of the thoracic spinous processes changes around the anticlinal vertebrae.

Thoracic vertebrae T3–T10 move mainly in flexion and extension with limited rotation and sidebending due to restriction by the ribs. As with the cervical spine, rotation occurs in the same direction as sidebending. Flexion is limited by the interspinous ligaments and the apposition of the vertebral bodies, while extension is limited by the articular facets and contact between adjacent spinous processes.[6]

Mobility Tests for the Thoracic Spine

Springing Test. This test is used to detect pain and muscle spasm. It has been used by greyhound trainers and "muscle men" since the inception of greyhound coursing and mechanical lure racing in Australia. With the greyhound standing, the thumbs are used to apply a short-amplitude thrust to the thoracic vertebrae, perpendicular to its body axis. The vertebral joint is mobilized into extension (Fig. 31–10). Strong paravertebral muscular spasm and discomfort are elicited if mobility faults exist. Further palpation may be required to accurately locate the lesion.[6]

Direct Palpation. Direct palpation is used to determine freedom of mobility. The greyhound is laid on its right side and the thorax flexed to give bilateral gapping of the articular facets. The fingers of the right hand support the right side of the spinous process of T2. The thumb of the left hand is used to rotate the spinous process of T1 to the greyhound's right. This process is continued through to L1 and then reversed for the contralateral side (Fig. 31–11). Direct palpation of the thoracic spine can also be performed on the standing patient.[6]

Manipulation of the Thoracic Spine

Direct vertebral manipulation is applied with the spine in flexion. A thrusting force is applied through the axis of the spinous processes of each thoracic vertebra. This is the only method available for adjustment of the thoracic spine.

Direct Vertebral Manipulation of T1–2 and T2–3. The thoracic joints are manipulated bilaterally. The greyhound is laid on a low table allowing the veterinarian to work over the dog. The spine is flexed. The left hand is placed on the sternum and the palm of the right hand on the dorsal tip of the spinous process of T1. Both forearms are held horizontal to the table and parallel to the direction of thrust, which is delivered when the greyhound exhales and is directed through the axis of the spinous processes (see Fig. 31–8A and B). In this manner the thoracic joints are induced to move to their full range of movement.[6]

Rib fixations are treated by pressing on the cranial surface of the angle of the rib (angulus costae), and rotating caudally[5] (Fig. 31–12).

CERVICOTHORACIC JUNCTION

Cervicothoracic Mobility Characteristics

The nerves of the brachial plexus (C6–8, T1–2) innervate the muscles of the forelimb[12] (see Fig. 31–1). The cervicothoracic junction extends from C6–T3 and is one of the two "transitional" or mobility zones of the spine. The cervical vertebrae have large amplitudes in their range of movement in flexion, extension, sidebending, and rotation. The thoracic vertebrae have significantly less capacity for these movements. It is the support provided by the rib cage to the thoracic spine that is largely responsible for the observed reduction of mobility.

The complex functional relationship between the cervicothoracic

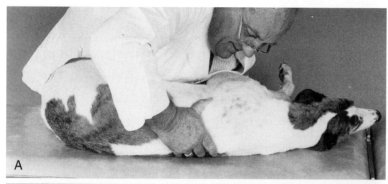

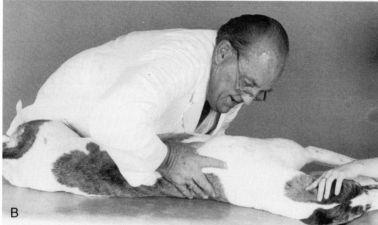

FIGURE 31–8. *A*, Direct thoracic vertebral manipulation with spine in flexion. *B*, Direct thoracic vertebral manipulation with spine in extension. Thrust directed through the axis of the spinous process.

FIGURE 31–9. Direct thoracic vertebral manipulation. With the dog standing, the palm of the hand is used to directly apply the thrusting force.

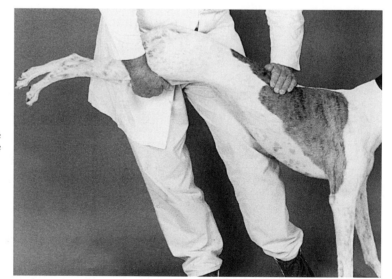

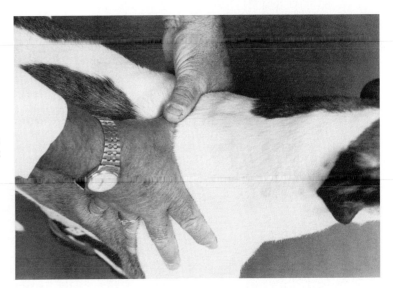

FIGURE 31–10. Springing test for T1–T3. Note that the thumbs are used jointly to deliver a short-amplitude perpendicular thrust through the axis of the vertebrae.

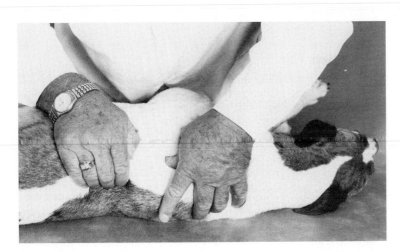

FIGURE 31–11. Direct palpation of thoracic vertebral mobility. Note dog in right lateral recumbency. The right hand supports the thoracic processes while the left thumb is used to rotate the T1 spinous process.

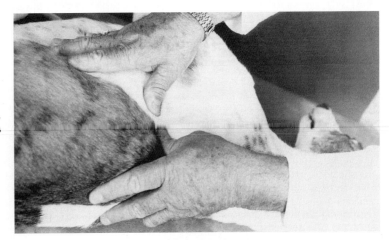

FIGURE 31–12. Rib fixation. With the dog in lateral recumbency, the thumbs are used to rotate the angle of the rib (angulus costae) caudally.

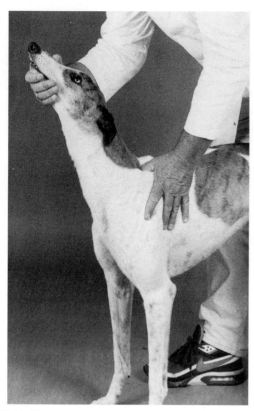

FIGURE 31–13. Direct palpation of the interscapular area. Note position of thumb.

junction and the forelimbs is reflected in pain referral, postural conformation, and balance of the greyhound.[6] Injury to this area significantly affects racing performance. Referred pain from the cervicothoracic junction is often mistaken for muscle soreness in the lateral muscles of the shoulder and forearm and for carpal pain.

Cervicothoracic Junction Spinal Mobility Tests

Direct Palpation. The neck is extended and the thumb or forefinger is used to apply pressure into the anterior interscapular area (Fig. 31–13). The area bounded by the thoracic spine, the vertebral border of the scapula, and the caudal trapezius musculature becomes intensely sensitive to deep palpation with cervicothoracic mobility faults.[6] Pain after corrective manipulation due to strain of the underlying musculature may be treated by injection or physiotherapy.

Flexion and Extension. As for the cervical spine, separation and apposition movement of dorsal spinous processes of T1–T3 during extension or flexion of the neck[6] may be detected with the thumb (Fig. 31–14). Restricted movement of dorsal spinous processes T1–T3 should not be confused with strain of the longissimus dorsi muscle that occurs in the greyhound.

Sidebending. Movement is tested as for cervical sidebending but continued until movement of T1–T3 is detected[6] (Fig. 31–15). Care should be taken to use firm, gentle, and controlled force to move the head and neck. Acute pain or discomfort should lead to abandonment of this test.

Springing Test. The thumbs, one on top of the other, are placed on the top of each spinous process (T1–T3) and used to produce force through the dorsoventral axis of the vertebrae (see Figure 31–10). Strong paravertebral muscular spasm and pain[6] are indica-

tive of restricted mobility. T2 is often the vertebral body involved with irritation of the nerve root. Pain may be referred to the lateral muscles of the shoulder and forearm.[12]

Combined Sidebending and Rotation During Extension. Extension of the neck with bilateral articular facet lock of the cervical spine allows the neck to be used as a lever to transmit force to the cervicothoracic area. To test the left-sided joints from C6–T3 the neck is extended until palpable facet apposition is detected at C6–7 joint. Then the neck is sidebent to the right and the head and neck rotated to the left. A shearing force is then directly applied from the concavity of the neck curvature to the C6–7 joint.

For the left C7–T1 joint, the procedure for the C6–7 is repeated until palpable tension and movement of the spinous process of T1 are detected (Fig. 31–16). This affects articular facet apposition in the right C7–T1 joint and ligamentous tension in the left C7–T1 joint. The thumb of the left hand is now used to lever the spinous process of T1 toward the left side, ie, a gapping force is applied to the left C7–T1 joint. Mobility restriction involving the left C7–T1 joint is detected in this manner.[6] The operator changes hands and carries out the procedure to test the right C6–T3 area.

NECK

Chiropractic treatment of the cervical spine has a relaxing effect on the spinal musculature and facilitates kinesis of the spinal articulations.[8]

Neck Pain

Greyhounds with neck pain are reluctant to shake, are hypersensitive to handling or patting around the head and neck, and are reluctant to drive into the first turn during a race, generally losing lengths. Trainers often describe the greyhound as a "sook" or "squib." These greyhounds invariably show pain and hypersensitivity with horizontal pressure applied bilaterally at the base of the neck. The pain on palpation may elicit spectacular aggression. The occasional greyhound will attempt to "take the veterinarian's arm, neck, and head off." Drug restraint may be necessary. However, the author prefers "traction" followed by normal manipulation.

In dogs, characteristic signs for neck pain are a cautious walk with lowered head, reluctance to jump and descend stairs, evidenced pain even as a result of movements, and in some cases lameness of one foreleg. Generally one can locate the cervical vertebra in question by digital palpation of the neck.[4]

Mobility Characteristics of the Cervical Spine

Occipitoatlantal Joint. Mobility fault is common in the occipitoatlantal joint. Contralateral rotation of this joint during sidebending allows the head to retain its neutral postural axis during sidebending of the neck. Rotation of the atlas, unlike that of the remaining cervical vertebrae, is contralateral during sidebending. The occipitoatlantal joint shows its greatest range of movement in flexion. Sidebending and rotation combine into flexion-extension movements of this joint.

Atlantoaxial Joint. Rotation is a marked feature and is ipsilateral to cervical sidebending. Extension, flexion, and sidebending are limited.

Cervical Vertebrae C2–C7. Cervical joint C2–3 demonstrates a range of both extension and flexion. There is limited sidebending and associated rotation. This is a joint of potential stress. Joints C3–4 through C5–6 are similar and show an additional gliding movement. In the occipitoatlantal, atlantoaxial, and C2–3 joints, sidebending can occur only with a strong component of rotation.

In the joints C3–4 through C5–6, sidebending can occur as a

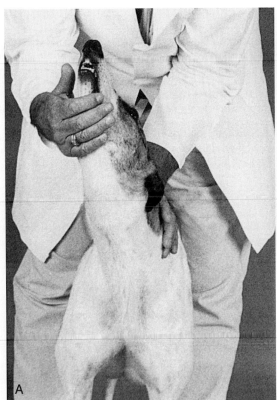

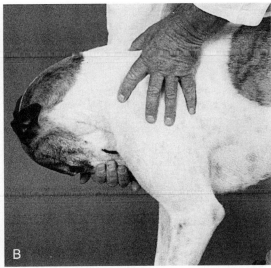

FIGURE 31–14. *A*, Movement of dorsal spinous processes T1–T3 with neck in extension. *B*, Movement of dorsal spinous processes T1–T3 with neck in flexion. The thumb of the palpating hand is used to detect spinous process movement.

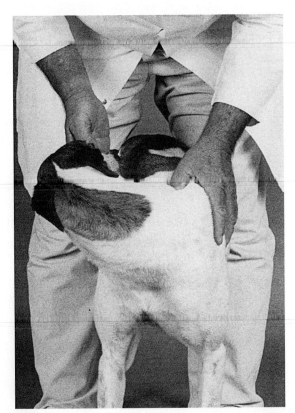

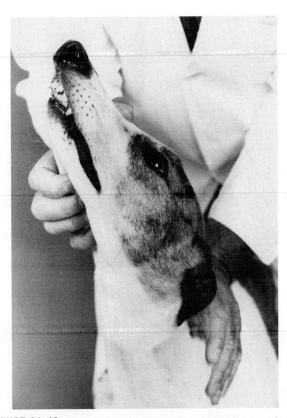

FIGURE 31–15. Sidebending of the cervical vertebrae to the right. Ensure that the greyhound is not subjected to excessive pain or frightened during the procedure.

FIGURE 31–16. Combined sidebending and rotation during extension for C7–T1. Extend the animal's neck using the right hand; sidebend the neck to the right while rotating the head and neck to the left. The left thumb levers spinous process C7 to the left side.

mode of movement while only a very small rotational movement occurs. The degree of flexion and extension movement progressively increases in each joint, moving down the cervical spine to the C5–6 joint.

Cervical joints C6–7 and C7–T1 show a return to rotation-sidebending movement. This is less pronounced at C7–T1 because of the restricted movement of the thoracic vertebrae. Extension and flexion movements are strongly represented at C6–7 and C7–T1; C6–7 is a stress region.[6]

Mobility Tests for the Cervical Spine

Extension and Flexion. The veterinarian straddles the greyhound and uses one hand to move the head of the patient. The thumb of the other hand is placed on the spinous process of T1. The thumb detects the point of flexion or extension at which movement of T1 occurs. Both the presence of discomfort of the dog and the range of flexion or extension are noted by the veterinarian[6] (Fig. 31–17A and B).

Sidebending. The convex side of the spinous process of T1 is palpated as the neck is drawn laterally. If the greyhound's neck is sidebent to the right, the palm of the veterinarian's right hand is placed on the left side of the greyhound's muzzle. The thumb of the left hand palpates between the spinous processes of T1 and T2 on the left side. The ease and extent of sidebending at which palpable movement of the T1 spinous process occurs are assessed[6] (Fig. 31–18).

Rotation. Rotation is assessed in the upper cervical spine. When one is assessing rotation to the right, the thumb of the left hand is placed to provide a pivot in the area of the right atlantoaxial joint. The palm of the right hand is placed on the left side of the greyhound's muzzle, and the ease or discomfort of rotation to the right is assessed[6] (Fig. 31–19).

Direct Specific Palpation. When the cervical spine is sidebent to the left, rotation of the vertebral bodies occurs to the left with joint gapping occurring to the left and articular facet apposition and lock to the right. The shearing force should be applied to the facet-locked joints from the concave side of the sidebent neck. To bring the articular facets on the left into apposition it is necessary to rotate the head and neck to the right. The right joints are then in a state of ligamentous tension. By increasing the extent of the sidebending to the left and simultaneously increasing the rotation of the head and neck to the right, the facet joints are progressively locked along the length of the left cervical spine. Shearing forces are now applied to the left cervical joints. The greyhound's jaw is cupped in the right hand and sidebending of the neck to the left progressed, while at the same time the head and neck are rotated to the right. The fingers of the left hand are used to palpate the articular processes of the left cervical spine. As each joint is felt to undergo facet apposition, a gentle thrust, directed transversely to the spinal axis, is applied to the joint. This effectively creates a gapping effect upon the contralateral joint at the level being examined[6] (Fig. 31–20).

Cervical Traction in Greyhounds

Traction, utilizing the greyhound's own body weight as the traction force, may be used to treat cervical adhesions. The assistant faces the veterinarian and supports the greyhound's forelimbs. The veterinarian places the hands under the mandible and behind the skull, ensuring that the throat is unrestricted. The greyhound is lifted and held suspended for 10 seconds (Fig. 31–21). Greyhounds in acute pain willingly tolerate this procedure. There is loss of pain with overall relaxation.

Occipitoatlantal Joint

Straddling the standing greyhound, the veterinarian places the palm of the left hand over the greyhound's left ear, with the left

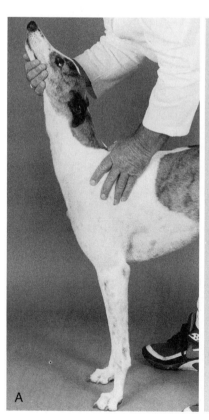
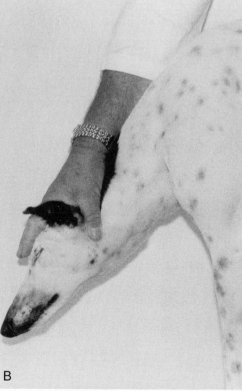

FIGURE 31–17. *A,* Extension of the neck. Note the position of the thumb on the spinous process of T1. *B,* Flexion of the neck.

left occipitoatlantal joint now in ligamentous tension, simultaneously the left thumb thrusts in a transverse plane to the occipitoatlantal joint as the right hand is used to apply a further short-amplitude flexion of the joint (Fig. 31–22). This manipulative technique is not specific to the occipitoatlantal joint as the atlantoaxial joint is fully mobilized.[6] This manipulation is difficult and requires coordination of the thrust between left and right hands; poor technique can injure the greyhound.

Cervical Manipulation (Lower Cervical Spine)

Indirect Cervical Vertebral Manipulation

Straddling the greyhound, the veterinarian passes the right hand through the greyhound's right axilla to grasp the left shoulder, and the left hand grasps under the mandible or under the wing of the atlas. The rotation and sidebending occur as the cervical spine is flexed.[6] Manipulation is achieved with a short-amplitude sharp thrust (Fig. 31–23).

Direct Cervical Vertebral Manipulation

With the greyhound in left lateral recumbency for a right-side cervical sidebending restriction, direct palpation reveals pain on gapping the left C7–T3 joints. The right hand is placed onto the occiput with the fingers and thumb spread from ear to ear behind the occipital protuberance. The thumb of the left hand is placed on the spinous process of T1. The cervical and cranial thoracic spine are brought into flexion. This grip is used to maintain the neck in flexion while sidebending to the greyhound's right. The head and neck of the greyhound are rotated to its left. The left thumb delivers a short thrust to the spinous process of T1. The force is directed perpendicular to the C7–T1 joint. Simultaneously a short sharp increase of sidebending and flexion with left rotation is delivered by the right hand[6] (Fig. 31–24).

Hauler[6] begins spinal manipulation at the neck, but one may

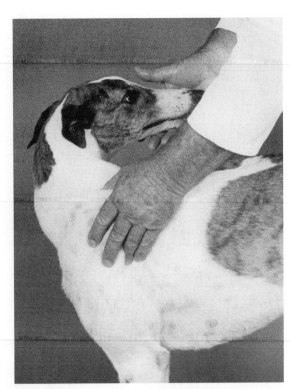

FIGURE 31–18. Sidebending to the right. Note the palm of the hand on the left side of the muzzle and the left thumb located between the spinous processes of T1–T2.

thumb under the angular process of the right mandible. The palm of the right hand is placed to lie along the left side of the greyhound's maxilla with the fingers extending toward the left ear. The head is flexed, sidebent, and rotated toward the right so that the left occipitoatlantal joint is fully flexed and rotated. With the

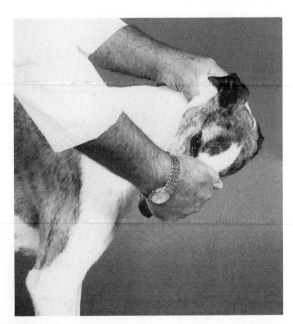

FIGURE 31–19. Rotation of the upper cervical spine to the left. Note that the thumb of the left hand is placed to provide a pivotal point in the area of the atlantoaxial joint.

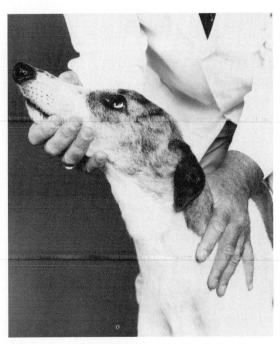

FIGURE 31–20. Direct palpation of cervical vertebrae. The right hand cups the greyhound's jaw, and the fingers of the left hand are used to palpate the articular processes of the left cervical spine. The thumb is used to direct a transverse thrust to each cervical joint.

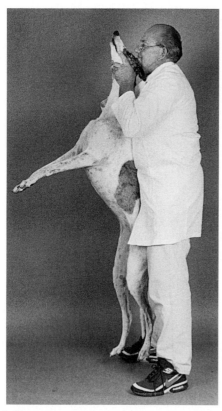

FIGURE 31–21. Traction to the cervical spine. Lift from under the mandible and from behind the skull with no restriction of the trachea for a period of 10 seconds. Note the fully relaxed greyhound. An assistant steadies the forelimbs until the lift is completed.

start at the sacrum and work cranially. Manipulation of the cervical spine in dogs has also been described.[4]

MOBILIZATION OF THE JOINTS OF THE LIMBS

Mobility fault in joints restricts stride length, leading to loss of speed. The veterinarian through manipulation may mobilize a joint and significantly increase the animal's performance. However, in normal greyhounds without joint mobility faults, performance may be improved further by extending the normal range of joint mobility. The author has found joint mobilization to be beneficial in other working dogs, such as German shepherds.

SHOULDER JOINT

Immobilization Syndrome

In 1988 the author surveyed more than 500 greyhounds in New South Wales and found the incidence of shoulder injury to be 21 per cent in the right shoulder and 79 per cent in the left. Greyhounds race anticlockwise, and shoulder injury is predominantly a left- or railing-side problem. Adhesions form around the joint causing pain and restricted movement. This is distinct from the referred pain of cervical mobility faults. Altered gait results in an increase in the incidence of carpal and metacarpal injury.

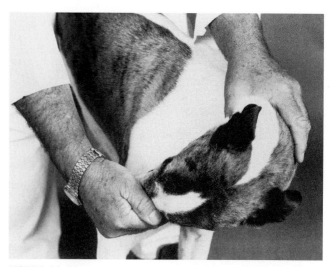

FIGURE 31–22. Manipulation of the occipitoatlantal joint. The head is flexed, sidebent, and rotated toward the right. The left thumb thrusts in a transverse plane to the occipitoatlantal joint as the right hand is used to apply a further short-amplitude flexion of the joint.

Mobilization of the Greyhound Shoulder Joint

Mobilization of the shoulder joint is carried out using a combination of stretch and manipulative procedures designed to release the shoulder joint without damaging the articular or periarticular surfaces. The greyhound must be held firmly by an attendant or its owner.

1. The shoulder joint is grasped with the corresponding hand of the veterinarian, eg, left shoulder joint, left hand. This hand holds the shoulder joint firmly, immobilizing the scapula. The right hand grasps the elbow joint, so that the index finger is

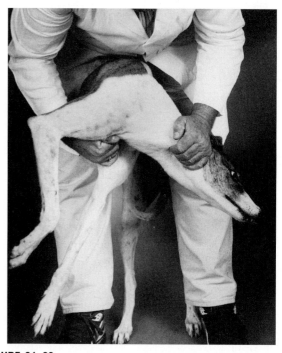

FIGURE 31–23. Manipulation of the cervical spine. The neck is rotated and sidebent in flexion, followed by a short-amplitude thrust.

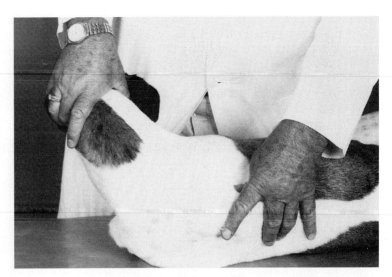

FIGURE 31–24. Manipulation of the cervical spine. Dog in left lateral recumbency with neck sidebent in flexion with left rotation. Note the position of the left thumb on the dorsal spinous process of T1.

over the top of the elbow and the elbow is held in a vise-like grip. This is important as the greyhound may injure itself if it struggles uncontrollably. Gradually the veterinarian firmly stretches the forelimb distally and toward the contralateral side to open the joint laterally (Fig. 31–25). This stretch manipulation is crucial to prevent damage to the joint and must precede the following manipulations.

2. The shoulder joint is further stretched. With the hands in their original position the antebrachium and manus are stretched distally. Once the distal forelimb is stretched it can be extended

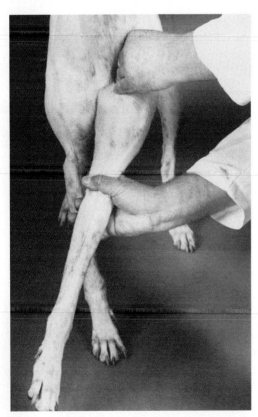

FIGURE 31–25. Mobilization of the shoulder joint. The forelimb is stretched distally and toward the contralateral side to open the joint laterally.

forward so that the scapula and humerus are in a straight line (Fig. 31–26). This manipulation fully opens up the posterior aspect of the shoulder joint.

3. This part of the manipulation should never be undertaken prior to the first two procedures or permanent damage may occur to the joint. It is a rotatory manipulation or mobilization of the joint and should be carried out only on a stretched joint. The scapula remains immobilized, and the elbow joint is raised and quickly rotated laterodorsally toward a horizontal position (Fig. 31–27). The elbow joint should never be raised above the level of the shoulder joint during this procedure.

The mobilization procedure is rotatory and frees adhesions on the medial aspect of the shoulder joint. Greyhounds may show minimal nonresidual pain.[5] Following this procedure the greyhound is allowed to move freely. The greyhound can be galloped immediately after this manipulation. If the greyhound is restricted from galloping, adhesions are likely to re-form, and little will have been achieved toward getting the animal back to peak performance.

A NSAID may be given for 24 hours following the procedure.

HIP JOINT

Anticlockwise racing results in the muscles of the right (off) hip frequently being injured. Atrophy occurs with reduced ability of the right hip to be fully extended as adhesions form in these muscles and in the joint capsule, severely restricting movement. Right hindlimb muscle atrophy may shorten the limb by 4 to 6 cm. Atrophy of the thigh musculature in "normal" raced greyhounds has been confirmed by dissection studies, with the gluteus medius, gracilis, pectineus, obturatorius internus, and quadratus femoris muscles[13] being involved.

This injury often has its beginnings during the breaking-in or schooling period and is perpetuated during subsequent racing. Early diagnosis and corrective therapy are essential to ensure a successful racing career.

The right thigh and peroneal muscles of the racing greyhound can be maintained free of atrophy using stretch mobilization. These techniques are useful in dealing with other working breeds such as German shepherds. Stretch mobilization significantly increases muscle mass and strength in the hindquarters, enabling dogs to work more efficiently.

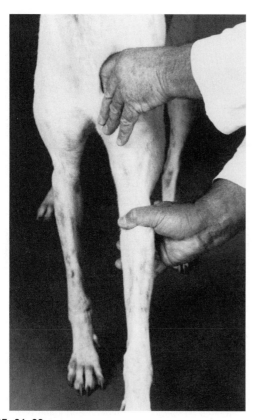

FIGURE 31–26. Mobilization of the shoulder joint. The forelimb is stretched distally and extended forward so that the scapula and humerus are in a straight line.

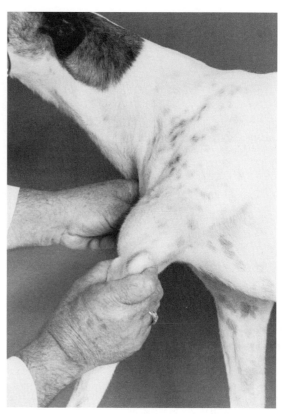

FIGURE 31–27. Mobilization of the shoulder joint. The scapula is immobilized, and the elbow joint is raised and quickly rotated laterodorsally toward a horizontal position.

Mobilization of the Hip Joint

The greyhound is held by the handler. The examining veterinarian lifts the hindquarters from the ground, trapping one hindlimb between the thighs (Fig. 31–28). The stifle and hip are extended and held so that the hindleg is overextended in a straight line with the dorsum of the back (Fig. 31–29). The opposite hand is then placed over the wing of the ilium (Fig. 31–30) and the palm pushed caudoventrally, over the gluteal muscles (Fig. 31–31). This stretches the gluteal muscles, breaks muscle adhesions, and loosens adhesions in and around the hip joint. The procedure is repeated on the opposite hip joint.

Next, the veterinarian stands behind the greyhound, grasping both anterior stifles and fully extending its hips by pulling the hindlegs caudally. The body of the greyhound and hindlimbs will then lie almost in a straight line (Fig. 31–32).

To flex the hindquarters, the veterinarian stands behind the greyhound, picks it up by the stifles, and cradles the hindquarters 18 inches off the ground. This fully flexes the hip joints, rotates the femoral heads in the acetabula, and stretches the flexor muscles of the hip joint[5] (Fig. 31–33).

These mobilizations maximize the greyhound's hindlimb reach, and stretch exercises are very important in maintaining performance.[5]

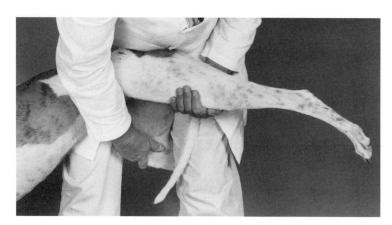

FIGURE 31–28. Mobilization of the hip joint. The hindquarters are lifted from the ground, with one hindlimb trapped between the clinician's thighs.

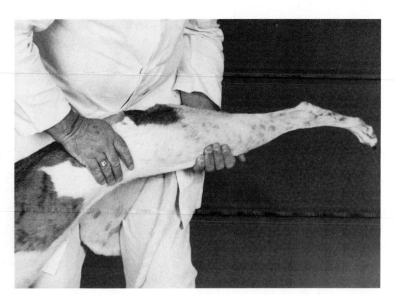

FIGURE 31–29. Mobilization of the hip joint. Hindleg fully extended.

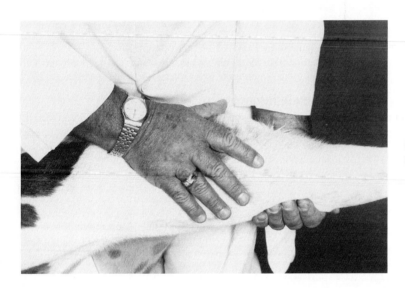

FIGURE 31–30. Mobilization of the hip joint. The hand is positioned over the ilium.

FIGURE 31–31. Mobilization of the hip joint. The palm is placed lateral to the gluteal muscles, and pressure is applied caudoventrally, in the direction of the arrow.

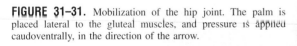

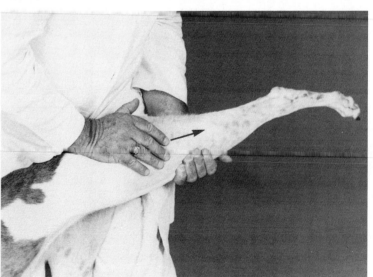

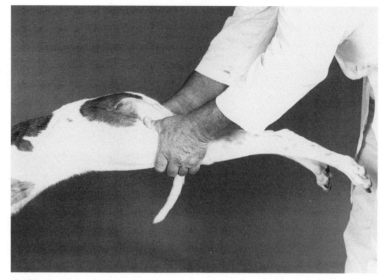

FIGURE 31–32. Mobilization of the hip joint. Hips fully extended with the dog standing.

FINAL SHOULDER JOINT CHECK

The veterinarian stands over the shoulders of the greyhound, taking each elbow and fully flexing the shoulder joints to stretch the extensor muscles of the shoulder (Fig. 31–34). Then the shoulder is fully extended parallel to the spinal column to further check that there is no restriction of forward movement of the shoulder and that the dog is free in its action (Fig. 31–35).

DISCUSSION

Manipulation may start from either the sacral or cervical end of the spinal column. Moltzen[4] and Hauler[6] prefer to begin manipulation from the head. The author prefers to begin in the sacral area as the dog is less apprehensive and easier to control. Dogs exhibiting pain from extreme spinal hypersensitivity are immediately given some relief with the first manipulation and are more amenable to further handling. It is a matter of personal preference.

Acknowledgments

I am indebted to George Hindle, who first introduced me to greyhound racing, and to the late George Sherwin, Geoff Watt, and the late Alf Wilkinson, for sharing their knowledge on greyhound manipulation. I would also like to acknowledge the assistance of my colleague and friend, Alex Hauler, for his help and expert advice on greyhound chiropractic. Thanks to Lois Scott and Tiffany Desborough of Veterinary Clinical Sciences for assistance with the manuscript; Tiffany Desborough for handling the greyhounds during photography; Pixie Maloney of the Camperdown Childrens Hospital for photographic illustrations; and to Bozena Jantulik of Veterinary Anatomy for drawing the anatomical illustrations.

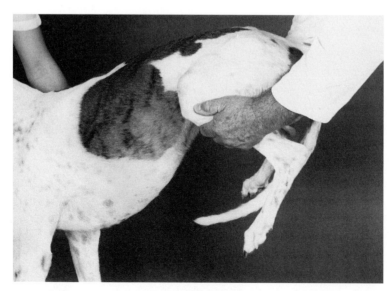

FIGURE 31–33. Mobilization of the hip joint. The hips are fully flexed, the femoral heads rotated, and the flexor muscles of the hip stretched.

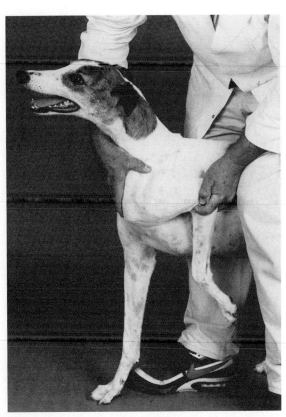

FIGURE 31–34. Flexed shoulder joint manipulation. While standing over the greyhound, fully flex its shoulder joint.

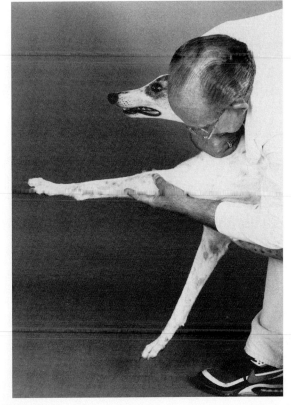

FIGURE 31–35. Extended shoulder joint manipulation. Fully extend the dog's shoulder parallel to the spinal column.

References

1. Withington ET: Hippocrates with an English Translation, 3rd ed. Howard University Press, 1959, p 299.
2. Schiotz EH, Cryiax J: Manipulation Past and Present. London, William Heinemann Medical Books, 1957, pp 5–45.
3. Boje Ove: Laerebog i Fysiurg. Kobenhavn, Munksgaard, 1958.
4. Moltzen H: Treatment of spinal disorders in dogs by manipulation. J Small Anim Pract 4:265–269, 1963.
5. Davis PE: Manipulation, traction, mobilization and stretch exercise in the racing greyhound. *In* Proceedings of the International Racing Greyhound Symposium, Florida Veterinary Medical Association, Orlando, Fla, 1989, pp 55–66.
6. Hauler A: Greyhound manipulation. Proc 140th Post Graduate Committee Refresher Course in Veterinary Science, University of Sydney, 1990, pp 1–34.
7. Lee M, Steven GP, Kelly DW: A finite element model to simulate spinal manipulation. *In* Valliappan S, Pulmano VA, Tin-Loi F (eds): Computational Mechanics. Balkema, Rotterdam, Brookfield, 1993, vol 2, pp 1207–1212.
8. Gatterman MI. Glossary: Chiropractic Management of Spine Related Disorders. Baltimore, Williams & Wilkins, 1990, p 410.
9. Cottrell GW: New, conservative, and exceptionally effective treatment of low back pain. Compr Ther 11(11):59–65, 1985.
10. Cottle LW: Traction in the treatment of canine spinal disorders. J Am Anim Hosp Assoc 8:332–333, 1972.
11. Johnson KA, Davis PE: Drug therapy in surgical musculoskeletal disease. *In* Bojrab MJ, Smeak DD, Bloomberg MS (eds): Disease Mechanisms in Small Animal Surgery, 2nd ed. Philadelphia, Lea & Febiger, 1993, pp 1105–1111.
12. DeLahunta A: Veterinary Neuroanatomy and Clinical Neurology, 2nd ed. Philadelphia, WB Saunders Co, 1983, pp 62–63.
13. Canfield RB: Anatomical Aspects of Perineal Hernia in the Dog. PhD thesis, University of Sydney, 1986, p 177.

CHAPTER 32

FIRST AID AND TRACK CARE OF RACING GREYHOUNDS AND OTHER SPORTING BREEDS

DESMOND P. FEGAN

FIRST AID PROCEDURES

The racing greyhound's pursuit of the lure is so intense that it disregards its health and well-being during its efforts. The desire to win and adrenaline and endorphin release combine to produce pain tolerance that is amazing to witness. Often a racing greyhound will complete the course after sustaining a major bone fracture early in the race. Its drive, discipline, and desire make it the most noble and heroic of the canine species.

When an accident or major trauma occurs, the attending veterinarian must provide, as soon as possible, for control of hemorrhage, relief of pain, tissue support, and control of infection.

Control of Hemorrhage. Hemorrhage is, unfortunately, a common occurrence in sporting dogs throughout the world. Prompt control of the hemorrhage is essential. A tourniquet can be helpful in controlling severe bleeding. Lesser bleeding can be controlled by a pressure bandage. The greyhound of approximately 30 kg has about 2 L of blood (7% of body weight). One of the difficulties faced by a veterinarian attending sports meetings is assessment of the total blood loss. Various indications used for this assessment are:

1. Packed cell volume. PCV of greyhounds is in the range of 68 to 75 per cent during racing and for a short time thereafter.
2. Capillary refill time and mucous membrane color. These are unreliable after exercise. If the animal is in shock, the peripheral circulation will be very poor.
3. General demeanor and physical appearance
4. Visual estimation of blood loss

Fortunately the incidence of hemostatic disorders is very low in most sporting breeds. The three essential components of the hemostatic process are the blood vessel, platelets, and coagulation factors. Vascular integrity in the racing greyhound may be compromised by the high incidence of hyperadrenocorticism.[1] Widespread use of nonsteroidal anti-inflammatory drugs (NSAIDs) can result in functional platelet disorders.

A suggested protocol for the control of hemorrhage is:

Assess nature of blood loss, ie, arterial or venous.
Apply tourniquet or pressure bandage immediately.
Investigate the injury site for blood vessels that can be clamped.
Begin intravenous fluid therapy with Ringer's solution and antibiotics; give blood transfusion, if required.
Débride and thoroughly clean the wound.
Remove tourniquet and examine site for hemorrhage.
Repair the wound with the appropriate suture materials; insert a drain in the most ventral aspect of the wound.
Bandage firmly for 24 hours if anatomically possible, and then change dressings and rebandage for an additional 5 days.

Relief of Pain. Reduction of pain as soon as possible is essential.

The dog should be given some pain-killing medication before it is moved from the track or other sporting arena. Because most sporting activities are public and, in the case of greyhound racing, are broadcasted, it is important that the veterinary profession have a caring and professional image.

Medications available for relief of pain include:

1. Xylazine (1 mg/kg IV or IM) offers poor pain relief but is a good muscle relaxant. It is acceptable to use xylazine in the case of suspected muscular damage.
2. Buprenorphine (0.1 mg/kg IV or IM) offers good pain relief for 8 to 12 hours. It can be given intramuscularly, intravenously, or sublingually for the control of acute pain.
3. Flunixin meglumine is a potent analgesic that is given intravenously or intramuscularly. It should not be used if there is hemorrhage or a possibility of surgical intervention within 24 hours of its administration.

Tissue Support. The initial trauma sustained during these high-level performances can be very severe. Prevention of further damage could be the difference between resumption of a career and euthanasia. The classic example is the distal humeral fracture that progressively serrates the radial nerve, causing permanent paralysis of the distal forelimb. An injured limb is immobilized to relieve pain. The type of support depends on the position and severity of the injury. General principles for supporting injured tissue are to:

1. Accurately diagnose the nature and extent of the injury
2. Cleanse open wounds or fractures before applying support dressing
3. Immobilize the injured area and the joints immediately above and below the injury by using a padded rigid splint, ideally one that will mold to the countours of the bandaged limb, eg, a modified Robert Jones type of bandage

Control of Infection. Many of the arenas where dogs perform are in continuous use, and the disinfection procedures in the kennel blocks and around the track area are often inadequate. Pathogenic bacteria thrive in these conditions. Open wounds sustained in these conditions should be treated as quickly as possible, as the tissue trauma and bacterial contamination rapidly cause infections. The wound contamination should be approached both systemically and locally. Parenteral administration of broad-spectrum antimicrobial drugs is advisable.

Locally, the wound should be cleansed. The surrounding hair may be removed by clipping; however, the wound should be packed with sterile sponges to prevent foreign bodies from causing further contamination. With the sterile pack still in place, the external wound should be thoroughly cleaned with a surgical disinfectant. Any contaminants—for example, clotted blood, sand, or hair—should be removed and the area irrigated liberally with warm isotonic saline. Detergents and skin disinfectants should be kept out of the wound as much as possible as these are irritating to the tissues. Once the external wound and surrounding skin are clean, a dressing or bandage can be applied to the area to await further surgical treatment.

MUSCULOSKELETAL INJURIES

Assuming that all the participants are healthy at the beginning of any canine sporting event, the most common problems are traumatic injuries, which can be categorized into three broad groups: (1) soft tissue, (2) bone, (3) and toe and ligament.

Soft Tissue Injuries. A defect in muscle or tendon is usually sudden in onset and causes a dramatic shortening of stride. However, even though an injury is obvious to the observer, the dog usually completes the race. Invariably this increases the severity of the injury. The positioning of marshals at strategic points around the course could help alleviate this problem. As soon as the injured dog has been restrained, it should be examined by the veterinarian. If the injury is not obvious immediately after the run, the dog should be reexamined 30 to 60 minutes later. It is quite common for a partial tear of the Achilles tendon, flexor carpi ulnaris tendon, or gracilis tendon to cause very little pain immediately after the run. In the case of Achilles tendon, the mild swelling that sometimes accompanies a partial tear is especially difficult to detect.

Rupture of muscle tissue, however, usually is obvious immediately, with extensive hemorrhage and swelling. Dogs develop a limp within minutes. It is imperative to employ the RICE principle—**r**est, **i**ce, **c**ompression, and **e**levation (if feasible). This will promote coagulation and diminish inflammation.

The animal should be restrained or the injured limb immobilized as soon as possible. Cold compresses consisting of a wet towel containing crushed ice can be applied. It should be applied for no longer than 10 minutes as vasoconstriction will not persist indefinitely. After 10 minutes the site can be bandaged, if applicable, until further measures are taken. The injured limb should be elevated. Care should be taken to ensure that drugs that increase blood pressure or cause vasodilation not be given in the first 48 hours after the initial injury as these tend to increase local swelling and pain and impair healing. Xylazine (1 mg/kg) is useful as it causes muscle relaxation, reduces blood pressure, and allows the animal to rest relatively peacefully, even with its leg elevated. An alternative to the use of ice is a magnetic therapy unit used on low frequency and low intensity for 10 minutes every 1 to 4 hours. This reduces inflammatory swelling and is a suitable alternative to ice packing.

Soft tissue injuries can be surgically repaired at the time of occurrence; however, conventional wisdom suggests that we leave these injuries for at least 48 hours before major surgical repair is attempted. The decision to intervene surgically at an early stage should be based on:

1. The severity of the injury
2. The site of injury, eg, some tensor fascia lata tears hemorrhage excessively after the initial first aid, and surgery to prevent this hemorrhage would be the most effective way to achieve an early return to exercise
3. The ability of the trainer or handler to perform basic home-care procedures

Trauma around the head and the eye is a special cause for concern. A severe contusion near the eye may appear as a minor bruise at the time of injury; however, after 24 hours exophthalmos may occur because of the limited space within the orbit. Trauma to the cranium may cause delayed neurological signs referable to head injury. (When such injury is suspected, a preventive intravenous injection of methylprednisolone sodium succinate [10 mg/kg]

is indicated.) Some clinicians also recommend the use of dimethyl sulfoxide (DMSO) in a dosage of 1 gm/kg intravenously twice daily to reduce cerebrospinal fluid pressure. A mannitol drip may prevent intraocular pressure elevation when there has been direct eye trauma.

Falls, collisions, and knocks are all part of competitive sports. Lacerations sustained on the race track or other sporting arena should be treated in accordance with the principles previously outlined. When reasonable cleanliness has been achieved and tissue trauma is minimal, healing by primary intention is likely. Abrasions from falls and subsequent friction burns result in some skin loss.

Toe pad lacerations are of particular concern because of the potential for foreign body penetration. A dog presented for a performance with a prior pad injury may be harboring a foreign body that, although not causing much discomfort during walking on an even surface such as concrete, may be manifested when the dog walks on gravel or is running in betting sports. To ensure that the dog is fit to perform to the best of its ability, these pad injuries must be examined thoroughly.

Bone Damage. Fractures are common in the sporting dog. Greyhound racing is usually conducted on a circular race track with the dogs racing counterclockwise. There are four areas of the skeleton that take much more strain and eventually succumb to fatigue fracture: metacarpal and metatarsal bones, right tarsus, and distal radius and ulna.*

If a veterinarian is available, the first step is to relieve pain. Pethidine (3 mg/kg IM or IV), buprenorphine (10 mg/kg IM or IV or sublingually), and flunixin (1.5 mg/kg IM or IV) are the drugs of choice. Dogs with fractures are likely to be suffering from some degree of hypovolemia, which is treated with warmed intravenous fluids.

The type of fracture determines the next step. Open fractures must be regarded as the most hazardous of wounds in which to control infection. For treatment of an open wound see the section Control of Infection under First Aid Procedures.

Most lower limb fractures lend themselves well to the application of a Robert Jones dressing. Fractures occurring in other areas where bandaging is not feasible require sedation to reduce movement and radiography to assess the long-term prognosis for both racing and retention for breeding or as household pets.

With suspected spinal trauma, a neurological examination is used to localize and assess the severity of the damage. It may not be possible to give a definite diagnosis and prognosis immediately after the race.

Toe and Ligament Damage. Injuries to the phalanges are common, especially on grass surfaces. These are presumably due to the greater torsional forces sustained by the animal on the track. Compared with bone injuries, ligament and tendon injuries are much greater on grass than on sand. Table 32–1 lists the common toe injuries and gives guidelines to the recovery period required for successful return to racing.

First aid procedures applied in the event of an accident may be the most exciting and at times challenging aspect of veterinary care at race and sporting meetings. However, equally important, but more mundane, for the health and well-being of the animal and the overall success of the event are the detection, treatment, and prevention of medical conditions either before the event begins or after exercise. In greyhound racing and in other sports, there is the important duty of reporting any detected injury or illness to the steward or other officials in charge of the meeting.

---

*Editor's Comment: Right metatarsals (especially the third) are more often affected then left metatarsals, and left radius and ulna more often than right.

TABLE 32–1. Common Toe Injuries in the Racing Greyhound

Injury	Recovery Time (Weeks)
P1–P2 collateral ligament rupture	6
Metatarsal–P1 collateral ligament rupture	8
Complete metatarsal–P1 dislocation	8
Sesamoid ligament damage	4
Sesamoid fracture	6
P2 fracture	8
Dorsal elastic ligament rupture	3
Dorsal elastic ligament rupture with avulsed chip from P3	6
Abductor digiti quinti rupture	4
P2–P3 collateral ligament rupture	4

CONDITIONS ENCOUNTERED BEFORE EXERCISE

Dehydration. The many and varied causes of dehydration are as diverse as simple lack of fluid to electrolyte, hormonal, or metabolic disturbances. Three major preventable factors contribute to dehydration in the otherwise healthy dog: travel, temperature, and temperament.

Long-distance travel, especially in inappropriate modes of transport without proper care and attention, will lead to loss of fluids and electrolytes. Dogs transported in the summertime, when environmental temperatures reach 30° C or greater, lose tremendous amounts of fluids through panting. They also exhale carbon dioxide with the water vapor, leaving them with respiratory alkalosis. This in turn leads to preservation of hydrogen ions by the kidney at the expense of potassium to correct this acid-base imbalance. Therefore, not only must the fluids lost in panting be replaced, but the potassium chloride that has been sacrificed by the renal tubules in an attempt to keep the body from becoming too alkaline must also be replaced. Travel over long distances should ideally be in air-conditioned vehicles. The animals should be allowed to have a drink of an isotonic electrolyte mixture or offered water. (Dogs performing in the summertime should have a daily supplement of potassium chloride.)

High environmental *temperature* will lead to dehydration, just as described. It is essential not only to protect animals traveling in heat but also dogs waiting to perform in excessive heat. Holding pens or kennels ideally should be air-conditioned when the environmental temperature is likely to be over 25° C during any meeting or event. Simple systems such as roof sprinklers or fans are sufficient in temperatures below 25° C. Ideally the rules of the competition should provide for administration of oral isotonic solutions of fluids before exercise is begun.

Temperament is often the difference between winning and losing. It has two essential components, inherent and learned: The more adapted an animal becomes to racing or competing, the more stress and dehydration are reduced. Excitable dogs pant, salivate, and bark before they perform. All these activities lead to loss of body fluids and electrolytes. Special care must be taken to ensure that these dogs receive supplements with electrolytes and water before they are kenneled, and the time they are kenneled should be kept to a minimum. In some cases the drug phenytoin has a positive effect on the canine temperament. A dose of 2 to 5 mg/kg may make a dog calmer and more at ease with the situation and surroundings. In most competitive sports the use of drugs is not permitted; however, they can be used while training or breaking in animals in an effort to change some bad habits.

Exertional Rhabdomyolysis; Diabetes Insipidus. Both of these conditions may be stress induced. Prevention of stress is the responsibility of the trainer or handler. Some of the common avoidable causes are: (1) racing a dog over a distance for which it has not been trained; (2) racing dogs in extreme environmental conditions; (3) allowing dogs of unsuitable temperament to progress to racing; (4) administering drugs, especially corticosteroids, that may affect stress tolerance.

With exertional rhabdomyolysis, acute stress causes loss of potassium through the renal tubules and a relative potassium deficit in the extracellular fluid after exercise. This leads to failure of the arteriolar circulation to dilate and adequately perfuse the muscle; consequently a build-up of toxic by-products occurs in the muscle. Even though the problem may be there for 3 days before it becomes clinically apparent, dogs that compete again in this period show dramatic loss of performance and the onset of clinical signs is accelerated. Subclinical rhabdomyolysis should always be part of the differential diagnosis in cases of unexplained poor performance.

Acute diabetes insipidus is seen at the time of racing with or without exertional rhabdomyolysis. Extreme stress, such as high environmental temperature, causes a temporary deficit of antidiuretic hormone (ADH). As soon as the dogs come off the track they develop an insatiable thirst. Volumes of 10 to 15 L can be consumed within minutes. As ADH is not available to reabsorb the electrolytes, there is washout of the renal medullary electrolytes. Unless the ADH and electrolytes are replaced within the first 6 hours after onset of the condition, the chances of survival drop dramatically.

A suggested protocol for treatment is:

Cold hosing, especially on the chest, in an attempt to drop body temperature as quickly as possible.
Do not allow the dog to drink plain water. Restrict drinking to about 2 L of isotonic solution with a sodium-potassium ratio of less than 20:1.
Begin intravenous administration of lactated Ringer's solution, monitor blood gases, and treat acidosis, if present.
Administer ADH (Pitressin) 5 IU for the average greyhound every 4 hours until its drinking habits have stabilized.
Frequently monitor the urinary specific gravity to determine renal concentration. Levels above 1.010 indicate that there is some urinary concentration.

Central Nervous System Abnormalities. Problems associated with the CNS, although relatively rare, are a challenge for the attending clinician. They are either induced by trauma or caused by other conditions associated with exercise. The sporting dog has a competitive and fairly hazardous lifestyle. Collisions with solid objects and other competitors lead to concussion, spinal trauma, or peripheral nerve damage such as radial nerve paralysis. The nature and extent of the trauma may not be immediately obvious; some cases of concussion take 24 hours to become apparent. Dogs with suspected spinal damage require careful handling during placement on a stretcher or blanket and removal to an examination table. A detailed neurological examination should be conducted and neurological injuries treated as needed.

Acute trauma to the spinal cord with paraplegia usually spells the end of an athletic career; however, intravenous use of anti-inflammatory drugs such as methylprednisolone sodium succinate may reduce the inflammation around the spinal cord and prevent serious neuronal damage. (I have seen intervertebral disc herniation occur during a race, creating a fall with transient paralysis, and a subsequent return to normal motor function.)

Other conditions associated with exercise:

1. Cramp is a syndrome with many causes that has confounded clinicians for decades. There appears to be a nervous component in which dogs with very excitable temperaments succumb to cramp during periods of intense exercise.

2. Idiopathic epilepsy may be triggered in states of excitement. Dogs with idiopathic epilepsy are usually excluded from competition.
3. Toxin-induced ataxia is induced by various substances such as the anticholine esterases, found in insecticidal washes, that affect transmission of the nerve impulse across the neuromuscular junction. The condition may be very subtle until the dog starts to exercise. A similar syndrome is found in dogs fed meats containing high levels of preservatives. The sulfur dioxide preservatives destroy vitamin B_1 (thiamine), and this leads to gradual loss of nervous function, similar to Chastek's disease.

Stranguria. Inability to pass urine is a condition suffered by some sporting dogs after intense exercise. The condition is caused by excessive stimulation of the sympathetic nerve supply to the urethral sphincter muscle. It may be present even before the dogs have exercised; more commonly it is apparent within a few hours after exercise. The condition causes dramatic loss of performance.

Treatment is twofold: decompressing the bladder and decreasing urethral resistance. The bladder should be catheterized three times daily and drug therapy (diazepam 2 to 10 mg/kg two or three times a day; phenoxybenzamine 0.5 mg/kg three times a day; dantrolene 1 to 5 mg/kg three times a day) used to control the sphincter spasm for the 2 to 3 days it takes for the condition to subside. Frequent urinalysis and appropriate antimicrobial therapy should be used if urinary infection occurs.

Hyperthermia. After exercise or excitement all dogs have some degree of temperature elevation. The normal temperature range is 37.8° C to 39.3° C. True fever causes elevation of this range. In true hyperthermia the thermoregulatory range remains unchanged. Various causes of hyperthermia seen in sporting dogs include heatstroke, hypothalamic lesions, malignant hyperthermia, seizures, thyrotoxicosis, drug reactions.[2]

Conditions due to increased environmental heat, which includes heatstroke, are the most commonly encountered after exercise. The dogs become distressed, pant excessively, and then go through a period of extreme agitation, presumably looking for some respite from the heat. The extreme body temperature (above 41° C) causes red blood cell disintegration and attempted renal excretion of hemoglobin. If the hyperthermia is uncontrolled, breathing will become loud and labored, and death is imminent.

Dogs with high body temperature before or after exercise may be suffering from one of the conditions just listed, or a febrile process may be present. Malignant hyperthermia is a very rare hereditary condition usually triggered by exposure to inhalant anesthetics or, rarely, caffeine. Prolonged status epilepticus elevates body temperature. Excessive thyroid hormone output or oversupplementation increases the metabolic rate and, in turn, elevates temperature.

The most vital aspect of treatment is the reduction of body temperature. Hosing down the dog with cool water will allow the greatest heat exchange between body fluids and the water. In extreme cases, cool water enemas will further reduce the body temperature. In most cases some dehydration occurs and intravenous fluid therapy is needed.

Tail Trauma. Working dogs are generally happy dogs. Their enthusiasm for the contest is usually expressed by excessive tail wagging, with no awareness for the damage they inflict on this poorly innervated extremity.

A light bandage is sometimes enough to cushion the blows; however, at times the trauma becomes so severe that the dog starts some self-mutilation by licking and/or biting. A key ring attached to the tail by tape and secured underneath the body with an elastic stocking will stop further wagging. Heavy bandages with or without solid splints tend to trigger more vigorous shaking and annoy the dog so much that it usually devours the dressing, splint, and the

underlying tail. Hanging fabric down the inside walls of the kennel will also reduce tail contact with the hard surface of the wall. If these conservative methods of management fail, the only alternative is amputation of the end of the tail.

Track Leg. Track leg, or ''Jack,'' is a hematoma and periosteal swelling on the medial aspect, usually of the left tibia. Track leg is caused by interference and injury in some part of the musculoskeletal structure causing abnormal gait whereby the medial tibia strikes the lateral condyle of the elbow or the lateral aspect of the lower front limb. About 50 per cent of cases are related to a left shoulder injury, 25 per cent to a right hindleg injury, and the remainder to other injuries or conformational disorders in the dog. Fresh track leg is soft, edematous, and painful. Chronic track leg is a hard, painless swelling and may be a legacy of a previous, corrected injury. Dogs with fresh track leg should not be performing as there is a strong likelihood that an undetected injury could be aggravated by further exercise. These dogs should be thoroughly examined, with particular attention being paid to the left shoulder and the right hindleg. If the dog is less than 2 years old, metacarpal soreness on either front leg may be the precipitating cause. It is always advisable to conduct another physical examination the next day to ensure that there are no further injuries needing treatment.

DUTIES OF VETERINARIANS ATTENDING GREYHOUND RACE MEETINGS

Veterinarians at these races are generally invited by the racing club, with the conduct of the meeting being controlled by the stipendiary stewards. The veterinarian invariably acts as an advisor to the stewards on animal welfare–related matters. The veterinarian's duty is to ensure that any pain or suffering endured by the racing dog is minimized and that the steward in charge is informed of any injury or illness that may detrimentally affect the dog's racing performance.

TABLE 32–2. Checklist for Veterinarians Attending Sporting Meetings

Anesthetic: ketamine, xylazine, and atropine or equivalent, lidocaine; portable oxygen cylinder
Sedatives: diazepam; acetylpromazine 2 mg/ml injectable, acetylpromazine tablets
Analgesic: flunixin meglumine, buprenorphine, pethidine; oral NSAIDs for dispensing
Antibiotic: lincomycin, amoxicillin, clavulanic acid; oral antibiotic for dispensing
Corticosteroids: dexamethasone, methylprednisolone sodium succinate
Bandage and splinting materials: elastic adhesive tape 2.5 cm, 5 cm, and 7.5 cm; cotton wool, crepe bandage, paraffin gauze, fiberglass casting material, bandage scissors
Syringes and needles
Euthanasia solution and disposal bag
Surgical kit and suture materials
Supportive therapy: Ringer's solution, mannitol solution, saline solution, whole blood, and plasma
Intravenous dripsets and intravenous catheters
Instruments for clinical examination: thermometer, stethoscope, otoscope, opthalmoscope, hematocrit, and centrifuge
Tourniquet
Disinfectant suitable for skin and wound cleansing
Antidotes: Vitamin K_1, atropine, pralidoxime (2-PAM)
Alligator forceps for removal of grass awns and foreign bodies

The veterinarian must have a kit so that he or she can provide basic first aid to any injured participant. Table 32–2 lists items included in such a kit. Any person undertaking racetrack duties has an obligation to become acquainted with the injuries common to racing greyhounds.

References

1. Watson ADJ: Proceedings 187. Post Graduate Committee of Veterinary Science, University of Sydney.
2. Zaslow JM: Trauma and Critical Care. Philadelphia, Lea & Febiger, 1984.

SECTION VII

REPRODUCTION

CHAPTER 33

BREEDING SOUNDNESS EXAMINATION OF THE WORKING DOG

PHILIP G. A. THOMAS \ NIGEL R. PERKINS

Unique among domestic animals, the working bitch has infrequent cycles and a short breeding life limited to a few estrous cycles following retirement from athletic activity. Establishment of breeding soundness in the working dog and brood bitch therefore must be rapid and thorough. This chapter details the procedures involved in breeding soundness examination (BSE) in the working dog and bitch. In each case, procedures are divided into those that are an essential part of the BSE and those that may be used as an adjunct in selected cases.

FEMALE BREEDING SOUNDNESS EXAMINATION

Minimum Data Base

History

Signalment. The breed, age, weight, and athletic history of the bitch should be recorded. Small breeds cycle more frequently than larger breeds. The mean age at the onset of cycling has been reported as 9.6 to 13.9 months; however, bitches may begin to cycle as late as 23 months.[1] Puberal estrus and the first estrus following retirement may be accompanied by few external signs and may not result in ovulation. Difficulty detecting this heat is compounded in the absence of an intact male dog.

Kennel management. The general health, diet, and exercise of the group should be noted. Parameters of kennel demographics include number of dogs in the kennel, number of breeding females, number of breeding males, numbers in each female or male group, and area devoted to each dog. Disease control and prevention, routine worming, vaccination, and heartworm protocols should be recorded along with hygiene and cleaning procedures, the isolation system for animals entering kennels, and whelping management. Relevant information regarding previous reproductive parameters that pertain to the population may allow the clinician to distinguish between specific problems of the individual and ''herd'' problems.

Parameters that might be recorded include average interestrus time, pregnancies per bred cycle, number of live pups per bred cycle, occurrence rates of reproductive conditions (eg, dystocia, eclampsia, mastitis, cesarean section, subinvolution), average litter size and weight, and neonatal morbidity and mortality rates.

Systemic health. A quantitative assessment should be made of the bitch's diet in light of requirements through various stages of the reproductive cycle. Note should be taken of supplements and additives and their relative levels. Few significant data pertaining to optimal nutritional programs for the brood bitch have been published; however, history taking should include close examination of feed additives, particularly those purported to ''promote fertility,'' because no feed additive has been shown to have this effect in male or female dogs. Prior or existing systemic and local diseases may have direct or indirect ramifications for the reproductive tract or the endocrine axes that control reproductive function. Although the effects of drugs on reproductive function are not well documented, some chemicals (including steroids, notably testosterone in greyhound bitches [Fig. 33–1], antimitotic agents, and some antimicrobials) have been shown to adversely affect cyclicity, fertility, and fetal development.[2] Vomiting, polydipsia, polyuria, skin and hair coat abnormalities, obesity or emaciation, altered exercise, or cold intolerance may herald an endocrine disease and should be noted.

Cycling history. Although variations in the regularity of estrus may occur in young and aged bitches, sudden increases or decreases in the period between heats in a mature bitch may indicate an endocrine abnormality.[1] If available, the average duration of estrus and proestrus and the interestrus interval should be recorded. Overt pseudopregnancy may be interpreted as a normal event in the bitch and is an indication that ovulation accompanied the previous estrus.[3] Results of previous diagnostic aids used in breeding management should be recorded. These may include changes in vulval morphology, nature of the vaginal discharge, vaginal cytology, vaginoscopy, and progesterone assays. Results provide obvious information about cyclicity and ovulation. Any exogenous

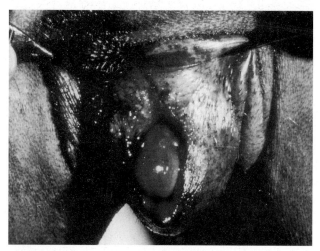

FIGURE 33–1. This greyhound bitch had been treated repeatedly with anabolic steroids. The swollen hyperemic clitoris protrudes between the vulval labia at the ventral commissure of the vulva.

steroid administration, including anabolics or drugs to suppress or induce estrus or ovulation, may affect subsequent reproductive function.

Breeding history. The rationale supporting the decision to begin breeding at previous heats should be scrutinized. Was the decision based on time from the beginning of clinical signs (the "day count"), receptivity, vaginal cytology, or progesterone assays? Canine spermatozoa have the ability to survive in the genital tract of the bitch for a period of 5 days or more, and conception can result from breedings that take place from the end of proestrus until the end of standing estrus.[4, 5] Nevertheless, the most common cause of

failure of conception is poor management resulting in mistimed breeding.[6]

Some of the clinical and endocrine events of the normal estrus cycle are summarized in Figure 33–2. Changes in vulvar morphology and discharge are unreliable.[5, 7] Some bitches may be receptive in late proestrus, while others, notably maidens and socially dominant bitches, may refuse to stand throughout estrus. Vaginal cytology provides useful information if the cytology samples are examined serially. Cornification index is the proportion of superficial and anuclear epithelial cells on a vaginal cytology assay (Fig. 33–2). Cornification of vaginal epithelial cells progresses until about the time of the onset of receptivity. No change will then be detected in cytology until diestrus. A single cytology assay is therefore meaningless in timing breeding.[8] Progesterone assays that predict the preovulatory luteinizing hormone (LH) surge give the most reliable method of establishing the best time to breed.[6, 7] Although a single well-timed mating will result in pregnancy and normal litter size, repeated breedings are more likely to produce desirable results. Because canine spermatozoa have a prolonged life within the genital tract of the female, it is not necessary to breed more frequently than every second day. In an expected receptive estrus of 7 to 9 days, three breedings at intervals of 2 to 3 days would be considered optimal for fertility.

The decision to stop breeding is equally important. The sudden cessation of receptivity and a marked change in vaginal cytology reliably indicates the onset of diestrus.[8] Counting days to determine when to stop breeding is unreliable.[9]

A record of the duration of the tie (see Chapter 35) and whether it was "inside" or "outside" should be made. The term *outside tie* refers to the instance when the swollen bulbus glandis is not within the vaginal vault. Outside ties may indicate the presence of strictures in the vestibule or vagina of the bitch. Because an anatomically "normal" breeding involves swelling of the bulbus glandis within the vaginal vault, it is reasonable to assume that fertility resulting from outside ties may be reduced, although this

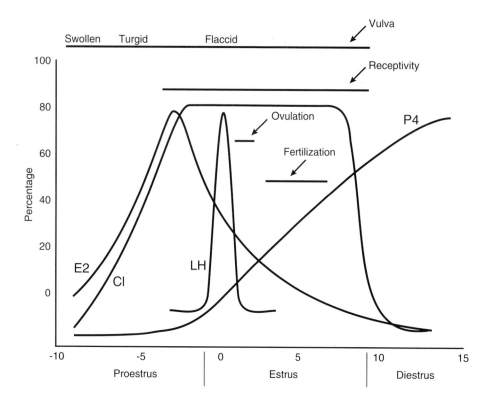

FIGURE 33–2. Representation of some of the endocrine and clinical events during estrus and proestrus in the bitch. Cornification index (CI) and hormonal values, including estrogen (E2), progesterone (P4), and luteinizing hormone (LH), are given as percentage of maximum levels attained. Days relative to the LH peak are shown on the x-axis.

premise has not been tested. The duration of the tie has not been linked with infertility. A tie of 10 to 50 minutes can be considered normal, and short instances of 1 to 3 minutes may indicate incomplete ejaculation.

If artificial insemination was used in previous breedings, the technique should be investigated and the number of motile spermatozoa used at each breeding recorded. Likewise, if frozen semen was used, the type of insemination (vaginal versus intrauterine) is pertinent, as are procedures for freezing, thawing, handling, and timing of insemination. Frozen-thawed semen has reduced ability to traverse the cervix and a life of 12 to 24 hours (reviewed by Concannon and Battista).[10] Artificial insemination is discussed in Chapter 36.

Pregnancy and parturition Previous litters and numbers of pups per litter should be recorded, as should numbers of stillborn, mummified, weakborn pups, or losses between birth and whelping along with any diagnostic examination of those pups. If pregnancy was diagnosed in the bitch with subsequent failure to whelp, the method and time of pregnancy diagnosis should be recorded. If clinical signs accompanied pregnancy loss, they are relevant. Aborted fetuses or vulvar discharge should be recorded, along with any diagnostic pathology.[11]

Individual reproductive parameters. Parameters can be recorded that keep track of the level of breeding efficiency in individual females, most of which are similar to group parameters. The most comprehensive of these for assessing female fertility is the number of live pups per bred cycle.[12]

Physical Examination. Systemic diseases and primary diseases of organs other than the reproductive system may influence reproductive performance. Cushing's disease, hypothyroidism, pituitary neoplasia, adrenal neoplasia, and severe debilitating diseases including parasitism and paraneoplastic syndromes are some conditions that can have ramifications for the reproductive system. Primary reproductive tract disorders such as pyometra may result in disease of other organs or systemic illness. Some infectious processes may be manifested in reproductive function while affecting multiple organs. Canine herpesvirus infection is an example.[11] For these reasons a physical examination is indicated in all infertile animals and should include the mammary glands, which must be inspected for abnormal discharge or enlargement.

Noninvasive examination of the posterior reproductive tract should precede invasive procedures. Vulval size, turgidity, conformation, integrity, and the presence or absence of discharge can provide information regarding stage of cycle, vaginitis, pyometra, vaginal foreign bodies, and space-occupying lesions.[13, 14] The clitoris may be swollen under the influence of large amounts of sex steroids or their analogues—for example, greyhound bitches receiving testosterone preparations to prevent estrus. Endogenous steroids from steroid-producing tumors may cause the same abnormality. Rarely an os clitoris may be present, or the clitoris may assume the appearance of the penis in intersex conditions. Digital examination should follow visual inspection and should precede passage of instruments or diagnostic tools into the anterior vagina. An exception to this rule may be made if uncontaminated cultures are to be obtained from the anterior vagina. Digital examination should include the vulva, vestibule, vestibulovaginal junction, and posterior and anterior vagina for mucosal consistency and degree of crenelation which may indicate stage of cycle. In addition, the vulva and vagina should be examined for strictures, adhesions, space-occupying lesions, and foreign bodies and to ensure patency prior to breeding or artificial insemination.

Transrectal digital palpation will allow examination of the reproductive tract to the pelvic brim of the bitch. The finger is swept from side to side across the bitch's anterior pubis. The cervix is located ventral to the rectum and used as a landmark by which to locate the remainder of the tubular tract posteriorly, and for exami-

nation of the uterine body. Transabdominal palpation using the thumb and fingers of one hand or the fingertips of both hands allows digital examination of the tubular tract. Palpation usually begins at the cervix or uterine body located ventral to the rectum and dorsal to the bladder. Palpation then extends forward to include the uterine horns. The ovaries are not commonly palpable unless grossly enlarged. A technique involving both transrectal palpation with the forefinger of one hand and transabdominal palpation with the other hand allows ready localization of the posterior tubular tract. Rectal and abdominal palpation alone or together provides information about the size, consistency, and tone of the vagina, cervix, and uterine body and horns and the presence of uterine distention with fluid, fetuses, or gas.

Clinical Pathology. A complete hemogram, urinalysis, and serum biochemistry profile may be obtained to isolate parameters indicating underlying disease, especially renal, adrenal, hepatic, and endocrine, that may affect reproductive function without necessarily showing signs in the reproductive system work-up. For example, the sex steroid hormones are metabolized by the liver. Hepatic disease may therefore effectively increase the life of circulating steroids.

Vaginal Cytology. Passage of any instrument into the vagina should adhere to the following protocol: The instrument or diagnostic tool must be sterile. The perineum must be cleaned and patted dry. Except in vaginal culture, passage of the instrument is preceded by vaginal examination. The instrument may be lubricated before being directed through the vulva at the level of the dorsal commissure and following the dorsalmost aspect of the vestibule and vagina. This avoids inadvertent irritation of the clitoris and bypasses the potential impediments of the clitoral fossa and the urethral orifice. Alternatively, a vaginal speculum may be used to avoid these structures. Slight resistance may be encountered at the vestibulovaginal junction.

Vaginal cells for cytological examination are obtained by sampling the anterior vagina with a saline-moistened cotton-tipped swab, transferring cells to a microscope slide and staining with new methylene blue, Wright-Geimsa, or trichrome stain. Serial sampling of exfoliated vaginal mucosal cells aid in identification of estrus cycle stage (Figs. 33–2 and 33–3). In addition, vaginal cytology provides information regarding vaginitis, vaginal neoplasia, and diseases of the uterus which discharge through an open cervix, including postpartum metritis, subinvolution of placental sites, cystic endometrial hyperplasia, and pyometra. Bitches with vaginitis yield vaginal smears that contain neutrophils and may contain red blood cells in addition to epithelial cells.[15] The neutrophils may be healthy or degenerate and often contain intracellular bacteria. In chronic vaginitides, macrophages or lymphocytes are occasionally seen. Bitches in proestrus or diestrus may show cytology patterns similar to vaginitis; however, in both cases the neutrophils present do not persist.[8]

Vaginal tumors such as fibropapillomas (polyps), leiomyomas, and transmissible venereal cell tumors exfoliate cells that can be present in vaginal cytology smears (Fig. 33–4). The vagina may be a site of secondary neoplastic invasion. For example, transitional cell tumors originating in the urinary tract may occasionally extend to the vagina. Draining pyometra will discharge through the cervix. Degenerate neutrophils, occasional vacuolated endometrial cells, and vaginal epithelial cells are present. The epithelial cells may be misshapen and have poorly defined borders. Bacteria are present on some but not all occasions.

Lochia will be discharged for up to 3 weeks after whelping. Cytological study may indicate vaginal epithelial cells as well as endometrial cells and large amounts of mucus with red blood cells and neutrophils. Uteroverdin, a metabolite of the marginal hematomas that form around the edges of the canine zonary placenta, may be present and may cause green discoloration of vaginal

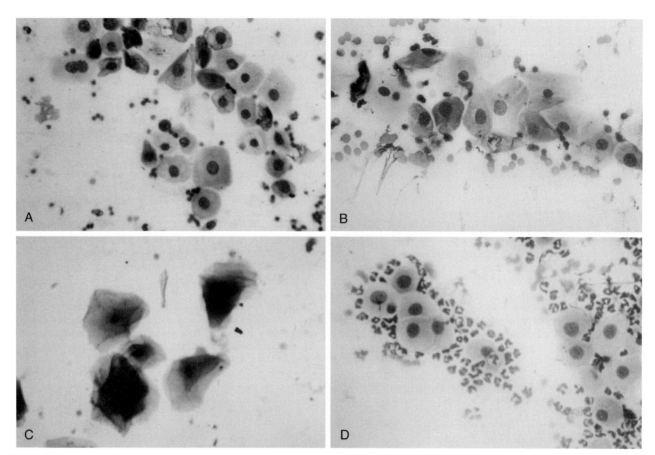

FIGURE 33–3. Representative vaginal cytologic findings. *A,* early proestrus with parabasal cells, intermediate cells, and plentiful erythrocytes. *B,* mid proestrus: epithelial cells showing condensing nuclear chromatin, increased cytoplasm, and angular edges. *C,* estrus: all epithelial cells superficial or anuclear; note debris is gone from the background. *D,* diestrus: note sudden reappearance of noncornified cells and dramatic neutrophil "shower."

discharge any time after placental separation begins. Postpartum bitches with metritis may have all the above cell types in vaginal cytology, especially neutrophils and bacteria, but in addition occasionally show muscle fibers if retained fetuses are the inciting factor. Subinvolution of placental sites is a postpartum disorder characterized by persistence of trophoblastic cells, which continue

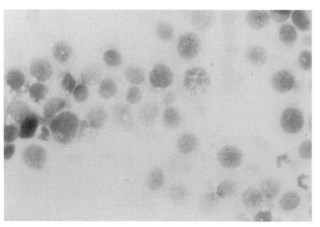

FIGURE 33–4. Example of the use of cytology in diagnosis of vaginal disease. In this case the characteristic chains of vacuolated cells indicate the presence of a transmissible venereal tumor.

to grow in the uterine mucosa. The bitch is healthy but has a persistent red vaginal discharge composed usually of red blood cells, occasional neutrophils, and possibly characteristic trophoblast cells.

Vaginal Culture. Obtaining of cultures, if necessary, should precede other invasive procedures. Samples for aerobic culture should be taken from the anterior vagina with a guarded culture swab. There is overwhelming evidence that normal, fertile bitches have bacterial flora colonizing the genital mucosa and that these bacteria include opportunistic pathogens.[16] Populations and numbers vary between breeds and between cycle stages and include *Pasteurella multocida, Escherichia coli, Mycoplasma* spp, and beta-hemolytic streptococci. The organisms may occur in mixed populations; however, it is possible to recover a pure culture from a fertile bitch. With the exception of open-cervix uterine disease such as discharging pyometra, there is no evidence to suggest that vaginal cultures represent uterine conditions. There is no rational justification for prebreeding vaginal culture in fertile bitches.[16]

Vaginal culture may be indicated in infertile bitches as part of a routine work-up. Aerobic culture is usually sufficient, although cultures for mycoplasma or ureaplasma may occasionally be necessary. To obtain some quantitative idea of organisms present, immediate plating is appropriate; however, if samples are to be held, transport media should be used. The results of vaginal cultures must be interpreted with caution. Consideration should be given to concurrent physical examination and vaginal cytology, in addition to the number and species of organism, when one is attempting to attach significance to the results of vaginal cultures.

Vaginoscopy. Reproductive tract inspection can be performed in two stages. The first involves evaluation of the clitoris, clitoral fossa, and vestibule with a duck-billed vaginal speculum. Vaginoscopy is then performed in the standing awake bitch or in the sedated bitch in ventral recumbency. The vaginoscope must be long enough to explore the far anterior vagina. The vagina of the greyhound bitch is 15 to 25 cm long. A pediatric proctoscope or a flexible or rigid endoscope is appropriate. There is some advantage in being able to insufflate with air or dilate the anterior vagina with sterile saline.

Commonly, the lubricated endoscope is passed forward to the anterior vagina and structures evaluated as the endoscope is withdrawn; however, the operator should be aware that submucosal hemorrhage will be induced by passage of the endoscope. As the endoscope is withdrawn the dorsal median postcervical fold will be apparent. This structure hangs down into the potential space that is the vaginal lumen and creates the appearance of a cervix.[17] The cervix may not be visible because of obstruction of the anterior vaginal lumen by this fold and the anatomy of the canine cervix, which lies at a 45-degree angle and opens almost ventrally into a ventral vaginal fornix. Vaginoscopic examination is used to evaluate mucosal integrity; to determine stage of estrus; to evaluate vaginal masses, lesions, and abnormalities; to obtain specimens for biopsy and culture; and to determine the source of a vulvar discharge.[13, 14, 16]

Elective and Invasive Procedures

Ultrasound Examination. Real-time ultrasonic examination may be performed with the bitch in dorsal recumbency or standing. The uterus is located dorsal to the bladder and the ovaries caudal to the kidneys.[19] Ovarian events such as the presence of follicles or corpora lutea accompanied by typical changes in uterine architecture may help the clinician establish cycle stage or aid in the management of reproductive diseases. Diagnostic and prognostic information can be gleaned in cystic endometrial hyperplasia, pyometra, postpartum metritis, subinvolution of placental sites, cysts of ovarian or parovarian structures, and ovarian tumors (Fig. 33–5).

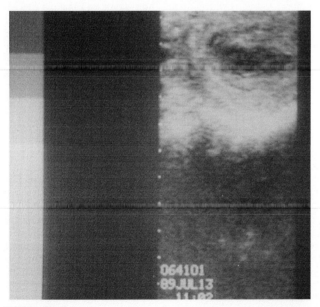

FIGURE 33–5. Sonogram of a canine uterus. The uterine horn is shown in transverse cross section. A hypoechoic or dark image in the center of the uterine cross section indicates presence of luminal fluid in this bitch.

Radiology. Radiology is useful in monitoring diseases of late pregnancy and is also used in identifying large space-occupying lesions of the female reproductive tract that grossly increase the size of the organ involved or that displace abdominal viscera. Closed pyometra is an example. Contrast studies may rarely be of use in determining the extent of vaginal anomalies and masses.

Thyroid Function Test. The role of thyroid hormones in canine reproduction is not fully understood. Hypothyroidism has been a scapegoat for a plethora of other causes of infertility and has been overdiagnosed. Caution is advised in the interpretation of test results.[20] Establishing a cause and effect between hypothyroidism and clinical infertility may be difficult. A deficiency of circulating thyroxine (T_4) or triiodothyronine (T_3) may result from abnormalities of the hypothalamus or the pituitary gland, although most cases originate in the thyroid gland.

Traditionally, basal levels of T_4 were considered a more useful indicator of thyroid function than T_3 concentration. However, in euthyroid dogs many factors can cause low T_4 results and lead to an incorrect diagnosis of hypothyroidism. These include age, breed, hourly fluctuations, obesity, starvation, concurrent disease or drug administration, corticosteroids, estrus, pregnancy, and antithyroid hormone antibodies. Low basal T_4 along with appropriate clinical signs provides only an indication for stimulation testing rather than a diagnosis. Stimulation testing with thyroid-stimulating hormone (TSH) is now considered mandatory to diagnose hypothyroidism.[20]

Endocrine Testing. Gonadotropin-releasing hormone (GnRH) from the hypothalamus drives reproductive function in bitches. In response to GnRH, pulses of the anterior pituitary hormones, follicle-stimulating hormone (FSH), and luteinizing hormone (LH) are responsible for follicular recruitment, development, and ovulation. Maintenance of the corpus luteum of pregnancy or diestrus is due to LH and prolactin. Estrogen and progesterone are produced by the developing follicle and the corpus luteum, respectively. Although often misused, peripheral hormonal levels may indicate reproductive dysfunction.[21] Reproductive hormones may be secreted in a pulsatile manner, making single samples and basal levels of limited value. Repetitive sampling for frequency, duration, and amplitude of pulses or stimulation testing to achieve maximal release is more informative.[21, 22]

Progesterone will rise above basal levels toward the end of proestrus (see Fig. 33–2) and remain elevated until about 2 months after ovulation and cannot be used to distinguish diestrus from pregnancy in bitches. Increased progesterone implies a functional corpus luteum and therefore usually indicates that both a normal LH peak and ovulation have occurred. Peripheral estradiol increases in late proestrus and again at the end of diestrus or pregnancy. Elevated estradiol levels may occur in bitches with follicular cysts or granulosa cell tumors. Testosterone also increases during proestrus and estrus in bitches. Elevated levels may occur in some intersex conditions. Relaxin is increased from midgestation and is specific to pregnancy.[23] Some reference values for commonly assayed steroid hormones are listed in Table 33–1.

Exploratory Laparotomy. The invasive nature and expense of this procedure may be justified by the knowledge gained. A ventral midline laparotomy is performed under general anesthetic, the tract

TABLE 33–1. Peripheral Single Sample Measurements of Reproductive Hormone Concentrations in the Normal Bitch

Steroid	Basal	Peak	Peak Occurs In
Progesterone	<2 ng/ml	10–85 ng/ml	Pregnancy diestrus
Estradiol	5–10 pg/ml	50–100 pg/ml	Late proestrus, late diestrus
Testosterone	<0.1 ng/ml	0.3–1.0 ng/ml	Early estrus

is gently raised to the incision, and isolated. The length of the tract may then be examined for abnormalities. Anatomical anomalies may be present, including absence of part or all of the tubular tract.[24] Varying degrees of intersex may be obvious. The ovary and vestments are examined for the presence of disease. The ovary is usually shrouded in the ovarian bursa, an extension of the mesosalpinx, which is the fold of peritoneum investing the ovary. The ovary is easily isolated; however, visualization may be impeded by this structure. Because the bursa is closely apposed to the delicate fimbriae of the infundibulum of the oviduct, handling should be done with great care. It is possible to ascertain ovarian status from gross examination. Cystic structures that may or may not contribute to infertility are occasionally present in and around the ovary. Following gross examination, samples for uterine luminal culture, cytological examination, and endometrial biopsy can be obtained through a small incision on the antimesometrial border of each uterine horn.

It has been suggested that oviductal patency be established by retrograde flushing of saline or dyes from the tip of each uterine horn into the ipsilateral oviduct. In our experience it is difficult to flush the oviduct in a retrograde manner at any stage of estrus; this procedure is fraught with potential dangers and the information obtained is of questionable value. Abdominal laparoscopy will be more widely used in the diagnosis of infertility as manipulation and sampling techniques improve.

Karyotype. The examination of peripheral lymphocytes for karyotype anomalies is indicated when the various forms of intersex are suspected. Abnormalities of sex chromosomes, including XO, XXX, XX/XY, and XY had all been described in phenotypic bitches. Such bitches may fail to have cycles or have irregular cycles, or may have a small vulva, enlarged clitoris, or ambiguous external genitalia.[24] Results of karyotyping should be used in conjunction with thorough examination of internal and external genitalia for anatomical abnormalities and, if necessary, biopsy of the gonad.

MALE BREEDING SOUNDNESS EXAMINATION

Minimum Data Base

History. Since many diseases of the reproductive system are secondary to or coincident with diseases of other organ systems, history that pertains to all organ systems is relevant, in addition to specific reproductive history. The following history should be recorded:

Signalment. Breed and age of the dog.

General history. Diet, medications, prior diseases, evidence of endocrine dysfunction (vomiting, polyuria, polydipsia, exercise intolerance, skin and coat abnormalities), and kennel demographics, including disease prevalence.

Reproductive history. Prior preputial discharge; preputial mass; scrotal redness, pain or swelling; signs of feminization and pain on urination or defecation.

Breeding history. Interest of the dog in estrous bitches, libido, details of the last mating (number of breedings, natural or artificial insemination) and the diagnostic tools used to manage breeding (for example, vaginal cytology or progesterone assays).

Conception history. Date of the last litter sired, conception rate (bitches pregnant/bitches bred), occurrence of abortion in bitches bred to this male, average litter size, and the occurrence of hereditary defects in offspring.

Clinical pathology. Results and dates of prior thyroid and adrenal function tests, *Brucella canis* titers, and semen evaluations.

Physical Examination. A complete examination of all body systems should precede specific reproductive tract examination, which may then be conducted by anatomical partitioning.

The canine testes are ovoid and aligned dorsocaudally within the scrotum. The scrotal skin is thin, may be pigmented and covered with hair, has many sweat glands and little subcutaneous fat. The testes are usually present in the scrotum 10 to 14 days after birth, although they may not be palpable until some weeks later. The normal dog has two scrotal testes that are bilaterally symmetrical and have a smooth, homogeneous, and elastic consistency. Testicular size may be recorded by measuring scrotal width with calipers or direct testicular measurement by ultrasonography. Testicular weight is highly correlated with sperm production. Testicular weight is also related to body weight, testes size, and scrotal width.[25] The epididymis, vas deferens, and spermatic cords should be palpated for evidence of abnormalities. The head of the epididymis lies dorsocranially, the body runs down the medial surface of the testes, and the tail of the epididymis is caudal.

The penis of the dog has muscular, cavernous, and bony components. The glans penis consists of two parts: the bulbus glandis containing erectile tissue surrounding the midpoint of the urethra and os penis, and the pars longa glandis with erectile tissue dorsally and laterally. The os penis reaches from the bulbus glandis almost to the tip of the glans. The penis and prepuce should be palpated in situ; the penis should then be extruded and, together with the internal lamina of the prepuce, examined for evidence of inflammation, discharge, trauma, foreign body, or masses. The examination may be repeated on the erect penis at the time of semen collection. The os penis is palpated through the nonerect penis for fractures or congenital anomalies.

The prostate gland is the only accessory sex organ in the dog. It lies on the cranial pelvic floor and surrounds the urethra just caudal to the neck of the bladder. It is symmetrical, globular, and divided into two halves by a median septum. Changes in size, consistency, and symmetry are detected by rectal palpation. Palpation is facilitated by elevating the forequarters of the dog and using the free hand to isolate the prostate in the abdomen and move it toward the rectum.

Clinical Pathology. Complete blood count, biochemistry profile, and urinalysis will aid in detection of primary reproductive tract diseases as well as underlying systemic illness, and are valuable prognostic tools. A *Brucella canis* titer should be obtained every 6 months in an active breeding dog. Disorders of the adrenal and thyroid glands have been linked to infertility in other species, although the relationship between hypothyroidism and subfertility has not been well established in the dog. Diagnosis of abnormal adrenal or thyroid function is contingent upon results of stimulation testing rather than resting hormone levels.[20]

Semen Collection and Evaluation. Semen is best collected in the presence of an estrous bitch with manual stimulation. Some dogs may ejaculate in the presence of a nonestrous bitch or absence of a bitch, particularly when trained to the procedure. In the absence of a bitch, use of the pheromone methyl *p*-hydroxybenzoate or swabs soaked in estrous vaginal fluid may act as a stimulus. A right-handed collector approaches the right side of the dog. The penis is gently massaged within the prepuce until penile engorgement begins. The dog's penis is then extruded from the prepuce and gentle pressure applied with the forefinger and thumb to the penis just proximal to the bulbus glandis. Ejaculation is induced by masturbation, with care taken to avoid hemorrhage from superficial vessels caused by vigorous manipulation. The presperm fraction is clear and small in volume (< 2 ml) and is rapidly followed by the cloudy, sperm-rich fraction (0.1 to 3 ml).[26] Pelvic thrusting will accompany the first and possibly the second fraction. The third fraction contains prostatic fluid. It is clear and voluminous (up to 40 ml). The dog may "step over" the arm of the operator during ejaculation of the third fraction. The collection apparatus may be changed between second and third fraction for separate collection of the prostatic fluid. It is not usually necessary to collect all the prostatic fraction. Care should be taken to ensure that the dog loses the erection and that the penis is retracted within the prepuce within 10 to 20 minutes. Semen collection apparatus and the collected sample should be held at 37C until processing is complete. Potential spermicidal agents such as detergents, some gels, dirt, and bacteria should be avoided. Exposure of the semen to lubricants and to latex should be minimized. Failure to collect an adequate sample may be caused by poor technique, inexperience of the dog, unfamiliar surroundings, excessive disturbance in the collection area, lack of an estrous bitch, or pain associated with reproductive or musculoskeletal lesions.

Semen should be evaluated immediately. Representative values for a normal spermiogram are given in Table 33–2. The evaluated ejaculate is usually composed of the first and second fractions with or without part of the third fraction. Volume is recorded for calculation of total numbers of spermatozoa. Color should be cloudy to milky white. Abnormal color may occur with urine contamination or the presence of red or white blood cells. pH of semen is normally in the range of 6.1 to 7.0 and is useful in selecting antibiotics with which to treat prostatitis,[27] because accumulation of high antibiotic concentrations in the prostate is facilitated if a basic antibiotic is administered to a dog with acidic prostatic fluid and vice versa.

A drop of the raw ejaculate is added to a prewarmed glass slide, coverslipped, and evaluated by phase contrast microscopy for progressive motility, spermatozoal agglutination, and the presence of debris. Progressive motility is the number of spermatozoa showing linear, progressive forward motion expressed as a percentage of all spermatozoa present. Debris and agglutination may be scored on an arbitrary scale. Concentrated ejaculates may be diluted for estimation of progressive motility by addition of isotonic saline, sodium citrate, or semen extender. A normal ejaculate has >70 per cent progressive motility.[28]

Total numbers of ejaculated spermatozoa are estimated by multiplying the concentration of spermatozoa (calculated from a sample of known dilution in a hemocytometer) with the volume of the ejaculate. Concentration of spermatozoa usually falls in the range of 10 to 300 million/ml of semen. Total semen numbers are dependent on testicular weight and are therefore influenced by body weight. From a dog weighing 20 to 50 kg, one would expect 300 million to 2 billion spermatozoa.[25]

Spermatozoal morphology should be examined by staining smears with modified Wright-Giemsa or nigrosin-eosin stain. Thin smears should be stained for 5 minutes in each of the Wright-Giemsa reagents. This stain has the advantage of staining somatic cells in addition to spermatozoa. Alternatively, 1 drop of nigrosin-eosin is mixed with a drop of semen, and a spreader slide is used to make an even smear of stained cells. The proportions of spermatozoa with normal and abnormal morphology are recorded. Abnormal spermatozoa may be recorded as specific defects or by the classifications major/minor (indicating the proposed effect of the defect on fertility) or primary/secondary (indicating the suspected site of origin of the defect). Abnormal head shape, nuclear vacuolations, double heads, midpieces or tail, midpiece structural abnormalities, coiling of the midpiece, and proximal cytoplasmic droplets are primary abnormalities. Secondary abnormalities include distal cytoplasmic droplets, detached heads, simple bent tails, and loosened or detached acrosomes. Much research is needed to determine which defects are associated with infertility in the dog. A normal ejaculate has >80 per cent morphologically normal cells.[28, 29]

Cytological examination of an air-dried smear stained with Wright-Giemsa or new methylene blue stain allows identification and quantification of epithelial and inflammatory cells and erythrocytes. Gram stain will identify bacteria, if they are present. Cells in the ejaculate may originate from the testes, excurrent ducts, urinary bladder, prostate, urethra, and penile surface. High numbers of white cells, particularly toxic neutrophils, or neutrophils containing phagocytosed bacteria, may be associated with infections.[28] Macrophages are not likely to be urethral contaminants and are associated with chronic infection.

Quantitative aerobic bacterial culture should be performed on the ejaculate. Greater than 10,000 bacteria per milliliter may be indicative of infection. Gram-positive bacteria are more likely to be urethral contaminants while gram-negative bacteria are more likely to represent infection. The role of anaerobes in male genital tract infection is thought to be minor. Semen should be transported in Ames Transport Medium for the isolation of *Ureaplasma* or *Mycoplasma* spp if they are believed to be a source of infection. Virus isolation for *Herpesvirus canis* is rarely performed. For both culture and cytology, the ejaculate may be fractionated to attempt to localize the site of a possible infection.[30]

Elective or Invasive Procedures

Endocrinology. Normal spermatogenesis in the dog requires the synergistic effects of testosterone and FSH, as well as LH, prolactin, androgens, and locally secreted factors. The hypothalamus secretes GnRH, which stimulates secretion of the gonadotropins, LH and FSH, from the anterior pituitary. Leydig cells in the testicular interstitium respond to LH with the production of testosterone. Testosterone is involved in the initiation of puberty and the maintenance of spermatogenesis in the adult. Testosterone has negative feedback effects on gonadotropin release. FSH is necessary for the initiation of spermatogenesis and exerts its effect on the Sertoli cells of the seminiferous epithelium. Under the influence of FSH, the Sertoli cell produces inhibin, androgen-binding protein (ABP), estrogens, and other substances. Inhibin has negative feedback effects on pituitary FSH, and ABP is involved in androgen transport within the testis.

Testosterone is essential for normal libido and spermatogenesis; however, levels vary in the normal dog from 0.1 to 5 ng/ml because of the pulsatile nature of secretion. Concentrations in castrates are usually <0.015 ng/ml. Testosterone-secreting ability is better measured by stimulation testing. One hour following administration of GnRH (2.2 μg/kg intramuscularly), testosterone concentrations can be expected to rise to 3.7 to 6.2 ng/ml.[22]

Gonadotropin secretion is episodic, so measurements of FSH or LH should be made three times at 20-minute intervals. Gonadotro-

TABLE 33–2. Normal Parameters of Canine Semen

Parameter	Normal Dog
Volume	0.5–40 ml
Presperm	<2 ml
Sperm rich	0.1–3 ml
Prostatic	2–40 ml
pH	6.1–7.0
Color	Cloudy
Motile (%)	>70%
Morphology (%)	
Normal	>80%
Primary defects	<10%
Secondary defects	<20%
Alkaline phosphatase (IU/L)	
Presperm	0–100
Sperm rich	>10,000
Prostatic	<5000
Total sperm numbers	100–3000 × 10⁶

pins are not often measured because assays are not routinely available but may be useful in the diagnosis of azoospermia. For example, FSH has been used as an indicator of spermatogenesis. Inhibin concentrations are reduced in the presence of testicular lesions, and FSH consequently rises. Concentrations in normal dogs range from 20 to 130 ng/ml while concentrations >250 ng/ml might indicate testicular damage. Peripheral LH concentration may fluctuate from 0.5 to 10 ng/ml.[22]

Semen Alkaline Phosphatase (SAP). Concentration of SAP is used as a marker for epididymal contribution to the ejaculate and is useful in distinguishing azoospermia from an incomplete ejaculate. The enzyme originates in the epididymis and is present at concentrations of 5000 to 40,000 IU/L in the ejaculate. Ejaculates with alkaline phosphatase concentrations less than 5000 IU/L are incomplete or may be delivered by dogs with bilateral outflow obstruction distal to the epididymis.[31]

Spermatozoal Ultrastructure. Scanning or transmission electron microscopy may be performed on spermatozoa if ultrastructural defects are suspected.[29]

Aspiration of Spermatozoa from the Epididymis. This invasive procedure may be indicated if the dog has a palpable abnormality affecting one or both epididymides or if the ejaculate is azoospermic. Aspiration may indicate the presence of obstructive lesions of the outflow tract, neoplasia, sperm granuloma, and epididymitis. In the standing or sedated dog, the scrotal skin over the tail of the epididymis is prepared aseptically and a 23- to 25-gauge needle used to aspirate epididymal contents. Microscopic examination of the aspirate indicates the presence of spermatozoa, inflammatory cells, or bacteria.

Testicular Biopsy. Biopsy will provide information regarding the etiology and severity of a testicular lesion and aid in prognosis. Biopsy is indicated in animals with oligospermia, azoospermia, and in those with high proportions of primary morphological abnormalities in the ejaculate. It is performed under general anesthesia. The scrotum is prepared aseptically and tissue may be obtained by fine-needle aspiration, split-needle biopsy, or wedge resection. Sequelae such as hematoma, adhesions, inflammation, and local autoimmune reactions are more likely with the more invasive techniques. Tissue samples may be cultured before being fixed in Zenker's or Bouin's solution for histological examination. Analysis should include the presence of germ cells and Sertoli cells; proliferation and maturation of the germinal epithelium; presence of spermatozoa in seminiferous tubule lumens; and presence of histologically normal Leydig cells. Quantitative measures such as germ cell to Sertoli cell ratio, seminiferous tubule diameter, and identification of maturational stage of germ cells may allow more accurate interpretation of the severity of a testicular lesion.[32]

Karyotype. Dogs with testicular hypoplasia or aplasia, abnormal external phenotype, or other signs consistent with intersex conditions should be karyotyped. Fresh whole blood in heparin is required by a cytogenetics laboratory.

Pelvic and Abdominal Radiography and Ultrasonography. Ultrasonography may be used to provide additional data in animals with testicular and epididymal lesions and tumors, retained testes, testicular torsion, inguinal hernia, and diseases of the prostate gland. Ultrasound can also be used for guided-needle biopsies and aspirates of the prostate gland.[33] Survey radiographs of the caudal abdomen are indicated for dogs with prostatic disease.

Isolation of *Mycoplasma* and *Ureaplasma* Species. These organisms may occasionally be cultured from the ejaculate or from preputial or urethral swabs. The association of these organisms with reproductive tract pathology is tenuous, and they are commonly recovered in normal fertile dogs.[30] A pure culture may be interpreted as suspect if isolated in association with cytological and clinical signs indicative of infection.

References

1. Johnston SD: Clinical approach to infertility in bitches with primary anestrus. Vet Clin North Am Small Anim Pract 21:421–425, 1991.
2. Papich MG: Effects of drugs on pregnancy. In Kirk RW (ed): Current Veterinary Therapy X Small Animal Practice. Philadelphia, WB Saunders Company, 1989, p 1291.
3. Concannon PW, Hansel W, Visek W: The ovarian cycle of the bitch: Plasma estrogen, LH and progesterone. Biol Reprod 12:112–117, 1975.
4. Doak RL, Hall A, Dale HE: Longevity of spermatozoa in the reproductive tract of the bitch. J Reprod Fertil 13:51–58, 1967.
5. Concannon PW, Whaley S, Lein D, et al: Canine gestation length: Variation related to time of mating and fertile life of sperm. Am J Vet Res 44:1819–1921, 1983.
6. Van Haaften B, Dieleman SJ, Okkens AC, et al: Timing the mating of dogs on the basis of blood progesterone concentration. Vet Rec 25:524–526, 1989.
7. Concannon PW, Hansel W, McEntee K: Changes in LH, progesterone and sexual behavior associated with preovulatory luteinization in the bitch. Biol Reprod 17:604–609, 1972.
8. Holst PA, Phemister RD: Onset of diestrus in the beagle bitch: Definition and significance. Am J Vet Res 35:401–408, 1974.
9. Concannon PW, Lein DH: Hormonal and clinical correlates of ovarian cycles, ovulation, pseudopregnancy and pregnancy in dogs. In Kirk RW (ed): Current Veterinary Therapy X Small Animal Practice. Philadelphia, WB Saunders Company, 1989, p 1269.
10. Concannon PW, Battista M: Canine semen freezing and artificial insemination. In Kirk RW (ed): Current Veterinary Therapy X Small Animal Practice, Philadelphia, WB Saunders Company, 1989, p 1247.
11. Purswell B: Differential diagnosis of canine abortion. In Kirk RW (ed): Current Veterinary Therapy XI Small Animal Practice. Philadelphia, WB Saunders Company, 1992, p 925.
12. Hillis GP: An examination of canine reproductive performance parameters. Proc Soc Theriogenology 288–294, 1898.
13. Romagnoli SE: A diagnostic approach to vulvar discharge in the canine patient. Proc Soc Theriogenology 295–306, 1898.
14. Manothaiudom K, Johnston S: Clinical approach to vaginal/vestibular masses in the bitch. Vet Clin North Am Small Anim Pract 21:509–522, 1991.
15. Johnson CA: Diagnosis and treatment of chronic vaginitis in the bitch. Vet Clin North Am Small Anim Pract 21:523–532, 1991.
16. Bjurstrom L, Linde-Forsberg C: Long-term study of aerobic bacteria of the genital tract in breeding bitches. Am J Vet Res 53:665, 1992.
17. Pineda MH, Kainer RA, Faulkner LC: Dorsal median post-cervical fold in the canine vagina. Am J Vet Res 34:1487–1489, 1973.
18. Lindsay FEF: The normal endoscopic appearance of the caudal reproductive tract of the cyclic and non-cyclic bitch. J Small Anim Practice 24:1–5, 1983.
19. Yeager AE, Mohammed HO, Meyers-Wallen VN, et al: Ultrasonographic appearance of the uterus, placenta, fetus and fetal membranes throughout accurately timed pregnancy in beagles. Am J Vet Res 53:342–351, 1992.
20. Nelson RW: Canine hypothyroidism: Establishing the diagnosis. Proc Soc Theriogenology 126–138, 1986.
21. Olsen PN, Bowen RA, Behrendt MD: Concentrations of reproductive hormones in canine serum throughout late anestrus, proestrus and estrus. Biol Reprod 27:1196, 1982.
22. Shille VM, Olsen PN: Dynamic testing in reproductive endocrinology. In Kirk KW (ed): Current Veterinary Therapy X Small Animal Practice. Philadelphia, WB Saunders Company, 1989, p 1282.
23. Steinetz BG, Goldsmith LT, Lust G: Plasma relaxin levels in pregnant and lactating dogs. Biol Reprod 37:719, 1987.
24. Meyers-Wallen VN, Patterson DF: Disorders of sexual development in dogs and cats. In Kirk RW (ed): Current Veterinary Therapy X Small Animal Practice. Philadelphia, WB Saunders Company, 1989, p 1261.
25. Olar TT, Amann RP, Pickett BW: Relationships among testicular size, daily production and output of spermatozoa and extragonadal sperm reserves of the dog. Biol Reprod 29:1114–1120, 1983.
26. Boucher JH, Foote RH, Kirk RW: The evaluation of semen quality in the dog and the effects of frequency of ejaculation upon semen quality, libido and depletion of sperm reserves. Cornell Vet 48:67–72, 1958.
27. Bartlett DJ: Studies on dog semen: II. Biochemical characteristics. J Reprod Fertil 3:190–205, 1962.

28. Olson PN: Collection and evaluation of canine semen. *In* Kirk RW (ed): Current Veterinary Therapy XI Small Animal Practice. Philadelphia, WB Saunders Company, 1992, p 938.
29. Oettle EE, Soley JT: Sperm abnormalities in the dog: A light and electron microscope study. Vet Med Rev 1:28–70, 1988.
30. Doig PA, Ruhnke HL, Bosu WTK: The genital mycoplasma and ureaplasma flora of healthy and diseased dogs. Can J Comp Med 45:223–238, 1981.
31. Frenette G, Dube JY, Tremblay RR: Origin of alkaline phosphatase of canine seminal plasma. Arch Androl 16:235–241, 1986.
32. Larsen RE: Testicular biopsy in the dog. Vet Clin North Am Small Anim Pract 7:747–755, 1977.
33. Finn ST, Wrigley RH: Ultrasonography and ultrasound-guided biopsy of the canine prostate. *In* Kirk RW (ed): Current Veterinary Therapy X Small Animal Practice. Philadelphia, WB Saunders Company, 1989, p 1227.

CHAPTER 34

SUPPRESSION OR PREVENTION OF ESTRUS IN RACING AND SPORTING DOGS

VICTOR M. SHILLE

Male and female racing, coursing, sled, and other sporting dogs are trained and raced together, so that the day-to-day proximity of the two sexes mandates that physical and behavioral signs of estrus must be suppressed. An estrous female may incite fights in the kennels and on the track and induce in males as well as other females a general lack of competitive concentration. It has been reported that pseudocyesis, which frequently follows estrus, has been associated with serious decline in performance; in some instances the affected bitches never recover their previous racing form. In addition, in some countries the estrous cycle affects racing eligibility; in the United Kingdom, for instance, a greyhound bitch is not allowed to race or take part in official trials for the 3 weeks of proestrus and estrus and also for an additional 10 weeks counting from the first day of reported proestrus.[1]

The ideal estrus-control agent should control all signs of estrus; it should require infrequent dosing, and it should be easily administered by a lay careperson. Because winning bitches are desirable for breeding, the compound, when discontinued, should leave no lasting effects on fertility. In addition, it would be desirable that the agent not be classified as a controlled substance, so that it could be acquired and used efficiently in a kennel environment on large numbers of dogs.

Effective 27 February, 1990, the United States Federal Drug Enforcement Administration (DEA) amended its regulations to place anabolic steroids into Schedule III of the Control Substances Act of 1990.[2] Anyone handling these substances must register with the DEA and comply with requirements for security of the inventory and for keeping of appropriate records. An anabolic steroid is defined as any substance that is chemically or biologically related to testosterone (other than estrogen, progesterone, and corticosteroids) or that promotes muscle growth. Certain anabolic steroids expressly prepared for administration as implants in non-human species are exempt from Schedule III requirements.

Individual states commonly develop additional rules to regulate substance abuse. At the time when anabolic steroids were included by federal law into the Schedule III category of compounds, in

Florida human chorionic gonadotropin (hCG) was also categorized as an anabolic steroid; however, recently hCG has been declassified in the state of Florida and is no longer a controlled substance.

A number of estrus-control products are available as human-labeled products (Table 34–1). The use of human-labeled drugs in veterinary medicine is regulated by the FDA. The Agency's intention is to (1) ensure that drugs are prescribed and administered by a veterinarian and (2) limit the use of these drugs to non–food-producing animals, except for some narrowly defined exceptions. Thus, use of human-labeled hormonal preparations in dogs is acceptable to the FDA under the two criteria stated above.

GENERAL PRINCIPLES OF ESTRUS CONTROL

Mechanisms That Regulate Reproductive Function

The reproductive cycle of the domestic bitch is unique among all the mammals studied so far. Estrus is not regulated by day length, yet it occurs approximately every 9 to 12 months, because the sexually active periods (proestrus, estrus, and diestrus) are separated by a long period of anestrus. The bitch does not require a coital stimulus for release of the eggs, yet ovulation occurs early in estrus so that the bitch remains receptive to the male in the presence of high blood concentrations of progesterone. The life span of the corpus luteum is relatively long and is the same whether the bitch is pregnant or not, while termination of the luteal phase does not trigger onset of folliculogenesis. In addition, the bitch is uncommonly sensitive to biological effects of both natural and synthetic gonadal steroid hormones (estrogen, progesterone, and testosterone).

In spite of the differences just stated, the mechanisms governing hypothalamic-pituitary-ovarian interaction in the bitch are essentially the same as in all mammals (see Chapter 35). Thus, the points at which reproductive function may be interrupted are similar to those found in other mammals. Among these are the release of GnRH, LH, and FSH, the binding of the gonadotropins to the follicle, and the response of the granulosa-theca cell system to gonadotropins.

The Logic of Estrus Control

Using the so-called long negative feedback loops that control release of GnRH, FSH, and LH, the gonadotropin release may be suppressed by progesterone or testosterone. It has been suggested that testosterone actually suppresses FSH and LH, while progesterone maintains the gonadotropins at the anestrous level, interfering with folliculotropic and preovulatory surges.[3] Estrogen is not useful because it not only stimulates the end-organs, producing vulval edema, vaginal cornification, endometrial hypertrophy, and estrous behavior but it also indirectly brings on the induction of LH receptors on the follicular cells,[4] thus initiating follicle maturation and estrus. In contrast to the long feedback loop activated by gonadal steroids, the short negative feedback loops are used when GnRH agonists are administered to suppress the release of GnRH, thus halting the gonadotropin release at its inception.

Two known methods are used to interfere with follicle growth without using the negative feedback loops. In one, using the principle of down regulation, a powerful GnRH agonist exhausts the GnRH receptors so that the endogenous GnRH cannot be bound to the target cells in the pituitary, thus reducing or eliminating FSH and LH release and synthesis. In the other method, biologically inactive GnRH antagonists bind to the GnRH receptor sites in the pituitary, preventing the biologically active endogenous GnRH from binding to the receptors. Thus, pituitary gonadotropin release and synthesis are again interrupted. Currently only compounds that act by means of long feedback loops are available commercially in the United States.

PRODUCTS FOR PREVENTION OR SUPPRESSION OF ESTRUS

Derivatives of Progesterone

In addition to the negative feedback on gonadotropins, there are other physiological effects of progesterone and its natural or synthetic derivatives (progestins). The effects appear to depend on the priming action of estrogens. The significant interrelationship of the two hormones is particularly demonstrated in the bitch by the cystic endometrial hyperplasia/pyometra syndrome.

Progesterone mediates the postovulatory maturation of the secretory glands of the endometrium and of oviductal lining. It also depresses the spontaneous activity of the myometrium so that the latter contracts less readily and frequently. Progesterone promotes secretion of viscous cervical mucus and desquamation of vaginal epithelium, thus hastening the onset of the diestrous appearance in the vaginal smear. Progestins have been shown to reduce libido and control aggressive behavior; some derivatives (megestrol acetate) have been used in behavior modification of male and female dogs. Progesterone appears to have an antiprolactin effect, resulting in an increase in prolactin when progesterone declines at the end of the luteal phase of the cycle. These endocrine changes are associated with mammary gland development and initiation of maternal behavior. A corollary phenomenon occurs when exogenous progestin treatment is stopped and the bitch experiences mammary hyperplasia, pseudolactation, and lassitude.

Apart from its effect on the reproductive organs, progesterone has a catabolic action and promotes negative nitrogen balance. These findings led to the supposition that progesterone affects

strength and stamina. In human athletes, neither the luteal phase of the cycle nor the use of progestin-containing contraceptives showed clear effects on women's athletic performance. Some investigators stated that peak performance is achieved in the estrogen-dominated follicular phase[5]; others refuted this finding,[6, 7] while still others showed that women can perform at their best regardless of cycle or type of contraceptive used.[8] In a study of 51 greyhound bitches the effect of a progestin was evaluated on racing performance.[1] Initially, best and worst running times were compared, but because worst times were overwhelmingly the result of running accidents (bumping, crowding), best running times were used as the performance criterion. The author recognized that running time was not necessarily a true measure of performance because it is influenced by the condition of the track and season of the year, but time is an objective measure, and different times may be conveniently compared. Comparison of running times showed that the effect of progestin was minimal, with a range of variation similar to that expected in bitches without it.[1] Anecdotal evidence seems to point to increased performance in bitches taking compounds used for human contraception, such as Nordette-21, which contains ethinyl estradiol and levonorgesterol, but the beneficial effect is most likely induced by the estrogen portion of the compound, not the progestin. Thus the effect of progestins on athletic performance in dogs remains equivocal, and the only prospective, controlled, published study seems to support this assumption.

Progestins that occur naturally in the body are of rather limited use as a source of therapeutically active material. Relatively little is stored in the ovaries, and administered compounds are rapidly inactivated by the liver. Oral compounds are particularly susceptible as they are carried directly to the liver via the hepatoportal system. Most commercially available estrus-control compounds have been designed to prolong their biological action by slowing the absorption from the injection site, using formulations suspended in oil, or deposited as crystals (repositol preparations), or by changing the structure of the molecule to make it more resistant to inactivation by liver enzymes.

Medroxyprogesterone Acetate (MPA). Primary use of this product is for behavior modification in intermale aggression and long-term estrus control in cats. In dogs, MPA has been recommended for progestin-responsive dermatitis[9] and was at one time used for long-term estrus control.

In dogs the long-acting injectable formulation has been associated with severe cases of hydrometra, mucometra, and pyometra. If MPA is administered subcutaneously, permanent local alopecia, atrophy, and depigmentation may result at the site of injection. Other side effects include polyphagia, polydipsia, polyuria, depression, lethargy, pseudolactation and mammary enlargement, mammary neoplasia, adrenocortical depression, and diabetes mellitus. Acromegaly and increased growth hormone concentrations were reported when it was used in dogs with preexisting diabetes mellitus.

Megestrol Acetate (MA). This product is approved by the FDA for estrus control in dogs. It is also used clinically for treatment of pseudolactation, and for dermatological and behavior-related conditions. To suppress an estrous cycle that has begun, treatment should be started no later than the third day of proestrus. The stage of proestrus should be confirmed by microscopic examination of exfoliated vaginal epithelium, which should show no more than 35 to 40 per cent superficial cells. The initial, suppressive dose is 2.2 mg/kg orally once a day for 8 days. If delay of the subsequent cycle is desired, treatment should be continued at the standard dose of 0.55 mg/kg orally once a day for 16 to 20 days. To postpone the onset of an anticipated cycle, 0.55 mg/kg orally once a day should be started at least a week before anticipated onset of proestrus and continued for 32 days. It is recommended that treatment should not be repeated to suppress two consecutive cycles.

TABLE 34–1. Products Used for Estrus Control in Dogs

Generic Name	Trade Name (Veterinary)	Trade Name (Human Use)	Suggested Dosage
Progestogens			
Medroxyprogesterone acetate	None	Provera, Depo-Provera	0.5–1 mg/kg po once weekly
Megestrol acetate	Ovaban	Megace	0.55 mg/kg po for 32 d
Androgens			
Methyltestosterone	None	Various trade and generic products	0.5–1 mg/kg po sid prn
Mibolerone	Cheque	None	30–180 µg/kg po sid (See insert)
Testosterone cypionate	None	Various trade and generic products	2.2 mg/kg IM once a month
Testosterone propionate	None	Various trade and generic products	2.2 mg/kg po every 2 to 3 d
Testosterone enanthate	None	Various trade and generic products	2.2 mg/kg po every 2 to 3 d

Adverse effects are similar to those mentioned for MPA, although the risk of inducing cystic endometrial hyperplasia and pyometra is reportedly less than for MPA and other progestins. When MA was administered during the embryonal period of pregnancy (before day 25 to 30), no effects on the bitch or the litter were observed. Reduced litter size and poor neonatal survival were reported when MA was given in the second half of pregnancy.

Some pharmaceuticals are incompatible with MA. Rifampin, an antifungal product used in systemic mycoses, may interfere with progestin action if given concomitantly, resulting in erratic but fertile cycles. Corticosteroid treatment given concurrently with MA will exacerbate adrenocortical suppression. If prolonged use is anticipated the dog should be monitored for weight gain, increase of blood glucose levels, development of mammary nodules, and changes in adrenocortical function.

Derivatives of Testosterone

It is important to remember that the effects of androgens are ubiquitous. For example, a general anabolic effect is seen as an increase in protein synthesis in the skeletal and cardiac muscles, a sparing effect on calcium in the bone, and stimulation of erythropoiesis. Effects on the embryo include masculinization of reproductive organs and development of the noncyclical male reproductive pattern. In the adult female the virilizing effects include reduction of subcutaneous fat, atrophy of vaginal epithelium (which may lead to chronic vaginitis), and hypertrophy of the clitoris, as well as suppression of lactation.

Intensive sports activity seems to produce an anabolic and virilizing effect in women athletes. The cause may be the increased testosterone production in the ovary.[10] No published studies were found on the effect of early exercise training and competitive running on estrous cycles of bitches. However, there is anecdotal evidence that racing bitches may remain anestrous for 2 to 3 years, and cycling will occur spontaneously when the bitch is rested because of an injury or traveling between tracks. In women early athletic training has been associated with delayed age at menarche and a masculine body type (lean body, long legs, narrow hips, low weight-height ratio). Menstrual disorders reportedly associated with exercise are luteal phase shortening, reduced plasma progesterone and estradiol in the presence of normal cycle length, and amenorrhea in the presence of reduced pulsatile LH, increased prolactin, and cortisol. It appears that there are no uniform miles/week or other exercise factors that delay menarche or induce amenorrhea—an individual threshold seems to be involved.[10]

Androgens that occur naturally in the body are of rather limited use as a source of therapeutically active material. Endogenous as well as exogenous compounds are rapidly inactivated and, similarly to progestins, oral androgens are particularly susceptible to inacti-

vation. In the plasma only about 1 to 3 per cent of the androgens are in a biologically active form, the remainder being bound specifically to sex hormone–binding globulin and transcortin, as well as nonspecifically to albumin. Most androgens are inactivated in the liver and excreted via the kidney. About 5 per cent are metabolized into the biologically active dihydrotestosterone or aromatized to estrogens in various tissues, such as liver, adipose tissue, adrenal cortex, and hypothalamus.

Methyltestosterone (MT) and other *testosterone esters (TE)* have been used as oral and injectable formulations to control estrus in dogs. Dosages and manner of administration vary with the particular compound and are best obtained from manufacturers' literature. Most commonly used compounds are listed (Table 34–1).

Adverse effects are reportedly uncommon, major problems being limited to clitoral hyperplasia and a viscous, mucous vaginal discharge. The latter is occasionally accompanied by inflammation of the vestibule and vulva, which may be due to the atrophy of the estrogen-dependent cornified epithelium. Polycythemia (packed cell volume > 50) is not uncommon during MT and TE administration. Diabetic animals receiving insulin will need to have the insulin dose adjusted (decreased). Thyroxine-binding globulin and total thyroxine concentrations may be decreased. Although no clinical signs related to the thyroid have been reported in dogs, it has been shown that racing greyhounds tend to have lower thyroxine levels than dogs that are not racing or receiving androgens.[11]

Mibolerone is effective for estrus prevention in adult bitches that are "not intended primarily for breeding purposes." Estrus is reliably controlled if administration is started at least 30 days before onset of anticipated proestrus. Efficacy is, however, breed related so that German shepherds and shepherd crosses require the maximal dose regardless of weight. Mibolerone is not recommended for use in prepubertal bitches because it induces premature epiphyseal closure as well as persistent atrophic vaginitis. When it is used longer than 2 years in adult bitches, side effects may include urinary incontinence, aggressive behavior, seborrhea oleosa, epiphora, and occasionally hepatic dysfunction. Because the drug causes masculinization of female fetuses, it is contraindicated in pregnant bitches.

References

1. Prole JHB: The effect of the use of norethisterone acetate to control oestrus in greyhound bitches on subsequent racing performance and fertility. J Small Anim Pract 15:221, 1974.
2. Federal Register: Amendments to the Federal Drug Enforcement Administration, 1990.
3. Concannon PA: Biology of gonadotropin secretion in adult and prepuberal female dogs. J Reprod Fert Suppl 47:3, 1993.

4. Richards JS: Maturation of ovarian follicles: Actions and interactions of pituitary and ovarian hormones on follicular cell differentiation. Physiol Rev 60(2):51, 1980.
5. Fraccaroli G: Li rendimento sportivo della donna durante il ciclo menstruale. Minerva Med 70:3557, 1980.
6. Wells CL, Horvath SM: Heat stress responses related to the menstrual cycle. J Appl Physiol 35:1, 1974.
7. Wells CL, Horvath SM: Responses to exercise in a hot environment as related to the menstrual cycle. J Appl Physiol 34:299, 1973.
8. Bale P, Davies J: Effects of menstruation and contraceptive pill on the performance of physical education students. Br J Sports Med 17:46, 1983.
9. Kunkle GA: Progestagens in Dermatology. In Kirk RW (ed): Current Veterinary Therapy IX: Small Animal Practice. Philadelphia, WB Saunders Company, 1986, p 601.
10. Bonen A, Belcastro AN: Effect of exercise and training on menstrual cycle hormones. Aust J Sports Med 10:39, 1978.
11. Bloomberg MS, Shille VM, Acre KE, et al.: Thyroid function of the racing greyhound. In Proc Intern Greyhound Sympos Orlando, Fla, 7, 1987.

CHAPTER 35

NATURAL BREEDING

DESMOND P. FEGAN

Breeding of sporting dogs is an important and responsible occupation. Unlike our counterparts in the show dog world, sporting dog breeders have objective parameters on which to base breeding decisions. We are selecting desirable features that we would like to have within the breed. The correctness or lack thereof of that decision is determined by the performance of the offspring. Like their counterparts in the wild we are creating a breeding program for these dogs that guarantees the survival of the fittest.

Dogs in the wild are pack animals, and as such breeding is a community event. There is usually one dominant male and female, the alpha pair, and a number of other females who, although they may experience cycling, are mated only when there is an abundance of food. The dominant female will produce puppies, and the lesser females will be enrolled as wet nurses for her offspring. False pregnancy is therefore a natural component of the canine breeding cycle. The length of the breeding cycle in pack dogs also varies between 6 and 12 months depending on the relative scarcity or abundance of food. This mimics what we see in domesticated dogs, ie, in those dogs that live in a stress-free environment as domestic pets cycles tend to occur every 6 months, whereas in more athletic dogs such as greyhounds adaptation results in cycling only once a year. Cycling in domestic pets will generally start much earlier—at 9 months compared to an average of 18 months for greyhounds. Breeding can continue until the female is approximately 12 years old. Bitches over age 10 tend to have reduced fertility and a much higher incidence of uterine inertia at parturition.

ESTROUS CYCLE

Even though athletic breeds tend to be slower to reach sexual maturity and cycling occurs with less regularity, the actual estrous cycle is the same. It is recognized as having four different parts.

Proestrus. from the first day of bleeding until the luteinizing hormone (LH) peak or when the bitch becomes receptive to the male.

Estrus. when the bitch is receptive to the male.

Metestrus. from the end of estrus until anestrus. (Also called diestrus.)

Anestrus. when the reproductive organs are largely dormant, from the end of metestrus to the beginning of proestrous.

The breeding cycle can be monitored in a number of different ways. No one method should be used in isolation, and best results are achieved by awareness of all the changes that are occurring in the bitch and her behavior. Ovulation has been recorded as occurring between the fifth day from the beginning of proestrous and the 35th.

MONITORING OF BREEDING CYCLE

Macroscopic. Observation of the bitch's response to the male is one of the most valuable guides to determination of optimal breeding time. It is usual for the dog and bitch to be introduced to each other about the 10th day after proestrus begins.

The bitch will tolerate sniffing and nuzzling from the male but will not allow mounting, and usually will retaliate aggressively to any attempts. As estrus begins the bitch will relent and gradually cooperate more and more with the male dog's agenda. When the time is right she will stand still for the dog, raise her tail to one side, and pout her vulva to allow penetration. Visual examination of the vulval discharge is also very helpful. There is a bright sanguineous discharge from the beginning of proestrus until the beginning of estrus. This is the discharge from uterine bleeding occurring as a result of estrogen stimulation. At the time of mating the discharge becomes much lighter and more serous. The color of the vulval discharge therefore changes from deep blood-red to light pink at the time of ovulation and then to yellow after the end of the estrus period.

Endoscopic. Endoscopic examination of the vaginal endothelium can reveal subtle changes in the vaginal folds. In anestrus the folds are flat and appear red because of the underlying capillaries; during proestrus they become larger, rounder, moister, and paler with a sanguineous discharge between the folds; during estrus the folds

FIGURE 35–1. Changes seen in epithelial cells as season progresses.

 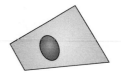 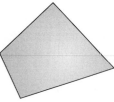

Early proestrus   Late proestrus   Estrus

gradually become more wrinkled and dry. In metestrus the folds are less distinct, and the mucosa appears patchy because of the loss of the cornified layer.[1]

None of the visual methods alone can be relied on to determine the optimal time of mating. Vaginal discharge is particularly unreliable, as some bitches will produce copious sanguineous discharge throughout the estrus period and others will cease bleeding long before the end of proestrus.

Olfactory. The human sense of smell is nowhere nearly sensitive enough to detect any subtle changes in odor emanating from the bitch. These odors are produced by chemicals, termed *pheromones.* However, the nasal passages of the dog are charged with a much more sensitive olfactory organ, and dogs can detect changes in the odor relating to the stage of estrus.

Cytological. Regular examination of the cells of the vaginal tract gives information on the stage of the cycle that the bitch has reached. A cotton swab inserted into the vagina and rotated three times will abrade cells from the vaginal wall to allow a microscopic examination. A "Diff-quik" stain or a Shorr stain are best used to demonstrate cell types. During anestrus the wall consists of columnar epithelial cells, further differentiated into parabasal and intermediate cells. When examined microscopically these are nucleated viable cells. As the bitch enters proestrus the vaginal wall begins to thicken and the outermost layers begin to die and are said to be cornified or keratinized. The ratio of cornified to viable cells, approximately 3:1, reaches a peak at the time of estrus. When estrus is over the vaginal wall reverts to its original thickness, and the vaginal smear will reveal a majority of viable cells and also a large number of white blood cells, mainly neutrophils, which "clean up" after the mating. The onset of metestrus is a valuable indicator of the time of ovulation. Ovulation will have occurred 6 days prior to the onset of metestrus. Representations of the cells are shown in Figure 35–1.

Biochemical. The hormonal changes that occur during the "season" are depicted in Figure 35–2. Progesterone is most readily monitored, with levels being very low during proestrus. As ovulation occurs the sites of the ruptured ova begin to produce progesterone and levels rise rapidly. In late proestrus the level rises from 0 to 3 ng/ml to 5 to 6 ng/ml at the time of ovulation. The level continues to rise for a further 20 days after the end of estrus. Insemination or breeding should be carried out 24 to 48 hours after predicted ovulation. Most clinicians in this area are now using one of the many available progesterone ELISA assays to monitor progesterone levels until they begin to rise and radioimmune assays are then utilized to give quantitative results.

Measurement of LH is used by some veterinarians to determine ovulation. However, the hormone must be assayed daily, and readings are reported to be extremely volatile. The hormone may have a diurnal rhythm, and the general trend tends to be toward progesterone assays. Nevertheless, levels of LH rise rapidly in late proestrus to reach a peak of 15 to 20 ng/ml 48 hours before the majority of ovulations. Therefore, insemination or breeding 72 to 96 hours after the LH peak should result in the ova and sperm meeting at the optimum time.

Progesterone testing should be performed on day 7 and every third day thereafter until the bitch has been bred. A progesterone level of 5 ng/ml indicates that ovulation has occurred. Mating can take place 48 hours after this level is reached, or if multiple inseminations are to take place, then 24 and 72 hours after. Progesterone levels greater than 12 ng/ml at the time of insemination usually result in pregnancy.[2]

Maturation of the ovum takes 48 hours, so mating should take place on day 4 after the LH peak. Metestrus occurs 8 days after the LH peak.

NORMAL COITAL BEHAVIOR

The bitch in estrus (standing heat) will allow the dog to sniff, nuzzle, lick, and eventually mount her. She will facilitate penetration by protruding the vulva and raising the tail to one side. Once the dog has mounted it will maintain a tight grip on the bitch with its forelegs. It will thrust to achieve penetration of the vulva. Once within the vulva the thrusting will be more forceful, and this will stimulate full erection and enlargement of the glans penis, which the bitch will clamp with the vulval muscles. The first fraction of the ejaculate is voided during this period before full erection is achieved. Ejaculation of the second fraction then occurs, and the dog will instinctively dismount. The bitch maintains a hold on the penis, and dog and bitch are facing in opposite directions with the dog's penis extending backward between its hind legs, 180 degrees from the normal position. This is called "the tie." The tie can be maintained for up to 30 minutes and is a normal part of coital behavior.

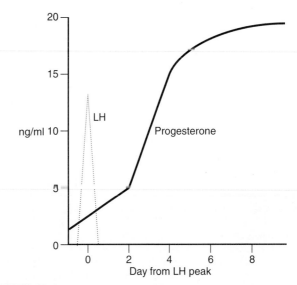

FIGURE 35–2. Hormonal changes occurring during the season. Summary of the important events of the estrus period and their correlation with progesterone levels.

After mating, if the tie has been released after a short period, the bitch should be held with hind quarters elevated and in a relaxed manner to allow gravity to aid the passage of the deposited semen into the anterior vagina. The male's penis and sheath should be douched with warm saline solution. Disinfectants should be avoided because these can be irritating to the mucous membrane of the sheath.

ANATOMICAL DEFECTS AFFECTING COPULATION

Female

Stenosis of the vulval vestibule or vaginal opening will cause failure of coital penetration. This condition is rare and diagnosis should not be made prematurely. In maiden bitches, the circulation of estrogen produces engorgement, enlargement, and relaxation of the vulval opening. Persistent remnants of the hymen can be digitally stretched under general anesthesia. If digital stretching fails, then episiotomy will be required.

Clitoral enlargement is a condition most commonly seen in the racing greyhound, the result of administration of large doses of anabolic steroids. The condition is usually temporary, and the enlargement subsides after the steroids are withdrawn. Persistent enlargement will require amputation before the bitch will tolerate a natural mating.

Vaginal tumors are, as a rule, benign. Usually they require surgical excision, and histopathological examination is recommended to ascertain whether viral transmissible tumor is involved. Vaginal prolapse is most commonly seen in bull terrier breeds. Prolapse occurs only during estrus. It is not clear why it occurs, but if it occurs once, it is likely to return each time the bitch is in estrus. It renders natural copulation almost impossible, and artificial insemination should be considered. Surgical excision of the prolapse will generally give permanent resolution.

Male

Phimosis is the condition in which the penis cannot be exteriorized through the preputial opening. Surgical correction is always necessary and very successful. Paraphimosis is the contrary condition in which the penis cannot be retracted back into the sheath after an erection. First aid with ice packs on the penis and a water-soluble lubricant such as K-Y jelly will enable the return of the penis to the sheath. Long-term resolution also involves enlargement of the preputial opening. Paraphimosis has been described after foreign body penetration of the penis, and in older dogs spinal lesions have been blamed for the condition.[1] Tumors of the penis are rare. Surgical excision is the treatment of choice, and histopathological examination is recommended.

Fracture of the os penis is a rare sequel to trauma. Conservative treatment with nonsteroidal anti-inflammatories and magnetic field therapy on *high* frequency is the best approach. Occlusion of the urethra may occur during the callous formation, necessitating urethrostomy of the proximal urethra. Cryptorchid dogs, in which both testes are retained in the abdomen or the inguinal area, are completely infertile. These dogs, however, have normal libido. Castration should be recommended, since the cryptorchid gonad is more likely to develop neoplasia. The breeder must be informed that this is a recessive genetic defect that will be transmitted to the next generation. Spondylitis in an older dog is a common cause of impotence. Treatment with a pain relief agent such as a nonsteroidal anti-inflammatory will usually help the dog endure the copulatory process. Chronic pain of any kind will reduce the overall sperm

output because of its negative feedback on the hypothalamo-pituitary axis.

OTHER PROBLEMS THAT MAY LEAD TO REDUCED FERTILITY AFTER NATURAL MATING

Semen Quality. Less than 100 million live motile sperm per ejaculate in stud dogs is generally regarded as below acceptable fertility. A regular monitoring procedure should be carried out for every active stud dog. The ejaculate of the dog contains three fractions: (1) A clear liquid emanating from the prostate gland, usually 1 ml in volume. It is expelled as the dog is thrusting. (2) A white cloudy liquid, the sperm-rich fraction, usually expelled just after the thrusting phase. If the operator holds the penis, this sperm-rich ejaculate can be felt as distinct urethral pulses, usually five to eight in number. The sperm-rich fraction emanates from the epididymis. (3) The third fraction also comes from the prostate gland. It is clear and can measure up to 20 ml.

If the semen quality is found to be inadequate at the time of mating, very little can be done to remedy this. Once poor semen production or quality has been diagnosed, there is generally a lag period of approximately 6 weeks after correction of the problem before viable semen will be produced.

Evaluation of canine semen is a simple process. An ejaculate can usually be collected in a jar or through an artificial vagina (AV), depending on individual preference. The temperature of the jar or AV should be 37°C. The semen should then be transferred to a water bath of the same temperature. A drop of semen placed on a prewarmed slide can be examined for motility, which is graded on a score of 0 through 5: If all sperm cells are dead, the score is 0; if there is slow side-to-side movement with no forward progression, the score is 1; if there is slow side-to-side movement and progression in spurts, the score is 2; rapid side-to-side movement, progression in spurts is graded 3; slow forward progression, grade 4; rapid forward progression, grade 5.

A calibrated test-tube can be used to measure the volume of semen collected. An effort should be made to collect only the second, sperm-rich, fraction and a small amount of the third fraction. The color should be recorded. It can vary from clear through milky to bloody. The pH of the semen can be measured with litmus paper; normal is 6.5.

A manual count using the "Unopette" system with a hemocytometer is the customary procedure. A 20-μl sample is taken from the semen and mixed with the unopette platelet/white blood cell chamber giving a dilution of 1:100. The chamber is allowed to stand for 5 minutes and the contents mixed well before being placed on the hemocytometer. Both sides of the hemocytometer are charged. The sperm are counted in the central area of small squares (Fig. 35–3; the red blood cell counting area) on both sides and a mean obtained. This is the average number of sperm in millions per milliliter.

Morphology can be studied by means of the "Diff-quik" stain in which a dried and fixed semen smear is immersed in part 1 and part 2 for 5 minutes each. Alternatively, nigrosin and eosin staining can be used to give better definition of the sperm head area and acrosome defects. Generally, 200 cells are counted, and the relative percentages of normal, bent, and immature sperm or other abnormal sperm are recorded. Evaluation of the semen sample is recorded as shown in Figure 35–4.

Stress Factors. Endogenous cortisol release at the time of mating can often be substantial, particularly in maiden bitches. The bitch may have been transported many kilometers, housed in a strange environment, had its diet and routine completely changed,

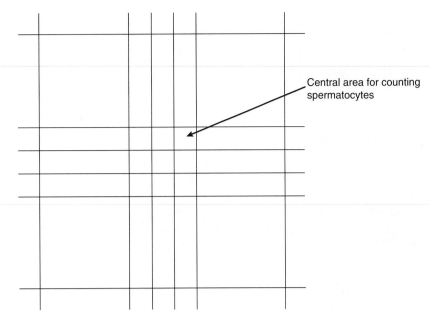

Central area for counting spermatocytes

FIGURE 35-3. Counting area for Neaubaurer counting chamber.

and then finally introduced to the male. The bitch must rely on an instinctual reaction rather than on knowledge gained from learned experience while growing up in the natural community of the canine—the pack. The cortisol release has negative feedback on the hypothalamus, which in turn has a depressant effect on the pituitary gland, which produces the hormones to stimulate the ovaries to produce follicles and corpora lutea and establish the pregnancy. A differential white blood cell reading at the time the bitch is mated will give an idea of the level of cortisol released into the bloodstream and provide an indicator of the animal's stress levels. Prevention is the only real solution here; however, monitoring of the bitch at each season may illuminate ways in which we can transport, house, and mate brood matrons to maximize chances of achieving a pregnancy.

Vaginal Infections. Low-grade vaginal infection can be a cause of canine infertility. Although this is a controversial area, many clinicians believe that the presence of bacteria is of no consequence providing there is no overt sign of disease. Other reports, especially in the human literature, place more importance on the presence of bacterial "infections" in the vaginal tract.[5] A recent study[1] found that the levels of intrauterine bacteria increase during proestrus and estrus, presumably because of transcervical migration of bacteria. This is also a time of increased vulnerability because the immune reaction of the uterus is suppressed to allow safe transit of the "foreign" spermatozoa to the ova. During metestrus and anestrus a healthy uterus should have a sterile environment. Bacterial growth in the uterus can lead to uterine disease and infertility, especially when the uterine lining is exposed to the stimulating effects of progesterone. Evidence in humans of dramatically increased fertility after broad-spectrum antibiotic treatment[5] suggests that the transcervical migration of bacteria at the time of ovulation and implantation may influence fertility adversely. Before mating, cultures can be grown from a sterile guarded swab inserted through the vulval lips and into the vestibule and vagina to ascertain bacterial flora of the vagina.

Uterine Problems. Each time the uterus is exposed to the stimulating effects of progesterone, it is being damaged. There is progression from endometritis to endometrial hyperplasia to hydrometra or mucometra as the uterus becomes more diseased. The condition can be reproduced by the use of progestogens such as

megestrol acetate, medroxyprogesterone acetate, and proligestone. Use of these products should not be considered in any breeding female. Low doses of injectable anabolic steroids such as norandrostenolone laurate (Laurabolin Intervet) 1 mg/kg each month intramuscularly, or milbolerone oral drops (Cheque drops) 30 mg/10 kg daily are effective alternatives to the progestin-type drugs. At these doses, continuous treatment for up to 5 years should not affect fertility.

Uterine disease should be suspected in bitches that continually fail to conceive. An ultrasonic examination during metestrus may reveal evidence of cystic hyperplasia. Vaginal swabbing and culturing as described above should be carried out. Cystic uterine hyperplasia can lead to pyometra if the hydrometra or mucometra becomes infected by vaginal bacteria. Treatment of choice consists of an appropriate antibiotic and prostaglandin $F_{2\alpha}$(Lutalyse) 50 to 100 mg/kg three times a day until the discharge ceases. If the uterus shows no sign of hyperplasia on ultrasonic examination, uterine biopsy should be the next step. Uterine disease is considered by many clinicians to be one of the most significant causes of canine infertility.[9] Biopsy is best conducted 60 to 70 days after the LH peak, as at this time the changes occurring in the uterine lining are at their most obvious, enabling the surgeon and the histopathologist to make a definitive diagnosis.

Ovarian Disorders. Ovarian disorders fall in two main categories: (1) Follicular cysts—failure of the ovulation process and continuation of the production of estrogen; (2) luteal cysts—failure of lysis of the corpus luteum and persistence of the progesterone phase of the cycle.

Follicular cysts are more common in bitches less than 3 years old. The cyst causes persistent vaginal bleeding, which may subside temporarily and then return, giving the owner the impression that the bitch is having a cycle every couple of weeks. Diagnosis can usually be confirmed by ultrasonic scan, as these cysts are often 2 to 3 cm in diameter. Treatment is either medical or surgical. Medical treatment by injection of human chorionic gonadotrophin hCG (Chorulon) 500 IU intravenously or intramuscularly every second day for three doses has proven effective. Surgical treatment physically removes the cyst and allows the bitch to enter metestrus. Persistent estrus in the older bitch is often a symptom of functional neoplasia of the ovary.

SEMEN EVALUATION FOR:

DATE:_____ VETERINARIAN: _____

DOG'S NAME: _____

BREED: _____

OWNER'S PHONE NUMBER _____ CONTACTED:_____

TEASER: _____ LIBIDO: _____ (0 being poor, up to 3 for dogs with high libido)

PER CENT MOTILITY: _____%

MOTILITY STATUS:
pH:_____ VOLUME:_____ml

COLOR:_____

SPERM COUNT/ml:_____x10^6 **TOTAL SPERM COUNT:** _____x10^6

MORPHOLOGY: NORMAL:_____%

HEAD ABNORMALITIES
  LIFTED ACROSOMES   _____% (early maturation of sperm)
  KNOBBED ACROSOME   _____% (abnormal sperm)
  CRATER DEFECT   _____% (genetic material malformed)

NECK ABNORMALITIES
  BENT NECK   _____% (handling defect)
  BROKEN NECK   _____% (handling defect)

MIDPIECE ABNORMALITIES
  PROXIMAL CYTOPLASMIC DROPLET
          _____% (usually regarded as normal)
  NECK TAG   _____% (abnormalities of mitochondria)

TAIL ABNORMALITIES
  DISTAL CYTOPLASMIC DROPLET
          _____% (usually regarded as normal)
  BENT TAIL   _____% (abnormal formation)
  COILED TAIL   _____% (abnormal formation)

TOTAL ABNORMAL   _____%

COMMENTS AND TREATMENT: _____
_____
_____

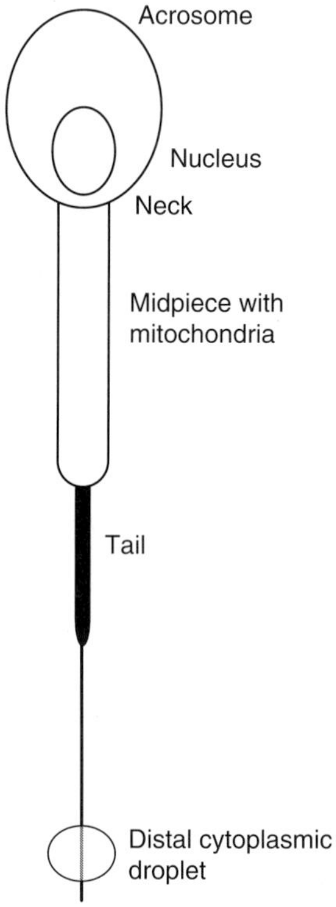

Acrosome

Nucleus

Neck

Midpiece with
mitochondria

Tail

Distal cytoplasmic
droplet

FIGURE 35–4. Evaluation form for the semen sample.

Luteal cysts are less common than follicular cysts and have the opposite effect, leading to prolonged intervals between cycles and often reduced external characteristics of estrus. Diagnosis is made by observing the clinical symptoms and by measurement of blood progesterone levels during anestrus. Levels in anestrus should be less than 2 ng/ml. Levels above 2 ng/ml are considered suspicious, and an exploratory laparatomy of the abdomen should be performed. Surgical removal is the only satisfactory treatment. Biopsy of the uterus is necessary because prolonged exposure to progesterone may have had an adverse effect on the uterus.

Thyroid Disorders. Hypothyroidism is the most commonly di-agnosed endocrine disease. Low thyroid levels have a depressant effect on many body systems. Bitches with the common symptoms of symmetrical bilateral alopecia, anemia, obesity, lethargy, and hyperpigmentation usually do not have cycles; however, there is a very high proportion of subclinical hypothyroidism, especially in racing greyhounds, that is affecting fertility. All breeding animals should have a free T_4 assay whether or not they show symptoms of hypothyroidism. Levels less than 10 ng/L require supplementation with sodium levothyroxine (Oroxine) 10 μg/kg on an empty stomach twice a day to ensure that low thyroid levels are not a contributing cause of infertility.

References

1. Allen WE: Fertility and Obstetrics in the Dog. Oxford, Blackwell Scientific Publications, 1992.
2. Van Hutchinson R: Personal communication.
3. Kurki T, Sivonen A, Renkomen OV, et al: Bacterial vaginosis in early pregnancy and pregnancy outcome. Obstet Gynecol 80:173–177, 1992.
4. Watts JR, Wright PJ, Whithear KC: Uterine, cervical and vaginal microflora of the normal bitch throughout the reproductive cycle. J Small Anim Pract 37(2):54–60, 1996.
5. McGregor JA, French JL, Parker R, et al: Prevention of premature birth by screening and treatment for common genital tract infections: Results of a prospective controlled evaluation. Am J Obstet Gynecol 173:157–167, 1995.

CHAPTER 36

CANINE INSEMINATION: ARTIFICIAL, CHILLED, AND FROZEN

ROBERT L. JOHNSON \ KATHERINE S. SETTLE

Artificial insemination (AI) has become a widely accepted and popular tool in the United States and most foreign breed registries (Ireland recently accepted AI). AI is a successful alternative to natural breeding and frequently the most prudent form of breeding since the development of extended, superior semen transport and hormonal estrous timing for optimal breeding. Both the American Kennel Club (AKC) and the National Greyhound Association (NGA) recognize AI, including insemination with fresh, chilled, and frozen semen.

Historically, early attempts at AI have been documented to the colonial period.[1] Any technique that deposited semen in the female reproductive tract and resulted in offspring has been described. Collection of semen in a myriad of containers (plastic bags, fruit jars, soda cans) and insemination by equally unusual mechanisms and equipment have been reported. A soundness examination should be completed for a stud dog and brood female before any breeding attempts.

WHY CHOOSE ARTIFICIAL INSEMINATION?

AI as a breeding technique has been employed primarily as an adequate substitute for natural breeding. Problems that arise and result in the need for AI are listed in Table 36–1.[2, 3]

WHAT FACTORS INFLUENCE AI?

Successful AI is the result of numerous factors, including: (1) semen quality, collection, and handling, (2) ovulation timing and insemination, and (3) differential insemination techniques associated with specific semen preparations. Following a male breeding soundness examination and semen evaluation (discussed in Chapter 33), collection of adequate fresh samples is not difficult.

WHAT EQUIPMENT IS NEEDED FOR AI?

Table 36–2 is a list of common equipment suggested for collection that can be purchased from many different vendors. The equipment must be handled with significant care. Different cleansing agents may be spermicidal, and it is therefore imperative to be very thorough in the preparation, use, and storage of the collection equipment.

HOW IS SEMEN COLLECTED AND EVALUATED?

Collection of the fresh semen for AI may be facilitated by use of a teaser female, but many studs require only manual manipulation. Canine semen is tri-fractionated. The first, a clear watery prostatic fraction (0.5 to 6.6 cc) is collected in the first few seconds. The second, a milky sperm-rich fraction (0.5 to 4 cc), likewise is collected over a few seconds. The third, the remaining prostatic fraction, is rather large in volume (3 to 40 cc) (breed dependent).

TABLE 36–1. Indications for Artificial Insemination

Environmental Factors
Risk of injury
Risk of infectious disease
Risk of commercial transportation
Cost of commercial transportation
Remote physical locations (international)
Desire to optimize genetic hybridization
Prolongation of offspring production beyond natural life
Increased offspring production, ie, split ejaculation
Behavioral and Physical Factors Preventing Natural Breeding
Altered libido
Aggression
Physical disability, anatomical abnormalities
Breed-specific limitations

Data from Feldman EC, Nelson RW: Canine female reproduction. In Feldman EC, Nelson RW (eds): Canine and Feline Endocrinology and Reproduction, 2nd ed. Philadelphia, WB Saunders Company, 1987, p 420; and Brown RM: An update of artificial insemination with fresh, chilled, and frozen semen. Probl Vet Med 4:445–452, 1992.

TABLE 36–2. Equipment for Collection of Canine Semen*

Item	Approximate Cost
Latex rubber collection funnel	5.00
Graduated collection tube	7.00
Compound microscope	200.00
Microscope slides and coverslips	5.00
Warming device (constant 37C)	—
Insemination pipettes (25/pkg)	2.50
Syringes (100/box)	15.00
Gloves (100/box)	7.00

*All can be obtained commercially by non-veterinarians.

It requires a longer collection interval and is not important to the actual insemination. Usual volumes desired for AI range from 2 to 10 cc. The entire ejaculate is used immediately if possible, or extended. Frequently, if large volumes are obtained, centrifugation to concentrate the sperm fraction is useful. A commercial vendor of semen should determine sperm concentration and morphology on each ejaculate to quantify the available breeding unit. Reasonable sperm concentrations are from 100 to 200 million viable motile sperm with 80 per cent normal morphology, but great variations occur.[4-6] Pregnancies with frozen breeding units have been achieved with 100 million or less, and with as few as 20 million in a fresh collection. Viability and fertilization capability differ greatly, depending on the environment, exposure, and handling. Recent extended chilled collections have maintained a 50-per cent viability at 4C on the seventh day post collection.[1]

HOW IS THE FEMALE INSEMINATED?

Once semen has been collected, fresh insemination into the female reproductive tract is a relatively simple procedure. A variety of insemination catheters is available, including bovine insemination catheters (0.5 cm × 45 cm), modified human uterine insufflation catheters, and specialized canine intrauterine catheters. Generally speaking, deposition and adequate retention of good-quality semen in the reproductive tract of a female after proper timing of ovulation should result in conception rates in excess of those of natural breedings (90% and 66%, respectively). After semen placement, elevation of the hindquarters and restriction of activity for a short time may facilitate breeding success. Live sperm have been observed in the uterus 11 days following breeding.[2, 7, 8]

Insemination techniques employing other than fresh semen require special handling, ie, semen extenders.

WHAT SEMEN EXTENDERS ARE AVAILABLE?

Most chilled semen extenders are available from local area professionals. Two common forms used are a tris-citrate buffer with 20 per cent egg yolk and antibiotics[9-11] (our favorite).[9-11] Also available is an extender with 80% homogenized and pasteurized cream (12% fat) and 20% (v/v) egg yolk with antibiotics.[3] Both are excellent chilled semen extenders and provide adequate environmental stability for transport.

HOW IS FRESH SEMEN CHILLED?

Following collection as previously described, we generally concentrate the ejaculate by centrifuge. Extender is added in 1:3 to 1:5 ratio (extender and semen must be at similar temperatures) until the proper volume is obtained. For multiple reasons, but primarily for shipping purposes, this procedure is best accomplished in a screw-top tube. Chilling can be accomplished by several methods:

1. Water bath method. The tube is placed in a water jacket that is the temperature of the semen, cooled for more than 1 hour in a 4C refrigerator, and then removed and stored in a refrigerator rack until packaged for shipping.
2. Whirl Pak method. Semen is put in a specialized package that is placed in a modular shipping container that gradually cools the semen to the proper temperature while in transit.
3. Commercially available kits. These generally include collection, extender, shipping kits, and instructions.

HOW IS CHILLED SEMEN INSEMINATED?

The most important component of this phase of AI is the planning and coordination between the stud master collector and the receiving inseminator. Because in today's fast-paced society most semen can be collected, shipped, and inseminated within 12 to 24 hours, small-package air freight is the most useful and economical destination-to-destination method. Therefore, ovulation timing, communication, collection, transport, and insemination require preplanning. Generally, an aliquot of semen is evaluated for quality on a 37-degree microscope slide before insemination. Each shipment of semen should include a quality report from the shipper. This allows comparisons by the inseminator. Usually the entire breeding unit is placed in the female and allowed to warm naturally to body temperature. The insemination technique is the same as with fresh AI.

ARE FROZEN SEMEN COLLECTION AND PROCESSING POSSIBLE?

Yes, but it is not feasible for the breeder who is not significantly experienced in this technology. Several factors make this process difficult: (1) costly equipment, (2) experience with semen handling, (3) proper training in specific techniques, (4) storage capacity with liquid nitrogen, (5) reliable extender, and (6) proper registry affiliation. We would suggest consultation with a professional in your area or at a state university. Additionally, many registries, such as the National Greyhound Association (NGA), require special application and approval before becoming recognized as a center for collection and insemination of semen. Contact with each registry should be completed before this project is undertaken.

Additionally, an important prerequisite to a successful AI program is impeccable record keeping. The NGA requires detailed collection, transportation, and insemination records, which are maintained by the registry. Fresh, chilled, and frozen insemination techniques have special designations that are required when a breeding is recorded.[12] Without these safeguards, confusion may exist in establishing parentage. DNA testing is now possible for additional reassurance of parentage.

Frozen canine semen has now become an international business with offspring of US stud dogs being produced in other countries such as Australia. Standardization of collection and insemination has allowed this progress. Deceased stud dogs are producing quality individuals today through frozen-semen technology.

HOW IS FROZEN SEMEN INSEMINATED?

Several insemination techniques have been employed with frozen semen: (1) anterior vaginal insemination, (2) transcervical insemination, (3) surgical intrauterine placement.[4] Each technique has been successful, with pregnancy rates from 40 to 80 per cent, but all rely on advanced training and technology to be successful. Success correlates well with experience of the inseminator in his or her chosen area.

The following is our procedure for surgical intrauterine insemination. The most critical aspects are proper timing and surgical intrauterine placement of the semen. It is important to determine the method that will ensure successful conception for the particular sire and dam that have been chosen. If the male is still alive, fertile, and accessible, chilled extended semen may be the better method. If frozen semen is chosen, high quality after thawing provides the best chance for success. In addition to fertility of the male, fertility of the female is important. Using frozen semen with a proven female rather than a maiden ensures that the female is capable of conceiving and carrying pups. Prior to insemination, a health physical examination and canine brucellosis test should be carried out. In females 7 years and older fertility tends to decline.

Prior to the insemination, the breed registry requirements for frozen semen should be known. Some registries for dogs require no extra paperwork, and others require the frozen straws or vial sent to them along with extensive documentation. If frozen semen from overseas is to be considered, it must be ascertained that the pups produced by such a breeding are eligible for registration by the desired organization. The American Kennel Club requires that certain paperwork be approved *before* deciding whether to approve the semen. The registry involved with the particular breeding planned should be consulted, and the bitch's owner advised accordingly.

Frozen semen *must* be stored in a special tank containing liquid nitrogen. Upon arrival, the semen should be transferred to a liquid nitrogen semen tank, or it may continue to be stored in the shipper for a short time. Be *sure* of the time that the semen will be safely held in the shipping container. It may be necessary to fill the tank with liquid nitrogen sometime during the storage. Ideally the semen should arrive close to the time of the insemination. However, early arrival helps avoid holidays, weekends, and shipping delays. Make sure instructions of how to handle and thaw the semen are obtained from the facility that froze the semen. Once again, commercial air freight is most feasible.

The collection facility should also recommend how many straws or vials of pellets will make up a breeding unit. A *breeding unit* should contain at least 100 million live, motile sperm *after* being thawed. Depending on how the freezing facility extended the semen, a *breeding unit* could mean one straw or eight straws. At least one *breeding unit* should be used for an insemination.

WHY IS TIMING SO CRUCIAL?

Sperm altered by chilling, freezing, and thawing have diminished fertility and viability. Sperm in fresh semen deposited from a male, as with natural breeding or proper artificial insemination, have been known to live for an *average* of 6 days in the female.[2] Some sperm have been known to live up to 11 days.[7, 8] Chilled extended semen has been reported to have 50 per cent live sperm after 2 to 8 days.[1] However, frozen semen, with the present freezing techniques, has a short survival time of 18 to 24 hours.[3] Because of this short life span, insemination should be as close as possible to the time that the egg is ready to be fertilized. Proper timing is very important in obtaining pups from insemination with frozen semen.

WHEN IS THE PROPER TIME TO INSEMINATE?

Unlike eggs of humans, horses, and some other species, those of the dog are not ready to be fertilized when they are ovulated. After ovulation, the eggs must mature for an average of 2 to 3 days (ranging from 1 to 5 days) before they are ready to be fertilized.[13] Therefore the best time to have the sperm in the oviduct is about 3 days after ovulation.

HOW IS THE PROPER TIME FOR INSEMINATION DETERMINED?

To know the third day after ovulation, it is necessary to determine the day of ovulation. Optimally, an assay detecting the pre-ovulatory luteinizing hormone (LH) peak is the preferred method of predicting ovulation. However, at present there are three practical ways to determine ovulation: (1) count *back* 63 days from whelping, (2) obtain vaginal smears and count *back* 6 days from the diestrus smear, and (3) use progesterone assays to *predict* ovulation. Obviously, the first two means of determining ovulation are after the fact. Ovulation has already occurred by the time whelping occurs or the diestrus vaginal smear is obtained.

At present, progesterone assay is the only way to estimate ovulation in advance (Fig. 36–1).[14, 15] The progesterone level is low during the beginning of a heat cycle. As the LH peak occurs, the progesterone level begins to rise. This initial increase in progesterone that correlates with the LH peak is the first indication of approaching ovulation. Ovulation occurs an *average* of 48 hours after the LH peak.[14, 15] When the progesterone level, which has been below 1.0 ng/ml, begins to rise, it will usually rise quickly. We define a progesterone level of 2.0 to 2.5 ng/ml as the LH peak. Therefore, 2 days later is assumed ovulation. The best time to inseminate with frozen semen is about 3 days after ovulation. Consequently, from LH peak, there are 5 days in which to prepare for insemination.

Several progesterone tests are available. Colormetric kits can be employed and completed by breeders; some must be sent to a laboratory by a veterinarian. Be aware that most test kits will give results that indicate a progesterone *range*, such as 2 to 5 ng/ml. Only RIA (radioimmune assays) done by a quality laboratory will provide quantification, such as 2.6 ng/ml. Although kits can be utilized in many instances for frozen insemination, as the progesterone approaches 1 ng/ml, we prefer the more precise results of RIA.[16]

Turn-around times for RIA progesterone tests vary from 12 hours to 7 days. Obviously, a long turn-around time will greatly affect the success of a frozen semen insemination. Check with the laboratory that will be completing the progesterone assay and establish a collection-to-result time. Remember also to find out the weekend and holiday schedules. To establish the characteristic increase of progesterone around the LH peak, tests must be done frequently. To document the progesterone value on any given day, blood can be drawn, centrifuged, and the serum frozen until it can be sent to the laboratory. We always obtain an RIA progesterone assay on the predicted day of ovulation. Ovulation progesterone should be about 5 to 10 ng/ml.[17]

Progesterone tests cost from $15 to $75 per test. If 10 progesterone tests are needed for timing for a particular female, it can be expensive. It is economical using the kits early in the heat cycle when progesterone is low. Frozen serum saved in the freezer may not need to be sent if the following day's progesterone is more significant. When progesterone assay was used to time insemination, most females were inseminated around day 16 after *observed* vaginal bleeding. However, individual females normally may vary. Successful pregnancies have also resulted when inseminations were carried out on day 8 and on day 23 of the heat cycle.

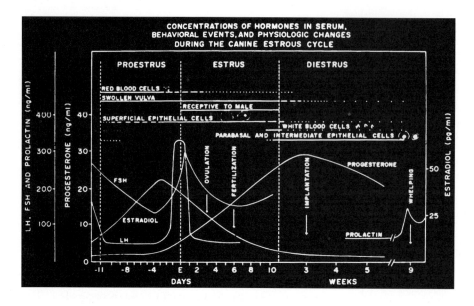

FIGURE 36–1. Concentrations of hormones in serum, behavioral events, and physiologic changes during the canine estrous cycle.

WHY PERFORM SURGICAL INSEMINATION?

With most species, thawed frozen semen must be deposited into the *uterus* through the cervix to achieve reasonable conception rates. Frozen semen has been used very successfully in cattle for years. The cervix is threaded with an insemination rod and the thawed semen pushed through the rod and into the uterus. With frozen semen, the number of sperm used for an insemination is less than the usual number inseminated with natural breedings. Also, the life span of thawed frozen sperm is decreased. Therefore the most success with frozen semen has been achieved when it was deposited directly into the uterus.

HOW IS THE SEMEN SURGICALLY PUT INTO THE UTERUS?

After a proper clinical work-up and physical examination for anesthesia, the female is anesthetized and prepared for an abdominal midline incision. (*Note*: Sodium barbiturate anesthetics should not be used in greyhounds.[18]) A qualified person begins preparation of the frozen semen when the surgeon begins the incision. Semen is frozen in straws or pellets, and thawing techniques vary. The facility that collected the semen should provide instructions for thawing it. The thawing instructions should be followed carefully. One common procedure with straw thaws is to thaw the straw in 98F water for 45 seconds. The thawed semen is then kept warm until deposited into the uterus.

After the semen is thawed, the "plug" end is cut (preferably with a special straw cutter). The straw end with cotton is not cut. Every time there is semen transfer, as from straw to syringe, there is a chance of semen loss. Therefore, the straw itself can be used as a syringe. A 22-gauge needle, a 0.5-inch piece of sterile intravenous tubing, and a wooden applicator stick are used. The intravenous tubing is placed into the needle. The straw is then placed into the other end of the tubing. The wooden applicator stick is used as the plunger by placing it into the cotton end of the straw. The semen is then inseminated into the uterus. The semen should be evaluated at the time of insemination. Therefore, a drop of semen left in the straw or syringe after the insemination is usually utilized. Once the semen is thawed in the syringe, handling should be minimized in order to avoid mistakes, such as dropping the semen, contamination of the needle, or too much time elapsing between thaw and insemination, causing the quality of semen to decline.

The practitioner should also be aware that the volume a uterus will hold is limited. If 6 cc of thawed semen is to be inseminated, the uterus will probably become full before all of the semen is used. The greyhound uterus will hold about 3 cc of semen. It may be necessary to ask the collection facility if the thaw procedure could be changed to keep the same number of sperm but to use less volume. (This is particularly applicable in insemination of small breeds.) Some facilities use a semen thaw medium that adds to the volume of the inseminating unit. Perhaps less medium could be used to reduce volume without compromising the sperm.

The surgical approach is similar to ovariohysterectomy (spaying). After the midline incision, one horn of the uterus is brought out for insemination. One-half the insemination dose is put into the uterus with a "syringe" and 22-gauge needle. The surgeon uses finger pressure across the uterus on the cervix side of the insemination injection area to help keep the semen from flowing toward the cervix. The inseminator deposits the semen in the uterus in the direction of the ovary. Semen is prevented from flowing out the cervix by digital pressure across the base of the uterine horn. As the needle is removed from the uterine wall, gentle pressure over the injection site will help seal the injection site and stop bleeding. Frequently the uterus will become slightly turgid when full of semen. Care should be taken not to fill the uterine horn too full, producing excessive pressure within the horn. Again, it is important not to use too much semen. If the surgeon releases the finger pressure on the uterus near the cervix, fluid capacity is increased; however, the semen can now flow out the cervix. Again, it is imperative that the practitioner determine the correct volume.

After the inseminated horn is replaced, the other horn of the uterus is inseminated by a similar procedure. The midline incision is then closed, and the female is allowed to recover from anesthesia. If a deep vaginal smear were to be taken after surgery, sperm frequently will be seen. This is a natural manifestation of sperm motility and should not be cause for alarm.

HOW SHOULD THE FEMALE BE CARED FOR AFTER INSEMINATION?

If possible, shipping and stressful situations for the bitch should be avoided until 21 days after ovulation. After 21 days, the embryos should be implanted in the uterus.[2] It is always helpful to diagnose pregnancy by expert palpation at 21 to 33 days or by ultrasound at 21 days. If the female was pregnant at 28 days and not at 63 days, then the problem was not with conception but with the female's ability to maintain the pregnancy.

CONCLUSIONS

Canine artificial insemination, whether with fresh, chilled, or frozen semen, has evolved significantly during the last decade. Secondary to the work of many researchers, the principles, science, theories, and techniques have been advanced, so success is now possible by well-trained non-veterinarians. The National Greyhound Association has seen a marked increase in inseminations with frozen semen (doubling in the past 24 months). To date, the show dog contingent has largely utilized the chilled semen process.

Exportation of frozen semen is now international business, with recent completion of successful insemination and birth of litters from US sires in Australia.

Further research is needed to eliminate the sperm mortality associated with cryopreservation. Development of an advanced cryoprotectant would vastly enhance conception rates. The type of insemination with frozen semen (vaginal vs intrauterine) continues to be debated frequently and is largely a preference of training and experience.

The serious breeder, with proper training and consultation, should be able to assist local professionals. Successful breeding programs generally exhibit dedication, teamwork, and attention to detail.

References

1. Concannon PW, Battiota M: Canine semen freezing and artificial insemination. *In* Kirk RW: Current Veterinary Therapy X. Philadelphia, WB Saunders Company, pp 1247–1258, 1989.
2. Feldman EC, Nelson RW: Canine female reproduction. *In* Canine and Feline Endocrinology and Reproduction. Philadelphia, WB Saunders Company, 1987, p 420.
3. Brown RM: An update of artificial insemination with fresh, chilled, and frozen semen. *In* Probl Vet Med 4:445–452, 1992.
4. Linde-Forsberg C: Achieving pregnancy by using frozen or chilled extended semen. Vet Clin North Am Small Anim Pract 21:467–485, 1991.
5. Morton, BSG: Semen evaluation, cryopreservation and factors relevant to the use of frozen semen in dogs. J Reprod Fertil (Suppl) 39:311, 1989.
6. Fougner JA, Forsberg M: Effect of different sperm numbers on fertility after artificial insemination of foxes. Acta Vet Scand 28:403, 1987.
7. Doak RL, Hall A, Dale HE: Longevity of spermatozoa in the reproductive tract of the bitch. J Reprod Fert 13:51–58, 1967.
8. Concannon PW, Whaley S, Lein D, et al: Canine gestation length: Variation related to time of mating and fertile life span of sperm. Am J Vet Res 44:1819, 1983.
9. Davis JS, Bratton RW, Foote RH: Livability of bovine spermatozoa at 5°, −25°, and −85°C in tris-buffered and citrate-buffered yolk-glycerol extenders. J Dairy Sci 46:57, 1963.
10. Olar TT: Cryopreservation of dog spermatozoa [dissertation]. Colorado State University, 1984.
11. Foote RH, Leonard EP: The influence of pH, osmotic pressure, glycine, and glycerol on the survival of dog sperm in buffered yolk extenders. Cornell Vet 54:78, 1964.
12. National Greyhound Association: Requirements for Participation in Frozen Semen Registry, 1997.
13. Concannon PW, McCann JP, Temple M: Biology and endocrinology of ovulation, pregnancy, and parturition in the dog. J Reprod Fertil (Suppl) 39:3, 1989.
14. Olson PN, Bowen RA, Behrendt M, et al: Concentrations of reproductive hormones in canine serum throughout late anestrus, metestrus, and estrus. Biol Reprod 23:1196, 1982.
15. Olson PN, Nett TM: Reproductive endocrinology and physiology of the bitch. *In* Morrow DA: Current Therapy in Theriogenology 2. Philadelphia, WB Saunders Company, 453–457, 1986.
16. Madej A, Linde-Fosberg C, Garmun F: A rapid radioimmunoassay for determination of LH in dogs. J Reprod Fertil (Suppl) 39:329, 1989.
17. Linde-Forsberg C: Fertility in dogs in relation to semen quality and the time and site of insemination with fresh and frozen semen. J Reprod Fert (Suppl) 39:307, 1989.
18. Robinson EP: Research in greyhound anesthesia. Greyhound Rev 37–39, 1987.

CHAPTER 37

MANAGEMENT OF PREGNANCY AND PARTURITION

FRANK R. JORDAN

GENERAL CONSIDERATIONS

It has been stated that good trainers, regardless of whether it be of man, dogs, or horses, must have common sense and be keen observers, not bound by the rules.[1] Historically, veterinary management of canine reproduction focused on the immediate concerns of the individual animal and was aimed at identification and resolution of the presenting problem. Greater attention must be paid to prevention of these problems and features of those operating systems that may result in such problems.

New diagnostic techniques and protocols allow a much more comprehensive assessment of reproductive problems. The availability of progesterone assays, ultrasonography, and fresh chilled and frozen semen have revolutionized reproductive management of the individual bitch. Practical knowledge of these clinical aids or techniques is imperative to meet the expectations of competitive breeder clients. Continued veterinary education, education of the breeder client regarding canine reproduction, and utilization of accurate record keeping are essential for successful reproductive management.

Bitches retired from competition or waiting for breeding must continue to receive individualized attention. Too often these bitches are subjected to (1) inadequate diet, both in quantity and quality, (2) lack of adequate exercise, (3) cessation or reduction in supplements such as thyroid replacement hormone, and (4) lack of dental care.

RECORDS

Historical information of previous cycles (with or without attempted breeding), breeding attempts, and whelping can be very useful. It is recommended that at least the following be recorded at each mating and whelping: (1) Signalment of the bitch (age, parity, general health, previous reproductive problems) and the stud dog (age, general health, reproductive history, results of semen evaluation). (2) The date of the first observed signs of heat (day 1 of cycle). (3) The date and results of supportive examination (progesterone assays, vaginal smears, *Brucella canis* testing, physical examination, complete blood count, biochemical profile). (4) The estimated day in the cycle of ovulation and the date (2 days following the estimated luteinizing hormone surge). (5) The recommended day or days in the cycle for mating and the date (2 to 4 days following the estimated ovulation day). (6) The day in the cycle of mating and the date. (7) The method and number of services (natural fresh semen; artificial insemination, fresh, chilled, or frozen semen; surgical implant, fresh, chilled, or frozen semen). (8) The semen quality and quantity (if known). (9) The estimated whelping date (65 days ± 1 day of luteinizing hormone (LH) surge).[2] (10) The actual whelping date. (11) The number of days from the last mating to whelping. (12) The number of days from the estimated date of ovulation to whelping. (13) The number of pups whelped (live-born, dead, normals, abnormals). (14) Problems observed at whelping.

DIET

Successful breeding programs result from optimal, not minimal, nutrition.[3] Feeding for maximal reproductive performance is simple. Only two types of food are needed: one for maintenance and one for late gestation, lactation, and growth. Any diet fed should be labeled as nutritionally complete and balanced for the appropriate life stage of the dog and should have claims supported by scientific research rather than analytical values only.

The nutritional requirements of reproducing bitches are as much as 2 to 4 times greater than that of the inactive adult dog.[4] Nutritional deprivation during pregnancy can compromise immunological competence of the offspring and may adversely affect the production of colostrum.[5] If the bitch becomes overweight or underweight, there may be problems in successfully gestating all pups to term, or the animal may suffer dystocia. Less than 30 per cent of fetal growth occurs during the first 5 to 6 weeks of gestation, and as a result, there is little or no change in the bitch's body weight or nutritional need during this period.[4] For this reason, a bitch in optimal body condition at time of mating should be fed the same amount needed for maintenance for the first 5 to 6 weeks of gestation.

It should be noted that bitches, like humans, may suffer from morning sickness. At about 3 weeks of gestation, many bitches undergo a short period of transient anorexia that typically lasts for 3 to 10 days. A slight transient weight loss may occur in some bitches. This refusal of a complete and balanced diet may represent a natural behavioral change in a healthy bitch during gestation.

The fetal size increases rapidly during the last 3 to 4 weeks of gestation. Thus, during this time, the amount fed should be gradually increased so that the bitch is receiving 15 to 25 per cent more food by the time of whelping. The body weight of the bitch should increase 15 to 25 per cent by the time of whelping. During this period, the caloric intake needed cannot be met by simply increasing the meal size. Meal frequency should also be increased, usually from one to two meals daily during midpregnancy, then to three to four meals daily by peak lactation.

As whelping nears, the bitch may lose appetite entirely. In many bitches, food refusal during the ninth week of gestation is a good indication that whelping will occur during the next 24 to 48 hours. Usually within 24 hours after whelping, appetite will return, and food consumption will increase dramatically. Failure of a bitch to regain a normal appetite after whelping signals abnormalities requiring intervention. Occasionally a very attentive or inexperienced bitch will be reluctant to leave a litter to feed herself for 24 to 48 hours after whelping. Bitches should be monitored for this behavior post partum as they will need more encouragement to eat and drink.

DRUGS AFFECTING PREGNANCY

Because of the availability and use of many drugs and medications by kennel managers, it is appropriate to carefully consider and question the use of drugs in the pregnant animal. Drug administration to the pregnant bitch should be avoided if at all possible. Unfortunately, little research has specifically addressed the administration of drugs to the pregnant bitch. Usually information must be extrapolated from studies performed on laboratory animals or from experience reported in humans. Virtually all drugs administered to a bitch have the potential to cross the placenta, just as nutrients and gases do. Thus, situations arise in which a developing embryo or fetus may become an inadvertent recipient of a drug administered to a pregnant bitch and raise questions as to the safety of that drug in pregnancy.

Drugs that would be contraindicated because they have been shown to cause congenital malformation or embryonic toxicity are: (1) ciprofloxacin, enrofloxacin, doxycycline, oxytetracycline, tetracycline, streptomycin; (2) griseofulvin; (3) gold (aurothioglucose); (4) pentobarbital; (5) misoprostol; (6) warfarin; (7) diethylstilbestrol (DES), estradiol cypionate (ECP), mitotane, stanozolol, and testosterone. Fortunately this list of drugs is relatively short and, in most cases, an alternative to a toxic drug can be selected. But if we include the drugs that may have potential risks to the embryo or fetus, the list becomes significantly longer. This list could include the antimicrobials chloramphenicol, metronidazole, and most of the aminoglycosides; virtually all of anticancer drugs and analgesics; many of the cardiovascular drugs, anticonvulsant drugs, and corticosteroids; and the antifungal drug amphotericin B. Also included would be the anesthetics methoxyflurane, halothane, thiopental; and the antiparasitics amitraz, trichlorfon, and thiacetarsamide. A complete listing can be found in reference 6. Clinicians and kennel managers should always question the safety of drugs administered during pregnancy in regard to the fetus and the bitch. Certain treatments or surgical procedures should be postponed until after parturition, if possible.

DIAGNOSIS OF PREGNANCY

The current methods of pregnancy diagnosis in the bitch include palpation, ultrasonography, and radiography. The reliability of pregnancy diagnosis by palpation can vary considerably, depending on

TABLE 37–1. Estimated Times of Various Events of Canine Pregnancy in Relation to Preovulatory LH Peak and Potential Times of Fertile Matings

Event of Pregnancy	Days after LH Peak	Days after Fertile Mating
Proestrus onset	−25 to +3	
Estrus onset	−4 to +5	
Preovulatory LH peak	0	−7 to +3
First of multiple matings	−5 to +7	−12 to 0
Fertile mating	−3 to +7	0
Ovulation of primary oocytes	2	−5 to +5
Oocyte maturation	4	−3 to +7
Fertilization	4 to 7	0 to 7
Vaginal cornification reduced	7 to 9	0 to 12
Morulae in distal oviducts	8 to 10	2 to 13
Blastocysts enter uterus	9 to 11	2 to 14
Zonae pellucidae shed	15 to 17	8 to 20
Attachment sites established	16 to 18	9 to 21
Swelling of implantation sites	18 to 20	11 to 23
Palpable 1 cm swellings	22 to 24	15 to 27
Pregnancy anemia onset	27 to 29	20 to 31
Uterine swellings detectable on x-ray	30 to 32	23 to 35
Reduced palpability of 3 cm swellings	32 to 34	25 to 37
Hematocrit below 40 per cent PCV	38 to 40	31 to 43
Fetal skull and spine radiopaque	44 to 46	37 to 49
Earliest x-ray pregnancy diagnosis	45 to 47	39 to 50
Hematocrit below 35 per cent PCV	48 to 50	41 to 53
Fetal pelvis radiopaque	53 to 57	46 to 60
Fetal teeth radiopaque	58 to 63	54 to 66
Prepartum luteolysis and hypothermia	63 to 65	56 to 68
Parturition	64 to 66	57 to 69

From Concannon PW: Physiology and Endocrinology of Canine Pregnancy. *In* Morrow RW (ed): Current Therapy in Theriogenology 2. Philadelphia, WB Saunders Company, 1986, p 492.

stage of pregnancy, the conformation of the bitch, and the expertise of the palpator. Palpation is generally performed most reliably between days 22 and 32 post LH peak (Table 37–1). Radiography is useful only during late pregnancy (day 45 post LH peak) (Table 37–1), and determination of fetal health is very difficult.

Ultrasound can effectively diagnose pregnancy and determine the stage of pregnancy and the viability of the fetus. The gestational sac and fetal heart beat may be visualized after 22 to 31 days of gestation.[7]

It should be noted that several hormone assays have been suggested for pregnancy diagnosis, but none has been used extensively in the dog. Serum progesterone assays cannot be used to diagnose pregnancy because the ranges in absolute progesterone levels in both pregnant and nonpregnant bitches are quite large (Fig. 37–1).

EVENTS OF PREGNANCY

See Table 37–1.

RADIOIMMUNOASSAY SERUM PROGESTERONE LEVEL ANALYSIS

The knowledge of serum progesterone concentration in the bitch can be a very useful tool. Radioimmunoassay (RIA) progesterone levels may be used before mating to estimate the date of the LH peak, ovulation date, recommended mating date, and the estimated normal whelping date.

If accurate records have been kept of previous estrous cycles and whelpings, it is much easier to identify problem bitches. Along with that information, strategically timed RIA progesterone assays can be used to determine the LH peak, estimated day of ovulation, recommended mating date, and the estimated whelping date. It often takes two or more tests, at 3- to 5-day intervals, to accurately make these predictions.

If RIA progesterone assays are unavailable, rapid ELISA serum progesterone assays and/or vaginal cytology may be used to determine the estimated date of ovulation. ELISA progesterone assays are generally less expensive, but much less accurate, than RIA. Vaginal smears only can be used retrospectively to predict the ovulation date and are very limited in prospective application.

PREPARATION FOR WHELPING

As previously noted, most bitches will stop eating 24 to 48 hours before whelping, and the rectal temperature will drop below 37°C (99°F). The major endocrine event of parturition is abrupt prepartum decline in serum progesterone levels (Fig. 37–1; Table 37–2) precipitated by maturation of the fetuses as they reach term development.

The prepartum decline in progesterone can also be predicted by

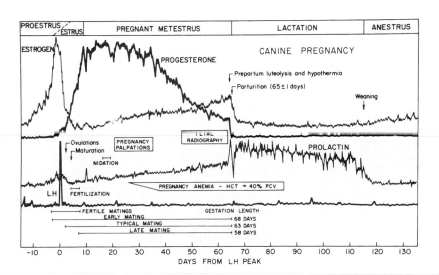

FIGURE 37–1. Typical endocrine changes reported to occur in association with ovulation, pregnancy, parturition, and lactation in the bitch, shown in relation to the day of the preovulatory peak in luteinizing hormone and various events of gestation. (From Concannon PW: *In* Kirk R [ed.]: Current Veterinary Therapy VIII, Small Animal Practice. Philadelphia, WB Saunders Company, 1983, pp 886–901.)

TABLE 37–2. RIA Progesterone Level Analysis in >4000 Bitches*

Prepartum Stage	Progesterone Level (ng/ml)
Proestrus and early estrus	0.1–1.0
Midestrus prior to LH surge	1.0–1.8
LH peak	1.8–2.5
Ovulation	4.0–8.0
Fertilization (3 days, Fig. 37–1)	8.0–25.0
Diestrus (whether pregnant or open)	15.0–to as high as 60.0
Last week of pregnancy	4.0–16.0
36–48 hours prepartum	Rapid decline in progesterone
24 hours prepartum	<2.0
8–12 hours prepartum	<1.0

*Author's personal experience.

measuring the rectal temperature, which parallels the decline in progesterone with a delay of about 12 hours.[8]

PARTURITION

Clinical management of canine parturition has traditionally relied on assessment of the bitch's health. A number of other aspects of the bitch's gestation should be evaluated, including fetal well-being. These include knowledge of gestation length, maternal rectal temperature, serum progesterone levels before mating and at term, radiographic and ultrasonic examination of the fetus, and knowledge of the duration of stages I and II of labor.

A most important tool is understanding the variation of gestation length, the time from mating to whelping, in the bitch. This variation not only affects determination of the estimated whelping date and the diagnosis of primary uterine inertia at term, but it also explains variable results with pregnancy diagnosis when gestational age is calculated from the first mating.

Motile sperm have been recovered in undiminished numbers from bitches 4 to 11 days after mating.[9] Some bitches even have been reported to conceive when bred as early as 10 to 11 days before ovulation. If the breeder does not know the date of LH peak and/or ovulation, gestation must be timed from the first service. With natural mating, the first service may occur as early as 9 to 11 days before or as late as 3 to 5 days after ovulation. This is due to the wide variation in the interval from onset of behavioral estrus to ovulation and diestrus. Conception from single matings at either of the extremes may result in an apparent gestation length (mating to whelping) of 58 to 71 days. Timing of gestation from the first mating may also influence pregnancy diagnosis by palpation and radiographic/sonographic examination of the fetus, because true fetal gestational age from fertilization may differ up to 11 days from the calculated fetal gestational age from the last mating.

The rectal temperature of the pregnant bitch should be monitored twice daily starting 55 days after the first mating, if the ovulation date is not known. A significant drop in the average normal temperature of 38C (101.5F) to 36 (98F) or 37C (99F) correlates with a decrease in serum progesterone, indicating that whelping should begin within the next 24 hours. If it does not, intervention is indicated.

If RIAs of serum progesterones are performed to assist in timing of mating, the whelping date can be predicted very accurately. Parturition occurs 63 days, ±1 day, from the day of ovulation. This accurately predicted date, calculated from the estimated ovulation date, can be very helpful in determining if and when intervention is indicated.

SIGNS AND STAGES OF PARTURITION[10]

For 2 to 3 days before parturition, bitches usually become restless, seek seclusion, and reduce their food intake. Uterine contraction and cervical dilation occur during stage I of parturition. External signs of stage I labor in the bitch are nonspecific and include increased restlessness, panting, scratching, chewing, and nesting behavior. Uterine contractions are not generally observed externally but may be palpated through the abdominal wall. This stage lasts 6 to 12 hours.

Stage II labor consists of fetal passage through the cervix and vagina. Mechanical dilation of cervix by the fetal head elicits a neuroendocrine reflex in the bitch resulting in increased oxytocin secretion, which strengthens uterine contractions. Cervical distention also causes the bitch to strain. Stage II labor can be recognized by (1) endoscopic visualization or palpation of a fetus through the dilated cervix, (2) observing contractions of the voluntary skeletal musculature of the bitch's abdomen (straining), and (3) observation of fetal membranes at the vulva.

Although the duration of stage II varies widely among bitches, in general, pup survival is optimal if no more than 4 hours elapse from onset of stage II labor to delivery, and no more than 2 hours elapse between delivery of pups. When there is failure to progress before or between deliveries in stage II labor, medical or surgical intervention is indicated for optimal pup survival. If cesarean section is performed more than 24 hours after the onset of stage II labor, one is likely to find dead fetuses and a septic uterus.

When parturition is thought to be completed, the bitch should be thoroughly examined for the presence of any remaining fetuses. This is particularly important in the greyhound and other large-breed dogs in which the last one or two fetuses of large bitches may be retained in the tip of the uterus. If there is any doubt whether the uterus has been emptied, a radiograph should be taken.

DYSTOCIA

Most often, when veterinarians have to intervene with a pregnant bitch at term, it is because of abnormal or difficult parturition (dystocia). This is a common and challenging problem, one for which each veterinarian must develop a philosophy that is best suited to his or her technical and diagnostic skills. The most difficult decision is choosing among medical therapy, manual delivery, and cesarean section or combination thereof. Factors to be considered include the nature of dystocia, physical condition of the bitch and pups, available equipment, and time. In addition, the utility of the bitch and economic value of the puppies is a consideration of the owners.

All cases of dystocia should receive immediate attention. A good history should be obtained, particularly of previous whelpings, and a quick but thorough physical examination (including abdominal palpation for pregnancy, approximate number of fetuses, fetal movement, and fetal heart beat) and vaginal examination should be performed. The vaginal examination should be performed with attention to antisepsis by careful cleaning of the vulva and the use of examining gloves. The examination should include evaluation of pelvic size, feathering (digital massage of the vaginal floor) to determine the presence or absence of uterine contractions, and determination of the location and position of the fetuses. Radiography of the bitch to determine the presence of, or number of, fetuses may be indicated.

There are many causes of dystocia in the sporting-breed bitch. Many cases can be prevented by proper care and planning before and during the gestational period. The bitch should have regular exercise, her diet regulated to prevent obesity, and a complete and accurate reproductive record kept. Classification of dystocia as maternal, fetal, or uterine inertia helps in the decision-making process.

Maternal dystocia factors can be subdivided by cause into anatomical, endocrine, and psychological (behavioral) types. Maternal anatomical factors may include inadequate size of the maternal birth canal due to vaginal stricture, prolapse, or neoplasia. This consideration comes into play with primiparous greyhound bitches that often have minimal vulvular enlargement and/or vaginal stricture, discouraging normal delivery. Once the first pup has been delivered, often with manual assistance, bitches may then deliver the remainder without further assistance. Endocrine dystocia may be seen in bitches carrying only one or two fetuses, possibly because of the lack of adequate fetal factors that initiate the abrupt decline in progesterone necessary for the onset of parturition. Psychological dystocia may be evidenced by nervous bitches that, with excessive interference, may fail to progress with parturition.

Fetal dystocia is associated with oversized fetuses (one-pup litters), fetal hydrocephalus, and abnormal position of the head, limbs, or buttocks at the pelvic inlet. *Maternal and fetal dystocia* are best handled by cesarean section or manual delivery. The latter is reserved for those cases in which there are one or two pups and economic considerations do not warrant cesarean section.

A lack of or inadequate uterine contractions *(uterine inertia)* is another cause of dystocia. The uterus itself is an amazing organ; the primary function of the uterine muscle is to contract and perform work. However, unlike the heart, the uterus must be dormant as well as active and perform different functions throughout different phases of reproduction. It must be able to propel contents in a caudal to cranial direction (semen at mating) and also in the opposite direction during parturition. The uterus is required to generate vigorous contractions during parturition and at estrus and yet remain quiescent during pregnancy to protect and nurture the developing fetuses.

Uterine inertia may be primary or secondary. Primary inertia may be caused by lack of tone or degenerative (geriatric) changes in the uterine musculature. It may occur in any breed. Secondary uterine inertia is primarily a result of exhaustion and is more common than primary. It is most often seen in bitches with large litters and in older or obese bitches. Lack of exercise, obesity, and excessive stretching of the uterus by fluid and/or fetuses are factors that cause or contribute to uterine inertia. Primary and secondary uterine inertia should be considered a medical problem initially. Oxytocin administration is the most commonly used therapy for uterine inertia during parturition. However, before oxytocin is administered, it is important to diagnose and treat any hypoglycemia or hypocalcemia present. Calcium plays an important role in the smooth muscle contraction-relaxation cycle of the uterus, and proper calcium concentration within the cells is necessary for effective myometrial contractility. Oxytocin stimulates contraction of the uterine myometrial cells and mammary myoepithelial cells.

When hypocalcemia is suspected with uterine inertia, the bitch is first given a calcium preparation intravenously, followed by 5 to 10 IU oxytocin intramuscularly in 10 to 15 minutes. The bitch should be kept in a quiet environment. A mature greyhound bitch can be given a calcium gluconate product containing 16.84 mg/ml calcium by intravenous titration until she vomits or a maximum of 30 ml is administered. The popular dose of oxytocin in dogs ranges from 5 to 20 IU given subcutaneously or intramuscularly; the duration of effect is approximately 20 minutes.[11] Therefore the oxytocin administration may be repeated at 20- to 30-minute intervals. If active labor and delivery are not initiated within 1 to 1½ hours, further medical therapy is not indicated. Excessive use of oxytocin contributes to myometrial fatigue and has the potential to exacerbate uterine inertia.

Instrument delivery may be used in selected cases, depending on the expertise of the clinician, number of pups remaining (one or two), and value of the pups. When this method fails, surgical intervention is indicated.

CESAREAN SECTION

When preparing for a cesarean section, the veterinarian has to deal with two patients, the bitch and the fetus/neonate, which are physiologically and pharmacologically vastly different from each other.[12] Only by understanding these differences can the veterinarian successfully deal with both.

Preoperative Preparation. Fluids should be given intravenously before induction of anesthesia, especially if dystocia has been of many hours' duration or if the bitch is suffering from pregnancy toxemia or septicemia, because these patients are frequently dehydrated. Placental blood flow may be reduced by dehydration, with reduced cardiac output and hypotension adversely affecting the fetus. The fluid of choice is a balanced electrolyte solution such as lactated Ringer's, or as in the case of pregnancy toxemia, one containing dextrose. A baseline administration rate of 10 ml/kg/hr may be increased as indicated by individual clinical needs.

Pregnant animals have a reduced requirement for inhalation anesthetics when compared to nonpregnant animals. Premedicants will further reduce anesthetic requirements, as does parturient hypothermia. The duration of general anesthesia before delivery should be as short as possible to minimize fetal depression. To accomplish this, the animal should be clipped and prepared for surgery prior to induction. The surgeon should be ready to start the operation immediately after induction and the final scrub are completed. Operative speed is important in cesarean section because long "incision-to-delivery" time is associated with increased fetal asphyxia and depression.

Induction and Anesthesia. Several factors should be taken into consideration when selecting a suitable anesthetic technique for cesarean section. These include the technical support staff and equipment available to the veterinarian, speed and skill of the veterinarian as a surgeon, veterinarian preference for and experience with a particular anesthetic technique, economic value of the dam and/or the neonates, whether the owner wants to have the dam bred again, and reversibility of the anesthetic.

By the judicious use (as few drugs as possible and in low doses) of injectables combined with a low concentration of an inhalation anesthetic, it is possible to deliver the neonate with minimal drug-induced depression. Numerous protocols are effective. One such would include the following. After determination that a cesarean section is required, an intravenous catheter is placed aseptically, taped in place, and administration of lactated Ringer's solution is started. As much as possible of the clipping and surgical scrubbing is completed. This is followed by atropine (0.02 mg/kg) and xylazine (1.1 mg/kg) by intravenous push. The rest of the surgical preparation is completed, and ketamine (5.5 mg/kg) is then given by intravenous push, an endotracheal tube passed and secured, the bitch placed on the surgical table, and oxygen flow started. Isoflurane or halothane gas anesthesia is usually started following delivery of the last pup. If a neonate is depressed by this anesthetic protocol, efforts to revive it are generally quite successful.

Surgical Procedure. The surgeon may choose between a flank or midline approach. Each has its advantages, and thought should be given to what might be encountered intraoperatively and postoperatively. The flank approach may be preferred by some because it does not interfere with lactation and it reduces the chance of wound dehiscence (a definite consideration in the greyhound breed).

The ventral midline provides better exposure of the uterus, generally requires less hemostasis, and is more familiar to most surgeons. This exposure may be necessary when dealing with the racing greyhound bitch or other sporting or working breeds that may be presented in prolonged labor (>24 hours) or with a large number of fetuses (8 to 13) and a friable uterus. One must either make a very lengthy incision to exteriorize the gravid horns or remove the pups with the uterus remaining in the abdomen. If dead fetuses and/or a septic uterus is found, combined hysterotomy and hysterectomy may be indicated.

Care of the Neonate. Weakened neonates are often delivered following dystocia and/or cesarean section. Birth ends the fetal life and initiates a sequence of events necessary for independent life of the neonate. Lung inflation is the first and most important step in the sequence of events that occurs at birth. It must occur within a few minutes of placental separation. The neonate with attached placenta is immediately handed to an assistant who removes the fluid and mucus from the nasal passages and oropharynx. The neonate is vigorously towel dried, its viability ascertained, and the umbilicus clamped and separated approximately 2 cm from the abdomen. The clamp may be removed after several minutes and the umbilical stump examined for hemorrhage. Vigorous rubbing of the neonate usually stimulates respiration. If further stimulation is necessary, doxapram (0.25 to 1.0 mg) may be administered to the neonate either sublingually or into the umbilical vein. Naloxone (0.001 mg/kg) may be given similarly for revival if opioid narcotics have been used in the bitch. The neonate may then be held firmly on its back in the palm of the hand, with its head supported by the fingers and its face and abdomen covered with the other hand. The neonate is then swung sharply up and down, helping to clear the nasal passage by centrifugal force and creating a pressure difference that will also stimulate respiration. The neonate should be breathing and crying by this stage. Other encouraging signs are pink mucous membranes and a strong pulse.

Neonates' body temperature is 34.5 to 36°C (94 to 97°F) for the first 2 weeks of life. They have no shivering reflex for the first 6 days and therefore depend on an external heat source such as the bitch to sustain normal body temperature.[4] An environmental temperature (32.5°C or 90°F) should be provided to ensure that the core temperature of the neonate is maintained after delivery. Factors that can continue to contribute to the compromise of the neonatal puppy include hypothermia, hypoxia, dehydration, hypoglycemia, deficient intake of nutrients (prenatal and postnatal), immune deficiencies, and inborn errors in metabolism.

Pups of lower than average birth weight may need supplemental feeding and close observation for hypothermia, dehydration, and sepsis. One of the more beneficial management practices is to weigh the pups daily for the first 2 weeks and then every 3 days until they are 1 month old. Periodic weight checks should be made thereafter, using a Gram scale. This scale is one of the best investments a breeder can make.[4] Diarrhea from any cause may rapidly lead to dehydration in the neonate. Weight loss is often the earliest sign of dehydration. Dryness of the mucous membranes is a more reliable test of dehydration in puppies than skin turgor. In early stages of dehydration, treatment with subcutaneous fluids may be sufficient. Management of environmental factors, including sanitation, vaccination, nutrition, and attended whelpings will improve the survival of the neonate.[13]

IMMEDIATE POSTPARTURIENT PROBLEMS IN THE BITCH

There are several disorders that can occur shortly after parturition in the bitch. Some disorders may be mild and due to psychological or physiological changes associated with pregnancy. For example, psychological anorexia may occur in very attentive bitches with large litters or primiparous bitches that refuse to leave the pups to feed themselves. They will need more encouragement to eat and

drink. It is important to be familiar with the normal physiological changes during pregnancy and alterations in laboratory values when attempting to evaluate a postpartum bitch. Physiological anemia occurs during pregnancy, and total protein, albumin, and calcium in serum decreases during late gestation.[14] Galactostasis, another normal physiological change disorder that may occur, is excessive accumulation of milk in the mammary glands. This often is seen in bitches following acute weaning or the sudden loss of a litter of puppies. Treatment is directed at decreasing the formation of secretion and reducing inflammation. Cold compresses, glucocorticoids, and diuretics may help resolve the condition. Reducing the food intake of the bitch will also aid in prevention of galactostasis.

There are other immediate postparturient disorders that may be severe and even life threatening, such as metritis or mastitis. Metritis generally occurs during the first week following parturition. Dystocia, obstetrical manipulations, retained placenta, and retained fetuses may predispose to the development of metritis. Any one of these events may delay involution of the uterus, resulting in an enlarged flaccid uterus, thus creating a favorable environment for bacterial growth. Bacteria from the vagina then invade the devitalized uterine/placental/fetal tissues and can accumulate in large numbers. Gram-negative bacteria, especially *Escherichia coli*, are the most common causative agent.[15] Streptococcal and staphylococcal infections also occur. Clinical signs may include fever, dehydration, depression, weakness, reduction of milk, anorexia, loss of maternal instincts, and a foul-smelling vaginal discharge.

Treatment should be prompt and aggressive because rapid deterioration is common and septicemia or endotoxemia results. Therapy consists of administration of intravenous fluids and antibiotics and evacuation of uterine contents.

Broad-spectrum, systemic antibiotics (chloramphenicol, cephalosporin, trimethoprim sulfate, ampicillin) should be instituted on presentation.[16] Samples from the cranial vagina should be obtained for bacterial culture and antibiotic sensitivity and therapy altered according to the results. Uterine ecbolic agents are utilized to promote uterine involution and evacuation. Oxytocin is most commonly used at 0.25 to 0.5 IU/pound (0.5 to 1.0 IU/kg), not to exceed 20 units.[16] This should be given intramuscularly and may be repeated in 1 to 2 hours. However, oxytocin may be ineffective in stimulating uterine contractions if several days have passed since whelping because of inappropriate sensitivity of the myometrium to oxytocin at this time.[16] Finally, in certain cases following stabilization of the bitch, an ovariohysterectomy remains the treatment of choice.

Acute mastitis, inflammation of one or more of the mammary glands, usually of bacterial origin, may occur as a complication of the postpartum period. The affected gland or glands are usually hot, swollen, and painful and sometimes discolored. The bitch may also display signs of systemic illness (depression, anorexia, fever, and failure to care for the pups). The presence of mastitis may also be evidenced in the behavior of the pups; they may be restless, dissatisfied, and crying frequently. Depending on the severity, they may need to be started on an orphan-puppy care routine.

Treatment is directed at overcoming the infection and inflammation. The first step should be to collect samples of the affected milk aseptically for culture, identification, and antibiotic sensitivity. Therapy using a broad-spectrum antibiotic should be instituted immediately. Chloramphenicol is a good initial choice for antimicrobial therapy because it is broad spectrum, and its concentration in the mammary gland and secretion are not affected by pH.[17] Local application of heat to the affected glands is of value. If an abscess develops, it should be incised rather than allowed to rupture and should be flushed with dilute povidone-iodine (1 per cent).

References

1. Davis PE: Greyhound Management. Proc. No. 64 Refresher Course in Greyhounds, p 34:237, 1983.

2. Concannon PW: Reproductive Physiology of the Bitch. Proc. of Canine Theriogenology Short Course, 1993, p 2.
3. Donoghue S: Nutritional Recommendation for Reproductive Performance. *In* Kirk RW and Bonagura JD (eds): Current Therapy XI Philadelphia, WB Saunders Company, 1992, p 971.
4. Lewis LD, Morris ML Jr, Hand MS: Feeding and Care during Reproduction, Small Animal. Clinical Nutrition III, Topeka, Mark Morris Associates, 1987, p 3:7.
5. Bebiak DM: Nutrition and the Reproductive Roller Coaster. Proc. of Annual Meeting, Society for Theriogenology. 1988, p 167.
6. Papich MG: Effects of Drugs on Pregnancy. *In* Kirk RW (ed): Current Therapy X. Philadelphia, WB Saunders Company, 1989, pp 1293–1296.
7. Memon MA, Mickelsen WD: Noninfectious Pregnancy Disease in the Bitch. Proc. of Annual Meeting, Society for Theriogenology. 1992, p 151.
8. Concannon PW: Physiology and Endocrinology of Canine Pregnancy. *In* Morrow DA (ed): Current Therapy in Theriogenology 2. Philadelphia, WB Saunders Company, 1986, p 496.
9. Olson PN, Husted PW: Breeding Management for Optimal Reproductive Efficiency in the Bitch and Stud Dog. *In* Morrow DA (ed): Current Therapy in Theriogenology 2. Philadelphia, WB Saunders Company, 1986, p 463.
10. Johnston SD, Smith FO, Balice NC, et al: Stages of Parturition. Comp. on Continuing Ed.
11. Wheaton L: Drugs Affecting Uterine Motility. *In* Kirk RW (ed): Current Therapy X. Philadelphia, WB Saunders Company, 1989, p 1299.
12. Ludders JW: Anesthesia for the Pregnant Patient. Proc. of Annual Meeting, Society for Theriogenology. 1988, p 39.
13. Chandler ML: Canine Neonatal Mortality. Proc. of Annual Meeting, Society for Theriogenology. 1990, p 243.
14. Olson PN: Parturient Diseases of the Bitch. Proc. of Annual Meeting, Society for Theriogenology. 1988, p 19.
15. Johnson CA: Uterine Diseases. *In* Ettinger SJ (ed): Textbook of Veterinary Internal Medicine, 3rd ed. Philadelphia, WB Saunders Company, 1989, p 1801.
16. Magne ML: Acute Metritis in the Bitch. *In* Morrow DA (ed): Current Therapy in Theriogenology 2. Philadelphia, WB Saunders Company, 1986, p 505.
17. Olson JD, Olson PN: Disorders of the Canine Mammary Gland. *In* Morrow DA (ed): Current Therapy in Theriogenology 2. Philadelphia, WB Saunders Company, 1986, p 507.

SECTION VIII

NUTRITION

CHAPTER 38

NUTRITION FOR THE RACING GREYHOUND

JOHN R. KOHNKE

The popularity of lure racing over set distances has resulted in major changes in the way greyhounds are selected, trained, housed, and fed, as compared with the original coursing bloodlines. A refined, faster strain of greyhound, with a narrower range of body weight, has been developed for lure racing. An adequate and well-balanced diet is paramount to the health, performance, and adaptation of the greyhound to the stress of repeated track racing. The performance grading and wagering systems require that racing greyhounds maintain body weight within set limits. This is achieved by careful management of energy and water balance in relation to training and climatic conditions and by monitoring of body weight and condition on a regular basis.

Although diets were traditionally based on fresh red meat and cereal meal, various other meats, meat by-products, offal, compounded dry foods, and vegetables can be incorporated into the ration. Recently, dry foods specially formulated to meet the needs of racing and working dogs, in which all or part of the meat base has been replaced, have been developed. These provide a convenient and economical alternative to traditional rations.

A number of reviews of greyhound nutrition and feeding have been published over the last decade, summarizing the scientific and practical aspects of dietary needs, ration formulation, and feeding methods.[1-8] The feeding and nutrition of greyhounds is both an art and a science, overshadowed by tradition and folklore.[2, 7, 8] The art is knowing how much to feed, when to feed, and the likes and dislikes of an individual animal.[2] The science is understanding the nutritional needs of the greyhound, the relative value of different feeds, and the benefits or disadvantages of individual ingredients or combinations.[2] This chapter is prepared for trainers and veterinarians as a practical guideline for feeding racing greyhounds.

NUTRITIONAL AIMS

In addition to maintaining health and vitality, the diet should meet the following criteria:

1. Provide an economical, palatable, low-bulk, highly digestible ration to maintain body weight within set limits and ensure optimal performance.[2, 7, 8]
2. Provide optimal proportions of carbohydrate, protein, fat, and fiber to maximize energy density while minimizing gut weight and volume compatible with efficient digestive function.[3, 7]
3. Maintain optimal electrolyte, anaerobic buffering capacity and fluid balance over a variety of climatic conditions and racing distances.[3, 6, 7]
4. Ensure energy and nutrient balance to counteract imbalances and inadequate levels in the diet and meet the specific metabolic demand for performance.[2]
5. Provide a diet formulated to counteract physical stress on the musculoskeletal system, ensure adaptation to and optimal recovery from racing and injury, and maintain the immune response and resistance against disease under high-stress situations of housing and repeated physical exercise.[5]

These aims can be achieved by careful selection of feed ingredients, regular monitoring of body weight, and use of specific supplements to correct low or inadequate feed levels relative to performance requirements and level of stress.

ENERGY AND ENERGY REQUIREMENT

Energy, with the exception of water, is the most important constituent of the greyhound diet.[2] Diets can be manipulated to improve oxidative yields and utilize short- and medium-chain carbohydrates and fatty acids over a wide range of race distances and climatic conditions.[2] Short-term, high-intensity exercise in the greyhound is fueled mainly from muscle glycogen and blood sugar to meet the predominantly anaerobic exercise demand.[3]

The energy supply and exercise duration, intensity, and frequency are all interrelated and can be influenced by the individual greyhound's temperament, kennel and environmental temperature, and efficiency of metabolism.[2] The total energy requirement for a racing greyhound is a summation of *maintenance, thermoregulation, exercise, and racing expenditure,* including behavioral influences and pre-race anticipation expenditure.[2, 4] Regular monitoring of body weight at least once weekly will assist in equating energy intake relative to expenditure.[2] All estimates are as metabolizable energy (ME) in kilocalories (kcal). To convert kcal to kilojoules (kj), multiply by 4.184.

Useful Energy Equivalents for Feed Adjustment[2]

Each 100 gm (3 1/3 oz) of:

- Lean raw beef (10 to 12 per cent fat) provides approximately 200 kcal ME.
- Dry food 24 to 28 per cent crude protein, 8 to 10 per cent crude fat provides approximately 300 to 310 kcal ME.
- Dry food 30 to 32 per cent crude protein, 15 per cent crude fat provides approximately 400 kcal ME.
- Each 17 gm (about 1/2 oz) or 20 ml (1 tablespoonful) of animal fat or vegetable oil provides approximately 150 kcal ME.

Maintenance. A greyhound requires approximately 132 kcal ME/kg body weight$^{0.75}$ daily under temperate (15 to 25°C or 60 to 77°F) conditions.[9] For greyhounds weighing between 25 and 35 kg, this equates to 55 to 60 kcal per kg body weight. An average 30-kg (66-pound) racing greyhound housed under temperate conditions requires approximately 1700 kcal ME/day.[2, 3] An excitable greyhound or one housed in a larger enclosure will have a higher basal metabolic expenditure because of panting, barking, or hyperactivity in the kennel, and may require up to 2100 kcal ME daily to maintain body weight and performance.[2, 3] In these greyhounds, additional fat included in the diet will increase energy input without significantly increasing ration bulk.[2] A weight check once weekly will enable adjustment of the fat intake to maintain body weight.

Thermoregulation. A greyhound housed and raced under *cold weather conditions,* between 10 and 15°C, will require an increase in energy at low-range ambient temperatures to maintain body warmth.[2, 5–7]

As a guide, for every 1°C (2°F) decrease in ambient temperature below 15°C (60°F), add 3 kcal ME/kg body weight$^{0.75}$, or approximately 40 kcal ME daily for a 30-kg (66-pound) greyhound.[6]

Under cold conditions, increasing the amount of dry food (see energy equivalents above) relative to the decrease in the ambient temperature will help to maintain body heat and body weight. Most greyhounds can consume up to a maximum of 100 gm extra dry food (about 3⅓ oz) daily without exceeding bulk or appetite limits. The greyhound should be weighed at least once weekly to ensure that it is maintaining body weight. If a greyhound loses weight or requires more energy under cold conditions, extra fat should be added to boost energy intake so as to avoid a significant increase in the volume of feed the animal has to consume above the additional 100 gm of dry food.[2, 6] The housing should be heated to a more comfortable temperature and a rug and adequate bedding provided under very cold ambient temperatures.

During *hot,* and especially humid, *weather,* the energy expended by panting to eliminate excess heat may increase daily requirements up to 3000 kcal ME for a 30-kg greyhound.[2] Exercise under these conditions may deplete glycogen stores more rapidly.[3] In addition, hot climates suppress appetite, and a more energy-dense diet boosted with fat will help limit the ration volume, provide a useful source of metabolic water, and minimize heat production from hindgut fiber fermentation.[6, 7]

High ambient temperatures for longer than 4 hours a day when a greyhound is panting will increase energy requirements. As a guide, for a 30-kg (66-pound) animal, each 1°C (2°F) increase

between 26 and 30°C (70 and 86°F), will require an extra 130 kcal ME daily and 160 kcal ME daily for a similar rise between 31 and 35°C (88 and 95°F). Under hot conditions, up to a maximum of 100 gm dry food will provide energy as well as fiber to maintain hindgut water reserves against panting losses.[6] However, for energy needs in excess of this input under hot conditions, as appetite and feed intake are often reduced, additional fat will meet the shortfall in energy requirement and provide a metabolic source of water to counteract dehydration.[2, 6] A weight check once a week will enable dietary adjustment, which should also be matched to weather conditions.[2, 6] Adequate electrolyte and fluid replenishment is also essential during hot weather to avoid dehydration and weight loss.

Racing Expenditure. Total energy expenditure for a greyhound in training and raced under temperate conditions ranges from 150 to 190 kcal ME/kg body weight$^{0.75}$, or approximately 1890 to 2390 kcal ME for a 30-kg (66-pound) greyhound.[5] It has been estimated that an additional 75 kcal ME is expended in each 30-second trial or race, or 4 to 5 per cent increase over maintenance requirements. Under temperate conditions the expenditure for racing can be provided by the standard diet.

Behavioral Influences. Excitable, barking, and "hard-walking" or hyperactive greyhounds may expend valuable energy reserves and dehydrate during training, and particularly during traveling or when kenneled in the pre-race period. Although the amount has not been quantified scientifically, a diet boosted with 30 to 60 gm (1 to 2 oz) of fat or vegetable oil in the pre-race meal about 6 to 8 hours before racing will provide extra energy expended in pre-race anticipation. Additional fat is recommended for nervous or hyperactive greyhounds that lose body weight, dehydrate, or perform below optimal levels.[2] Regular body weight and condition assessment with appropriate dietary adjustment are essential to maintain racing weight limits.

ENERGY SOURCES

Carbohydrates, proteins, and fat included in the ration blend provide the major sources of energy to meet requirements.

Carbohydrates

Energy Yield and Food Content. Carbohydrates (sugars and starches) yield 3.5 kcal ME gm,[3, 9] and, on average, contribute 40 to 45 per cent of the energy in traditional racing diets.[2] Meat is low in carbohydrates, contributing only 4 to 5 per cent of the total carbohydrate intake from the traditional 70 per cent meat-by-weight diets.[2] Dry foods contribute varying amounts of carbohydrates, mainly from cereal grains, ranging from 35 to 40 per cent carbohydrates in dry foods containing 27 to 30 per cent crude protein and 15 per cent crude fat, to 55 per cent carbohydrates in lower protein (13 per cent crude protein, 2 to 3 per cent crude fat), dry foods, or kibbles.[2] Other foods, such as vegetables, provide additional carbohydrates, with human breakfast cereals containing up to 70 per cent, bran 53 per cent, bread 45 per cent, rice 30 per cent, pasta 25 per cent, and potatoes 20 per cent.[2]

Excess Carbohydrates. Excess intake of carbohydrates in the form of cereal grain starches can have a number of adverse effects in racing greyhounds. High starch intake may increase potential glycogen overstorage in muscles, with resultant accumulation of higher lactate levels and lower clearance rates, and ultimate earlier onset of metabolic fatigue and risk of exercise rhabdomyolysis or cramping.[1, 2, 5, 8]

High intakes of poorly digested carbohydrates, particularly in the form of cereal-based lower-protein human breakfast or dry dog foods, may also reduce protein and fat digestibility and uptake of sodium, potassium, and calcium because of their higher fiber content.[5] The higher fiber, while helpful in maintaining fecal bulk, increases iliocecal water flow and results in wetter feces,[5, 6] with less retained as an intestinal reservoir against dehydration during hot weather.[6]

As a guide, carbohydrate sources, such as human breakfast cereals, should be limited to 75 gm (2½ oz) daily, bread to 100 gm (3 1/3 oz, 4 slices), and rice to 150 gm (5 oz) daily and pasta and mashed potatoes to 200 gm (7 oz) daily to avoid excess carbohydrate intake, as part substitution or in addition to that provided by dry foods.

Feeding pre-race snacks containing soluble short-chain sugars, such as sucrose (sugar) and glucose (dextrose), can lead to increased insulin sensitivity.[2, 7] When excess amounts are ingested in the immediate pre-race period, rebound hyperinsulinemia may be triggered, leading to lowering of blood sugar levels. The combined hypoglycemia and the effect of insulin decrease on mobilization of fatty acids and glycerol from lipid stores may also delay liver and muscle glycogen replenishment during the pre-race kennel period.[2, 7] Both these effects, in theory, can cause a risk of earlier metabolic fatigue and reduced race performance. In practice, it is widely recommended to avoid feeding large amounts of soluble sugars in a pre-race "snack" feed, limiting to 15 gm (½ oz) glucose or 60 ml (2 oz) honey within 4 to 6 hours before racing.[2, 6, 7]

Proteins

Energy Yield and Food Content. Proteins yield 3.5 kcal ME per gram.[3, 9] Proteins provide a source of energy, as well as essential amino acids, for protein synthesis. As a source of available amino acids, greyhound diets should contain 30 to 35 per cent high-quality crude protein on a dry matter basis.[2, 4] Protein sources contribute, on average, between 35 and 40 per cent of the total energy needs for a racing greyhound.[2, 4] Lean meat ranges from 17 to 21 per cent crude protein on an as-fed basis, or approximately 60 per cent crude protein on a dry-matter basis.[2, 9] Dry foods contain a wide range of crude protein, depending on the content of meat by-products and oilseed protein sources, and commercial products range from 17 to 35 per cent on a dry-matter basis.[2] Most greyhound diets based on meat and/or dry foods to satisfy energy demands contain adequate protein to meet daily requirements.

Excess Protein. High intakes of protein increase the cost of the ration blend, and the elimination of excess poor-quality protein, such as contained in cereal-based dry foods, is an energy-consuming process. It is much more economical, and metabolically more efficient, to feed a diet containing adequate protein, with additional energy provided by fat to greyhounds during hot weather or those competing in longer-distance races.[2]

Fats or Lipids

Energy Yield and Food Content. Fat or lipids yield 8.5 kcal ME/gram, or approximately 2.25 times that of carbohydrates or protein.[3, 9] Fats are a useful energy-dense feed that provide an energy boost without adding excessive volume or weight to the ration.[2] The lipids in fats and oils are a palatable, highly digestible source of energy; greyhound diets should contain at least 12 to 15 per cent fat on an as-fed basis, and greyhounds can tolerate up to 25 to 30 per cent fat on a dry-matter basis.[2] Higher fat intake is recommended for excitable, hyperactive greyhounds and during hot or very cold weather conditions.[2]

Both animal and plant oils and fats are highly digestible. Lipids with a high percentage of short-chain (unsaturated) fatty acids remain liquid (oils) at room temperature.[2] As the percentage of long-chain fatty acids increases, the lipid becomes solid at room temperature as a fat, and digestibility is reduced in fats with high long-chain saturated content.[2, 6] Short- to medium-chain saturated

triglycerides, as contained in coconut, canola, palm, and copha, are considered better utilized, as these lipids are digested by pancreatic enzymes without need for bile emulsification.[4] Although it is suggested that up to 25 per cent of the total fat be provided by these sources of short- to medium-chain triglycerides,[4] greyhounds may not readily accept these items in their diet. Stepwise introduction over 7 to 10 days may be necessary to obtain acceptance.[6]

Excess Fat. High intakes of long-chain saturated fats, such as beef and mutton fat (trimmings or suet) or butter fat, can reduce overall lipid digestibility, although greyhounds find these animal fats naturally more acceptable.[2, 4] Animal fat sources are generally cheap to purchase as trimmed fat or omental fat from carcasses. However, if more than 60 gm (2 oz) of animal-derived fat is required to boost energy content in the ration during hot weather, or in dehydrated greyhounds, it is preferable to provide additional fat in the form of vegetable oil.[2]

Essential Fatty Acids. Greyhounds require essential fatty acids. The diet should contain at least 1 per cent of linoleic acid, an omega-6 fatty acid, on a dry-matter basis, or 2 per cent of ME intake, to prevent the characteristic dry, flaking dermatitis associated with a deficiency in dogs.[9] Linoleic acid is the precursor of other linoleic acid family members, linolenic and arachidonic acid, if adequate linoleic acid is available in the diet. Linoleic acid is the main unsaturated fatty acid (omega-6) in vegetable oils, such as safflower (78 per cent), corn (70 per cent), sunflower (69 per cent), cottonseed (54 per cent), soybean (54 per cent), and wheat germ oil (48 per cent).[2, 10] The highest amounts in animal fat forms are contained in pork lard (15 per cent), and chicken fat (16 per cent).[2, 10] Beef tallow (4.3 per cent), horse fat (6 per cent), and fish oils (2.7 per cent) contribute only small amounts.[2] Therefore, a lean meat–based diet should ideally be fortified by approximately 10 ml (2 teaspoonsful or 1/3 oz) per greyhound of a rich linoleic acid source, such as corn oil or safflower oil, to ensure adequate intake of this essential fatty acid.[2]

Some oils and fats also provide omega-3 fatty acids. Alpha linolenic and other omega-3 fatty acids are provided by linseed (flax) (57 per cent), canola (rapeseed) (8 per cent), and soybean (7 per cent) oils and cold water fish oils.[2, 4, 10]

Although purified fish oils are poor sources of the linoleic acid and omega-6 family of essential fatty acids, they contain high levels of omega-3 fatty acids, including arachidonic, eicosapentaenoic, and docosahexaenoic acids.[2, 10] These fatty acids are considered to act as precursors to the body's natural anti-inflammatory compounds and may be of benefit to counteract the inflammatory reactions initiated in muscles by intense exercise, as well as protect the intestinal mucosa.[2, 4, 10] Recent reviews suggest an optimal range of omega-6 to omega-3 fatty acids of 6–10:1 for racing greyhound diets to promote skin health, intestinal mucosal activity, and beneficial natural anti-inflammatory activity following intense exercise.[10] Some complete dry foods developed for racing greyhounds contain this ratio of fatty acid within the fat profile, and additional amounts do not have to be added to the diet.[10] Excess omega-3 fatty acid intake has been associated with rectal bleeding in sled dogs.[10] Alternatively, 20 ml (1 tablespoonful or 2/3 oz) of a mixture of 6 parts sunflower or corn oil, 1 part linseed oil, and 1 part fish oil (not cod liver oil) will provide an omega-6 to omega-3 fatty acid ratio within the optimal range to satisfy linoleic acid requirements in lean meat–based diets. However, because of the characteristic odor of fish oils, it is best to introduce this oil blend to the main meal in a stepwise manner over 5 to 7 days, depending on acceptance.

Storage of Oils and Fats. Ideally, fats and oils should be stored under refrigeration to reduce oxidation and rancidity, which reduce palatability and digestibility. Rancid fat also catalyzes the destruction of vitamin E in the ration. It is also important to avoid shaking oils before use, as shaking causes aeration and increases the risk of oxidation. Vegetable oils, even at refrigerated temperatures, do not settle out.[6]

When polyunsaturated oils are added in amounts exceeding 1 per cent of the total diet as fed (approximately 10 to 15 ml or ⅓ to ½ oz), then additional vitamin E should be fed to limit peroxidation of muscle membrane phospholipids, as the requirement for vitamin E is related to the dietary concentration of polyunsaturated fatty acids (PUFA).[9] An optimal tocopherol (vitamin E) to PUFA ratio of at least 50 per cent, or 1.0 mg (or IU) of vitamin E per 2 gm PUFA added to the diet is suggested.[2] As the majority of racing greyhounds' diets are supplemented with vitamin E, extra vitamin E above the supplementary amounts of 50 to 100 IU, is not required in practical feeding to compensate for the higher PUFA level in the diet.[2] However, if high fat levels are being fed and vitamin E is not already being supplemented, then provision of additional vitamin E should be considered.[2] As a practical guideline, for racing greyhounds, it may be beneficial to supplement 10 mg vitamin E for every 1 per cent increase in PUFA fat sources added above 10 per cent fat in the ration as fed.[2] Alternatively, for every additional tablespoonful (17 gm) of polyunsaturated oil, an additional 10 IU of vitamin E should be provided.[2, 6]

Fiber

Greyhounds require from 3 to 5 per cent of moderately fermentable crude fiber in their diet for efficient digestion.[2, 4, 11] Meat contains relatively small amounts of fiber, so most of the fiber is provided by dry foods or, in some cases, when cereals or vegetables are fed.[2] Recent studies of dietary fiber needs and composition suggest that lower solubility, moderately fermentable fiber sources from beet pulp and rice bran incorporated into dry foods provide optimal fermentation to produce short-chain fatty acids, optimize nutrient absorption, and add stool bulk and moisture content.[10] Not only greyhounds are unable to digest large amounts of fiber effectively but also levels of fiber in the diet above 10 per cent increase fecal bulk and water loss.[2, 6] High dietary fiber levels also direct water excretion from the kidneys to the feces.[6] Excessively fibrous rations may also interfere with absorption of calcium and decrease the digestibility of fats in the diet by shortening gut transit time.[2, 7] A cup of cooked leafy fibrous vegetables or 1 tablespoonful of beet pulp, wheat, or rice bran is a practical way to provide a mild laxative effect in constipated greyhounds, as well as to increase hindgut water reserves.[2]

Water

Greyhounds must be provided with an adequate supply of clean fresh water at all times. The requirement for water is approximately 1 ml/kcal ME consumed per day,[9] or a total of 2 L in a racing greyhound housed and raced under temperate conditions.[9] Water must be available during hot weather, after exercise or traveling, or when electrolyte supplements are added to the diet.[2] The requirement for water depends on the amount supplied in the feed, the environmental temperature, the type of exercise, and the individual animal's electrolyte balance.[2, 7] Most adult racing greyhounds on a high meat-based diet, with dry food soaked before feeding to provide additional fluid intake, will drink about 350 to 500 ml (⅔ to ¾ pint) of water per day in cool weather.[2] However, some greyhounds are naturally poor drinkers and often develop a mild, chronic form of dehydration. In these animals, water intake can be encouraged by adding recommended doses of electrolyte supplements to the feed. Alternatively, fluid intake of the diet can be increased by soaking dry food for 10 to 15 minutes before feeding, or feeding an extra 30 to 60 gm (1 to 2 oz) of fat, such as suet or lard, as a metabolic source of water in excitable, chronically dehydrated greyhounds. Although it is common practice to withdraw water 6 hours before racing to minimize racing weight fluctuations,[2] during hot weather water should be offered prior to race kenneling to excitable, dehydrated greyhounds.

COMMON DIETARY CONSTITUENTS

Meats

Traditionally, meat-based diets contain 50 to 70 per cent by weight of meat, supplemented with dry food and, in some cases, offal meats and cooked vegetables to make up the shortfall of energy, protein, and fiber.[2] Muscle meat itself is deficient in a number of vitamins and minerals, particularly calcium, and is low in carbohydrates.[2] Most of the energy contained in meat is provided by the protein content, with increasing amounts contributed by fat, as the fat content is increased.[2]

Many authorities believe that raw meat is a natural food for dogs, and it is best fed coarsely minced or in small cubes, rather than minced to a fine paste.[2] Although cooking tends to make meat more tender and attractive to greyhounds that are poor eaters, overcooking at high temperatures (above 200C [420F]) can destroy some of the protein and fat and inactivates many of the vitamins.[2] Cooking by boiling at 100C (210F) as in preparing stews, or at extrusion temperatures of up to 140C (310F) during gelatinization of dry foods, is less damaging than grilling or roasting meat, for this reason. In larger kennels, bulk meat is stored frozen, then thawed and coarsely minced as required each day. Individual trainers with smaller operations usually purchase frozen, chilled or freshly minced meat from meat suppliers or butcher shops weekly.

A number of meats are used as a base for greyhound diets. Of these, beef and horse meat are the most common worldwide.

Beef. Traditionally, lean beef has provided the basis for the greyhound diet in most countries. Beef can vary in fat content; in practice, therefore, visual assessment of every batch of meat for its fat should be made before feeding. In American racing kennels, pre-minced and frozen salvaged meat from dying, diseased, disabled (3-D), or dead livestock (4-D) that is unsuitable for human consumption is widely available and used because of its lower cost relative to higher-grade beef or horse meat.[8] An average fat level of 7 per cent for racing kennels and 15 per cent for breeding and training farms is available.[8] Most trainers provide additional fat as vegetable oil or suet to boost the fat content of the standard racing beef. Although the use of 4-D grade beef increases the economic feasibility of training greyhounds in large kennels, the presence of antibiotic and other drug residues from treated or euthanatized animals salvaged for meat can result in excretion of residues of regulated drugs in the urine of racing greyhounds.[8] Salvaged 4-D meat also often contains high bacterial contamination, which can cause acute and debilitating gastroenteritis in greyhounds fed on this meat.[8]

As a guide, if the amount of fat in the meat visually appears to be less than 10 per cent, fat should be added to the diet to boost it to 12 to 15 per cent fat, particularly during hot weather. Excess fat on non-minced meat can be trimmed off, frozen, and later used as a fat boost to very lean batches of meat. However, when pre-minced meat contains more than 15 per cent fat and there is no alternative, the amount of meat provided should be reduced. As a guide, for every 1 per cent (10 gm/kg) increase in fat above 15 per cent the weight of meat fed should be reduced by 50 gm (about 2 oz) daily. The animal's body weight should be monitored at least once weekly, and feed intake adjusted accordingly to achieve an energy-exercise equilibrium.

Horse Meat. Horse meat can be substituted in part, or completely, to replace beef when beef is relatively more expensive. Horse meat usually has a lower fat content than other meats and hence is lower in energy for equivalent weight of standard lean beef.[2] When horse meat is substituted for lean beef on an equal-weight basis in a diet, there may be a shortfall of up to 35 per cent in energy content in lean horse meat compared to lean to medium-fat beef.[2] Therefore, horse meat should be fed either mixed with beef or boosted with additional fat to increase the energy density and reduce the amount required.[2] Horse protein is only 80 to 85 per cent digestible as compared with beef, and therefore, when the low fat content and reduced digestibility are considered, it is recommended to feed up to 25 per cent more horse meat for the equivalent amount of lean to medium-fat beef.[2] Some greyhounds may also develop a digestive allergy to a full horse meat diet, exhibited as a chronic, mild digestive upset with low-grade diarrhea.[2] When introducing a greyhound to horse meat, it is best to substitute horse meat for lean beef or other meat in a stepwise manner over a 5 to 7 days. Fat at the rate of 1 tablespoonful (17 gm or ½ oz) per 200 gm (7 oz) horse meat should be added as a direct substitute on a weight basis for standard lean beef. Alternatively, the amount of horse meat can be limited to 25 to 50 per cent of the diet, with the remainder provided by lean to medium-fat beef, or other types of meat. It is unwise to change to horse meat within 7 days of racing, in case it causes mild digestive upset until the animal becomes accustomed to the increased amounts of horse meat in the diet.[2]

Other Meats. The energy content of most meats containing 10 to 12 per cent fat, such as chicken and lamb, is similar to that of lean beef. Extra fat added in increments of 10 gm (⅓ oz) per kg (about 2½ pounds) will raise the fat content by 1 percentage point. Average fat content in other meats is beef heart 3 per cent, sheep heart 5 per cent, kangaroo (Australia only) 1 per cent, fish 1 per cent. Chicken and fish are low in iron and copper, minerals important for blood formation, and a supplement containing these minerals should be given when these meats form the base of the regular diet.[2, 6] Raw, bone-free fish should be lightly cooked to inactivate thiaminase enzymes in certain types of fish (carp) that destroy thiamine (vitamin B₁) in the diet.[2, 8] Cooking fish also improves its acceptance in most greyhounds when it is used in an after-race meal as a protein source.[2]

Dry Foods

In most countries, dry foods are becoming more widely used as a staple diet for greyhounds. Traditionally, cereal-based dry foods were added to the predominantly meat diet to make up the shortfall of carbohydrates, protein, and fiber. A large variety of dry food formulations have been developed to meet the specific needs of racing greyhounds, providing a palatable, convenient, economic, scientifically balanced, and easily stored dietary base.

Generally, dry foods fall into four categories. Some dry foods are formulated to supplement meat-based diets, while others contain a higher density of energy and protein as a complete ration for the racing greyhound. A practical guide to the selection of dry foods is summarized in Table 38–1. Dry foods are easy to store, and on the basis of cost per unit of energy complete dry food rations are often cheaper than meat-based diets. Well-formulated dry foods also have selected antioxidants included to minimize the risk of oxidation of their fat and vitamin content during storage. As dry foods contain a maximum of 15 per cent moisture, they should be moistened before feeding, either in the meat and dry food mix with added water or in the complete dry food ration by soaking for at least 10 to 15 minutes. Shape and form of the dry food should be maintained to achieve a soft, but not sloppy, consistency.[2] It is particularly important that the dry food be soaked before feeding, particularly during hot weather or when a greyhound is dehydrated. As most dry foods contain up to 1 per cent salt as a preservative, generally, in amounts in excess of 300 to 400 gm/day, additional sodium chloride (salt) does not need to be added to the greyhound's ration.[2, 6] Many dry foods contain added vitamins and minerals, including calcium, as a complete feed for greyhounds.

Vegetables

Vegetables are a useful source of carbohydrates, fiber, and moisture.[2] Cooked vegetables can be mixed into dry food to increase the moisture content and used in meaty stews to increase the bulk. In large kennels, cooked vegetables may not be fed at all because of the time required for preparation, and with the advent of high-quality complete dry foods, the need to add vegetables to the diet is minimized. Excess vegetables can increase the fiber level, bulking the stools and diluting the energy content of the diet.[6] Therefore, when vegetables are added to the diet, at least 25 per cent of the vegetable bulk should be made up of diced potatoes, pasta, or rice, with another 25 per cent from protein-rich vegetables such as peas, beans, and soybean (cooked), and the remainder of high-moisture vegetables such as carrots, pumpkin, and celery.[8] This mix of vegetables will provide nutritional benefit other than fiber and moisture to the diet.[8]

The cooking water from vegetables should not be discarded, as it contains many soluble minerals and electrolytes leached out during cooking.[2] There is no need to peel vegetables, and they should not be overcooked by excessive boiling. It is preferable to blanch, steam, or microwave cook to soften vegetables and dice them into small pieces before feeding to retain their soluble nutrient content. Small toppings of raw vegetables or fruits, such as carrots and apples, can be fed but are best grated for better digestibility.

TABLE 38–1. Dry Foods for Greyhounds (Values per 100 gm as Fed)

	Use	Energy (kcal ME)	Crude Protein (%)	Fat (%)	Approx. Daily Amounts (30 kg [66 pound] greyhound)
Group 1 Kibbles Dry foods	Meat-based diets High-carbohydrate content	270	13	2–3	200–250 gm (7–8 oz) daily mixed with 700 gm meat
Group 2	Minimum meat diets	290–300	17–20	8–10	250–300 gm (8–10 oz) daily mixed with 500–600 gm meat
Group 3	Complete feeds	330–340	20–24	8–10	Complete feeds 500–550 gm (16–18 oz) daily, or 250–300 gm (8–10 oz) mixed with 200–250 gm meat
Group 4	High-energy complete feeds	400	30	15–18	Complete food. Refer to feeding guidelines on bag

These are guidelines only; check manufacturer's recommendations on individual brands for feed amounts and mixing instructions.

TABLE 38–2. Daily Vitamin and Mineral Requirements in 30-kg (66-pound) Racing Greyhound:[2, 6] Practical Guidelines

Nutrient	Recommended Daily Intake (RDI)		Practical Guidelines for Supplementation in Racing Greyhounds
	Resting[9]	Racing[6]	
Calcium	3570 mg	6000–8000 mg	Supplement meat-based diets to 75% of RDI, dry food diets to 30% RDI; essential in all young greyhounds in training
Phosphorus	2670 mg	5000 mg	
Magnesium	246 mg	800–900 mg	Add 50% RDI in nervy, cramping greyhounds or hot weather
Iron	20 mg	60 mg maximum	Add 50% RDI, especially to chicken- and fish-based diets
Copper	1.8 mg	50 mg	Add 50% RDI, especially to chicken- and fish-based diets
Zinc	21.6 mg	65 mg maximum	Add 50% RDI to dry foods if calcium is supplemented
Manganese	3.0 mg	6.0 mg	Add 50% RDI in meat-based diets
Iodine	0.36 mg	1.0 mg	Add 50% RDI to high carbohydrate diets
Sodium	330 mg	3000–5000 mg maximum	Do not add extra if more than 300 gm dry food with 1% salt is fed; do not supplement horse or human salt mixes containing high sodium
Potassium	2670 mg	4500 mg maximum	Add 50% RDI in hot weather, cramping, nervy greyhounds in slow-release tablets
Vitamin A (retinol)	2250 IU (0.675 mg)	3375 IU (1.0 mg)	Add 50% RDI to lean-meat diets
Vitamin D (cholecalciferol)	240 IU (0.06 µg)	260 IU (0.09 µg)	Add 50% RDI to lean-meat diets, or when calcium is supplemented
Vitamin E (tocopherol)	15 IU (15 mg)	30–100 IU (30–100 mg)	Freezing meat destroys vitamin E—add 50% RDI to meat diets and up to 100% RDI in fat-boosted diets
Thiamine (vitamin B₁)	600 µg	1.8 mg	Add at least 50% RDI to meat-based diets
Riboflavin (vitamin B₂)	1.5 mg	4.5 mg	Add 100% RDI to fat-boosted diets
Niacin	6.75 mg	20 mg	Add 50% RDI daily when racing regularly
Pantothenate	6.0 mg	18 mg	Add 50% RDI to cooked foods (stews)
Pyridoxine (vitamin B₆)	0.6 mg	2.0 mg	Add 50% RDI to high-protein dry foods
Cyanocobalamin (vitamin B₁₂)	15 µg	45 µg	Add 100% RDI to chicken- and fish-based diets
Folic acid (folacin)	120 µg	360 µg	Add 50% RDI to all racing diets
Vitamin C	Enterosynthesis	250–300 mg	Add 100% RDI when racing regularly

Minerals and Vitamins

Generally, minerals should comprise about 2 to 3 per cent of the dry matter of the diet.[2, 9] The exact mineral requirements of racing greyhounds are not established, but increased levels of certain minerals, such as calcium, phosphorus, magnesium, iron, zinc, copper, and iodine, are considered essential for muscular exercise, metabolism, maintenance of the musculoskeletal system, and formation of blood.[2, 6–8]

Of all the minerals, the macrominerals calcium and phosphorus are important in the maintenance and structural integrity of the musculoskeletal system. Traditional high-meat diets should be supplemented with calcium and phosphorus to balance the meat component. The ideal Ca-P ratio in racing greyhounds is 1.2 to 1.4:1.0.[2] Commercial supplements are available that are formulated to balance the calcium-phosphorus ratio of meat when fed in measured amounts in direct proportion to the weight of meat in the diet. Many of these supplements also contain vitamin A, vitamin D, and trace minerals to help regulate the calcium and phosphorus balance. Alternatively, as a guide, the calcium and phosphorus balance can be optimized in meat so that for every 100 gm (3⅓ oz) meat, approximately 400 mg elemental calcium and 45 mg elemental phosphorus must be added to achieve a 1.3:1.0 calcium-phosphorus balance. This can be achieved by a mix of 3 parts calcium carbonate to 1 part dicalcium phosphate or steamed bone meal, added at the rate of 10 gm (⅓ oz or 2 level teaspoonfuls)/kg (about 2½ pounds) of meat. As the requirement for calcium in racing greyhounds is considered to be higher than in other dogs, often this mixture is added at the rate of 10 gm (⅓ oz) per 500 gm (about 1 pound) of meat.[2] A supplement of vitamin D according to National Research Council (NRC)[9] recommendations should be included in the diet if calcium in addition to that contained in the dry food component is included. Other important minerals that may require supplementation are iron and copper to at least 50 per cent of the recommended daily intake in diets containing white meats, such as chicken, pork, and fish, and the electrolytes sodium, potassium, magnesium, and chloride during hot weather, in conjunction with adequate water.

The vitamin requirements for racing greyhounds are considered to be elevated above those required for maintenance animals.[2, 5, 7, 8] Although the NRC[9] recommends levels for mineral and vitamin intake for maintenance, various other estimates have been provided as a guide to daily supplementation for racing greyhounds.[1, 2, 5–8] The American Association of Feed Control Officials (AAFCO) recommends higher levels of certain minerals to allow for bioavailability from food sources. The recommended daily intakes (RDIs) of minerals and vitamins that are provided as a practical guide to supplementation in Table 38–2 are based on an average of published recommendations.[1, 2, 5, 6] Higher intakes for conditions of stress, disease, or injury are recommended by various authors.[5, 6, 8]

ERGOGENIC AIDS

In greyhound racing, as in other athletic sports, nutriceutical or metabolic active compounds are supplemented in an effort to enhance exercise capacity and increase speed, stamina, and endurance. It is claimed that feeding these supplements will improve performance without the risk of drug detection. While many of these compounds have a role in energy production or utilization, mimic vitamin activity, or are claimed to reduce pain or modify behavior, there are few controlled studies to support their benefits in racing greyhounds.

Often the published claims are based on clinical evaluation in winning races, without scientifically controlled dose titration studies, placebo comparison trials, or results that are based on uniform track conditions, grade of greyhound, or the effect of increasing fitness over the time of supplementation. When evaluated under controlled conditions, many have failed to be of benefit at recommended dose rates used in racing greyhounds.[8] The proposed mode of action, suggested oral dose rates, and claimed benefits of a range of ergogenic compounds are summarized in Table 38–3. Of these compounds, creatine, a constituent in raw skeletal muscle, has been shown to increase muscle stores in greyhound and human athletes.[12] Studies indicate that supplementation enhances the capacity to sustain intense exercise in human athletes. A number of other compounds, including probiotic digestive aids, aspartic salts, inosine, adenosine triphosphate, inositol, superoxide dismutase, and direct alkalinizing compounds such as sodium bicarbonate in increased dosages have been promoted as ergogenic aids in greyhounds. No controlled scientific studies have been carried out to support their use as performance-enhancing compounds, and it is doubtful that they have any direct performance benefit in greyhounds.[8]

FEEDING PRACTICES

The composition of the diet and frequency of feeding are influenced by tradition, number of greyhounds in a kennel group, race start times, availability and cost of base foods, and racing practices. Surveys indicate wide variation in the composition of traditional meat and dry food diets between countries in which greyhound racing is established.[8] However, the energy intakes remain relatively constant on a body weight basis, with allowances for race distances and climatic conditions to maintain an ideal body weight for competitive racing.[2] Body weights range from as low as 25 kg (55 pounds) for bitches up to 37 to 40 kg (81 to 88 pounds) for larger males racing on Irish and British tracks.

In Australia, Ireland, New Zealand, and the United Kingdom, where racing is organized on a club basis, the average private greyhound trainer has two to five greyhounds in full-time training. Race meetings are held locally once or twice a week at night. Two meals are normally provided each day. A low-bulk morning meal, higher in carbohydrates provided by cereal biscuits or kibbles with milk or other fluid, is complemented by a larger evening meal including meat, dry foods, vegetables, or a meaty boiled stew, with supplements based on the individual greyhound's likes and dislikes, body weight, stage of training, and climatic conditions.[2]

In the United States, where approximately 20 per cent of the world population of racing greyhounds are housed in crate units in larger kennel groups, one meal commonly is fed in mid-morning. This practice allows easier kennel management of large groups of up to 80 greyhounds, as well as enabling pre-race feeding of greyhounds competing in matinee and evening races. All greyhounds are fed to individual need and weight with a standard mix of meat and dry food with added fat, water, and supplements, weighed on scales at the time of feeding. Greyhounds in early training, or those that are underweight or recovering from injury or illness, may be fed twice daily.[8]

Examples of greyhound diets in Australia, Ireland, New Zealand, and United Kingdom are shown in Table 38–4. Amounts are based on a 27- to 33-kg greyhound trialing or racing every 5 to 7 days, handslips twice weekly over 200 meters, walked 1½ km daily,

TABLE 38–3. Ergogenic Aids: Practical Guidelines

Compound (Nutrient Source)	Theoretical Metabolic Activity	Suggested Dose Rate	Claims/Benefits
Dimethylglycine (DMG; metabolic cofactor)	Increases oxygen utilization and reduces lactate accumulation in muscles	0.8–1.2 mg/kg orally daily[2, 8]	Increased endurance by a glycogen-sparing effect; controlled studies have failed to demonstrate benefit[8]
Methylsulfonylmethane (MSM; sulfur source)	Bioavailable sulfur for metabolic and anti-inflammatory activity[8]	7–80 mg/kg orally daily[8]	Little scientific verification[8]; practical use as natural anti-inflammatory nutrient[8]
Carnitine (amino acid)	Aids transport of long-chain fatty acids into muscle cells to provide energy source	20–50 mg/kg body weight orally daily[1, 8]	Increased endurance in sled dogs[5]; no controlled studies in greyhounds
L-Tryptophan (amino acid)	Precursor of brain neurotransmitter, serotonin; suppresses CNS hyperactivity	500 mg/15 kg orally in two equal doses 30 minutes prior to feeding[8]	Clinical use to reduce anxiety and pain perception in apprehensive, nervous greyhounds in pre-race period[8]; 5 mg/kg orally may enhance endurance.[13] No controlled studies in greyhounds
Phenylalanine (amino acid)	Precursor of CNS neurotransmitter activity	500 mg/15 kg orally in two equal doses 30 minutes prior to feeding	Increased alertness and mood elevation;[8] no controlled studies in greyhounds
Arginine (amino acid)	Creatine formation and ammonia detoxification	15 mg/kg orally or by injection for 2–3 days prior to race	Improved race performance and recovery.[8] No controlled studies in greyhounds
Creatine (high-energy source)	Stored as phosphocreatine used during high-intensity exercise	Rapid uptake from food or supplement 2–3 gm daily;[12] each 100 gm raw meat contains 0.5 gm creatine	Increased creatine muscle stores in greyhounds[12]; improved capacity for sustained intense exercise in human athletes.[12] No controlled studies in greyhounds

TABLE 38–4. Greyhound Diets in Australia, Ireland, New Zealand, and United Kingdom

Morning Meal	Body Weight (kg)	Food Need
Dry food 310–330 kcal ME/ 100 gm	27–29	75 gm
	30–31	100 gm
	32–33	125 gm
OR	27–30	2 biscuits
Dry dog biscuits 150 kcal ME per biscuit	31–33	3 biscuits
OR	27–30	2 biscuits
Breakfast cereal (Weetabix or Wheatbix) 340 kcal ME/100 gm (40 gm/ biscuit)	31–33	2–3 biscuits
OR	27–30	2–3 slices
Whole-meal bread toasted 216 kcal ME/100 gm (35 gm/ slice)	31–33	3–4 slices

This meal is soaked with water, milk, thin vegetable soup, or meat stock cube broth. Supplements of vitamin E, electrolytes, and calcium are often used as top dressings.

Evening Meal	Body Weight (kg)	Food Need
Raw lean 10% fat beef or other meat	27–30	600–650 gm
	31–33	700–750 gm
Dry food 310–330 kcal ME/ 100 gm	27–30	200 gm
	31–33	250 gm

The following are added to this meal: cooked diced mixed vegetables (optional), 1–1½ cups; fat (lard, chicken, beef), 1½ tablespoonfuls relative to climate or type of meat.

housed in 3-square-meter kennel area under temperate conditions. Adjustments are made according to manufacturer's recommendations relative to the energy content of the dry food and the climatic conditions.

Water or vegetable-cooking water is added to soak the dry food for 15 to 20 minutes to a moist consistency. Supplements include vitamins and minerals, electrolytes, and calcium, when necessary, as top dressings. Small amounts of up to 50 gm chopped fresh liver or kidney or 150 gm cooked tripe may be added once or twice weekly. Fresh water is available at all times.

Over recent years the availability of high-quality dry foods, formulated for minimal meat diets or as complete diets, has changed traditional feeding practices, with greyhounds being fed the manufacturer's recommended amounts. Regular body weight checks every 5 to 7 days are essential to allow ration adjustment for maintenance of an optimum racing weight.

In American race kennels the ration is prepared usually in bulk, and then weighed out at the time of feeding according to each greyhound's individual need, body weight, or time of racing.

A typical bulk mix for 80 greyhounds would include 100 pounds of 4-D beef (7 per cent fat), (or alternatively 80 pounds 4-D beef and 25 pounds horse meat [5 per cent fat]), 50 to 55 pounds of dry food 310 to 330 kcal ME/100 gm (3⅓ oz), 2 to 3 pints of corn oil, soaked for 30 minutes in 5 to 7 gallons of water to produce a soft, moist consistency ideal for measuring out at feeding. The exact amount of bulk mix depends on the average size of the greyhounds in the kennel group, weather conditions, and relative energy needs.

The feed blend is mixed by hand or paddle in a large trough or bathtub. Calcium powder and electrolyte supplements are added at the appropriate rate for 80 dogs, or measured individually at feeding. Often a table on wheels is used to transport the bulk meal mix through the kennel room at feeding time. Each greyhound receives a weighed portion of the meal mix relative to needs and body weight, usually ranging from 1½ pounds for small bitches up to 3 pounds for large dogs.[8] Supplements of vitamin E, iron, and vitamins are often added to each measured feed portion as required. Additional fat or oil is added, depending on weather conditions, and up to ½ pint of vegetables, warm meat stew or cooked barley grain is added in cold weather. Water is provided at each of the 4 or 5 turnouts each day.[8] A number of other alternatives, including individual feeding with minced meat, dry food, and supplements measured out for each greyhound, providing a complete dry food diet, are also adopted in some kennels.[8]

Pre-Race Feeding. In most countries, greyhounds are given their larger main meal the evening before racing, and a small meal 6 to 8 hours before the start time of the race. These meals vary, but usually include about a quarter portion of the main meal mixture or soaked high-energy greyhound dry food. Pre-race additives include higher doses of B complex vitamins, vitamin C, vitamin E, electrolytes, and ergogenic aids.

Post-Race Feeding. Greyhounds are often fed a meal of cooked meaty stew or about half the portion of the main meal mix on return to the kennel. Supplements after racing include B complex vitamins and electrolytes to aid recovery and interest in food. Many trainers feed a higher protein meal topped with one to two lightly cooked eggs, or half a cupful of high-protein dry food added as a top dressing. Replacement of electrolytes is important after racing, and higher protein meals are fed for two meals after racing to provide an increased level of amino acids that are considered helpful to counteract muscle damage during racing.

Food Hygiene and Food Safety. At all times, strict hygiene and correct storage must be adhered to in the preparation of meat and meat by-products used in greyhound diets. Meat that is purchased already minced may contain bacterial contamination or preservative compounds to extend the storage life under refrigeration. Preservatives such as nitrite compounds and sulfur dioxide used in minced meat may induce diarrhea and destroy thiamine (vitamin B_1) in the large intestine, with symptoms of incoordination, excitement, weakness, and even seizures if the treated meat is fed on a regular basis.[8] It is essential that each new batch of fresh meat or thawed meat be thoroughly inspected prior to feeding. Normally, spoiled meat has a distinct "rotting" odor, with brown to black fluid seepage and a mushy, friable consistency. This meat should not be used, even to prepare cooked stews. Strict hygiene must be adopted in food preparation, including cleaning and sanitation of mincing machinery, mixing vessels, knives, cutting boards, and bench tops. Minimal handling and storage times for meat once it is thawed or minced before mixing and final portioning at mealtime will help reduce risk of spoiling or contamination.[8]

Salvaged meat, such as 3-D and 4-D meat, may be contaminated with *Salmonella* spp and *Escherichia coli* bacteria, causing gastroenteritis in greyhounds and in personnel preparing the food or cleaning up kennels, turnout areas, and the affected greyhounds.[8] To avoid risk of gastric "blowouts," it is recommended to thaw and use the meat within a short time, wear clean gloves when handling and mixing the meat, and remove any meat or food that is not consumed promptly.[8] Hygiene measures include thorough cleaning and disinfection of affected greyhounds and kennels. Affected greyhounds should be left until last at turnout and their droppings promptly removed from the pens or yards.[8] Personnel handling animals should wear gloves and exercise strict hygiene at all times.[8] Feed dishes should be soaked and washed in hot soapy water and rinsed after each meal.

Meat from dead or diseased livestock that were treated with antibiotics, such as procaine penicillin or sulfonamides, or were destroyed by barbiturate drugs should be avoided because of drug residues in the meat. In a recent survey, up to 85 per cent of randomly selected samples of 4-D meat tested positive for procaine penicillin.[8] There is a high risk of drug residues being detected in the urine of greyhounds fed meat containing these therapeutic drugs. Much more research must be carried out within the regulatory system of greyhound racing to determine urinary limits and thresholds of drug residues that affect performance.

Meat can also become contaminated with organic matter, skin, hair, and other foreign material during processing. Some common examples are mincing chicken skin, which commonly carries *Salmonella* spp and *E. coli* bacterial contamination, with fresh chicken mince. Chicken skin should not be used in mince, but it may be more safely used in well-cooked stews. Likewise, whole eggs should be thoroughly washed with hot soapy water and rinsed before blending and mixing into a meal.

References

1. Grandjean M: Nutrition and performance in the racing greyhound. *In* Proceedings of Fourth Annual International Racing Greyhound Symposium, pp 1–25. Florida, Eastern States Veterinary Conference. Jan 12–13 1988.
2. Kohnke J: Feeds and feeding of greyhounds. *In* Greyhound Medicine and Surgery. Proceedings No. 122, Sydney. Post Graduate Committee of Veterinary Science, 1989, pp 421–466.
3. Grandjean D, Paragon BM: Nutrition of racing and working dogs: I. Energy metabolism of dogs. Compend Contin Ed 14:1608–1615, 1992.
4. Grandjean D, Paragon BM: Nutrition of racing and working dogs: II. Determination of energy requirements and the nutritional impact of stress. Compend Contin Ed 15:45–57, 76, 1993.
5. Grandjean D, Paragon BM: Nutrition of racing and working dogs: III. Dehydration, mineral and vitamin adaptations, and practical feeding guidelines. Compend Contin Ed 15:203–211, 1993.
6. Kohnke J: Nutrition for the racing Greyhound. *In* Proceedings of Tenth Annual International Racing Greyhound Symposium, pp 11–20. Florida, Eastern States Veterinary Conference Jan 15–16, 1994.
7. Britton S: The role of nutrition in maximising the performance of the racing greyhound. *In* Proceedings of Annual Conference. pp 1–26. Canberra. Australian Greyhound Veterinary Association. March 9, 1994.
8. Blythe LL, Gannon JR, Craig AM: Digestive system and nutrition. *In* Care of the Racing Greyhound. American Greyhound Council, Inc. 1994, pp 107–125.
9. National Research Council: Nutrient Requirements of Dogs. Revised ed. Washington DC, National Academy of Sciences, National Academy Press, 1985.
10. Reinhart GA: Fat for the performance dog. *In* Proceedings of Performance Dog Nutrition Symposium, pp. 23–20. Colorado State University. Iams Co. April 18, 1995.
11. Reinhart GA: Fiber for the performance dog. *In* Proceedings of Performance Dog Nutrition Symposium, pp 30–35. Colorado State University. Iams Co. April 18, 1995.
12. Harris RC, Lowe JA: Absorption of creatine from meat or other dietary sources by the dog. Vet Rec 137:595, 1995.
13. Grandjean D: Nutritional peculiarities of racing greyhounds. *In* Proceedings of Seventh Annual International Racing Greyhound Symposium, Florida, Eastern States Veterinary Conference. Jan 12–13 1991.
14. Ferguson R: Greyhound Enteropathies. *In* Proceedings of Annual Conference. pp. 2–12. Sydney. Australian Greyhound Veterinary Association, No. 7, 1987.

CHAPTER 39

NUTRITION FOR SLED DOGS

DOMINIQUE GRANDJEAN

Heavy work and competition induce both organic and psychological stress in dogs, just as in humans and horses. The nutritional adaptation produced must take into account not only the specific energy requirement of the muscular effort itself but also the nutritional needs caused by the animal's state of stress. Thus, along with genetics, training, and psychology, diet is one of the basic foundations of sporting performance. Of these four areas, diet undoubtedly gives rise to the greatest amount of scientific research in view of its potential economic repercussions. Most racing dogs are prime athletes, and an understanding of the racing dog as a nutritional model has potential implications for pet animals. In practice, food adapted to racing dogs should meet the following criteria. It must:

- Provide energy of optimal quality in adequate amounts
- Minimize the weight and volume of the intestinal bolus insofar as possible
- Help to maintain a suitable state of hydration in the animal
- Have a possible buffer effect on any metabolic acidosis induced by running
- Aid in optimizing the result of training activity
- Make up for any physiological shortages brought about by stress

METABOLIC BASES

In addition to having a direct effect on the nature and amount of energy requirements, muscle work also has a major influence on the nutritional balance of food intake via induced stress. The following discussion is restricted to fundamental or novel aspects of knowledge concerning the physiological bases of exercise in the dog.

Energy Mechanism During Exercise

The chemical energy released during muscle contractions is derived solely from the high-energy bonds in adenosine triphosphate (ATP). Intracellular ATP is, or tends to be, decreased during exercise and is then reconstituted instantaneously in situ by means of four processes: transfer from phosphocreatine (PCr), destruction of glycogen, oxidation of glucose, and oxidation of fatty acids (Table 39–1). The metabolic specificity of each type of exercise is determined by the relative contribution of each process in reconstituting the store of ATP.

Phosphagens. Phosphocreatine allows such rapid reconstitution of ATP within the muscle cell itself that ATP and phosphocreatine form an indissociable system known as the phosphagen system. This energy system predominates during supramaximal exercise not lasting more than a few seconds (jumping, start of a race). The bioavailability of muscle phosphagens is not affected by training or diet.

Glycogenolysis. ATP can also be regenerated by anaerobic glycogenolysis, which leads to the release of lactic acid. The rate of ATP renewal by anaerobic glycogenolysis represents only a third to one half of that generated by the phosphagen system. Consequently, the lactic anaerobic system can only create half the maximum power (work/time) generated by the alactic anaerobic system (phosphagens). The power induced by lactic anaerobiosis is probably at its peak after 3 to 10 seconds and remains predominant for 30 or so seconds at the most.

Oxidation of Glucose. Glucose is transported in the blood and then penetrates the muscle cells, where it undergoes oxidation in the mitochondria. Its degree of oxidation depends largely on its ability to enter muscle cells, which is linked to the blood glucose level and corresponding regulatory hormones such as insulin, glucagon, growth hormone, and cortisol. The rate of ATP renewal from the oxidation of glucose is approximately 50 per cent of that obtained via anaerobic glycolysis, with an equivalent power ratio. The anaerobic metabolism of glucose, like that of glycogen, produces lactic acid; both have one important point in common, that is, the conversion of pyruvate to lactate or acetyl-CoA. This conversion is catalyzed by a pyruvate dehydrogenase complex, an enzyme controlled by cofactors derived from thiamine, lipoic acid, pantothenic acid, pyridoxine, and niacin. It is also affected by dichloroacetic acid (a presumably toxic compound) and doubtless by N,N-dimethylglycine (DMG). Glucose oxidation is probably the main source of muscle energy during any exercise lasting 60 seconds to a few minutes; it is enhanced by the ingestion of slow carbohydrates and can be decreased by an intake with an excessive fat content or by fasting.

Lipid Oxidation. While the oxidative metabolisms of glucose and fatty acids are closely interlinked in muscle cell function, they are nevertheless two distinct metabolic pathways for energy production. The fatty acids oxidized in the muscle cell are derived from long chain free fatty acids (FFAs) circulating in the plasma. There are several potential limiting factors during the stages leading to their oxidation. FFAs enter the cells by a process of diffusion; consequently, their entry is increased when their plasma concentration rises. Once inside the muscle cells, carnitine plays a very important role in their transportation (linked to acylCoa) across the mitochondrial membrane. Intramitochondrial enzyme activity constitutes the final step prior to the β-oxidation of fatty acids. At the same time, FFAs can be removed by the liver, converted into ketone bodies, and released into the blood, with acetoacetate and β-hydroxybutyrate subsequently being oxidized in muscle.

The oxidation of FFAs acts as the principal energy source for muscle during low to moderate exercise continuing for some time, i.e., approximately semi-maximal. As with the oxidation of ketone bodies, FFA oxidation is augmented by fasting, undernourishment, and training, especially when the latter involves feedings with a high fat content (adaptive phenomenon).

Protein Catabolism. Branch-chain amino acids (leucine, isoleucine, and valine) can supply 5 to 10 per cent of oxidative energy to the muscles. Their amino groups are transferred to the pyruvate, forming alanine, and to glutamic acid, forming glutamine. Alanine and glutamine are released into the blood and then removed by the liver and used for glucose synthesis. In its turn, glucose is released into the blood and becomes available for intramuscular oxidation. At the same time, alanine transferase, aspartate aminotransferase, and glutamate dihydroaminotransferase activities are raised by 80 per cent. Urinary excretion of urea increases and the nitrogen balance drops. The level of 3-methylhistidine is raised in blood and decreased in muscle following exercise; this indicates a limitation of actin and myosin synthesis during muscle work.[1, 2] These processes can be quantified by determining serum levels of amino acids, ammonia, and urea,[2] or even by assays of urinary urea and proteins.[3, 4]

Roles of the Aerobic Energy System

This energy pathway is undoubtedly the most important to keep in mind in relation to sled dogs. When exercise is prolonged (more than a few minutes) and of moderate intensity (50 to 70 per cent of the maximum oxygen consumption, still poorly quantified in the dog), aerobiosis becomes the system used in covering muscular energy requirements. Data already published concerning aerobic metabolism can be found elsewhere.[5, 6] During endurance testing, fatty acids—in considerable measure derived from tissue lipolysis[7]—form the principal energy source of muscle cells when the animal undergoes suitable basic training, food intake has a high fat content, and the FFA level is high.

Prolonged muscle work is therefore responsible for a marked increase in FFAs,[8–11] occurring earlier and more effectively during cold weather. In fact, adipose tissue supplies the dog with most of its energy for combating the cold. At low temperatures, blood levels of FFAs can be multiplied by 1.88:[12] the renewal of these acids and their rate of oxidation are increased 4.5 and 8.3 times, respectively, while at the same time the relative participation of FFAs in carbon dioxide formation rises from 36 to 64 per cent. This observation is confirmed in huskies, in which an increase of close to 50 per cent is noted in blood concentrations of lipids during winter.[13] Apart from supplying energy to muscle cells, the aerobic system thus makes it possible for full advantage to be taken of the preexisting metabolic adaptation and above all to spare the animal's glycogen reserves. The exhaustion of glycogen reserves is the chief factor limiting any continued effort.

Metabolic Fatigue

These metabolic considerations are among those determining fatigue: substances whose concentrations drop as a result of exercise (ATP, glycogen) and substances that accumulate during exer-

TABLE 39–1. Production of ATP Per Unit of Substrate Consumed, Depending on Metabolic Pathway

Reaction		ATP/mol Substrate	O_2	Resp Quotient
Glycogen	→ Lactate	3	—	—
Glucose	→ Lactate	2	—	—
Lactate	→ $CO_2 + H_2O$	17	5.7	1.00
Glycogen	→ $CO_2 + H_2O$	37	6.2	1.00
Glucose	→ $CO_2 + H_2O$	36	6.0	1.00
FFA	→ $CO_2 + H_2O$	138	5.6	0.71
Acetoacetate	→ $CO_2 + H_2O$	23	5.7	0.73
β-hydroxybutyrate	→ $CO_2 + H_2O$	26	5.8	0.80

cise (lactates, hydrogen ion). The transition of lactic acid from muscle into blood is enhanced by the rapid circulation of blood and by the presence of bicarbonates in the blood. The accumulation of lactates in the blood (hyperlactatemia) is traditionally associated with anaerobic metabolism and an oxygen debt. It is not restricted to dogs making short, intensive efforts. In fact, hyperlactatemia associated with hyperglycemia can be found in huskies, the combination of the two indicating the animal's excitation and the fatigue that it induces by encouraging anaerobic glucose metabolism. On the basis of such observations, it is recommended that huskies (and any other dogs exerting a relatively prolonged effort) be kept quiet before competing. This is, in fact, the opposite of what usually occurs.

Muscle glycogen is another major determining factor in fatigue. Its concentration may be appreciably increased before a competition by loading with carbohydrate intake,[14, 15] or even by the implementation of dissociated diets that are counterproductive in the dog because they increase its risk of muscle disease.[5] At the same time, it is known that the oxidation of fatty acids spares muscle glycogen, especially after long metabolic adaptation to fatty acids. Consequently, rival nutritional strategies that consist of carbohydrate loading and fat adaptation must be adjusted (in terms of their respective intake) to the various exercise intensity levels and duration.

Power versus Speed

As in humans and horses, a balance is created between power and speed during exercise in dogs that affects the choice of nutrition. The relationship between power and speed varies as a function of external factors specific to the nature of the ground, the corresponding tractive force and air resistance. In the case of dogs whose speed exceeds 50 km/h, speed varies in proportion to the square root of the power,[16] and this corresponds to the metabolic considerations previously discussed. Thus, if the power developed is doubled, the speed is multiplied by 1.4 (approximately the square root of 2); when there is a threefold increase in power, the speed is multiplied by a factor of 1.7. The power developed, and hence the type of metabolism involved, can be assessed from an analysis of an animal's racing speed.

Given the various types of competition available (speed, middle distance, long distance), the dog sled illustrates these theoretical concepts. Sled dogs trained for endurance can keep up an "Iditarod" type of trot (approximately 16 km/h) for 10 to 14 hours per day for several days in succession; this is only possible when their diet consists predominantly of lipids. It is therefore reasonable to assume that the preferred energy source in such dogs is the oxidation of fatty acids and to assign it a power factor of 1. (Compared with muscle in humans, this is equivalent to approximately 0.25 mmol of ATP/kg/sec.) Glucose can in turn be oxidized and, as previously described, generate twice as much developed power (power factor 2), and consequently increase the speed by a factor of 1.4; i.e., approximately 23 km/h. This speed corresponds to a moderate gallop or a rapid trot, which good dogs can keep up for several hours per day for several days (middle distance races of the "Alpirod" type). As for glycogen utilization, it ensures a yield twice that obtained from the oxidation of glucose in terms of developed power. It is used by sled dogs when racing at speeds above 30 km/h (32 to 34 km/h for the best teams). This speed is maintained by good teams in speed trials carried out over two or three legs of 25 to 35 kilometers.

Finally, the phosphagens can generate two to three times as much power as that released by anaerobic glycolysis. This enables sled dogs to attain maximum speeds close to 45 km/h for 30 seconds, or even peaks of 50 to 55 km/h for a few seconds.

This highlights the fact that, in practice, the three clearly distinct theoretical energy metabolic pathways are superimposed on one another, and this must be taken into account when deciding on nutritional requirements. Strictly aerobic metabolism under pure endurance conditions can give way to aerobic-anaerobic metabolism once the trial decreases in length. However, the zone of aerobic–anaerobic transition, corresponding to the appearance of the anaerobic threshold, is still ill-defined in the dog. It can even give way to the enhancement of lactic (glycogen) or alactic (phosphagen) anaerobic catabolism during peaks in speed in sprint racing. Accordingly, canine athletes can be fed and trained to improve oxidative yields and the required balance between the use of fatty acids or glucose as energy fuels. Various similar methods can be used to increase the storage of glycogen in muscle and anaerobic glycolysis. However, there is currently no known method of modifying the metabolic behavior and stores of phosphagens.

SPECIFIC NUTRITIONAL APPROACH

There are three groups of factors that affect the nutritional needs of racing dogs: (1) the provoked energy expenditure, which is highly variable quantitatively but basic qualitatively; (2) stress induced by training and competition and its requisite nutritional adaptation; and (3) dehydration, which can be avoided appreciably by suitable nutrition. Specific nutritional recommendations can be defined on the basis of such information, while bearing in mind that the only scientific data currently available relate to greyhounds (sprinter prototype) and huskies (prolonged effort prototype).

Quantitative Change in Energy Requirements

The daily energy requirements of racing dogs depend on numerous variables and are still sometimes difficult to predict. Each owner must ascertain the dog's in-form weight by weighing it every week when possible and must adjust the amount of food provided. Huskies tend to be distinctly different from other types of racing dogs as far as changes in energy requirements are concerned. First, these needs are lower for any given effort under maintenance conditions; this is especially true in Siberian huskies (100 to 110 kcal $ME/kg^{0.75}$ weight compared with 132 for other breeds). This is undoubtedly due to an improved metabolic energy yield and also to decreased expenditure on thermoregulation because of thermal insulation by the animal's fur and a body temperature slightly lower than is normal in the breed. During training and racing, energy requirements alter in accordance with the type and length of exercise involved, and the external temperature. Examples of such changes are shown in Table 39–2. A more precise approach should consider that the total daily energy requirement is the summation of: maintenance energy requirement (MER) + thermoregulation energy requirement (TER) + racing energy requirement (RER).

TABLE 39–2. Changes in Energy Requirements of a Husky in Harness (Weighing 20 kg)

Period	Energy Requirements (in kcal ME)
Maintenance	1000–1200
Training (5 to 8 km/d)	1300–1400
Training (10 to 20 km/d)	1700–1800
Training (30 km/d)	2000–2400
Speed racing	1400–1800
Long-distance race (Alpirod)	2500–3000
Iditarod	7000–8000

It seems possible to approximate these components for a 20-kg Alaskan husky:

- **Maintenance:** MER # $(20 \text{ kg})^{0.75} \times 132$ # 1250 kcal ME
- **Thermoregulation:** According to Mac Namara,[17] the TER is around 3 kcal ME/kg$^{0.75}$/° C under a temperature of 20° C. Therefore, for a 20-Kg Alaskan husky, the approximate TER would be (1) 0° C (Alpirod): # 570 kcal ME, and (2) −50° C (Iditarod): # 2000 kcal ME.
- **Racing:** The RER can be determined as a result of the following equation:

$$RER = O_2 \text{ consumption} \times \text{thermal coefficient}$$

- **Oxygen consumption:** With a $\dot{V}O_2$ max close to 200 ml/min/kg:

Iditarod: 12 hours of race per day (= 720 minutes) at a level of 30 per cent $\dot{V}O_2$ max → $720 \times 20 \times 0.07$ L # 1000 L O_2 per day
Alpirod: 2 hours of race per day (= 120 minutes) at a level of 60 per cent $\dot{V}O_2$ max → $120 \times 120 \times 0.14$ L # 300 L O_2 per day.

- **Thermal coefficient** (TC): The TC of oxygen is the quantity of heart (kcal) produced by the consumption of one L of oxygen. During aerobiosis in the sled dog, oxygen oxidizes around 80 per cent of fat (TC — 4.72), 10 per cent of glycogen (TC — 5.05), and 10 per cent of amino acids (TC = 4.60). Therefore, the mean thermal coefficient can be estimated around 4.73 kcal per L O_2.
- **Racing energy requirement:** (1) Iditarod → RER # 1000 L O_2 × 4.73 kcal # 5000 kcal, (2) Alpirod → RER # 300 L O_2 × 4.73 kcal # 1500 kcal.
- **Total daily energy requirement:** For Iditarod, MER, 1250; TER, 2000; RER, 5000; DER, 8250 kcal EM. For Alpirod, MER, 1250; TER, 570; RER, 1500, DER, 3320 kcal EM.

This determination must be considered only theoretical because some information will be lacking, but practical experience shows it is realistic.

Qualitative Aspects of Energy Requirements

The quality of the energy supplied to dogs during effort is of primary importance, and hence *optimal energy* criteria have been defined for racing dogs. Apart from the nature of the nutrients used, these qualitative considerations must be borne in mind: (1) the energy must be readily and rapidly available at the site of use (muscle cells), and (2) the balance of the energy components must be such that their combustion is accomplished with maximum efficiency, minimum waste, and without risk of metabolic blockade.

Energy Availability. Primarily, nutrients supplying energy must be digested and then metabolized. Given the alterations in gastrointestinal motility and physiological adaptations of racing dogs, it is important to briefly consider the behavior of various nutrient groups that provide energy, i.e., lipids (approximately 8.5 kcal ME/g), nitrogen free extract (NFE) (approximately 3.5 kcal ME/g), and proteins (approximately 3.5 kcal/g).

Gastrointestinal Utilization of Nutrients. The acceleration in *gastrointestinal transit time* brought about by exercise must be taken into account. First, the *gastric transit time* must be optimized. Diarrhea is caused by poor predigestion of proteins and accentuated by stress when transit time is too short, while gastric stasis, which may cause vomiting and especially twisting of the stomach, can occur when it is too long. While no reliable scientific study has yet been made of the problem, experience shows that the physical form of the food provided is important. The best results are obtained in racing dogs when dry, extruded foods are lightly rehydrated 10

minutes or so before meals. Kibbles, which keep their initial shape after rehydration and do not become souplike, are desirable.

The *digestibility* of food sources must also be considered. In fact, the time available for gastrointestinal enzyme attack is limited when the rate of transit is increased. Table 39–3 shows the mean apparent digestibility of the principal carbohydrate, lipid, and protein starting materials in the dog. For starches (the predominant share of nitrogen free extract), digestion often levels off because amylase activity is sometimes inefficient in the dog, especially in working breeds such as German shepherds and Nordic dogs. In the intestine, the rapidity with which amylase attacks starches depends essentially on the botanical origin of the starches.

The physicochemical treatments used in food processing can destroy certain bonds and thus increase the surface exposed to amylase attack;[10] the efficacy of amylase digestion can thus be increased up to 100 times (as in the case of boiled starch). Dextrinization refers to dry thermal treatment, which reduces amyloses and amylopectins to short chain compounds known as dextrins.[19] This term is not altogether suitable for the starches (boiled or extruded) used for feeding domestic animals because processing alters only their physical structure.[20]

It is vital that the starch sources used in racing dogs be hyperdigestible. In fact, compared with fats (with a calorific value approximately two and a half times higher), starches notably increase the volume of food intake in animals requiring high energy levels for racing purposes. But even a small increase in the volume ingested results in lowered digestibility and wetter feces, which

TABLE 39–3. Apparent Total (and Prececal) Digestibility of Food Materials in the Dog

	Raw Materials	CUDa (%)
Protein sources	Fresh meat	98 (96)
	Lung	95 (93)
	Belly	93 (88)
	Liver	95 (93)
	Fish meal	85
	Powdered meat	90 (86)
	Casein	94
	Egg	89
	Powdered horn	58
	Powdered feathers	46
	Soy bean protein	84 (80)
	Bean	74 (65)
Starches	Potato	15.0
	Corn	99.3
	Tapioca	91.5–93.4
	Boiled	93.7–99.8
	Extruded	
	Infra-red cooked	99.4–100
Sources of fat	Lung fat	86–87
	Chicken fat	84–99
	Pig fat	96
	Goose fat	98
	Fish oil	97
	Butter	95–97
	Crude soy bean oil	96
	Cooked soy bean oil	93
	Peanut oil	97
	Linseed oil	97–99
	Cottonseed oil	97–99
	Corn oil	97
	Olive oil	98
	Coconut oil	97

From Meyer H, Kienzle E: Dietary proteins and carbohydrates: Relationship to clinical disease. Eastern States Veterinary Conference, 1991, pp 13–26.

can lead to softening of stools.[21] In addition, carbohydrate digestion can alter the absorption of other ingredients in the food intake, such as proteins, certain electrolytes, and water. Poor starch digestibility reduces prececal and total digestibility of proteins in the dog (Table 39–4), while at the same time a sharp drop in sodium and potassium absorption is observed.[22–24] Finally, a highly negative factor in racing dogs is that water turnover in the intestine is also altered by the ingestion of poorly digestible carbohydrates, with an increase in ileocecal water flow,[24] and increase in hydration of feces.

The dog can digest large amounts of *proteins,* especially those of animal origin. (Proteins of plant origin pose difficulties, with the exception of antitrypsin factors, due to accompanying carbohydrates.) While the gastrointestinal problems raised by protein intake are relatively rare in domestic breeds, they can be more extensive in racing dogs. Thus the consumption of proteins that are resistant to pancreatic proteases but biodegradable (scleroproteins in feathers, collagen in tendons and udders, inadequately cooked eggs) may lead to microbial abnormalities in the intestine. These can compromise the overall digestibility of the food intake, increase fecal volume, and contribute to production of diarrhea.

Lipids are mentioned because they constitute, in most cases, the preferential source of energy in racing dogs. They combine the advantages of being extremely appetizing and highly digestible, and, with their optimal organoleptic quality, they are well tolerated by the dog. Two groups of fatty acids have a qualitative advantage in racing dogs: (1) short or medium chain fatty acids (coconut, copra, and palm fats), whose digestion is facilitated because it occurs passively and without the participation of bile salts; and (2) essential fatty acids of the n-3 series (basically purified fish oils), which help maintain the integrity of the intestinal mucosa by their local anti-inflammatory properties.[25] When the alimentary bolus is too large or has an excessive fiber content, the intestinal mucosa of racing dogs can undergo traumatic microerosion.

Because energy must be made easily available and rapidly convertible by the body during exercise, it seems essential to utilize low-bulk hyperdigestible foods, which occupy little space in the feces. The optimal volume of feces is 40 to 50 gm per 100 gm of ingested dry matter for a racing dog. This objective is difficult to attain with a domestic food intake and is rarely achieved by processed foods.

Metabolic Fate of the Energy. The hormonal control of energy metabolism during physical exercise must be considered within the scope of the energy supply to muscle cells. Hormonal factors actually play a determining role in the mobilization and utilization of various energy substrates. Hormonal factors act either at membrane receptors by stimulating the production of a second hormonal

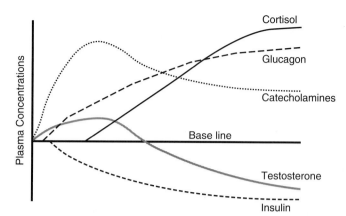

FIGURE 39–1. Changes in plasma concentrations of various hormones involved in metabolic regulation as a function of muscle exercise time. (From Rieu M: Bioénergétique de l'exercice musculaire et de l'entraînment physique. Paris, Presses Universitaires de France, 1988.)

messenger or by crossing the membrane and binding to a cytosol receptor. The first mode of action is a modification of the activity of certain enzyme or other reactions (a short-term process), whereas the second increases the amount of enzyme material and produces effects over the long term. All of the hormonal messages are called into play during physical exercise, the degree of variation depending on intensity and duration (Fig. 39–1).[26] It should be noted that the drop in serum insulin and the increase in glucagon and catecholamines during exercise can increase the production and utilization of carbohydrate reserves, with the mobilization of adipocyte lipid reserves controlled only by an increase in plasma catecholamines and a drop in serum insulin levels.[27]

While the mobilization of lipid reserves from adipose tissue is controlled by several hormones, the utilization of FFAs appears to be subject to the effect of relationships between metabolites which are relatively independent of hormones. FFAs penetrate into muscle cells by diffusion and their oxidation in the cell is controlled by enzyme stages, whose function is regulated by the activity of other metabolic pathways, such as glycolysis. From the metabolic viewpoint, endocrine and enzyme adaptative data must be taken into account for energy optimization. An excessive supply of nonmembrane carbohydrates (starches and sugars) to racing dogs can aggravate glycogen overstorage, promoting lactic anaerobiosis during exercise accompanied by excessive lactate production. In addition, the distribution of fast sugars before training or races causes marked secondary hypoglycemia at the start of the exercise due to a rebound hyperinsulin reaction. During prolonged exercise, the food energy supply is derived mainly from fats. The fats must be incorporated progressively into the food intake for reasons of hormone and enzyme adaptation as previously mentioned. Under these conditions, high levels of fats can produce a considerable improvement in the performance of dogs during endurance exercise, while at the same time enabling reduction of the volume of the daily food intake and limiting the impact of stress-induced diarrhea.[13, 28, 29]

Factors Determining Variations in the Energy Yield. The energy supplied to dogs must be qualitatively adjusted to the required physiological objective and the type of energy metabolism involved. Accordingly, the muscle energy yield can be considerably reduced by an accumulation of metabolic waste or by metabolic blockade. The nitrogenous hypercatabolism due to exercise may exaggerate the release of ammonia and increase muscle fatigue.[30] A collapse in blood glucose or deficiency in glucose-forming amino acids (global insufficiency in protein intake) can, during severe endurance exercise, lead to actual metabolic blockade resulting

TABLE 39–4. Effect of Carbohydrates on Total and Prececal Digestibility of Proteins in the Dog

Protein Sources	Carbohydrate Supplementation (5–10 g/kg BW/d)	Changes (% Total)	
		Prececal dig	Total dig
Powdered meat	Rice	− 6.7	− 2.5
	Corn starch	− 7.9	− 1.9
	Sucrose	− 10.2	+ 1.2
	Potato starch	− 19.6	− 6.9
Meat	Rice	− 4.6	− 4.1
	Tapioca starch	− 9.3	− 5.7
Soy bean cake	Rice	− 4.0	− 0.9
	Tapioca starch	− 8.3	−12.2

From Meyer H, Kienzle E: Dietary proteins and carbohydrates: Relationship to clinical disease. Eastern States Veterinary Conference, 1991, pp 13–26.

from the accumulation of ketone bodies. However, this risk is minor in the dog, given its capacity for putting ketone bodies to good use in energy production. Adaptation of the qualitative energy intakes should therefore offset these risks, especially since certain ergogenic nutrients improve the muscle energy yield:

- L-Carnitine, which transports long fatty acids across the mitochondrial membrane
- Fatty acids of the n-3 series, which improve erythrocyte deformability and the permeability of the membrane to oxygen[31]
- Arginine, an amino acid that prevents hyperammonemia
- Vitamin B complex, which plays a recognized, vital role in the correct functioning of the cell energy mechanism

Application to Huskies. The husky is the prototype for endurance racing and its energy metabolism is geared to aerobiosis. However, given the changes occurring in this sport and the levels of competition encountered, distinction must be made between various nutritional approaches. During *long-distance races* (Iditarod, Yukon Quest, Beargrease), the dogs run at a rapid trot or even a limited gallop, probably between 30 to 40 per cent of their $\dot{V}O_2$ max, using a totally aerobic energy metabolism. During *middle-distance races,* or races in stages (Alpirod), the teams can momentarily increase their speed (in the zone of aerobic-anaerobic transition in energy terms) and exceed their anaerobic threshold for short periods. During *speed racing* (7 to 20 kilometers per leg), particularly in small categories (only a few entrants) or Scandinavian pulka, lactic anaerobiosis can play a significant role, estimated at 10 to 15 per cent coverage of total energy expenditure. It is immediately obvious that, as the length of the race increases, the fat content of the food intake assumes increasing importance at the expense of residual starches.

In overall terms, carbohydrate oxidation covers only 10 to 15 per cent of the energy supply to muscles in huskies, whereas plasma FFAs account for 70 to 90 per cent.[32, 33] A reversal in the lipid:carbohydrate ratio of the food intake results, to the detriment of the carbohydrates, with the oxidation of amino acids constituting 8 to 12 per cent of the energy supplied to muscle. Kronfeld and Dunlap[34] studied food intakes containing (on the basis of metabolizable energy) 0.23 or 38 per cent of NFE and 61, 45, or 34 per cent of lipids, respectively. They reported that no pathological disturbances were seen in harnessed huskies fed on the first of these diets (high fat and carbohydrate deficient), and that performance endurance improved, combined with a better response by the body, both in hematological and metabolic terms. Moreover, Kronfeld had carried out unpublished trials in 1971 whose failure had led him to permanently abandon high carbohydrate diets ("carbohydrates loading") in huskies.[35] In addition, work conducted by Hammel[31] using the same diets showed that that there was a greater capacity for mobilizing fatty acids in dogs receiving food containing 0 per cent NFE and 61 per cent fats. This obviously confers a certain advantage on such dogs during prolonged effort, when there is a predominance of FFA oxidation.

Methodology that produced reproducible, programmable, and quantifiable exercise in the dog,[36] employing treadmill walking and a latin square experimental protocol, showed that an increase in fat content (to 50 per cent of the dry material) in food intake led to a marked improvement in the dog's sporting performance and the biological repercussions during endurance exercise.[28]

Philip[37] studied a team of seven Siberian huskies throughout one racing season and showed that the shift from 45 per cent of fats (based on dry matter) to a diet with a 33 per cent fat content, without any gradual transition, decreased the part played by fatty acids in energy metabolism during exercise and decreased that of glucose by means of an increase in protein gluconeogenesis.[38]

To summarize, the inclusion of too high a proportion of carbohydrates as energy source in the food intake of dogs undergoing

endurance exercise leads to a drop in performance[39] and may cause clinical signs such as muscular stiffness, malaise, myositis, and coprophagy.[40, 41]

Although not ideal from the gastrointestinal point of view, working dogs can quite happily tolerate a food intake entirely deficient in carbohydrates without any lowering of blood glucose (by means of an increase in gluconeogenesis from glucose-forming amino acids) or pathological complications.[35] This is in contrast to humans, who require 15 per cent of carbohydrates in the diet at the very least. In practice, the acceptable minimum content of NFE in the food intake of huskies is 30 per cent: This ensures that a high energy concentration is maintained in the intake and any problems are avoided. This figure of 30 per cent is used in suitably treated carbohydrate sources (e.g. extruded dry food) under maintenance or racing conditions (such as speed racing in "small" categories [3 to 6 dogs]). Any augmentation in carbohydrate intake above this threshold triggers an episode of acute diarrhea; however, this is not serious because it regresses immediately after the food intake is corrected.

Between 25 to 40 per cent of fats should be incorporated in the dry material, the optimum being 35 per cent under normal racing conditions; this has been confirmed by all our field trials. Lipids thus occupy a large percentage of the food intake with a decrease of carbohydrates. This was recently confirmed by Querengässer et al[42] Attention should also be paid to the quality of the fats employed, i.e., saturated long chain fatty acids, short and medium chain fatty acids, and essential polyunsaturated fatty acids of the n-3 and n-6 series.

The supply of fats with a high concentration of long chain saturated fatty acids in the diet allows the dog to build or rebuild stores of adipose tissue from empty calories. Utilization of aerobic metabolism during exercise leads to tissue lipolysis: this increases plasma FFA concentration. The latter are finally oxidized in muscle cells to provide ATP. It is easy to understand the latency period observed in "getting up to power" in aerobic energy metabolism using such a route. In this connection, it was recently shown that hypothyroid dogs had higher postprandial concentrations of triglycerides than did normal dogs; this is due to a lower transfer of plasma triglycerides to adipose tissue, based on diminished lipoprotein-lipase activity (insulin- and thyroid-dependent) in adipose tissue.[4] Given the large percentage of huskies who are either clinically hypothyroid or have a tendency to hypothyroidism[43] (Fig. 39–2), the question of a long-term interrelationship between dietary fats and thyroid hormones might be raised at this point. Short or medium chain fatty acids can be defined[44] as a mixture of fatty acids with 6 carbon atoms (1 to 2 per cent), 8 carbon atoms (65 to 75 per cent), and 12 carbon atoms (1 to 2 per cent) obtained by the hydrolysis of coconut oil followed by fractionation of the various fatty acids. These are of obvious nutritional value in huskies. The digestive action of pancreatic lipase is facilitated by their low molecular weight, and they require no solubilization by bile.

Triglycerides containing short or medium chain fatty acids are thus hydrolyzed more rapidly and more completely than those with long chains; they are released preferentially if the triglyceride is mixed.[45] In metabolic terms, a second advantage derives from the low incorporation of these fatty acids into adipose tissue.[46] In addition, they do not require carnitine to penetrate mitochondrial membranes;[47] in this way, intramuscular oxidation is more rapid than in the case of long chain fatty acids. Finally, they have a restraining effect on the synthesis of fatty acids from scratch in adipose tissue.[48] The inclusion of short chain fatty acids into the food intake conserves carnitine and thus improves the global energy yield, while at the same time preventing certain forms of muscle disease frequently found in huskies. In practical terms, short or medium chain triglycerides should be incorporated into the food intake, with an optimum of up to 25 per cent of fats.

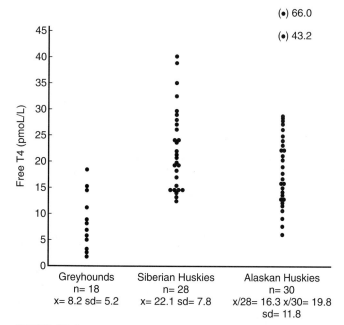

FIGURE 39–2. Serum thyroxine levels of various categories of trained dogs (greyhounds, Siberian huskies, Alaskan huskies). (Hellemann and Grandjean, unpublished data.)

The intake of essential fatty acids should be doubled (in comparison with maintenance standards) for EFAs in the n-6 series because of their role in membrane structures. It is vital that provision be made for an adequate intake of fatty acids in the n-3 series, given their anti-inflammatory properties and the points already mentioned. A dose of 50 mg/kg should be supplied, care being taken to maintain an n-6:n-3 ratio of around 5 to 6. Figure 39–3 shows diagrammatically the various qualitative contributions made by energy sources in huskies.

As far as other racing dogs are concerned, qualitative energy

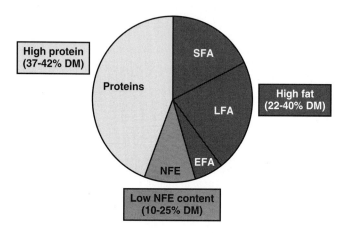

SFA: Short chain fatty acids

LFA: Long chain fatty acids

EFA: Essential fatty acids (n-6 / n-3 = 5 to 6)

FIGURE 39–3. Optimal distribution of dietary energy in huskies.

intakes must in fact be derived from the two extreme models represented by racing greyhounds and huskies. The fat concentration should take precedence over nonmembrane carbohydrate intakes as the exercise becomes more prolonged and consequently less intense. The fat content should thus rise from 14 per cent for relatively brief exercise to 22 per cent for competitions or prolonged work, while the protein content should similarly increase, rising from 33–34 to 40 per cent of the dry material to preserve a high protein:calorie ratio (more than 30 per cent of calories of protein origin).

Nutritional Impact of Stress

While the sources of stress as defined by Selye[49] are vast, it is certain that racing dogs, like any other sporting animals, experience both organic stress (training, competition) and psychological stress (transportation, psychological environment, spectators, temperature, noise). Just as with the energy expenditure strictly due to exercise, such stress contributes to alterations in the animal's nutritional requirements.

Some authors would like to extend the concept of stress to include more than the body's central response (Fig. 39–4). The catecholaminergic central response characteristically corresponds to various emotional disturbances and can be diminished by the reduction or elimination of the emotional component of any stressful situation. In fact, the relative importance of the central component in stress decreases when any given situation is repeated, and in sporting dogs can be one of the noteworthy consequences of suitable training.

Stress and Proteins. Stress due to exercise has a modifying effect on the regulation of cerebral serotonin (5-hydroxytryptamine [5-HT]) synthesis and activity.[50] This neurotransmitter participates in the regulation of numerous physiological functions (digestion, sleep, blood pressure, energy metabolism). The precursor of serotonin is tryptophan. Exercise increases the transport of tryptophan to the brain, due to the effect of catecholamines released.[3] Tryptophan penetrates the cephalic compartment through a saturable stereospecific transporter,[51] which is itself controlled by the supply of neutral amino acids (valine, leucine, isoleucine, methionine, tyrosine, phenylalanine, threosine and histidine).[39, 45] The overall cerebral metabolism of serotonin is increased by exercise, to an extent depending on the type of training.[52]

In dogs, the first nutritional consequence of exercise stress is an

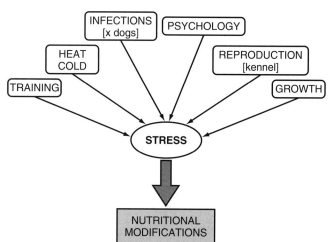

FIGURE 39–4. Sources of stress in racing dogs. (From Kronfeld DS: Stress supplements: Protein and vitamin C. Kennel Gazette 100(10):8–9, 1983.)

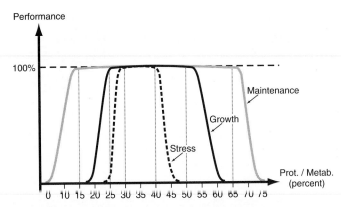

FIGURE 39–5. Concept of "optimum protein level": the range of variation in proven requirements narrows under conditions of stress.

increased demand for neutral amino acids and tryptophan, i.e., for good-quality protein with a high essential amino acids content (high biological value). It is not yet possible to be more specific in quantitative terms. Numerous studies conducted in dogs.[29, 35, 53–56] have demonstrated that stress is linked to the appearance of anemia, which can sometimes be serious. It can be prevented by a minimum dietary intake of protein corresponding to at least 30 per cent of the metabolizable energy in the food intake, in the form of good-quality proteins.[35, 55, 56] A recent study by Billerey[57] involving the annual monitoring of laboratory parameters in greyhounds showed that there was a progressive drop in the hemoglobin concentration (less than 18 g/dl), hematocrit level, and number of red blood cells after 5 months of training and racing.

Regarding the energy concentration of the food intake, the protein content must therefore account for more than 35 per cent with respect to the dry material in the case of racing dogs. In dogs, the range of protein requirements—which is very broad under maintenance conditions—is narrowed (Fig. 39–5).

Stress and Vitamins. Ascorbic acid (vitamin C), although synthesized physiologically by the dog, induces a marked improvement in their organic and metabolic response to exercise stress at a dosage of 1 mg/kcal ME.[58] Ascorbic acid derivatives are cofactors for numerous hydrolases.[59] One such derivative participates in the synthesis of carnitine, which facilitates the transport of fatty acids across the mitochondrial membrane. In one trial, performance was correlated with the plasma concentration of ascorbic acid,[56] and a concurrent decrease in serum levels of vitamins C and E was noted in huskies with the cumulative stress of a racing season (Fig. 39–6).

On the other hand, the dietary intake of pyridoxine (vitamin B_6) is usually boosted when the protein intake is increased (as in racing dogs), so as to bring about transamination.[60] But because of the role assumed by vitamin B_6 in gluconeogenesis, the concentrations of energy substrates might be altered if this vitamin is too readily available during exercise. An exaggerated pyridoxine intake increases the concentration of glycogen-phosphorylase in muscle, and this may give rise to excessively rapid utilization of muscle glycogen.[61] Defective energy metabolism may result with unwanted overproduction of lactic acid, particularly during brief exercise.[62] On the basis of these data, it is recommended that pyridoxine supplements not be exaggerated in racing dogs undertaking brief exercise and receiving a diet containing a high concentration of nonmembrane carbohydrates.

Stress and Cell Membranes. The stress of intensive exercise brings about the release of peroxides and free radicals that affect the integrity of cell membranes of the mitochondria, endoplasmic reticulum, and sarcoplasmic reticulum. The membranes contain polyunsaturated fatty acids, and their oxidation is prevented by

selenium in conjunction with vitamin E. Selenium and vitamin E preserve the membranes intact, especially in the muscles. This doubtless explains why vitamin E is the vitamin most frequently employed as a single nutritional supplement in racing dogs. Its reputation is based on its antioxidant effect in the tissues (skeletal muscles and myocardium), on the clinical improvement it produces in performance capability, and on the reduced muscle fatigability it induces.

Biological membranes contain numerous essential fatty acids; the permeability of the membranes is increased according to their degree of polyunsaturation, and the intensity of energy metabolism and sporting capability is consequently improved.[63] As already stated, these should be incorporated into the diet of racing dogs, in the proportions previously mentioned. It is evident that the nutritional impact of stress must always be taken into consideration and should make it possible to prevent many specific pathological disturbances—such as rhabdomyolysis, anemia due to racing, and stress diarrhea—which lead to an inferior performance.

Required Vitamin and Mineral Adaptations

High-fat diets given to dogs engaged in prolonged exercise can stimulate fecal losses of calcium and magnesium (soap formation). It therefore appears necessary to establish a relationship between the fat content of the food intake and its calcium concentration (Table 39–5). Unpublished trials conducted in French husky teams showed that serum calcium dropped considerably (from 120 mg/L to 80 mg/L) when the proportion of lipids was increased from 30 to 40 per cent of the dry matter while maintaining a constant calcium intake of 2.2 per cent with respect to the dry matter. Such trials are certainly worth describing, especially taking into account the hormonal regulation of calcium. They lead to the recommendation of a calcium concentration close to 2.5 per cent when the lipid content of food exceeds 30 per cent.

The changes observed in plasma magnesium during long-term exercise show that its concentration should be increased in food, especially when the food has a high fat content. Chronic magnesium deficiency in racing dogs results in decreased endurance and resistance, less habituation to heat and cold, loss of motivation, changes in neuromuscular excitability, asthenia associated with cramps, and ligamentous laxity.

Sodium chloride intake must be restricted because the dog sweats

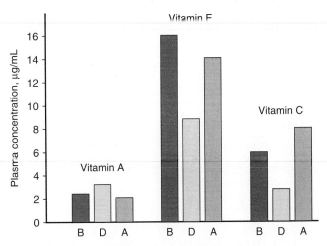

FIGURE 39–6. Serum vitamin levels: before (B), during (D), and after (A) a period of stress in the dog. Significant drops in serum (but not retinal) levels of alphatocopherol and ascorbic acid occur during season in a top class husky team. (Donoghue and Kronfeld, unpublished data.)

TABLE 39–5. Phosphorus and Calcium Requirements in Racing Dogs

Type of Exercise	Ca/P Ratio		Mg/kg Body Weight	g/1000 kcal/ME	Per Cent DM*
Brief exercise	1.3/1.6	Ca	250–300	3.2–4.0	1.25–1.50
(greyhounds, agility, ring)		P	190–240	2.5–3.0	1.0–1.2
Prolonged effort or stress	1.4/1.6	Ca	300–400	3.5–4	1.4–1.5
(sled dog sprint races)		P	200–250	2.7–3.1	1.0–1.3
Prolonged endurance	1.5/2.0	Ca	400–500	4.0–5.0	1.8–3.0
(sled dog distance races)		P	200–300	2.7–3.1	1.0–1.5

*The increase in fat content, and hence in the energy concentration, is partially responsible for the increase in calcium and phosphorus concentrations in the food.

very little through interdigital spaces. Overconsumption of salt, based on the use of quantities recommended for humans or horses, readily leads to polyuria associated with polydipsia.[64–68] Extracellular dehydration and collapse can ensue in both hot and very cold climates. Diarrhea can also occur when solutions of electrolytes intended for horses are used (as frequently happens in the world of dog racing).

The intake of all trace elements should be doubled compared with intake under maintenance conditions. This allows a margin of safety, takes into account the higher energy concentration of foods, and compensates for the antagonistic effects of calcium on their digestibility. Special attention should be paid to the following trace elements:

- Iron, which helps to prevent anemia, and should be avoided for strictly digestive reasons, since salts of iron are frequently responsible for the hemorrhagic appearance of stress diarrhea and rectal bleeding
- Copper, which can also help in preventing certain types of anemia,[69] and improves the solidity of bone framework and cartilage
- Zinc, which is involved in muscle contraction[70] and is the active metal in the enzyme LDH and the plasma protein that transports vitamin A
- Iodine, which activates thyroid function and can help in preventing myodystrophy
- Selenium, which in combination with vitamin E preserves muscle cell integrity

As far as vitamins are concerned, two different aspects must be considered, i.e., long-term biological preparation and a kind of "doping" often carried out at the actual time of the race. While the former practice has a sound basis, vitamin overdosage before a race is of little or no value. Vitamins C, B, and E alone appear to be of some slight occasional value, although this has only been demonstrated empirically. Much work has been published concerning the effect (or lack thereof) of any given vitamin on exercise metabolism and physical performance. However, there are numerous obstacles to the objective interpretation of such work because the subjects were nutritionally saturated with the vitamin being tested; vitamin action requires chronic and repeated administration (action latency period); a vitamin is often a cofactor in metabolic pathways, without value in the process itself, and generally influences only one of the steps in a metabolic pathway; and vitamins may, depending on the dose employed, cause unwanted pharmacological effects. In general, the intake of vitamins A, D, and K can be doubled, while that of vitamin E may be tripled compared with maintenance standards. The same is true for vitamin B complex, and this is applied most of the time in practice.

An understanding of metabolism, physiological changes and nutritional requirements (shown in Tables 39–6, 39–7, and 39–8) in the various categories of racing dogs should enable one to develop a formula for food intakes in practice.

PRACTICAL FEEDING

Any practical diet formulation for racing dogs must be nutritionally balanced, concentrated and easy to digest, and suitably adapted to and eaten by the dogs concerned.

Diets for racing dogs can be adapted to provide coverage of maintenance requirements, increase in energy and nutrient concen-

TABLE 39–6. Nutritional Recommendations for Racing Dogs

	Maintenance	Brief Exercise	Prolonged Exercise	Endurance
Energy (kcal ME/kg$^{0.75}$)	132	150–190	200–400	400–800
Proteins (g/1000 kcal ME)	50	70–80	80–90	80–90
Proteins (per cent ME)	20	30	35	35–40
Proteins (per cent DM)	20–27	30–35	35–40	35–40
Fats (per cent DM)	5–10	12–20	20–30	35–40
FA n-6 (per cent DM)	1	2	3	3
FA n-3 (per cent DM)	0.2	0.4	0,6	0.6
Short chain FA (per cent DM)	—	2.5–5	5–7	8–10
Fibers (per cent DM)	2–5	3	2.5	2
Calcium (mg/kg)	200	250–300	300–400	400–500
Calcium (per cent DM)	0.9–1.1	1.25–1.5	1.4–1.5	1.8–3.0
Phosphorus (mg/kg)	170	190–240	200–250	200–300
Phosphorus (per cent DM)	0.7–0.9	1.0–1.2	1.0–1.3	1.0–1.5
Potassium (mg/kg)	130	130–150	150	150
NaCl (mg/kg)	240	240	240	240
Magnesium (mg/kg)	8	20–25	25–30	25–30
Magnesium (per cent DM)	0.04	0.10	0.15	0.15

TABLE 39–7. Limits and Optimal Daily Intake of Vitamins in the Dog (mg/kg)

Vitamin		Limit	Optimum	Supplement
A	min	61	76	45
	max	610	110	–
D	min	550	700	375
	max	5500	1050	–
E	min	1200	1900	1500
	max	24000	3600	–
K	min	–	0	30
	max	–	105	–
Thiamine	min	54	100	24
	max	1620	210	–
Riboflavin	min	100	160	65
	max	2000	290	–
Niacin	min	450	850	340
	max	13500	1800	–
Pantothenic acid	min	400	750	68
	max	12000	1600	–
Pyridoxine	min	60	110	25
	max	1800	230	–
Folic acid	min	8	15	6
	max	240	31	–
B_{12}	min	1	1.9	0.7
	max	30	3.9	–
Biotin	min	–	0	–
	max	–	14	–
Ascorbic acid	min	–	0	–
	max	–	150	–
Choline	min	50	53	5
	max	150	60	–

From Kronfeld DS, Ferrante PL: Evaluation of ergonomic diets and nutrients for stressed dogs. *In* Colloque International Medecine Sportive Canine. Blagnac, 1990.

tration of the food and decrease in the amount of fecal material, enrichment of the food for exercise purposes (provision of empty carbohydrate or lipid calories) and to meet the demands of exercise and induced stress. The choice or evaluation of any type of food depends on its energy concentration, insofar as energy requirements are significantly affected by the amount and intensity of exercise required, making the volume of the food intake a limiting factor. Under these circumstances it is clear that there is a place only for those manufactured dry, complete feeds to which supplements adapted to the specific requirements of each sport can be added

TABLE 39–8. Limits and Optimum Daily Intake of Trace Elements in the Dog (mg/kg)

Trace Elements		Limit	Optimum	Supplement
Iron	min	1.7	2.3	0.600
	max	20.0	3.5	–
Copper	min	0.16	0.5	0.005
	max	12.5	1.4	–
Zinc	min	1.9	3.3	0.150
	max	50.0	6.7	–
Iodine	min	0.03	0.05	0.005
	max	0.64	0.09	–
Manganese	min	0.28	1.00	0.006
	max	25.00	2.80	–
Selenium	min	0.006	0.013	–
	max	0.250	0.025	–

From Kronfeld DS, Ferrante PL: Evaluation of ergonomic diets and nutrients for stressed dogs. In Colloque International Medecine Sportive Canine. Blagnac, 1990.

(home-made feeds being irrelevant and wet food excluded). The user must bear in mind that, while nutrients fulfill energy requirements, they are also the animal's sole means of preventing the effects of stress.

The Relationship Between Training and Diet

A training schedule for racing dogs should include the concept of customized basic training, taking into account specific sequences (speed, resistance, power). When the racing season is over, the dog should not be allowed to rest immediately but should be put through a progressive de-escalation of training. Consequently, the diet should be finely attuned to changes in training:

- Rest period: good quality maintenance diet
- Training period: progressive transition to a working food intake (allowing one week for each change), or progressive addition of a working diet supplement to the maintenance diet
- Racing period: stress is added to work and may require additional nutritional adjustments; quantitatively, food intake is adjusted to changes in the animal's weight
- Detraining period: progressive return to the maintenance diet

In qualitative terms, it is possible to define the adjustments required by specifically adapting the amount of fats to the length of the aerobic training sessions.

Choice of Foods

In racing sled dogs, the quality of starting materials or complete foods used to satisfy nutritional requirements is of prime importance. The food intake must be very easy to digest, provide an optimal energy yield, and optimize detoxification processes.

Sources of Proteins. Any source of protein with low amino acid bioavailability and poor biological value (essential amino acid equilibrium) should be avoided. The same is true of poorly digestible, collagen-rich proteins (the collagen:total protein ratio must not exceed 15 per cent). Accordingly, the following are recommended: meats (red or white); fish meal and meat flour with a protein content of at least 55 to 60 per cent with respect to the dry material; powdered whole eggs; and lactose-free casein (to which approximately 2 per cent of methionine should be added for perfect balance).

Sources of Carbohydrates. Foods or starting materials with a high starch content should be selected on the basis of quality and undergo optimal heat treatment so as not to produce microbial infection in the intestine. Rapidly absorbed sugars should be banned. Fibers should be introduced in reduced amounts (2 to 3 per cent of cellulose in the food) because they are bulky, they lower the global digestibility of the food intake, and they lead to water retention in the feces, adversely affecting hydration in the dog.

Lipid Sources. These should be considered as the vehicles of particular fatty acids, and great care must be taken to avoid oxidation and rancidity: pork fat, suet, poultry fat (saturated long chain fatty acids); coconut, copra, and palm oils (short or medium chain fatty acids); sunflower, soya bean, and corn oils (essential fatty acids in the n-6 series); and purified fish oils (essential fatty acids in the n-3 series).

Mineral and Vitamin Sources. Mineral sources that are perfectly assimilated, such as calcium phosphates and carbonates, should be used. Yeasts can be used systematically as an excellent source of vitamin B complex. Fat-soluble vitamins should be provided in commercially available forms. Table 39–9 gives an example of a formulation for a vitamin and mineral supplement suitable for racing dogs eating home-made feed.

Manufactured Complete Feeds. For reasons already mentioned,

TABLE 39–9. Example of a Formulation for a Vitamin and Mineral Supplement for Home-made Feed Suitable for Racing Dogs

Formula (g pour 120 g)		Analysis	
Magnesium sulfate	3	Minerals	42%
Iron sulfate	1.08	Calcium	10%
Copper sulfate	0.025	Phosphorus	6%
Manganese sulfate	0.5	NaCl	6%
Zinc sulfate	0.003	Magnesium	3500 ppm
Potassium iodide	0.0002	Iron	1800 ppm
Sodium chloride	2	Copper	75 ppm
Vit. A (500)	0.04	Manganese	60 ppm
Vit. D_3 (500)	0.001	Zinc	1500 ppm
Vit. E (acetate)	0.1		
Calcium phosphate	30	Vit. A	200,000 IU/kg
Calcium carbonate	13	Vit. D_3	5,000 IU/kg
Brewer's yeast	42	Vit. E	500 IU/kg
Vit. B_1	0.02		
Vit. B_2	0.04		
Vit. B_6	0.02		
Vit. B_{12} (1000 μg/g)	0.2		
Fish hydrolysate	0.6		

only complete feeds in a dry or even semimoist form should be employed in racing dogs.

Maintenance Diet. Some owners adopt the simplest approach of increasing the daily food intake in proportion to increasing energy requirements, without changing the feed. In this case, there is no special approach to diet, and the resulting performance is inferior. Two alternatives might conceivably be more effective: *first, the same maintenance diet is used throughout the year,* simply progressively supplemented during training and the racing period. In this case, the best basis is provided by a "25:10" type feed (25 per cent protein and 10 per cent fat in the raw product, corresponding to approximately 27 per cent of protein and 11 per cent of fat with respect to the dry material), with high digestibility (optimum of 50 gm of feces passed per 100 gm of dry material ingested). By retaining this feeding program throughout the year, training supplements and then racing supplements can consist of lean meat or fish for brief exercise and fat meat or fish for prolonged exercise. In this way, a food intake containing one quarter to one third of dry feed and three quarters to two thirds of meat or fish can progressively be attained at the peak of training. A suitable vitamin and mineral supplement is then mandatory at this point.

Second, the maintenance diet is only used during the rest period. It should satisfy the qualitative conditions mentioned and be replaced by a specific complete feed once training becomes intensive.

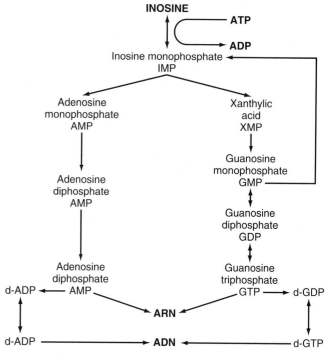

FIGURE 39–7. Simplified metabolic pathway of inosine.

Transitions in diet should be made over a period of one to two weeks.

Specific Diets. Ideally, a 30:15 type food should be aimed at for short to medium exercise, and 35:20 type food for prolonged exercise. Once again, high digestibility and low intestinal and fecal volume are required, while quantities must be adapted to weight changes in the dog. For huskies, 35:20 type food is perfectly suitable for most of the training period as well as for team races in the "small" categories.

Otherwise, specific protein, fat, mineral and vitamin supplements appear to be necessary, either in home-made or manufactured form (Fig. 39–7 and Table 39–10).[71] For long distance purposes, the progressive transition to a semimoist complete feed of the 35:36 type appears to be an excellent solution. However, the problem for manufacturers is a market that is still small and does not warrant the necessary investment.

A rationing schedule in which the proportion of specific supplement included in the daily food intake is progressively increased is feasible.

TABLE 39–10. Composition of a Work Supplement for Brief Exercise in Racing Dogs

Semi-manufactured feed	
Powdered meat (60% proteins)	#50%–60%
Powdered egg	#15%
Fats	#10%–20% ← f (anaerobic training)
Yeast	#5%
Calcium carbonate	#2%
Calcium phosphate	#1%
Minerals, trace elements, vitamins	qsp
Energy	#3500 kcal ME/kg

$$\text{Average quantity} = \frac{\text{Energy requirements linked to training} - 1700 \text{ (maintenance energy requirements)}}{3500} \text{ Kg}$$

Useful Supplements

Details of possible nutritional supplements (ergogenic acids) for racing are beyond the scope of this chapter. Those that now appear to be of real value, especially in terms of improving energy yield and combating stress, are L-carnitine (50 mg/kg), ascorbic acid (vitamin C, 1 mg/kg, i.e. 100 mg/kcal on average), and vitamin B$_{12}$.[72]

References

1. Poortmans J: Influence of physical exercise on proteins in biological fluids. *In* Biochemistry of Exercise. Medicine and Sport, vol 3. Basel, Karger, 1969, pp. 312–327.
2. Poortmans J: Métabolisme des protéines pendant l'effort. *In* 2ème cours international de physiologie and de biochimie de l'exercice et de l'entraînement physique. Nice, 29 Oct–1 Nov 1982.
3. Dominici G, Rottini E, Milia U, Cozzolino G: Protéinurie de fatigue: Détermination quantitative de certaines fractions protéiques. *In* Biochemistry of Exercise. Medicine and Sport, vol. 3. Basel, Karger, 1969, pp 365–370.
4. Segers A: Répercussions des activités physiques modérées sur le taux de la protéinurie intermittente des adolescents. *In* Biochemistry of Exercise. Medicine and Sport, vol 3. Basel, Karger, 1969, pp 361–364.
5. Grandjean D, Paragon B: Alimentation du chien de traîneau. 1. Bases physiologiques et métaboliques. Rec Med Vet 162:1167–1180, 1986.
6. Grandjean D, Paragon BM: Alimentation du chien de traîneau. 3. Rationnement pratique. Rec Med Vet 163:213–240, 1987.
7. Gazzola A, Valette JP, Grandjean D, Wolter R: Les acides gras libres plasmatiques chez le poney et le chien en effort prolongé. Rec Méd Vét 160:69–77, 1984.
8. Brzezinska Z, Kaciuba-Uscilko H, Nazar K: Physiologic responses to prolonged physical exercise in dogs. Arch Int Physiol Bioch 88:285–291, 1980.
9. Issekutz B: Energy mobilization in exercising dogs. Diabetes 28:Suppl. 1, 39–44, 1979.
10. Issekutz B, Miller H, Paul P, Rodahl K: Aerobic work capacity and the plasma free fatty acid turnover. J Appl Physiol 20:293–296, 1965.
11. Rodahl K: Plasma free fatty acids in exercise. J Appl Physiol 19:489–492, 1964.
12. Vincent Falquet JC, Pernod A, Forichon J, Minaire Y: Les acides gras libres comme source majeure d'énergie pour la thermogénèse chez les chiens. Life Science 14:725–732, 1972.
13. Wolter R, Grandjean D, Valette JP: Nutrition lipidique et aptitudes sportives en effort d'endurance. Sci Vet Med Comp 85:183–193, 1983.
14. Blom P: Régime alimentaire et processus de récupération. *In* 2ème cours international de physiologie et de biochimie de l'exercie et de l'entraînement physique. Nice, 29 Oct–1 Nov, 1982.
15. Lacour JR: Facteurs limitants de l'exercice de longue durée. 3ème Congrès National Scientifique de la Société Française de Médecine du Sport. Toulouse, 12–14 May 1983.
16. Kronfeld DS, Ferrante PL: Evaluation of ergonomic diets and nutrients for stressed dogs. *In* Colloque International Medicine Sportive Canine. Royal Canin ed. Blagnac, 1990.
17. McNamara JH: La nutrition des chiens de travail militaires soumis à des conditions de tension. Vet Med Small Animal Clin 67:615, 1972.
18. Kienzle E: Eine in vitro Methode zum Vergleich der Abbaubarkeit verschiedener Stärkevarianten durch Pankreasamylase. J Am Phys An Nutr 60:12–13, 1988.
19. Radley JA: Starch and Its Derivatives. London, Chapman and Hall, 1960.
20. Meyer H, Kienzle E: Dietary proteins and carbohydrates: Relationship to clinical disease. Eastern States Veterinary Conference, 13–26, 1991.
21. Pibot P: La digestibilité des aliments pour chiens. Forum Européen de Nutrition. Annecy, 23–24 Feb 1991.
22. Hammel EP, Kronfeld DS, Ganjan YK, Dunlap HL: Metabolic responses to exhaustive exercise in racing sled dogs fed diets containing medium, low or zero carbohydrate. Am J Clin Nutr 30:409–418, 1977.
23. Kienzle E, Schneider R, Meyer H: Investigations on palatability, digestibility and tolerance of low digestible food components in cats. Int Symp Nutr Small Comp Anim, Davis, CA, 1990.
24. Meyer H, Behfeld T, Schünemann C, Mühlum A: Intestinaler Wasser,

Natrium, and Kalium Stoffwechsel. Adv An Phys An Nutr 19:109–119, 1989.
25. Grandjean D: Diététique clinique et diarrhées chroniques chez le chien. Forum Européen de Nutrition. Annecy 23–24 Feb 1991.
26. Rieu M: Bioénergétique de l'exercice musculaire et de l'entraînement physique. Presses Universitaires de France, 1988.
27. Gollnick PD, Soule RG, Taylor AW, Williams C, Ianuzzo D: Exercise induced glycogenolysis and lipolysis in the rat: Hormonal influence. Am J Physiol 219:729–733, 1970.
28. Grandjean D: Nutrition hyperlipidique et aptitudes sportives à l'effort d'endurance chez le chien; étude des paramètres physiologiques, plasmatiques et hématologiques. Thèse Doct Nutrition. Université del Paris VI; 1983.
29. Grandjean D, Mateo R: Aspects métaboliques de l'exercice musculaire chez le chien. *In* Première Journée de Médecine Sportive Canine. Alfort, Point Vet, 1985, pp 1–67.
30. Wolter R: L'alimentation du chien de sport. Rec Med Vet 165:585–604, 1989.
31. Guezennec CY: Influence d'un régime riche en acides gras polyinsaturés sur la réponse hémorragique à l'exercice physique en hypoxie. Med Armées 16:583–588, 1982.
32. Issautier-Limonne MN: Notions de physiologie sportive appliquée à la surveillance biologique et fonctionnelle des chiens d'avalanche. Thèse Doct Vet. Lyon n° 30, 1976.
33. Paul P, Issekutz B: Role of extramuscular energy sources in the metabolism of exercising dogs. Am J Physiol 22:615–622, 1967.
34. Kronfeld DS, Dunlap HL: Common clinical and nutritional problems in racing sled dogs. Team and Trail 14(7):16–17, 1977.
35. Kronfeld DS, Hammel EP, Ramberg CF, Dunlap HL: Hematological and metabolic responses to training in racing sled dogs fed diets containing medium, low and zero carbohydrates. Am J Clin Nutr 30:419–430, 1976.
36. Wolter R, Grandjean D, Valette JP: Relations nutrition-aptitudes sportives en effort d'endurance. Sci Vet Med Comp 160:657–668, 1983.
37. Philip J: Comparaison de deux régimes alimentaires chez le chien de traîneau en situation. Applications en nutrition comparée. Thèse Doct Med, Université de Paris XI; 1984, 173 pp.
38. Paul P, Issekutz B, Miller H: Interrelationship of free fatty acids and glucose metabolism in the dog. Am J Physiol 21:615–622, 1966.
39. Downey RL, Kronfeld DS, Banta CA: Diet of beagles affects stamina. J Am Anim Hosp Assn 16:273–277, 1980.
40. Kronfeld DS: Diet and the perfromance of racing sled dogs. JAVMA 162:470–473, 1973.
41. Wyatt HT: Further experiment on the nutrition of sledge dogs. Br J Nutr 17:273–280, 1963.
42. Querengässer A, Iben C, Leibetseder J: Optimization of protein and fat in diets for racing sled dogs. Proc. Waltham Symposium on the nutrition of companion animals. Adelaide, 1993, p 113.
43. Simpson JW, Van den Broeck AH: Fat absorption in diabetic and hypothyroid dogs. Res Vet Sci 50:346, 1991.
44. Bach A, Schirardin H, Weryha A, Bauer M: Ketogenic response to medium chain triglyceride load in the rat. J Nutr 107:1863–1870, 1977.
45. Mott CV, Sarles H, Tiscornia O: Action differente des triglycerides à chains courtes, moyennes ou longues sur la sécrétion pancréatique exocrine de l'homme. Biol Gastro Enterol 5:79–84, 1972.
46. Scheig R: Hepatic and extrahepatic metabolism of medium chain fatty acids. In Senior JR (ed.): Medium Chain Triglycerides. Philadelphia, University of Pennsylvania Press, 1968, pp 39–49.
47. Groot PHE, Hulsmann WC: The activation and oxidation of octanoate and palmitate by rat skeletal muscle mitochondria. Biochim Biophys Acta 316:124–135, 1973.
48. Lavau MM, Hashim SA: Effects of medium chain triglyceride on lipogenesis and body fat in the rat. J Nutr 108:613–620, 1978.
49. Selye H: The Stress of Life. New York, McGraw-Hill, 1976.
50. Fernstrom JD, Wurtan RJ: Brain serotonin content: Physiological regulation by plasma neutral amino acids. Science 178:414–416, 1972.
51. Pardridge WM: Kinetics of competitive inhibition of neutral amino acid transport across the blood brain barrier. J Neurochem 28:103–108, 1977.
52. Chaouloff F, Laude D, Serrurier B, Merino D, Guezennec Y, Elgozi JL: Brain serotonin response to exercise in the rat; the influence of training duration. Biogenic Amines 4:99–106, 1987.
53. Adkins TO, Kronfeld DS: Diet of racing sled dogs affects erythrocyte depression by stress. Can Vet J 23:260–263, 1982.

54. Kronfeld DS, Dunlap HL, Adkins T: The red blood cell connection. Team and Trail 18(9):4–6, 1981.

55. Kronfeld DS, Downey RL: Nutritional strategies for stamina in dogs and horses. Proc Nutr Soc Austr 6:21–29, 1981.

56. Kronfeld DS: Stress supplements: Protein and vitamin C. Pure bred dogs. Kennel Gazette 100(10):8–9, 1983.

57. Billerey E: Contribution à l'étude des paramètres biologiques chez le lévrier de course: Variations chez le greyhound et le whippet au cours d'une saison course. Thèse Doc Vet; Alfort, 7 July 1989, 118 pp.

58. Donoghue S, Kronfeld DS, Banta CA: A possible vitamin C requirement in racing sledge dogs trained on a high fat diet. *In* Nutrition, Malnutrition, and Dietetics in the Dog and Cat. Hanover, 1987, pp 57–59.

59. Hornig D, Glatthaar B, Moser U: General aspects of ascorbic acid function and metabolism. *In* Ascorbic Acid in Domestic Animals. Copenhagen, Royal Danish Agricultural Society, 1984, pp 3–23.

60. Kohnke JR: Nutrition of the racing greyhounds: Vitamins, amino acids, additives. Proc Greyhound Course, University of Sydney, 64:681–684, 718, 1983.

61. Black AL, Guirard BM, Snell EE: Increased muscle phosphorylase in rats fed high levels of vitamin B_6. J Nutr 107:1962–1968, 1977.

62. Manore MM, Leklem JE: Effect of carbohydrate and vitamin B_6 on fuel substrates during exercise. Med Sci Sport Exerc 20:233–241, 1988.

63. Bourre JM, Dumont O, Piciotti M, Pascal G, Durand G: Controle par les acides gras polyinsaturés de la composition des membranes. Mini-

64. mum alimentaire nécessaire en acide linoléique et linolénique. Bull Soc Sci Hyg Alim 73(4):43–50, 1988.

64. Brossard JJ: Influence de l'apport luquide sur la capacité physique. Plan de réhydration à l'effort. Colloque Médico-Sportif FFC-FFHB. Paris, 22 Feb 1975.

65. De Mondenard JP: L'alimentation de l'effort; bases physiologiques. Can Nutr Diet 15:285–294, 1980.

66. De Mondenard JP: La diététique du sportif. Ann Kines 8:103–111, 1981.

67. Kjeldsen B, Stromme SB, AasMundrud O: Sport et diététique. *In* Étude sur l'alimentation du sportif. Documents sonulate de Norvège à Lyon, 1980.

68. Robinson S, Robinson A: Chemical composition of the sweat. Physiol Rev 54:202–220, 1954.

69. Griess D: L'alimentation particulière à l'effort bref. *In* Société Française de Cynotechnie: Séminaire sur le chien au travail. Toulouse, 1 March 1987, pp 138–158.

70. Richardson JH, Drake PD: The effects of zinc on fatigue of striated muscle. J Sports Med Phys Fitn 19:133–134, 1979.

71. Sarret O: Contribution à l'étude des précurseurs d'ATP en médecine sportive canine. Étude de l'inosine lors d'épreuves standardisées. Thèse, École Nat Vét Alfort.

72. Grandjean D, Valette JP, Jouglin M, Gabillard C, Bacque H, Bene M, Guillaud JP: Intérêt d'une supplémentation nutritionnelle en L. Carnitine, vitamine C et vitamine B_{12} chez le chien de sport. Étude expérimentale conduite chez le chien de traîneau en situation. Rec Med Vet 169:543–551, 1993.

CHAPTER 40

NUTRITION FOR SPORTING DOGS

GREGORY A. REINHART

Diet and good nutrition play a crucial role in sporting dog performance. Incorporating new nutritional findings into a practical feeding program can improve the dogs' athletic success and enhance overall well-being. A manageable feeding program will also reduce stress on the handler/owner by easing the labor-intensive burden typical in common feeding regimens.

WHAT MAKES A SUCCESSFUL FEEDING PROGRAM?

A balanced diet for sporting dogs should:

- be rich in nutrients required by the dog
- meet energy requirements when fed in acceptable amounts
- include optimal protein levels
- include optimal fat levels
- have a fat profile that minimizes inflammation
- allow for repletion (replacement) of muscle glycogen
- contain the amount and type of fiber that promotes a healthy gut
- be palatable and readily accepted during training and especially while under the stress of competition

- be easy to prepare
- be stable at normal temperatures to avoid rancidity

SOURCES OF ENERGY

Exercise has a profound impact on the amount of energy required by dogs to maintain basal metabolic functions as well as perform muscle work. Different types (aerobic vs anaerobic, speed vs power) of exercise utilize different metabolic pathways to support muscle contraction (for review of this topic see reference 1). These metabolic energy requirements are ultimately provided by three primary dietary sources: fat, protein, and carbohydrates. Nutritional programs designed for canine athletes should provide ample energy to support muscle contraction during athletic bouts while allowing the dog to benefit from training over the course of a season. Both the immediate needs of the muscle as well as longer-term concerns such as aerobic capacity, proneness to injury, blood volume, and palatability can be met with the proper nutritional strategy.

Fat. Fat provides the most concentrated form of energy of all nutrients, is a source of essential fatty acids, and allows absorption of essential fat-soluble vitamins. Dietary fat contains 8.5 kcal of metabolizable energy (ME)/gm and is over twofold more calorically dense than either dietary protein or carbohydrate. As fat content in a diet increases, the energy density (number of calories provided by the food in a given weight or volume) of the diet also increases. Fat also contributes to the palatability and acceptable texture of commercially prepared canine foods. Common sources of fat include chicken fat, tallow, lard, corn oil, safflower oil, soybean oil, sunflower oil, fish oils, and full-fat flax/flax oil.

Protein. Dietary protein can be supplied by animal sources, plant sources (grains), or a combination of the two. In general, high-quality animal-source proteins provide superior digestibility, amino acid balances, and palatability. However, animal-protein sources can range from excellent quality to poor quality. Nutritional quality of dietary protein sources is determined by protein digestibility and amino acid availability, which can be ascertained only through feeding trials. Animal-protein sources commonly included in commercially prepared dog foods include chicken, chicken by-product meal, chicken meal, beef, dried egg, fish meal, meat and bone meal, meat by-products, meat meal, lamb, and lamb meal. The term *meat* can represent any species of slaughtered mammal but typically represents the striated muscle of pork, beef, sheep, or horse. *By-products* may include secondary carcass components that can vary greatly in their nutritional quality. Depending on the supplier, by-product meals can have exceptional nutritional quality or be low in nutritional quality because of higher amounts of indigestible ingredients.

Protein is one of the least desirable muscle fuels. All proteins in the muscle cell have a function and cannot be stored like fat or carbohydrate for energy. Proteins consumed in excess of requirement are deaminated, and the remaining carbon structure is utilized for energy. Protein contains 3.5 kcal ME/gm and is less energy dense than fat. Fed in excess, high-quality animal proteins are an expensive source of carbon intermediates for ATP generation. However, athletic dogs have a higher protein requirement than sedentary animals, so this component of the diet should also not be underfed.

Carbohydrates. Ingredients that contribute dietary carbohydrates in the sporting dog's diet include various forms of corn, rice, wheat, sorghum, barley, potato, and oats. These ingredients contribute complex carbohydrates in the form of starch that is highly available when properly cooked. Feeding uncooked grains often results in loose stools and flatulence, an indication of poor nutrient availability. Other sources of carbohydrates include molasses and certain types of hydrolyzed starches. Dietary carbohydrates provide sporting dogs with a source of energy. A limited amount of carbohydrate can be stored in the body as glycogen with excess metabolized to body fat for energy storage. Carbohydrates provide 3.5 kcal ME/gm and are less nutrient dense than fat.

ENERGY REQUIREMENTS

Athletic canine diets need to have dietary sources of fat, protein, and carbohydrates in appropriate proportions to meet energy needs and optimize athletic performance. Achieving energy balance is very important in any dog and critically important from a competitive standpoint in sporting dogs. The ideal situation is for energy expenditure to equal energy intake and avoid large variations in body weight. Positive energy balance occurs when caloric intake exceeds energy expenditure and results in an increase in the quantity of fat stored by the body. Negative energy balance occurs when caloric intake is lower than energy expenditure, resulting in weight loss and a decrease in both fat and muscle mass. Either of these latter two situations will compromise athletic performance.

Both physical and environmental stresses result in increased energy needs in sporting dogs. Short bouts of intense physical activity may cause only a small increase in energy needs while long-distance training and/or prolonged sporting events can substantially increase energy needs. Environmental conditions commonly associated with sporting dogs will also increase energy demands, with additional energy expenditure required to enhance cooling mechanisms in warm conditions or support normal body temperature in cold conditions. The total energy needs of a sporting dog consist of a maintenance energy requirement, a voluntary muscular activity requirement (exercise), and a thermoregulation energy requirement. The 1974 National Research Council recommends 132 kcal ME/kg body weight (see reference 3 for more details) for maintenance energy needs.[2] However, the preferred calculation of energy requirements of adult sporting dogs at maintenance is as follows[3]:

Maintenance metabolizable energy requirement = $K \times W_{kg}$ (see reference 3 for more details).

$$
\begin{aligned}
K &= 132 \text{ Inactive} \qquad W = \text{weight (kilograms)}\\
&\quad\ 145 \text{ Active}\\
&\quad\ 200 \text{ Very active}\\
&\quad\ 300 \text{ Endurance performance}
\end{aligned}
$$

This equation takes into consideration the increased proportion of muscle mass and increased metabolic activity of highly trained athletes. However, the energy requirements predicted by either of these proposed equations are specific for adult maintenance, and periods of strenuous physical work and/or exposure to environmental extremes will require much greater energy intakes to maintain energy balance. For example, a conditioned greyhound may require an additional 10 to 20 per cent above maintenance energy requirements, while a sled dog has been proposed to require two to four times maintenance requirements to avert significant weight loss.[4] The energy needs of sled dogs have been estimated to be 2500 to 3000 kcal ME/day for mid-distance stage races and 7000 to 8000 kcal ME/day for long-distance sled dog racing.[5] The other extreme involves working dogs in hot humid environments in which 50 to 100 per cent more energy is required than in similar dogs in less environmentally stressful conditions.[6]

Recent scientific studies have quantified the energy expenditure and energy intake of Alaskan sled dogs.[7] Energy expenditure was measured by the double-labeled water technique and energy intake by dietary analysis in eight Alaskan sled dogs during a 490-km sled dog race. Energy expenditure was also measured in four other trained dogs that did not run, and changes in background abundance of ^{2}H and ^{18}O were monitored in five unlabeled dogs. The dogs completed the 490 km at an average speed of 7 km/hr with ambient temperatures ranging from -10C to -35C. Total energy expenditure, measured by the double-labeled water technique, was 11,253 $\pm$ 1410 kcal and metabolizable energy intake was 10,655 $\pm$ 980 for the exercising dogs. There was more than a 4.5-fold increase in energy expenditure due to physical exercise (Fig. 40–1). The dogs that exercised also lost 4.5 per cent of body weight while the nonexercising dogs did not lose weight during the duration of the trial. This study validated the double-labeled water technique for determining energy expenditure in dogs associated with prolonged exercise in the cold. The trail conditions were excellent, and there was little wind during this particular event. Colder temperatures, deep snow, and/or high winds are often present and would be expected to impose greater environmental stress than the conditions encountered during this race. Future studies need to address the energy expenditures of sporting dogs involved in other types of athletic performance and environmental conditions (including heat/humidity).

In summary, systematic equations to determine feeding amounts that meet energy requirements of sporting dogs participating in a wide range of activities are impractical and can be misleading.

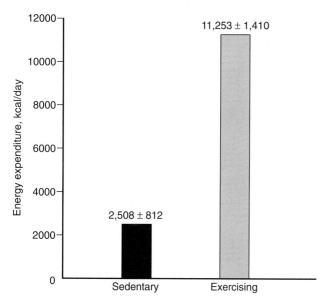

FIGURE 40–1. Effect of exercise on daily energy expenditure of Alaskan sled dogs.

Nevertheless, a useful approach is to determine the maintenance energy requirements (taking into account activity level) and increase this maintenance amount approximately 10 per cent for each hour of work the dog performs. However, the best recommendation remains to feed each individual animal to a body condition that is appropriate for the sport and environmental conditions in which it is participating.

WATER REQUIREMENTS

Water is the single most important nutrient for survival in sporting dogs as well as any terrestrial animal. While animals can survive after losing nearly all of their adipose tissue and over half of their body protein, a 10 per cent loss in body water can result in death. Approximately 70 per cent of lean adult body weight is water, with intracellular fluid comprising 40 to 45 per cent and extracellular fluid accounting for 20 to 25 per cent of the body's mass. The aqueous medium inside the cell is essential for the metabolic processes and chemical reactions that fuel muscle contraction as well as other maintenance activities that sustain life. Because of its high specific heat, water is also able to absorb the heat generated by metabolic reactions associated with exercise with a minimal increase in body temperature. Extracellular fluids are then able to transport the heat away from the working muscles as well as remove metabolic waste products.

Water is lost from the body of exercising dogs by three major routes. Elimination of waste products from the kidneys results in a large amount of obligatory water loss via the urine. Urinary water loss has been speculated to be directly related to the solute load of the diet, which in turn is affected by diet composition and quantity.[8] Consumption of high-protein diets and/or high caloric intakes would be expected to increase obligatory urinary water loss. Fecal water loss accounts for a much smaller portion of water excretion, and becomes substantial only when aberrations occur in intestinal capacity to absorb water. Stress-induced diarrhea is common in performance dogs and may contribute to excessive water loss via the feces. A third route of water loss is evaporation from the lungs during respiration and panting. Exercise results in high respiration rates and is an important consideration in most practical situations.

Sustained exercise in cold ambient temperatures results in a high water loss due to the low relative humidity of the inhaled air, while high-intensity exercise at any temperature or moderate exercise in warmer ambient temperatures promotes panting as a thermoregulatory mechanism.

Field studies in Alaskan sled dogs have demonstrated the very high water needs of exercising dogs. Sled dogs competing in the mid-distance race, the 1993 Copper Basin 300, had daily water turnovers in excess of 5.0 L per day (Fig. 40–2).[9] These dogs weighed 24.2 kg, completed the 490-km race in 70 hours, and consumed an average of 890 gm of protein, 750 gm of fat, and 450 gm of nitrogen-free extract (carbohydrate) per 24-hour period. The ambient temperature during the study ranged from −10C to −35C.

Diet-induced obligatory urinary losses, exercise-induced thermoregulatory panting, respiratory evaporation, and stress-induced diarrheas are all significant contributors to the increased water needs of sporting dogs. Future scientific efforts need to focus on type of exercise and the effect of ambient temperature on specific water needs for different sporting events.

DIETARY FAT

Dietary fat is a concentrated source of readily available energy, provides essential fatty acids, and enhances palatability. Dietary fat is in a classification of compounds known as lipids. The most common source of dietary fat is the simple lipid, which includes the triglyceride. Triglycerides are composed of three fatty acids linked to one molecule of glycerol. Dietary fats (triglycerides) in the diet can be differentiated according to the type of fatty acids that each triglyceride contains. Recent scientific findings from canine nutritional studies have revealed new concepts on how much and what types of fat (fatty acids) to feed to athletic dogs.

Quantity of Fat. It is generally accepted that energy is the nutrient of most concern for sporting dogs, yet the ''optimal'' method of supplying this energy in the diet has been controversial. It is well recognized in human athletic events that an important limiting factor in prolonged exercise is the amount of glycogen present in the working muscles and that onset of fatigue is highly

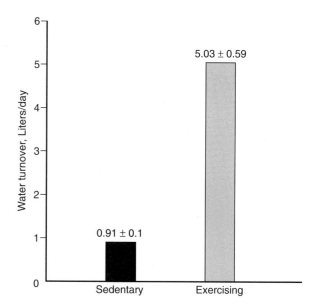

FIGURE 40–2. Water turnover of exercising and sedentary trained Alaskan sled dogs.

correlated with muscle glycogen depletion.[10] However, unlike the human, the dog derives approximately 70 to 90 per cent of the energy for muscle contraction from fat metabolism and only a small amount from carbohydrate metabolism.[11, 12] These laboratory findings are consistent with research in sled dogs[13, 14] and beagles,[15] in which the ability to use fatty acids through aerobic pathways for energy is more important for performance than the use of muscle glycogen through anaerobic pathways. In work conducted by Reynolds and coworkers,[14] 16 Alaskan huskies were fed either a high-fat (60%, fat, 25% protein, 15% carbohydrate on an energy basis) or a high-carbohydrate (15% fat, 25% protein, 60% carbohydrate) diet for a 1-month acclimation period followed by 6 months of exercise tests. At the beginning of the exercise tests, the high-fat–fed animals had significantly higher levels of circulating free fatty acids (FFA) during aerobic exercise tests than dogs fed the high-carbohydrate diet.[16] One of the major determinants of the rate of free fatty acid utilization in working muscle is the concentration of FFA in the bloodstream. By promoting increased plasma FFA levels, the high-fat diet facilitated FFA utilization during exercise. This phenomenon has been further documented in Labrador retrievers, which have a 45-per cent increase in maximal fat oxidation when fed a high-fat (65% of energy) compared to a low-fat (25% of energy) diet.[17] These same dogs also had nearly a 50-per cent increase in VO_{2max} (Fig. 40–3) and a 40-per cent increase in mitochondrial volume in biopsies of the triceps brachii (Fig. 40–4) when fed a high-fat diet. It is proposed that feeding a high-fat diet stimulates growth of mitochondria and thereby increases maximal rates of fat oxidation, aerobic capacity, and endurance in Labrador retrievers until they reach the high endurance levels of sled dogs. In essence, feeding a high-fat diet to a Labrador retriever produces an animal that has an aerobic capacity and mitochondrial volume density indistinguishable from that of a sled dog. This strongly suggests that the legendary endurance of sled dogs may be due to diet and not to generations of selective breeding. These results further imply that diet may have been underestimated in its importance on stamina and performance from a practical standpoint, because training is typically associated with only a 15- to 20-per cent increase in VO_2 max and maximal fat oxidation.[18]

Type of Fat. The benefits of dietary fatty acid supplementation is receiving increased attention in the veterinary[19] and sports exercise physiology fields. Recently the ability of dietary omega-3 fatty acids to reduce the concentrations of inflammatory compounds in canine skin, plasma, and neutrophils has been reported.[20] The reduction in the inflammatory response is due to the competitive

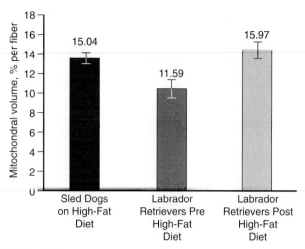

FIGURE 40–4. Dietary fat increases mitochondrial volume in sporting dogs.

inhibition of omega-3 fatty acids on the production of omega-6 fatty acid metabolites (proinflammatory eicosanoids).

Omega-3 (n-3) fatty acids are found in high concentrations in marine oil (cold-water fish) and certain terrestrial plant oils (flax). Enriched sources of omega-6 (n-6) fatty acids include terrestrial plant oils (corn, safflower, canola, soy) and animal fats (Table 40–1). Polyunsaturated fatty acid terminology is determined by the number and location of the double bonds (by counting back from the terminal methyl group). Omega-3 fatty acids have the first double bond at the third carbon while n-6 fatty acids have the first double bond at the sixth carbon (Fig. 40–5). Animals are unable to synthesize n-6 or n-3 fatty acids de novo or interconvert one series of fatty acids to another. (If an n-6 fatty acid is ingested, its methyl end remains the same, and all metabolites from it will be n-6.)

Eicosanoids are derivatives of 20-carbon fatty acid metabolism and modulate inflammation. Both n-6 and n-3 fatty acids are precursors of eicosanoids and compete for the same enzyme systems. Cell injury activates membrane phospholipases and initiates the lipid inflammatory cascade in which both n-3 and n-6 fatty acids are metabolized. Metabolism of n-6 and n-3 fatty acids produces eicosanoids with vastly different inflammatory capabilities. For example, dietary supplementation of the marine n-3 lipids eicosapentaenoic acid (20:5n-3) and docosahexaenoic acid (22:6n-3) resulted in the enrichment of n-3 fatty acids in membrane phospholip-

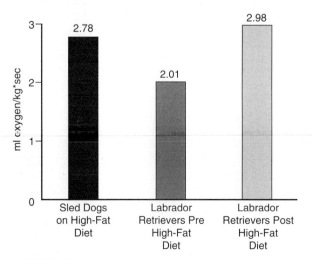

FIGURE 40–3. Dietary fat increases VO_{2max} in sporting dogs.

TABLE 40–1. Dietary Omega-3 and Omega-6 Fatty Acid Sources

Omega-3 Fatty Acid Sources and Concentrations (%)	
Cold water fish oils	12–15 eicosapentaenoic acid (20:5n-3)
	8–10 docosahexaenoic acid (22:6n-3)
Flax oil (linseed)	57 alpha-linolenic acid (18:3n-3)
Canola oil (rapeseed)	8 alpha-linolenic acid (18:3n-3)
Soybean oil	7 alpha-linolenic acid (18:3n-3)
Omega-6 Fatty Acid Sources and Concentrations (%)	
Corn oil	70 linoleic acid (18:3n-6)
Safflower oil	78 linoleic acid (18:3n-6)
Sunflower oil	69 linoleic acid (18:3n-6)
Cottonseed oil	54 linoleic acid (18:3n-6)
Soybean oil	54 linoleic acid (18:3n-6)
Chicken fat	16 linoleic acid (18:3n-6)
Pork fat (lard)	15 linoleic acid (18:3n-6)

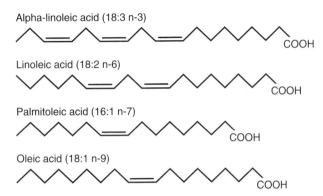

FIGURE 40–5. Fatty acid nomenclature and structure.

TABLE 40–2. Effect of Decreasing Dietary Omega-6:Omega-3 Fatty Acid Ratio on Canine Plasma and Skin Fatty Acid Profiles

		Plasma	Skin
Linoleic	(18:2n-6)	↓	↓
Gamma-linolenic	(18:3n-6)	↓	ND
Alpha-linolenic	(18:3n-3)	↑	ND
Stearidonic	(18:4n-3)	↑	↑
Arachidonic	(20:4n-6)	↓	↓
Eicosapentaenoic	(20:5n-3)	↑	↑
Docosatetraenoic	(22:4n-6)	↓	ND
Docosapentaenoic	(22:5n-3)	↑	ND
Docosahexaenoic	(22:6n-3)	↑	ND

ND = no difference detected

ids of the skin,[21] plasma,[22] and neutrophils.[21] Omega-3 fatty acids are converted into isomers of leukotriene B, prostaglandin E, and thromboxane A that are much less inflammatory than their corresponding n-6 fatty acid isomers, which tends to decrease the inflammatory response (Fig. 40–6). Overall, the net effect of arachidonic acid (n-6) metabolism is production of eicosanoids that promote proinflammatory, proaggregatory, and thrombotic reactions. Conversely, eicosapentaenoic acid (n-3) metabolism produces eicosanoids that are much less inflammatory, vasodilatory, and antiaggregatory.[23]

Because the n-6 and n-3 fatty acids compete for the same enzyme systems, the ratio between these two types of fatty acids in the diet is very important. This ratio determines the relative proportions of the respective n-6 (proinflammatory) and n-3 (less inflammatory) metabolites that are produced. Dietary omega-6:omega-3 fatty acid ratios between 5:1 and 10:1 also meet the essential n-6 fatty acid requirement but do not alter blood clotting parameters.[24]

Canine plasma fatty acid profiles are very diet responsive, with dietary omega-6:omega-3 fatty acid ratios of 5:1 and 10:1 resulting in increased plasma omega-3 fatty acids and decreased plasma omega-6 fatty acids (Table 40–2). Skin fatty acid profiles were not as diet responsive as plasma; however, dietary omega-6:omega-3 fatty acid ratios of 5:1 and 10:1 resulted in increases in certain omega-3 fatty acids and decreases in certain omega-6 fatty acids (Table 40–2). Although the magnitude of response was not as great as the plasma, skin fatty acid concentrations were influenced by diet. Dietary omega-6:omega-3 fatty acid ratios of 5:1 and 10:1 resulted in increases of certain long-chain omega-3 fatty acids in both the small intestinal and colonic mucosa. Conversely, a decrease in arachidonic acid (20:4n-6) was observed in the small intestine and colon after dogs were fed dietary omega-6:omega-3 fatty acid ratios of 5:1 and 10:1 (Table 40–3).

Research in the dog has demonstrated that a dietary omega-6:omega-3 fatty acid ratio between 5:1 and 10:1 reduces the production of inflammatory mediators in canine skin, plasma, and neutrophils. Dietary omega-6:omega-3 fatty acid ratios between 5:1 and 10:1 meet the canine essential omega-6 fatty acid requirement (2 to 6% of metabolizable energy and/or 1% of dry matter)[25] but do not alter blood clotting, neutrophil reactivity, or wound-healing parameters.[26]

Preservatives. One of the primary concerns in feeding a sporting dog is safety. A nutritional product or feeding regimen must be both nutritious and safe. The nutrition must be supplied in a form that is stable, free of harmful bacterial contamination and/or harmful toxins, and protected from degradation and loss of nutrients during storage. A primary nutrient in pet foods that requires protection during storage is dietary fat and the fat-soluble vitamins A, D, E, and K. These nutrients all have the potential to undergo oxidative destruction during storage. Commercially prepared nutritional products are likely to contain an antioxidant to prevent this harmful oxidative process. Unprotected fats in the diet result in decomposition and production of offensive odors and tastes as well as formation of toxic peroxides and free radicals, which are documented to be harmful to the health of the animal. Common synthetic antioxidants include ethoxyquin, butylated hydroxytoluene (BHT), and butylated hydroxyanisole (BHA). Ethoxyquin has been approved for use in animal feeds for nearly 40 years and is approved for limited use in human foods. Ethoxyquin is more efficient in preventing fat rancidity than BHA or BHT, which allows lower inclusion levels. Ethoxyquin is also very effective at protecting polyunsaturated fatty acids (ie, omega-3 fatty acids), which are prone to oxidative damage if not properly preserved. However, a wide variety of unsubstantiated health concerns have been raised about the safety of ethoxyquin. The United States Food and Drug Administration maintains that ethoxyquin has a "safe tolerance level" of 150 parts per million,[27] with most levels of ethoxyquin in commer-

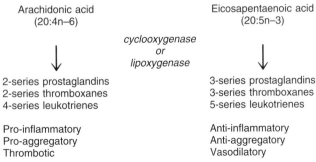

FIGURE 40–6. Metabolic fate of omega-6 and omega-3 fatty acids.

TABLE 40–3. Effect of Decreasing Dietary Omega-6:Omega-3 Fatty Acid Ratio on Canine Small Intestinal and Colonic Mucosa Fatty Acid Profiles

		Plasma	Skin
Arachidonic	(20:4n-6)	↓	↓
Eicosapentaenoic	(20:5n-3)	↑	↑
Docosatetraenoic	(22:4n-6)	ND	↓
Docosapentaenoic	(22:5n-3)	↑	↑
Docosahexaenoic	(22:6n-3)	↑	↑

ND = no difference detected

cial products many times lower than this level. It is currently recommended that commercially prepared diets be chosen that have incorporated a proven antioxidant system. This becomes even more important if the benefits of feeding a high-fat diet and/or omega-3 fatty acids are being considered. The documented health benefits of consuming stable, nonrancid fats and fatty acids far outweigh the unsubstantiated negative claims concerning synthetic antioxidants.

DIETARY PROTEIN

There is the currently held belief that exercise increases an athlete's protein requirement. There is also a commonly held supposition that these increased protein needs can be met solely by the increased nutrient intakes of exercising dogs and that specific dietary modifications are not required. Because strenuous exercise involves damage to tissues, which then must repair and remodel itself, it has been recommended that the guidelines for feeding adult athletic dogs use the nutrient requirements for growth rather than maintenance.[28] The question remains regarding what level of protein to feed sporting dogs. A study involving 32 sled dogs compared the metabolic responses to training in dogs fed diets deriving 16, 24, 32, and 40 per cent of their calories from high-quality animal protein. Fat levels were kept constant at 50 per cent, and the source of protein did not differ between diets. It was observed that dogs fed the highest protein level maintained a larger plasma volume and red blood cell mass during strenuous training.[18] It was also observed during this study that all of the dogs consuming the low-protein diet had at least one injury during the racing season that resulted in its being removed from training for a minimum of 1 week (Table 40–4). Only two of eight dogs fed the 24 per cent of calories from protein diet had serious injuries, while none of the dogs fed the higher protein level diets had injuries.[18] It appears from this research that an adult athletic dog may have a *minimum* protein requirement of 24 per cent of ME calories. This is substantially different from the 11.4 per cent minimum requirement for canine growth established by the National Research Council[25] and 18 per cent of ME calories for adult maintenance and 22 per cent of ME calories for growth recommended by the Association of American Feed Control Officials 1994 guidelines.[29]

DIETARY CARBOHYDRATE

If an excessive amount of dietary carbohydrate is fed to a sporting dog, it will dilute out the calories derived from protein and fat and not allow for the injury reduction associated with higher protein intakes or the stamina improvement associated with higher fat intakes. High-carbohydrate diets have also been associated with exertional rhabdomyolysis in dogs,[4] presumably from glycogen overstorage resulting in excessive lactate production during exercise. The goal is to strategically feed carbohydrates to achieve targeted metabolic benefits without compromising other aspects of the athlete's overall nutritional program. However, the

TABLE 40–4. Effect of Increased Dietary Protein on Injury Rate in Sled Dogs

Injuries per Group	Calories from Protein (%)
No injuries	40
No injuries	32
2 of 8 dogs injured	24
At least 1 injury in every dog	16

practice of feeding simple sugars before training or a sporting event can actually lead to marked secondary hypoglycemia at the initiation of exercise due to "rebound hyperinsulinemia." In these cases, the attempts to increase blood sugar levels have actually resulted in hypoglycemia. It is recommended to avoid quick energy sources, such as simple sugars and candies, 2 hours or less before a race or training bout and focus on strategic carbohydrate feeding immediately post exercise to restore muscle glycogen.

IMPORTANCE OF MUSCLE GLYCOGEN

Glycogen is the storehouse for carbohydrates in the body. The glycogen found in the muscles, including the heart muscle, supply "fuel" to the muscle cells. Muscle glycogen levels can decrease dramatically during endurance exercise in athletic dogs. The ability and desire for canine athletes to resume exercise after a rest period (whether hours or days) is often related to muscle glycogen levels. Therefore, a major goal when feeding endurance athletes is to increase muscle glycogen stores and/or delay muscle glycogen depletion during exercise.

The conventional approach of "glycogen loading" by feeding high-carbohydrate diets has not resulted in positive results to date. This performance failure in exercising dogs fed high-carbohydrate diets has been attributed to excessive lactate production during the rest-to-exercise transition[30] and a decrease in food energy density.[15] Recently, when sled dogs fed high-carbohydrate diets were compared with animals fed high-fat diets, both higher resting muscle glycogen levels and accelerated muscle glycogen utilization during exercise were observed.[14] The potential benefits of higher resting glycogen levels were offset by the rapid utilization of these carbohydrate stores during exercise. Conversely, dogs fed the high-fat diet were able to "spare" muscle glycogen levels and maintain adequate muscle glycogen throughout both anaerobic and aerobic exercise tests.

Although glycogen sparing may be a more sound strategy for endurance than glycogen loading in sporting dogs, glycogen depletion remains a major factor associated with fatigue. Therefore the challenge is to nutritionally up-regulate muscle glycogen storage while feeding diets enriched in fat and protein. This novel approach was tested in a field research study with 24 Alaskan sled dogs because they typically consume diets low in carbohydrates (< 15% of ME kcal during racing events) and would not be expected to fully replete muscle glycogen levels because of diet and short rest periods between exercise bouts. The sled dogs participated in an exhaustive training run designed to significantly decrease muscle glycogen levels and were then provided either glucose polymers in water (targeted total dose of 1.5 gm carbohydrate/kg body weight) or plain water immediately post exercise. The sled dogs receiving the glucose polymer (partially hydrolyzed starch) supplementation demonstrated significantly greater muscle glycogen repletion during the first 4 hours of recovery than nonsupplemented dogs (Fig. 40–7). Carbohydrate supplementation immediately after exercise also increased plasma glucose concentrations 100 minutes after exercise.[18]

Thus it appears that two nutritional strategies are beneficial for improving endurance and delaying fatigue. Feeding to enhance the ability of working muscles to preferentially use fatty acids for energy (and spare muscle glycogen) and postexercise supplementation of small amounts of carbohydrate to increase muscle glycogen stores. Strategic feeding of readily available carbohydrates immediately after exercise allows repletion of muscle glycogen without significantly diluting the diet with carbohydrate calories.

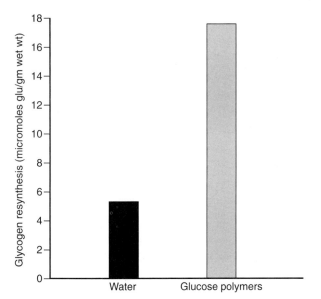

FIGURE 40–7. Postexercise carbohydrate supplementation increases muscle glycogen resynthesis.

DIETARY FIBER

Three vitally important aspects of the sporting dog's health are affected by fiber in the diet: (1) maintaining proper amounts of water in the body (hydration status); (2) functionality of the gastrointestinal tract; and (3) the performance effects of "going on the fly." These factors can all be controlled by balancing the conservation of fecal water, promoting easy defecation, and maintaining gut health. Clearly, a healthy intestinal tract is essential for optimal nutrient absorption and peak performance of sporting dogs. The source of dietary fiber plays an important role in intestinal function and stool quality.[31]

Dietary fiber is the portion of the diet that is not digested by endogenous secretions of the digestive tract. Fiber is a chemically heterogeneous substance that may be composed of cellulose, hemicellulose, pectin, gums, mucilages, and lignin. Cellulose, hemicellulose, pectin, and lignin are structural components of plant cell walls, while other components are plant or seed storage polysaccharides or plant exudates. Fiber has many physiological functions: increasing water-holding capacity, altering food transit in the gastrointestinal tract, delaying gastric emptying, providing bulk, impacting nutrient absorption and adsorption, and maintaining structural integrity of the gastrointestinal mucosa. The response as well as the magnitude of the response that fiber elicits in the identified physiological processes are dependent on fiber type. Because dietary fibers are diverse in chemical structure and origin, they vary considerably in water-holding capacity, adsorption of organic materials, effects on chyme viscosity and transit, and fermentation by bacteria. Fiber characteristics (ie, fermentable vs nonfermentable, soluble vs insoluble) can be determined and utilized effectively in clinical treatment. Understanding the role of fiber in maintenance of normal intestinal function has become the focus of increased emphasis in canine nutrition.

The epithelium of the gastrointestinal tract is a dynamic and rapidly renewing tissue. The gastrointestinal mucosa must be a resilient interface between the body's internal and external environments, while acting as the site of secretory and absorptive transport of nutrients and water. These functions require very high metabolic activity, which also makes these epithelial cells depend on a con-

stant supply of nutrients and oxygen. Enterocytes and colonocytes depend upon respiratory fuels to maintain cellular turnover and function. These respiratory fuels can be derived from either the bowel lumen or the systemic circulation. Colonocytes derive more than 70 per cent of their energy from luminal nutrition supplied by short-chain fatty acids (SCFAs).[32] Short-chain fatty acids are produced by bacterial fermentation of carbohydrates and are the preferred energy source of colonocytes.[33] In the dog, SCFAs and/or dietary fermentable fiber have also been reported to increase colonic blood flow,[34, 35] promote sodium and water absorption,[36] stimulate colonocyte hypertrophy,[37] increase colonic tissue mass,[38] and decrease the incidence of colonic lesions.[38]

Provision of specific bowel nutrients has been demonstrated to both protect and promote restoration of normal intestinal function in other animal models. Such fuels include the SCFAs produced by the colonic fermentation of fiber. Rather than restricting fiber altogether or providing a relatively inert fiber source, such as cellulose or peanut hulls, dietary incorporation of fermentable substrates that will yield SCFAs seems prudent. There is mounting evidence that inadequate SCFA provision may be involved in abnormal intestinal conditions.[39]

Current knowledge suggests that the optimal fiber system for dogs should contain a fermentable component to facilitate SCFA generation and a nonfermentable component to provide form to the stools. Research has demonstrated that beet pulp provides both of these attributes and is an excellent fiber source for dogs.[40, 41] The total fiber level in the diet should be at a moderate level (3 to 7%) to achieve the desired results. Excessive fiber (especially of a nonfermentable variety) should not be used in sporting dog diets. Several prominent nutritional effects are noted as dietary fiber increases: protein digestibility decreases,[42, 43] energy digestibility decreases,[42–44] fat digestibility decreases,[42] mineral absorption decreases selectively,[42] dry matter digestibility decreases,[42–44] fecal volume increases,[42–44] and defecation frequency increases.[42, 44] These phenomena are all actions that work in the opposite direction desired for the gastrointestinal tract of a canine athlete.

A diet for a sporting dog should provide the gut with substrates to maintain normal intestinal function without overloading the tract with unnecessary bulk. This is best accomplished through a high-quality nutritional matrix that includes moderately fermentable fiber. The end result is a diet that specifically "feeds" the gut while providing excellent overall nutrition for the animal. Total dietary fiber between 3 and 7 per cent with a moderately fermentable fiber source keeps fecal consistency normal with 25 to 35 per cent dry matter, eases defecation, and provides SCFAs necessary for gut health. Higher levels of nonfermentable fiber produce drier feces (harder to pass) and few SCFAs (reduced energy source for intestinal cells).

TRAINING AND DIET

Commercial diets formulated for athletic performance should be energy dense and highly palatable. Overfeeding this type of ration to a sporting dog not in heavy training will invariably lead to loss of condition and even obesity. However, this does not imply that the recommended nutritional approach used for training and athletic competition should be altered in the off-season or during periods of lower work output. Transitioning a well-conditioned sporting dog to a diet lower in fat and protein and/or lower quality ingredients is the metabolic equivalent to "detraining" that animal. Higher dietary fat levels are needed to maintain aerobic capacity, endurance, and resistance to fatigue. Changing to lower fat diets will decrease the stamina and endurance of canine athletes. When this decrease in metabolic capacity is coupled with decreased training, the sporting dog will experience rapid decline in fitness. Wide fluctuations in fitness are best avoided when possible; feeding a high-quality diet year round is an easy method of minimizing the decrease in fitness associated with the off-season. This does, however, create increased emphasis for attention to detail when feeding the sporting dog and the importance of observing body condition. Remember, it is always best to feed athletic dogs on the basis of body condition. It is more appropriate to make adjustments in the amount that is fed and not to decrease the quality or energy density of the diet. Maintaining an animal on a fairly constant nutritional program is also less likely to induce gastrointestinal stress that is common during changeovers in feeding practices.

It takes approximately 6 weeks for the increase in VO_{2max}, mitochondrial volume increases, and increases in maximal fat oxidation to occur after feeding high-fat diets to dogs. For this reason, a higher plane of nutrition should be implemented a minimum of 6 weeks prior to the beginning of training. Failure to metabolically adapt canine athletes before training will drastically reduce the animals' ability to benefit from training and perform at peak capacity.

ERGOGENIC AIDS

The major nutritional considerations for sporting dogs experiencing physical stress are energy density, diet digestibility, and caloric distribution. It has been suggested that many other nutrients benefit the health and performance of performance dogs. Elevated levels of vitamin C, selenium, β-carotene, medium-chain triglycerides, B vitamins, and iron have all been alleged to boost performance, but no controlled studies have been done to support these theories. Extensive hematological monitoring of several elite, world-class sled dog teams has failed to show anemia or serum chemical abnormalities. *These supplements are not recommended at this time, pending investigations.* Selecting a dry, extruded food that has been formulated to be complete and balanced in essential nutrients remains the most prudent and cost-effective approach.

PRACTICAL RECOMMENDATIONS

An overall nutritional matrix for enhancing performance, based on numerous studies with canine athletes, is shown in Table 40–5.

The nutritional program in Table 40–5 has been scientifically demonstrated to provide the following benefits: (1) increased aerobic capacity and endurance; (2) increased utilization of fatty acids to provide energy for muscle contraction; (3) decreased level of inflammatory reactions in body; (4) decreased injury rate; (5) improved intestinal health, including small firm stools; and (6) reduced feeding volumes.

Strategic carbohydrate feeding should be utilized with this nutritional program and can increase muscle glycogen repletion (or restoration). A postexercise intake of 1.5 gm glucose polymers/kg body weight is suggested for every training and/or competition

TABLE 40–5. Nutritional Recommendations for Health and Performance

Energy density	= 4,000 kcal ME/kg or greater
Fat	= 50–65% of calories
Protein	= 30–35% of calories; animal based sources
Fatty acid profile	= omega-6:omega-3 ratio between 5–10:1
Carbohydrate	= 10–15% of calories
Total dietary fiber	= 3–7% of dry matter; moderately fermentable

bout. Polycose or a similar carbohydrate is mixed with water (roughly a pint). This should be offered to the dogs within 30 minutes after the end of the exercise; to wait longer misses the benefit. It is also recommended that this be used only during rests of 2 hours or longer.

In addition to selecting a proper nutritional program, the following practices may also be helpful: (1) Select dogs that eat readily and maintain their weight; (2) avoid baiting during training; save special "baits" for stressful competitions; (3) add water to food to increase voluntary consumption of nutrients and water; (4) select and care for fresh/frozen ingredients very carefully; and (5) use dry food when possible; it prepares easily and frees time for other functions.

Meat and bone meal use should be approached with caution; the amount of bone that is contained in the product can affect its quality as a protein source, as well as the mineral balance of the entire diet. Bone contains high levels of collagen, which analyzes as protein, but is very poorly digested by dogs. In addition, inexpensive meat and bone meals often contain excess levels of minerals that can cause the diets to be too high in calcium, phosphorus, and magnesium. Very high calcium levels in a pet food are a good indication that the protein source was of poor quality and contained excessively high amounts of bone.

Feeding high levels of meats can cause a different type of mineral imbalance if the diet is not adjusted. Meat tends to be very low in calcium yet contains moderate amounts of phosphorus. This can result in an overall dietary calcium–phosphorus imbalance. The adult sporting dog should be fed 0.9 to 1.3 per cent calcium and 0.7 to 1.0 per cent phosphorus on a dry-matter basis with a calcium-phosphorus ratio of approximately 1.3:1.

The recommendations forwarded by these recent research findings have applications to dogs that participate in:

- trials (retriever, herding dog, coonhound, beagle, Schutzhund, agility, obedience, shooting)
- search and rescue missions
- races (greyhound, foxhound)
- military and police dog operations
- competitions (bloodhound, German obedience, frisbee)

The performance of any sporting dog is only as good as genetics, training, and diet can support. Any one of the three can have sufficient influence to make or break an effort. Diet is crucial, and several factors have been shown to improve performance and enhance well-being under physical stress. If nutrition is used properly, it provides a foundation for effective training and performance; if abused, it will undermine the benefits of training and ultimately affect performance.

References

1. Grandjean D, Paragon BM: Nutrition of racing and working dogs: I. Energy metabolism of dogs. Compendium 14:1608-1615, 1992.
2. NRC, 1974. National Research Council. Nutrient Requirements of Dogs. Washington, DC, National Academy Press, 1974.
3. Case LP, Carey DP, Hirakawa DA: Canine and Feline Nutrition. A Resource For Companion Animal Professionals. St. Louis, Mosby-Year Book, Inc, 1995.
4. Kronfeld DA, Hammel EP, Romberg CF Jr, Dunlap HL Jr: Hematological and metabolic responses to training in racing sled dogs fed diets containing medium, low or zero carbohydrate. Am J Clin Nutr 30:419, 1977.
5. Grandjean D, Paragon BM: Nutrition of racing and working dogs: II. Determination of energy requirements and the nutritional impact of stress. Compendium 15:45-57, 1993.
6. McNamara JH: Nutrition for military working dogs under stress. Vet Med Small Anim Clin 67:615-623, 1972.
7. Hinchcliff KW, Reinhart GA, Burr JR, et al: Metabolizable energy

intake, total energy expenditure and metabolic scope of Alaskan sled dogs during prolonged exertion. FASEB J 8II:A791, 1994.

8. Hinchcliff KW, Reinhart GA, Burr JR, et al: Energy metabolism and water turnover in Alaskan sled dogs during running. Recent Advances in Canine and Feline Nutritional Research: Proceedings of the 1996 Iams International Nutrition Symposium. Wilmington, Ohio, Orange Frazer Press, 1996, pp 199-206.

9. Hinchcliff KW, Reinhart GA, Burr JR, Swenson RA: Water metabolism of Alaskan sled dogs. Comp Phys Soc 37:5 P. A-81, 1994.

10. Bergstom J, Hermansen L, Hultman E, Saltin B: Diet, muscle glycogen, and physical performance. Acta Physiol Scand 71:140-150, 1967.

11. Theriault DG, Beller GA, Smoake JA, et al: Intramuscular energy sources in dogs during physical work. J Lipid Res 14:54-61, 1973.

12. Paul P, Issekutz B: Role of extramuscular energy sources in the metabolism of the exercising dog. Am J Physiol 22:615-622, 1976.

13. Hammel EP, Kronfeld DS, Ganjan VK, Dunlap HL: Metabolic responses to exhaustive exercise in racing sled dogs fed diets containing medium, low, or zero carbohydrate. Am J Clin Nutr 30:409-418, 1976.

14. Reynolds AJ, Fuhrer L, Dunlap HL et al: Effect of diet and training on muscle glycogen storage and utilization in sled dogs. J Appl Physiol 79:1601-1607, 1995.

15. Downey RL, Kronfeld DS, Banta CA: Diet of beagles affects stamina. J Am Anim Hosp Assoc 16:273-277, 1980.

16. Reynolds AJ, Fuhrer L, Dunlop HL, et al: Lipid metabolic responses to diet and training in sled dogs. J Nutr 124:2754S-2759S, 1994.

17. Reynolds A, Hoppeler H, Reinhart G, et al: Sled dog endurance: A result of high fat diet or selective breeding? FASEB J 9:A996, 1995.

18. Reynolds AJ, Taylor CR, Hoppler H, et al: The effect of diet on sled dog performance, oxidative capacity, skeletal muscle microstructure, and muscle glycogen metabolism. Recent Advances in Canine and Feline Nutritional Research: Proceedings of the 1996 Iams International Nutrition Symposium. Wilmington, Ohio, Orange Frazer Press, 1996, pp 181-198.

19. Logas D, Beale KM, Bauer JE: Potential clinical benefits of dietary supplementation with marine-life oil. JAVMA 199:1631-1636, 1991.

20. Vaughn DM, Reinhart GA, Swaim SF, et al: Evaluation of effects of dietary n-6 to n-3 fatty acid ratios on leukotriene B synthesis in dog skin and neutrophils. Vet Dermatol 5(4):163-173, 1995.

21. Savic MS, Yager JA, Holub BJ: Effect of n-3 and n-6 fatty acid dietary supplementation on canine neutrophil and keratinocyte phospholipid composition. Proc Sec World Congr Vet Derm 1992, p 77.

22. Reinhart GA: Review of omega-3 fatty acids and dietary influences on tissue concentrations. Recent Advances in Canine and Feline Nutritional Research: Proceedings of the 1996 Iams International Nutrition Symposium. Wilmington, Ohio, Orange Frazer Press, 1996, pp 235-242.

23. Lewis PA, Austen KF, Soberman RJ: Leukotrienes and other products of the 5-lipoxygenase pathway: Biochemistry and relation to pathobiology in human diseases. N Engl J Med 323:645-655, 1990.

24. Vaughn DM, Reinhart GA: Influence of dietary fatty acid ratios on tissue eicosanoid production and blood coagulation parameters in dogs. Recent Advances in Canine and Feline Nutritional Research: Proceedings of the 1996 Iams International Nutrition Symposium. Wilmington, Ohio, Orange Frazer Press, 1996, pp 243-255.

25. NRC: Nutrient Requirements of Domestic Animals. Nutrient Requirements of Dogs. Washington, DC, National Academy Press, 1985.

26. Vaughn DM, Reinhart GA: Dietary fatty acid ratios and eicosanoid production. Proc. 13th Am. Coll. Vet. Int. Med. Forum, 1995, pp 464-465.

27. Dzanis DA: Safety of ethoxyquin in dog food. J Nutr 121:S163-164, 1991.

28. Kronfeld DS, Ferrante PL, Granjean D: Optimal nutrition for athletic performance, with emphasis on fat adaptation in dogs and horses. J Nutr 124:2745S-2753S, 1994.

29. Association of American Feed Control Officials: Nutrient profiles for dog foods. Official Publication, AAFCO, 1994.

30. Kronfeld DS: Diet and performance of racing sled dogs. JAVMA 162:470-473, 1973.

31. Reinhart GA, Sunvold GD: In vitro fermentation as a predictor of fiber utilization. Recent Advances in Canine and Feline Nutritional Research: Proceedings of the 1996 Iams International Nutrition Symposium. pp. 15-24. Wilmington, Ohio, Orange Frazer Press, 1996.

32. Roediger WEW: Role of anaerobic bacteria in the metabolic welfare of the colonic mucosa in man. Gut 21:793, 1980.

33. Roediger WEW: Utilization of nutrients by isolated epithelial cells of the rat colon. Gastroenterology 83:424, 1982.

34. Kvietys PR, Gronger DN: Effects of volatile fatty acids on blood flow and oxygen uptake by the dog colon. Am J Physiol 80:962, 1981.

35. Howard MD, Sunvold GD, Reinhart GA, Kerley MS: Effect of fermentable fiber consumption by the dog on nitrogen balance and focal microbial nitrogen excretion. FASEB J 10:A257, 1996.

36. Hallman JE, Reinhart GA, Wallace EA, et al: Colonic mucosal tissue energetics and electroylyte transport in dogs fed cellulose, beet pulp or pectin/gum arabic as their primary fiber source. Nutr Res 16:303-313, 1996.

37. Hallman JE, Moxely RA, Reinhart GA et al: Cellulose, beet pulp and pectin/gum arabic effects on canine colonic microstructure and histopathology. J Vet Clin Nutr 2(4):137-142, 1995.

38. Reinhart GA, Moxely RA, Clemens ET: Source of dietary fiber and its effects on colonic microstructure, function and histopathology of beagle dogs. J Nutr 124:2701S-2703S, 1994.

39. Sunvold GD: Dietary fiber for dogs and cats: An historical perspective. Recent Advances in Canine and Feline Nutritional Research: Proceedings of the 1996 Iams International Nutrition Symposium. pp. 3-14. Wilmington, Ohio, Orange Frazer Press, 1996.

40. Sunvold GD, Fahey GC, Jr, Merchen NR, Reinhart GA: In vitro fermentation of selected fibrous substrates by dog and cat focal inoculum: Influence of diet composition on substrate organic matter disappearance and short-chain fatty acid production. J Anim Sci 73:1110-1122, 1995.

41. Sunvold GD, Fahey GC, Jr, Merchen NR, et al: Dietary fiber for dogs: IV. In vitro fermentation of selected fiber sources by dog fecal inoculum and in vivo digestion and metabolism of fiber-supplemented diets. J Anim Sci 73:1099-1109, 1995.

42. Fahey GC, Jr, Merchen NR, Corbin JE, et al: Dietary fiber for dogs: I. Effects of graded levels of dietary beet pulp on nutrient intake, digestibility, metabolizable energy and digesta mean retention time. J Anim Sci 68:4221, 1990.

43. Fahey GC, Jr, Merchen NR, Corbin JE, et al: Dietary fiber for dogs: II. Iso-total dietary fiber (TDF) additions of divergent fiber sources to dog diets and their effects on nutrient intake, digestibility, metabolizable energy and digesta mean retention time. J Anim Sci 68:4221, 1990.

44. Fahey GC, Jr, Merchen NR, Corbin JE, et al: Dietary fiber for dogs: III. Effects of beet pulp and oat fiber additions to dog diets on nutrient intake, digestibility, metabolizable energy, and digesta mean retention time. J Anim Sci 70:1169, 1992.

SECTION IX

EXERCISE AND TRAINING

CHAPTER 41

THE EXERCISE PHYSIOLOGY OF SPORTING DOGS

ROSS V. STAADEN

ENERGY SOURCES

Knowledge of energy sources is necessary to understand many aspects of training and racing. Muscle fiber contraction runs on the basic cellular fuel unit, a molecule called ATP (adenosine triphosphate). Only a tiny amount of this is available, but as it is broken down, it is constantly re-formed using energy from other fuels. The contractile meshwork cannot directly use other fuels such as glucose, glycogen, or fat. These other fuels have different characteristics and limitations: time to reach maximum supply rate, maximum energy supply rates, maximum total energy supply, and time to replenish stores.

Aerobic and Anaerobic Energy Sources

Aerobic means requiring air. Actually one component of air, namely oxygen, is required. The chemical reactions of some of the energy sources require oxygen, so they are termed aerobic. The end products of burning with oxygen are water and carbon dioxide, both of which are produced in easily managed quantities. The carbon dioxide is carried away from the muscle in the blood that delivered the oxygen. The blood returns to the lungs to be reoxygenated, and the carbon dioxide escapes into the air. Consequently, aerobic energy can be supplied for hours or days. Anaerobic means *not* requiring oxygen. Anaerobic energy sources can operate for only a few minutes.

FATS

Fat is burned with oxygen so it is classified as an aerobic energy source. Fat can be stored in a cell as fat droplets or in special fat storage cells that are little more than a cell membrane around a giant fat droplet. Aggregates of fat cells are called fat depots. Fat has some advantages: It can be spread over the body surface where it can be a mechanical buffer, it can form attractive secondary sex characteristics, and coupled with a good blood supply, it can form an insulator. It can insulate like asbestos when the vessels are closed off but allow heat in or out if the blood vessels are open. The insulating properties of fat have allowed warm-blooded mammals such as seals and whales to live in the cold polar seas.

Because fat can store the most energy per gram of weight carried (9600 calories) and because of its variable insulating properties, fat is the fuel of choice for large-scale storage. It is the bulk fuel store for getting through snowbound winters and summer droughts. Most animals have enough fat for days or weeks of running at low speed. Racing greyhounds are something of an exception—they carry very low fat reserves, much lower than do wild hunting dogs. This is probably due to artificial selection for sprint speed, coupled with the reduced need for fat reserves because of a steady supplied diet.

The main features of fat as an energy source are that (1) it is very slow to reach peak rate (probably a minute or two); (2) the peak rate of energy supply is very low; (3) the total stored is enormous; and (4) it is replenished after a meal of fat, protein, or carbohydrate. Fat stores are so large compared with the cost of a run, that it is not usual to speak of depletion except in very long runs such as the 1000-mile-plus sled dog races, when it may take many meals to fully restock the fat stores.

GLYCOGEN

Glycogen granules consist of millions of glucose molecules strung together. The string is structurally combined with water and potassium and the enzymes necessary to split off glucose in readily usable form. Glycogen can be used in two entirely different ways.

Glycogen Burned with Oxygen. Because this process requires oxygen, it is classified as an aerobic fuel. The muscles store only enough for a few hours of running at aerobic (long distance) speeds in humans. The amount of glycogen stored is similar in large and small animals, but because of the greater biomechanical efficiency of larger muscles and limbs, the stored amount lasts longer in larger animals. The peak rate is higher than the burning of fat and faster in its time-to-peak rate (probably something like 5 to 60 seconds depending on body size, mouse to whale). Its major limitation is the rate of oxygen supply to the muscles.

The main features of the burning of carbohydrate as an energy source are that (1) it is slow to reach peak rate; (2) the peak rate of energy supply is low; (3) the total stored is moderate; and (4) it is not replenished until carbohydrate is eaten—although some excess protein can be used. In most species, fat intake cannot be converted to glycogen, but bears and other hibernators just may be exceptions.

Glycogen Broken Down to Lactic Acid. Because this process does *not* require oxygen, glycogen is classified as an *an*aerobic fuel. The glycogen is converted to lactic acid, which at high levels begins to damage the muscle cell. When produced at a moderate rate, it diffuses or is possibly actively transported out of the cell at a rate sufficient to avoid damage. However, at very high rates of production, enough can accumulate to damage the muscle cell. Minor damage causes mild ''acidosis,'' characterized by dullness, dehydration in spite of increased thirst, and urine changes. Severe muscle cell damage causes severe muscle pain, dehydration, and release of large amounts of myoglobin from the cells. The myoglobin colors the urine dark port-wine red.

When greyhounds are allowed to go round the racetrack twice instead of the usual once, rapidly fatal rhabdomyolysis may result. A similar rapid death has been seen when greyhounds bred for ''tin hare'' racing have been released after a coyote and failed to catch the coyote in a minute or two.

In the catching of wild animals—darted or roped or corralled—the chase, or even just the thrashing of capture, may generate sufficient lactic acid to damage the muscle cells. This is known as *capture myopathy*. Lactic acidosis and capture myopathy both come under the medical classification of exertional rhabdomyolysis, ie, exercise-induced muscle cell breakdown. After severe muscle damage, a large percentage of the muscle cells may be lost. Because of poor regenerative properties, few new muscle cells appear, and the muscle suffers some permanent loss of cells and cannot recover its former strength.

The muscle glycogen store is more than enough for repeated bouts of sprinting; indeed, it is hard to deplete the muscle glycogen stores by sprinting. Dogs in events lasting over 10 minutes would not generate much lactic acid, and in sled dog races the amount generated is small—an equilibrium level leaking from some muscles and being burned by others—unless the team has a sprint or a fight.

The liver also stores some glycogen, but this is usually only ''leaked'' into the circulation at a low rate. It is not readily available for short bursts of high-speed work and may represent a store inaccessible to the muscles that has evolved to provide glucose for brain function.

The main features of the breakdown of carbohydrate to lactic acid as an energy source are that (1) it reaches its peak rate in less than a second, (2) the peak rate of energy supply is high, (3) the total stored is moderate, and (4) as mentioned before, glycogen is not replenished until carbohydrate is eaten—although some excess protein can be used.

PHOSPHAGENS

These are the ATP mentioned earlier and a compound called *creatine phosphate* (CP). CP rapidly re-forms any used ATP. The two are in solution in the muscle meshwork. They contribute only enough energy for a few seconds of all-out exercise. Creatine phosphate use is proportional to the power output of the muscle: rapid use at acceleration and high speed, but little involvement at low speeds. Consequently its greatest importance is in power events such as jumping and events requiring rapid acceleration such as racing.

The main features of the breakdown of phosphagens as an energy source are: (1) The peak rate is reached virtually instantly; (2) the peak rate of energy supply is very high; (3) the total energy stored is tiny; and (4) CP is replenished from other energy stores as soon as the rate of exercise drops.

PROTEINS, AMINO ACIDS, AND OTHER MOLECULES

These are seldom used as a way to store energy, except perhaps in fish, in which storage as fat might cause the fish to float! However, after meals containing abundant protein, protein is oxidized, and some may be converted to carbohydrate or fat. Also, in starved animals, when all other fuels have been used up, muscle protein is mobilized and oxidized. Amino acids in the blood and in the muscle cell at the time of exercise may also be oxidized.

MUSCLE PHYSIOLOGY

Characteristics of Fast- and Slow-Twitch Muscle Fibers. There is a great range of muscle fiber types. In racing, we can divide those in skeletal muscle into two broad groups—fast twitch and slow twitch. Compared to slow-twitch fibers, fast-twitch fibers begin contracting more quickly after a nerve stimulus, reach a higher peak of contractile strength per cross-sectional area, reach that peak sooner, and relax sooner. They have greater power and can contract more often per minute. However, the nervous system controls the rate and degree of contraction, within the fiber type's capability. Fast twitch can be made to contract just as slowly as a slow twitch.

If the nervous system can make fast-twitch fibers contract as *slowly* as slow twitch, but slow twitch cannot deliver the really fast contractions, why have slow twitch? Surely as prey or predator, you would prefer to be 100 per cent fast twitch. Well, perhaps not—the big advantage of slow-twitch fibers is that they are very economical. In one experiment in guinea pigs, the fast-twitch fibers required up to three times as much energy to do the same work. In the wild, where calories are often in short supply, just about every animal seems to have some slow-twitch fibers for such low-speed activities as walking.

Some other advantages of slow twitch are endurance—they can usually contract many more times before fatiguing—and more rapid recovery. The stamina and rapid recovery are due to greater use of aerobic fuels and better blood supply than fast twitch. Slow-twitch fibers, because they rely on getting oxygen in and carbon dioxide out, are usually of lesser diameter than fast-twitch fibers and have more capillaries around them. Lactic acid build-up is consequently much less likely; indeed, some slow-twitch fibers take in lactic acid from neighboring fast-twitch fibers (during high-speed work) and oxidize it!

For Sprints, the More Fast Twitch the Better. Clearly the advantage of fast twitch is rapid contractions of great power—ie, speed—but the disadvantages are inefficiency and lack of stamina. This is why one animal with the highest percentage of fast twitch does not win at all distances. (Remember the margin between first and last is often only 2 or 3 per cent of the race time.) With similar anaerobic energy reserves and aerobic supplies, there is an ideal mix of fast and slow fibers for any particular race distance. In muscle samples from winners at a particular distance, however, a surprising amount of variation exists, because other factors, eg, biomechanics, heart size, and temperament, also have big roles in determining winners at a particular distance.

Slow-twitch fibers rely almost entirely on aerobic energy supplies. Fast-twitch fibers in the human have little oxidative capacity relying mainly on anaerobic energy. In the horse and dog there are two subtypes of fast-twitch fibers—some rely almost entirely on anaerobic sources (called *fast-twitch high anaerobic*) while others make considerable use of aerobic energy (called *fast-twitch high aerobic*).

THE HIERARCHY OF FUEL AND MUSCLE FIBER USE

The fuels are used strategically, with the organism attempting to use the abundant fat and foods just eaten, and so preserving CP and glycogen for moderate to all-out efforts. The fuels are used aerobically if possible, because then there is no accumulation of limiting end products. This means using slow-twitch fibers at low speeds. The usual order of use of fuels for muscles is as follows:

1. At rest and low level exercise: After eating, excess food is burned, whether carbohydrates, fats, or even proteins. The energy supply is 100 per cent aerobic, and slow-twitch fibers are used. In fasting animals, a mix of mainly fat and a little glucose is burned.

2. At medium levels of exercise: As speed increases there is a tendency to burn an increased proportion of carbohydrate and a decreased proportion of fat. Energy supply is still 100 per cent aerobic, and some fast-twitch fibers are used.

3. At high exercise levels: Above the point at which adequate energy can be obtained from the aerobic sources (ie, at a speed above the anaerobic threshold), the muscles begin to rely more on the breakdown of glycogen to lactic acid. Some energy is from anaerobic use of glycogen, and many fast-twitch fibers are contributing in addition to almost all slow-twitch fibers.

4. At all-out levels of exercise: Phosphagens are used up in 1 or 2 seconds of acceleration. Glycogen is broken down to lactic acid at its peak rate and is also burned at whatever rate the highest oxygen uptake will allow. Fat oxidation is very low. The aerobic energy production is as high as it can go, but much more energy is required, and this comes from anaerobic sources. Almost all muscle fibers, including slow-twitch, are contributing.

Why the Progressive Switch from Burning Fat to Burning Carbohydrate? Fat is abundant in food and is light to store, so why does not the greyhound, like the sled dog, oxidize a lot of fat? It could simply be that the fat cannot be mobilized at a fast enough rate, that the glycogen granules outstrip the fat droplets as substrate suppliers. However, if that was the only reason, surely evolution would simply provide more droplets, probably more smaller droplets to give more surface area for rapid release of fat molecules.

The other reason seems to be that per unit of oxygen, the body can get about 10 per cent more energy from glycogen than from fat. In greyhound racing, a sport of tiny margins, the difference in the race times between the winning dog and the last dog in the field is often less than 2 or 3 per cent of the race time. Ten per cent more meters from the same lungful of air is therefore a very useful advantage. Because greyhound racing is over sprint distances, there is more than enough glycogen in the muscles. The result, I believe, has been genetic selection for greyhounds that slowed fat oxidation in favor of increased glucose oxidation.

Would Carbohydrate Loading Help Greyhounds or Sled Dogs? Carbohydrate loading is a practice of human athletes to increase muscle glycogen. First the athlete depletes the muscle of glycogen by a long run—15 to 25 miles. Then the athlete eats large amounts of carbohydrate-rich foods. The muscle fibers respond to the depletion by storing extra glycogen. The theoretical benefit in distance events is readily apparent—the athlete can run 10 per cent faster on the limited oxygen supply than if he or she burned fat. In practice, most coaches seem to think that it has proven beneficial to athletes in middle-distance to marathon-length events. No clear benefit to sprinters or ultramarathoners (who go farther than the marathon, eg, 500 km) has been shown, although some individuals and coaches believe there is an advantage. One problem for sprinters is that the effort required to deplete the fibers has a dampening effect mentally. For ultramarathoners, 15 to 20 miles often does not produce depletion—ultramarathoners are natural fat oxidizers.

Sled dogs in long races are virtually doing a depletion run every day, but do not have the luxury of several days' light exercise or rest to let glycogen build up to an extra high level. If they oxidized glycogen by preference it would soon run out, because of the sheer distances they cover per day. Probably the biggest limitation for sled dogs is obtaining enough calories from the food-holding capacity of the stomach. A cubic measure of fat contains little else. The same volume of meat will be 80 per cent water, and the 20 per cent protein has only half the calories per gram as fat. The result is that fat has some eight or ten times the calories per kilogram as red meat. The fat on the edge of a chop often has more calories than the rest of the chop. So sled dogs have to eat high levels of fat to fit in enough calories per day.

Greyhounds would probably be worn out by the effort required for the depletion run. Repletion (in humans, anyway) can be delayed by eating fats and proteins for a few days before the great carbohydrate feed. So in spite of its success in humans, it has not surfaced as a training practice, to my knowledge, in either greyhounds or sled dogs.

Would Dietary Fat Restriction Make any Difference? Work done almost 70 years ago found that increasing the ratio of fat to carbohydrate in the dietary intake did increase the percentage of fat burned.[1] Modern work has verified this, and it fits well with the almost world-wide practice of restricted fat-feeding among greyhound trainers. If it is correct, greyhound trainers are on a tightrope: Feed too much fat and you can decrease the dog's race performance. Feed too little and you run down the dog's health (and performance) through a deficiency of essential fatty acids. The first obvious sign of fatty acid deficiency is dry flaky skin. I do not know if race performance is affected before this skin change appears, but if it is, I suspect that trainers would have noticed.

Some top greyhound trainers remove almost all the fat from the meat but substitute an amount of vegetable oil. This way they give the dog the essential fatty acids in a minimum amount of fat. (Vegetable oils usually have a greater percentage of the essential fatty acids than do animal fats.)

PHYSIOLOGY OF EXERCISE

The Respiratory System of the Dog. The family Canidae includes some of the great aerobic athletes of the animal kingdom. The wolf and Cape hunting dog are capable of running at speeds of the order of 20 to 30 mph for half an hour. In the wide open savannah or tundra, they rely more on wearing their prey down rather than ambushing, like most members of the cat family. Some of the canine prey, eg, pronghorn antelopes, caribou, and zebras, have similar outstanding aerobic capability.

The exact lineage of the domestic dog is still disputed, but some breeds show clear resemblance to the wolf and have its huge aerobic capacity. Sled dogs cover thousands of miles in a matter of days. Cattle dogs and sheepherding breeds can cover many tens of miles and perhaps over a hundred miles per day, at considerable speed.

$\dot{V}_{O_2max}$. The measure of aerobic capacity is the volume of oxygen taken in and burned per kilogram per minute, called the $\dot{V}O_{2max}$. In humans it is easily measured by having the subject run at progressively higher speeds, until there is a step-up in speed but no increase in oxygen uptake. The subject wears a mask, and the test usually involves running for more than a minute at each speed level.

Dogs have proven very unwilling to run at or above their $\dot{V}O_{2max}$. Of 180 references to dogs running on treadmills, only one study demonstrated leveling off of oxygen uptake—at 159 ml/kg/min.[2] This compares with typical figures of 30 to 80 ml/kg/min in a range of humans and a record of 94 for a cross-country skier.[3]

Cardiac Function. The dog has a very large heart as a percentage of body weight, averaging 0.77 per cent in one study[4] and 0.80 per cent in another,[5] for mongrel dogs compared with 0.5 per cent for humans,[6] but the racing greyhound has an even larger heart at about 1.18 to 1.34 per cent of body weight.[7-9] The maximal heart rate of the dog is in the range 310 to 340 beats/min.[10-12] Greyhounds racing had an average maximal heart rate of 311.[13] This compares with 170 in athletes, up to 210 for unfit young people.[3] Presumably the human heart has more slow-twitch characteristics, ie, less contractile power per gram, and is slower to contract and relax but more economical.

Greyhound Treadmill Studies. In the mid 1970s the general belief was that large animals such as horses had to synchronize respiration with stride, but smaller animals (humans) could escape this restriction. Racing greyhounds, the popular wisdom went, held their breath during races, like a human does in a 100 m sprint. The evidence was bluish gums immediately after a run. Their giant heart, one of the largest in the animal kingdom, was considered to be an interesting example of nonpathological hypertrophy—increased size for no apparent reason. In 1975 I began a study of the greyhound running on a high-speed treadmill at sprint race speeds.[14] A summary of findings for a range of parameters is presented in Table 41–1.

RESPIRATORY SYSTEM OF THE GREYHOUND

The greyhound, far from holding its breath, turned around a phenomenal volume of air per minute. A mask with very large valves had to be developed to cope. Respiration and stride were found to be very tightly linked.

$\dot{V}O_{2max}$. The figures were not of the steady-state type usually given for the human, in whom exercise is increased in a series of steps and the exhaled gases collected over a minute or more of exercise at a runner's peak effort. Rather, the gases were collected over 15-second periods during runs of 15 to 60 seconds. The highest average figure was 143 ml/kg/min in the last 15 seconds of 45-second runs. There were considerable differences between dogs: One well-performing dog donated because it was a fighter was vastly superior to the rest, which were mainly donated because they were too slow to win races.

TABLE 41–1. Effects of Exercise on Some Parameters in the Racing Greyhound

	VE	Vo₂	Vco₂	RR	V_T	RER	Lac	pH	BE	PCV	HR	CO	SV
Rest	0.2	5	5	16	15	0.95	8	7.42	−0.5	46			
Pre										58		552	2.8
During 30-sec run:													
0–15 sec	4.0	86	77	188	20	0.95							
15–30 sec	4.3	114	141	188	23	1.2					318	914	2.9
±	1.9	68	100	8	12	0.2					8	209	0.6
Post 30-sec run:													
0–0.5 min											258		
0.5–1 min											172		
0–1 min	3.8	62	129	76	54	2.0	85	7.11	−16				
1–2 min	3.2	22	51	92	35	2.3					157		
2–3 min	3.0	21	39	92	34	1.9	125	7.11	−21		64	164	
3–4 min	3.1	23	39	95	36	1.6					176		
4–5 min	2.9	20	34	98	33	1.6	164	7.09	−23		64	184	
5–6 min	2.9	21	30	97	33	1.4					188		
6–7 min	2.7	22	28	89	30	1.3	154	7.09	−23		194		
7–8 min	2.6	22	29	82	38	1.3					198		
8–9 min											198		
9–10 min							150	7.14	−22		63	199	
15 min											184		
20 min											170		
30 min							50	7.45	−2.2		59	142	
60 min							6	7.43	−0.7		56	108	181	2.2

VE = Ventilation—Volume of gas exhaled in L/kg/min
Vo₂ = Oxygen consumed in ml/kg/min
Vco₂ = Carbon dioxide produced in ml/kg/min
RR = Respiration rate in breaths/min
V_T = Tidal volume or volume per breath in ml/kg
RER = Respiratory exchange ratio = VCO₂/VO₂
Lac = Lactic acid in mEq/L
pH = Measure of acidity vs alkalinity, 7.0 = neutral, above alkaline
BE = Base excess—a measure of alkalinity, mEq/L, negative if acidic
PCV = Packed cell volume—hematocrit in % red cells
HR = Heart rate in beats/min
CO = Cardiac output—blood pumped by the heart in ml/kg/min
SV = Stroke volume in ml/kg body weight

THE CARDIOVASCULAR SYSTEM OF THE GREYHOUND

Although the greyhound heart and the human heart are of similar size, the greyhound heart in this study beat 318 times/min during runs compared with 170 in top athletes and 200 in nonathletes.[3]

Cardiac output during runs was almost 1 L/kg/min—914 ml. The best dog did achieve 1 L/kg/min. Cardiac output was determined by the thermodilution method. Electromagnetic flowmeter cuffs proved very unreliable—large "flow" waves could be made by simply fluctuating the pressure in the aorta when it was clamped.

Stroke volume is the amount of blood pumped with each beat of the heart. It might be expected that at high heart rates there would be insufficient time for the ventricle to refill or perhaps insufficient time to contract fully. In the human there was a long-standing controversy whether stroke volume increased from rest to exercise or not. Of a large number of studies in the human, some found up to 30-per cent increases in stroke volume from rest to exercise, while others found small increases, no change, or small decreases. (Some of these differences, it later proved, were due to the body position in which the resting studies were done.[3]) In this study the change in stroke volume from rest to racing was an increase of 32 per cent.

Most mammalian blood is about 30 to 45 per cent red cells by volume. Studies of blood viscosity by various methods indicate a slow rise in blood viscosity as the percentage of red cells increases—to about 60 per cent—then an increasingly steep rise with further increases in red cell percentage. The blood stored in the greyhound spleen was typically 81 per cent red cells. The greyhound can release this thick "spleen milk" to increase the percentage of red cells in the general circulation.

The packed cell volume (PCV) in sleeping greyhounds was as low as 42 per cent, rising with the level of excitement to 61 to 63 per cent when viewing the lure, and 63 to 66 per cent after a run. The extra rise in PCV to 63 to 66 per cent required a run; excitement alone could not do it. This can be interpreted as follows: maximal splenic storage during sleep; graded splenic emptying with excitement up to 61 to 63 per cent; water drawn from the blood during a run by the osmotic pull of lactic acid in the muscle fibers lifted it to 63 to 66 per cent.

One of the things that makes the cardiac output and heart rate of the greyhound during a race even more extraordinary is that they are achieved while pumping blood with a PCV around 63 to 66 per cent (even 72 per cent in some samples at one racetrack).

If this high PCV has some benefit, why does the greyhound not have this high PCV all the time? The answer seems to lie in changes that occur in the blood viscosity with increasing rates of flow. For blood of any given PCV, the viscosity falls as the speed of blood flow (shear rate) increases. Aggregation of cells, a dangerous precursor to clotting, is decreased. The circulating PCV of the greyhound is lowered when it is sleeping, because at the low flow rates, blood with a high PCV would be very viscous, hard to pump, and inclined to clot. During high-speed exercise, the blood is flowing much faster, and the heart is capable of pumping blood with a much higher PCV. This carries more oxygen per milliliter, with obvious benefits. During recovery, blood is moved back into the spleen, lowering the PCV, so that "clot up" does not occur. Obviously there are some special controls to prevent clotting in the spleen with its PCV of 81 per cent.

Decreased Arterial Oxygen Pressure (PaO₂) During Running. The greyhounds had catheters implanted into the aorta and pulmonary artery, about 4 cm above the heart. The aortic blood sample taken during runs was so deoxygenated it was at first thought that the sample had been erroneously taken from the pulmonary artery. Repeat runs soon made it clear that indeed the arterial blood was poorly oxygenated. It was easy to see how catchers in the catching pen had concluded that greyhounds held their breath during races.

Because it was known that the greyhounds had a huge oxygen uptake, this finding was a surprise. In the literature to 1978, there were two reports of a drop in arterial PO₂ during running. A 10-mm Hg drop was found in athletes, but the same studies found no drop in nonathletes[15, 16] (excluding pathological conditions, of course). On viewing an oxygen dissociation curve, it became readily apparent that this big drop in oxygen pressure did not significantly decrease the *amount* of oxygen carried per milliliter of blood. Enough blood was simply passing through the lungs to strip out more oxygen, down to a critical PO₂, around 60 mm Hg. It seemed to be an athletic adaptation.

Presumably the volume of air turned around is limited by the chest size, and by the stride rate, which determines respiratory rate at the gallop. By passing more blood through a given volume of air, it is possible to get more oxygen from it. There has been a report of the same phenomenon in horses.[17]

Acid-Base Changes—Right to the Edge. The highest average venous lactate values in this study were 181 mg/dl, about 8 minutes after the 60-second runs. These were slightly lower than the highest values reported in humans and horses, but the greyhounds were not running against each other, which may have produced higher readings.

The lowest jugular venous pH values were 6.7 to 7.00 after runs by the most motivated dog. Arterial values were not as low, but presumably muscle pH must have been considerably lower at the end of exercise. Certainly these values approached those at which cardiac muscle have been shown to begin to lose contractility.[18–20]

ACID DAMAGE, "ACIDOSIS," AND TREATMENT

In considering damage done by lactic acid, it is worth noting that even 1 minute after exercise the buffering by H₂CO₃ has removed the peak H⁺. Once the muscle damage is done it progresses, and the clinical signs of "acidosis" develop over hours or days without further acid damage. By 30 minutes after exercise, the acid having been metabolized, the blood is alkalotic with pH of the order of 7.40 to 7.55. One hour after running, the pH is moving back down toward normal. Consequently there is no indication for the use of intravenous alkaline solutions to counter lactic acid hours after a race. Rather, the focus should be on helping to move myoglobin through the kidneys and supporting the damaged muscle cells.

THE ENERGETIC BASIS OF GREYHOUND RACING

How much of the total energy for a race comes from aerobic sources? The contribution of aerobic energy sources rose from under 20 per cent for 15-second runs to about 75 per cent during the last 15 seconds of the 60-second runs.

Energy Cost of Acceleration. One of the major achievements of the study was the quantification of the cost of acceleration. This was quite high, three times as much per meter as running at top speed. With data from the literature it was possible to show a similar cost in humans. Little wonder that severe checking in a race is so costly.

Success Secrets of the Greyhound—Why so Much Faster Than Humans? The amount of lactic acid tolerated is similar, so the amount of anaerobic energy per kilogram is similar. The greyhound has greater oxygen stores in the body at the start of a race.

but the main difference is that the greyhound can muster an oxygen uptake of some 140 ml/kg/min during an all-out sprint, whereas a human fixes the torso, and oxygen uptake is minimal. Even when compared with average human athletes running at a slower speed, at which they can manage an oxygen uptake of 60 ml/kg/min, 140 is vastly superior.

The greyhound has about double the human ratio of heart to body weight, and it pumps 50 per cent more times per minute. The greyhound heart pumps blood with a higher PCV, ie, is able to carry 50 per cent more oxygen per milliliter. And while human arm and leg movements are no help in respiration, the greyhound exploits the galloping action to help force air in and out of the lungs.

The much larger heart of the horse can beat 220 to 250 times per minute at the gallop,[21] so the question becomes, Why is the maximal heart rate of the human so low? Possibly it has to do with the lack of opportunity for all-out sprints in the tree life of our ancestors, or perhaps it is because we do not have the gallop-assisted breathing requiring greater blood flow to remove the oxygen, or perhaps it is for economical work over a prolonged period.

PRINCIPLES OF TRAINING

The Overload Principle

The most fundamental principle of training is that if an increased work load is imposed on a muscle fiber, bone, ligament, or enzyme chain, it will—if it can—change itself to better cope with that load.

Specificity of Training

In general, training should resemble the event to produce the best results. However, many training programs simply get the dog to approach race fitness, and then trials and races provide highly specific "training" to finish off the preparation. There are four important aspects of specificity:

Rate Specificity. The running speed in some of the training should be similar to the race speed. Different muscle fibers and different fuel mixes are used at different running speeds. The fuels are produced by biochemical pathways that are sped up by agents called enzymes. These are very specific, and enzyme production is increased only if their pathway is used.

Duration Specificity. In training, some of the running, at or near race speed, should approach the race duration. Duration specificity is seldom directly related to fuel reserves. When the body runs low on one fuel, it simply switches to another source. Duration specificity relates more to feelings of fatigue. The "fatigue system" is there to limit the production of lactic acid in sprints, to limit wear and tear damage to structures, and to limit the wastage of fuel resources—an "Is this really necessary?" system. Feelings of fatigue may also relate to depletion of reserves of substances that stimulate release of endorphins, cortisone, etc. Suffice to say, to win an event going for 30 seconds, some of the training, trials, or lead-up races should be of the same order; to win a 24-hour event, some training, trials, or lead-up races must be of a similar duration.

Interval training can be viewed as a series of shorter runs, which have the same duration specificity effect as a longer run, simply because of the short rest periods. The rests mean that lactic acid is less likely to reach dangerous levels.

Functional Specificity. Some of the training must use exactly the same limb and body movements. In dogs it may have some role in cornering, recovering from bumps, etc. Perhaps the best example is the use of a lure on a fishing pole for training coursing greyhounds. Coursing in Great Britain consists of two greyhounds chasing a hare flushed from brush. There is a lot of zigging and zagging, which puts a great deal of strain on the joints and ligaments. Frequent changes in direction without stumbling and losing speed require coordination and skill. Chasing a lure flicked about on the end of a fishing line has great functional and structural specificity for coursing.

Structural Specificity. This is easy: Training develops the muscle, fibers, bones, and ligaments used. Very little leg development is obtained from working the arm muscles.

Timing and Training: The Essence of the Art?

How often should a dog train? Many factors have to be considered.

Response Time and Weeks to Racing. The response time of something being trained is the time it takes to undergo the necessary adaptive changes. The enzymes on the energy pathways have been shown to react very quickly and can be brought to a peak in 3 weeks. At the other extreme are the bones, joints, and muscle-to-bone attachments, which can take many months. Long periods of walking will strengthen these slow responders. This is why many training programs start with a period of walking—to get the bone remodeling under way. The response time for increased muscle bulk falls between the muscle enzyme and bone response times.

Training programs that start immediately with sprint training tend to lead to muscle strength outstripping the strength of the muscle-to-bone attachments, with consequent soreness and increased frequency of muscle tears, shin soreness, and fractures. It can also use up some inapparent reserves in the system, causing early loss of interest. Failure to stay well inside these reserves in the first weeks of a training program account for the failure of many people and animals to keep an exercise program going.

Training Frequency and Increments

Increments are the step-ups in the load. A training program of small steps will avoid injury but take a long time to bring the dog to a peak. Very large increments, while saving time, are a strain on the animal, predisposing it to injury or to mental jading. The spacing of the runs is also a factor. Spaced too far apart, the adaptation is partially or totally lost. Too close, the animal cannot cope, again predisposing it to injury or to mental jading. The ideal increments and frequency are obviously interrelated, and top trainers will set the next work only when they see how the animal has coped with its last run. They will increase the step-up or increase the frequency if they see that the animal has coped well. Conversely, they will give a longer rest between works and/or lessen the work load if it has not.

Poor trainers have little idea of the increments and frequency or poor control. Of course, dogs can get carried away and perform above what the trainer intended them to do, but nevertheless the art of training athletic animals is in avoiding sudden large step-ups in the work load. Letting the dog get too fresh is one pitfall. Trialing dogs together that have large differences in ability is another. Having a dog escape in the bush or having the catching pen operator caught napping can lead to the most extreme forms of "too large a step-up" problems.

Careful management of increments matters much more in sprint events, in which a large amount of lactic acid is produced, than in true staying events, in which little lactic acid is produced.

References

1. Rapport D, Ralli EP: The type of fuel used in muscular exercise. Proc Soc Exp Biol Med 24:964, 1926/7.
2. Seeherman HJ, Taylor CR, Maloiy GMO: Recruitment of metabolic power during running: A general mammalian pattern based upon maximum aerobic power. *In* PhD thesis, Harvard University, 1977.

3. Astrand P-O, Rodahl K: Textbook of Work Physiology. New York, McGraw-Hill Book Co, 1977.

4. Northrup DW, Van Liere EJ, Stickney JC: The effect of age, sex and body size on the heart weight-body weight ratio in the dog. Anat Rec 128:411, 1957.

5. Herrmann GR: Experimental heart disease. I: Methods of dividing hearts; with sectional and proportional weights and ratios for 200 normal dogs' hearts. Am Heart J 1:213, 1925.

6. Stahl WR: Organ weights in primates and other animals. Science 150:1039, 1965.

7. Herrmann GR: The heart of the racing greyhound. Hypertrophy of the heart. Proc Soc Exp Biol Med 23:856, 1926.

8. Schneider HP, Truex RC, Knowles JO: Comparative observations of the hearts of mongrel and greyhound dogs. Anat Rec 149:173, 1964.

9. Steel JD, Taylor RI, Davis PE, et al: Relationships between heart score, heart weight and body weight in greyhound dogs. Aust Vet J 52:561, 1976.

10. Wang Y, Marshall R, Shepherd J: Stroke volume in the dog during graded exercise. Circ Res 8:558, 1960.

11. Sanders TM, Werner RA, Bloor CM: Visceral blood flow distribution during exercise to exhaustion in conscious dogs. J Appl Physiol 40:927, 1976.

12. Erickson HH, Bishop VS, Kardon MB, et al: Left ventricular internal diameter and cardiac function during exercise. J Appl Physiol 30:473, 1971.

13. Donald DE, Milburn SE, Shepherd JT: Effect of cardiac denervation on maximal capacity for exercise in the racing greyhound. J Appl Physiol 19:849, 1964.

14. Staaden RV: The Exercise Physiology of the Racing Greyhound. PhD Thesis, Murdoch University Veterinary School, Perth, 1984.

15. Holmgren A, Linderholm H: Oxygen and carbon dioxide tensions of arterial blood during heavy and exhaustive exercise. Acta Physiol Scand 44:203, 1958.

16. Doll E: Oxygen pressure and content in the blood during physical exercise and hypoxia. In Keul J (ed): Limiting Factors of Physical Performance. Stuttgart, Georg Thieme, 1973.

17. Bayly WM, Grant BD: The effects of maximal exercise on acid-base balance and arterial blood gas tensions in thoroughbred horses. In Snow DH, Persson SGB, Rose RJ (eds): Proc First Int Conf Equine Ex Phys, Oxford, 1982.

18. McElroy WT Jr, Gerdes AJ, Brown EB Jr: Effects of CO_2, bicarbonate and pH on the performance of isolated perfused guinea pig hearts. Am J Physiol 195:412, 1958.

19. Wang H-h, Katz RL: Effects of changes in coronary blood pH on the heart. Circ Res 17:114, 1965.

20. Cingolani HE, Mattiazzi AR, Bloon ES, et al: Contractility in isolated mammalian heart muscle after acid-base changes. Circ Res 26:269, 1970.

21. Fregin GF, Thomas DP: Cardiovascular response to exercise in the horse. In Snow DH, Persson SGB, Rose RJ (eds): Proc First Int Conf Equine Ex Phys, Oxford, 1982.

Suggested Readings

Staaden RV: Exercise physiology. In Electrocardiography and Cardiology. Proceedings no 50, p 261. Post Graduate Committee in Veterinary Science, University of Sydney, 1980.

Staaden RV: The Exercise Physiology of the racing greyhound. In Greyhound Medicine and Surgery, Proceedings no 122, p 71. Post Graduate Committee in Veterinary Science, University of Sydney, 1989.

CHAPTER 42

PERSPECTIVES ON RAISING, TRAINING, AND RACING THE RACING GREYHOUND

A. RAISING, TRAINING, AND CONDITIONING THE RACING GREYHOUND

HERB "DUTCH" KOERNER

People often ask, What is the most important element in developing successful racing greyhounds? Is it breeding and bloodlines? Is it the raising of pups? Or is it the training and conditioning?

They might as well be asking, What is the most important element in sustaining life itself: food, air, or water? Of course, all are vitally important. The same is true about raising greyhounds. Remove any one of the key elements of breeding, raising, or training, and there can be no successful greyhound development program.

In this business of producing top-quality greyhounds, no one ever has all the answers. If they did, they would win every kennel-standings title wherever they raced, they would capture every major

stake, and their stock would perennially be the most prized in the sport. That just doesn't happen—which is one of the things that makes our sport so intriguing.

After more than 30 years in the business of breeding, raising, and racing greyhounds, I am still constantly discovering new ideas that will improve our operation. At times, our operation has been blessed with periods of such great success that we are tempted to believe that we have found all the trade secrets, and that no one will ever outperform us again. Eventually (and all too soon), we are brought back to reality, and the humility of defeat reminds us that there are still mountains to climb, truths to be learned, and new techniques to be tried.

Through it all, there are some absolutes, some constants, in all successful greyhound programs. Sometimes these constants are discovered and implemented into our individual programs only after years of trial and error. Sadly, many will not implement them upon discovery, either because of lack of commitment to excellence or unwillingness to put forth the hard work that is required. There may be some variance in the specifics of how individual owners utilize these constants, but, in general, all must fall back on these basics if they expect to be successful over the long term.

A book the size of this one could not begin to contain all of the good ideas there are about breeding, raising, and training greyhounds. It would take many years to compile such a text. In this chapter, I am able to touch only upon some of the more key ideas that I feel have brought me some success over the years. I do not claim that my way is the only way to do it. In fact, I would encourage every newcomer to seek out the methods of as many successful owners as possible and adopt what he or she feels are the best in that collection. I believe that one finds, however, that many of the major principles mentioned here—the constants, the absolutes—are the same for almost everyone who has enjoyed long-term success in our sport.

BREEDING PROGRAM

Every successful breeding program begins with the discriminating selection of brood stock. I know of no successful greyhound person who does not emphatically believe that. We may all have different criteria, or prioritize the criteria differently, but we all agree that starting out right in this business requires the careful selection of breeding stock.

All respected breeders agree that the primary criteria for selecting a female include (1) outstanding bloodlines, (2) track performance (either in the specific female or in her litter), and (3) outstanding temperament and conformation.

All bloodlines are good if tracing goes back far enough, but that is not necessarily justification for breeding. What separates good stock from mediocre, as far as bloodlines are concerned, is the presence of quality stock up close (in the first two generations) and a pedigree that is loaded with classic families with great winning traditions.

As for performance—a female that showed she had the class to race in the upper grades at a major track is my preference. If there was good reason why she did not have that kind of performance record (eg, injury), but her littermates were excellent racers, the female is given consideration as brood stock.

A female with good temperament is one that is not too "spooky" or nervous and does not fret too much. Another important criterion of mine, when it comes to selecting brood stock—and it ties in with good conformation—is balance. I am sure I give this more attention than most other breeders. It is very important that the female have a well-proportioned, balanced body. Her legs must be in proportion with her body—not too short, nor too long.

Next comes the selection of a sire. All good breeders give serious consideration to a sire's bloodlines and, of course, his track performance. I agree with those breeders who, in the sire-selection process, pay attention to what the female-to-be-bred and her lines have been working with effectively in the immediate past. It is only common sense to go with what is working. There is also much to be said for using proven sires most of the time. It is certainly unwise to take an unproven female to a young, unproven sire.

FEMALE CARE

Care of the female before and after breeding is absolutely essential in the development of good pups. The female should be wormed before she is bred and again 30 days into her pregnancy. She should be given a booster shot prior to being bred. While in whelp, she should have a good vitamin- and calcium-enriched diet. While she is whelping, someone should stay with her throughout the event in case any problems develop. Two days after the pups are born, the infant pups' nails should be clipped. If the pups' nails are allowed to get too long, the mother will stop producing milk.

The pups should begin to be fed at about 3 weeks of age. Their diet should consist of an instant baby formula with milk, more solid foods being added as they get older. They should be given a high-protein, fatty diet with milk. Most puppy chows are very good to include in the young pups' feed.

The pups should be wormed at 3 weeks of age for roundworms only and given a follow-up at 5 weeks. I use a medication that is used for control of roundworms and hookworms. Beginning at 8 weeks of age, they are given a wormer once a month for the control of all worms except tapeworms. Medication for tapeworms is administered as needed.

I vaccinate pups for distemper and measles at 5 to 6 weeks of age, at which time they also receive a killed parvovirus inoculation. At 9 to 10 weeks of age and again at 16 weeks, they are inoculated for distemper, hepatitis, parainfluenza, leptospirosis, parvovirus, and coronavirus. I recommend annual revaccination.

As soon as possible, the young pups should be placed on a solid-food diet, gradually cutting back the milk. They should be fed twice a day, with regular cows' milk given between feedings. This feeding schedule should continue until the pups are about 8 months old, at which time they are switched to a once-a-day feeding schedule. Milk continues to be given to them once daily, until they go into the kennels at about 13 or 14 months of age.

HANDLING YOUNG PUPS

A young pup should be leash trained (taught to lead) by the time it is 4 months old. This is very important at our farm, and we actually start lead-breaking our pups at 3 months of age. We stress this because much that we do ties into the philosophy of adequately preparing the pup for what is to follow by not overwhelming it with too much at any of the various learning stages. If the pup is taught to lead early, it does not have to be distracted by this later when it is being taken through other training regimens. The job at hand at that particular stage can then be an easier, more positive learning experience for the pup rather than a negative or intimidating one.

More needs to be said about paying attention to the mental attitude of the pup. For example, some owners pick up pups and handle them only when they get their shots or are administered worm pills. At our farm the pups are constantly being handled. This leads to a positive mental attitude in them and is important in their development, helping them to learn quicker and more effectively.

From the age of 3 months until the pups are ready to go into the kennel, they should be routinely exercised in fields. Some owners raise their pups in long runs (500 to 600 ft); others raise their pups in runs that I believe are too short (200 to 300 ft). My preference is 200-ft runs that open up to large exercise fields (eg, 200 × 1000 ft) where they can romp and twist and develop their agility. The pups should be out in the exercise field no less than every other day, running strictly on their own. We turn ours out for 12-hour periods, during which time they still have access back into their smaller runs and pens.

If exercise fields are not available, an owner should take the pups out into the open. This is an extremely vital aspect in the pups' development. It is here, in the large exercise fields or in the open, that greyhound pups learn to run and develop their potential to become great racers.

EARLY TRAINING

The pups at our farm enter into their first stages of training when they are 6 to 8 months of age. They are allowed to punch an artificial lure—a coyote hide equipped with a predator call—three or four times during this period. It is toward the end of this period that the pups are moved to runs where they have kennel crates in their pup house. The pups are placed in the crates when they are fed—a positive reinforcement that prepares them to mentally accept the kennel crate long before they go into the kennel house. This minimizes the adjustment when they are brought into the kennel. Obviously, if a pup has been constantly handled, leash trained at a young age, and is already accustomed to kennel crates, it is not such an intimidating exercise to be taken through the extensive levels of training or moved into a different environment, such as the kennel, when that time comes. When the pups are moved from the exercise fields into the kennel house at 13 or 14 months of age, they are taken out and sprinted every other day until they have totally accepted the new life-style in the kennel. This exercise will help in that adjustment by giving the pups something to do and by getting their minds off their former farm life-style. No other extensive training should be carried out during this period.

After the pups are adjusted to the kennel, they are ready for drag-lure training. The drag-lure course should be at least 1000 feet long. My preference of artificial lures is a coyote hide. A jacked-up truck is the means I use to pull a nylon cord, with the hide attached to the cord. At the end of the pursuit, a predator call is used to further instill interest by the pups. Depending on how well they perform, this exercise should be carried out five to eight times. When the pup is running hard and attacking the lure, it is ready for the next stage, the whirlygig, a small, circular track. The arm is about 25 feet long and is pushed by hand from the center of the track, with the lure attached to a mechanism that rides on the rail. It is used to familiarize the pups with running a lure above the ground around a rail that is to their left—as it will be at the track. Greyhounds are sighthounds and are bred to sight and chase, and this exercise magnifies that instinct. The same coyote hide and predator call used in the drag-lure training should be used here. On the first trial, the pups should be taken on a lead to the lure and allowed to punch it, so they will know what they will be chasing. After two or three trials on the whirlygig, the pups should be ready for the training track.

Once again the same lure—the coyote hide and predator call—should be used on the training track. Every trainer has his own method of bringing the pups along on the training track. Again, on the first trial, I take them on a lead to the lure and allow them to punch it, so they are familiar with what they will be chasing. For the first two schoolings, I start my pups by handslipping them going into the first turn. For these initial schoolings, I release them close to the lure so they can see it clearly. I then move them to the "short box," which is about 100 ft from the first turn, and handslip them from there. I then put the pups in the short box for their next 10 schoolings. The next step is to handslip them from about halfway between the short box and the 5/16-mile box. I then move them back to the 5/16 box for a handslip. Finally, I will put the pups in the 5/16 box for 8 to 10 schoolings. By now, the pups should be ready for the track.

During this long process, I make certain the pups are paired according to their ability, matching pups that are fairly equal. To safeguard their mental attitude, I make certain that no pup is severely outrun or that no pup runs back more than twice in a row before it is allowed to win.

TRANSITION TO THE TRACK

An important step in the pup's development is the transition from training to the actual racetrack. Here the pup needs to be monitored more closely than ever. Too often, trainers pay attention only to the older dogs when it comes to soreness and are not concerned about the young pups. These pups have not yet adjusted to the track and the track kennel, and any soreness is going to hurt their performance. If a pup is sore, it is important that the trainer let the pup recuperate (even if it means missing a schooling or two) and get back in top condition. The trainer can assist by using ultrasound, whirlpooling, or other methods to help alleviate the soreness. One important way for a trainer to prevent soreness and injury is to make sure racers are properly "cooled out" after every race. In addition, the trainer should see to it that a greyhound is worked between starts, whether in the sprint pen, through unofficial schooling, or by walking. Between starts, the trainer must have them doing something.

Every kennel should have a walker. They are especially good for the morning after a race or for racers working their way back from injuries. If a kennel does not have a walker, it has no choice but to sprint the greyhounds, and sometimes that can overextend them and cause more injury.

Conditioning of racing greyhounds has much to do with feed (see Chapter 38). The diet in the racing kennel should have high vitamin content, good meat and meal, and enough fat so that the racers do not "dry up." A sound diet goes a long way in preventing soreness in racing greyhounds.

RACING DIET

For a successful kennel operation, a trainer must have good feed and conditioning programs. The trainer must also constantly check for injury and soreness and take all measures to prevent both. For the sake of the racers, trainers should do all they can to bring about a safe racing environment for the greyhounds. This includes working together with each other and with track and state officials to ensure the greyhounds are always competing on a safe racing surface. A racing greyhound cannot easily be replaced. The loss, due to injury, of a top-grade greyhound in the prime of life at a major track is probably the greatest tragedy that a kennel must sustain. Anything that can reduce that awful occurrence should be pursued by everyone in the industry.

CONCLUSION

Finally, trainers must remember that greyhounds are not robots, and a good, happy mental attitude must exist in the racing kennel. This starts with the trainers and their assistants.

If all the pieces fall into place, and the owner has done his or her homework in all facets of development—from breeding, raising, training, right on up to proper conditioning and care at the track—then the owner will enjoy the fruits of his or her labors. A healthy, top-quality racing greyhound is the goal of all owners and breeders. When the goal is achieved, it makes our efforts (trying as they are) all worthwhile.

B. WHELPING, RAISING, AND TRAINING OF RACING GREYHOUNDS

DONALD CUDDY \ PATRICK DALTON

Greyhound bitches are selected for breeding on the basis of performance, ability, temperament, and genetic background. The female selected for breeding should be free from all internal and external parasites, fully vaccinated, and receiving a good balanced diet that maintains body weight within 2 to 6 pounds of her racing weight.

A culture and sensitivity test taken by the veterinarian will eliminate the possibility of any vaginal infection, which could be responsible for reduction or loss of fertility.

Details of the estrus cycle and the timing of ovulation were discussed previously; the period of gestation lasts an average of 63 days, ranging from 60 to 67 days.

SIGNS OF PREGNANCY

In the first trimester the bitch may show mood changes and variable appetite and may become "picky" with her food. There is no real change in her body shape during this period despite the fact that all the body organ systems of the puppies are being formed—quite a complex series of events. In the first week of the second trimester, the pups may be felt for the first time with gentle pressure in the lower abdomen; they are about the size of Ping-Pong balls or small eggs. Toward the latter half of the second trimester the abdominal wall begins to sag and enlarge and the mammary glands begin to develop. The third trimester is the period of maximum growth of the puppies and of the greatest demands on the bitch. The abdomen swells to its maximum size, becoming pendulous toward the end of the period. The mammary glands enlarge and fill with milk and may begin to excrete milk 12 to 24 hours before term.

FALSE PREGNANCY

This hormonal condition is possible in a bitch that has been mated but has not conceived. All signs of pregnancy, including mammary development, weight gain, abdominal enlargement, and nest making, are present, but no pups are forthcoming. Various hormonal treatments exist to deal with this condition.

FEEDING DURING PREGNANCY

A bitch tends to put on weight during pregnancy more readily than when nonpregnant. In the first 6 weeks, no added food intake is necessary; she should be fed a balanced diet. It is wise not to give any additives or medicines in the first trimester without first consulting the veterinarian, as some drugs can interfere with normal development of the various organ systems.

The growth of the pups is most rapid in the last trimester. It is during this time that the bitch should be given more to eat; up to about 1½ times normal. In the latter stages of the pregnancy there is less space in the abdomen for a large amount of food at any one time; consequently, she must be given a number of small meals during the day rather than one large meal daily. There must be an increase in calcium intake to attain normal bone development in the puppies and to maintain normal blood calcium levels in the

bitch (large amounts of calcium are utilized in uterine contractions and in milk production); 2 teaspoonfuls of dicalcium phosphate or equivalent per 500 gm meat is adequate. The bitch should be wormed to reduce environmental contamination during the second trimester.

THE LAST WEEK OF PREGNANCY

During these last 7 days, the bitch should be placed in her whelping box, or the area where she will whelp, to acclimatize her to the new environment. The area should be clean and quiet with good lighting and ventilation and provision for heating. The bitch should be whelped down on sheets of newspaper, which are more easily disposed of and replaced when soiled during the birth process. Two to five days before giving birth, the bitch becomes more sunken in the loin area, with a pendulous abdomen. The spines on the vertebrae along the back may become more prominent. The vulva will become enlarged, the ligaments around the tail base slacken, and a straw-colored mucous discharge may be seen from the vulva. Within 24 hours of whelping, the bitch's body temperature will drop from normal (approximately 38.5C) to below 38.0C, usually close to 37.0, so monitoring her temperature during the last few days would be worthwhile.

During the last week a visit to the veterinarian would be beneficial so that he or she is aware of the imminent whelp and may supply a number of injections to give the bitch to assist with the birth—calcium, oxytocin, and possibly some prophylactic antibiotic.

THE WHELP—THE NORMAL PROCESS; PROBLEMS AND WHAT TO DO

Stage of Excitation—Before the Pups Arrive

Close to the time of giving birth, the bitch becomes restless, pants, tears up bedding (newspaper is cheaper to replace than the family's best blanket), and engages in nest-making behavior. Maiden bitches may do this for up to a week before time, but usually this behavior is seen only for 16 to 24 hours before birth of the first pup.

Stage of Contractions—Birth of the Pups

After this initial period of excitation, abdominal contractions begin—usually six to eight at a time followed by a period of rest. The first pup should be born within 2 to 2½ hours. As whelping continues, a further bout of contractions will cause a gray-green fluid-filled bag to appear from the vulva, and further contractions will cause the pup to be expelled from the birth canal. The bag of fluid (placenta) may be burst by the force of the contractions. The fluid then lubricates the birth canal for delivery of the pup. The pup may appear head first or tail first—both of these presentations are *normal* in greyhounds. Some maiden bitches may become distressed with the onset of labor—an experience they have not had before. Normally the bitch will chew the bag open, chew through the umbilical cord (the blood vessels and structures leading from the belly of the pup), and lick the pup, stimulating it to breathe, squeal, and move toward the teats. If the bitch appears to be unaware of what to do, or if, toward the end of whelp, she is tired and unable to clean the pup, the bag should be broken open and the pup's mouth cleared of fluid. The pup should be rubbed vigorously with a towel or a piece of sheet, and the bitch made aware that there is a pup there for her to tend by placing the pup near her face. The bitch may then respond and lick and clean the pup. The pup should not be cleaned overzealously because its smell is important for recognition by the bitch. If the bitch fails to chew the cord and clean the pup, the umbilical cord should be broken, leaving approximately 4 to 6 inches of cord attached to the pup. *Sharp instruments should not be used* because a straight cut will cause the blood vessels to bleed freely (and the pup to lose vital blood volume), whereas vessels that are manually broken will contract and prevent further blood loss. If the vessels continue to bleed, the umbilical cord may be tied off with some cotton, preferably soaked in diluted iodophor or similar antiseptic.

Sometimes a pup will be born and the afterbirth will remain attached to the bitch for a short time, especially if the gray-green bag bursts during the phase of active contractions. The afterbirth is usually expelled by further contractions shortly afterward, or the bitch may chew and swallow the placenta, pulling it free as she does. There is no reason to stop the bitch from eating the placenta, as it is a good source of iron for her.

Once the abdominal contractions begin, a pup and its placenta should be born quickly, usually in 10 to 15 minutes; if more than 2 hours goes by without a pup, something is seriously wrong, and the veterinarian should be contacted. Pups may be born singly or in pairs (one quickly after another), usually one from each horn of the uterus.

After the Pups Arrive

After the birth of each pup, a period of uterine rest occurs. During this period the bitch will be actively cleaning and feeding the pups and disposing of the afterbirth. Following a suitable rest period of 10 to 60 minutes, abdominal and uterine contractions begin again, and the whole process will be repeated until all the pups are born.

Discharges

The normal discharge accompanying the birth is dark green-black. A discharge of this color always signifies separation of the pup's blood supply from the wall of the uterus. The initial blood discharge may continue after the whelp for 10 to 21 days, becoming darker and reducing in volume with time. In some bitches there may be recurrence of a blood-tinged discharge for 3 to 7 days, 5 to 8 weeks after the whelp.

Assistance to be Offered

It is preferable to supervise the entire whelping period with the assistance offered, depending on the experience of the person supervising the bitch. If one is unsure, uncertain, or worried about the situation, the veterinarian should be called for appropriate advice and guidance, and the correct course of action can then be taken.

If no pups are born after prolonged and repeated contractions, the following may exist: (1) a pup that is dead, malformed, or incorrectly positioned and wedged at the front of the pelvis; (2) abnormal pelvic conformation (which may be genetic—size and shape—or traumatic—pelvic fracture) resulting in insufficient room for passage of the pups; (3) incomplete cervical dilation (the cervix,

which normally acts to close off the uterus, fails to dilate and relax fully as a result of hormonal imbalances); (4) uterine inertia (the muscles of the uterus fail to contract in the normal manner or have become exhausted [especially with large litters and/or low blood calcium levels]).

If a pup is visible but appears to be stuck in the vagina, gentle traction (gentle pulling) on the pup as the bitch contracts will assist her in expelling it. Also, sliding a finger along the dorsal (top) wall of the vagina will gently stimulate stronger contractions. If the bitch is tired or does not know how to clean or stimulate the pup, proceed as mentioned before.

After Whelping Is Completed

(1) The bitch should be taken out to urinate or defecate since she may be reluctant to leave her pups. (2) Her anus should be cleaned with warm water; strong-smelling antiseptics should be avoided. (3) The whelping area should be cleaned and bedding replaced. (4) The bitch should have free access to food and fluids. If she is reluctant to leave the pups to feed, she should be encouraged to do so. (5) Adequate ventilation and/or heating as required should be ensured; 21 to 23C is optimal for the bitch, and the bitch will keep the puppies warm. If the temperature is too high, the bitch will move away and leave the pups.

What to Do in the First Days Afterward

The Bitch. The mother should be fed as much as she wants, her food intake being increased to three to four times what she normally eats. Some may eat 3 kg of meat plus kibble/bread, milk, and so on each day and still lose weight, especially with a large litter and good milk flow. A balanced diet is necessary with a large amount of calcium (2 teaspoonfuls of dicalcium phosphate or equivalent per 500 gm meat). Nipples and mammary glands should be observed for any signs of insufficient milk, or redness and swelling and pain with abnormal milk (mastitis). She should be watched carefully for signs of shivering and incoordination, which may be due to milk fever or low blood calcium levels.

The Pups. The pups should always feel warm to the touch. They should drink from the teat, pushing on the mammary glands with their front feet; they fall asleep, only to wake up several hours later, cry, be licked by the bitch (to stimulate them to urinate and defecate), drink again and fall back to sleep. If the dew claws are to be removed, the procedure (quite simple) should be performed within the first week of life. It is most important that all the puppies drink well during the first 24 to 72 hours after birth (to ensure adequate intake of colostrum antibodies), and it is important to note if the pups are acting abnormally.

SELECTION OF A YOUNG PUP AFTER WEANING

If one decides to buy a pup shortly after weaning, then the responsibility and expense of rearing the greyhound to racing age will have to be accepted. Rearing the pup at home will require facilities such as a kennel and a puppy yard; one must also be prepared to take the pup to a larger area for free galloping (park or beach) daily.

The health of the pup will also be a prime consideration. The pup must have a regular worming program, vaccinations must be up to date, the kennel and yard must be kept clean (removal of droppings daily), and other parasites (fleas, flies) must be kept under control.

The option is having the pup reared on a rearing farm. Here the greyhound will probably be in long runs with several others of the same age. The pup will get the necessary diet and exercise but not the individual care it would get at home. It will therefore be necessary for the owner to visit the pup frequently, to check on its health and progress and to handle it. The pup's association with people as it grows older is very important, to prevent its growing into a very timid, crowd-shy greyhound. During racing the greyhound will be handled by many people who are complete strangers (veterinarians, stewards, catchers), and it is essential that the dog is used to people and not fearful of anyone who approaches. While the pup is on the farm, it will still be the owner's responsibility to check on vaccinations, worming programs, calcium supplementation, and the like.

WHEN TO START SCHOOLING AND PREPARING FOR RACING

Age. I believe that a greyhound should not be broken-in until it has reached 14 to 16 months of age. This gives it a chance to mature physically and mentally and results in fewer problems with metacarpals and hocks.

Broken-in to Lead. The greyhound must be trained to lead before "breaking-in" is attempted, to give it confidence, which makes it easier to handle and break-in. Also, before breaking-in the greyhound should be checked by a competent veterinarian to ensure freedom from musculoskeletal injury.

THE BREAKING-IN PROCEDURE

Initially the greyhound should be teased with an artificial lure and allowed to watch trials before being allowed to run on the track. The next step is to slip the greyhound behind the lure for approximately 150 meters before catching it. The distance is increased over the next three or four times, at 2- to 3-day intervals, until the greyhound has completed a full lap of the track and is chasing keenly.

When progressing to box practice, we prefer to back the greyhound into the boxes through the front door. This gives it the impression that there is only one way out, "through the front." This procedure should be carried out at least three times or until the pup is familiar with all aspects of entering and leaving the starting box in the normal racing manner. The greyhound is now ready to race with other dogs. This will give it added confidence and the experience of racing with another greyhound. Begin by introducing one other competitor in a trial, and progress to half and full trials over the next few weeks. The breaking-in program usually takes 6 to 8 weeks.

COMMON PROBLEMS

Not Chasing. If the greyhound fails to chase, slip the dog behind another greyhound that has already completed one lap. It will then chase after that greyhound and observe what that dog is doing. Complete this procedure three or four times, then gradually progress as above.

Running Past Objects. Some greyhounds will stop or balk at objects near the track, eg, driving tower, motors, people, wire, fences. If this occurs, slip the greyhound 5 to 10 meters in front of the object.

Running Wide. While some greyhounds are naturally wide-runners, ie, keep a few feet from the inside rail, any greyhound that consistently runs wide or is not true in its action should be checked for injuries, as muscle and lower-limb bone problems are the most common cause of running wide.

Turning in the Boxes. Greyhounds that turn in the boxes should be held firmly by the bridge of the tail until the box opens. Repeat this procedure three or four times until the undesirable behavior is corrected.

HEALTH PROGRAM

Worming. After breaking-in has been completed, the greyhound should be dewormed thoroughly as detailed in Chapter 13.

Veterinary Examination. Most greyhounds will sustain some degree of bone and muscle injury during the breaking-in program. It is essential that the dog receive a thorough examination for injury.

TRIALING OR SCHOOLING

When the greyhound starts racing year-round, it is necessary to make sure it is fit enough and confident enough to handle the situation. The owner should try to place it in weak fields with greyhounds of similar age and keep it in low grade races for as long as possible, ie, *build and maintain confidence in the greyhound.*

FEED

Feed is basic in all kennels: meat, meal, vegetables, vitamins, and minerals. Greyhounds must have access to fresh clean water at all times, and approximately 1 to 1½ lb of meat daily, 8 oz dry feed, and liquids.

CONCLUSIONS

There are no secrets in training. The dogs should be kept clean and comfortable. For physiotherapy, I recommend ultrasound, magnetic field therapy, laser, and hydrobath.

Most greyhounds race for 2 to 3 years, or until they reach 5 years of age. They are then retired for breeding or as pets. Several groups are now involved in placing retired greyhounds as pets in homes across the United States.

C. RACING AND TRAINING GREYHOUNDS

JOHN R. STEPHENS

BACKGROUND

Greyhound racing began in Australia in the late nineteenth century when greyhounds were imported primarily from England and Ireland. Greyhound racing existed as open-field coursing, whereby the participants raced in twos in the pursuit of live hares. The greyhounds, released simultaneously from a leather harness known as a slip lead, pursued their quarry, obtaining points for speed, and causing the hare to turn, but rarely actually caught it. The hare, bred and reared specifically for this purpose, and being on its home ground, most often led its enemy on a course that lasted up to 3 minutes before the hare escaped. In live-hare coursing, the greyhound that accumulated the most points proceeded in the contest, while the loser was eliminated. The contest continued on a last-greyhound-standing basis, whereby one greyhound was pronounced the winner. Therefore, 128 greyhound stakes saw the greyhounds compete four times on a Friday, which reduced the number of winners to eight. These eight greyhounds then coursed three times on Saturday to determine the winner of the event.

MECHANICAL HARE RACING

Mechanical-hare racing was introduced to Australia in 1926, based on the American invention. Since that time, there has been a rapid decline in coursing; realistically it is now conducted in only two states of Australia, Victoria and South Australia. (Live hare coursing was banned in Australia in 1970; since then, coursing has existed with the same basic rules but the contestants chase a "drag lure" along an approximately 300-yard straight course.)

Speed tracks quickly multiplied, basically in New South Wales and Victoria, through the 1930s; they proved to be a very popular attraction. The tracks were privately owned, rules and regulations varied, and the sport obtained dubious recognition. During the mid 1950s, state governments legislated for *nonproprietary* mechanical hare racing, with the legislation providing for a Greyhound Racing Control Board. Since that time, combined with the development of the Totalizator Agency Board (TAB) or off-track tote betting, greyhound racing has developed into a multimillion dollar business, providing about 40 million dollars in stakes annually, while creating a regulatory nightmare for owners and trainers.

PROFESSIONAL AND HOBBY TRAINERS

Since the huge explosion in greyhound breeding, following the popularity of the sport and its subsequent lucrative prize monies during the 1970s, many individuals began training greyhounds. People with a basic knowledge of fitness in human terms, gamblers, retired sportsmen, and general money seekers attempted what appeared to be a fairly simple vocation. As a result, in Australia today, a typical race program would have ten races involving 80 greyhounds. Of these about 80 per cent would be trained by hobby trainers, defined as persons training four or fewer greyhounds. The remaining 20 per cent are trained by professionals who are defined as persons earning their income from greyhound racing. Obviously, professional trainers in Australia are more along the American

lines. In basic terms, large numbers, quality greyhounds, strong turnovers, and incentive-based contracts allow their kennels to succeed. A top Australian professional trainer will charge about $50 Australian per week for each greyhound he or she trains, plus all veterinary costs, plus 33 per cent of all stakes $100 and above. The trainer retains *all* stakes below $100.00. A high profile trainer would have his kennel set up as follows: racing greyhounds, 30; greyhounds in pretraining, 40; breaking-in greyhounds, 30; pups, 40; brood bitches, 5; stud greyhounds, 4; staff, 5.

Such a trainer would train most of the greyhounds on a 50:50 basis. That is, they are bred and reared by various breeders to the age of 14 months. After schooling, the greyhounds of the desired ability are retained under a 50:50 split of all prize money from this time. No other charges are involved. In a normal year, greyhounds trained by a high profile trainer would win in excess of $250,000 Australian.

RULES AND REGULATIONS

All persons involved in the greyhound racing industry are registered by their respective state authorities, or the Greyhound Racing Control Board (GRCB). Each state has a Control Board that is responsible for the absolute control of greyhound racing within the state. Rules involve training, racing, training tracks, swabbing, appeals, registration, fees, and promotion.

GREYHOUND RACING CONTROL BOARD FUNCTION

The GRCB must function with respect to:

1. **The Government**—via the Racing Act.
2. **The TAB**—the off-track betting system, which also is government regulated.
3. **The Greyhound Racing Grounds Development Board (GRGDB)**—a body responsible for the provision of permanent fixtures on a course, necessary for the conduct of a meeting. Grandstands, kennels, hire equipment, starting boxes, and the like are all funded via the GRGDB, which receives its finance as a fixed percentage of government deductions from all bets.
4. **The Greyhound Owners Trainers and Breeders Association**—a body representing the interests of all greyhound owners, trainers, and breeders.
5. **The Clubs.** Although overseeing the total operations of all clubs or tracks, the GRCB has wide ranging powers that allow it to closely monitor the total performance of any club.

FINANCE

To allow for a simple summation of the industry finance is difficult, but shown in Table 42–1 is an example from the state of Victoria (Sandown Greyhound Racing Club). Total turnover for the year is measured in distinct amounts.

TABLE 42–1. Sandown Greyhound Racing Club, 1992–1993

	Total Turnover
TAB off course betting turnover	$25,000,000.00
TAB on course betting turnover	10,000,000.00
Bookmakers	11,000,000.00
Total	**$46,000,000.00**
Number of meetings conducted	53
	Total Return
Return from off-track	$1,420,000.00
Return from on-track (net)	334,000.00
Return from bookmakers (net)	93,000.00
Total	**$1,847,000.00**

SELECTION OF PUPPY

Personal choice is the guiding principle of greyhound racing: Natural opinion allows the dream of success pending the reality of the eventual race track performance. There will be many conflicting ideas regarding selection.

Breeding Lines. A puppy should be selected from sound breeding lines. An unbroken dam line of proven winners is preferred, and ability must be considered. Strong preference is to breed with a sister to a well-performed track greyhound, where, because of injury or other misfortune, the dam did *not* have many race starts. Some breeders prefer not to race a female at all when the rest of the litter shows ability; rather they prefer to keep her solely as a brood matron. The sire line is *not* as dominant as the dam line; however, proven crosses or nicks should be followed for obvious reasons.

Conformation. A good-looking, well-conformed pup is not guaranteed to have pace; however, a poor looking, poorly conformed pup will not have pace. Some of the characteristics I look for in a greyhound puppy are: a fine, intelligent-looking head; appearance of confidence and character; straight legs, slightly turned in at the front; a straight line down the back legs; solid muscle development; a sense of strength; good feet, and cat-like, sound toes.

An ideal greyhound should have perfect symmetry in all directions. In selection of a pup, the conformation is determined by viewing the animal from five differing cross sections.

The owner looks the animal straight in the eyes, imagining a plumb line running down in a vertical manner. Perfect symmetry is preferable. A variation of symmetry is usually a sign that the greyhound has had a problem during rearing. Obviously if it has taken weight off a limb through soreness, the associated muscle mass can wither. In many cases this muscle withering leads to further injury when the greyhound is put into full work.

The owner goes to the rear of the animal for a *back view* and checks for ''dropped hips.'' Although many greyhounds race successfully with dropped hips, the success rate is usually proportional to the associated muscle around the lower hip muscle. If the muscle has grown well and is strong, the dropped hip (or skeletal deformity) will not present problems; however, if the muscle is weak, usually the greyhound develops consistent injuries. From behind, the major muscles in the back legs should be symmetrically identical.

The *astride view* is from a position as if a camera were above the greyhound. Of particular notice, the muscle mass around the front and back legs.

The greyhound should be examined *rail side* and *offside* on both a skeletal and muscular basis. In some cases, skeletal problems in young pups follow a natural healing curve, whereby the build-up

of calcium causes protrusions or ugly growths in the bone. These asymmetrical growths are regarded as a good thing—Mother nature has done her job, and the resultant bond usually never worries the animal, unless it causes irritation with another limb.

In general, experience will tell whether a pup has good conformation. Only time will tell if this idea of good conformation proves to be beneficial on the race track. When one is selecting a puppy, and assuming that the work has been done with respect to breeding, conformation, inoculation, and registration, the following should be looked for: a keen, happy pup that shows some sort of character to separate it from the rest, not lacking in aggression, possessing alertness to sound and movement, and having a desire to compete.

Inoculations. In Australia, the present regular inoculation of puppies has virtually wiped out the major diseases—distemper, hepatitis, and parvovirus. There are variations in the administration of inoculations, which in my view are again dependent on past experience. Where disease had *not* been a problem over many years, the pups can be allowed to develop their own immunity up until the age of 12 to 14 weeks. The pups are then inoculated against the three main disease groups; they are *not* permitted contact with any other greyhounds for at least another 2 weeks following inoculation. If the mother and pups are separated from all other canine contact during the first 16 weeks, disease is nonexistent, provided the ground on which they are raised has had a long disease-free history. Parvovirus in particular seems to ''rise up'' from the ground and can be very hard to control. Many other inoculation programs are available, but basically we follow this procedure: major inoculations: distemper, hepatitis, parvovirus 12–14 weeks; follow-up booster: 13 months; then annually.

In general, disease can be eliminated with consistent cleanliness and a regular proven inoculation program.

Registration Papers. The poor attitude shown in some to regulatory procedures is amazing. Organization is paramount. It is absolutely essential that all regulatory procedures be followed and records kept in a safe place and duplicated if possible. Partnerships, breeding agreements, ownerships, and other agreements can all be in dispute if not finalized prior to whelping.

REARING

Rearing of pups at home is preferred, simply because someone is available to look after them. They are reared in a 2-acre paddock, are continuously handled, galloped as much as possible, and educated to skin lures from an early age. The personal touch allows consistency in feeding, regular worming and veterinary attention, proper attention to feet, and generally better rearing. Many will argue that rearing farms allow the pups to develop in their natural environment. Success with both farm-reared and home-reared pups is possible, but personal attention is best. The home-reared pup has its pre-training spread over 5 to 14 months, rather than concentrated over 4 to 6 weeks. All pups are rested for 2 to 3 months following breaking-in to allow maturity and development. Greyhounds are put into full training at about 16 months of age.

FULL TRAINING

Housing. Given the fact that in Australia the majority of greyhounds are ''hobby trained,'' housing is relatively cheap and easy to manage. Most hobby kennels consist of about three partitions, usually inside a garage or outbuilding. Consequently they are relatively easy to keep clean. A typical hobby setup is a concrete floor with bedding raised about 1 foot from the flooring. Wire separations define individual kennel units. The basis of sound housing must be warmth, ventilation, and cleanliness. In Australia, variations in temperature can be extreme; hence, some trainers prefer a complete air-conditioning system. There is a strong belief that the greyhound thrives in a natural environment; therefore the "seasons" are actually beneficial to the greyhound's makeup. To have a greyhound lose its coat because it is hot in winter is completely unnatural and will affect its performance. The greyhound should be kept at the seasonal temperature at which a human would be comfortable. It is hoped that most greyhounds can be housed where cleanliness is of major concern. Bedding should be changed regularly, and the basic unit kept free from anything that could promote ill health.

Feeding. Obviously, feeding varies between trainers, but a basic diet consists of: (1) breakfast: roughage (Weetbix or biscuits), 500 ml liquid (honey, water, milk); (2) dinner: 1½ lb beef (fat included), 6 oz whole meal bread, kibble, 6 oz cooked vegetables, 400 ml liquid. The diet is varied every second day with fish, pasta, or chicken substituting for the meat; a stew is provided at least once a week, usually following a race.

Galloping. During pretraining, greyhounds gallop beside the car to monitor pace. They are rested for 5 to 10 minutes and then repeat this gallop. As a fitness routine, they gallop twice at three-quarter pace over 350 meters, every other day for 3 to 4 weeks. The galloping routine allows muscles to develop and harden, thus reducing the incidence of track injuries.

Once fit, the greyhound is hand-slipped into the bend, possibly 40 meters before the bend. This allows it to "roll" into the turn because it has not attained full pace. It should hand-slip into the turn on *all* occasions when it is young, and then go back to the boxes because it is fit enough to run the distance without stress, and it is acquainted with the surroundings and knows when to lean into the turns.

Once it has knowledge of the track, the greyhound is introduced to other runners in field trials. Extreme care is taken to avoid interference, which may cause a youngster to become field-shy. Railers should be mixed with wide-runners and strength with weakness to allow a youngster to be confident in passing its opponents.

Trialing. The biggest single factor involved in the surface of a track is consistency. Many injuries occur when the track surface is inconsistent, as the greyhound moves laterally. It is not good for a greyhound to have two legs on soft ground while its other legs are on a firm or a slippery surface. Proper track conditions are likely to save many greyhounds from serious injury during the year, so, given the value of top greyhounds, the cost of proper track preparation is small. Trialing should be considered only in ideal temperatures because cold conditions can leave the animal susceptible to injury when it is not properly warmed-up and hot conditions can lead to overexcitement and urinary problems.

A general rule of thumb—Would a true athlete consider these conditions ideal to perform in and show maximum ability?

Symmetry. After all gallops, the greyhound should be examined for injury. Symmetry is the key. Serious injury will be noted by a lack of symmetry. Pending injuries will become obvious to the trained eye. It is important that trainers learn and continue to learn as the years go by. The "keen eye" of a trainer will tell him or her many things, but the most important things the eyes look for are symmetry and consistency. The walk, gallop, action, breathing, recuperation, eating, sleeping, every little movement of the greyhound, is a sign. From minor lameness to major skeletal damage, one learns from all variations of the normal. The keen eye will then be able to distinguish between "basic" and "veterinary" injuries. Basic injuries or problems can be treated by the trainer, who must know what he or she can or cannot achieve in injury treatment. Regular consultation with the veterinarian is an absolute necessity.

Sight and Mind. Top trainers never cease to use their sight and mind to analyze the greyhound. The *galloping* action will reveal injuries, timidness in a field, and ability to seek distance variation. A well-balanced greyhound will traverse the track with a sense of elegance and beauty. Abnormalities such as lateral movement, uncontrolled tailspin, and variation in the position of the head usually mean the greyhound is *not* performing to maximum ability. Some greyhounds destroy their own ability from an overzealous desire to rail or run wide. These characteristics are often hereditary and not desirable in the pursuit of clean racing. Wide-runners cause accidents on the track, and really they are not favored if consistency is required. Erratic chasers, fighters, and inconsistent types generally should not be continued in training or racing. Often they have excellent ability, but in the long run they are simply poor greyhounds, lacking in concentration and desire to do their best.

Sectional Timing. The times a greyhound runs are of particular significance. When a greyhound is fit and chasing well, and the track surface is consistent, it will run almost identical times to various points of the track. Of particular significance is the first section, or the time to run from the boxes to the post. This distance is usually about 80 meters, and at Sandown Park requires about 6 seconds. This guide to a greyhound's early speed can, in fact, indicate hindlimb injury or soreness when the time to reach this point increases. The second section, from the post to the top of the backstretch, takes 12 more seconds to complete the 200-meter distance. Deterioration in time in this section could indicate that the greyhound has trouble handling the turn or may have front limb soreness or injury. The last section, from the top of the backstretch to the finish line (about 200 meters), also takes about 12 seconds for a *strong* greyhound to complete. Weakness in the last section can indicate stamina or breathing problems or, in fact, that further blood testing is required. The main point in sectional timing is that it provides valuable information as the greyhound performs.

PRESENTATION AND RESPONSIBILITY TO PEERS

It is often said that we are our own greatest opponents. People within our industry *must* realize that they are in the entertainment industry. The participants of the greyhound industry are our performers to our customers. Therefore the production of fine athletes on a regular basis shows our industry to the world. There is little doubt that the end product or race night is the culmination of many facets of our industry. If the manner in which we produce our pups, house our youngsters, and train our champions is of paramount performance from day one, our industry will grow. If the participants do not strive for excellence at every stage of the racing greyhounds' career, then the overall effect is diminished.

CHAPTER 43

ARTIFICIAL LURES

KEITH DILLON

Greyhounds were first imported to America to help reduce the huge jackrabbit population in the Midwest in the latter half of the 1800s. Jackrabbits were so numerous that they could wipe out a sizable alfalfa field overnight. It is also claimed by early settlers that 20 jackrabbits could collectively consume as much food as a single cow. As far as farmers were concerned, jackrabbits were a scourge on the land.

Jackrabbit drives were traditionally held on Sundays. People would surround a section of land, then drive the jacks to the center of the section and kill them in any manner they could—anything to lessen the numbers of those harmful rodents. The importation of a few greyhounds from England and Ireland actually did little to rid the farmers of their problem with jackrabbits.

No sooner had the greyhound arrived in America than farmers discovered that they were also a great source of sport. One farmer would match his greyhound against another in pursuit of a jackrabbit to see who had the faster greyhound—nothing more than the perpetuation (American style) of the ancient sport of *coursing*, which had been practiced in the Old World for centuries. Sometimes small side bets were made. These challenges soon evolved into regular coursing meets in the open fields. The winner of a course would advance to meet the winner of the next course. Winner would meet winner until only two greyhounds were left for the final race. So it was that a champion would eventually be crowned.

Races were sometimes very long and took much out of the greyhounds, which led to the development of park coursing. In park coursing, a large field was enclosed with rabbit-proof fence. At one end were rabbit pens, a runway on which a jackrabbit was released, and two greyhounds held behind a blind. After a long lead was given the jack, the greyhounds were released from a pair of slips to provide an even start. At the other end of the park were escapes, made so the jackrabbits could get through but the greyhounds could not. Depending on which greyhound led in the run-up to the jack and the number of times each greyhound turned the rabbit, a winner was determined by the judge, who would wave either a red or white flag, corresponding to the color of the collar worn by the winning greyhound.

Coursing greyhounds was a part of the Old West and Midwest tradition of that era and would remain a popular pastime for more than half a century. It was the immediate forerunner to track racing and eventually to the use of artificial lures. About 1919, O. P. Smith came up with the idea of greyhounds running on a circular track with an artificial lure. A circular track would allow spectators to view the entire race, and a wagering system on the races could be implemented, as in horse racing. Ideas like Smith's had been tried before, but he was the first person to make it work. Greyhound track racing as we know it today was born.

From the start, there was reluctance by many greyhounds to chase this type of lure. Greyhounds were still being trained on live lures, but most would immediately adjust to the artificial lure, not realizing the difference. A large percentage of the greyhounds, however, could not be fooled. Many turned their heads or quit, so were of no value as far as a racetrack was concerned. Something needed to be done to improve the breed of greyhounds for track racing. Consequently, greyhounds that performed well on the track were used for breeding. This eventually resulted in development of what was called a track greyhound or track dog. Those people who were still more interested in coursing bred strictly good coursing dogs. So, for a while, there were actually two distinct strains of greyhounds in the United States—the track greyhounds and the rabbit or coursing dogs.

After many years, the time came to train track greyhounds only by artificial means. The jackrabbit population was nearly gone—not from coursing them with greyhounds, because that practice had marginal impact on the huge numbers of jacks. Rather, they were killed off by the fertilizers and insecticides used by the farmers in their farming operations. Public and media pressure were also brought to bear against the sport, coupled with protests by the humane societies. Racetracks took a "dim view" of live-lure training because of adverse publicity in the print media and later the broadcast media. Some tracks included in their contracts with kennels a provision that would not allow any greyhounds trained on live lures to race at their tracks. Practically every state eventually passed animal protection statutes that in effect banned coursing and live-lure training.

For years, young greyhounds were trained first on live lures, then switched to an artificial lure as they matured and were nearing the age to race at the tracks. The time had come to develop some kind of system to train track-bred greyhounds exclusively by artificial means from the outset of training to the final stages. At first, there was much resentment toward artificial-lure training by owners and trainers. They thought that too many greyhounds would not respond to this type of training and that a large percentage of the young greyhounds would not qualify at the tracks.

Developing an artificial lure that would appeal to the greyhound was a problem. One of the first functional lures involved the use of a coonskin cap. It was an artificially made cap, with fur and color that greatly resembled a jackrabbit's. Inside this cap was placed a predator call so that every movement of the lure produced a squeaky sound. Because greyhounds run by sight and are attracted by sound, this seemed like a good idea. The device was named the Jack-A-Lure (Fig. 43–1). It was introduced in the mid 1970s and became the first successful and widely used artificial lure in greyhound racing. As artificial-lure (track) greyhounds continued to be mated to one another, that seemed to produce greyhounds that more readily adapted to this means of training.

As time passed, many different types of lures were used. They ranged from coyote hides to Clorox bottles with predator calls placed in them or tied alongside.

A machine to drag an artificial lure was first used by the whippet owners and trainers. It consisted of an automobile starter run by a battery and a simple push-button control. Many used a tractor takeoff; some used attachments to an automobile wheel. Many

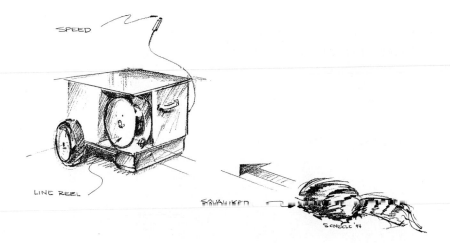

FIGURE 43–1. Jack-A-Lure and drag machine.

other methods were employed—even one that used a manually driven bicycle pedal for power.

As for specific techniques in the training process—it is best to start the greyhounds running in a straight line in pursuit of the artificial lure. This is done by using a long, strong string to pull the lure on the ground. Greyhounds adapt more readily to something moving along the ground; it is a greyhound's instinct to chase anything that moves. So, encouraged by both the moving lure and the noise of the predator call, most greyhounds will chase the artificial lure in their first attempt. They improve with each training session, so that by about the fifth time out they are running hard and driving into the lure aggressively. Muzzles are left on the greyhounds so the lure is not torn to pieces and can be reused many times. If possible, it is best here to use a starting box each time. This teaches the greyhounds to leave a box properly and will avoid problems later on.

It is almost imperative that the lure be pulled on the ground in a straight line before any circular attempts are made. Usually after about five training sessions on the drag, the greyhounds are ready to be tried on a small circular track called a whirlygig. There are many types of whirlygigs—from elaborate power-driven gigs to simple, inexpensive hand-pushed gigs (Fig. 43–2). All seem to do the job very well if good judgment and handling are used.

The same artificial lure used in the early training should be used at the whirlygig. The greyhounds are accustomed to it and know that it is to be chased. At this juncture in training, the lure is tied to the arm of the whirlygig. This teaches the greyhounds to chase something off the ground, which is important because lures on the racetracks are about 24 inches from the ground. Again, a starting box should be used.

Now that the greyhound is acquainted with the lure and the starting box, it must grasp the idea of pursuing something off the ground in a circle. Usually a greyhound will chase the first time. However, if it hesitates or refuses to chase, running it with another pup that does chase will help. Sometimes it is necessary to tie the lure low or even let it drag on the ground the first time to create more interest. Usually the greyhound is muzzled so it can catch and hit the lure, thereby activating the predator call. It is helpful if the lure is sturdy enough to allow the greyhound to bite and pull on it. Also, having the pup watch a few races on the gig will quite often create more interest in chasing the lure.

All the preliminary training should occur between the ages of 10 and 14 months. By this time the greyhound should be ready for the training track.

Most training tracks are very similar to an official track in size and structure. Many are operated by electric motors, while some

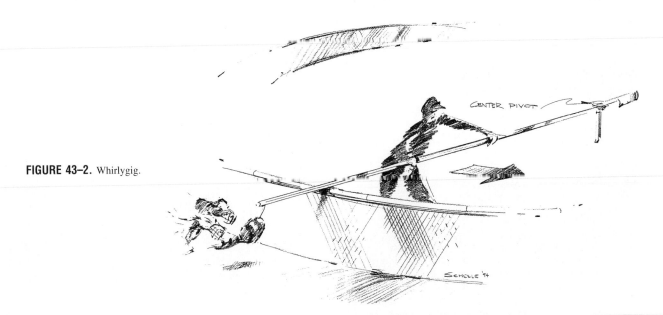

FIGURE 43–2. Whirlygig.

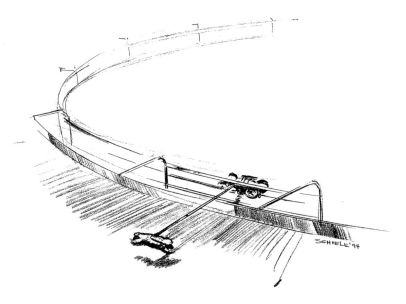

FIGURE 43–3. Training track.

are powered by old autos placed in the infield with ropes or cables to pull the lure. However, as with the whirlygigs, most do the job and prepare the young greyhounds to run on an official racetrack.

Practically the same procedure used at the whirlygig should be used at the training track (Fig. 43–3). The "green" pup should be allowed to watch a few races at first. This shows the pup what is going on and intensifies its desire to run. A starting box should be used; the greyhound knows what it is by now and why it is placed in it. The same lure used on the whirlygig should be used on the training track for the first two or three times around. If the greyhound goes around aggressively, the lure can be replaced by the regular track lure. If the greyhound does not go well the first time or two, it should be taken back to the early training track for a short period. After five or six schoolings, the young greyhound should be running the training track very well. Now would be the time to switch it to a disappearing lure if one is available.

The disappearing lure at the end of the race is now used by all official racetracks. So now the pups should be schooled on a regulation training track, perhaps twice a week, until they are running well enough to participate in unofficial schooling at an official racetrack. Some pups can do this in a dozen or so schoolings, while others may take many more trials to prepare for this type of schooling. After several unofficial times around the official track, they should be ready for official schooling. Most tracks require three official schoolings before a greyhound can start in an official race. These schoolings must meet the track's qualifications before entry into official races.

Finally, it should be understood that before any training occurs, the pups must be in the best of health and in condition to run. This can be accomplished by walking and sprinting, along with the use of a large exercise field.

Many people thought that the end of live-lure training would eventually result in the demise of track racing. The feeling was that not enough greyhounds could be developed by artificial means to supply the tracks. However, this has not been the case. Greyhounds are participating as well as or better than ever.

CHAPTER 44

TRAINING SLED DOGS

KATHRYN J. FROST

Alaska- or Nome-style mushing is the oldest form of sled dog sports in the world, where teams of 3 to more than 20 dogs, usually harnessed in pairs, pull a driver and a sled. In the far north, working dog teams have been used for at least 1500 years to haul wood, water, and other supplies; to run traplines; and in the last century to haul mail and support expeditions for exploration of polar regions. More recently, as the need for working dogs has diminished, recreational teams have been used for such diverse activities as afternoon outings and camping trips, or supporting adventure expeditions. At some point, as with other activities utilizing working animals (such as sheep herding or cattle ranching), the routine of necessary daily tasks was broken by sporting competition

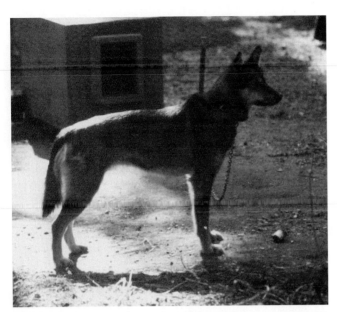

FIGURE 44–1. This is a typical racing sled dog built for speed and endurance. Note angulation of the front shoulders and the long pelvis.

to see whose animals were the best or the strongest or the fastest (Fig. 44–1). These early competitions were the beginning of sled dog racing as we know it today.

Nome-style dog racing occurs as sprint, middle-distance, and long-distance events. Sprint, or speed, racing is the Kentucky Derby of the dog world. Teams sustain speeds of 20 miles per hour (32 km/hr) for distances of more than 20 miles, depending on team size. Common classes in most competitive events today consist of 4 dogs, 6 dogs, 8 dogs, 10 dogs, and unlimited teams (usually 12–22 dogs). Although there is no standard, teams often race approximately 1 mile (2 km) for every dog in the team. Dogs run or lope for the entire duration of sprint races. Championship sprint races are run in heats on 2 or 3 consecutive days. Two of today's most prestigious sprint races are the Fairbanks Open North American and the Anchorage Fur Rendezvous, where unlimited class teams race 70 miles over 3 days.

Long-distance racing is best known in the form of the Iditarod, an 1100- to 1250-mile (1800 to 2000 km) race from Anchorage to Nome, Alaska. A variety of these endurance marathons have developed around the world to test not only the dogs' ability but to provide the musher (the driver) with a wilderness experience and a test of his or her personal fortitude. Long-distance races usually extend over more than 500 miles (800 km). The dogs travel at average speeds of 6 to 12 mph (10 to 20 km/hr) and spend most of the time trotting. Some loping occurs, depending on the stage of the race and the musher's style. Races may last 10 to 20 days.

Mid-distance racing has for the most part developed in the last 10 years as a form intermediate between sprint and long-distance events. Typical distances are 50 to 300 miles (80 to 480 km) at speeds of 12 to 17 mph (20 to 27 km/hr). These races seldom exceed 2 to 4 days. Mid-distance competition entails neither the top speeds of sprint mushing nor the extreme endurance required by distance events, but requires that the dogs be able to maintain a lope over a long period across irregular trails.

The newest arrival on the dog racing scene is stage racing. The best known of these is the Alpirod, which is run through the mountains of Europe. Stage races often consist of 6 to 16 heats or stages that range from 15 to more than 75 miles (24 to 120 km). Dogs and drivers usually sleep in the comfort of a dog truck and

motel, although some stages may require camping out. Each stage begins as if it were a new race, with teams starting at regular intervals from an established starting line. The shorter a team's time on the trail, the longer it can rest before the next stage. Drivers are usually required to carry some minimum amount of camping and survival gear and to drive a sled of a specified minimum size. A variety of dogs are used for this type of racing. Some drivers adapt sprint teams to a somewhat slower pace and longer distance. Others use distance-type dogs accustomed to many consecutive days of racing, and speed them up somewhat.

Traditionally, dog mushing has been a winter activity. Dogs pulling sleds were used to transport people and supplies across snow-covered country when rivers, lakes, and other transportation corridors were otherwise difficult to travel. Dog racing was purely a winter sport. Training began in autumn after the first snow fell and when it was possible to use a sled. As dog mushing spread to other, more southern regions and as racers looked for any competitive edge, training began to occur before there was snow. Mushers adapted a variety of wheeled carts, automobiles, or other vehicles to be pulled by their dogs (Fig. 44–2). With the development of all-terrain vehicles, or four-wheelers, yet another tool became available to mushers. Unlike nonmotorized wheeled carts, which are generally light weight with poor braking ability, four-wheelers offer almost total control of a dog team. The motor can be used to assist the dogs in climbing very steep hills, to establish a "pace," to teach speed cues, and most importantly the brakes make it possible to stop at any time to work with dogs in the team.

During the last decade, dog mushing has expanded rapidly around the world, and is now practiced in more than 30 countries. Some of these (such as South Africa, Australia, and England) have little or no snow at any time of year. In these countries, the sport is practiced almost entirely using wheeled carts and gigs. Races occur on trails through the forest, along sandy beaches, or on dirt roads. Although the type of vehicle pulled by the dogs is different, the rest of the mechanics of the sport remain largely the same.

The most standard dog team configuration is a tandem hitch that

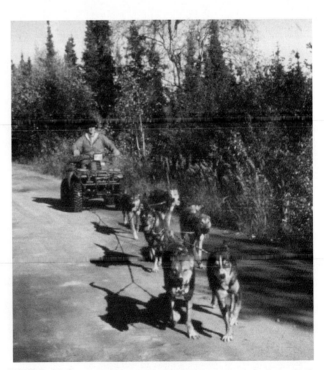

FIGURE 44–2. Early season training using an all-terrain four-wheeler. Note small team and dogs hitched in tandem.

employs a single, central towline running from the sled up through the pairs of dogs in the team (Fig. 44–3). Each dog is connected to the central towline by a tugline to the back of its harness and a neckline to its collar. The tugline must be long enough to allow free movement as the dog runs and not pull downward on its hips and back. The sled is functionally designed either to carry a load over often irregular trails or to carry a single driver during a race. Working or distance racing sleds may be designed either as toboggan-style or basket sleds, and often weigh 35 to 75 pounds (20 to 35 kg). Sprint sleds are normally basket-type sleds weighing 17 to 30 pounds (8 to 14 kg) with a basket length less than 3 feet (1 m).

Dog mushing is as variable as the people who practice it. However, whether the dogs will be sprint speedsters, long-distance marathoners, or working dogs, the key to success is consistent, regular conditioning and training. This chapter describes conditioning activities that enhance a dog's physical performance—exercise to build muscle tone, aerobic conditioning, and speed—and training activities that affect behavior—instilling mental discipline and toughness, teaching behavioral cues, and achieving responses to commands. The training techniques described here pertain particularly to sprint mushing, but many are applicable to all aspects of the sport.

WHAT IS A SLED DOG?

A sled dog is any dog (male or female, neutered or not) that can do the job, regardless of breed. Traditionally, northern husky-type breeds were used as sled dogs. Examples of these breeds include Alaskan, Siberian, and Greenland huskies and Alaska malamutes. These dogs were developed in northern regions and had the attributes necessary for living in the cold. In general, they had coats with thick underfur; densely furred, thick ears that would not be affected by frost-bite; coarse and thickly furred, tough feet that did not split and crack in the severe cold; and the physical conformation and gait that allowed them to run and pull efficiently. These dogs also had to have the desire to run and the mental toughness necessary to survive under often extreme conditions. These same traits are necessary today for sled dogs that live and work in the north.

As mushing has spread to more southern regions, other types of dogs have come into common use as sled dogs. Body type is no

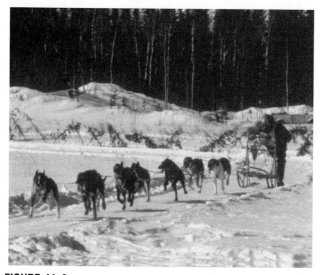

FIGURE 44–3. Typical sprint sled and team hitched in race configuration.

longer determined by the ability to withstand severe cold. Selection of breeds is based on the ability and desire to run and pull, suitable temperament, and perhaps the ability to perform in warm temperatures. Through this very different selection process, breeds such as German shorthair pointers have emerged as viable sled dogs in southern regions.

Whatever the breed, sled dogs must be able to pull a sled and driver, with or without an additional load, over a variety of trails under a wide range of environmental conditions. In Alaska, dogs are trained and raced in temperatures ranging from −60 to +45° F (−50 to +7° C). In Europe, the range is more often 14 to 45° F (−10 to +7° C). Trails range from flat, perfectly packed, and groomed race "highways" to barely broken trails in unpacked snow through mountainous terrain. The dogs must be selected for the conditions in which they will be expected to work and the type of performance the driver desires. A sprint-racing dog must have a near-perfect running gait and be built to run effortlessly at top speed for 15 to over 90 minutes. Sprint-racing dogs are usually of medium size (35 to 55 pounds; 17–27 kg) and are of light to medium build. Dogs used for distance-type racing must have an efficient, smooth trot and be able to maintain a comfortable gait over many miles of irregular terrain while pulling a load. In distance races in which the dogs do not pull heavy loads, average dog size is similar to that for sprint racing. For dogs that regularly pull heavier loads, average size is somewhat larger, 55 to 75 pounds (25 to 35 kg).

Regardless of the task at hand, sled dogs must be mentally suited to the job they perform. They must truly love to run and pull. In the northern breeds that were developed as sled dogs, pulling is as natural and inborn as retrieving or pointing is to a bird dog. Small husky-type puppies do not need to be taught to pull; they must only learn the rules about how to behave in the dog team. A good sled dog must be mentally tough, responsive to the commands of the driver, able to cope with new situations, and unstressed by repetitive training and conditioning.

EARLY SEASON TRAINING AND CONDITIONING

Because dog mushing is practiced in so many different climates, early season training is highly variable. Whatever the methods and means, the goal is to produce a well-muscled, aerobically conditioned, properly behaved team of dogs and to achieve this while keeping the dogs healthy, happy, and uninjured. Most competitive mushers today use a motorized, four-wheeled all-terrain vehicle for early training. Others may use wheeled carts, a bicycle, or even an automobile. For mushers without access to some sort of wheeled vehicle, training generally begins with a sled. While the steps involved in training with a sled are similar, the musher's control over the dogs is considerably less and extra care must be taken to avoid injury to dogs or musher.

Early season conditioning must occur at moderate pace with gradually increasing distance so as not to injure dogs before they have built up the muscle mass necessary for running at high speeds or pulling heavy weights. Most sled dogs are rested during the summer months. When training begins, the dogs' muscles are soft; aerobic conditioning is poor; and they are not prepared for long, uninterrupted runs. Nonetheless, they are extremely enthusiastic and want to run as fast and hard as they can. It is the musher's responsibility to prevent injury during this period by controlling speed and duration of training while the dogs gradually build strength and stamina.

The first training runs should be 2 to 3 miles (3 to 5 km) at speeds not more than 13 to 16 mph (20 to 25 km/hr), usually with several stops. Initially the dogs may be exercised only twice a week, increasing soon to 3 days a week. The dogs should be running 3 to 4 days per week by 3 to 6 weeks into training, depending on the condition of their feet, the weather, and the rate at which they are progressing. While sprint-racing teams are seldom trained more than 4 days a week, distance teams may sometimes be trained 4 or 5 consecutive days, then rested for several days. An increase of approximately 1 mile (2 km) per week, after about the second week, is common for sprint training. Increments may be somewhat greater for distance training. Four-wheeler training usually lasts 4 to 6 weeks for sprint mushers living in areas with regular winter snow (6 to 10 weeks for distance mushers) so the maximum distance dogs will train in this manner is 5 to 7 miles (8 to 12 km).

Teaching Manners and Commands. Early season training with a four-wheeler provides an unparalleled opportunity to teach manners and reinforce control. The musher may speed up or slow down at will, teach cues associated with these speed changes, and stop at any time. A training team should never be so large that it can overpower the musher and equipment. Training in small teams has many advantages. It is easier to see how each dog in the team is performing, and it is far easier to correct problems, no matter how small. Even though a large training vehicle is capable of stopping and holding a large team, it is often tempting to ignore small behavioral problems to keep the rest of the team moving.

Early season training is a time of physical stress. Muscles may be slightly stiff and sore as the dogs come into condition. Dogs progress at different rates, and some require much more training than others. If a dog is progressing more slowly than other dogs in the team, it should be moved into another smaller, slower team until it is more easily able to contribute. This is the time to instill manners and good habits more than commands. Commands to the dogs during this period should be simple and only the most essential. It is important to let the dog—particularly a sensitive one—concentrate on one thing at a time. Once the running has become easy and the dog is in condition, then the commands may become more complicated and expectations more rigorous. This should wait, however, until the dog is running easily and without physical stress.

Sled dogs are taught a variety of commands. At a minimum, all dogs in the team must be taught to stop (Whoa) and go (Hike) on command, to pass by another team or distraction without interruption, and to stand or work in the team without becoming tangled, chewing lines, or bothering an adjacent dog. Because sled dogs are directed by voice command rather than by physical cues, the lead dogs in the team must also know directional commands (Gee for right, Haw for left, and Straight ahead or On by). Depending on a musher's personal needs and desires, other commands may be added to change speed, finish hard at the end of a race, or go "easy" through difficult terrain. Although commands may be taught or reinforced at any time, it is most beneficial for the dogs to get in the habit of doing things right at the beginning of training. It is far easier to spend a little extra time early in the year instilling the proper responses to commands than to undo incorrect or inconsistent behavior later in the season.

Allowing sled dogs to run free and teaching them to come when called builds confidence. Whether the dogs are taught to run free from their houses to the dog truck or the sled, or dropped free for a break when they are traveling in the truck, it will improve their attitude. There are other practical advantages also. It is often very difficult to detect an injury in a dog that is clipped on a short drop chain to a truck or walked on a leash. However, such an injury may be quite easy to see in a dog that is playing around the truck and oblivious to the musher's scrutiny. When dogs are trained to stay near their teammates and truck, losing a dog during the harnessing or hookup process is no longer a worry. The dog can simply be called back to the team.

Rest. The importance of rest is often underestimated in a training schedule. At any time, but particularly during early training, adequate rest is essential. The dogs need time to recover from minor injuries that will occur to poorly conditioned muscles. Their muscles need time to build and rebuild tissue after strenuous training runs. Equally important as the number of times and distance a dog is trained are the number and pattern of the days it has rested. Dogs that become cumulatively tired are more susceptible to injury. They are more likely to develop behavioral problems and be less than enthusiastic about training. Older dogs often need less physical training but more mental rest than young dogs. In contrast, yearling dogs may require additional physical training and recover more quickly from heavy training both mentally and physically. However, because years of experience have not yet tempered youthful enthusiasm, it is possible to overtrain young dogs and not know it until acute problems develop. Overtrained (and overstressed) young dogs are likely to become sick more often and to develop sports (stress) anemia as the season progresses.

Variety. No matter how well rested and healthy dogs are during training, they may still develop attitude problems. This is often a function of boredom. Dogs get tired of doing the same thing on the same trail. Their training regimen should include variety. Dogs should be intentionally trained where they will be exposed to a variety of distractions. The team must be under complete control when taken into these situations, and the situation must be safe for dogs and driver, so that they are positive rather than negative learning experiences.

Foot Problems. Early in the season, dogs may be trained on gravel roads, icy paths, or other trail surfaces that wear the feet. At some point, the frequency of training may be determined by the health of the dogs' feet. Poor trail conditions coupled with too-frequent runs may simply wear the pads and nails to the point that training becomes counterproductive. The feet will toughen as the dogs are run, but worn nails or pads can continue to be a problem if the trail surface is abrasive. Dogs can be booted to protect sore feet, but the life of a boot is very short on dirt and gravel roads. Feet and toenails should be checked regularly during all aspects of training.

Work Ethic. Early season training is the time to teach a group of dogs to function as a team and to work together. Most huskies pull naturally from the time they are first harnessed, but even the most naturally pulling dog must learn to pull even when it is distracted or thinking about other things. The musher must teach a dog that it is expected to work but must watch carefully to ensure that the dog is not asked to do more than it can. For example, the musher may require the dogs to pull the weight of a training vehicle without the assistance of a motor for all or part of the training run. At every stop, the dogs should be required to start the vehicle or sled again without help, thus teaching them to pull together in a coordinated manner. If the terrain is hilly, the dogs should be encouraged to pull up hills without motorized assistance, and enthusiastically congratulated when they succeed. If it is clear that the dogs will not succeed, the musher should give the command to stop. The dogs should not be allowed to stop on their own. Care should be taken not to overdo work to the point that attitude suffers or the dogs hurt themselves.

Speed Development. Early season training is not the time to train for speed. Speed comes when everything else is right. When muscles are strong, bodies conditioned, and aerobic endurance has been developed, then speed will come. Emphasis on speed rather than the ability to work will likely result in a poorly conditioned team that is unable to perform satisfactorily under less than perfect conditions. Cues for more or less speed can be effectively taught during early training by taking advantage of the ability to slow down or speed up at will while using a motorized vehicle. However, maximum speeds should be carefully controlled, especially in young dogs that are very enthusiastic but lack the musculature to support extreme speed. The failure to do so will almost certainly result in injuries to poorly developed front shoulders or to back muscles and may inhibit the dog's ability to perform for the entire race season.

SNOW TRAINING

Early Season. Most mushers look forward to the transition from four-wheeler to sled. The power of the team is no longer absorbed in the frame of the four-wheeler but can be felt through towline and sled. The surge of response as a dog team charges down the trail is exhilarating, and the dogs love it too. But this speed and freedom from the heavy training vehicle can be the start of problems. Early season snow trails are often rough and sometimes icy. The dogs are still learning to find their footing on irregular surfaces, and as the speed increases a simple misstep can precipitate a fall that could injure a dog for weeks. At this time of year, even the most experienced musher is a little rusty driving the sled. This puts additional stress on the dogs, especially those closest to the sled. However, as long as the dogs are moving slowly enough to concentrate on their footing and adjust to irregularities in the trail, these conditions can be beneficial to the dogs. They will learn to pay attention to where they put their feet and to cope with a variety of trail surfaces.

The transition from four-wheeler to sled allows the training distance to increase substantially with little additional effort by the dogs. If the dogs were training 4 miles (6 km) on the four-wheeler, they should easily be able to accomplish 6 to 8 miles (10 to 12 km) pulling a sled. For the first time since very early training, however, the dogs may be limited by aerobic conditioning rather than muscle strength. Dogs pulling a sled will run somewhat faster than they did with the four-wheeler. They may become winded, necessitating stops to catch their breath. The goal is to increase aerobic endurance, but this should not be done by overtiring the dogs. Stops provide an excellent opportunity to go up into the team and praise dogs that are doing particularly well.

Benchmarks. The time the dogs spend running and the regularity with which they are run is far more important than the distance run on a particular day or the total distance per season. Temperature, humidity, and trail conditions greatly affect the amount of work performed on a particular training run, and a driver must always focus on what the dogs are experiencing rather than what the training book says the day's run should be. Performance will not be the same for all dogs on all days. Dogs have good days and bad days, just as mushers do.

The total distance run during a season provides a general guideline by which to measure expectations for a team. It is a guideline only and may vary considerably by dog, depending on age, past training history, and the individual. There are several benchmarks along the way to a fully conditioned and race-ready team. As a general rule, early season (four-wheeler) training should entail 10 to 20 training runs totaling about 50 miles (80 km). Most will be less than 5 miles (8 km). Their purpose is to toughen soft muscles, begin aerobic conditioning, and teach manners and work ethic. By the time the dogs have at least 50 miles (80 km) of training, their muscles should be tough enough (and their manners remembered) so that the transition to sleds is smooth and safe. The next benchmarks come at approximately 100, 300, and 500 miles (160, 480, and 800 km).

Early snow training will entail runs of 6 to 8 miles (10 to 13 km) and generally extend from the time the dogs first begin to pull a sled at about 50 miles (80 km) until they have about 100 miles (160 km) of training. These runs primarily build strong muscles and develop aerobic capacity. By the time adult dogs are trained for 100 miles they reach a first level of conditioning. After this, the dogs are somewhat more resistant to injury, are once again used to the routine of running, and are ready for additional distance and challenges. During the next phase, between 100 and 300 miles (160 and 480 km), distance will be increased from 6 to 8 miles (10 to 13 km) per run to up to 10 to 12 miles (16 to 19 km). Speed may be increased somewhat but should still be carefully controlled. This is the stage in training that will provide the foundation upon which the rest of the season is built. Dogs that are carefully and regularly trained during this period will be ready for whatever additional training the musher decides to do. That may be as diverse as maintaining conditioning and racing distances of 6 to 12 miles (10 to 19 km) or increasing distance and eventually racing 20 miles (32 km) or more. The foundation is basically the same.

Mid Season. Mid-season snow training (usually late October to early December in Alaska) is the time to emphasize aerobic conditioning. The goal is to increase the time that the team can run and work hard without becoming exhausted. Such training is usually characterized by periods of hard work and faster pace interspersed with periods of rest, either through stops or reduced speed. Without some form of repeated burst exercise, it is unlikely that a dog will fully develop its aerobic capacity. It is for this reason that sprint dogs trained for relatively short distances, but in excellent aerobic condition, can be readily adapted to run distances of 50 or more miles (80 km) in a short time. It is far more difficult to move a dog trained for distance into a sprint team, because of both the lack of aerobic capacity to sustain the exertion at top speed and the different musculature developed in training.

Mid-season snow training is the time when work ethic should be engrained. Dogs should be trained in small teams with a heavier training sled to provide control, limit speed, and require that the dogs work. The dogs become accustomed to and comfortable working. If at all possible, some training should take place in hilly terrain where the dogs must work hard and learn that they can pull up moderately steep hills if they work together. With practice, a well-trained team will run steadily and willingly to the top of hills or through deep snow.

Late Season. By the time dogs have been trained for 300 miles (480 km), they should have well-developed muscles, good aerobic capacity, and be ready to perform sustained exercise. At this stage, most dogs should run 10 to 12 miles (16 to 20 km) with ease. It is now time to develop endurance and speed. If the conditioning foundation has been well laid, distance can be increased much more rapidly than it was early in the season. An additional 2 miles (3 km) per week is not unreasonable. The more slowly distance is increased, the less likely the dogs are to slow their pace with the increased distance. It is important to evaluate carefully each dog's need for rest at this time, since some dogs will add distance very easily while others will need time to build to it.

This is the time to allow speed. If the proper foundation has been laid, strength built slowly and steadily, and aerobic fitness adequately developed, speed will follow. Speed can be encouraged by changing to a lighter sled, assisting the dogs by kicking the sled, and adding more dogs to the team. When the dogs run faster, the musher should signal encouragement and approval. If the dogs tire and lack speed at this stage of training, the driver has misjudged their conditioning. They are either being asked to run too far before they are ready or are otherwise not prepared.

Proper training and conditioning are essential for a dog to realize its natural potential to run fast, but a musher cannot change a dog's inherent physical ability. If a dog is physically constrained by poor build, rough gait, or some other physical flaw, it will not be able to run as fast as other dogs, no matter how it is trained. It is the trainer's responsibility to learn to evaluate a dog's ability and to determine its potential for top speed. A driver may not know which is the fastest dog in the team, but it is essential to know which is the slowest and consider this dog in all aspects of training and racing. The dog must be able to trust the musher not to ask it to do more than it can.

Attitude is a good measure of whether training methods are adequately addressing a dog's limitations. Enthusiasm to run is generally one of the best measures of the success of a training program. If a dog becomes unhappy, doesn't want to leave its house, or is reluctant to go to the team, something is amiss. The dog may be tired, injured, asked to do more than it can, or otherwise stressed. Such a dog should be carefully observed in the team, given extra attention, extra rest, and a thorough medical examination to make sure it is physically healthy. Good dogs do not become poor dogs for no reason. The musher must learn to diagnose sore, injured muscles, anemia, and illnesses or infections that translate into behavioral and performance problems.

Almost all demands for particular standards of performance, except for routine team manners, should wait until after the dogs are strong and fit in about late November or early December. It is essential that the driver know that a dog is physically able to perform a task before requesting it. Dogs that are regularly asked to do more than they can will soon learn to distrust their trainer and hold something back at all times just in case more is demanded—or they will simply quit.

The vast majority of all "discipline" should be positive reinforcement. Sled dogs quickly learn to repeat behavior that brings praise. However, when it is necessary to negatively reinforce undesirable behavior, the trainer must be absolutely sure that the dog understands what it has been asked to do. A trainer's failure to communicate properly is no excuse for reprimanding a dog. Willful disobedience may occur in dogs, but it is usually a sign of poor training. If a trainer is inconsistent about whether a particular set of verbal cues is a suggestion or a command, the dogs will also be inconsistent. Before any command is given, the trainer should know what response is expected and within what time frame. The same response must be required every time.

TRAINING PUPS

Training pups is one of the most gratifying parts of owning and training a dog team. Mushers are often asked how they teach or make their puppies run. There is no "make" involved. Sled dog puppies are bred and born to run—they pull in harness as naturally as a Labrador retriever pup chases a ball or an Australian shepherd pup herds the family pets. (But just try to teach a husky pup to retrieve a ball!) The musher's job is to teach the manners and discipline that must accompany the pulling so that the team goes forward in a coordinated, organized manner with lines untangled and harnesses unchewed.

Training begins well before pups are first harnessed. From shortly after birth, pups should be regularly handled and socialized. Ideally they will be exposed to a variety of people. Nothing is better for producing well-adjusted, adaptable dogs than exposure to young children. The more pups are held on their backs, rubbed, and handled, the easier they will be to work with as adults. A pup that has its toes played with when it is small will be easy to check for foot injuries or to put boots on as an adult. A pup that is dressed in doll clothes will be easy to harness. Pups should be exposed to new things. They should be allowed to run around the dog yard (under supervision), go for walks, come in the house, or ride in the truck. The more new things pups encounter when they are young, the more confident they will be in new situations as adults. Pups should learn to learn when they are young so that learning becomes a habit.

Although often considered by mushers to be unnecessary, and certainly time consuming to teach, standard obedience commands such as Come, Sit, Down, and Stay, as well as house training, are all useful in the context of dog mushing. Whatever commands are taught to puppies should be taught gently and with far more positive than negative reinforcement. Pups are so impressionable and so eager to please that almost any lesson can be taught with very little negative feedback. Positive feedback should take a variety of forms—petting, play behavior, verbal praise, or a snack. This same sequence of praise can then be used when the dog is an adult in the dog team.

There is no set age at which sled dog pups should first be harnessed, but it should occur in the first year. Pups may be harnessed as young as 4 to 5 months, if the musher goes slowly and does not expect too much too soon. Timing will vary according to the pace at which particular breeds mature, personality of the individual pups, the time of year the pups were born, and when the musher has the time available to work with pups. A pup that is harnessed at 5 months and does not pull may simply not be ready. If a pup is harnessed two or three times and is still frightened, it may be necessary to wait a month—or more—before trying again. Just because a pup does not pull at first does not mean it will fail as a sled dog. Dogs mature at different paces. Some dogs never really do much as pups but are outstanding as early-season yearlings. The more a musher is familiar with a particular breed of dogs, the easier it is to interpret this pup behavior.

When pups are first harnessed, things should be set up to go right. Harness-breaking should occur on a good trail with good leaders and a patient musher. The first time a pup is run in harness, it should be placed in a small team, usually with two or three other pups and at least two well-behaved, strong adults to get them going. Ideally the musher will have at least one helper to untangle jumping, squirming pups that do not know whether they should go forward or backward. The first runs should be quite short, often just a mile or two, with several stops to pet and reassure the pups that everything is OK. Pups learn remarkably fast from experience and from other dogs. If they are placed in the team with well-behaved adults that pass well, run across overflow ice or through puddles, and do not jump and scream, the puppies will also learn these manners. If things go right the first time, there is increasing likelihood that they will continue to go right. Similarly, pups that are run with rowdy, poorly behaved adults will develop all of the same bad habits. It requires hard work to undo bad habits learned by careless training. It may take many repetitions to undo bad behavior learned in one disorganized moment. Consequently it is important to train pups with the best possible leaders.

Pups should always be run in circumstances in which the musher has complete control. Teams should be small enough so that each pup is required to work steadily and so that the musher can stop and anchor the sled ("hook down") at any time. There should be enough adults in the team to ensure forward momentum, but not so many that the speed is too great.

No matter how good or how maturely a pup acts, the musher must always remember that it is still a pup. Pups are capable of many things but must not be pressured to perform. There is no reason why pups cannot run in lead, learn to pass, and learn other basic commands. However, their attention span is short, and they tire easily. A pup team will respond wonderfully to regular training. Pups, like adults, can be run three or four times a week. For the first month or so, runs should be 1 to 3 miles (2 to 5 km). After that, distance can be increased gradually until the pups are running 5 to 7 miles (8 to 11 km), depending on age and maturity. If the pups get tired during a longer run, the driver should simply stop and rest for a few minutes. This is an ideal time to teach pups that stopping is a good experience and to encourage good manners during stops. With such a schedule, pups that are harnessed in October or November may have 300 miles (480 km) or more of training by spring.

As long as pups are run with other pups of similar age and size, and there are not more than one or two adults in the team, speed is usually not a problem. The pups will run at a speed that is comfortable for them. This is especially true when team size is kept small. If training is done in a hilly area where speed downhill may be too great for some of the pups, the driver should watch carefully and slow the team so that all pups are comfortable. Too much speed too soon can frighten pups and make them worry about running fast, even as adults.

AGE AND TRAINING

Yearlings. Most mushers owning a modest number of dogs do not have the luxury of strictly segregating dogs by age class during training and racing. They must blend the young and the old with prime-age dogs to create their team. Consequently it is necessary to understand how physical ability and mental toughness are affected by age and to build these factors into a training and racing program. There are periods during training, particularly early in the year, when the differences between yearlings and adults or adults and ''senior'' appear minimal. It is easy to believe this apparent equality will persist. If age is subsequently ignored as a factor in training, it will likely lead to poor performance in both young and old dogs and to an increased incidence of injuries and illness.

During four-wheeler and early sled training, runs are short. Yearling dogs, full of energy and enthusiasm, often excel. They recover quickly from these short runs and are enthusiastic about training again soon. Because speed is carefully controlled during this period, the young dogs are not stressed by running with older, more physically capable animals. It is easy to confuse this early season exuberance with true conditioning, endurance, and toughness.

The first indication that adolescent dogs are not as tough as they feel often comes with the transition to sleds, when distance and speed are increased and the trail becomes more challenging. For the first time, yearlings may become tired and somewhat insecure. If they are treated with care, this phase should pass quickly as the young dogs become more confident on the trail and familiar with the routine. The degree to which this occurs, if at all, depends a great deal on their training as pups. If they were trained regularly and learn to encounter new situations and succeed, it is likely that yearlings will sail through early sled training with ease. Nonetheless, it is necessary to increase distance and speed more slowly than for adults. While adults may proceed quite quickly from 6 to 8 to 10 miles, it may take additional runs and several weeks to a month longer for the yearlings to make these same increases. Training yearlings for an extra day every week or two can help to increase toughness. Always, however, this must be balanced by the need for adequate rest.

The differences between yearlings and adults are usually most apparent in the 300- to 500-mile (480 to 800 km) range, or about January. By 300 miles the adults are quite tough. They have built on a muscle base developed in previous years and are thoroughly familiar with the routine. The increased intensity of training and the demands for additional speed, distance, and response to driver cues are familiar and expected. For yearlings, however, this is a time of stress. Their bodies are not yet as tough as those of adults. Many yearlings require about 500 miles (800 km) of training to achieve the toughness attained by adults in 300 miles (480 km). The first races of the year usually occur in late December or January, when adults are adequately conditioned and tough but when the yearlings may not be quite ready. Consequently the yearlings may be performing near the limits of their ability, while the adults are well within their comfort range. Young dogs may worry about whether they are performing satisfactorily, which

aggravates stress. This is the most common time for young dogs to develop stress anemia. The most important tool for dealing with yearlings is patience. It is necessary to take the long view and to give young dogs adequate time to develop. Yearlings that are not able to run with the adult team may be outstanding dogs by the time they are 2 or 3 years old.

For all dogs, but particularly for young dogs, training should be enjoyable. A trainer should take the time to reward the dogs by petting, verbal reinforcement, or play behavior for a job well done. A young dog must also learn to trust its trainer. The dog must know that the musher will not ask more than the dog can give and that the musher will help it through difficult situations. The seeds of this trust should be planted when the dog is a pup and nurtured as it grows older, but especially during the yearling training year. An insecure dog should be held, reassured, complimented on its performance, and encouraged when it is asked to perform a difficult task. Special one-on-one time with a young dog, when it is not in harness and not being trained, can be one of the most effective ways to alleviate stress and build trust and confidence.

Veterans. In today's world of improved nutrition and veterinary care, it is not uncommon for dogs that are 7, 8, or even 9 years old to race in competitive sprint teams. However, like young dogs, these veterans require special attention and care. Older dogs that have been well trained all of their adult lives need less training to come into and maintain condition than do younger dogs. Too many training miles may diminish their interest and cause them to ''sour.'' For many older dogs, maintaining attitude and interest is far more challenging than maintaining good condition. Attitude can often be improved by added days of rest, occasional short runs on new trails, and extra personal attention. Extra care should be taken to ensure that older dogs are not overweight and that their diet is suited to their age. Some older dogs may develop mineral or vitamin deficiencies that can be remedied by simple, inexpensive dietary supplements. Many older dogs develop some slight stiffness in legs and back when they first get up or when they come out of their dog box. Care should be taken to limber up these dogs before they race, either by massage or light exercise.

Most older dogs are less enthusiastic about running at top speed than they were as youngsters. They may hold back at high speed or on downhill sections of a trail. However, they are also incredibly tough and seemingly tireless. A good musher must learn to observe carefully, accommodate these differences in pace, and balance the team so that the differences become a strength rather than a weakness. During training, care should be taken to put these older dogs in slower teams so that they are not continually stressed. They are likely to be willing to run fast during races if they are not also required to run at top speed during every training run. It is particularly useful to run these veteran dogs in mixed teams with yearlings, which should also run somewhat slower during training. These older dogs know the commands for speed control, have good passing and stopping habits, and in general are exactly what the musher desires in a race dog. When trained with the younger dogs, these veterans will teach almost all of the basic commands and manners with surprisingly little input required from the musher!

Many older race dogs do not seem to enjoy training but still enjoy racing. They may pull halfheartedly in training, yet become the pacesetters in a race. It is the musher's job to understand these attitudinal differences and insist on performance when it is necessary, not simply on principle. The dogs do understand the difference. If a musher is unwilling to compromise, it is likely that the dog may simply decide to retire as a useful race dog. Most veteran race dogs develop minds of their own. They become far more opinionated about what they will and will not do, and about how promptly and which commands they choose to obey. Although these dogs cannot be allowed to forget all of their manners and discipline, it is likely that a middle ground can be reached where age has some privileges but the basic rules are obeyed.

LEADER TRAINING

Truly exceptional leaders are born with the mental and physical potential necessary to lead a winning dog team. However, no matter how much natural aptitude a young leader possesses, it must be nutured and developed with care to ensure that the dog reaches its full potential. A truly gifted young leader can be spoiled by inappropriate expectations and poor timing. Developing leaders is one of the most challenging and gratifying parts of training sled dogs, but like almost all other aspects of training, it requires patience, consistency, and thorough familiarity with the strengths and weaknesses of the dog.

Leaders come in all varieties, and thus there is no set formula for when and how to train a dog to run up front. Until a dog is at least 3 or 4 years old, it is generally a good idea to try it in front of the team at least several times a year to determine whether it is willing to run in lead. Yearlings that do not have the confidence to run in lead, often because their bodies are not yet fully developed and running is not as easy as it is for the adults, may be competent leaders at age 2. Alternatively, some dogs that run comfortably in lead as puppies or yearlings in slower teams may not be happy later when they must run in front of a race team.

Pups. Pups may be tried in lead within the first few runs after they are harnessed, so long as it is done carefully and with a well-behaved adult leader. Some pups naturally run up front. From the first day they are placed in lead, they look straight ahead, are resistant to distractions, seem comfortable with other dogs behind them, and run and pull whenever the team is under way. More commonly, pups in lead for the first time will look over their shoulders, turn around, and try to come back into the team. If the adult leader is confident and assertive, the pup will usually start down the trail. Many of these pups will learn to be comfortable in lead. The more they do it, the more accustomed they become to being in front, and the less likely they are to turn around. The better behaved the leader next to it, the better behaved the pup will be.

If a young, newly harnessed pup is comfortable running up front, it may be allowed to do so. Such a pup should never be pushed too hard or expected to have the manners of an adult. If a pup is run in lead, the trainer must make sure it is regularly praised and never pressured. The pup should gently be taught basic trail manners, but most of its early education should be left to the adult leader running with it. Puppies trained with seasoned adults will quickly learn to pass other teams, run across ice or flowing water, cross roads, and ignore distractions. However, any bad habits the adult leader has will be just as quickly transferred to the pup, and it will take the trainer much time and effort to erase these bad habits. If the leaders available for puppy training are not very well behaved, it is probably better not to train young pups in lead with them, unless the musher is willing to live with the bad habits they transmit.

Yearlings. Early season training is an excellent time to try yearlings in lead. After the first few runs, when the dogs have had a chance to remember their manners and get used to the routine, yearlings may be harnessed in front of small teams. They should be placed with a well-trained, confident adult to ensure that things go smoothly. The relatively slow pace used during four-wheeler training allows the young dog to concentrate solely on the demands of being in lead. The almost total control afforded by a four-wheeler makes it possible to teach manners such as starting and stopping, increasing or decreasing speed, and to a lesser extent, turning.

When training leaders, it is essential for the musher to ensure that it is no less pleasant for a dog to be in lead than in the team. Running in lead should not mean more discipline, more stress, more nagging, and fewer pets. If a dog hears only praise when it runs in the team, then moves into lead and is constantly corrected, it will associate being in lead with more stress. It will soon learn to do whatever is necessary to be taken out of lead and placed back in the team where life is fun and easy. The musher must make running in lead a special job that brings special praise. A leader should never be taken for granted. It should be singled out for attention and always told when it does the right thing. For all but the most exceptional dogs, being in lead does bring extra responsibility and stress, and there must be extra reward to make it worthwhile.

Some dogs will run in lead day in and day out, during training and racing, for their entire lives. For these special dogs, being anywhere else in the team is not relief but punishment. They belong in lead. Most leaders, however, need occasional rest. This may be because of cumulative stress, illness, or a heavy racing schedule. It is important for the trainer to anticipate the need for rest before the leaders balk or misbehave in lead. These dogs may hold back when being led to the team or turn around or come back into the team when they are hooked up. Leaders that are allowed to run free during hookup may show stress by refusing to run to the front of the team to be hooked up, standing in the middle of the team, or running back to the truck even when called. If at all possible, dogs in this condition should not be placed in lead but rotated back into the team for the needed rest and relief. Usually they will be ready to go back in lead within a few runs. If there is no other choice but to run such a dog in lead, it should receive extra praise and encouragement, and as little pressure as possible. It may be necessary to shorten or skip several training runs, run smaller teams (dogs can count!), adjust the diet, check for illness, and generally reexamine one's training schedule to determine what is causing the stress.

Leader training in some form can occur during all phases of training. However, intensive leader training (teaching commands) should occur only after the dogs are in condition. A dog should not be expected to concentrate on learning commands at the same time it has sore muscles from working hard to get into shape.

RACING

By the time the racing season begins, basic conditioning and training should be complete. Training distances may increase as race distances increase, and response to commands may be fine-tuned, but the foundation upon which race performance is built should be in place before serious racing begins. Because it takes less exercise to maintain conditioning than to build it, the dogs may need to be run only 3 days a week rather than the 4 more common during training. The musher should concentrate on variety and rest (for body and mind). Races themselves provide some diversity, but it is also important to seek out new trails and new situations to keep things interesting and enjoyable for dogs and musher. The dogs must have adequate rest both before and after a race. As a general rule in sprint competitions, the team should be rested 1 day before and after the race for each day of racing.

Racing and training must not be confused. Races are generally more stressful for the dogs than training, and a musher must take care to not make racing miserable. Racing should be accompanied by some extra reward such as extra attention or an extra treat. Training should not occur during a race. The musher must live with whatever habits (good or bad) that have been instilled beforehand. Similarly the musher must not "race" during training. Training during the race season should be enjoyable and as stress free as possible to avoid aggravating the unavoidable stress of racing itself. A dog team should never be pushed to its limit during training.

MUSHER AND DOG BOND

Ultimately the success or failure of a musher depends on how well he or she understands each dog in the team and accommodates its individual needs, and the ability to develop trust and confidence in each and every dog. There must be teamwork between musher and dogs. A musher must have clear, consistent expectations, and the dogs must be praised and rewarded when they meet these expectations. There should be an abundance of positive reinforce-

ment and a minimum amount of discipline. The best dog drivers and their teams are bound by a bond of respect, trust, and affection.

Suggested Readings

Collins M, Collins J: Dog Driver: A Guide for the Serious Musher. Loveland, Colo, Alpine Publications, 1991.
Dogs of the North. Alaska Geographic 14:1, 1987.
Høe-Raitto M, Kaynor C: Skijor with Your Dog. Fairbanks, Alaska, OK Publishing, 1991.
Levorsen B (ed): Mush! A Beginner's Manual of Sled Dog Training. Westmoreland, NY, American Publications, Inc, 1976.
Welch J: The Speed Mushing Manual. Eagle River, Alaska, Sirius Publishing, 1989, 127 pp.

SECTION X

DRUGS AND MEDICATIONS: QUALITY ASSURANCE/TESTING PROGRAMS

CHAPTER 45

DRUG TESTING IN SPORTING DOGS

A. MORRIE CRAIG

HISTORY OF DRUG TESTING IN ANIMALS

The use of drugs or other perceived performance enhancers in athletic events is as old as history itself. Romans could be crucified for using a mixture of honey and water called hydromel. However, suspecting and proving "doping" remained without scientific basis until Russian chemist Bukowski demonstrated in 1910 that it was possible to detect drugs in a horse's saliva. A Professor Frankel in Vienna confirmed Bukowski's findings, and the science of using analytical chemistry for drug testing for compounds such as strychnine, morphine, cocaine, and caffeine was born. The first animal disqualified for doping was a horse named Bourbon Rose who won the French Gold Cup at Maisons Lafitte in 1912. In the United States in the early 1940s, the greyhound was the first sporting dog in this country to undergo this surveillance.

Prior to 1932 in the United States, betting on races was legal in only eight states, but a law passed in that year expanded legalized racing and betting to another 20 states, which increased interest in keeping racing honest. In response, the Florida Racing Commission sent a veterinarian, Dr. Catlett, and a chemist, Dr. Morgan, to France to learn the new saliva-testing techniques and to bring them back to America. From these humble beginnings, drug testing came to America. From 1932 to 1947, a number of racing laboratories were set up across the United States and Canada to do routine testing of race horses. Testing initially focused on saliva, but urine and blood were later found to be more effective substances in which to test for drugs. In 1947, the Association of Official Racing Chemists (AORC) came into being. This group, in conjunction with each state's racing commissioners, serves as the monitor of performance animals.

While there are varying laws as to which legitimate medications, if any, can be used in horse racing, greyhounds are required by laws throughout the United States and most of the world to race "drug free." Still followed in Ireland is an age-old custom of allowing greyhounds tea prior to a race, which results in trace levels of caffeine and its metabolites in their urine. This, however, is a unique situation in the world of greyhound racing. In the United States there are some complications to enforcement of this drug-free law in greyhounds that will be discussed in the section, Inadvertent Drugs.

Drug testing for sled dog racing began only in the last 4 years, starting with the famous Alaskan Iditarod race. The officials of the Iditarod Racing Committee decided that a drug-testing program was needed to ensure fair competition and to forestall possible critics of this arduous race. Sled dogs are allowed certain medications to care for them over this long, 1200-mile endurance race. However, those medications are restricted by the race committee, and no known performance-enhancement drugs are allowed. Official drug testing of sled dog races throughout the world is increasing. Table 45–1 lists the sled dog events currently being monitored for drugs.

CRUCIAL FACTORS IN SETTING UP A DRUG-TESTING PROGRAM

Currently in the United States there are two ways of drug testing sporting dogs. For greyhound racing where there is public pari-mutuel wagering, there are state regulations with appointed racing commissioners trying to guarantee a "level playing field." The commissioners are responsible for collecting samples with a proper chain of evidence and contracting with a racing laboratory for sample analysis. Results are sent to the commission veterinarians and stewards, the latter of which level the appropriate penalty for

383

TABLE 45–1. Sled Dog Races Being Monitored for Drug Use in the 1996–97 Racing Season

Iditarod	Alaska, USA
Yukon Quest	Alaska, USA
Caribou Classic	Northwest Territories, Canada
Can-Am 300	USA
Race to the Sky	Montana, USA
John Beargrease Sled Dog Marathon	Minnesota, USA
World Sled Dog Spring Championship	New York, USA
European Championship	Europe
Upper Zoo	Michigan, USA
Stage Stop	Wyoming, USA
Open North American	Alaska, USA
Kusko	Alaska, USA

"positives." Appeals of these decisions are handled by the state's racing commissioners, and if need be, final appeals can go through civil courts. Fines and penalties are often part of legislated laws of the state.

In contrast, in private sporting organizations the organizing committee needs (1) to decide which, if any, drugs are allowed; (2) to establish collection, storage, and transport procedures that will support an unbroken "chain of evidence" that will withstand legal scrutiny; and (3) to determine the penalties to be levied against offenders. These penalties may include public identification of dogs with drug-positive tests, elimination of dogs from future contests, and withholding of purses. There may be conflict within a sporting organization regarding the need for drug testing. There may be members who believe that there are no problems and that the organization committee is over-reacting to a few accusations. There may be other individuals threatening to leave the sport because they believe that some dogs have "unfair" advantages as a result of drug use. Once the organization has a consensus, they can establish a drug-testing program in conjunction with one of the official racing laboratories in the United States.

DRUG-TESTING METHODS

In the United States there are a number of drug-testing laboratories with AORC-certified racing chemists that contract with state officials or private canine sporting clubs to test participants in athletic events. While most of these are commercial companies, there are several universities with personnel, often in the veterinary college faculty, that provide this service to the industry. Examples would be the University of Connecticut and the veterinary colleges in Iowa, Louisiana, and New York (Cornell). The Racing Commissioners International (RCI), which is the official organization for coordination of efforts between state racing commissions, has strived to promote uniform drug testing in the United States, but the final authority rests with each state's officials. The result of this is that different laboratories bid for drug-testing contracts, offering specific levels of testing relative to the degree of financial commitment being considered. The basic philosophy in American USA greyhound racing is to test one to three greyhounds per race for every race in a day's program. This method of testing results in many samples being collected and forwarded each day to the testing laboratory. This is in marked contrast to the philosophy of drug testing in Australia, in which samples may be taken from one to two greyhounds from the entire racing program.

The handling of large numbers of samples necessitates rapid drug-screening methods in the initial testing of samples. Two independent surveys in 1994 found that thin-layer chromatography (TLC) and immunoassays were the number one and two, respectively, drug-testing methods used for screening urine in racing greyhounds throughout the world.[1, 2] A suspected positive finding is then confirmed by gas chromatography/mass spectrometry (GC/MS) or other highly sophisticated chromatography methods. An overview of these drug-testing methods is useful in understanding why a drug can sometimes be missed and why trace amounts of legitimate medications can be found days after administration when their therapeutic effects have long ceased.

Thin-Layer Chromatography. This is the most common drug screen used in the United States and throughout many drug-testing laboratories in the world. It is a chromatographic technique that uses a glass plate covered with a thin silicon layer. Urine samples undergo one or more liquid extraction techniques to selectively compartmentalize any drugs present into an organic phase. The extracted material is then spotted onto the bottom of the TLC plate (origin) in minute amounts (Fig. 45–1). Multiple urine samples can be tested along the horizontal length of one TLC plate, as well as pure drug standards that serve as controls. Once drug extracts have been spotted on the plate, the plate is then placed into a developing tank with a small amount of solvent on the bottom (Fig. 45–2; see Fig. 45–1). Any drugs contained in the extracted sample are separated by a rising liquid solvent front according to a variety of physical characteristics of the drug. The TLC plates are then sprayed with one or more chemicals to make the drugs visible by

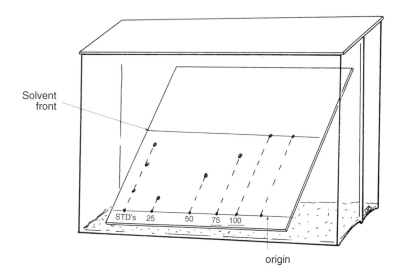

FIGURE 45–1. Schematic of a urine-extract-spotted TLC plate in a developing tank. Note the solvent rising on the plate (solvent front) and different relative separation (R_f) of different drugs.

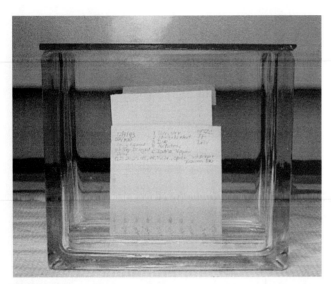

FIGURE 45–2. A TLC plate in a development tank with the solvent front approximately halfway up the plate. Spots of extracted urine can be seen at the lower section of the plate.

specific colors on the plate. The height to which a drug separates from the initial spotting site on the plate is measured and defined as the R_f value. These values are unique and characteristic of individual drugs and can be compared to the R_f values of concurrently run or known drug standards. Any spot that can be chemically detected on the TLC plate can be "scraped off" and subjected to futher analysis for identification by the more sensitive and specific GC/MS.

The advantages of TLC are its relative quickness and capability to test many samples at low cost, which is often essential when screening large numbers of samples. Several different extraction procedures are required for each urine sample to isolate basic, neutral, and acidic drugs. Some drugs are protein bound in the urine, and these often need to undergo an enzyme hydrolysis step to be detected. The disadvantage of TLC as a screening method is that low concentrations of potent drugs, eg, narcotics, may be missed because with this chromatographic technique it is difficult to detect drugs below concentrations of 0.05 µg/ml. In addition, there are some drugs that simply will be missed with TLC screening. As a consequence, racing chemists have developed the more sensitive immunoassays to detect many of these drugs.

Immunoassays for Drug Screening. Immunoassays all use drug-specific antibodies obtained from serum of drug–sensitized experimental animals to attach to any of that drug present in the urine sample. Enzyme-linked immunosorbent assay (ELISA) is the most commonly used immunoassay in racing laboratories. These assays are used to identify potent and hard to detect drugs, especially narcotics, steroids, and bronchodilators. Common use of ELISA is to *target* specific drugs in certain time periods to determine if any usage is occurring, since racing jurisdictions could not logically afford to run all of the ELISA tests on every urine sample.

Gas Chromatography/Mass Spectrometry (GC/MS) Confirmation. GC/MS is a sophisticated analytical tool that determines a molecular "fingerprint" of suspect compounds in urine (Fig. 45–3). There are 700,000 compounds known to organic chemists; GC/MS can individually identify each one. The judicial system has recognized GC/MS as giving irrefutable evidence of the identity of a drug. For this reason, all the suspected drug positives with TLC or ELISA screening techniques must be confirmed with GC/MS. Figure 45–4 is a GC/MS chromatogram for the drug flunixin meglumine (Banamine).

CLASSIFICATION OF DRUGS

While there are many ways to classify all the known drugs, from pharmacological action to molecular structure, in racing and performance animals a breakdown of drugs into the following categories is a highly workable method for racing authorities: (1) performance-altering drugs, (2) legitimate medications and/or their residues, (3) inadvertent drugs from feed or environmental sources, and (4) masking agents.

Performance-Altering Drugs. Performance-altering drugs, whether stimulants to enhance performance, depressants or tranquilizers to diminish performance, narcotics and analgesics to reduce or mask painful lesions, or mood enhancers, all attempt to directly affect the athletic performance of the dog. Use of drugs to reduce performance has its greatest potential for abuse when people wager on the outcome of the event, as occurs with pari-mutuel betting in racing greyhounds. Dogs with painful lesions that would reduce performance should not be in competition until the problems are resolved. The other types of stimulant or performance-enhancing drugs run counter to the essence of the sport in which the wish is for the best dog or dog team to win on its own inherent abilities.

Legitimate Medications. Legitimate medications may be needed at times for the proper medical care of racing or performance injuries or stress-related problems of canine athletes. By law, these medications must be cleared from the greyhound prior to racing. In sled dogs, use of select medications is permitted; any medications not on the approved list must be cleared from the dog's system.

It is this concept of "clearance" that can result in dilemmas for both the racing authorities and the dog owners/trainers. Theoretically, once a medication is put into the body, its pharmacological elimination is an exponential function, and in theory, never reaches zero. However, current clearance times are based on that time when the drug or its metabolites can no longer be detected by the analytical chemists in samples of fluids from the animal, most commonly urine in dogs. Thus, clearance times depend on the sensitivity of the analyst's assay for that medication, and these vary between analysts and are often relative to the type of analytical assay being used to detect the drug. TLC can detect levels of drugs in the 0.05 µg/ml range, while immunoassays can detect nanogram (10^{-9}) and smaller drug concentrations. The problems that can result when immunoassays are used to detect residues of legitimate medications comprise one of the major controversial issues in racing today in both the greyhound and horse racing industries. Minute levels of these medications or their metabolites may be present and detected by these very sensitive techniques. However, based on pharmacological data, the therapeutic or physiological effects of these medications at these residual levels are long past. Flunixin meglumine can be used as a good example. This nonsteroidal anti-inflammatory drug is commonly used to treat muscle soreness or traumatic injuries from falls or collisions. Analytical chemists can now detect traces of this medication in urine with immunoassay at 10^{-9} parts, a level that is still present in urine 72 hours post administration. The pharmacological data for flunixin meglumine cites 3.7 hours as the half life in dogs. Pharmacologists often recommend the general rule of 7 times the half-life as an estimate for drug clearance time in animals. With flunixin meglumine, this would be 25.9 hours. Thus, there is a threefold difference between analytical detection limits and theoretical clearance times and an even wider discrepancy between time of pharmacological effect and detection time in urine with immunoassays.

Clearance times have been studied in racing greyhounds and published by the American Greyhound Council in the text *Care of the Racing Greyhound*.[3] These approximate withdrawal times were determined using the current TLC screening methods at Harris

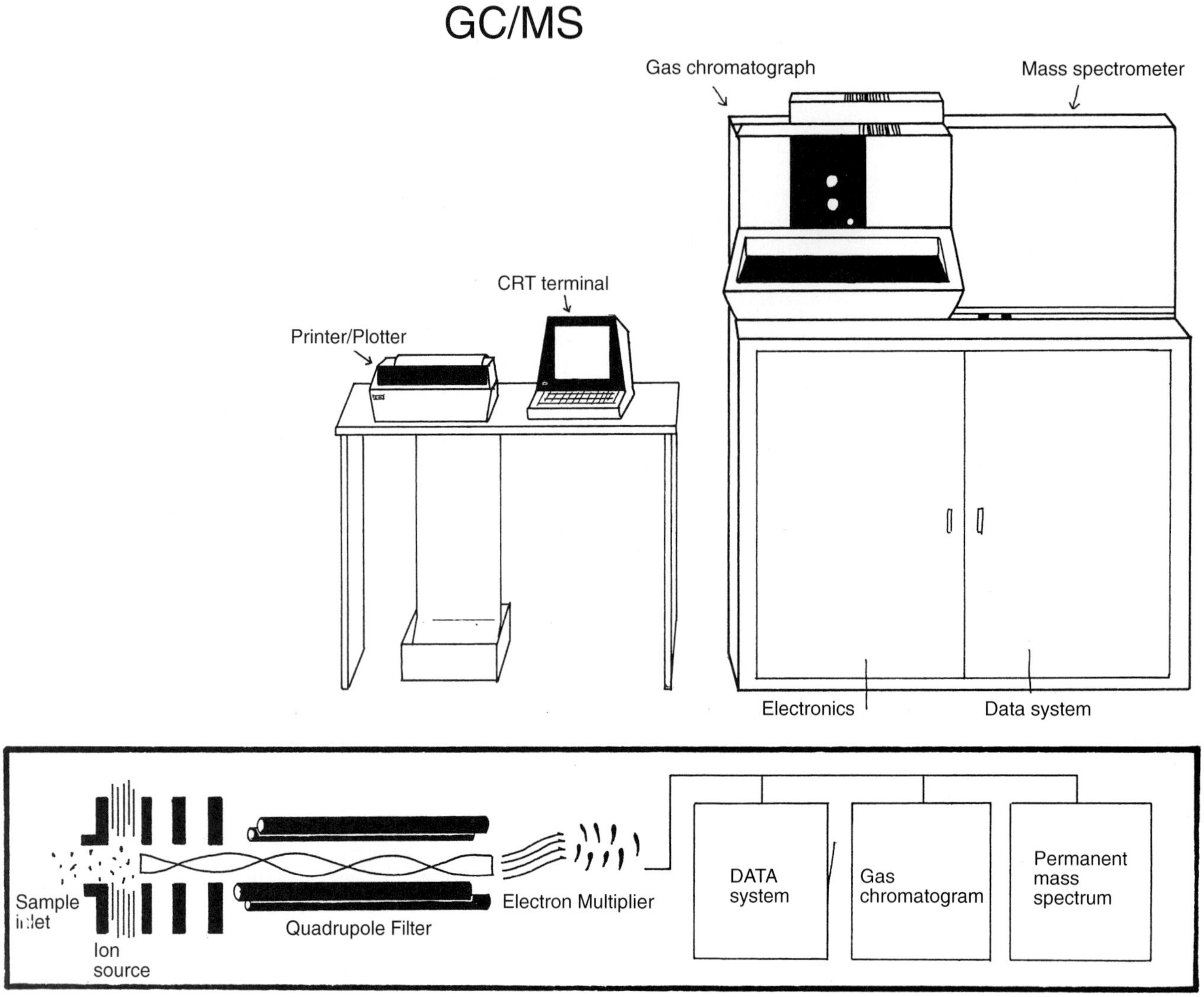

GC/MS

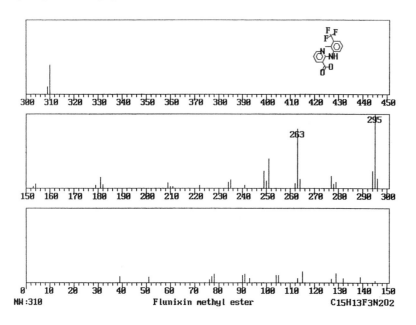

FIGURE 45–3. Schematic of a gas chromatograph/mass spectrometer (GC/MS) instrument. In the bottom box, one sees how drug molecules are separated by the gas chromatograph.

FIGURE 45–4. GC/MS chromatogram of flunixin meglumine (Banamine).

Laboratories, Inc., and at my laboratory. If more sensitive detection methods are applied to these legitimate medications, then problems can be anticipated.

This dilemma of detection sensitivity vs pharmacological or physiological activity when the drug in question is a legitimate medication is a serious one for regulators, trainers, and veterinarians. In Australia, this problem is circumvented by the racing jurisdictions working with the analytical laboratories to set threshold levels of detection for legitimate medications, below which "positives" are not reported. Racing authorities in the United States are currently addressing this problem at the national level.

Inadvertent Drugs. Medications or drugs inadvertently present in natural feed sources of racing animals have recently come to the forefront in horse racing with detection of hordenine from sprouting barley and scopolamine in alfalfa hay. However, this problem of inadvertent drugs in food has been a major controversy in greyhound racing for the past 10 years. Procaine from procaine penicillin and sulfonamides are both very common antibiotic residues in the meat fed to greyhounds. Class 4-D meat, from commercial sources, which originates primarily from cattle that were diseased, disabled, dying, or dead, often is contaminated with residues of procaine. Surveys across the United States have identified percentages of procaine-positive meat ranging between 31 and 49 per cent.[3] Sulfa antibiotics are common contaminants of poultry that is fed to greyhounds.

The crises over antibiotic residues began when a new ion pair extraction procedure for TLC chromatography was introduced in racing laboratories testing greyhound urine.[4] It became evident that this assay was particularly sensitive in the detection of procaine on TLC screens, as many states began reporting an increasing number of positives for traces of procaine. Procaine can be classified as a stimulant and as a local anesthetic, but the drug would have to be present in very high doses to be effective for the former and given very close to the time of the race to be effective as the latter. In fact, utilization of procaine hydrochloride subcutaneously over a nerve as an anesthetic agent was effective for only approximately half an hour in experiments I conducted on greyhounds. Thus the use of procaine in any nefarious manner would be highly unlikely.

Trainers have no way of telling which meat has antibiotic residues and have resorted to altering their feeding of meat to avoid any possible chance of a positive drug test. Studies have shown that if greyhounds ate low levels of procaine in contaminated meat, it would take up to 36 hours to clear 100 per cent of the procaine from the dogs. With most greyhounds racing twice a week to three times every 2 weeks, this change of diet to avoid trace positives of antibiotic residues is a major dietary disruption and not in the best interest of the dogs. Then there is also the possibility of the greyhound eating meat from an injection site, which would result in considerably higher levels of procaine in the urine, since each milliliter of procaine penicillin contains 246 mg of procaine. Some state officials have partially resolved this dilemma by setting threshold levels for procaine, below which they do not penalize the trainer. However, this does not have universal acceptance, and greyhound trainers have to be aware of each state's rules in this regard. Work is ongoing at the national level to reduce the impact of traces of drugs known to be contaminants of feed in both horses and dogs.

Masking Agents. Analysts utilizing TLC drug-testing screening methods can have problems when certain chemical compounds are present in the animal's urine. Polyethylene glycol (PEG), thiabendazole worming medications, and vitamin B_1 are examples of compounds that can interfere with or mask an illicit drug. Chemists used to solve this interference by utilizing different extraction techniques and solvent and spray development to detect possible hidden drugs. However, with the advent of ELISA immunoassay techniques, masking agents are far less of an analytical problem.

References

1. Dyke TM, Sams RA: Analytical methods used by racing laboratories: An international survey. Proceedings, 10th International Conference of Racing Analysts and Veterinarians. Stockholm, July 1994. R & W Publications Ltd, Newmarket, Suffolk, 344–347.
2. Hill DW: Tests used in greyhound urine drug screening in 1994. Proceedings, 48th Meeting Assoc of Official Racing Chemists. Oklahoma City, April 1995.
3. Blythe LL, Gannon JR, Craig AM: Care of the Racing Greyhound: A Guide for Trainers, Breeders and Veterinarians. American Greyhound Council, Abilene, Kan, 1994.
4. Hill DW, Kelley TR, Matiuck SW, et al: Single extraction for recovery of basic, neutral and weakly acidic drugs from greyhound dog urine. Anal Letters. 15(B2):193–204, 1982.

CHAPTER 46

DRUG CONTROL PROGRAMS IN CANINE SPORTS MEDICINE

JAMES R. GANNON

Charles Dickens immortalized the first Artful Dodger in the tale of Oliver Twist in 1837. This character lives on in the hearts and souls of those who would seek to use illicit drugs to modify performance, or use regular medications to modify behavior, in the hope of influencing the outcome of a sporting event or competition. Administrators of such events and competitions, when seeking to punish the transgressors and deter the tempted, must introduce an effective drug control program. This requires a precise and comprehensive set of regulations and the services of a laboratory competent in drug detection chemistry.

DRUG DEFINITION

The first step in the introduction of the drug control program and the formulation of its rules involves defining what a "drug" is for the purposes of that particular sport. While there is a pervading philosophy worldwide that all athletes—human, equine, or canine—must be presented for competition drug free, there is remarkable variation in the definition of what constitutes a drug. This ranges from "a chemical medicine or substance that may affect or may be capable of affecting the speed, stamina, courage, or conduct of a contestant" to the most comprehensive Australian definition, namely:

a. Any substance capable of affecting a contestant by its action on the central or peripheral nervous system or any part of that system (such as the autonomic nervous system), cardiovascular system, respiratory system, alimentary digestive system, musculoskeletal system or genitourinary system and includes without limitation analgesics, antihistamines, anti-inflammatory agents, blood coagulants, diuretics, hormones and their synthetic counterparts, stimulants, corticosteroids, anabolic steroids, local anesthetics, muscle relaxants, tranquilizers, and antibiotics.

b. Substances administered to disguise or make undetectable, or attempt to disguise or make undetectable, the administration of any of the substances referred to in paragraph *a.*

c. A metabolite or artifact of any of the substances referred to in paragraphs *a* and *b*, irrespective of whether such metabolite or artifact has any pharmacological effect.

d. Unusual or abnormal amounts of endogenous substances including but not limited to cortisol and testosterone; or

e. Any substance specified in Schedules 1–8 (inclusive) of the Drugs, Poisons and Controlled Substances Act.

There is no rule or regulation that prevents, or is intended to prevent, the use any registered therapeutic substance for the treatment of illness or injury in a competitor of a sporting event. The only stipulation is that the competitor must be drug free when presented for the event.

PURPOSE OF DRUG CONTROL

The first purpose is to maintain the credibility and image of the sporting activity. In the racing industry there is enormous pressure

on the gambling dollar, which is being spread over casinos, lotteries, slot machines, and between the equine and canine codes. In the show ring and other canine sporting venues, there is equal pressure to gain the glory and financial benefits that come from winning. Any sporting event tarnished by drug abuse soon loses its supporters and followers.

Second, the welfare of the competing dog should receive top priority. Animals requiring medication to mask pain or modify behavior during events represent an unacceptable risk to the other contestants as well as to themselves, because there is no way of verifying the effectiveness of the medication employed.

Third, a drug control program is essential for protection of the genetic pool. Contestants whose success depends on performance-enhancing medication may well be selected for breeding on retirement. Offspring from these matings will most likely exhibit the same undesirable characteristics as their parents, resulting in an ever-increasing group whose performance will require similar performance-enabling medications. Finally, an effective drug control program ensures an "even playing field" for all contestants, because competitors must perform on their own merits without performance-enhancing or enabling medical aid.

SWABBING

The term *swabbing* refers to the collection of a body fluid from a competitor. Invariably this is a urine sample from the sporting dog. Occasionally a blood sample may be requested, but urine is preferred as medications and drugs have a relatively short timespan in the circulation because of their loss to a target organ, their metabolism by the liver, and their concentration and removal by the kidney.

In Australia, chemically clean sterile sample collection kits are supplied by the analytical laboratory. The kit consists of three screw-top plastic bottles sealed in a clear plastic bag upon which collection instructions are plainly printed—This ensures that a standard uniform collection procedure is maintained on all occasions. Tamper-proof seals and security documents relating to the identification of the contestant, the event, and the location accompany the kit.

Throughout the entire collection procedure the rights of the owner/trainer/breeder are protected by ensuring that this person witnesses all the facets of the swabbing and signs the security documents. There must be no denial of natural justice at any stage. The sealed sample is then transported to the laboratory, which should have in place an unbroken chain of security up to and including its acceptance and analysis. In addition there is the right to appoint an independent analyst to witness the confirmatory retesting of a reported positive result.

SAMPLE ANALYSES

Samples packs are usually delivered directly to the laboratory by the stewards controlling the racing or sporting event. At the time of delivery the sample number, date, time, and the steward's signature are recorded in the laboratory logbook and the sample is allocated a serial laboratory number. Samples are also inspected carefully to ensure that the seals are intact and that they have not been tampered with in any way. Samples are then refrigerated until required for analysis.

A set of analytical tests is allocated to each sample. These tests combine two distinct approaches to drug screening. The first of these uses open-ended drug detection methods such as gas and liquid chromatography and gas chromatography mass spectrometry (GC/MS). These wide-ranging methods are intended to discover any unusual component in the urine that may indicate the presence of a drug. The second approach is based on target screening in which relatively specific tests are used to detect particular drugs or groups of drugs. The available target screens are randomly rotated to achieve wider coverage of the drugs that may be detected.

If the presence of drug is suspected after this preliminary analysis, the particular test that indicated it is repeated on a fresh portion of the original urine. If this also proves positive for the drug, a further portion of urine is subjected to confirmatory analysis using a definitive technique such as GC/MS. If the presence of the drug is confirmed by this method, the control sample is then analyzed to ascertain that the drug detected in the urine sample did not result from contamination of the collection vessel or the storage bottles. The control sample should therefore show no trace of the drug in question.

In some cases enough urine may have been obtained to be divided into two portions at the time of collection. These portions are referred to as the first and reserve samples of split samples. If a drug is detected in the first sample, the trainer of the animal concerned is invited to have the analysis of the reserve and control samples witnessed by his or her nominated analyst. The results of all analyses are reported to the controlling body in the form of a weekly summary of negative samples and individual reports for positive samples. Laboratory staff may subsequently be required to give evidence at stewards' inquiries into positive drug reports.

THE LABORATORY

The physical attributes and technological procedures of an analytical laboratory are covered in detail in Chapter 45. Philosophically, the laboratory should:

- Be dedicated to analytical and racing chemistry as distinct from toxicology or forensic pathology.
- Be independent, functioning without fear or favor politically, and standing alone, with adequate financial resources.
- Be objective and impartial, having no vested interests in the result of the analyses.
- Have its own research and development facilities for the ongoing generation of new methods and improved analytical sensitivities when deemed necessary.
- Have internal and external quality control to maintain efficiency in analyses and to encourage and motivate staff performance and equipment maintenance.
- Function only to analyze and report on samples submitted. The laboratory has no role in the imposition of fines or penalties other than to provide analyses that can withstand legal appeal and challenge.

PERFORMANCE MODIFICATION

In the sporting canid, three categories of behavioral change are dealt with:

1. Enhancement—by the use of ergogenic aids popularly called *stimulants* or *goers*.
2. Reduction—by the use of depressants or suppressants popularly called *stoppers*.
3. Normalization—to suppress unwanted physiological responses to excitement, eg, salivary drooling, or minimize localized pain and discomfort.

Administrators in different sports, and indeed in different countries, encounter varying degrees of sophistication in terms of drug abuse and behavioral modification in racing and other sporting canids. In this realm of drug abuse, there is a ladder of sophistication as regards the types of drugs used and the extent of knowledge of the user. This ladder of dubious drug use has three distinct phases.

Phase One—The Unsophisticated Stage. This phase prevails when there is no, or virtually no, drug testing program in operation. Examples of drugs given are caffeine, ephedrine, strychnine, arsenic, barbiturates, local anesthetics, aspirin, and phenylbutazone. All, or most, of the compounds used during this phase can be detected by relatively simple analytical procedures, eg, thin-layer chromatography.

Phase Two—The Sophisticated Stage. It soon becomes clear that introduction of a drug-testing program, which detects the commonly available drugs of phase one, does not mean an end to drug abuse. Rather, there is a focusing of the mind of the greedy and the desperate toward the use of drugs that are more difficult to detect, but that are nonetheless capable of detection given suitable circumstances. The problems now facing the sporting administrators and the laboratory analysts are awareness of the increasing range of medications requiring detection and development of suitable analytical techniques to detect these newer compounds or their metabolites. Examples are prolintane, methylphenidate, amphetamine, tricyclic antidepressants, benzodiazepines, corticosteroids, anabolic steroids, beta-blockers, reserpine, hyoscine, quinine, nicotine, chenbutarol, heptaminol, and bronchodilators. All of these have been detected, but they require an equivalent degree of sophistication of analytical technology, incorporating GC, high-performance liquid chromatography (HPLC), mass spectrometry (MS), radioimmunoassay, enzyme-linked immunosorbent assay (ELISA), and particle concentration fluoresence immunoassay (PCFIA).

Phase Three—The Avante Garde Stage. Next is the realm of top-level sophistication requiring, on the part of the perpetrators, access to a source of intimate knowledge of pharmacology. This user group is very small in number so far but is dangerous, dedicated to its goals (with large financial resources capable of manipulating larger wagers) and very unwilling to share its medication and knowledge, both of which are jealously guarded. Included are scarce physiological extracts such as erythropoietin and designer drugs. Although most of these compounds are undetectable in the current state of technology and equipment, there is clear unequivocal evidence of their use. Consequently, sporting administrators and laboratory analysts face an enormous challenge from this wily, well-informed coterie with strong financial resources.

The term *designer drug* can be used in several contexts, namely, (1) computer-assisted molecular modeling to design drugs with specific medicinal properties. In fact, drug companies have been doing this for years—making small molecular structural changes to a particular medication to improve its function or to avoid an opposition company's patent. (2) The other context in which designer drugs are used was coined by Prof. Henderson of the Pharmacology Department at the University of California, Davis, in

1960, when he referred to the illicit substances synthesized outside the pharmaceutical industry. For example, from amphetamine comes methamphetamine (ice), methylenedioxymethamphetamine (MDMA or ecstasy); from morphine comes methylfentanyl (china white), sufentanil, carfentanil, alfentanil, lofentanil—each representing a minor structural change but each with a profound effect on sporting performance at a dose rate of 0.25 to 0.5 μg. Another example is the development of crack from cocaine free base.

Currently our laboratories have the capability to detect the drugs in the phase one and phase two categories. A few of the simpler compounds from phase three have been detected (cocaine, fentanyl). However, there seems little doubt that the problem of extremely low dose designer drugs must qualify for integration into international research and development programs.

CONCLUSION

A drug control program to combat deliberate performance modification will require a coordinated effort by all sections of each sporting fraternity. There is no end to the battle, so there is no room for complacency or relaxation of standards. Rather there is an ongoing need for:

1. The laboratory to continually diversify and expand the routine screening procedures, to strive for continued improvement in detection techniques, and to maintain awareness of the limitations of existing equipment with a view to periodic upgrading or replacement.
2. Sport administrators to be astute in the selection of candidates for swabbing so that the criteria used incorporate performance variation, random selection, and targeted sampling in addition to the customary winning contestant.
3. Communication between laboratory analysts, administrators, and participating owners/trainers/breeders by providing them with as much information as possible in relation to guidelines for withholding periods for registered therapeutic substances.
4. Research and development so that laboratories nationally and internationally can coordinate programs to meet mutual and specific needs.

Suggested Readings

Blythe L, Craig M: International Greyhound Research Database. Miami, American Greyhound Council, 1994.
Blythe L, Gannon J, Craig M: Care of the Racing Greyhound. Miami, American Greyhound Council, 1994.

MISCELLANEOUS TOPICS

CHAPTER 47

RACE TRACK BIOMECHANICS AND DESIGN

BEDE W. IRELAND

This chapter addresses the significant factors that control the speed potential of a racing greyhound. (It is important to remember that an ounce of prevention is worth a "ton" of cure.) These factors are (1) speed and strain (musculoskeletal system of the greyhound); (2) track geometry; (3) racing surface of the track (materials, drainage, preparation and maintenance).

The chapter is supported by my research and the acknowledged success of the tracks that I have designed in Australia, New Zealand, and Macao. The principles outlined in this chapter are applied to the design of the successful Australian tracks.

COMPARISON OF TRACK RECORDS: QUARTER-MILE SAND (LOAM) TRACKS

It is helpful to compare the track records set on American tracks with those set on these designed Australian tracks. The comparison is made on tracks of similar size and racing surface material and over comparable race distances.

At Albion Park, Queensland, Australia, 520 meters distance, Flying Amy won in 29.73 seconds. The world record is comparable to 5/16 mile (509.2 meters) in 28.73 seconds. The American record for 5/16 mile was set at Bonita Springs, Florida, by Tiki's Ace in 29.61 seconds (claimed to be a world record). In 1993, Pilgrim's Star, racing at Albion Park, set the Australian record for 710 meters in 41.88 seconds, adjusted to the American 7/16 distance (704.1 meters) in 41.53 seconds. In 1973 Old Bill Dozd set the current American record for 7/16 mile of 42.83 seconds, at Tucson, Arizona. It is assumed that the 1.30-second differential is due to the design of the tracks.

SPEED AND STRAIN

Greyhounds are subjected to centrifugal, gravitational, and frictional forces when racing around circular curves. To balance these

forces and maintain speed, the greyhound "leans" toward the inside lure rail (Fig. 47–1). As the greyhound supports its mass on the support leg and is in the leaning position that is necessary for its speed to be maintained, the support leg joints are subjected to strain (Figs. 47–2 and 47–3). On the tracks where the racing is in a counterclockwise direction, the center of gravity is located to the inside (left side) of the support. It is also noted that the animal closest to the inside rail or lure (in the case of greyhound racing) is required to lean more if it is to remain competitive with the animal to its outside. Other common examples are those of motorcycle and harness racing (Figs. 47–4 and 47–5). Clearly the supporting joints of the greyhound are subjected to strain. In particular, the strain to the knee and wrist joints as the greyhound is required to lean should be noted, and also that the greater the speed generated, the greater the required amount of lean. With this, there is the greater strain on the joints. The musculoskeletal system places a limit on the maximum amount of lean available to any greyhound. As this limit is exceeded, the greyhound takes protective actions that will reduce the centrifugal force (CF).

$$CF = \frac{Mv^2}{r}$$

M = Mass of greyhound
v = Velocity (speed)
r = Radius of the track turn

The greyhound will either slow down (reduce v) or attempt to race on a larger radius (increase r). For these reasons, the leader, racing at top speed on a poorly designed track (small radius and flat banking), will slow down as it enters into the turn. This slowing causes interference to the greyhound following. In searching for the larger radius, it will continue on a straight path past the "tangent point" of the turn. This results in the interference that is common to the tracks of small radius and flat banking. Figure 47–6, "*into the turn*," is a reproduction of a post race, on track (small radius and flat banking) measurements of the actual path

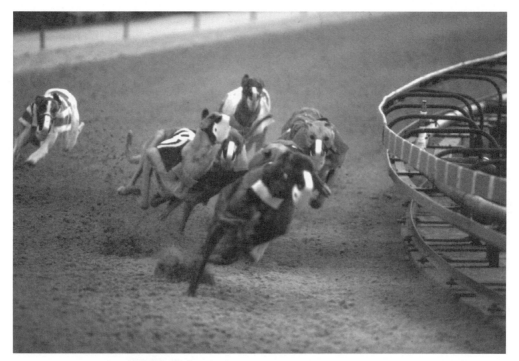

FIGURE 47–1. Greyhound "leaning" toward inside lure rail.

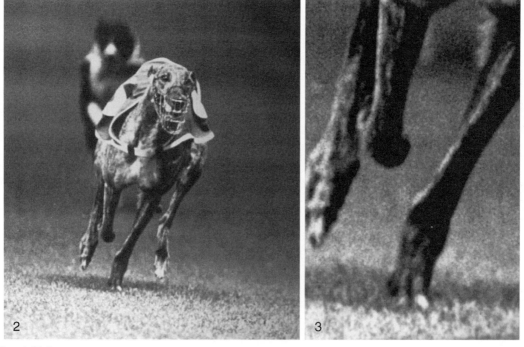

FIGURES 47–2 and 47–3. Greyhound support leg in the leaning position necessary for its speed to be maintained. Illustrates how leg joints are subjected to strain.

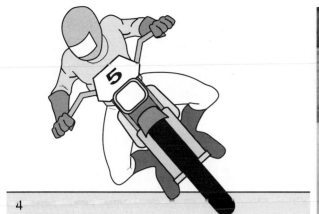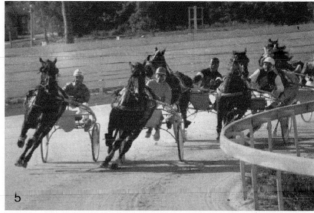

FIGURES 47–4 and 47–5. Clockwise racing "lean" required in motorcycle and counterclockwise racing "lean" required in harness racing.

traced by the greyhounds. In the illustration, note greyhound no. 2 runs past the tangent point of the curve and greyhound No. 1, in searching for a larger radius, runs toward the lure rail. The predictable outcome is interference. A track should be designed to minimize interference and injury and at the same time allow the greyhound to attain its best speed.

The speed car, on the other hand, has its center of gravity fixed in relation to its support and therefore cannot balance the forces by "leaning" and remain with all of the support wheels in touch with the ground (Fig. 47–7). For this reason the application of highway engineering principles to the design of greyhound, harness, and flat horse racing seems to be inappropriate.

TRACK GEOMETRY: (Radius of Track Turn, Slope of Track Banking, and Transition Curves)

The size of the radius of the turns and the steepness of the slope of the banking of the turns are important design factors. The variation in the maximum speed of a greyhound when racing on different sizes of turn radius and steepness of slope confirms conclusively that (1) steeper track banking combined with a larger track turn radius will allow for greater speed, and (2) a reduced amount of lean results from an increase in the size of the track turns. A reduced lean will allow for greater speed. The anatomy of the joints fixes the upper limit to the amount of lean for any particular greyhound (Fig. 47–8).

Because of their superior speed, champions are the first to be injured when racing on a track of poor design and are restricted from reaching their best speed. Poor track design has a serious adverse and costly effect on the industry. The racing life, and therefore the earning capacity of the valuable champion, is diminished by injury or breakdown. Poor track design indicates scant regard for the welfare of the animal. Tragically, a poorly designed track costs no less than a track of good design. The measured speed of a greyhound will improve dramatically when that greyhound races on a better combination of turn radius and turn banking. The larger the radius and the steeper the banking, the better the outcome. *This is a matter that is commended to the breeding, racing, and training industries for serious and urgent consideration.*

Transition Curves

Early work by the Australian land surveyor W. Tibbs (1954), my work (1969, 1973), and that of Dr. I. Fredricson (1975), and others forms the foundation for our current knowledge of track design. The banking required to eliminate the necessity for any lean, according to the 1975 work, was 1:3 for the half-mile and 1:5 for

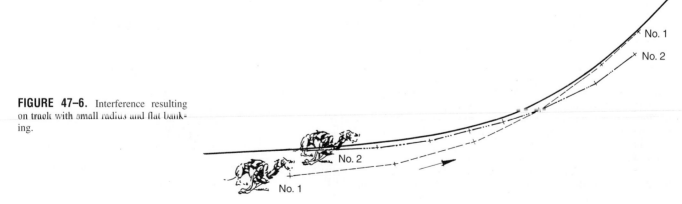

FIGURE 47–6. Interference resulting on track with small radius and flat banking.

INTO THE TURN

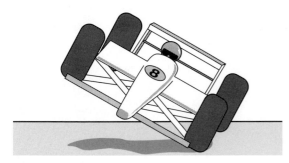

FIGURE 47–7. Speed car's inability to "lean" and keep all of the support wheels in touch with the ground.

TABLE 47–1. Recommended Gradings in Material Selection

Australian Sieve Size	% Passing
Loam	
1.18 mm	100
600 μm	98
300 μm	80
150 μm	50
75 μm	35
Sand	
1.18 mm	100
600 μm	99
300 μm	90
150 μm	10
75 μm	5

the 1000-meter harness racing tracks. Dr. George Pratt of MIT is reported to have suggested a banking of 1:2 for the elimination of lean for a greyhound racing on an American quarter-mile greyhound track.

RACING SURFACE OF THE TRACK

In regions of heavy rainfall, the use of the steep banking suggested by Dr. George Pratt presents an expensive maintenance problem. Heavy storms may scour the sand and loam of the track surface and move it down the slope, transporting it from the track to under the lure rail and then onto the inner field area. The regular replacement of this racing surface material is prohibitively expensive.

Design of Track Drainage. The scour and movement of the surface material may be reduced by controlling the volume and velocity of storm runoff across the track surface. With calculated permeability of the surface material, some of the storm water may be taken through the track and drained away below the surface of the track via a subtrack drainage system.

Figure 47–9 demonstrates the method used with success at the Parklands Track Southport, Queensland, Australia. Note the use of the Geofabrics separating the layers of track materials. The base layer of this track is pervious to allow for the required drainage. The concrete sidestone (marked "1st pour") is constructed to the inside of the track. It supports the pavement materials and maintains the design levels for the inside of the track. It also ensures swift removal of the across the track storm water from the surface of the track in storm conditions. Continuity of racing, even in heavy storm conditions, is ensured with these design principles. The harness racing track built to these principles in 1979 in Macao confirmed their effectiveness. This track withstood 575 mm of rain over a 2-day period without any interruption to the racing program.

Track Surface Materials. The forces exerted by the greyhound on the track surface are both forward and downward. The material of the surface must allow controlled compression of and forward sliding through the surface layer. The compressive strength, the shear strength, moisture content, permeability, and coefficient of friction must be carefully calculated for the material. It is important that the material be "resilient," so that impact forces can be dissipated as the material compresses. It is also important that the material be at "optimum moisture content."

The mixture of light-colored loam with white sand is ideal for the racing surface. The gradings shown in Table 47–1 are recommended as points of commencement in the process of material selection. A mixture of 2 parts loam with 1 part sand will provide a suitable racing surface for banking as steep as 1 in 7, ie, one unit of banking for each 7 units of track width, or 1¾ inches/

foot. A track 7 meters wide, approximately 23 feet, would have a banking of 1 meter, approximately 3 feet 3 inches. The loam and sand should be as light-colored as possible. The permeability of this design mix is rapid even at high rates of compactness. The particle shape of the materials is important. The particles should not be sharp or pointed.

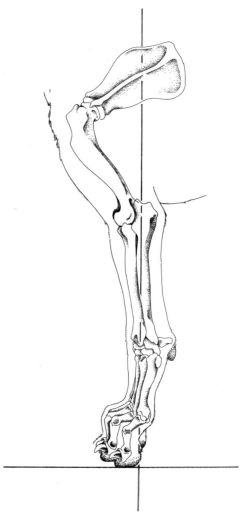

FIGURE 47–8. Anatomy of foreleg combined with track design allows for maximum potential speed.

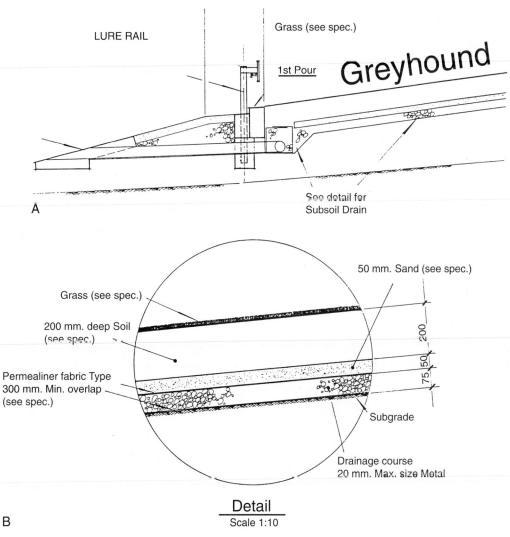

LURE RAIL

Grass (see spec.)

1st Pour

Greyhound

See detail for
Subsoil Drain

A

Grass (see spec.)

200 mm. deep Soil
(see spec.)

Permealiner fabric Type
300 mm. Min. overlap
(see spec.)

50 mm. Sand (see spec.)

200

75 50

Subgrade

Drainage course
20 mm. Max. size Metal

Detail
Scale 1:10

B

FIGURE 47–9. *A* and *B*, These demonstrate the method used with success at the Parklands Track Southport, Queensland, Australia. (Note the use of the Geofabrics separating the layers of track materials.)

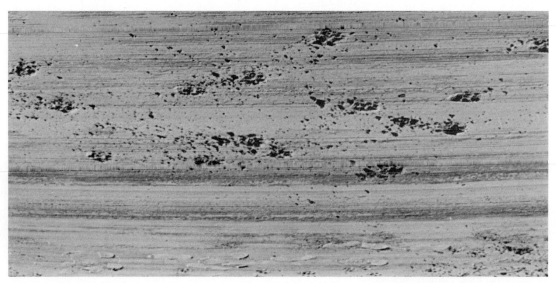

FIGURE 47–10. A good racing surface; indentation of the material by the foot in the support process.

It is important that the subsurface layer, the layer immediately below the surface (the force dissipation layer), is of the correct compactness and optimal moisture content and provides the friction necessary for the greyhound to run at a smooth gait. The compressive strength (the strength of the material necessary to withstand the forces of impact) and the shear strength (the strength of the material that allows the support foot to slide into the surface and take up a position prior to the impact forces being dissipated and the material to be ready for the propulsion) depend on the moisture content being consistent and at optimal value. Generally, the moisture should be maintained within 2 per cent above or below the optimal value. The strengths of the material will be adversely affected by moisture greater than the optimum (a sloppy track). When the track is drier than ideal it may become unacceptably hard and the all-important ''fines'' may be blown away and lost from the track surface. Figure 47–10 indicates a surface considered to be ideal. The material has allowed a movement forward of the support foot before the support takes place. The indentation of the material by the foot in the support process is clean and sharp. It will be noted further that there is little disturbance of the material as a result of the propulsion process. In these circumstances surface will not be thrown into the dogs' eyes during racing. In contrast, Figure 47–11 indicates the outcome of racing on a surface of lesser quality. Here the surface has insufficient shear strength, with the result that the material is dragged out and propelled into the greyhounds that follow. Further, the ''sliding'' of the support foot is more marked, and the mounding formed as the material fails in shear following the propulsion process should be noted.

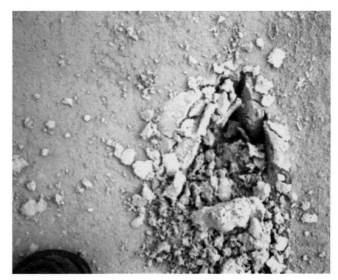

FIGURE 47–11. Outcome of racing on a surface of lesser quality. Surface has insufficient shear strength, which results in material being dragged out and propelled into the greyhounds that follow.

Preparation and Maintenance. The best of design and material selection will be of little value if the pre-race track preparation and ongoing maintenance are wanting. The track manager is a significant contributor to the success of any racing circuit.

CHAPTER 48

IMAGING TECHNIQUES AND RADIOGRAPHIC EXAMINATION OF THE APPENDICULAR SKELETAL SYSTEM

RICHARD D. PARK

IMAGING MODALITIES AND TECHNIQUES

Radiology has been used in veterinary medicine since the early part of the twentieth century. Within the last two decades several new imaging modalities have been developed to complement and add to radiographic imaging. As these new imaging methods are incorporated into diagnostic regimens, advantages and disadvantages of each for diagnosing diseases within specific systems need documenting. Selecting the proper modality for the most expeditious and accurate diagnosis is most important. A knowledge of technical aspects and information that may be obtained with each imaging process is necessary.

Radiology

Radiology is the oldest diagnostic imaging procedure and serves as the base imaging method in veterinary medicine today. Radiology provides bone images with excellent spatial resolution. Contrast resolution is relatively poor on radiographs; therefore, specific soft tissue structures are not well visualized. Radiographs are two-dimensional images of three-dimensional structures, thus limiting the three-dimensional concept of structures and pathological processes. Radiographic examinations are fast and relatively simple to perform. Equipment and knowledge to provide the studies are widely available. Radiographic examination protocols for the appendicular skeletal system[1, 2] and diagnostic criteria (radiographic signs) have been established, thus providing a reliable diagnostic modality. Knowledge of examination techniques, normal radiographic anatomy, and radiographic signs of disease is essential to effectively use radiology for diagnosing disease conditions of the appendicular skeletal system.

X-ray Machines

A 300-mA x-ray machine is recommended for radiographic studies of the appendicular skeletal system. Smaller mA machines can be used for examinations of the distal extremities, but for large-dog stifles, shoulders, and pelves, a 300-mA machine is recommended to perform adequate studies. High–frequency generator-equipped machines are now available. These machines provide a higher kV during a given exposure, thus increasing the exposure for specific kV(p) and mAs settings compared to single- or three-phase generators. High-frequency generators are comparable to three-phase, 12-pulse generators and may have the added advantage of running on a single-phase power line.

Accessory Radiographic Equipment

Good-quality, properly functioning accessory radiographic equipment is an absolute necessity for performing high-quality radiographic examinations. Grids, cassettes with an ideally matched rare-earth screen-film system, a legible and reliable film-marking system, and miscellaneous positioning aids are some of the necessary accessory equipment.

Grids. A focused or nonfocused parallel grid, with at least an 8:1 ratio and over 100 lines/inch, is recommended for parts thicker than 8 cm. Ratios higher than 8:1 could also be used, if needed. With grids having over 100 lines/inch, grid lines are difficult to see but are still visible. A movable bucky will obliterate visible grid lines from the radiograph.

Screen-Film Combinations. Rare-earth screen-film combinations are available that provide a variety of speeds, resolution, and latitude. For extremity examinations of the carpus, tarsus, and distal, a slow-speed, high-detail system is best. An approximately 100-speed system provides excellent spatial resolution for these smaller structures. For structures more proximal, ie, structures proximal to the carpus and tarsus, a 400- to 600-speed system provides good detail. The 400- to 600-speed systems are also faster to accommodate the larger exposure factors needed in the more proximal structures. Radiographs with a higher spatial resolution can be obtained with single emulsion film and a single intensifying

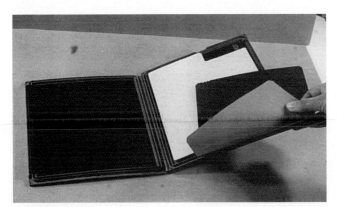

FIGURE 48–1. X-ray cassette with a single-fine-screen and single-emulsion film. This film-screen combination produces excellent detail for extremity examinations, but requires a higher exposure.

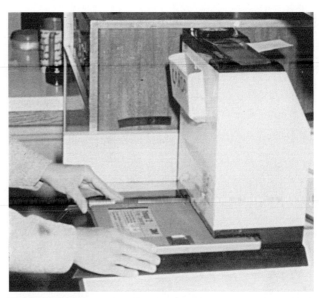

FIGURE 48–2. Film identification is added to the film by inserting the cassette into the photoflash machine. Information is transferred by light from a pretyped card to the x-ray film.

screen (Fig. 48–1). This system can be used for examinations of the carpus and tarsus distally. The system has the disadvantage of needing approximately three times the exposure of a 100-speed rare earth system to produce an acceptable radiograph.

Film Marking Systems. Radiographs should be marked with the date, animal identification, practice, or veterinarian's name, and the part being examined, ie, left or right. The system should provide permanent marking exposed on the x-ray film before film processing (Fig. 48–2). Several systems are available; lead impregnated tape, lead markers, and photoflash systems (Fig. 48–3). Markers placed on the cassette prior to an exposure that are not acceptable for marking are coins, nails, hypodermic needles, or other such objects. Similarly, adhesive tape is also unacceptable for marking radiographs after processing.

Miscellaneous Positioning Aids. Many positioning devices are available (Fig. 48–4). Personal preference and the examination to be performed may determine which is used. Adhesive tape, gauze, sandbags, sponges, paddles, and other holding devices are all helpful for positioning animals during the radiographic examination. The goal is to use such positioning devices so that personnel may vacate the examination room while the exposure is made. Heavy tranquilization or general anesthesia is necessary for most animals in order for the positioning devices to be used effectively.

Storage Phosphor Digital (Computed) Radiography

Computed radiography (CR) is an imaging modality that produces a radiographic image from digital information. Storage phos-

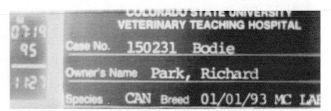

FIGURE 48–3. Photoflash identification marked on the film. All necessary identification information is in a small concise area.

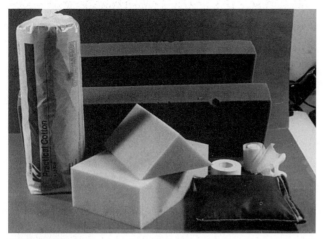

FIGURE 48–4. Positioning aids consist of sponges, tape, gauze, and sandbags.

phor imaging plates made of Europia-doped barium flurohalide (BaFBr:Eu) (Fig. 48–5) are used to record the image much the same as a traditional screen-film system. The storage phosphor imaging plates store the absorbed energy from the x-ray beam. The plates are then placed in a laser reader where energy in the storage phosphor plate is released when excited by a laser beam. The emitted energy released from the plate is detected and digitized. The digitized information can be viewed on a monitor and the density, latitude, and other parameters adjusted before printing a radiograph (hard copy).

Disadvantages of Computed Radiography. The primary disadvantages of CR are the high monetary cost and the technical complexity and difficult procedures necessary to produce consistent diagnostic images. Both disadvantages have to be eliminated or minimized if the imaging method is to receive routine use. Another less restricting disadvantage is seen on low-frequency, edge-enhanced images. A lucent halo may be produced in areas where there is a transition between high- and low-density tissues. These lucent halos may simulate fractures. The lucent halo effect may also be seen around metallic implants, producing a pseudoperi-implant lytic zone. This may be confused with bone lysis.[3] Decreased spatial resolution may also occur at an unacceptable level if exposure levels are too low.

Advantages of Computed Radiography. CR has several advantages: A single exposure can provide more than one image. The digital information can be changed to optimize visualization of bone or soft tissue structures or compensate for overexposure or underexposure (Fig. 48–6). The image can be edge enhanced to accentuate sharp margins such as hairline fractures or other subtle bone changes, or better define periarticular soft tissue structures and changes. Since the number of exposures necessary because of poor or unacceptable radiographs is decreased, attending personnel are exposed to less radiation. Because of image manipulation capabilities, CR provides tremendous potential for improving the quality of radiographic examinations. In the future digital radiography may replace conventional screen-film systems.

Arthrography

Arthrography is a simple, safe procedure for examining joints.[4–7] It is used almost exclusively in the shoulder, but its use has been reported in the stifle and elbow.[8, 9] Arthrography consists of placing contrast material intra-articularly and recording the image on radiographs. This provides visualization of intra-articular structures not seen on survey radiographs. The extent of the joint capsule and outline of synovial and cartilage surfaces can be evaluated on arthrograms. The location of opaque bodies can be positively identified as intracapsular or extracapsular. The cranial and caudal cruciate ligaments and menisci can also be visualized in the stifle in normal dogs.[8] Arthrography provides important diagnostic information, particularly in the shoulder joint, is complementary to other imaging methods, and is simple to perform. Newer imaging procedures—arthroscopy, magnetic resonance imaging, and to a limited extent ultrasonography—also provide visualization of intra-articular structures and may decrease the need for arthrography.

Arthrographic Technique. Arthrography is performed by means of aseptic joint centesis. Synovial fluid can be withdrawn if joint capsule distention is present but is not necessary before injection of contrast material. Positive contrast (iodinated contrast medium) arthrography is most diagnostic in dogs.

Positive contrast arthrography is performed by injecting iodinated contrast material intra-articularly. A dose of approximately 2 to 4 cc of iodinated contrast material (approximately 33 mg-I/cc) is sufficient for most joints.[10] This dose is varied depending on the specific joint and size of the animal. The joint should be flexed and extended after the injection to mix contrast material and joint fluid. Radiographs should be made immediately or at least within 2 to 3 minutes after injection because contrast material is absorbed from the joint and diluted by fluid drawn into the joint due to the higher intra-articular osmotic pressure. These two processes make

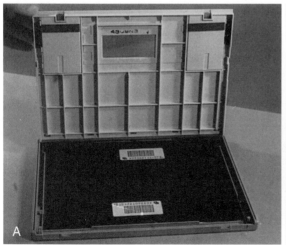

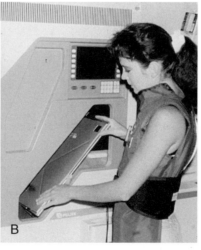

FIGURE 48–5. *A,* Computed radiographic (CR) cassette with a storage phosphor imaging plate in the cassette. *B,* CR cassette is being placed into the laser reader where information from the CR plate will be digitized.

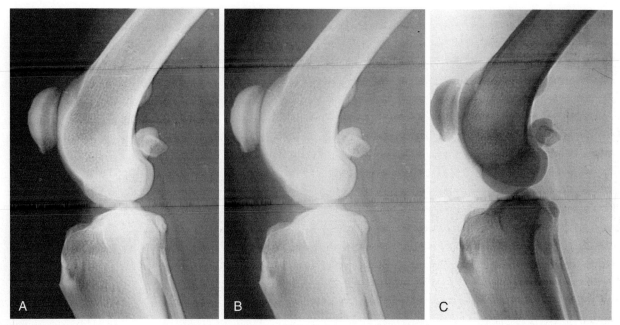

FIGURE 48–6. Mediolateral computed radiographic images of a dog stifle. Window levels and widths and other viewing parameters can be changed to facilitate visualization of anatomic structures. *A,* Relatively high window level and narrow window width, good for bone. *B,* Relatively low window level and wide window width, good for soft tissue visualization. *C,* Inverse image good for demonstrating more subtle bone lesions.

the arthrogram nondiagnostic after a short time (usually 5 minutes). Nonionic contrast materials, such as iohexol and iopamidol, have greater opacification with time (up to 15 minutes) than ionic contrast material.[5, 8, 9] Newer dimer contrast materials remain opacified longer with less severe inflammatory reactions than ionic or nonionic contrast material.[7, 11] Radiographic exposure can be optimized with iodine-containing contrast material by setting kV(p) in the range of 75 to 80.[12] This kV(p) range takes advantage of the photoelectric absorption in iodine, thus producing more contrast on the arthrogram.

Interpretation Principles and Clinical Uses. Arthrograms are used to evaluate articular cartilage, the joint capsule, and free joint bodies. Cartilage fragmentation as occurs with osteochondrosis is demonstrated with positive contrast arthrography and is identified as contrast material infiltrates or dissects beneath the articular cartilage (Fig. 48–7). Joint capsule proliferation, tears, hernias, and abnormal communications are also demonstrated with positive contrast arthrography. Synovial proliferation may take the form of an irregular synovial outline with decreased distention of the synovial membrane involved. Joint capsule tears are easily identified as

contrast material extravasates into the surrounding soft tissues.[13] This should not be confused with a small amount of contrast material leaking from the centesis site. Arthrography is useful to determine if an opacified body is intra-articular or extra-articular and if a nonossified joint body is present within the joint (Fig. 48–8). Ossified and nonossified joint bodies will appear as radiolucent filling defects surrounded by the positive contrast material.

Shoulder arthrograms provide valuable diagnostic information. Mediolateral and caudocranial views of the shoulder should be routinely obtained. A traction mediolateral radiograph provides better visualization of articular cartilage, and pronated and supinated mediolateral views provide better visualization of the bicipital tendon.[10] Arthrograms can be used to identify surgical osteochondrosis lesions,[13, 14] (see Fig. 48–7) rupture of the joint capsule[13] (Fig. 48–9), and bicipital tendon and synovial sheath problems (Fig. 48–10).[15, 16] Dissection of contrast material beneath cartilaginous flaps is diagnostic of a surgical osteochondrosis lesion, whereas a thick articular cartilage area is not an indication for surgery.[14] Arthrographic changes associated with bicipital tendinitis or inflammatory changes within the tendon sheath include incom-

FIGURE 48–7. *A,* Mediolateral radiographic view of the shoulder, and *B,* a shoulder arthrogram. On the survey radiograph (*A*), a subchondral bone defect is present on the caudal humeral head (arrows). The caudal circumflex humeral artery (*open arrows*) is outlined with fat. On the arthrogram (*B*), a free cartilaginous flap (*arrows*) appears radiolucent as it is outlined with contrast material.

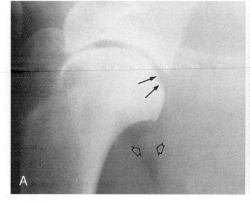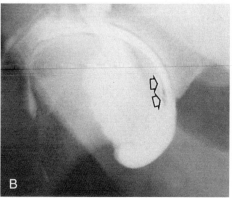

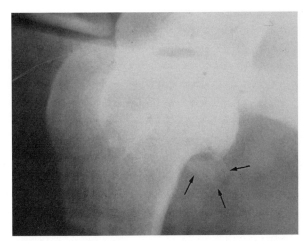

FIGURE 48–8. A mediolateral shoulder radiograph. A round radiopaque "joint body" is present within the cul-de-sac on the caudal aspect of the joint (arrows). These round joint bodies are usually synovial osteochondromas.

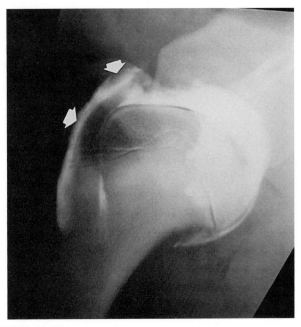

FIGURE 48–10. Mediolateral view of a shoulder arthrogram. There is a mildly irregular outline to the bicipital tendon sheath (*arrows*) with small filling defects present within the sheath. These changes are seen in association with inflammatory changes within the tendon sheath and/or tendon.

plete filling of the sheath, irregular synovial outline, and filling defects within the sheath[15, 17, 18] (Fig. 48–10). Although arthrograms may appear normal with bicipital disease,[13] arthrography has proven to be a valuable technique for diagnosing bicipital disease when corresponding clinical signs are present.[15]

Stifle arthrography and elbow arthrography have not proven to be clinically valuable techniques in dogs.[8, 9] Interarticular pathological changes such as meniscal damage and cranial and caudal cruciate ligament rupture are not readily identified on most stifle arthrograms. This technique does not provide good diagnostic information in cases of stifle trauma. Outline of articular cartilage and joint capsule can be demonstrated in the elbow with arthrography, but the technique does not help delineate fragments from the medial coronoid process.[9]

Computed Tomography

Computerized tomography (CT) is best used in the appendicular skeleton for better defining bone pathology in complex bony struc-

tures not identifiable or well defined on radiographs or by other imaging modalities.

Technique

A CT scanner consists of an x-ray tube and sensors in a circular gantry, an incrementable table, x-ray generator, computer, and video monitor. The image is made as x-rays penetrate the part examined and interact with sensors as the x-ray tube travels around the circular gantry. Direct images are acquired in a transverse or axial plane at specified slice thicknesses and intervals, thus producing an image in the third dimension. With appropriate software this

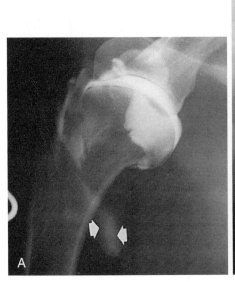

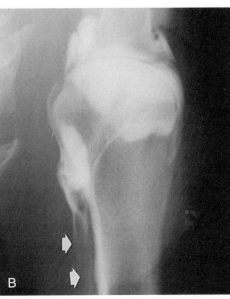

FIGURE 48–9. Mediolateral (*A*) and caudocranial (*B*) views of a shoulder arthrogram. Contrast material is leaking from the bicipital synovial sheath and extending distally in the limb (*arrows*). This is diagnostic of a joint capsule tear in the bicipital synovial sheath (*arrows*).

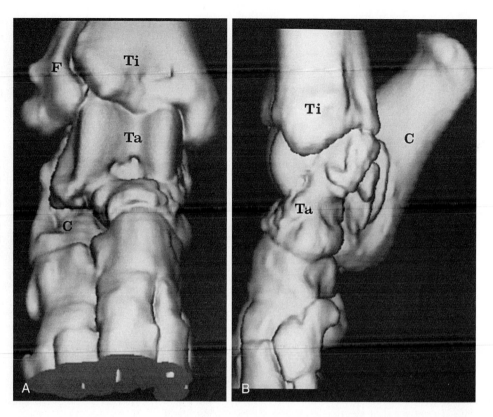

FIGURE 48-11. Three-dimensional image of a dog tarsus. The images were constructed from a CT scan with three-dimensional software. The image can be rotated to view different surfaces. The dorsal surface (A) and medial surface (B) are illustrated. The tibia (Ti), fibula (F), talus (Ta), and calcaneus (C) are labeled for orientation.

information can be reformatted into sagittal and dorsal planes or three-dimensional images (Fig. 48–11). When compared with routine radiographs, the spatial resolution on CT images is poor. The contrast resolution, however, is superior to radiographs, and the image contrast level and width can be adjusted to visualize bone or soft tissue structures. To optimize a bone image, a wide window width (1500 to 2000 ct number) and high window levels (250 to 350 ct number) are used. Appendicular soft tissue structures can best be visualized with lower window levels and widths, ie, 60 window level and 200 to 350 width. By selecting different window settings and imaging algorithms, CT images can be used to show bone and soft tissue lesions. Bone lesions that cannot be adequately defined on radiographs because of superimposition are easily visualized with CT.

Clinical Uses

CT is most helpful in examining the appendicular skeletal system when preceded by a radiographic examination. CT is good for defining complex intra-articular fractures, fractures not visualized on radiographs, subchondral bone sclerosis, and other subchondral bone lesions such as subtle defects or small articular bone fragments. CT is particularly helpful in more complex joints such as the carpus, tarsus, and elbow. It is useful for defining the extent of bone or soft tissue neoplasia involving bone. The extent of the tumor within the medullary cavity (Fig. 48–12) and externally within the soft tissue can be approximated. Neurofibromas, if external to the cervical musculature, can also be imaged (Fig. 48–13). These lesions can be defined better with CT because of images produced in the third dimension, the ability to reformat in other planes, and the increased contrast resolution. In most cases the CT study is generated from unanswered questions on the routine radiographic examination or when further information is needed to diagnose or define a pathological condition more accurately.

Computed Tomography of the Elbow. The elbow is a complex joint with a potential for multiple subtle changes associated with elbow dysplasia. This combination makes radiographic evaluation difficult. CT with capabilities for reformatting in parasagittal and dorsal planes provides a thorough examination of the elbow joint. Changes that may be detected by CT are fragmented medial coronoid processes, osteochondrosis of the medial aspect of the distal humeral condyle, subchondral defects in other joint surfaces, sub-

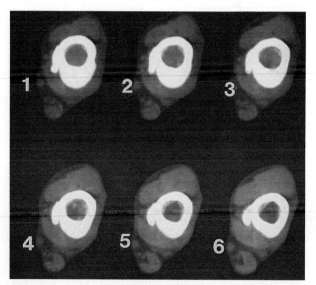

FIGURE 48-12. Contiguous 3-mm thick transverse CT images of a primary bone tumor border in the tibial diaphysis. Soft tissue density is present within the medullary cavity representing tumor and/or inflammation (slices 1 and 2). The soft tissue density gradually ends and is replaced with normal fat density on slices 3 through 6.

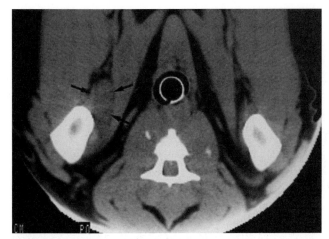

FIGURE 48–13. Transverse CT scan through the caudal cervical area and the proximal humeri. The dog was positioned in dorsal recumbency for the examination. A soft tissue mass is present adjacent to the medial surface of the right humerus (*arrows*) within the area of the vascular/nerve bundle. The mass was a neurofibroma.

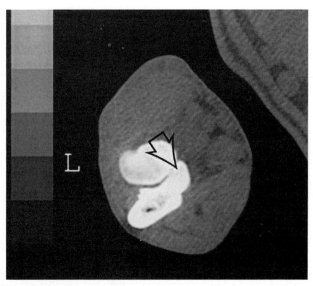

FIGURE 48–15. Transverse CT scan of the proximal radius and ulna. A faint lucent line is present on the lateral cranial aspect of the medial coronoid process (*arrow*). This is an in situ medial coronoid process fragment.

chondral bone sclerosis, periarticular osteophytes, and incongruity in the humeroulnar, humeroradial, and radioulnar joints. In one study, accuracy of detection of medial coronoid process fragments (Fig. 48–14) was 86.7 per cent with CT and 56.7 per cent with radiography, compared with findings at surgery.[19] Subchondral bone defects and cleavage lines without a separate fragment can also be detected with CT (Fig. 48–15). These changes are not evident on radiographic studies. Osteochondrosis and other subchondral bone defects on the medial portion of the humeral condyle are easily diagnosed with CT (Fig. 48–16), but they could be missed on radiographs if the x-ray beam is not tangent to the subchondral bone lesion. "Wear lesions" appear as subchondral bone defects with surrounding bone sclerosis and are associated with fragmentation and other changes on the medial coronoid processes. These changes are not easily appreciated on radiographs, but can be easily demonstrated on a CT study with dorsal plane reformatted images. Other subchondral bone defects can be seen with CT in the medial coronoid process and on the radial incisure of the ulna in the radioulnar joint (Fig. 48–17). Joint incongruity is easily demonstrated with CT (Fig. 48–18), but if severe enough it can also be seen on a routine radiographic study. Subluxation or

wide joint spaces and relative displacement between the lateral coronoid process and the radial head are seen on CT. CT is a superior imaging technique for detecting all changes associated with elbow dysplasia.

Magnetic Resonance (MR) Imaging

Magnetic resonance imaging provides sectional images much the same as CT images. They are produced in machines similar in configuration to CT scanners. The images have high contrast and spatial resolution and are produced from protons, mainly from hydrogen nuclei. The images provide exceptionally good anatomical, pathoanatomical, and pathophysiological information about soft tissue structures. MR has the potential to provide information not provided by any other imaging modality, including arthroscopy.

Technique

An MR scanner consists of a strong magnet, transmit/receive radiofrequency coils, gradient magnets, a computer, gantry, table,

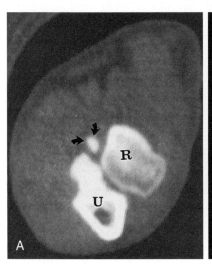

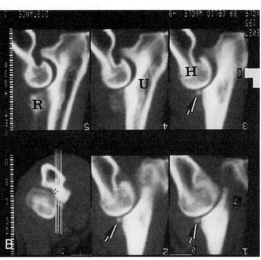

FIGURE 48–14. Direct transverse (*A*) and reformatted sagittal (*B*) CT images of an elbow. A fragmented medial coronoid process is apparent on both image planes (*arrows*). There is also bone sclerosis within the medial coronoid process noted best on the transverse scan. The radius (R), ulna (U), and humerus (H) are marked for orientation.

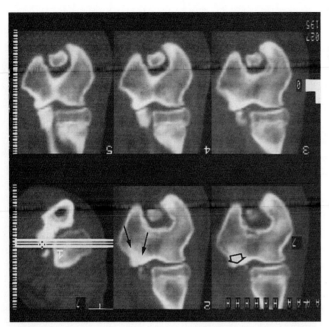

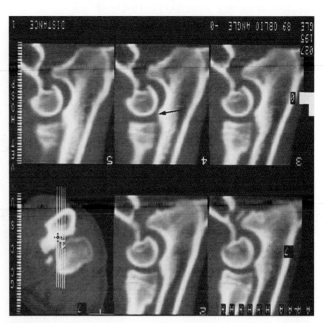

FIGURE 48–16. Dorsal plane 1-mm thick contiguous reformatted CT images of the elbow. Subchondral bone sclerosis (*solid arrows*) and a subchondral bone defect (*open arrow*) are present on the medial aspect of the humeral condyle. This may represent an osteochondrosis lesion or a "wear lesion" caused by pressure from the medial coronoid process.

FIGURE 48–18. Sagittal reformatted contiguous 1-mm thick CT images of the elbow. The elbow joint is incongruent. There is increased width to the humeroulnar and humeroradial joints. The lateral coronoid process (*arrow*) is proximal to the normal position adjacent to the radial head.

and video monitor. A detailed description of MR scanners and the mechanism of image production is beyond the scope of this chapter. A simple description of image production follows. Nuclei that have an asymmetrical spinning charge are imaged. The proton from the hydrogen nucleus is imaged for most diagnostic studies. These spinning charged nuclei are aligned in the strong magnetic field of the scanner. The spinning aligned nuclei also precess around an axis in the magnetic field much the same as a spinning top. A

radiofrequency (RF) wave is used to bombard the precessing nucleus, tilting the precessing axis 90 degrees. The signal from the precessing nucleus or proton then produces an electric signal in the RF receiver coil that is transmitted to the computer for image construction. A signal for image construction is produced as the nuclei relax into their demagnetized states. By varying the RF pulse, the time for protons to become magnetized before the RF pulse (TR) and the time after the RF pulse (TE), images with different information can be produced. These images are termed T1-weighted, T2-weighted, and proton density images. Direct images can be obtained in any plane by adjusting the magnetic gradient coils.

Interpretation Principles

Signal intensity from tissues and structures varies with the imaging sequence, ie, T1- or T2-weighted or proton density images. T1-weighted images are the most commonly used for imaging musculoskeletal structures; however, T2-weighted images provide different tissue contrast and therefore may add information in some cases.[20, 21] T2-weighted images are best to demonstrate lesions in periarticular muscles and to identify synovial fluid. A knowledge of tissue intensities on T1- and T2-weighted images is necessary for interpreting the examinations. On T1-weighted images subcutaneous and fascial plane fat and bone marrow have the brightest signal (white), hyaline cartilage is less bright (white-gray), followed by muscle (gray-white). Fluid, ligaments, tendons, and bone have little or no signal intensity (black).[20] Synovial fluid sometimes produces some signal and can be seen (gray) adjacent to articular cartilage. On T2-weighted images, fluid has the highest intensity (white) followed by fat, bone marrow, and muscle in decreasing order of intensity. Ligaments, tendons, and bone have little or no signal intensity (black).[20] Newer imaging sequences, such as a fat-suppressed SPGR sequence, have provided increased definition of articular cartilage, which has a trilaminar appearance. This sequence also has increased sensitivity for detecting cartilaginous erosion and degeneration.[22]

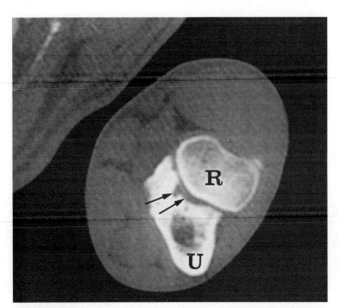

FIGURE 48–17. A transverse CT scan through the proximal radius (R) and ulna (U). The medial coronoid process is malformed, has bone sclerosis and a defect along the radial incisure of the ulna (*arrows*).

MR imaging is an effective imaging means to evaluate and detect pathological changes in articular cartilage, menisci, and bone marrow. Alterations in bone marrow due to bone sclerosis, neoplasia, fluid accumulation secondary to infection or inflammation, and ligament, tendon, joint capsule, and muscle injury can be detected and diagnosed with MR imaging. Hyperintense or hypointense defects may be observed in injured ligaments, tendons, and muscle. The signal intensity will be hyperintense on T2 and hypointense on T1 with edema or fluid accumulation. Signal intensity of blood or hemorrhage changes with time. Acute hemorrhage is isointense with muscle on T1 and hyperintense on T2. After 2 days, the signal on T1 images will be more intense, and in several days the hemorrhage will be hyperintense on both T1- and T2-weighted images.[20]

Clinical Uses

MR imaging has been used in preliminary studies to image the stifle[23-25] and shoulder[26] in the dog. It is superior for imaging meniscal changes, capsular fibrosis, and early osteophyte productions in the stifle.[23, 24] Detection of lesions can also be done earlier. With osteoarthritis, changes can be detected at 4 weeks of age as compared with 12 weeks by radiology. Subchondral bone changes were effectively demonstrated in the humeral head of dogs affected with osteochondrosis.[26] Cartilaginous lesions or fragments were not demonstrated in these osteochondrosis lesions using a T1-weighted imaging sequence,[26] but with newer imaging sequences, cartilaginous lesions can be demonstrated.[22]

Future Development

Drawbacks at present to MR are the cost and availability of equipment, including equipment maintenance, and the complexity of imaging sequences to obtain diagnostic examinations. As constraints are overcome, MRI of appendicular structures will add a new dimension to in vivo diagnostic imaging of the appendicular skeletal system.

Ultrasound

Ultrasound has received only limited attention for imaging the appendicular musculoskeletal structures in the dog. It has been used to evaluate the bicipital tendon and synovial sheath in dogs with a histopathological diagnosis of synovitis or tendinitis of the synovial sheath and bicipital tendon.[15] A linear array, 7.5-MHz transducer with an acoustic standoff was used to image the bicipital structures. Increased fluid was identified within the synovial sheath of some dogs, but no tendon changes were observed. Increased fluid within the synovial sheath may be unassociated with specific pathological findings in the bicipital structures. Any cause of increased joint effusion may result in bicipital sheath distention. The bicipital tendon was difficult to image consistently because of off-incidence artifacts produced within the tendon and the difficulty of positioning the transducer within the bicipital groove for good transverse images.[15]

Tendons (Fig. 48–19) and muscles can be imaged to diagnose acute and chronic injuries and monitor healing. Foreign bodies embedded in soft tissue structures can also be identified. Ultrasound is particularly helpful for diagnosing nonradiopaque foreign bodies, eg, large segments of porcupine quills and wood splinters. These will usually appear as a hyperechoic area with shadowing deep to the foreign body.

Nuclear Medicine

The nuclear medicine image is produced by ionizing radiation (gamma rays) originating from a radionuclide injected intravenously into the patient; it is a physiological map of the radiopharmaceutical uptake. The uptake pattern of the radiopharmaceutical is increased in areas with higher blood flow and/or increased osteoblastic activity.[27] The three recorded phases are a flow phase (vascular), pool phase (soft tissue), and bone phase. The flow phase is recorded 1 to 2 minutes after injection, the pool phase 10 to 20 minutes after the flow phase, and the bone phase 2 to 4 hours or longer after the flow phase.

Clinical Uses

Nuclear medicine imaging is more sensitive for detecting pathological conditions than other imaging methods. It can be used to find the activity of radiographic lesions or to detect lesions not apparent on radiographs. Potential candidates for a nuclear medicine scan are lame animals in which a lesion cannot be localized

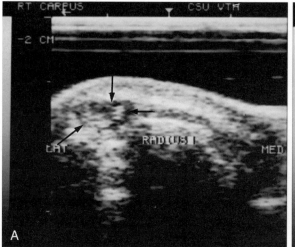
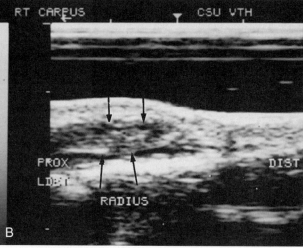

FIGURE 48–19. Transverse (*A*) and sagittal (*B*) ultrasound scan of the lateral digital extensor tendon in a dog at the level of the distal radius and ulna. On the transverse image the lateral digital extensor tendon is large with an inhomogeneous echo pattern (*arrows*). On the sagittal (longitudinal image) the tendon is large, and the tendon fibers are disrupted with an inhomogeneous echo pattern (*arrows*). The changes are chronic and have resulted from traumatic incomplete disruption of the lateral digital extensor tendon.

at physical examination or identified on radiographs. Nuclear medicine is also sensitive for identifying metastatic neoplastic lesions in the appendicular skeletal system. This is particularly useful as a screening examination before treatment is started for the primary neoplasm.

RADIOGRAPHIC EXAMINATIONS

Radiographic examinations consist of routine views for each part or area examined and additional views necessary to better demonstrate a suspected disease condition in a specific anatomical location. The routine radiographic views have been illustrated in other textbooks,[1, 2] and so will only be listed here. Additional or supplemental radiographic views are often necessary to make or confirm a suspected diagnosis. Additional radiographic views may consist of stress radiographic studies or projections of an anatomical part that provides better visualization of the part or area where a lesion may be present. Stress radiography has been defined as "the application of controlled force to a joint to demonstrate an abnormal spatial relationship between two or more of its components."[28] Stress radiographs are made by applying shear, wedge, rotary, and traction maneuvers.[28] Stress views are helpful to demonstrate subluxation or joint instability caused by ligamentous injuries. Stress views can be made, using a horizontal x-ray beam (Fig. 48–20), with the animal bearing weight, or stress can be applied to the medial, lateral, or dorsal surface of the joint with the animal in a recumbent position (Fig. 48–21).

Fore and Hind Paws

Routine Radiographic Views. Mediolateral, dorsopalmar-plantar, dorsolateral-palmaroplantaromedial and dorsomedial-palmaroplantarolateral views should be routinely made to thoroughly examine the fore and hind paws. "Spacers" such as cotton can be placed between the digits to decrease superimposition of bony structures on radiographs of the paw (Fig. 48–22).

Additional Views. If a more thorough examination of one digit

is necessary, gauze can be used to extend and isolate the digit for a lateral view (Fig. 48–23).

Metacarpus and Metatarsus

Routine Radiographic Views. Four views of the metacarpus-tarsus are recommended for a routine radiographic examination: mediolateral, dorsopalmar-plantar, dorsolateral-palmaroplantaromedial, and dorsomedial-palmaroplantarolateral views. Superimposition of the proximal metacarpal and metatarsal bones will occur in all views. Pseudofracture lines may be created by superimposition of the cortex from adjacent metacarpal or metatarsal bones (Fig. 48–24).

Carpus

Routine Radiographic Views. Routine views of the carpus are a mediolateral, dorsopalmar, dorsomedial-palmarolateral, and dorsolateral-palmaromedial views.

Additional Views. A flexed mediolateral view is helpful to evaluate the articular margins of the radius and carpal bones. It is also helpful to evaluate small fractures of the accessory carpal bone that occur at the dorsal proximal and distal margins and instability in the carpometacarpal joint from ligamentous injury. With stress radiographic views, a specific joint can be identified within the carpus that is unstable or subluxating (see Fig. 48–21). Once it is identified, possible treatment regimens can be formulated.

Elbow

Routine Radiographic Views. Mediolateral, flexed mediolateral, and craniocaudal views are routine for evaluating the elbow. A flexed mediolateral view is necessary to evaluate the entire anconeal process. A nonflexed lateral view provides good visualization of articular margins on the radius, ulna, and humerus, as well as good visualization of the humeroulnar, humeroradial, and radioulnar joint spaces. The craniocaudal view is necessary for joint space and subchondral bone evaluation.

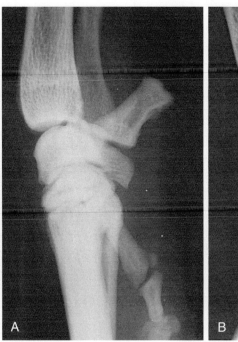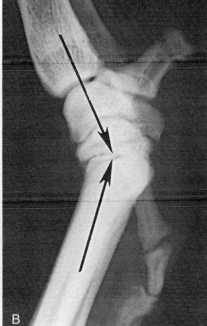

FIGURE 48–20. Non-weight-bearing mediolateral (*A*) and hyperextended mediolateral (*B*) views of the carpus. The hyperextended view demonstrates excess extension occurring in the carpometacarpal joint (*arrows*) indicative of instability from ligament and/or tendon injury.

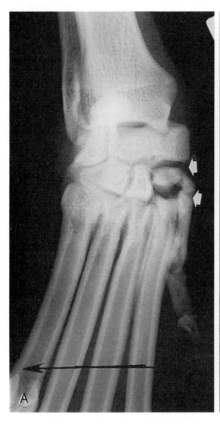 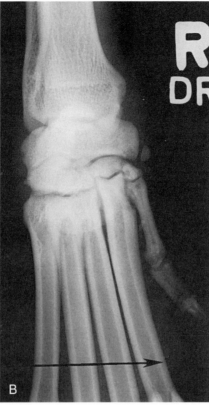

FIGURE 48–21. Dorsopalmar views of the carpus with stress applied to detect possible joint instability. *A,* Force is applied on the paw in a lateral direction (*long arrow*). Increased joint space width is produced in the middle and carpometacarpal joints (*white arrows*). Medial subluxation of the middle carpal and carpometacarpal joints occurs after disruption of the dorsal ligament from the radial carpal bone to the second carpal bone and/or the ligament from the palmar process of the radial carpal bone to metacarpal bones II and III. *B,* Force is applied on the paw in a medial direction (*long arrow*). No significant joint space widening is produced on the lateral aspect of the carpal and metacarpal joints.

Additional Views. A caudal 75 medial-craniolateral oblique view (mediolateral 15 degrees supinated) has been proposed[29] as a view to better identify fragmented medial coronoid processes; however, another study[19] found the view of no benefit for identification of fragmented medial coronoid processes. A cranial 20 lateral-caudomedial oblique view is helpful to better outline the medial portion of the humeral condyle when checking for osteochondrosis lesions or other subchondral bone changes that may occur in this area.[29]

Shoulder

Routine Radiographic Views. A mediolateral view and a craniocaudal view are routinely made to study the shoulder joint. When evaluating only for osteochondrosis of the humeral head, a mediolateral view may be sufficient.

Additional Views. A supinated mediolateral view of the shoulder is helpful in some cases to demonstrate osteochondrosis lesions located on the medial-caudal aspect of the humeral head. With

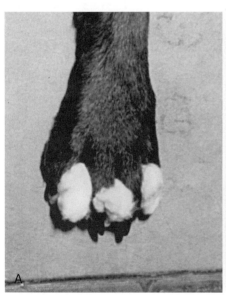 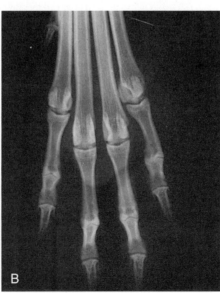

FIGURE 48–22. *A,* Cotton has been placed between the digits of the forepaw. *B,* Dorsopalmar view of the forepaw. The digits are straight and separated by the cotton.

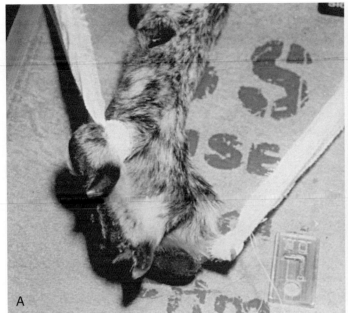 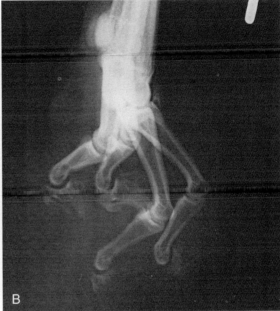

FIGURE 48–23. *A*, Gauze has been placed on the digits and traction applied to separate the toes and prevent superimposition. *B*, Lateromedial radiographic view of the forepaw. The digits are separated so that each can be visualized without superimposition.

this view, osteochondrosis lesions are more easily detected, and mineralized cartilage flaps are more consistently demonstrated.[30] Occasionally a lesion can be demonstrated on the supinated mediolateral view that was not apparent on the straight mediolateral view (Fig. 48–25). A flexed cranioproximal-craniodistal view of the intertubercular groove on the proximal humerus is helpful to localize bone fragments or mineralization located in the bicipital bursa or tendon area on the mediolateral view.[31] Mineralization of the biceps brachii tendon and the supraspinatus tendon can be differen-

tiated on this view based on location relative to the intertubercular groove. Bone fragment location within the intertubercular groove or lateral or medial to the groove can also be determined (Fig. 48–26). Radiographs of the shoulder made with traction on the forelimb and medial stress on the humeral head have been proposed as a technique to diagnose instability in the shoulder and specifically medial subluxation of the humeral head.[32] This condition is most often congenital in small dogs and traumatic in large dogs. Severe soft tissue injury and disruption are necessary with traumatic injuries to produce medial subluxation of the humerus.

Tarsus

Routine Radiographic Views. Mediolateral, dorsoplantar, dorsomedial-plantarolateral, and dorsolateral-plantaromedial views are recommended to study the tarsus.

Additional Radiographic Views. A flexed mediolateral view is helpful to observe the plantar aspect of the talus, ie, the trochlea. A dorsoplantar view with the tarsocrural joint in different degrees of flexion is helpful to demonstrate osteochondrosis lesions on the trochlear ridges that might not be tangential to the x-ray beam on a standard dorsoplantar view (Fig. 48–27). Stress views as applied in the carpus may also be used to demonstrate subluxation from ligamentous instability in the tarsus.

Stifle

Routine Radiographic Views. Mediolateral and craniocaudal views of the stifle provide sufficient information for a routine radiographic examination.

Additional Radiographic Views. A flexed cranioproximal-craniodistal view can be used to evaluate the patella and femoral trochlear groove in cases of patellar luxation. This view will demonstrate the position of the patella and the size, shape, and depth of the femoral trochlea. With chronic medial patellar luxation, the medial trochlear ridge is smaller and the femoral trochlea more shallow.[33] A mediolateral radiographic view with stress applied in a cranial and caudal direction can be used to demonstrate cruciate

FIGURE 48–24. Dorsopalmar view of the carpus and proximal metacarpal bones. A longitudinal pseudofracture line (*arrows*) is caused by superimposed bone cortices from the second and third metacarpal bones.

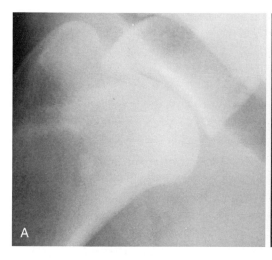 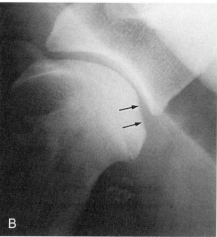

FIGURE 48–25. *A,* Straight mediolateral and, *B,* supinated mediolateral views of the shoulder. The contour of the humeral head appears normal on the straight mediolateral view (*A*). A subchondral bone defect (flattening) is demonstrated in the caudal humeral head on the supinated mediolateral view (*arrows, B*).

ligament ruptures, but this is usually not necessary because the instability can be characterized clinically in those cases in which it would also be apparent on stress radiographic views. Craniocaudal views with stress applied from either a medial or lateral direction are helpful in documenting ruptured collateral ligaments.

Pelvis

Routine Radiographic Views. The pelvis can be evaluated with a ventrodorsal and lateral radiograph. A ventrodorsal view with the hind limbs extended and parallel is necessary when the coxofemoral joints are being evaluated for hip dysplasia.

Additional Radiographic Views. A ventrodorsal view with the hind limbs in a flexed frog-leg position is useful for evaluating the femoral heads and necks for subtle fractures that may be suspected only on the extended ventrodorsal view or from the clinical examination.

Ventrodorsal radiographs with the hind limbs in extension and under traction to detect possible instability or laxity have been proposed for diagnosing hip dysplasia at an early age.[34] A view has also been described to evaluate the dorsal rim of the acetabulum[35] (Fig. 48–28). This view is a craniocaudal view of the dorsal

acetabular rim. This view has been reported to coincide with hip joint palpation in detecting joint laxity and dysplasia.[35]

GENERAL MISCELLANEOUS BONE CONDITIONS—YOUNG DOGS

Panosteitis

Panosteitis is an idiopathic disease generally of young large-breed dogs. It affects the long bones in the appendicular skeleton and produces lameness of varying severity and duration. The disease is self-limiting and requires a radiographic examination for diagnostic confirmation. The disease was first recognized in Europe and described as hematogenic purulent osteomyelitis[36] and as eosinophilic panosteitis.[37] It has also been described as juvenile osteomyelitis[38] and given the name enostosis.[39] Numerous other reports and descriptions have been given.[40–49] Large-breed male dogs are affected most commonly, with a high incidence reported in German shepherd dogs.[39, 43, 45] Clinical onset of the disease is usually between 5 and 12 months of age, but may occasionally occur in dogs up to 5 years of age or older. The course of the disease is usually

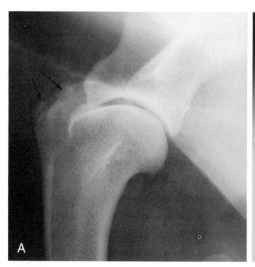 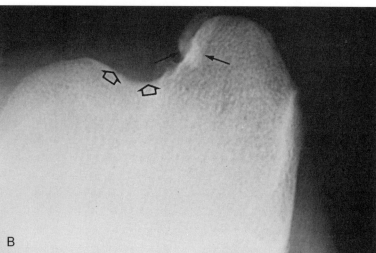

FIGURE 48–26. *A,* Mediolateral view of the shoulder and, *B,* cranioproximal-cranial distal (skyline) view of the proximal humerus. Bone fragments are present in the area of the greater tuberosity and intertubercular groove on the mediolateral view (*arrows, A*). On the (skyline) view the bone fragments are present on the greater tuberosity (*arrows, B*). The intertubercular groove (*open arrows*) and lesser tuberosity are normal.

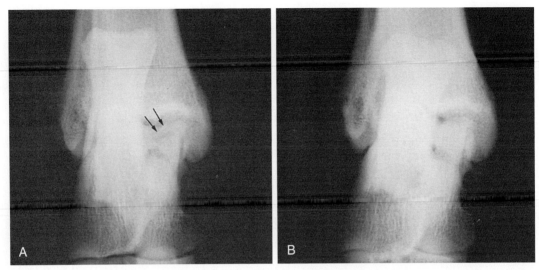

FIGURE 48–27. Dorsoplantar views of the tarsus, in extension, *A*, and in flexion, *B*. The medial aspect of the tarsocural joint is wide. On the dorsoplantar view made with the joint in extension (*A*) a small bone fragment and subchondral defect is present (*arrows*). The fragment is not identifiable on the dorsoplantar view made in flexion (*B*).

2 to 3 months but may range from 6 to 8 months. Clinically dogs have a shifting limb lameness. Intervals of no lameness may occur between lameness episodes as the lameness shifts from one limb to another. Pain may be elicited when local digital pressure is applied to long bones. Although numerous etiological factors have been proposed (osteomyelitis, vitamin deficiencies, mineral imbalance, allergy, viruses, parasites, vascularity, metabolic dysfunction, and genetic), no specific cause has yet been identified.

Scintigraphy has been shown to be more sensitive than radiography for diagnosing early lesions and correlates most accurately with lameness.[46] Radiography is necessary to confirm a specific diagnosis of panosteitis. In some late case of panosteitis, radiographs may be positive for the disease, scintigraphy negative, and the animal may have no clinical lameness.[46] Radiographic changes consist of increased trabecular pattern, endosteal proliferation, poorly marginated areas of increased medullary opacity usually located first in the area of the nutrient foramen, distinct focal or diffuse medullary opacities, and smooth periosteal reaction[39, 44, 48] (Fig. 48–29). All or any combination of these changes may be present in one bone or in several bones of the same animal. Early, middle, and late phases of panosteitis have been described relative to the radiographic appearance. The early phase has poorly marginated areas of increased opacity and accentuation of the trabecular pattern in the medullary cavity. In the middle phase, medullary opacities appear first in the region of the nutrient foramen, then progress to mottling and eventual opacification. The cortices may be thick, and a smooth periosteal reaction may be present. The late phase has a coarse trabecular pattern that may persist after clinical signs of lameness disappear.[42] High-contrast, high-detail radiographs will increase the diagnostic potential of radiographic views. Mediolateral views of long bones are best, and comparison radiographs of the contralateral bone are helpful if one is unsure of the diagnosis.

Hypertrophic Osteodystrophy

Hypertrophic osteodystrophy (HOD) is a systematically debilitating disease involving long bones of medium- and large-breed dogs.

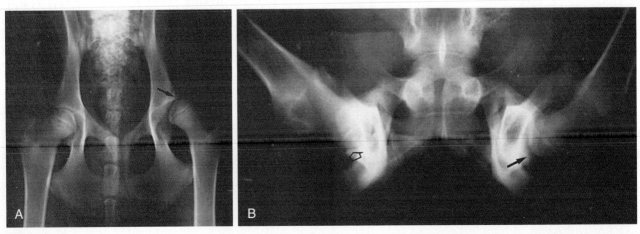

FIGURE 48–28. *A*, Ventrodorsal and, *B*, dorsal acetabular rim view of the pelvis. On the ventrodorsal view the left femoral head is subluxated and the left acetabulum is shallow with abnormal conformation of the dorsal acetabular rim (*arrow*). On the dorsal acetabular rim view the left acetabular rim is incomplete (*solid arrow*) compared with the right acetabular rim (*open arrow*).

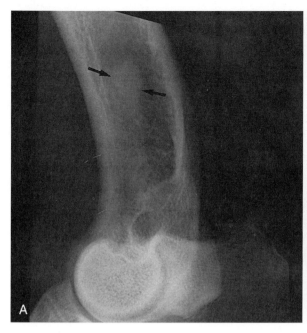

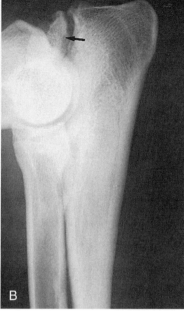

FIGURE 48–29. *A,* Lateral view of the distal humerus. A nodular medullary opacity (*arrows*) is present in the distal humerus, diagnostic of panosteitis. *B,* Lateral view of the proximal radius and ulna. There is a diffuse opacity within the medullary cavity of the proximal ulna typical of panosteitis. An ununited anconeal process is also present (*arrow*).

The disease is bilaterally symmetrical, and more severe in the distal aspect of long bones and limbs. It has been given several names over the years: Barlow's disease,[50] skeletal scurvy,[51] hypertrophic osteodystrophy,[52, 53] osteodystrophy II,[53] and metaphyseal osteopathy.[54]

The clinical onset of the disease is usually at 3 to 6 months of age with no sex predilection reported. Clinical signs consist of lameness, generalized soreness, fever, depression, inappetence, and reluctance to move.[55] On physical examination the long-bone metaphyseal areas are firm, warm, and swollen, and pain can be elicited on palpation.[54] The disease may also involve costochondral junctions,[55–57] teeth,[57] and the skull.[58] Several causes have been

proposed, but none has been proven. The most popular etiological considerations are vitamin C deficiency,[51, 52, 59] overnutrition,[53, 60, 61] and infection.[57, 62, 63] At present, considering the systemic manifestations and the histological and radiographic appearance of the lesions, infection appears to be the most logical causative factor. Specific organisms have not been cultured from the bony lesions.

Radiography is the imaging procedure of choice for diagnosing HOD in vivo. Although the radiographic appearance is not specific for determining an etiological agent, it is specific for diagnosing the syndrome of HOD.[54–56, 64] The radiographic changes consist of a radiopaque zone on the diaphyseal side of the physis with an adjacent radiolucent zone (Fig. 48–30). The radiopaque zone is

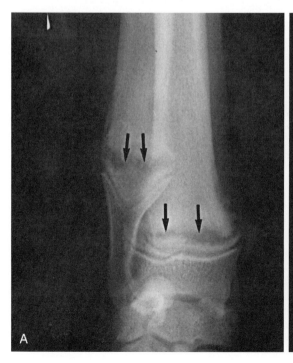

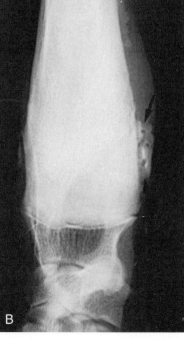

FIGURE 48–30. Radiographic changes of hypertrophic osteodystrophy (HOD) are present in the distal radius and ulna. *A,* Proximal to the distal radial and ulnar physes, a zone of bone adjacent to a lytic zone (*arrows*) is present in the metaphyses typical of the more acute stages of HOD. *B,* A wide, bone-dense metaphysis is present in the distal radius with a cuff of new bone production in the adjacent soft tissue (*arrows*) typical of the late or healing stages of HOD.

reported histologically to consist of an elongated calcified cartilage lattice of the primary spongiosa and impacted trabeculae from infraction.[57] The radiolucent zone has been reported to represent accumulation of erythrocytes[54] or inflammatory cells.[57] Other radiographic changes that may also be seen are increased metaphyseal opacity and widening, periosteal reaction, and a metaphyseal cuff of bone within the surrounding soft tissues (Fig. 48–30).[57] The increased metaphyseal bone density may represent a healing phase of the bone disease and the bone production in the soft tissue, a response to suppurative inflammation.[57] It has been suggested that HOD has phases that are recognizable radiographically.[54, 56] The phases that occur in a time sequence are soft tissue phase, alterations in metaphyseal bone structure (sclerotic and lytic zones), and a healing phase consisting of increased bone density and soft tissue bone production. Since the disease has systemic signs, radiographic identification of the disease using the above-listed signs is important.

References

1. Ticer JW: Radiographic Technique in Veterinary Practice, 2nd ed. Philadelphia, WB Saunders Company, 1984.
2. Morgan JP, Silverman S: Techniques of Veterinary Radiography, 4th ed., Ames, Iowa, State University Press, 1984.
3. Galanski M, Oestmann JW, Kattapuram SV, et al: Digital radiography in bone and joint disease. In Greene RE, Oestmann JW (eds): Computed Digital Radiography in Clinical Practice. New York, Thieme Medical Publishers, 1992, p 126.
4. Dik KJ: Equine arthrography. Vet Rad 25:93–96, 1984.
5. Wright JD, Wood AKW: Arthrography of the equine tarsus: A comparison between iohexol and sodium and meglumine diatrizoate. Vet Rad 29:191, 1988.
6. Nixon AJ, Spencer CP: Arthrography of the equine shoulder joint. Equine Vet J 22:107–113, 1990.
7. van Bree H, Van Rijssen B, Tshamala M, et al: Comparison of the nonionic contrast agents, iopromide and iotrolan, for positive-contrast arthrography of the scapulohumeral joint in dogs. Am J Vet Res. 53:1622–1626, 1992.
8. Atilola MA, Pennock PW, Summer-Smith G: Evaluation of analytical grade of metrizamide for canine stifle arthrography. JAVMA 185:436–439, 1984.
9. Lowry JE, Carpenter LG, Park RD, et al: Radiographic anatomy and technique for arthrography of the cubital joint in clinically normal dogs. JAVMA 203:72–77, 1993.
10. Muhumuza L, Morgan JP, Miyabayashi T, et al: Positive-contrast arthrography—A study of the humeral joints in normal beagle dogs. Vet Radiol 29:157–161, 1988.
11. van Bree H, Van Russen B, Peremans K, Peremans J: A comparison of diatrizoate and ioxaglate for positive contrast shoulder arthrography in dogs. Vet Radiol 32:291–296, 1991.
12. Lamb CR: Contrast radiography of equine joints, tendon sheaths and draining tracts. Vet Clin North Am Equine Pract 7:241–257, 1991.
13. Suter PF, Carb AV: Shoulder arthrography in dogs—Radiographic anatomy and clinical application. J Small Anim Pract 10:407–413, 1969.
14. van Bree H: Evaluation of the prognostic value of positive-contrast shoulder arthrography for bilateral osteochondrosis lesions in dogs. Am J Vet Res 51:1121–1125, 1990.
15. Rivers B, Wallace L, Johnston GR: Biceps tenosynovitis in the dog: Radiographic and sonographic findings. Vet Comparative Orthopaed Traumatol 5:51–57, 1992.
16. Barthez PY, Morgan JP: Bicipital tenosynovitis in the dog—Evaluation with positive contrast arthrography. Vet Rad Ultrasound 34:325–330, 1993.
17. Lincoln JD, Potter K: Tenosynovitis of the biceps brachii tendon in dogs. J Am Anim Hosp Assoc 20:385–392, 1984.
18. LaHue TR, Brown SG, Roush JC, et al: Entrapment of joint mice in the bicipital tendon sheath as a sequela to osteochondritis dissecans of the proximal humerus in dogs. J Am Anim Hosp Assoc 24:99–105, 1988.
19. Carpenter LG, Schwarz PD, Lowry JE, et al: Comparison of radiologic imaging techniques for the diagnosis of fragmented medial coronoid process of the cubital joint in dogs. JAVMA 203:78–83, 1993.
20. Murphy WA: Magnetic resonance imaging. In Resnick D (ed): Bone and Joint Imaging, Philadelphia, WB Saunders Company, 1989, p 120.
21. Kang HS, Resnick D: MRI of the Extremities; An Anatomic Atlas. Philadelphia, WB Saunders Company, 1991.
22. Recht MP, Kramer J, Marcelis S, et al: Abnormalities of articular cartilage in the knee: Analysis of available MR techniques. Radiology 187:473–478, 1993.
23. Sabiston CP, Adams ME, David KBL: Magnetic resonance imaging of osteoarthritis; Correlation with gross pathology using an experimental model. J Orthop Res 5:164–172, 1987.
24. Widmer WR, Buckwalter KA, Braunstein EM, et al: Principles of magnetic resonance imaging and application to the stifle joint in dogs. JAVMA 198:1914–22, 1991.
25. Widmer WR, Buckwalter KA, Braunstein EM, et al: Radiographic and magnetic resonance imaging of the stifle joint in experimental osteoarthritis of dogs. Vet Rad Ultrasound 35:371–393, 1994.
26. van Bree H, Degryse H, Van Ryssen B, et al: Pathologic correlations with magnetic resonance images of ostechondrosis lesions in canine shoulders. JAVMA 202:1099–1105, 1993.
27. Lamb CR: Non-skeletal distribution of bone-seeking radiopharmaceuticals. Vet Rad 31:246–253, 1990.
28. Farrow CS: Stress radiography: Application in small animal practice. JAVMA 181:777–784, 1982.
29. Voorhout G, Hazewindel HAW: Radiographic evaluation of the canine elbow joint with special reference to the medial humeral condyle and the medial coronoid process. Vet Rad 28:158–165, 1987.
30. Callahan TH, Ackerman N: The supinated mediolateral radiograph for detection of humeral head osteochondrosis in the dog. Vet Rad 26:144–148, 1985.
31. Flo GL, Middleton D: Mineralization of the supraspinatus tendon in dogs. JAVMA 197:95–97, 1990.
32. Puglisi TA, Tangner CH, Green RW, et al: Stress radiography of the canine humeral joint. J Am Anim Hosp Assoc 24:235–240, 1988.
33. Owens JM, Ackerman N, Nyland T: Roentgenology of joint trauma. Vet Clin North Am 8:419–451, 1978.
34. Smith GK, Biery DN, Gregor TP: New concepts of coxofemoral joint stability and the development of a clinical stress-radiographic method for quantitating hip joint laxity in the dog. JAVMA 196:59–70, 1990.
35. Slocum B, Devome TM: Dorsal acetabular rim radiographic view for evaluation of the canine hip. J Am Anim Hosp Assoc 26:289–296, 1990.
36. Baumann R, Pommer A: Die chronische osteomyelitis der jungen schaferhunde. Tierarztl Mschr 38:670, 1951.
37. Gratzl E: Die eosinophile panostitis der junghunde (Osteomyelitis der jungen schaferhunde). Wien terarztl Mschr 38:629, 1951.
38. Wamberg K: Atlas Radiologica. Copenhagen, Medical Book Company, 1966.
39. Cotter SM, Griffiths RC, Leav I: Enostosis of young dogs. JAVMA 153:401, 1960.
40. Barrett RB, Schall WD, Lewis RE: Clinical and radiographic features of canine eosinophilic panosteitis. J Am Anim Hosp Assoc 4:94, 1968.
41. Evers WH: Enostosis in a dog. JAMA 154:799–803, 1969.
42. Bohning RH Jr, Suter PF, Horn RB, et al: Clinical and radiologic survey of canine panosteitis. JAVMA 156:870–883, 1970.
43. Burt JK, Wilson GP III: A study of eosinophilic panosteitis (enostosis) in German shepherd dogs. Prog Vet Radiol Acta Radiol Suppl 319, pp 7–13, 1972.
44. Kaastrom H, Olsson SE, Suter PF: Panosteitis in the dog: A radiographic, scintimetric and trifluorochrome investigation. Progress in Vet Radiol, Act Radiol Suppl 319, pp 15–23, 1972.
45. Van Sickle D: Canine panosteitis. Selected orthopedic problems in the growing dog. AAHA Publication 20–28, 1975.
46. Turnier JC, Silverman S: A case study of canine panosteitis: Comparison of radiographic and radioisotopic studies. Am J Vet Res 39:1550–1552, 1978.
47. Bone DL: Canine panosteitis. Canine Pract 7:61–68, 1980.
48. Stead AC, Stead MCP, Galloway FH: Panosteitis in dogs. J Small Anim Pract 24:623–635, 1983.
49. Grondalen J, Sjaastad O, Teige J: Enostosis (panosteitis) in three dogs suffering from hemophilia A. Canine Pract 16:10–14, 1991.
50. Merillat LA: Barlow's disease of the dog. Vet Med 31:304, 1936.

51. Holmes JR: Suspected skeletal scurvy in the dog. Vet Rec 74:801, 1962.
52. Meier H, Clark ST, Schnelle GB, Will DH: Hypertrophic osteodystrophy associated with disturbance of vitamin C synthesis in dogs. JAVMA 130:483, 1957.
53. Riser WH: Radiographic differential diagnosis of skeletal diseases of young dogs. J Am Vet Radiol Soc 5:26, 1964.
54. Grondalen J: Metaphyseal osteopathy (hypertrophic osteodystrophy) in growing dogs. A clinical study. J Small Anim Pract 17:721–735, 1976.
55. La Croix JA: Osteochondrosis dissecans, enostosis (eosinophilic panosteitis) and hypertrophic osteodystrophy (lameness). *In* Kirk RW (ed): Current Veterinary Therapy. Small Animal Practice. Philadelphia, WB Saunders Company, 1977, pp 874–878.
56. Rendano VT, Dueland R, Sifferman RL: Metaphyseal osteopathy: (Hypertrophic osteopathy). Letter to the editor. J Small Anim Pract 18:679–683, 1977.
57. Woodard JC: Canine hypertrophic osteodystrophy, A study of the spontaneous disease in littermates. Vet Pathol 19:337–354, 1982.
58. Watson ADJ, Blair RC, Farrow BRH, et al: Hypertrophic osteodystrophy in the dog. Aust Vet J 49:433–439, 1973.
59. Vaananen M, Wikman L: Scurvy as a cause of osteodystrophy. J Small Anim Pract 20:491–500, 1979.
60. Hedhammar A, Wu FM, Krook L: Overnutrition and skeletal disease, An experimental study in growing great Dane dogs. Cornell Vet (Suppl) 5:64, 1974.
61. Teare JA, Krook L, Kallfelz FA, et al: Ascorbic acid deficiency and hypertrophic osteodystrophy in the dog: A rebuttal. Cornell Vet 69:384–401, 1979.
62. Clarke RE: Hypertrophic osteodystrophy in the canine associated with a lowered resistance to infection—An unusual case history. Aust Vet Pract 8:39–43, 1978.
63. Schulz KS, Payne JT, Aronson E: *Escherichia coli* bacteremia associated with hypertrophic osteodystrophy in a dog. JAVMA 199:1170–1173, 1991.
64. Alexander JW: Hypertrophic osteodystrophy. Canine Pract 5:48–52, 1978.

CHAPTER 49

GREYHOUND RACING INJURIES: RACETRACK INJURY SURVEY

MARK S. BLOOMBERG \ WILLIAM W. DUGGER

Beginning in 1990, the racing greyhound injury survey program at the University of Florida's Center for Veterinary Sports Medicine (CVSM) was converted from a manual collecting format to a "fill in the bubble" optical scan sheet combined with a summary sheet for each meet or specific time period. The survey sheets are completed by the track veterinarian and then forwarded along with a summary sheet to the CVSM. The survey sheets are optically scanned and transferred to a high-density 3.5-inch diskette from which the data are entered into a Paradox 3.5 spreadsheet for preparation of reports and statistical evaluation. Sixteen racing greyhound tracks are presently submitting injury survey sheets for data collection.

The initial injury survey took place in January, 1984, and ran through June, 1990. A total of 761 injuries was reported from 47,323 races. Only those injuries that occurred during the actual race and were recognized by the track veterinarian were recorded. Table 49–1 represents the distribution of the injuries reported. Tables 49–2 and 49–3 represent the relationship of racing injuries to box number and race number, respectively.

The new racing injury survey system has identified 1269 racing injuries in 5 years at 16 greyhound tracks (these are not necessarily the same tracks as in the earlier study). Table 49–4 represents the distribution of these injuries. We have expanded the list of injuries to reflect the anatomical location of the injury more accurately. There appear to be some interesting changes in the distribution of the injuries using the present format. The number of tarsal injuries has decreased from 52.2 to 44.3 per cent. The number of metatarsal and metacarpal (quarter-bone) injuries has increased from 8.3 to 15.4 per cent. This may be a reflection of the effect of increased banking of the turns and faster or more firm racing surfaces resulting in more vertical stress forces being placed on these bones.

TABLE 49–1. Injuries at Six Racing Greyhound Tracks 1984–1990

Injury	Total (%)
Tarsal	397 (52.2)
Muscle	85 (11.2)
Foot	63 (8.3)
Toe	63 (8.3)
Other	58 (7.6)
Ankle	49 (6.4)
Foreleg	46 (6.0)
Total	761

Tabulated from 47,323 races involving approximately 378,584 dogs.

TABLE 49–2. Tarsal Injuries at Six Greyhound Tracks Relative to Post Position 1984–1990

Post position	1	2	3	4	5	6	7	8
Tarsal injuries	31	48	34	49	36	51	47	50
Total other injuries	32	35	42	29	51	29	34	29
Total	63	83	76	78	87	80	81	79

134 did not have post position.
Tabulated from 47,323 races involving approximately 378,584 dogs.

Greyhound Racing Injuries / **413**

TABLE 49–3. Relationship of Tarsal and Muscle Injuries to Race Number at Six Racing Greyhound Tracks 1984–1990

Type of Injury	1	2	3	4	5	6	7	8	9	10	11	12	13
						Race Number							
Tarsal	13	21	22	23	37	35	30	33	36	39	29	43	35
Muscle	6	7	7	6	7	7	7	8	5	8	7	4	4
Total	32	48	54	47	57	59	62	62	64	76	63	54	50

TABLE 49–4. Injuries at 16 Racing Greyhound Tracks from 1990–1995

Injury	Total (%)
Muscle	125 (9.85)
Long-bone fracture	78 (6.15)
Tarsus	562 (44.29)
Metatarsus	167 (13.16)
Carpus	63 (4.96)
Metacarpus	28 (2.21)
Toe	99 (7.80)
Laceration	31 (2.44)
Cramping	10 (.79)
Other	97 (7.64)
?	9 (.71)
Total	1269

TABLE 49–5. Location of Injuries at 12 Racing Greyhound Tracks 1990–1995

5/16

Injury	Box	First Turn	Backstretch	Second Turn	Homestretch	Escape
Muscle	9	24	7	10	24	1
Long bone fracture		58	3	7	1	
Tarsus	6	224	35	83	27	9
Metatarsus		71	13	18	9	4
Carpus	1	20	4	8	4	1
Metacarpus		12	2	1	6	1
Toe	1	21	3	9	3	2
Laceration		7		3	2	1
Cramping		2		3	2	2
Other	5	31	1	10	13	3
?		1		1	1	
Total	22	471	68	153	92	24

3/8 and 7/16

Injury	Box	First Turn	Backstretch	Second Turn	Homestretch	Escape
Muscle	1	3		2	5	
Long bone fracture		2	1	1		
Tarsus	2	44	9	20	13	
Metatarsus	1	10	3	8	1	
Carpus	1	1	1		1	
Metacarpus		2	1			
Toe			2			
Laceration		3		3		
Cramping						
Other		3	1	5	4	
?						
Total	5	68	18	39	24	0

126 injuries occurred in races with unreported length.

TABLE 49–6. Injuries per Grade of Race

Race Grades	% of Total Races	% of Total Injuries
Stakes	.4	1
AA	.2	1
A	12	18
B	17	17
C	21	24
D	24	22
Maiden	8	3
Schooling	17	7

TABLE 49–7. Type of Injury vs Race Number at 16 Greyhound Race Tracks from 1990–1995

Injury	1	2	3	4	5	6	7	8
Muscle	16	8	5	8	6	10	8	8
Long-bone fracture	3	10	8	2	6	7	2	3
Tarsus	20	33	29	40	37	38	36	41
Metatarsus	10	15	6	2	12	11	18	7
Carpus	5	6	3	5	4	5	5	4
Metacarpus	1		2	4	2	3	2	1
Toe	10	7	4	7	8	5	9	7
Laceration	5			2	2	3	3	2
Cramping	2		2	1		2		
Other	4	11	6	8	11	10	8	4
?	2	1		1	1	1		
Total	78	91	65	80	89	95	91	77

Injury	9	10	11	12	13	14	15	?
Muscle	5	8	10	10	6	5	2	10
Long-bone fracture	6	9	6	6	3	2	1	4
Tarsus	37	43	44	47	34	24	11	48
Metatarsus	11	15	11	12	14	8	3	12
Carpus	3	5	8	2	2	1		5
Metacarpus	1	2	2	4		2		2
Toe	9	8	6	4	3			12
Laceration	2	2	2	2	1	2		3
Cramping	1		1		1			
Other	6	6	2	6	4	2	2	7
?		1	1		1			1
Total	81	98	93	93	69	46	19	104

TABLE 49–8. Type of Injury vs Box Position at 16 Greyhound Race Tracks 1/1/90–8/30/95

Injury	1	2	3	4	5	6	7	8	?
Muscle	15	6	16	16	10	15	19	18	10
Long bone fracture	10	11	9	11	9	5	8	11	4
Tarsus	55	67	80	58	79	47	61	76	39
Metatarsus	17	17	18	24	20	16	17	28	10
Carpus	6	7	6	5	7	11	10	6	5
Metacarpus	1	3	4	3	5	5	3	2	2
Toe	20	13	4	12	11	7	15	6	11
Laceration	1	5	9	3	3	4	2	1	3
Cramping	1	1	1	2		2	2	1	
Other	12	11	6	10	15	8	16	12	7
?		1	1	3		1	2		1
Total	138	142	154	147	159	121	155	161	92

This would be in contrast to the torsional forces placed on the tarsus on the lower banked tracks that often resulted in tarsal fractures. The percentage of the injuries that occurred on the turns (74%) has remained constant (Table 49–5). This emphasizes that important research still remains to be obtained relative to the ideal construction of the racing surface in the turns and its biomechanical relationship to injuries.

The addition of the completed summary sheets has provided crucial information to evaluate the incidence of injuries per grade of race and injuries per performance. Distribution of grades of races during a meet at a typical racing greyhound track is shown in Table 49–6.

There appears to be a trend toward a higher incidence of injuries in the higher grades of races. This may be a reflection of the speed, competitive spirit, or the intense physical contact these greyhounds face in these very competitive races.

The previous surveys identified a trend for more injuries to occur in the later races of a performance, but this does not seem to be represented by the data in Table 49–7. There does not appear to be a difference in the number of injuries relative to box number (Table 49–8). This information has been utilized to calculate the incidence of racing injuries per performance in an attempt to inform the racetrack management if a problem is developing. We documented

the incidence of injuries at one track from 1 injury per 5 performances to 1 per 14 performances following major reconstruction of the racing surface. Subsequently we have seen the incidence of injuries at that particular track increase to 1 per 8 performances. This indicates that a causal relationship may be present and should be investigated, especially relative to maintenance of the original racing surface. It is noteworthy that the injury incidence in this track's 3/8th races were twice that of the 5/16th races. This may be a reflection of the greyhounds' having to negotiate an extra turn in the 3/8th races.

In 1995 we began to look at a new statistic. We began comparing the number of mishaps or collisions and falls per race at approximately 20 greyhound tracks. This information is being gathered from the racing programs as entered by the respective track's chart writer. The incidence of mishaps and falls per race ranges from a low of 25 per cent to a high of 83 per cent. Looking at this information monthly allows the evaluator to determine if problems are developing at a certain track or if a track is consistently having a high incidence of mishaps and falls.

All of the aforementioned data are kept confidential inasmuch as only the greyhound track involved in the survey program knows its code number. If comparison data are shared it is done only as a total of all injury information and resultant averages.

CHAPTER 50

VETERINARY PROBLEMS OF RACING SLED DOGS

DOMINIQUE GRANDJEAN \ KENNETH W. HINCHCLIFF \ STUART NELSON \ KARIN A. SCHMIDT \ PETER D. CONSTABLE \ ROBERT SEPT \ ALBERT S. TOWNSHEND

The increasing popularity of sled dog racing highlights the importance of veterinary involvement in this sport. Veterinarians are responsible for educating dog drivers (mushers) on kennel care, preventive medicine, and minor medical care of dogs; providing care of dogs during and after races; and for overseeing drug (doping) control programs. Therefore, a veterinarian on a sled dog race should have a good knowledge of the specific problems of sled dogs, an understanding of the race rules, and an appreciation of the musher's role in the sport.[1]

There are three types of sled dog races: sprint races, which are usually organized over 3 days (one heat per day: 5 to 20 miles per heat depending on the number of dogs), for example, the Fur Rendevous in Anchorage, Alaska; and long distance or stage races, in which teams of 12 to 20 dogs race for days to weeks, such as the Iditarod Trail Race in Alaska. Sprint races are usually run at high speed (20–30 mph), whereas endurance races are run at a much slower speed (8–10 mph). A third category of races appeared

10 years ago in Europe (stage races including 10 to 20 stages, each from 40 to 80 miles per day) and is now seen in Alaska, Wyoming, and Scandinavia. Because of the different speeds at which the dogs run, medical problems in sprint races differ from those found in longer races. The approach is quite different in long-distance races, as the veterinarian is one of the officials (with race judges and the race marshal) sharing the life of the dog teams from the starting line to the finish. It becomes possible on these races to handle and follow more "chronic" disorders and to adapt decisions as problems develop. The following is a brief description of common problems found in sled dogs.

MUSCULOSKELETAL CONDITIONS

Foot Problems. Care of the feet is a vital part of the overall maintenance of a racing sled dog. Neglected feet may lead to lameness, infection, depressed appetite, and poor performance. Years of improvement in breeding, nutrition, treatment, and prevention now allow a dog to travel thousands of miles in a racing season with healthy feet. The basics of foot care are the prevention

This chapter is dedicated to the memory of Tom Cooley, DVM, a founding member of the International Sled Dog Veterinary Medical Association.

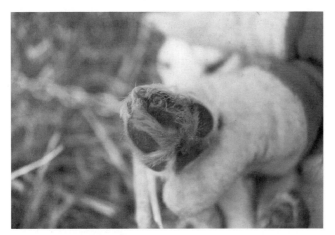

FIGURE 50–1. Circular abrasion on a pad.

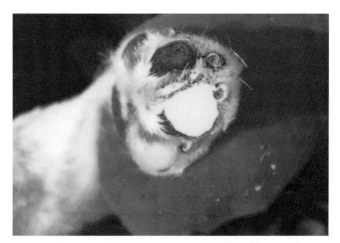

FIGURE 50–3. Gluing of a moleskin patch on the pad abrasion seen in Figure 50–2.

and early recognition of potential problems, accurate assessment of any developing problems, and prompt and adequate treatment. Foot conditions can be categorized as involving the pads or palmar or plantar interdigital areas (webs).

Pad Injuries. Pad injuries are the easiest to recognize and are usually cuts, slices, and/or abrasions. Cuts and slices are usually caused by ice, frozen rough ground, or sharp objects. Worn pads are often associated with gravel or road surfaces not covered by snow. Deep cuts into the pad must be sutured as soon as possible. Slices off the pad have to be protected by glueing a patch of soft material such as moleskin over the raw pad. Worn pads should be protected with booties (Figs. 50–1 through 50–5).

Web Disorders. Web (palmar or plantar interdigital space) disorders are harder to recognize than are injuries to the pads. To visualize these injuries, the toes are separated and the area between them is examined in good light or with the aid of a flashlight. Both the top and the bottom of the foot are examined thoroughly for cracks, splits, and abrasions, although these lesions are much more common on the palmar or plantar surface. Common interdigital lesions include irritation or splits in the skin deep between the toes and friction burns or blisters between the toes. Without prompt recognition and care, the foot tends to become moist and swollen, aggravating the condition. Web injuries may require diligent care to heal initially. The accumulation of snow or soft ice between the toes (''snowballs'') may cause inflammation of soft interdigital

tissues and depilation of hair. The resulting loss of interdigital fur appears to hasten the progress of infection. Wind-blown or granular snow and booties with holes in them often cause serious web problems.

Interdigital lesions may be graded[2] as follows: Grade 1, interdigital irritation and the area pink and swollen (Figs. 50–6 and 50–7); Grade 2, splits in the skin between the toes and the pads (Fig. 50–8); Grade 3, cracks and cuts (Figs. 50–9 through 50–11); Grade 4, inflammation and accumulation of pus; and Grade 5, infection affecting the whole foot and producing fever, depression, and malaise, which can quickly progress to septicemia.

In sprint or stage races, only Grades 1 or 2 occur during the competition. On long-distance races such as the Iditarod or the Yukon Quest in Alaska and Canada, it is not uncommon to see interdigital problems up to Grades 3 or 4. Grade 5 lesions are rare but should be treated aggressively. This is particularly true when the delay between consecutive checkpoints exceeds 24 hours and the musher is inexperienced. Up to Grade 3, the treatment mainly consists of soothing foot ointments and wearing of booties. Basic treatment of foot injuries begins with cleaning deep wounds with a mild disinfectant such as tamed iodine or chlorhexadine solutions. An efficient prevention and treatment is the use of liniment enriched with hyperoxygenated fatty acids, which have strong antiinflammatory effects and are not drugs (APgyval). Systemic antibiot-

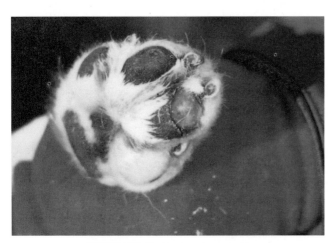

FIGURE 50–2. Circular cut on a pad.

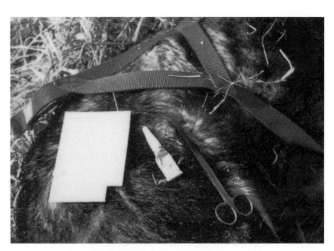

FIGURE 50–4. Pad cuts: necessary equipment.

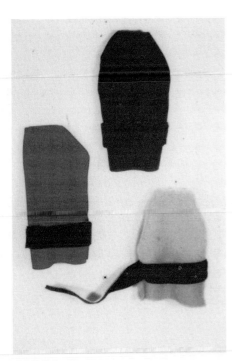

FIGURE 50–5. Different types of booties utilized on sled dogs.

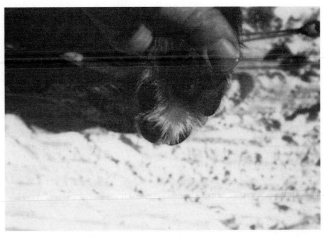

FIGURE 50–7. Starting "strawberry" lesion.

ics should be used for deep or infected lesions. Amoxicillin works well on most problems; however, clindamycin may be more effective for more serious (Grade 5) infections. Untreated infections beginning in the feet have developed to fatal systemic infection in less than 24 hours under race conditions.

A wide variety of home remedy foot ointments have been developed. A basic ointment using a drying agent such as zinc oxide mixed with an antibiotic ointment such as bacitracin-neomycin-polymyxin is considered a good initial foot ointment (proportion 1 to 10). Dexamethasone (when no cuts are present), scarlet oil, aloe vera, and the "skin cocktail" of vitamins are some of the ingredients added to some homemade ointments. Betadine ointment may be used for severely infected feet. Furacin ointment has been used extensively in the past but is now being replaced by these newer ointments.

Good conditioning, good nutrition, and genetics are important in preventing foot problems. A poorly trained, tired, or overly stressed dog may be more likely to develop foot problems than is a dog that is well trained. During the training period, when there is no snow, gravel roads must be avoided. Dogs that have been bred for good feet have fewer problems than do dogs with poor foot conformation. Good foot conformation includes small or "tight" feet with hair between the pads for distance races, whereas for sprint races it is better not to use dogs with too much hair between the toes.

The diet must be balanced, with high-quality protein, fat, and adequate amounts of minerals and vitamins. Chronic foot problems sometimes improve with zinc supplementation. Pads become thicker with a supplementation of 2.5 g per day per 10 ounces of gelatin in the food.

Booties are often and effectively used on racing sled dogs (Figs. 50–5 and 50–12 through 50–15). They can be made of any one of several materials, including Cordura, nylon, Polar Fleece, ballistics nylon, trigger cloth, cotton duck, and polypropylene fabrics, with

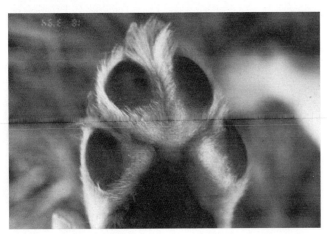

FIGURE 50–6. Grade 1 interdigital irritation.

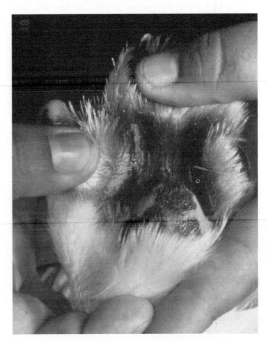

FIGURE 50–8. Grade 2 interdigital problem.

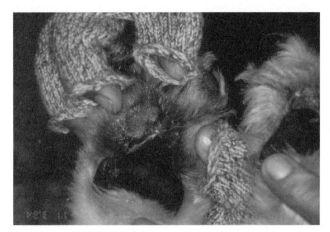

FIGURE 50–9. Grade 3 interdigital problem.

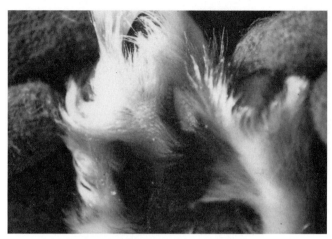

FIGURE 50–10. Grade 3 cuts between the toes.

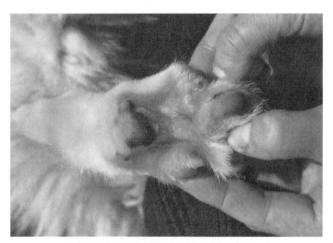

FIGURE 50–11. Grade 3 cuts laterally to the pad.

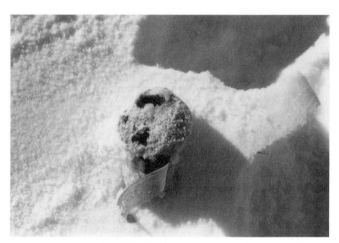

FIGURE 50–12. Misused booty.

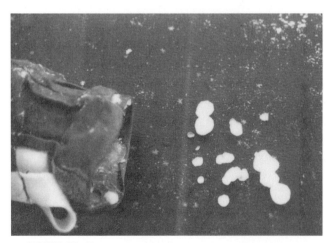

FIGURE 50–13. Ice balls inside the Velcro of a waterproof bootie.

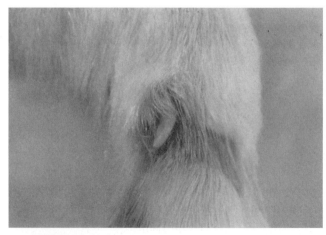

FIGURE 50–14. Consequence of misused Velcro on the booty.

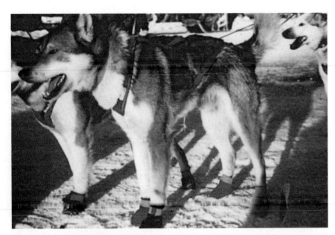

FIGURE 50–15. Sled dogs with booties on.

Velcro closing straps. Cordura and ballistics nylon are waterproof and very resistant to abrasion but provide poor traction on ice, whereas polar fleece provides excellent traction. A dog team may use as many as 1500 to 2000 booties over an entire long-distance race. During the race water will be trapped inside the bootie, which, on freezing, causes abrasion of the foot. Booties must be intact (no holes) and applied so that they fit snugly but not so tightly that they impede the circulation. Tight booties do not let the feet expand naturally and overly large booties hamper the dog's gait. Booties should be removed or loosened during rest periods to restore normal circulation and to allow the dog to clean its feet. Many mushers recommend the use of booties whenever the temperatures drop below −20 to −30 degrees F. Cold temperatures delay healing, and at these temperatures prevention of foot lesions is very important. Under the right conditions, such as soft, clean snow, it is beneficial to remove the booties shortly before coming into a checkpoint to allow some cleansing of the feet. Swollen toes or feet (without splits or other problems) are rarely seen except under racing conditions (Fig. 50–16). They occur after long periods of running on hard trails. Ointments may help reduce swelling while the dog rests.

Nails and Toes. Conditions in which the dog's feet break through the snow or ice on the trail (especially crusty snow) injure nailbeds. Nail and nailbed injuries include periungual infections, broken nails, and accidental or traumatic loss of the nail. Signs of nailbed injuries and infection include swelling and redness of the

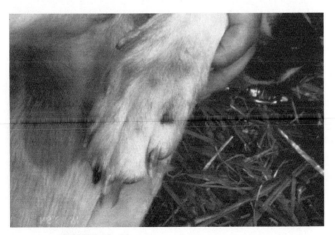

FIGURE 50–16. Inflammation on top of the toes.

tissue, often with serum or pus around the base of the nail. Lost nails are readily apparent on careful examination. These lesions may be easy to miss in a dog with long dark hair on its feet. Long toenails are prone to being torn or being pulled out. Nailbed disorders are treated with use of booties, ointments, and/or antibiotics. Keeping toenails trimmed reduces the chance of nail loss or fracture.

Dewclaws can be problematic in sled dogs. Dewclaws are prone to injury or to irritation when booties are worn. When irritation develops under dewclaws, the booties are removed unless needed to treat more serious conditions. If booties are needed, the area between the dewclaw and the foot should be protected with tape or other bandage material. Antibiotics are used, if necessary. Removal of dewclaws on newborn puppies is the best prevention for these problems. Adult dogs prone to dewclaw irritation should also have them removed.

Orthopedic Injuries. Lameness is one of the most common afflictions of sled dogs. Assessment of its cause depends on a clinical examination and knowledge of common conditions.

Physical Examination of the Racing Sled Dog. Examination of the musculoskeletal system of sled dogs can be learned quickly and provides valuable information about the cause of the lameness and often provides a likely prognosis. A skilled evaluator can recognize incipient orthopedic problems, which can aid in the early diagnosis and treatment of injuries, preventing unnecessary pain and allowing full return to function as soon as possible. It is recommended that the musher perform complete examinations regularly throughout the year to familiarize the dogs with the examination process and to increase the musher's familiarity with each dog. Physical examination of sled dogs should focus on three important elements: observation, gait analysis, and palpation.

Physical examinations are more detailed before and after the race than are those done during the race. Although it is difficult to assess a large team as they come into a checkpoint, veterinarians should examine every dog at every checkpoint. When the team enters the checkpoint or crosses the finish line, the veterinarian should assess the attitude of the dog and note any individuals with gait abnormalities. One must watch for subtle lameness, which will increase when the bad leg is on the inside of a turn. The dogs must then be observed in a normal standing position, and the veterinarian should assess symmetry and conformation. It is sometimes helpful to walk the dog in a straight line and then in a circle. Finally, a thorough orthopedic examination should be performed, including examination of cervical and lumbar spine.

Metacarpus. Hairline (incomplete stress fractures) and chip fractures involving the metacarpals, and more rarely metatarsals and digits, occur mainly on sprint races. They are a minor problem but require the dog to be eliminated (dropped) from the race. Accumulation of stress, poor training, and diets insufficient in calcium may produce metacarpal lameness and stress fractures as a manifestation of secondary nutritional hyperparathyroidism.[3]

Carpus. The main foreleg problem of racing sled dogs involves the carpus and flexor tendons. Severe cold temperatures and winds often produce hardened trails that cause an increased incidence of diffuse carpal joint swelling, joint fluid effusion, and ligamentous/tendon tearing (sprain). This is attributable to the fact that 75 per cent of the dog's body weight goes to the forelimbs when it runs. This is more significant in the Alps, where trails very often go downhill.

The two principal goals of treatment of synovitis and tenosynovitis are to stop inflammation before permanent damage to the joint capsule and cartilage occurs, and to return the joint fluid to a more normal state. Synovitis can be treated with physical therapy or drugs.[4] The most commonly used form of physical therapy is rest. The stress and strain that caused the synovitis is then removed, and the joint is allowed to heal. Fortunately, during a race, mild cases of carpal/flexor tendon strain can be treated to avoid dropping the dog from the race. Cold therapy (applying snow or ice packs) is useful in treating acute, early cases of synovitis. During a long-distance race, the best treatment for mild cases is to put a soft compressive wrap (Fig. 50–17) on the wrist, with or without the use of an anti-inflammatory ointment, during rest stops. Due to doping rules, it is often forbidden to use corticosteroids, nonsteroidal anti-inflammatory drugs, or dimethyl sulfoxide on dogs immediately before or during the race, but ointments containing hyperoxygenated fatty acids can be used.

Elbow. The elbow joint is very rarely a problem in racing sled dogs, unless there is specific trauma.[5]

Shoulder. An important foreleg problem in sled dogs is bicipital tenosynovitis. This injury is often the result of work on hard trails and downhill runs. Moderate flexion of the shoulder joint easily elicits a painful response because of the inflamed bursa. This injury does not respond to treatment while the dog continues to run. Dogs with bicipital tenosynovitis should be retired from the race. Treatment consists of rest.

Deep palpation of the muscular joint, which exists between the scapula, humerus, and the thoracic wall, is very important. Caudal flexion with palpation of the neck muscles may indicate pain coming from the lower muscular attachments and may be demonstrated during abduction of the pectoral muscles. Injuries to this area include muscle bruising and rubs. This area is the primary contact pressure point and the area of maximum biomechanical stress. Therefore, the configuration of harnesses may also aid in reduction of injuries. A change in harness size and type can protect against shoulder injuries. The optimum, according to Rooks,[6] would be to change harness type depending on terrain, because some harnesses seem to cause more injuries. The key is prevention, as both of these conditions tend to occur when dogs are run for too long a period of time without sufficient rest.

Hind Leg. Lameness involving the hip and stifle joints is seen much less often than are injuries to the foreleg. The most commonly seen hindlimb problem involves rupture of the Achilles tendon and/or avulsion of the gastrocnemius muscle from its origin on the distal femur. These dogs require surgical repair and are removed from the race. The prognosis for future racing is guarded, and these dogs are often used for training pups and breeding.[5]

Muscle and Tendon Injuries. Muscle injuries are quite common in athletic dogs, including sled dogs. Bruising or contusion of the muscle is a common injury. It is frequently associated with tearing of muscle fibers, a condition known as muscle strain. The clinical signs of bruising—swelling, heat, localized pain, and discoloration of the skin—may or may not be obvious. Lameness may occur

depending on the location of the injury. In racing sled dogs, these types of injuries are common in the muscles of the neck, back, and shoulder. Treatment for muscle injury should be initiated as soon as possible and includes rest, use of nonsteroidal anti-inflammatory drugs, and ice packs.

Exercise-induced rhabdomyolysis (''sled dog myopathy'') appears to be quite common in dogs participating in long-distance sled races. Cases are most frequently encountered in the first 400 miles of the race (J. Blake, personal communication). We have noted that elevations in serum creatine kinase (CK) activity in dropped dogs are greatest within the first 400 miles of the Iditarod, whereas serum CK activity is only mildly elevated in dogs at the end of the race (K.W. Hinchcliff, K.E. Schmidt, unpublished information). The cause of sled dog myopathy may be related to exercise-induced cellular oxidative stress, responsible for a decreased antioxidant status of the muscle cell and an induced vitamin E deficiency. Recent unpublished data from Grandjean, obtained during the Alaska Come Back Race 97, tend to show a preventive role of vitamin E supplementation at a level of 0.75 IU per fat kcal in the diet. Treatment includes rest, fluid therapy, and analgesics.

Tendon injuries are less common than are muscle injuries. Racing or training on soft or uneven terrain can predispose a dog to tendon injury. Tendinitis can result in lameness, but observable swelling and bruising is usually minimal. The treatment is conservative and healing may take three to six weeks, after which time the dog should be exercised lightly for three to six weeks. Prognosis for return to function is good.[7] Partial or complete rupture of a tendon is possible, and must be seen as a severe injury causing lameness and loss of function of the muscle.

THERMAL INJURIES

Physiology. Racing sled dogs are vulnerable to abnormalities owing to temperature extremes, both hypothermia and hyperthermia. Very low ambient temperatures, combined with low wind-chill temperatures and the risk of becoming wet (such as in overflow conditions), can quickly result in hypothermia. In contrast, calm and sunny days on a snow-covered (reflective) landscape with moderate temperatures create an environment conducive to hyperthermia.

Cooling of the dog results from decreased heat production and/or increased heat loss. The former typically is a response to lowered metabolic rate, ie, reduced energy intake (anorexia), or diminished muscular activity (resting). In the quiet animal, skeletal muscle contributes about 25 per cent of the total heat produced. Other metabolic heat sources are primarily the liver, brain, and heart. In a running sled dog insufficient heat production is unlikely to be a problem, although in extreme conditions or if the dog is wet, it may occur. Resting dogs, particularly if they are anorexic, may be at greater risk of hypothermia because of inadequate heat production. Heat loss occurs by four basic forms: radiation, evaporation, convection, and conduction. The physiological functions designed to enhance heat loss include panting, vascular alterations (vasodilation), and sweating.

Simply defined, radiative loss involves the transfer of heat as electromagnetic energy (infrared) from the sled dog to the atmosphere. Radiation is usually the greatest type of heat loss and normally amounts to about 60 per cent of the total. However, this can be highly variable. Cold, clear nights result in much greater radiative loss than do bright days. The second major method of heat dissipation is through evaporation. This is accomplished primarily by panting and salivation, as water is lost from the airways of the dog. Since sweat glands of the dog are mostly limited to the foot pad, their role in thermoregulation is minimal. A situation that results in the animal becoming wet will greatly increase the

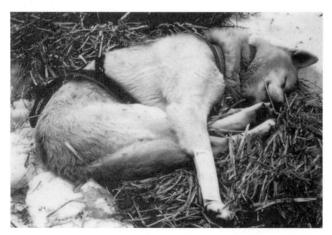

FIGURE 50–17. Strap on a wrist inflammation.

significance of evaporative heat loss. Some breeds have been banned from marathon races because of inadequate coats. In poodles, for example, there is a propensity for collecting ice balls on the hair, and when melting occurs, the wet animal becomes vulnerable to hypothermia.

Convective heat loss is highly variable, depending primarily on air movement around the dog, and therefore on wind conditions and speed of travel. This type of heat loss ordinarily amounts to 12 per cent in a static condition. Heat lost through conduction is usually relatively small (3 per cent) but will become more significant as temperatures drop (atmospheric) and is most critical in cases of water immersion. Vasodilation is the physiological response operative in utilizing these last two forms of heat transfer when cooling is required.

For the sake of avoiding redundancy, it may be assumed that factors contributing to warming of the sled dog are inversely related to those that create cooling. However, some specific points should be emphasized. In response to cooling body temperatures, the hypothalamus enhances heat production through appetite stimulation, increased metabolism (assuming adequate caloric availability), and greater muscular activity (shivering, restlessness). This may help explain why many dogs eat poorly upon arrival at checkpoint but have hearty appetites after resting (cooling) for 1 to 2 hours. Muscular exertion may increase metabolic heat production by as much as 60-fold.

One of the best methods of reducing heat loss is through body posture. As the dog rests in a tight curl, surface area is greatly reduced, which diminishes convective and conductive heat loss. The nose tucked under the tail serves to allow pre-heated air to enter the respiratory tract. The straw bedding that is almost universally utilized by mushers serves as an effective insulator from the snow surface, thus reducing conductive heat loss.

Injuries. Hypothermic injuries may be classified as local or systemic. Local injuries include freezing (frostbite) wherein a portion of tissue, usually the skin, cools to 0 degrees C (32° F) or less. Areas most vulnerable include the vulva, mammae, prepuce, penis, scrotum, flank folds, and chafing-induced hairless regions as seen around harness and bootie rubs (Figs. 50–18 and 50–19). It is interesting to note that, in contrast to humans, the dog is not susceptible to freezing of feet or toes, except in extreme cases of vascular compromise. Rectal temperatures below 37.8° C (100° F) are indicative of systemic hypothermia.

Treatment approaches vary depending on severity of the lesion, but if refreezing cannot be prevented, the animal must be dropped from the race. Superficial lesions with minimal swelling can be thawed using warm water (40.6° C/105° F) if needed and medicated

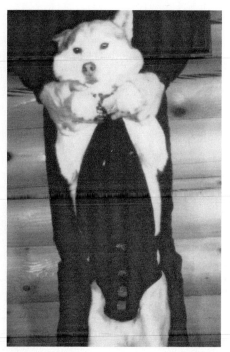
FIGURE 50–19. Abdomen protection against cold.

with nonaqueous antibiotic ointments. Aqueous ointments may actually make tissue more vulnerable to cooling via evaporation. The area must be protected as needed from further exposure with jackets, bandages, or sheath protectors. Lesions demonstrating substantial edema are more serious and require aggressive treatment. Prepucial swelling can be severe enough to cause phimosis or paraphimosis. Broad-spectrum antibiotics and nonaqueous ointments are indicated.

Danger Zone. A patient's condition becomes critical as the core temperature drops below 35.5° C (96° F). These animals are often dehydrated, which contributes significantly to development of the hypothermic state. Rapid infusion of warm fluids intravenously (38.9° C [102° F]), preferably normal saline (0.9% NaCl), is a priority. Water baths heated to similar temperatures will significantly enhance rewarming. Sleeping bags and space blankets are good when baths are not available. In a survival situation, warm bodies—human or canine—may provide needed warmth. In less severe cases, accompanied by shivering and lethargy, and in patients that have responded to the above, a hot meal will provide energy and thermal mass to enhance recovery. Even after apparent recovery, urine production and cardiac function should be closely monitored for 24 hours. Life-threatening serum potassium abnormalities may be present.

Hyperthermia may also be local and systemic, although local injuries (burns) are rare. Systemic hyperthermia may be further classified as pyogenic or exertional. Pyogenic hyperthermia is typically associated with the release of endogenous pyrogens as the result of illness. The febrile state has numerous potential causes, but most commonly is associated with infected bite wounds, abscessed foot lesions, or pneumonia. Exertional hyperthermia may be "normal" or pathological. Upon arrival at a checkpoint, the dogs may display a rectal temperature of 41.4° C (109.5° F), particularly after sprints. In such cases, the animal is alert and the temperature returns to the normal range within 15 to 20 minutes. Pathological exertional hyperthermia (heat exhaustion/stroke) is the most immediately life-threatening of all temperature abnormalities, requiring prompt medical intervention.

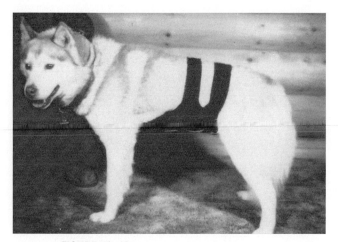
FIGURE 50–18. Abdomen protection against cold.

Ample data are available on the treatment of burn injuries. Mild lesions would be treated similarly to superficial frostbite after a return to normal tissue temperature. Life-threatening hyperthermia (sustained temperature greater than 41.7° C/107° F) typically occurs as the result of overexertion on warmer days (greater than −7° C/20° F). Early signs include increased respiratory rate, excessive salivation, rapid heart rate, and bright-red gingiva. Assuming good health otherwise, dark-colored, heavy-coated and hard-working dogs are usually the first to have a problem. If the problem is caught early, merely stopping and offering cold water will suffice. As the condition progresses, heat exhaustion/stroke develop, as evidenced by collapse and shock. Lowering the body temperature becomes an immediate priority. This is best accomplished by cold water immersion. An IV catheter should be established and lactated Ringer's solution (24.0° C/75° F) administered.

Cerebral edema may develop, as indicated by a state of stupor or coma, in which case mannitol (20%, 2 mg/kg) and dexamethasone (1–2 mg/kg) are appropriate treatments. Urine production must be closely monitored. Should oliguria develop, furosemide (2 mg/kg) and intravenous fluids are used. The patient should be observed closely for at least 24 hours after correcting the temperature, as renal complications and/or DIC may develop.

Racing sled dogs are susceptible to a wide variety of thermal injuries. Fortunately, most can be prevented by close observation and applying common sense solutions. In the event that injury occurs, treatment is typically successful with the application of readily available resources and medications. Injuries should be prevented whenever possible and treatment begun promptly when they occur.

CARDIOVASCULAR SYSTEM

George Hermann described the greyhound's heart as larger, relative to the dog's body weight, than those of mongrel dogs.[8–11] He also observed that the largest heart was found in the most successful racing dog and speculated that the greyhound's heart responds to training by hypertrophying to an unusual degree.

Physiology. That species of animals classically regarded as athletic have hearts that are larger than expected for their body size has been recognized at least since 1628.[8] Dogs as a species have comparatively large hearts. The average mammalian heart comprises 0.6 per cent of the body weight,[12] whereas the mean heart weight of dogs is 0.8 per cent of body weight. A marked breed variation in relative heart size exists among dogs, with athletic breeds having proportionately larger hearts than do sedentary breeds: greyhounds have hearts of approximately 1.2 per cent of their body weight,[13, 14] whereas the hearts of mongrel dogs are smaller (0.8 per cent).[8] In our experience (KWH, PDC), hearts of trained Alaskan sled dogs average about 1 per cent of body weight.

What is not so readily appreciated is that the size of the heart can be increased through training for endurance exercise.[15] Human endurance athletes have larger hearts than do untrained people, with cardiac size regressing upon cessation of training.[16] Similarly, the heart of dogs increases in size in response to physical training.[17] The nature of this training-induced increase was a subject of debate for many years. It was originally regarded by some as a pathological change indicative of the noxious nature of repetitive exercise and carried a prognosis for a shortened life span, while others recognized it, correctly, as normal.[18]

Enlargement of the heart as a consequence of endurance training is a normal response to the volume load to which the heart is subjected during exercise.[16, 19] Endurance exercise is characteristically low to moderate intensity exercise that is performed for considerable periods of time (tens of minutes to hours). The cardiovascular responses to such exercise include an increase in cardiac output, a redistribution of cardiac output, and a decrease in systemic resistance. Mean arterial blood pressure increases only slightly during prolonged exercise and may actually decrease.[20] Endurance exercise therefore imposes a volume load on the heart, as opposed to the pressure load associated with weight lifting or sprinting. The physiological response to volume load is an increase in heart size achieved through both an increase in left and right ventricular cavity dimensions and an increase in myocardial wall thickness.[16] In contrast to weight lifters and bodybuilders, who have large hearts with normal cavity dimensions, human endurance athletes have large hearts with large ventricular cavities. The concomitant increases in ventricular capacity and wall thickness of the heart permit a larger stroke volume while maintaining the mechanical efficiency of systole.

Clinical Examination. Training-induced cardiac enlargement in humans is apparent clinically as bradycardia at rest, a physiologic or "flow" murmur, an increase in the size of the cardiac silhouette on thoracic radiographs, changes in the electrocardiogram characteristic of cardiac enlargement, and an increase in cardiac dimensions on echocardiographic examination.[18, 21] Similar findings are reported for greyhounds[22] and trained Alaskan sled dogs (Fig. 50–20). It is important that the physical and ancillary diagnostic findings be interpreted in the appropriate context because, taken in isolation, they may be mistaken for evidence of heart disease. Conversely, knowledge of the normal findings on physical examination of a highly trained dog permits identification of dogs with cardiac abnormalities.

Bradycardia may not be an unusual finding in highly trained Alaskan sled dogs, although it may be difficult to demonstrate on an electrocardiographic examination because of apprehension of the dog. Van Citters and Franklin recorded telemetered heart rates of 40 to 60 beats per minute in sleeping sled dogs.[23] The authors have recorded femoral pulse rates as low as 35 beats per minute in highly trained sled dogs. Heart rate increases to 80 to 100 beats per minute when the dogs stand, and to 120 to 150 beats per minute in anticipation of running.[23] Heart rates of 250 to 300 beats per minute are recorded in running sled dogs.[23]

Physiological murmurs are present in 30 to 50 per cent of human dynamic athletes. Similarly, low-intensity systolic murmurs were detected in 40 per cent of 48 highly trained Alaskan sled dogs, but none were detected in 14 similarly sized mongrel dogs. The prevalence of these murmurs increases with increasing training in Alaskan sled dogs, and there is a trend for an increase in prevalence of murmurs in dogs rated as better athletes by their trainers.[24] Physiological murmurs in endurance athletes are characterized as low-grade (1–3/6) systolic, cresendo-decrescendo murmurs that do not include either the first or second heart sound, with a point of maximal intensity over the left heart base. Important factors in differentiating physiological murmurs from those associated with cardiac disease is the timing of the murmur, the fact that it does not include either the first or second heart sound, its point of maximal intensity, and its relatively low intensity. The cause of the murmur is likely related to the enhanced stroke volume, but maintained ejection period, of the trained heart. The ejection velocity of blood into the aorta is therefore higher in endurance-trained dogs than in untrained animals. The probability that the critical Reynolds' number is exceeded with subsequent development of turbulent flow and a murmur is therefore greater in the athlete.

Highly trained Alaskan sled dogs often have electrocardiograms consistent with cardiac enlargement (Fig. 50–21). The prevalence of electrocardiographic changes consistent with right and left atrial enlargement increases with more training of sled dogs.[24] The electrocardiograms of trained sled dogs are characterized by a long QRS duration, an increase in R wave amplitude in leads II, aVF, V3, and V10, a rightward shift of the mean electrical axis in the frontal plane and long QT intervals.[24, 24a] Indeed, there is a signifi-

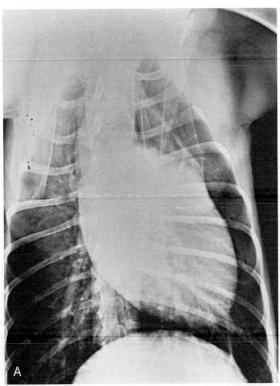
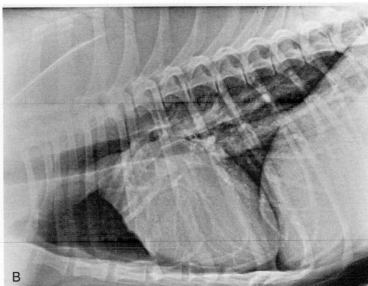

FIGURE 50–20. Dorsoventral *(A)* and lateral *(B)* radiographs of thorax of a trained Alaskan sled dog. The cardiac silhouette is consistent with left ventricular enlargement.

cant but weak association between QRS duration and finishing status in the Iditarod.[25]

Recognition that the physical examination of highly trained Alaskan sled dogs may reveal a higher prevalence of low-intensity systolic murmurs than in sedentary dogs may prevent expensive and often unwarranted ancillary diagnostic testing. Conversely, an understanding of the type of murmur expected will allow potentially important abnormalities to be detected at routine or pre-race examination. Subsequent ancillary testing may include electrocardiography, radiography, and echography. Again, it should be recognized that the thoracic radiograph (Fig. 50–20) and electrocardio-

gram (Fig. 50–21) of the highly trained sled dog probably varies from that of an untrained dog.

DIGESTIVE PROBLEMS

Vomiting and diarrhea associated with racing are common problems in sled dogs.

Noninfectious Problems

Vomiting. During the first races of the season, vomiting may occur following the consumption of snow by the dog when running.

FIGURE 50–21. Electrocardiogram of a trained Alaskan sled dog (different dog from that in Fig. 50–19). The electrocardiogram was made with the dog standing and demonstrates changes consistent with left ventricular hypertrophy (R wave amplitude of 5.00 mV in lead II). The mean electrical axis was +86 degrees and the QRS duration was 72 msec. Calibration signal is 1 mV and 200 msec.

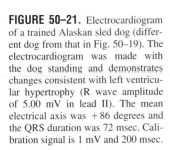
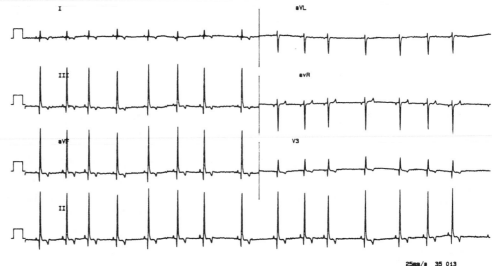

25mm/s 35 013

This phenomenon is prevented by watering the dogs ad libitum approximately three hours before the starting time, and in providing limited amounts (100 ml) of water 30 to 40 minutes before the start of the race. Generally, mushers know that, in sprint races, they must not feed the dogs within the three hours preceding starting time. It is advised to mix one quarter of the daily ration with water and feed the mixture to the dogs three to five hours prior to the start. In long-distance races, dogs are generally fed two main meals per 24 hours and given snacks and water more frequently, often during each stop.

Diarrhea-Dehydration-Stress Syndrome. Diarrhea problems often plague some dog teams and can be difficult to control. Initially described by Adkins,[26] the diarrhea-dehydration-stress syndrome (DDSS) is often seen in the first two days of the race and is associated with diarrhea, partial anorexia, and dehydration. The dog team may be running well, then suddenly the majority of the team is affected within a 12-hour period. Diet and training leading up to the race coupled with the musher's ability to pace the dog team play the most important role in the prevention of this stress-induced diarrhea.[10] Clinical observations at numerous competitions indicate that in spite of major improvements in preparation and methods of feeding, there are still frequent cases of acute diarrhea associated with racing.

Recovery from this type of diarrhea is extremely variable, as a protocol that works with one team may not work for another. Increased resting time, divided meals, and restored level of hydration are the keys to treatment. The use of gastrointestinal absorbents and protectants is often encouraged, although of unproved efficacy. The use of motility modifiers is controversial. In most diarrheal disease, information about changes in motility is minimal or absent, and, without this knowledge, rational use of drugs that affect intestinal motility is not possible. A trial was carried out at the 1992 Alpirod race to test the curative effect of an argile (clay) medication on acute diarrhea. Smectite (12.5 g/d) in two doses, an antidiarrheic similar to the opioid loperamide (2 mg/d) or a combination of the two at the same dosage were used.[27] One hundred and twelve cases were tested. There was no control group because of the high level of competition. Following 36 hours of treatment, 91 per cent of dogs in the smectite group no longer suffered from diarrhea, compared with 65 per cent and 88 per cent in the loperamide and combination groups, respectively. Whether smectite reduced fecal water loss or simply improved fecal consistency through a bulk effect is unclear.

There is no indication for the routine use of antimicrobials in the treatment of acute diarrhea of sled dogs.

Infectious Diarrhea

With infectious diarrhea there are no factors specifically related to sled dogs, except the potential for transmission when many dogs are racing on the same trail and in constant contact. Dog teams originating in isolated regions may have more vomiting and diarrhea problems during races as they are exposed to gastrointestinal viruses (parvo-, corona-, and rotaviruses). This problem becomes more important each year, with more teams competing in international races.

Concerning bacterial diarrhea, *Campylobacter* sp. seems to be the most frequently isolated bacterium in chronic cases of diarrhea during training.

DEHYDRATION

Dehydration is a very common disabling condition affecting racing sled dogs. There have been few studies of the actual losses of electrolytes and fluids experienced by the stressed and exercising canine athlete under racing conditions.[28] But there are few instances in canine sports in which these losses are more evident than in long-distance sled dog racing in cold environments. As described by Leach,[29] sprint dogs may run distances of 3 to 30 miles and normally have an opportunity to rest and replenish after a day or two of racing or hard training. Distance or stage-race dogs, on the other hand, run a minimum of 200 miles up to 1200 miles, or 10 to 20 days, with minimal recovery time for replenishment. During such long-duration activity evaporation and water loss from the tongue and upper respiratory passages occurs at 10 to 20 times more than normal. High-fat diets provide the opportunity for an increased production of metabolic water (107 g per 100 g of fat oxidized), especially as sled dogs may use over 10,000 kcal per day.[30]

The racing sled dog is trained to run at ambient temperatures below 0° F. At −10° F, the daily water requirement is approximately 1 liter per 5 kilograms of body weight (1 gallon for an average dog),[28] although biochemical evidence of dehydration is not evident in most dogs during a long-distance race.[31] In cold temperatures, a dog can become dehydrated in less than 12 hours. The problem usually originates from a dog refusing to eat and drink when it becomes tired or stressed, or from severe diarrhea. During the race, an experienced veterinarian must be able to quickly evaluate the hydration of each dog. At the earliest sign of dehydration, the musher must be made aware of the problem so that the water intake can be increased. Sometimes a musher must make the decision to either drop a dog or to prolong its stay at a checkpoint until it is well enough rested to resume eating and drinking. When the dehydration is greater than 7 per cent, the dog is normally not allowed to continue racing until rehydration has occurred. Dehydration may not be able to be remedied with oral fluids alone and may require intravenous fluid therapy.

To help prevent dehydration, sled dogs need to be taught to drink during the training period and must be given water immediately prior to exercise and frequently during exercise of two hours or longer. If dehydration is allowed to develop, the sensation of thirst may be depressed, and the dog may not drink, potentiating the early hydration deficit. The addition of electrolyte powders to the water might be helpful, but these should be isotonic or hypotonic.[29]

By encouraging and increasing water intake as well as maintaining or replacing electrolytes losses, dehydration can be avoided and the aerobic performance of the sled dog enhanced.

OTHER MEDICAL PROBLEMS

Respiratory Disease. Respiratory diseases are generally associated with two main problems: infectious tracheobronchitis and bacterial bronchopneumonia. The etiology of infectious bronchitis commonly involves parainfluenza virus, adenovirus type II, and/or *Bordetella bronchiseptica*. Despite vaccination programs, dog teams have experienced a sharp rise in infectious bronchitis during the racing season when exposure is at its highest. *Bordetella* sp. is a bacterium that attaches to the cilia of the respiratory tract as a primary or a secondary invader following viral infection, and is generally susceptible to chloramphenicol, gentamicin, kanamycin, and tetracyclines. Bronchopneumonia becomes a problem in the second or third week of the races. Fever, anorexia, harsh deep cough, and an inability to pull characterize this syndrome, which is generally responsive to broad-spectrum antibiotics. The majority of dogs with infectious bronchitis continue to eat and work well, but dogs with bronchopneumonia should be pulled from the race.

Metabolic Disorders. Two common metabolic disorders are being diagnosed more frequently in Alaskan huskies, Siberian huskies, and Alaskan malamutes: hypothyroidism and zinc-responsive dermatoses.

Hypothyroidism. Hypothyroidism is first revealed as a decrease in pulling power, lethargy, and alopecia. It is a primary hypothyroidism, and produces clinical signs only when the dog is placed under the stress of the race. If genetics are involved, we still lack information on the origin and transmission of the disease. Treatment consists of daily supplemental thyroxine.[32]

Zinc-responsive Dermatosis. As this is not a sport disease, we only mention the existence of this ''Nordic breed's affection.'' The skin lesions of the zinc-responsive dermatosis are now well known, and treatment consists of a supplement with 100 to 300 mg zinc sulfate twice daily.

NECROPSY EXAMINATION

As veterinarians concerned with the welfare of the canine athlete, we are obligated to use every available source of information to better understand the medical and disease processes peculiar to the athletic animal. To that end, the necropsy is one of our most valuable tools in trying to answer the question of why the animal died. In answering that question we must rely on every source of information available. This includes a complete history, clinical signs, necropsy findings, and laboratory tests.

The history is valuable in many cases but rarely will it alone provide the complete answer. For example, the history could suggest a fatal fall, which could be confirmed only by the necropsy results. Diagnosis of death due to hypothermia or hyperthermia may be difficult to confirm on necropsy examination but may be obvious from the history.

A saying in sled dog racing is "You are only as fast as your slowest dog." Signs observed by the musher that affect the dog's performance will cause the musher to either carry the dog in the sled bag or drop the dog from the race. When a death occurs, it is most often sudden and without obvious premonitory signs.

The necropsy may provide the most objective information available about the dog's condition. It must be done properly and completely. Also, all information must be compiled centrally so that significant statistics and patterns can be determined. In each necropsy a proper chain of evidence is considered: properly identifying the animal and owner, logging witnesses, taking photographs, legally identifying tissues, and sealing them in preservatives so as to ensure that results are accurate and reliable. The gross necropsy must be conducted under favorable conditions of proper lighting, ventilation, and with the necessary equipment. It must be done as soon as possible so as to reduce postmortem change.

In all cases multiple histopathology specimens must be collected and preserved properly for further evaluation in the laboratory. Recently, athletic myopathies have been discovered that can be diagnosed only with multiple muscle tissue samples. It may also be necessary to submit whole organs for evaluation. To properly evaluate the heart, the whole organ must be submitted, and, if the cardiac conduction system is to be evaluated, serial sections must be examined.

During the necropsy the material necessary to conduct further laboratory testing must be collected. If bacterial or viral culturing is to be performed, the proper samples must be preserved at the time of the gross necropsy. Feces for parasite identification, cerebrospinal fluid, urine, and stomach contents all may be necessary to properly make a diagnosis. The ultimate goal is to better understand the mechanisms leading to the death and thus prevent these incidents from recurring. We can do this only by expanding our knowledge through every source available. The necropsy is essential if we are to achieve success. (The ISDVMA recently published *1995 ISDVMA Guide to Sled Dog Necropsy* by Dr. A. Cantor.)

References

1. Schmidt K: Iditarod Sled Dog Race Musher's-Veterinarian's Handbook. Wassila AK, Iditarod Trail Committee, 1995.
2. Grandjean D, Sept RJ: Spécificités pathologiques du chien de traîneau en situation de course. Rec Med Vet 167:763–773, 1991.
3. Sept B: Problèmes médicaux et chirurgicaux chez les chiens de traîneau en course de fond. Colloque Int Med Sport canine. GERMES-CNVSPA, Blagnac, October 1990.
4. Rooks B: Synovitis in racing sled dogs. Vet Check 1:2–4, 1994.
5. Sept B: Pathologic particularities of sled dogs during long distance races. In Proceedings of the 11th World Congress WSAVA. Paris, December 1986, pp. 4–13.
6. Rooks B: Physical examination of racing sled dogs. Vet Check 3:8–10, 1994.
7. Rooks B: Muscle and tendon injuries. Vet Check 2:2–3, 1994.
8. Harvey W: Anatomical studies on the motion of the heart and blood. (Translated by CD Leakes.) Springfield, Charles C Thomas, 1930.
9. Hermann GR: Experimental heart disease. Am Heart J 1:213–231, 1925.
10. Kronfeld D, Dunlap H: Common clinical and nutritional problems in racing sled dogs. First Nordic Symposium. Small An Med Oslo, 1982, pp 360–367.
11. Hermann GR: The heart of the racing greyhound. Hypertrophy of the heart. Proc Soc Exp Biol Med XXIII:856–857, 1925.
12. Stahl WR: Organ weights of primates and other animals. Science 150:1039–1042, 1965.
13. Schneider HP, Truex RC, Knowles JO: Comparative observations of the hearts of mongrel and greyhound dogs. Anat Rec 149:173–180, 1964.
14. Steel JD, Taylor RI, Davis PE, Stewart GA, Salmon PW: Relationship between heart score, heart weight and body weight in greyhound dogs. Aust Vet J 52:561–564, 1976.
15. Steinhaus AH: Chronic effects of exercise. Physiol Rev 13:103–147, 1933.
16. Shapiro LM, Smith RG: Effect of training on left ventricular structure and function. Br Heart J 50:534–539, 1983.
17. Wyatt HL, Mitchell JH: Influences of physical training on the heart of dogs. Circ Res 35:883–889, 1974.
18. Rost R: The athlete's heart. Historical perspectives. Cardiol Clin 10:197–207, 1992.
19. Shapiro LM: Morphologic consequences of systematic training. Cardiology Clin 10:219–226, 1992.
20. Ekelund L: Circulatory and respiratory adaptation during prolonged exercise. Acta Physiol Scand 70 (Supp.292):5–33, 1967.
21. Huston TP, Puffer JC, Rodney WM: The athletic heart syndrome. N Engl J Med 313:24–32, 1985.
22. Page A, Edmunds A, Atwell RB: Echocardiographic values in the Greyhound. Aust Vet J 70:361–364, 1993.
23. Van Citters RL, Franklin DL: Cardiovascular performance of Alaskan sled dogs during exercise. Circ Res 24:33–42, 1969.
24. Constable PD, Hinchcliff KW, Olson J, Hamlin RL: Athletic heart syndrome in dogs competing in a long-distance sled race. J Appl Physiol 76:433–438, 1994.
24a. Hinchcliff KW, Constable PD, Farris JW, Schmidt KE, Hamlin RL. Electrocardiographic characteristics of endurance-trained Alaskan sled dog. JAVMA 211:1138–1141, 1997.
25. Constable PD, Hinchcliff KW, Farris J, Schmidt KE. Factors associated with finishing status for dogs competing in a long distance sled race. JAVMA 208:879–882, 1996.
26. Adkins T, Morris J: The Iditarod sled dogs and DVMs. Med Vet Pract 56:456–461, 1975.
27. Grandjean D, Crepin F, Paragon BM: Intérêt de la smectite dans les diarrhées aigües du chien de traîneau. Rec Med Vet 168:323–329, 1992.
28. Hinchcliff KW, Reinhart GA, Burr JR, Swenson RA: Exercise-associated hyponatremia in Alaskan sled dogs: Urinary and hormonal responses. J Appl Physiol 83:824–829, 1997.
29. Leach JB: Electrolytes-fluid losses in the long distance canine athlete.

In Turner A (ed): Arctic Sports Medicine Performance Guide. American College of Sports Medicine, 1989, pp 200–213.
30. Hinchcliff KW, Reinhart GA, Burr JR, Schreier CJ, Swenson RA: Metabolizable energy intake and sustained energy expenditure of Alaskan sled dogs during heavy exertion in the cold. Am J Vet Res 58:1457–1462, 1997.

31. Hinchcliff KW, Olson J, Crusberg C, et al: Blood chemistry changes in dogs competing in a long distance sled dog race. JAVMA 202:401–405, 1993.
32. Coady S, Sept J: Racing sled dogs: Injury care and prevention. *In* Turner A (ed): Arctic Sport Medicine Performance Guide. American College of Sports Medicine, 1989, pp 199–212.

CHAPTER 51

UNIQUE VETERINARY PROBLEMS OF COURSING DOGS

S. GARY BROWN

Coursing is a field event in which sighthounds chase, turn, and try to capture either a live hare (a practice that is waning on the West Coast and still popular in England) or an imitation bunny, pulled by ropes attached to a mechanical system that darts and turns quickly over the ground. *Lure coursing*, as it is called, maintains its popularity while satisfying animal rights' concerns. These concerns, as well as the sport's history, date back to the Greek author Flavius Arrianus (Arrian) writing in Rome, who noted that the sport was to test the running, turning, and agility of the dogs, and it was better for the hare to escape. In fact, less than 5 per cent of live hares are actually caught.

The manner of running and the unevenness of the terrain are the primary factors that contribute to the kinds of injuries seen today. Firmness of soil itself is a secondary factor that also contributes to these types of injuries. Most enthusiasts postpone training until the first rain has softened the hard clods of a plowed field. Imagine a greyhound running and turning at breakneck speed having to make instantaneous and bizarre adjustments to the ground immediately ahead. Speeds achieved in the "run-up" (when the hound pair is released behind the running hare) can approach 45 mph. One can imagine the forces generated on the dog's limbs at the first turn.

Understanding the physical dynamics of the *turn* helps to understand how these stresses can cause limb injuries. The small ligaments and bones of the carpus, tarsus, and more distal limbs and joints undergo great angular stresses during high-speed cutting and turning and commonly sustain injuries.[1]

Each turn has three discrete parts: the entry, the curve, and the exit.[1,2] To enter the turn, all animals that run must slow down. The reduced speed usually involves a shift from the double suspension gallop to a modified gait and subsequent return to the gallop. During the double-suspension gallop, the powerful rear legs drive the body forward. Then, like a swimmer's racing entry into the pool, the flexed spine extends and the front legs reach forward into the air to gain distance. For the moment before the front legs reach the ground, both front and rear legs are suspended in the air. The transition, downshift, and return to the gallop are extremely demanding. The ability of the racers to "singletrack" when running a straight line is of little coursing consequence. However, in the turn it is absolutely essential to singletrack to maintain top speed. During the walk or slow trot, the width of the front feet and rear

feet approximates the width of the body. As speed increases, the imprints of the feet narrow and tend to make a single track, slightly more so in the front than the rear. If the hound is running and leaning at a 45-degree angle, it must singletrack to keep its legs the same effective length. If it runs with them apart, the inside leg must be shortened by a considerable amount. Some hounds can run without singletracking, but they are usually slow and inept, and frequently stumble or overrun a turn. Uneven ground can cause the same performance. Coursing greyhounds and whippets rarely run through a turn planting one foot after another in a precise manner. Instead, they *drive* their bodies or slide through the turn, either more esthetically with a *controlled slide* or with a *power slide*, throwing up sprays of flying dirt and debris.[2,3] It is during these slides that distal limb injuries can occur (Figs. 51–1 to 51–6).

COMMON INJURIES

Proximal and Distal Interphalangeal Joint Instabilities. These joint injuries have been divided into three types. Type I injuries

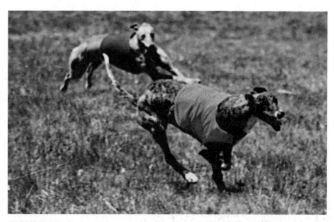

FIGURE 51–1. Beginning of the turn. (Courtesy of Leaping Lizards Action Photography, Halley, ID.)

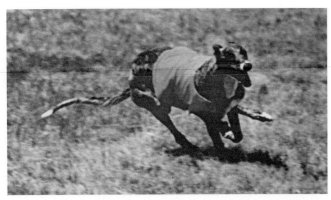

FIGURE 51–2. Middle of the turn, the curve. The front feet are singletracking. The rear feet never track as close, but close up more in the exit. (Courtesy of Leaping Lizards Action Photography, Halley, ID.)

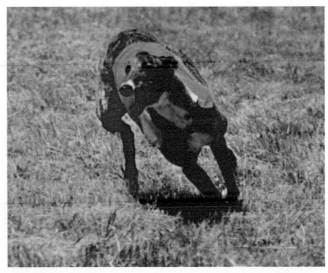

FIGURE 51–3. "Pete" beginning his exit. (Courtesy of Leaping Lizards Action Photography, Halley, ID.)

involve stretching of the collateral ligament. Type II injuries involve complete disruption with angular dislocation (Fig. 51–7), while type III injuries involve bilateral collateral ligament damage, frequently with avulsion chips.

Type I injuries can occasionally be coapted, but more consistent results are obtained with surgery. Type II injuries require surgery, and surgery is preferred over coaptation even if the delay is as long as 2 weeks. Usually two mattress sutures are placed side by side, using 4/0 polypropylene, or occasionally 3/0 polypropylene. Some surgeons prefer Polydek or polyglycolic acid. The distal aspect of the limb is supported by a special wrap for 6 weeks and the patient is confined. The dog may begin carefully controlled progressive ambulation after 6 weeks. Many of these injuries are medial collateral ligament tears caused by sudden outward deviation of the foot. This outward force needs to be prevented during healing by the support wrap, while movement in the cranial caudal direction is permitted. A shorter walking wrap may be used after 6 weeks. The toenail on the operated digit is cut back and covered by a dab of hobbyist's acrylic glue or nail polish. Amputation of this nail prevents it from acting as a long lever arm. (One dog became so habituated to his wrap that he refused to course without it.) Type III injuries are very severe. For these, most surgeons have recommended amputation or arthrodesis; however, some injuries are amenable to primary surgery repair.[4] Coursing dogs, however, *cannot turn quickly* when the front *digit 5 is missing*. This digit seems to act somehow as an outrigger in a power turn and protects the distal interphalangeal and proximal interphalangeal collaterals on digits 3 and 4. One case of "blown collaterals" in digits 3 and 4 occurred following digit 5 removal in a big whippet.

Metatarsal and Metacarpal Bone Fractures. These fractures are usually seen in dogs whose physes are not closed. They are also more common as the younger dog begins training. There is a tendency for the outside (fifth metacarpal) to be involved, perhaps because it bears the load during the curve part of a power turn. Additional metacarpal-metatarsal bones may be fractured if the foot was jammed or stuck into a small opening or crevice. Stress fractures develop in the young dog because its muscles increase in strength faster than its bones can remodel to accept the additional stresses generated.[5, 6]

Acute metacarpal-metatarsal fractures should be subjected to open reduction and rigid internal fixation with small plates and screws. These fractures can be stabilized with 1.5 or 2.0 mm ASIF cortical screws in neutral or lagged manner and veterinary cuttable (VC) plates (Figs. 51–8 and 51–9). Excessive callus (second-intention healing) should be prevented. Coaptation should be used for 5 weeks in the adult.

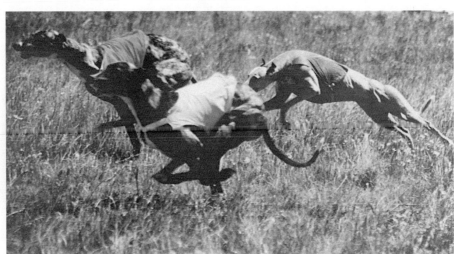

FIGURE 51–4. Double-suspension gallop: Hound on the right is suspended, middle dog is "cocked." (Courtesy of Leaping Lizards Action Photography, Halley, ID.)

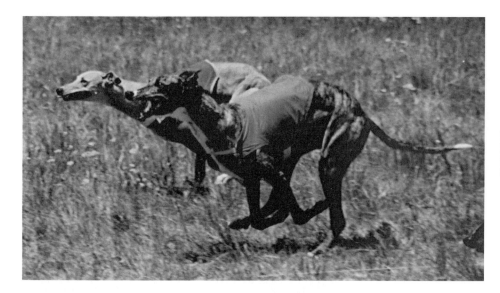

FIGURE 51–5. Double-suspension gallop: near dog is starting to "unload." (Courtesy of Leaping Lizards Action Photography, Halley, ID.)

Limb splinting has caused flattened, weblike toes (due to weakening of the flexor musculotendinous unit) if applied for longer than 2 weeks. This problem is more likely to occur in young dogs, particularly immature dogs in which the front forelimb is splinted. To prevent this, some *slight amount of stretch* on the flexor tendon units (toes) seems to be advantageous during the growth phase. Use of coaptation from below the elbow to the metacarpal pad allows the digital pads to bear weight. A medial and a lateral partial shell (one-third approximately) should be constructed, using a resin-cast material conforming to the limb, which is prewrapped with cast padding. These can slip distally and require close monitoring.

Metacarpal or metatarsal 2 or 5 may be approached surgically medially or laterally, respectively, directly over the fracture. If 2 and 3 or 4 and 5 are fractured, a simple longitudinal incision may be considered on the dorsum of the foot between 2 and 3 and another between 4 and 5, thus exposing both fractures through one incision.

Wire Cuts. Barbed wire cuts are a hazard. Depending on the amount of tissue trauma, contamination, and time elapsed before treatment, they are usually best debrided, flushed, and closed primarily. If debridement and flushing are by necessity incomplete, delayed primary closure within 48 hours or occasionally 72 hours usually is satisfactory.

Lacerations. Proper management of tendon laceration requires knowledge of the regional anatomy. The repair should be supported to relieve tension for 5 to 6 weeks. An additional 5 to 6 weeks should be allocated for closely controlled and slowly progressive ambulation. The small superficial digital flexor tendons below the bifurcation are difficult to repair, because the sutures pull out of the small flat tendon. Achilles tendon repairs need to be supported by a screw from the calcaneus to the distal tibia plus a Jorgenson splint, or a more rigid double-bar external fixator spanning the tarsocrural joint from the tibia to the metatarsals. This rigid support should be maintained for 5 to 6 weeks. (The reader is referred to Chapter 16 for a detailed discussion of tendon repair and healing.)

OCCASIONAL INJURIES

Metacarpal-Phalangeal and Metatarsal-Phalangeal Joint Instabilities. In the coursing dog (and field trial dogs), the outside digit is snagged at high speed, causing valgus angular stress, rupturing the axial collateral ligament, and producing type II injuries, which should be surgically repaired. With careful palpation, these injuries can be felt (valgus instability). The joints are best approached medially. Providing medial-lateral support while encouraging early return to full range of motion to prevent metacarpal-phalangeal and metatarsal-phalangeal joint stiffness is recommended for 5 weeks. A walking wrap is used for an additional 5 weeks.

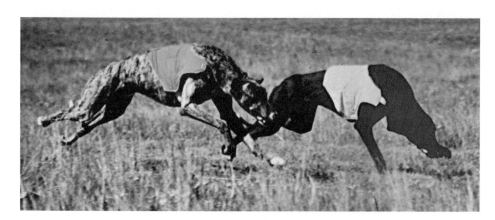

FIGURE 51–6. Double-suspension gallop: "coming down"—right dog more than the left; head down, driving hard. (Courtesy of Leaping Lizards Action Photography, Halley, ID.)

Distal Radius-Ulnar Fractures. These are caused by high-speed power turns over uneven ground. In the coursing dog they are usually closed but on occasion may be open fractures. These are class 2/3 open fractures.

For the distal fracture of the greyhound, the double plating method is recommended.[9] This decreases callus formation, produces the best range of motion, and allows early return to function. The contoured 2.7 dynamic compression plate (DCP) is applied medially to the radius and the ulna is fixed separately with a 1.5/2.0 VC plate (Figs. 51–10 to 51–12). Plates are removed in 7 to 12 weeks; however, optimal time is not certain.

For smaller hounds and whippets, stacked 1.5/2.0 VC plates using 2.0 screws are placed cranially on the radius while the ulna is plated separately with a 1.5/2.0 VC plate. Plate placement on the radial fracture is important because the 1.5/2.0 plate is beneath the 2.0/2.7 VC plate and is two screw holes longer on the diaphyseal side and perhaps one screw hole longer in the metaphysis. The stacked configuration is not as rigid as 2.7 DC plates and the 2.0 screws' holes are not as large. The risk of refracture through the top screw hole after removal of a 2.7 DC plate is greatly diminished. In open fractures there is dirt contamination, even into the medullary canal, with lesser tissue trauma. An open fracture protocol is used; the fragments, the wound, and medullary canal are strictly cleaned. Usually the skin penetration is medial and the surgical approach cranial. In the stacked VC plate method, the medial wound and the cranial incision are left open, both under a petroleum jelly gauze dressing. The dressing is changed daily until the cranial skin incision is managed by delayed primary closure in 60 to 72 hours.

Splints have not been used, but strict cage confinement and tranquilization have been used frequently. Plates are always removed after healing of open fractures.

Collision Injuries. Because the hounds' primary attention is on the hare, they may collide with one another at high speed, produc-

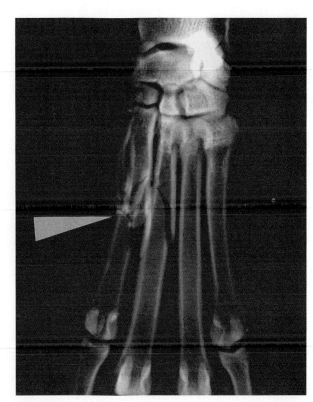

FIGURE 51–8. Comminuted fracture of metacarpal 2; comminuted fracture of metacarpal 3 with butterfly fragment.

ing a variety of injuries. The cervical spine is vulnerable, and cervical sprains can be seen occasionally. Direct shoulder injuries can also occur. Collisions may be averted only for the dog to run into an unseen rock or post. From this kind of direct trauma, one case of fractured patella and one case of patellar tendon detachment from the superior pole of the patella have been seen.

Superficial Digital Flexor Tendon Tears. A flattening of the phalanx (P1–P2) joint may occur, without laceration, because of tearing of a superficial digital flexor (SDF) tendon (Figs. 51–13 to 51–15). Although repair has not been attempted in the few cases seen, the dogs were able to course successfully. The nail was kept trimmed short. Toenail on floor indicates integrity of the deep digital flexor (DDF) tendon.

Phalanx 1–Phalanx 2 Fractures. Whenever possible lagged 1.5 screws and miniplates have been used. This promotes primary bone healing and a more predictable outcome. Coaptation is used.

Tibial Tubercle Physeal Separations. This injury can be devastating if it occurs early. Repairs in a 5- to 6-month old dog often result in "patella baja" (low patella). If the injury occurs at 8 months or older, the slightly lower patella may not be so significant. Unrepaired, however, the injury at this age leads to "patella alta" (high patella). Owners of coursing dogs believe that this impairs top performance. Objective data are lacking.

Repairs should be made but should not compress the physis but merely replace the epiphysis (apophysis) in its anatomical position. I use one small .045 Kirschner wire at a 45-degree angle to the tibial long axis and a noncompressing tension band wire that is removed in 14 days. Knowledge of what this injury can do to the tibial plateau, either alone or in combination with a proximal tibial physeal injury, is incomplete. The effect of tibial plateau–leveling osteotomies and the effect of tibial tubercle–repositioning osteotomies are under scrutiny[8] (Fig. 51–16).

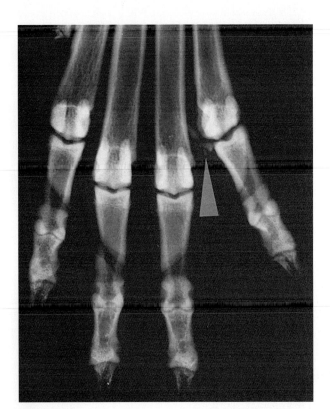

FIGURE 51–7. Type II medial collateral ligament injury. Notice the small avulsed pieces of bone.

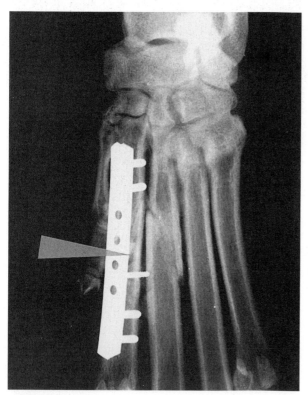

FIGURE 51–9. Metacarpal 2 fixed with 2.0–2.7 VC plate, lagged 1.5 screw beneath plate. Mainly primary healing. Metacarpal 3, mainly oblique, treated by closed reduction, splintage, 6 weeks.

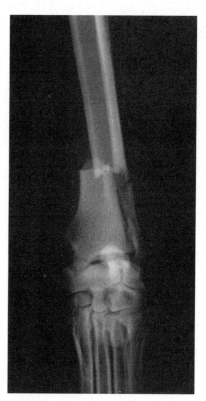

FIGURE 51–10. Distal radius and ulnar fracture—saluki.

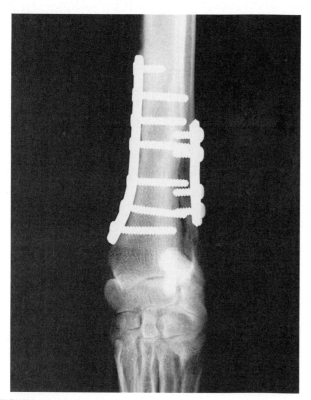

FIGURE 51–11. 2.7 D.C.P. medially on radius. 2.0–2.7 VC plate laterally on ulna. Note primary bone healing.

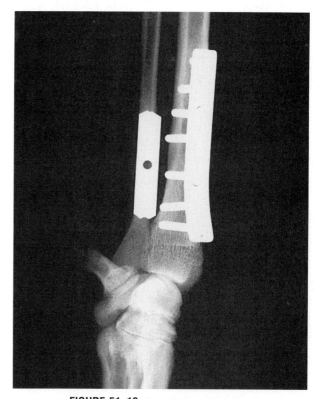

FIGURE 51–12. Lateral view of 2.7 plate.

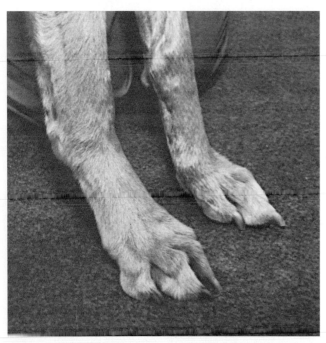

FIGURE 51–13. SDF tendon tears of digits 2 and 3. Note toenail on floor, indicating integrity of deep digital flexor tendon (DDF)—whippet.

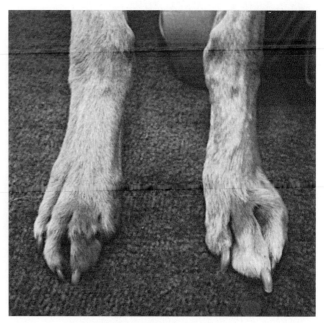

FIGURE 51–14. Same whippet.

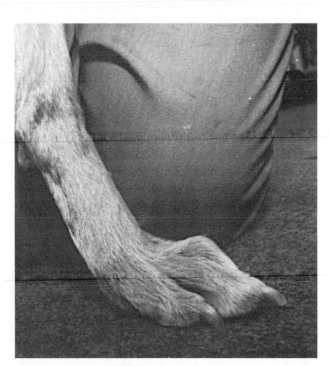

FIGURE 51–15. Same whippet.

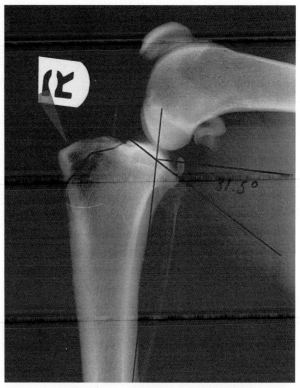

FIGURE 51–16. Unrepaired tibial tubercle avulsion; possible injury to proximal tibial physis. Tubercle sits higher than it should. Tibial plateau is more than the usual 22 to 24 degrees. Dog quit after 250 yards.

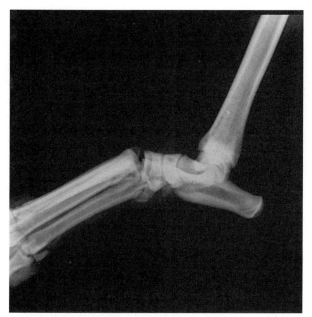

FIGURE 51–17. Tarsometatarsal subluxation, cranial and medial collateral ligament disruption.

UNCOMMON INJURIES

Proximal Intertarsal Instability (Plantar). Good radiographs and stress radiographs are necessary. I have seen only the plantar subluxation with plantar ligament rupture, although dorsal subluxa-

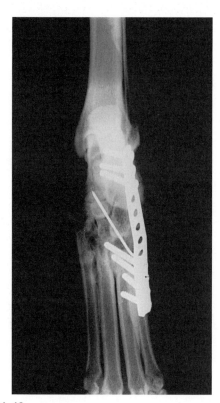

FIGURE 51–18. Arthrodesis of tarsometatarsal and intertarsal joints. Similar idea to proximal intertarsal fusion.

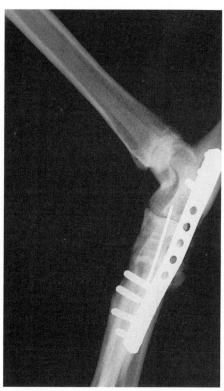

FIGURE 51–19. Healed. Metal was removed.

tion has been reported.[10] The only possibly effective treatment for athletic dogs is arthrodesis of the calcaneoquartal and talocalcaneocentral joints. A lateral approach is used with a 1.5/2.0 mm VC plate or a reconstruction plate contoured and used caudolaterally from calcaneus to proximal metatarsus. The calcaneus faces caudolaterally and the metatarsal faces laterally; therefore, careful contouring and torsion of the plate are necessary. A small temporary K-wire may transfix the calcaneal base across the tarsals exiting at metacarpal base 2. The K-wire holds the anatomical position while the plate or template is being molded to the lateral face. The smaller 1.5/2.0 mm VC plate may be easier to contour and twist. A cancellous graft from the proximal tibia is always used; this weaker fixation must be supported externally 6 to 8 weeks and then removed. The hound may or may not course again. An injured Chesapeake retriever and a Labrador retriever, however, took birds the season following this method of treatment.

Spiral Fracture of Femur. A spiral fracture can occur as the result of torsional forces. This was seen to occur in one greyhound who jerked its foot, which was stuck in a crevice. Spiral fractures can be successfully plated with a 3.5 plate. In two cases that were seen, the plate was removed 11 and 12 weeks after surgery.

Tear of Spinal Head of Deltoid Muscle. The insertion may partially tear at the deltoid crest. It can be resutured, and the hound can regain racing form.

Gracilis Muscle Origin Tear. A single case was seen. A classic finger-trough indentation was palpable high in the groin. Abduction under anesthesia showed the separation from the ventral midline. A primary repair was done 3 days post injury. The rear legs were then bandaged in hobble manner to allow standing and walking but with no abduction, for 3 weeks. Activity was then limited for an additional 3 weeks. This whippet did return to racing form.

Tear of Flexor Carpi Ulnaris Tendon. The actual tendon itself may tear. The oval humeral head tendon of insertion on the accessory carpal bone lies beneath the SDF muscle at the dorsal palmar

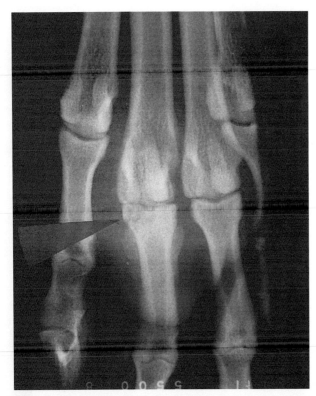
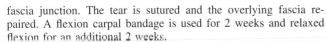

FIGURE 51–20. Fractured tubercle of articular surface of P1 removed. Dog did well early but was lost to follow-up.

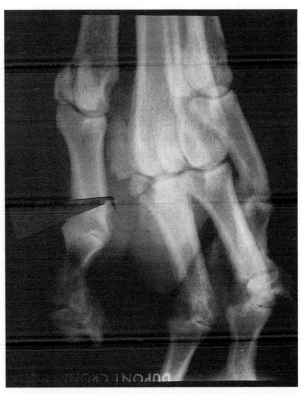

FIGURE 51–21. Same fractured tubercle—oblique view.

fascia junction. The tear is sutured and the overlying fascia repaired. A flexion carpal bandage is used for 2 weeks and relaxed flexion for an additional 2 weeks.

Fractured Tubercle of Proximal Phalanx 1 Articular Surface. The fracture occurred in a turn. This tubercle was successfully removed (Figs. 51–20 and 51–21). Larger fragments may be successfully managed via a pin and figure-of-eight wire.

CONCLUSIONS

Carpal and tarsal bone fractures that occur on the outside limbs of racing greyhounds do not occur as frequently in coursing dogs, nor do the accessory carpal injuries. The stress-type midcaudal acetabular fractures have not been seen. There also seems to be a greater prevalence of distal limb ligament injuries in coursing dogs. The manner of the high-speed run and turn, the hardness of the ground, and the unevenness of the terrain contribute to such injuries.

References

1. Eaton-Wells R: Canine Sports Medicine and Surgery. WB Saunders Company, 1998
2. Copold, S: The Gazehound. A periodical of the National Coursing Club. 1978, p. 38.
3. Netboy D: Personal communication.
4. Brown S: Analysis of videotapes of Waterloo Cup, 1993.
5. Dee JF, Hungerford TG: Short Course Proceedings 122:607–613, 1989.
6. Taylor RA, Dee JF: *In* Slatter D (ed): Textbook of Small Animal Surgery, 2nd ed. Philadelphia, WB Saunders Company, 1993, p 1881.
7. Dee JF: Personal communication.
8. Dee JF, Dee LG: Fractures and dislocations in racing greyhounds, *In* Newton CD, Nunmaker DM: Textbook of Small Animal Orthopedics. Philadelphia, JB Lippencott Co. 1985, pp 467–477.
9. Eaton-Wells R: Specialized treatment of radius-ulnar fractures in racing greyhounds. *Aus Vet Pract* 13:175, 1983.
10. Slocum B: Personal communication.
11. Taylor RA, Dee JF: *In* Slatter D (ed): Textbook of Small Animal Surgery, 2nd ed. Philadelphia, WB Saunders Company, 1993, p 1876.

CHAPTER 52

VETERINARY PROBLEMS UNIQUE TO SECURITY AND DETECTOR DOGS

PAUL B. JENNINGS, Jr. \ JAMES R. FREEMAN, Jr.

Because of the variety of tasks and environments to which working dogs are subjected, unique medical, surgical, training, and behavioral problems do occur. This section begins with selection of working dogs. Then, specific injuries and diseases unique to working dogs today are presented, with historical vignettes, when applicable.

Modern police use of working dogs has progressed hand in hand with military use, because the major assignment for which dogs are used today (detection of illegal drugs, explosives) was a major military concern before society at large was affected by these problems. In addition, many civilian police dog trainers and handlers received their schooling in the military and applied these skills to establishing viable canine programs for federal, state, and local law enforcement agencies.

SELECTION OF WORKING DOGS

As noted in Chapter 5, the German shepherd is the standard animal for all of the duties required of a working dog. With the desire of most agencies to have a dual-trained dog (patrol-explosive or patrol-drug), this breed has been the most successful, because of a relatively good nose for detection and the strength and stamina for security duties.

In 1984, the Belgian malinois was introduced into the Military Working Dog Program, on the basis of experiences and recommendations of European military and police agencies[1-4] (Fig. 52–1). This dog adapted well to the rigors of training. The Belgian malinois breed has also become popular with civilian police agencies, and these dogs are gaining recognition from the general public.

Other dog breeds have been used as working dogs with varying success, including giant schnauzers, Bouvier des Flandres, and rottweilers (for patrol and detection duties). For standard detection work, Labrador and golden retrievers and pointers have worked well. Some agencies have requested small-breed detector dogs, and Cairn terriers and beagles have been trained. Only males and ovariohysterectomized females are selected for training.

Prospective canine candidates are subjected to temperament testing prior to selection. The dog is observed as it is walked on a leash by the owner and again with a handler. Next, inquisitiveness is tested. If the dog is willing to follow a ball or respond to a "squeaky" toy or food, this suggests a degree of curiosity that may be exploited. The animal's response to gunfire is then evaluated. With the dog on a leash with an experienced handler, the dog is selectively tested for its response to 38-caliber blank pistol fire from gradually decreasing distances of 100, 50, and 25 yards. If the dog cowers or tries to hide or pull the handler away, it is disqualified. If the dog's curiosity is stimulated by the noise of gunfire and if it stands its ground, it has passed this portion of the evaluation. Finally, with the dog on a leash, it is agitated by an evaluator wearing an attack sleeve. The dog should stand its ground when agitated and bite and hold the sleeve for 5 seconds (Fig. 52–2).

The dog should not be over or under aggressive. If a dog wants to attack everything, including the handler at the end of the leash, or responds to stimuli by hiding behind the handler or cowering, it is not suitable.

Dogs in their own environment may pass these tests successfully and nevertheless subsequently perform poorly in the training environment. Such dogs are rejected early, do not undergo training, and are sold or given away.

Following successful completion of the temperament test, dogs are subjected to a complete veterinary examination. An important facet of this examination includes sedation and radiography of the coxofemoral and elbow joints for hip and elbow dysplasia. A thorough evaluation of the hips (plus the maturity to be "trainable") has dictated that the youngest age that a dog can be accepted as a worker is 1 year. In the ideal situation, only dogs

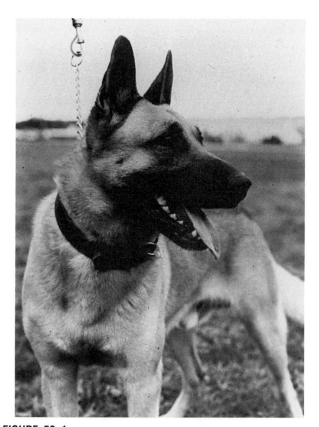

FIGURE 52–1. The Belgian malinois breed has gained popularity as a security–detector dog and is now used by many agencies.

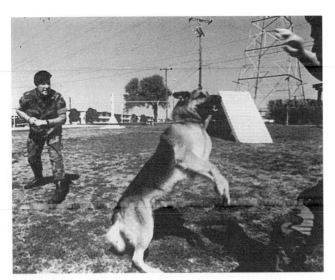

FIGURE 52–2. The prospective canine candidate should stand its ground and actively challenge an aggressor.

with perfect hips would be selected. Reality, however, depends on supply and demand, so some degree of mild hip dysplasia may have to be accepted in order to get enough trainable dogs. The veterinarian has to be somewhat clairvoyant in his or her estimation of whether the rigors of training will exacerbate a mild degree of hip dysplasia in a "marginal" animal. Annual radiographs of all dogs identified with hip dysplasia are obtained to follow the progress of the disease.[5]

Radiographic evidence of ununited anconeal process or fragmented coronoid process is grounds for rejection. Some dogs with ununited anconeal process have slipped through into the program, and the process has been surgically removed. Most of these dogs have worked effectively only 1 or 2 years before developing debilitating arthritis.

As will be discussed later, dental disease is the most common cause of morbidity in working dogs. Thus, a clean, healthy oral cavity is essential in a dog entering training. All four canine teeth must be intact and not chipped or cracked, tartar accumulation should be minimal, and there should be no evidence of oral bony or soft tissue lesions.

Unresolved medical problems include infectious or parasitic diseases and wounds, fractures, and the like. Dogs should be treated for external and intestinal parasites and heart worms before acceptance. All infectious processes and traumatic wounds should be resolved.

Watching the dog in a kennel situation, with its handler or with other dogs, may reveal bad habits that invariably will worsen in the kennels or in a training setting. Examination of the mouth may reveal metal abrasions and wear on teeth, indicating nervous chewing on fences or metal water or feed pans. A raw, denuded tail may signify a tail beater or chaser, again a nervous habit that is disqualifying. Finally, the finding of lick granulomas on the extremities denotes a chronic medical or behavioral problem that *always* gets worse. These dogs should not be selected.

Conditions such as heart murmurs, deafness, ocular defects, and bite abnormalities dictate nonselection.

The veterinarian's role in the selection process is to watch for dog responses that may be behaviorally or medically motivated. In many cases the veterinarian proves to be the "bad guy," because some of the best dogs, in regard to temperament, have medical problems that prohibit selection. The veterinarian must have the welfare of the animal plus the good of the total working dog program in mind when selecting or rejecting a dog.

The veterinarian also can assist the evaluators by monitoring the vendors and suppliers to see the types and quality of dogs they offer for sale. A visit to the vendors' kennels with observation of the physical facilities and sanitation and any pretraining activity that the dogs undergo before offering can often be very enlightening.

VETERINARY PROBLEMS UNIQUE TO WORKING DOGS

The Head and Neck

Cracked and Fractured Teeth. Except for straight detector dogs, working dogs must have a good set of teeth. The canine teeth, especially, must be intact and pain free to allow the dog to apprehend a suspect, to bite the attack sleeve, and, of course, to grasp and ingest food. Dental problems are *the* most common reasons for seeking veterinary care.

Dogs may crack or fracture their canine teeth by chewing on kennel fences and steel water and feed pans, or when biting and twisting while training on the attack sleeve. Side-to-side movement of the attack sleeve by the handler may place undue stresses on the dog's teeth, leading to fracture (Figs. 52–3 and 52–4). The Belgian malinois has seemed more prone to fractured canine teeth than the German shepherd dog.[4] The nonagressive smaller breeds of dogs rarely have tooth fractures.

The pain of a broken or infected tooth or both can distract a working dog to the point that it cannot perform normal duties. Endodontic therapy of such fractured canine teeth has been success-

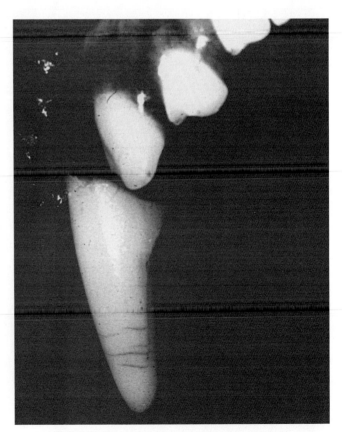

FIGURE 52–3. Cracked canine tooth, the result of trauma.

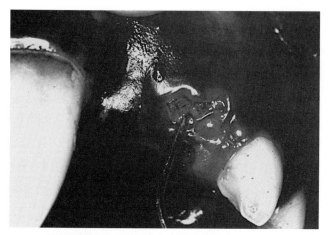

FIGURE 52–4. Worn incisor teeth and gum lacerations.

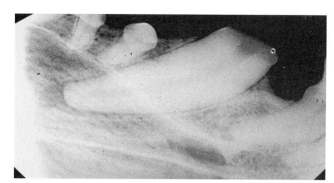

FIGURE 52–6. Radiograph of fractured canine tooth following root canal therapy, prior to filling of the canal.

ful in working dogs and has allowed the dogs to continue to have a good bite. Root canal treatment removes the pain and, even if one half of the total exposed tooth is absent, the dog still can bite well.[6]

The actual technique used for endodontic treatment seems to have very little overall effect on the outcome of the treatment. The majority of military working dogs have been treated using an injection technique, with a liquid restorative material that hardens into a solid state.[7] This technique can be easier to perform than the classic method that uses cones of gutta–percha. There have been no known complications in any military working dog in which this injection method has been used over the past 10 years (Figs. 52–5 to 52–8).

Attempts to apply caps or crowns to endodontically treated canine teeth have been relatively ineffective, because of the tremendous forces applied to the prosthesis by the dog's biting and chewing. Some dogs with severely worn canine teeth may have a very serviceable bite and still can perform their duties.

An alloy filling is the preferred material to seal the endodontically treated tooth in the working dog. It has the highest degree of compressibility and holds up well to the stresses placed upon it.[8, 9] In addition, it is easy to visualize during dental cleaning and is therefore easier to avoid. Composite and glass isomer restorative materials can be damaged easily during dental prophylaxis if proper care is not given to cleaning around them.

Canine teeth that have fractures extending below the gum line

should be extracted. These teeth rarely do well if treated otherwise. The preferred method is the buccal flap technique.[10] This technique avoids an oral-nasal fistula and is tolerated very well by dogs.

Premolar and molar teeth, with their multiple roots, also may be treated endodontically.

Carnassial tooth (upper fourth premolar) abscesses are not common in the working dog population, possibly because dental prophylaxis is performed at least every 6 months.

Periodontal Disease. The dog seems to accumulate plaque readily, and working dogs on a soft diet will develop excess calculus unless dental prophylaxis is performed regularly. Softer diets seem to deposit around the gingival sulcus more readily than hard diets and are not easily cleared away by the action of the tongue. Brushing of teeth can be carried out daily and has proven to be beneficial. However, one must weigh the positive effects of brushing against the liklihood of handler injury from a dog trained to bite. Therefore, great care should be taken to acclimate the working dog to the brushing procedure.

Removal of calculus with an ultrasonic scaler and polishing (to smooth out the scratches made by the scaler) are necessary on a frequent basis. The smaller-breed dogs (Cairn terriers, beagles) have more calculus and gingival disease than the larger breeds[11] (Fig. 52–9). Regular periodontal probing is the best method of assessing the severity of periodontal disease and should be performed during each dental cleaning.[12]

Older dogs may develop gingivitis, gingival recession, and tooth loosening. Gum resection sometimes has been necessary to remove hyperplastic tissue. The good vascular supply has allowed healing to progress rapidly in most cases.

Gingival trauma, usually a result of biting the attack sleeve, occasionally requires suturing.

The Tongue. Dogs occasionally get their tongues between their

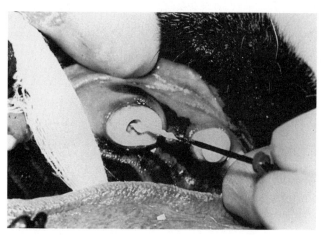

FIGURE 52–5. Preparation of canine tooth for root canal therapy.

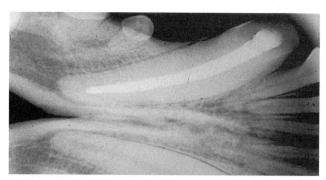

FIGURE 52–7. Root canal filled with liquid filler, prior to placement of alloy filling.

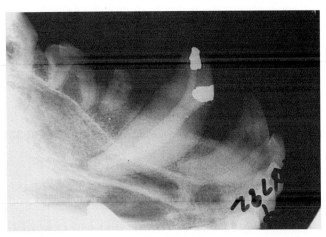

FIGURE 52–8. Completed endodontic procedure, with alloy filling of canal and access opening.

teeth and the object they are biting, resulting in varying degrees of laceration. The animal usually has a mouthful of blood. The dog should be anesthetized and intubated as soon as possible to allow a complete examination and to prevent aspiration of blood. Partial amputation of the tongue may be necessary if necrosis has occurred.

A unique lingual condition of military working dogs in Vietnam, which first appeared in 1968 and produced more lost working days for dogs than any other medical condition, was known as acute glossitis, or ''red tongue.''[13] Clinical signs included excessive salivation and inability to lap water. The anterior one third of the tongue was red and smooth, with evidence of loss of papillae. Dogs would develop permanent scarring of the anterior tongue, and recurrences of the acute disease were frequent.[14] The common denominator of this condition seemed to be sunlight, and removal of affected dogs from direct exposure to the sun resolved the acute condition, at least temporarily. In an experimental study, exposure of the tongues of dogs to intense ultraviolet light produced lesions that were microscopically identical to the natural cases.[15] Why this condition occurred in epidemic proportions in Vietnam and not in the training areas of Georgia and Texas was never determined.

Epistaxis. Epistaxis may be unilateral or bilateral and usually occurs during agitation or when the dog is excited. Some dogs may

be susceptible to this condition because of nasal blood vessel anatomy. Foreign bodies, such as grass awns, lodged in the nose, may stimulate excessive sneezing and discomfort, leading to epistaxis. Treatment includes cold packs, nasal epinephrine flushes, and hypotensive agents. Anesthesia and intubation will eliminate nasal breathing and allow a thorough examination.

Choke Chain Trauma. Restraint and training of working dogs requires liberal use of the smooth metal choke chain. Tightening down on the choke chain usually is all the reprimand a working dog needs for enforcement of commands. Occasionally, overly vigorous use of the choke chain, or tying a dog via a long leash and choke chain to a tree or fence, will result in hair loss and skin abrasions under the chain, or even serious musculoskeletal damage to the neck.[16] One Belgian malinois had oral hemorrhage following liberal use of the choke chain, when the dog apparently climbed up the leash to attack the handler. Attempts to stop the bleeding under general anesthesia were not successful, and the dog died from aspiration of blood. Tissue sections of the pharynx revealed abnormalities of the blood vessel walls (seen usually in much older dogs) that may have resulted in friability of the vessels and uncontrollable hemorrhage.

Atrophic Myopathy of the Belgian Malinois. We have noted a muscle-wasting syndrome in this breed, in which the muscles over the frontal, parietal, zygomatic, and temporal bones atrophy, resulting in a gaunt appearance and prominence of the sagittal crest and zygomatic bones. Unlike the classic descriptions of eosinophilic or atrophic myositis, in which the primary involvement was in the muscles of mastication, these dogs did not have problems in chewing, swallowing, or attacking and holding an attack sleeve, nor did they exhibit pain or swelling before the muscle atrophy. No abnormalities have been noted in blood or clinical chemistry profiles. These dogs have continued to work, but their appearance has not escaped comment.[17–20] No treatment has been necessary (Figs. 52–10 and 52–11).

Gastrointestinal System

Gastric Dilatation–Volvulus. Gastric dilatation–volvulus (GDV) has been the most frequent life-threatening condition seen in working dogs.[21] Dogs with GDV often have a clinical history of ''not acting right,'' trying to vomit, salivating profusely, and

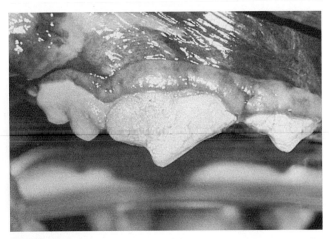

FIGURE 52–9. Excess calculus and gingivitis in a working dog. Routine dental prophylaxis is needed to prevent gum disease.

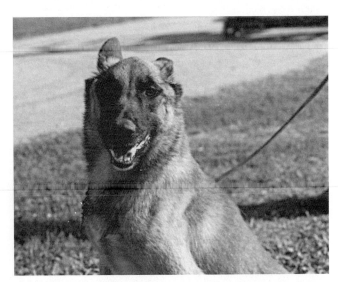

FIGURE 52–10. A Belgian malinois with atrophic myopathy. Note prominence of sagittal crest and zygomatic bones and atrophy of musculature over the frontal, parietal, and temporal bones.

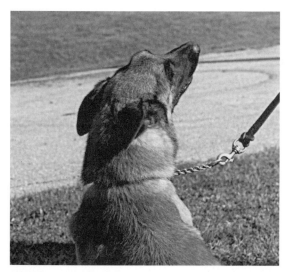

FIGURE 52–11. Dorsal view of the same dog showing extent of muscle wasting in this condition. This dog had no problems in mastication and worked well.

staggering, and frequently the abdomen is tense and swollen. These dogs received prompt veterinary care, and the results usually were good. If the aforementioned clinical signs are not observed, the dog may die and be found moribund in its kennel.[4]

One of the reasons for development of the Maximum Stress Diet, Medicated was its digestibility, high energy, and low bulk and that it did not expand appreciably in water.[22] The fact that most of the dogs until 1992 were on this diet and that GDV still appeared suggests that this ration alone had not solved the problem.

Most working dogs are fed once a day, with the only addition being food rewarded as "treats" given during training or duty. An exception has been large dogs that need more than 1¼ pounds of food per day. The ration is usually divided into two meals for these animals. The once-per-day feedings are more for the convenience of the training schedule than for the dog. Frequent small feedings might be more beneficial and less conducive to acute GDV.

Our treatment protocol for working dogs with acute GDV has been to recommend initial passage of a stomach tube and aspiration of gastric contents, if possible. A tape roll is used as a mouth gag, and a feeding tube is measured and marked prior to its passage. If the tube will not pass, placing the dog in different positions may help (sitting, on side). A little ketamine/diazepam administered intravenously often will relax the dog enough to allow the tube to pass.[21] In our experience, we have been unable to pass the stomach tube in 75 per cent of cases.

If passage of a stomach tube is impossible, the stomach must be decompressed by another method. Surgical preparation of the right paralumbar fossa, just behind the last rib, allows the stomach to be trocarized, using an 8–12 gauge, 4″ needle. Attach suction and aspirate contents. Very often following this form of decompression, the stomach tube can be passed.

Shock therapy is begun; this includes rapid administration of intravenous crystalloid solutions, corticosteroids, antibiotics, as indicated. The cardiovascular system is monitored, and if arrythmias appear, they should be treated appropriately with antiarrhythmic drugs.

When the dog's condition is stabilized, abdominal radiography may be performed. If the pyloric shadow indicates a volvulus is present, surgery should be performed immediately.

As a surgical procedure, our staff has prefered the tube gastrostomy because it provides open access to the gastrointestinal tract (for drainage, feeding) and produces a good gastropexy. Even in dogs that have simple gastric dilatation without volvulus, we recommend performing a "pexy" (circumcostal, belt-loop, and the like), if not immediately after the stomach has been decompressed, then as soon as possible after the dog has returned to normal. In our experience, once the dog has become "bloated," the condition will invariably recur and the next time may progress to GDV. A fairly recent survey demonstrated that dogs that had one or more episodes of acute gastric dilatation that were treated by stomach tube decompression and medical supportive therapy only eventually died from GDV. Those animals in which surgery was performed (and in which the "pexy" was still intact), survived.[22] In our opinion, the stretching of suspensory ligaments, sphincters, or musculature, which is produced by the first occurrence of acute gastric dilatation or GDV, produces irreversible damage that will predispose to future episodes.

Occasional complications have occurred with tube gastrostomy, including necessity for premature tube removal and delayed gastric emptying.[23]

Nervous System

Seizures in the Belgian Malinois. Some of these dogs in training have developed seizures, usually associated with aggression training.[4, 24] The dogs would attack and then suddenly roll to one side, exhibit a "glassy stare," and fall to the ground. These episodes would last for 30 seconds or less. The dog would then apparently recover and return to normal. Recurrences of the seizure frequently were noted if the dog attacked the sleeve again (see Chapter 11). In a litter of five pups born to a Belgian malinois with a history of seizures, two of the pups began exhibiting seizure activity at 13 months of age.

Degenerative Myelopathy. This condition is mentioned only because it is a leading reason for euthanasia of working dogs, together with hip dysplasia[25] (see Chapter 11).

THE SKIN AND ADNEXA

Aural Hematoma. Aural hematomas in shepherds usually are related to the presence of otitis externa. In our experience, highly excitable, aggressive dogs that shake their heads vigorously are more likely to have aural hematomas than are dogs of similar breeds with a more relaxed temperament.[14]

One method of treatment with which we have had success is incision and drainage of the hematoma and through-and-through suturing of skin to cartilage, using 0 nonabsorbable sutures in an interrupted horizontal mattress suture pattern, to obliterate all dead space. Following surgery, the ears are taped together over the dorsum of the head and the head is bandaged. A plastic bucket, which is attached to the dog's collar, is used to encase the bandage and prevent self-multilation (Fig. 52–12). (Note: We have not found success with the use of Elizabethan collars in these high-strung dogs.) Bandages are changed every 2 to 3 days and can be removed 10 to 14 days after surgery. This condition may recur in the same ear or appear in the contralateral ear in the future. Regular ear cleaning by handlers and prompt attention to signs of otitis externa will prevent the otitis externa that predisposes these dogs to aural hematomas.[26] Chronic otitis and its complications may require lateral ear canal resection to resolve the drainage problem.

Sternal Exuberant Granulation. This term was first used in Vietnam to describe the reaction of military working dogs to grass awns embedded in the skin and subcutaneous tissue over the midventral sternum.[14, 27] Hard cores of fibrous tissue and draining fistulous tracts were created by the antigenic stimulus of the awns. Attempts to remove the fibrous tissue and tracts were frustrating,

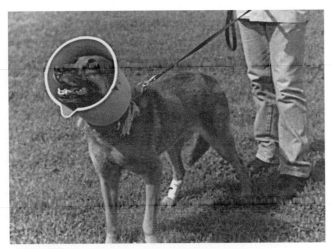

FIGURE 52–12. Plastic head bucket, attached to the dog's collar, will prevent self-mutilation in the aggressive dog and allow it to eat and drink normally.

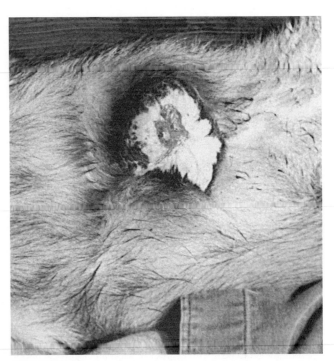

FIGURE 52–14. Chronic sternal exuberant granulation. This dog underwent three surgical procedures and had a chronic mushroom-appearing dormant lesion on its sternum.

because the response to incision, debridement, and use of buried absorbable ligatures and sutures—plus the lack of mobilizable skin over the sternum—frequently resulted in dehiscence, poor healing, and production of an open ulcerated sternal wound that would granulate excessively.

We have seen similar lesions in working dogs today with comparable results (Figs. 52–13 and 52–14). In the Belgian malinois, whose skin is soft and thin, the sternal area will develop black pigmentation and fibrous cores, and fistulous tracts will be present. Some of the methods of treating these lesions that have been moderately successful include refraining from use of any absorbable ligatures or sutures subcutaneously. Instead, we have used electrocoagulation for all bleeders and use the electrosurgical unit exclusively to incise muscle and fascia and for removal of fistulous tracts.

Tension-relieving skin incisions are then used on the lower right and left sides of the thorax to ensure that the skin closure over the

sternum will be tension free. The skin over the midventral sternum is then closed with interrupted horizontal mattress sutures of 3/0 stainless steel wire, with rubber dams to relieve skin pressure. The skin edges are then closed with simple interrupted sutures of 3/0 wire.

A large pressure bandage is placed over the incision area, and the entire chest is covered with 12-inch stockinette. Two holes are placed in the stockinette for the dog's front limbs, the "sweater" is pulled over the thorax, and the entire stockinette is wrapped with 2- or 3-inch adhesive tape. The bandage should be changed at least every 2 days. We have used silver sulfadiazine (Silvadene) as a wound dressing and believe that this product has kept the tissue moist while encouraging healing.[28]

Tail Beating in the Belgian Malinois. Many of the veterinary problems in the Belgian malinois relate to kenneling.[1] The dogs will circle rapidly while in a kennel and when agitated (or merely when someone walks by the kennel), will spin and climb the walls, barking constantly. In many cases, these dogs will abrade the tip and sides of their tails, filling the kennel with blood and exposing the last coccygeal vertebrae. The abrasions along the length of the tail have prompted us to call this a "piccolo" tail. These lesions will heal if the dog can be taken out of a conventional kennel and staked on a large kennel chain in an enclosure without walls. However, the condition will recur as soon as the dog returns to conventional kennels. Amputation of only the affected portion will not work, for the remaining tail will develop the same lesions and hemorrhage (Fig. 52–15).

Complete tail amputation between cy 2 and 3 has been curative. The stump heals to the contour of the dog's perineum and, in this breed, is cosmetically acceptable[29] (Fig. 52–16).

Soft Pads. The Belgian malinois seems to have more problems with tender foot-pad than do other working-dog breeds. Standard treatments, including application of tincture of benzoin or copper sulfate, have been only partially successful. Placing a rubber mat in kennels and working the dogs on grass or dirt does help.

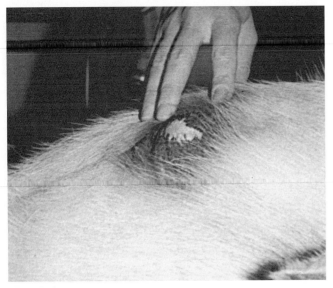

FIGURE 52–13. Small area of sternal exuberant granulation. Note pigment change around margins of lesion.

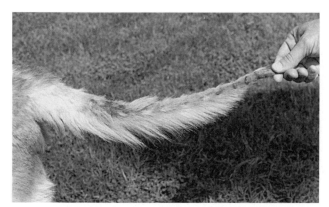

FIGURE 52–15. "Piccolo tail" in Belgian malinois.

Occasionally, dogs have to be eliminated from training for this condition.

Perianal Fistulas in German Shepherd Dogs. German shepherd working dogs may develop perianal fistulas. We have treated these dogs, using all of the conventional treatments.[30] Recurrence has been frequent, and on occasion, the fistulas have been unresponsive to therapy, resulting in the dogs' being euthanatized.

Elbow Hygromas. The Belgian malinois is predisposed to elbow hygromas[4] (Fig. 52–17). Medical treatment (aspiration of fluid, instillation of corticosteroids) has been ineffective.[31] The lesions invariably return and are best treated surgically.

A 1.5 to 2.0-cm horizontal skin incision is made proximal and distal to the hygroma. A stab incision is then made into the false

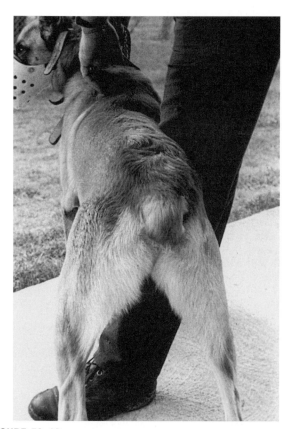

FIGURE 52–16. Appearance of Belgian malinois following tail amputation.

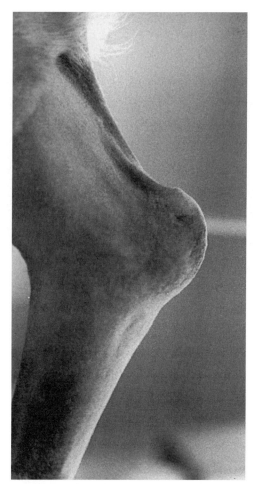

FIGURE 52–17. Elbow hygroma in Belgian malinois.

bursa at both ends of the incision, and fluid is aspirated. All fibrous cores are resected and the cavity is flushed with sterile isotonic saline. A 1-inch Penrose drain is folded in half, placed into the cavity, and the ends of the drain are sutured to the proximal and distal skin incisions (Fig. 52–18). The elbow is next wrapped with a soft bandage. Early attempts to use a postoperative bandage alone to apply even pressure to the hygroma site in this breed were ineffective because of the animals' highly nervous temperament and exuberance. Thus, to keep even pressure on the elbow, we devised a light fiberglass cast, used with an extension over the elbow, applied in a clamshell manner, over the soft bandage (Fig. 52–19). The cast could be opened every 3 days, the bandage replaced, and the cast reapplied. The drain was removed when it was ready. As healing progressed, the distal portion of the cast was removed, leaving a firm support of bandage and fiber glass over the elbow until healing was complete.[4]

Scrotal Dermatitis. Although seen sometimes in German shepherd dogs, Bouvier des Flandres, giant schnauzers, and other working-dog breeds, scrotal dermatitis has been an especially debilitating problem in the Belgian malinois. Conventional medical treatment, including a variety of ointments and keeping the dog in a dry kennel, have provided only temporary remission. Because this condition will recur in individual dogs and these dogs may be required to work in parts of the world where moisture, heat, and cold may produce relapses, castration and surgical ablation of the scrotum have been necessary to resolve the condition.[32] Because scrotal dermatitis has been such a problem in this breed, we have

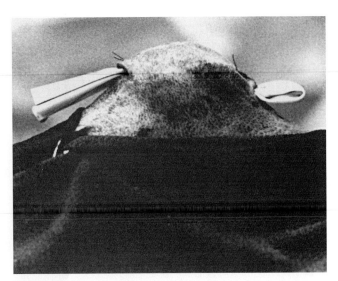

FIGURE 52–18. A 1-inch Penrose drain is folded, placed into the hygroma cavity, and sutured at the proximal and distal skin incisions.

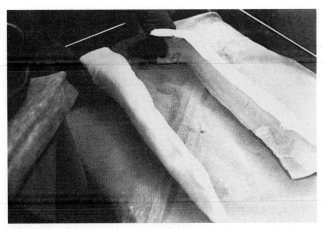

FIGURE 52–19. Fiber glass "clamshell" cast used over bandage to cover draining elbow hygroma. Note the extension to maintain pressure over the elbow.

performed castration plus scrotal ablation routinely, including those performed for temperament or prostatic disease.

Calcinosis Circumscripta. The Belgian malinois may have calcinosis circumscripta associated with the lateral or medial aspects of the distal metacarpal and metatarsal areas (Fig. 52–20).

Neoplastic Disease. A 1-year survey of death or euthanasia in 444 military working dogs revealed that 10.81 per cent were the result of neoplastic disease. Most neoplasms were lymphosarcomas and hemangiosarcomas, and the mean age at death for these dogs was 8.8 years.

Salvaging the Older Dog. Once a dog has been selected and trained to work, the value of the animal appreciates ($10,000 to $20,000). The goal of the handlers, trainers, kennel masters, and veterinary personnel is to continue the dog's useful life for as long

as possible. Although the mean age of death/euthanasia of working dogs has averaged 8.7 years, many 12- to 14-year-old dogs have continued to work well.

As dogs age, existing medical conditions may worsen, ie, hip dysplasia. Modification in the training and use of these animals may be necessary. For example, a dual-trained dog is required to maintain proficiency in both patrol and detection capabilities. Patrol training includes climbing and jumping through an obstacle course. Various modifications of patrol training are possible, and the dog may still be usable. The other option is to decertify the dog from patrol work and use it as a detector dog only.

Returning the older working dog to the training school to act as a training aid for new students is another method of increasing the dog's useful life. The dog can be used by successive classes of students and can be rested when medical problems erupt.

Veterinary input to increasing the dog's usefulness to the pro-

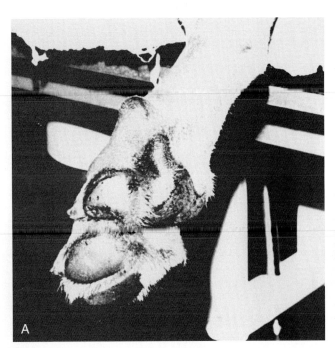
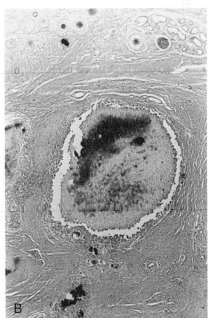

FIGURE 52–20. Gross *(A)* and microscopic *(B)* appearance of calcinosis circumscripta lesion on the medial metatarsal area of a Belgian malinois.

gram involves clinical evaluation, medical or surgical treatment, evaluation of response to treatment, and final judgment as to when humane considerations should override further continuation as a working dog.

When a dog is no longer able to work and is decertified, some options still exist. Older nonaggressive dogs (beagles, retrievers) that have not received any aggression training can be given away to the public. Usually, former handlers want these dogs to finish out their lives in the comforts of their homes and yards. Because of their aggressive nature, patrol-trained dogs are usually given or sold to police agencies.

References

1. The Belgian Malinois. *In* American Kennel Club: The Complete Dog Book, 17th ed. New York, Howell Book House, Inc., 1989, pp 584–587.
2. Jiles ML: A history of the Belgian shepherd dogs. Pure Bred Dogs/ American Kennel Gazette 109(1):40, 1992.
3. Foster C: The versatile sheepdogs of Belgium. Dog World 75(7):18, 1990.
4. Jennings PB: Veterinary care of the Belgian Malinois military working dog. Mil Med 156(1):36, 1991.
5. Townsend LR: Hip dysplasia in canine military candidates. Proceedings of the Canine Hip Dysplasia Symposium and Workshop, St. Louis, Mo, Oct 19, 1992, pp 127–130.
6. Rosman LE, Garber DA, Harvey CE: Disorders of teeth. *In* Harvey CE (ed): Veterinary Dentistry. Philadelphia, WB Saunders Company, 1985, pp 79–105.
7. Schindler WG, Doran JE: Nonsurgical endodontic therapy on the canine tooth of the dog. J Endodontics 12:573, 1986.
8. Ridgway RL, Zielke DR: Nonsurgical endodontic technique for dogs. JAVMA 174:82, 1970.
9. Eisenmenger E, Zetner K: Veterinary Dentistry. Philadelphia, Lea & Febiger, 1985, pp 83–112.
10. Holstrom SE, Frost P, Gammon RL: Veterinary Dental Techniques. Philadelphia, WB Saunders Company, 1992, pp 192–194.
11. Kertesz P: Veterinary Dentistry and Oral Surgery. London, Wolfe Publishing, 1993, pp 73–99.
12. Holstrom SE, Frost P, Gammon RL: Veterinary Dental Techniques. Philadelphia, WB Saunders Company, 1992, pp 128–129.
13. Stedham MA, Jennings PB, Moe JB, et al: Glossitis of military working dogs in South Vietnam: History and clinical characteristics. JAVMA 163:272, 1973.
14. Jennings PB, Moe JB, Elwell PA, et al: A survey of diseases of military dogs in the Republic of Vietnam. JAVMA 159:434, 1971.
15. Jennings PB, Lewis GE, Crumrine MH, et al: Glossitis of military working dogs in Vietnam: Experimental production of tongue lesions. Am J Vet Res 35:1295, 1974.
16. Medford MA: The choke chain; more than a correction? Dog World 69(2):12, 1984.
17. Averill DR: Diseases of the muscle. Vet Clin North Am 10:223, 1980.
18. Whitney JC: Atrophic myositis in the dog; the differentiation of this disease from eosinophilic myositis. Vet Rec 69(2):130, 1957.
19. Fainbach GC: Canine myositis. *In* Kirk RW (ed): Current Veterinary Therapy VIII. Philadelphia, WB Saunders Company, 1983, pp 681–686.
20. Brogden JD, Brightman AH, McLaughlin SA: Diagnosing and treating masticatory myositis. Vet Med 86:1164, 1991.
21. Jennings PB: The gastric dilatation–volvulus syndrome in the military working dog. Mil Med 152:636, 1987.
22. Jennings PB, Butzin CA: Epidemiology of gastric dilatation-volvulus in the military working dog program. Mil Med 157:369, 1992.
23. Jennings PB, Mathey WS, Ehler WJ: Intermittent gastric dilatation after gastropexy in a dog. JAVMA 200:1707, 1992.
24. Clark RD, Teinquist M: The Belgian sheepdog. *In* Clark R, Stainer JR (eds): Medical and Genetic Aspects of Purebred Dogs. Edwardsville, Kan, Veterinary Medicine Publishing Co, 1983, pp 65–66.
25. Dutton RE, Moore GE: Clinical review of death/euthanasia in 123 military working dog necropsies. Mil Med 152:489, 1987.
26. Bright RM, Buchard SJ: Nasal cavity, paranasal sinuses, larynx and ears. *In* Gourley IM, Vasseur PB (eds): General Small Animal Surgery. Philadelphia, JB Lippincott Co, 1985, pp 189–190.
27. Jennings PB, Elwell PA, Moe JB, et al: A coding system for the epidemiological study of military dog diseases in Vietnam. Am J Public Health 62:1317, 1972.
28. Heggers JP: Personal communication, 1992.
29. Newton CD, Olmstead ML: Reconstructive surgery. *In* Harvey CE, Newton CD, Schwartz A (eds): Small Animal Surgery. Philadelphia, JB Lippincott Co, 1990, pp 621–622.
30. Johnston DE: Surgical diseases of the rectum and anus. *In* Slatter DH (ed): Textbook of Small Animal Surgery. Philadelphia, WB Saunders Company, 1985, pp 777–785.
31. Pope ER: Surgical treatment of hygroma of the elbow. *In* Bojrab MJ (ed): Current Techniques in Small Animal Surgery, 3rd ed. Philadelphia, Lea & Febiger, 1990, pp 486–487.
32. Boothe HW: Testes, epididymis and spermatic cord. *In* Slatter DH (ed): Textbook of Small Animal Surgery. Philadelphia, WB Saunders Company, 1985, pp 1623–1626.

CHAPTER 53

What's New on the Horizon for Comparative Orthopedic Sports Medicine

WILLIAM G. RODKEY \ C. WAYNE McILWRAITH \ J. RICHARD STEADMAN

Any effort to predict the future, especially in the field of medicine, inevitably is fraught with mistakes. One is almost certain to make both overstatements and understatements. With our extremely rapid changing technology, we are likely to miss certain areas completely. Nonetheless, in this chapter we venture down that treacherous path and speculate on what is new and what we believe may be important in the future to the art and science of veterinary orthopedic sports medicine.

Before the evolution and development of orthopedic sports medicine as a recognized subspecialty and discipline, orthopedic surgeons were trained to treat athletic injuries, but few had the training or recognized the need to treat injured athletes.[1] In only the past 20 years have specialty societies of sports medicine and specialized training programs been developed to help recognize these needs. As a result, the individual orthopedic surgeons and the societies have worked together to ensure the integration of the care of sports injuries into the overall context of the rigors and demands of the individual athlete's training and competition. In the very recent past, a similar trend has developed within the veterinary profession that has led to various efforts, including this textbook, to help be sure that the subspecialty of veterinary orthopedic sports medicine includes a great deal of concern for the need of the individual patient, not just treating certain types of injuries.

The concept of orthopedic sports medicine, whether it involves human patients or animal patients, must make certain assumptions. For instance, we believe that orthopedic sports medicine assumes a patient (or the patient's owner or trainer) for whom participation in a given sport presents special significance, and that such a patient has specific achievement goals and a strong desire to return to training and competition. Considering the current social and athletic trends, both human and animal athletes have been pushed to a level of serious training and advanced competition never before seen. The optimal care of these athletes requires thorough understanding and a high level of competency by more than just a few orthopedic sports medicine specialists.

This need now is well recognized for human athletes, and there are numerous orthopedic sports medicine fellowship training programs throughout the United States that are providing these necessary orthopedic sports medicine specialists to provide these necessary services. The veterinary profession, on the other hand, is at a stage at which human medicine was perhaps 20 years ago. It is therefore essential that veterinarians with a specific interest in orthopedic sports medicine continue to become professionally organized and truly dedicated to this subspecialty so that our animal athletes will be provided the best medical care and be offered the best opportunity for long and successful careers in their own athletic endeavors.

SPORTS MEDICINE INJURIES AND PROBLEMS

While animal athletes suffer many problems, most of the injuries and conditions by themselves are not unique to athletes. However, the way these injuries and illnesses are managed requires unique considerations in athletes. The most prevalent and career threatening of these were described in the earlier chapters of this textbook. Therefore, this chapter emphasizes how these injuries and pathological conditions might be better managed in the future as we look beyond our current capabilities and predict new methods of diagnoses, instrumentation, and treatment that will provide special benefit to animal athletes.

Inflammation

While inflammation is a commonly observed tissue response to musculoskeletal injury, sports-induced inflammation appears unique because of the circumstances surrounding its etiology.[2–5] Additionally, the treatment of sports-induced inflammation must be administered in the context of patients who are eager to return to and, it is hoped, exceed their pre-injury performance levels. Consequently, various inflammatory responses are among the most common conditions for which treatment is sought and given in all types of athletes.[2, 3, 5] As a result, such terms as *myositis, fibrositis, fibrocystic nodule,* and *tendinitis* are too frequently used to justify a therapeutic regimen, while attempting to satisfy the patient's (or owner's or trainer's) expectations of a definitive diagnosis, while at the same time relieving the attending medical professional of admitting the limits of his knowledge. Thus, it is essential that the orthopedic sports medicine specialist place the highest emphasis on understanding the pathophysiology of inflammation at the cellular level to diagnose accurately and treat effectively these common injuries.

Sports injury is the loss of cells and/or extracellular matrix resulting from sports induced trauma. Sports trauma results from an injury from some mechanical force applied externally that causes structural stress or strain and that results in a cellular or tissue response.[1, 2, 5] The biomechanical effect of load on tissue is typically described as strain and stress, in which strain is the deformation of a tissue or structure in response to an external load, and stress is the internal resistance to such deformation.[5] As a signal of distress by the tissues or structures under stress and strain, inflammatory responses may be initiated whenever the biomechanical forces and loads applied to the tissue exceed the individual biomechanical and/or metabolic limits.[2, 3]

Many of the conditions that result in sports-induced inflammation are directly attributable to the so-called overuse syndrome[6] or microtrauma-associated injuries.[4, 6] A major limitation in gaining a better understanding of such injuries stems from the fact that only a limited number of research models exist for this type of inflammation, and essentially none of these is directly applicable to the mechanisms of overuse. Similarly, little research on sports-induced injury exists that focuses on microtrauma at the cellular level. Furthermore, there is a lack of published data on the analysis of tissue biopsies that correlate directly with a specific stage of a clinical diagnosis of sports-induced inflammatory processes because the majority of such injuries are not treated surgically. One potential future method to overcome the necessity for such biopsies involves the use of advanced spectroscopic and physiological data acquisition methods as an adjunct to magnetic resonance imaging as discussed below. This entire area of the study of sports-induced inflammation is one that must be pursued in the future as we move forward to gain better understanding of the pathophysiology and, in turn, to formulate better methods of management and treatment for these injuries.

Sports-induced inflammation typically is a localized tissue response that results from injury or destruction of vascularized tissue exposed to excessive mechanical loads as described above.[2] This process evolves over time and is characterized by vascular, chemical, and cellular events that lead to eventual tissue repair or regeneration or to scar formation.[2, 4, 7] A part of this overall process is the phenomenon of pain. Pain must be given appropriate attention because it frequently is the defining factor of the state of the injury. The injured athlete with soft tissue pain often is faced with inability to perform the sports activity. Because the classic signs of inflammation are not always present, especially in deep-lying structures, it often is difficult or impossible to identify the exact location and source of the pain, especially in animal athletes. Therefore, the orthopedic sports medicine specialist must be very thorough and competent to ensure an accurate physical diagnosis in these cases. This specific area is one that must receive greater attention in the future as the subspecialty of veterinary orthopedic sports medicine continues to develop. These enhanced skills must come as a combination of improvement in both physical diagnosis and instrumented techniques, some of which are described below.

To diagnose and prescribe the most appropriate therapy for sports-induced injuries, the sports medicine specialist should first answer three specific questions.[2] (1) Accurate definition of the injury must be established, that is, the knowledge and understanding of how different tissues react to different injuries is essential. (2) The seriousness of the injury must be made. Methods to assess soft tissue injuries objectively continue to be limited, and determining the seriousness of the injury remains a clinical dilemma in many cases. (3) One must determine the relationship between the cause of the injury and its effect. Understanding this relationship further helps define the injury itself and may provide insight on how to prevent future re-injuries. With these three questions answered, the most ideal treatment then can be administered. Such treatment should include positively influencing the process of inflammation and repair and expediting recovery of function; minimizing the early negative effects of excessive inflammation such as pain, edema, and loss of function; returning the athlete to the pre-injury level of activity; and preventing or at least minimizing the recurrence of the injury by positively influencing the structural integrity of the injured tissue to resist future biomechanical overloads[7, 8]; that is, the goal and philosophy in the treatment of sports-induced inflammation and injury are the same as for all wound care, specifically to assist the natural processes of the body while doing no harm.

A number of both clinical and basic science studies would be useful to enhance our overall understanding of the pathophysiology of sports-induced inflammation and to better understand the ramification of overuse injuries. These studies might provide more information of the interaction of training and conditioning programs and how they can best prevent or overcome sports-induced injuries and inflammation. A clinical study to determine the probability of injury in a given population of athletes performing a specific sport would be useful to aid in prevention and early intervention and also to help reduce the risk and impact of sports-induced injuries. It would also be useful to identify the various physiological responses to different exercise protocols that would be used in training programs so that orthopedic sports medicine specialists could better recommend specific training regimens that might also help minimize injuries. Studies are also needed to identify and refine various chemical markers that would help to characterize various injuries, especially those related to the chronic aspects of overtraining and overuse syndromes. It is anticipated that ongoing studies will further define the value of markers in synovial fluid and serum to signify both inflammation and articular cartilage degradation following injury. For example, serum hyaluronate levels can serve as an indicator of soft tissue inflammation in rheumatoid arthritis. At present, it is difficult to predict an exact state of inflammation or degradation from a single sample, but as more monoclonal antibodies against specific components are developed, we believe that markers will provide an accurate reflection of the state of disease deep within the tissues. Since the immune system may play an important role in inflammation and overuse injuries, it would be very useful to conduct a clinical study to measure circulating immunological mediators and then correlate these factors with the local immune environment in which the inflammation and healing occur. Such a study might lend itself to determination of the appropriate recovery period between exercise events based on the presence or absence of these circulating immunological mediators.

A number of basic science studies might also be performed to provide more information on how training influences musculoskeletal tissues and their inflammatory response to injury. One area in particular would be to identify the effects of inflammation on ligaments in both acute and chronic sports-induced inflammation. There are a number of biochemical and biomechanical determinations that should be made to answer these questions. There is also a need for more thorough understanding of the effects of nonsteroidal anti-inflammatory drugs (NSAIDs) on the healing of musculoskeletal tissues following injury and inflammation. The relatively recent identification that NSAIDs can be divided into two groups that (1) inhibit normal physiological prostaglandin production (Cox-1 inhibitors) and (2) inhibit abnormal or inflammatory production of prostaglandin (Cox-2) offers exciting possibilities in terms of therapeutic modulation of inflammation without adverse side effects on the gastrointestinal tract and kidneys. Major efforts continue to identify the perfect chondroprotective agent. We still do not have an ideal drug that inhibits all deleterious processes associated with trauma but prevents articular cartilage damage in the joint. Extensive work has already been done in the horse to identify differential therapeutic values of corticosteroids as well as the therapeutic effects of intra-articular or intravenous hyaluronan and intramuscular glycosaminoglycan. Scientific validation of the beneficial effects of oral glycosaminoglycan still needs to be done. Finally, the development of gene sequences for interleukin-1 receptor antagonists as well as metalloproteinase inhibitors such as tissue inhibitor of metalloproteinase (TIMP) also offer exciting therapeutic alternatives and the possibility of modulation of disease by gene therapy. Another broad basic science area that should be studied is determination of the role of repetitive microtrauma in training-induced injuries and sports-induced inflammation. At present, we are unaware of any good research models to study the cumulative effect of microtrauma and overuse injuries. Finally, it is important to determine the effect of increased loads on tendons so that we may have better understanding of the specific adaptation of tendon as a structure and to enhance our knowledge of how mature collagenous structures respond to increased loading states. This knowledge would help develop training programs that would increase the threshold and baseline of tissue strength while simultaneously preventing or lessening the chance of failure under high tissue loads that occur doing athletic activities.

IMAGING TECHNIQUES

Over the past several years, improvements in radiographic equipment, techniques, and special contrast studies have significantly enhanced the practitioner's ability to assess the anatomical structures associated with the musculoskeletal system. In the more recent past, the advent of magnetic resonance (MR) imaging has provided an entire new dimension for imaging. MR has been especially useful in the practice of human medicine because of its capability to image soft tissues with a high degree of resolution. While other modalities such as ultrasound and scintigraphy have proven useful for specific purposes, it is MR that has the most utility and capabilities.

The technology associated with MR has expanded greatly, and it continues to evolve at a rapid pace. The result has been ever increasing diagnostic capability in human medicine because of this one tool. As the technology continues to improve, the cost of MR continues to drop. As a consequence, MR imaging is becoming much more accessible for veterinary use. We believe that in the near future MR will become a much more commonly used diagnostic imaging tool in comparative orthopedic sports medicine, especially for those patients that are the elite athletes. However, until MR is fully accessible for veterinary use, ultrasound and scintigraphy remain useful and necessary for specialized imaging.

It is also interesting to note that MR now has greater potential for monitoring physiological changes as well as anatomical ones. The newer technology for the MR units include physiological data acquisition components. As a result, new bioassays and nondestructive tissue tests can be done to further understand the cellular processes that are ongoing in any given condition. Coupled with magnetic resonance spectroscopy, the enhanced MR techniques should contribute to the overall information that will be integrated into the training and rehabilitation of patients with sports-induced inflammation and injuries.

Finally, a significant recent adjunct to MR permits real-time imaging of extremities. That is, a limb can be taken through a range of motion and imaged simultaneously in a manner similar to the way fluoroscopy is used at present. This real-time MR imaging will provide the ability for true assessment of mechanical function of the limbs.

ARTHROSCOPY AND SURGICAL TECHNIQUES

The advent of the arthroscope clearly has provided significant advances in surgical techniques in the treatment of orthopedic injuries, especially those involving articular joints. As surgeons have become more proficient with the arthroscope and performing arthroscopic procedures, the postoperative recovery period has been reduced dramatically. Instead of disabilities lasting many weeks or months following arthrotomy, a similar procedure performed arthroscopically may require that the patient be limited in activity for only a few days. The surgical instrumentation that has been developed for use in conjunction with the arthroscope has also changed dramatically in recent years. The techniques and instrumentation permit major reconstructive surgery of joints to be performed through two to four small stab incisions.

Although the arthroscope is now used extensively in equine surgery, its use in the dog has been relatively limited. The technique of canine arthroscopy (diagnostic) was first presented in 1978.[9, 10] Techniques for arthroscopy of the shoulder, hip, tarsus, stifle, and elbow have been described.[11–14] Most of these discussions have been limited to diagnostic arthroscopy, but arthroscopic surgery for the treatment of osteochondritis dissecans of the shoulder has been reported in the literature,[15] and McIlwraith has operated on one patient. Canine arthroscopy has been the subject of a seminar in the United States,[16] and a course has been given in Europe.[17] The principles of arthroscopic surgery are the same as have been well documented in the horse. Special problems of note in the dog

include difficulties associated with working in a small joint as well as the fine balance between sufficient distention of the joint for visualization and excessive fluid pressure causing extravasation of fluid (with consequent closure of the visible joint space). The recent trend in human medicine for development of small arthroscopes and instruments for working in the smaller joints has helped the development of techniques in the dog. An arthroscope with an angled field of view was critical, and the wide-angled lenses now available permit excellent visualization of the entire joint without the need for extreme joint motion or repositioning.

We believe that the technology will continue to permit further miniaturization of both the arthroscope itself and the surgical instrumentation. As these changes occur, arthroscopic procedures will become much more commonplace for the canine sports medicine specialist. Just as has occurred with human athletes, animal athletes then will be able to undergo surgical procedures with minimal morbidity, and their return to full activity will be accelerated far beyond what might be imagined at present.

TISSUE REPAIR, REGENERATION, AND ENGINEERING

Tissue repair involves replacement of damaged or lost cells and the accompanying extracellular matrix with new cells and matrices.[18] Tissue regeneration, on the other hand, is a form of repair that results in new tissue that is essentially structurally and functionally identical to normal tissue.[18] Clearly, tissue repair is a much less complicated and far less valuable process than is tissue regeneration. Unfortunately, most higher mammals lack the ability truly to regenerate lost or damaged tissue. Fortunately, new methods and techniques are under development through a discipline referred to as tissue engineering that will permit the eventual regeneration of many musculoskeletal tissues.[18, 19]

Tissue engineering, a relatively new discipline, has provided fundamental understanding and technology that has permitted development of structures derived from biological tissues. One such product of tissue engineering is reconstituted bioresorbable collagen structures.[20, 21] These materials have many positive features for use in supporting tissue regeneration to include a variable rate of resorption controlled by the degree of cross-linking, the immune response can be minimized through enzymatic treatment of the collagen, and the extremely complex biochemical composition of various joint tissues can be closely approximated in the reconstituted structure. Rodkey and Steadman have taken this approach as a concept that might be exploited to provide a possible solution to support the regrowth and regeneration of the irreparably damaged meniscus cartilage of the knee.[21–23] This same technology for collagen-based bioresorbable materials has also been used successfully for the production of nerve conduits and skin replacements.[20]

The definition of tissue engineering continues to evolve as more is learned about this new discipline. However, the definition that we have found most practical is "the application of principles and methods of engineering and life sciences toward the fundamental understanding of structure-function relationships in normal and pathological mammalian tissues and the development of biological substitutes to restore, maintain, or improve tissue functions."[18, 19] We believe that this evolving technology will eventually permit the successful regeneration of various musculoskeletal tissues to include the meniscus cartilage, articular cartilage, and intra-articular ligaments. As the level of success continues to improve, this technology will provide the orthopedic sports medicine specialist a powerful new tool to treat many injuries that in the past have been career-ending for their patient athletes.

BIOCHEMICAL MODULATORS OF HEALING

During the past 20 years, an explosion of new knowledge has occurred in the fields of molecular and cellular biology. Application of this new knowledge to studies of tissue organization is having a major impact on our understanding of the molecular and cellular processes that interact to produce living tissues. Furthermore, from this new basic knowledge we have learned a great deal more about how tissues heal, and we have gained new understanding of the extremely complex interaction of various biochemical modulators of healing.[7] Some of these most important biochemical factors of healing include the cytokines, basic fibroblast growth factor (bFGF), transforming growth factor–beta (TGF-β), insulin-like growth factor–1 (IGF-1), and interleukin-1 (IL-1). All of these factors stimulate many different cell activities that are consistent with a central role in the control of cell application and tissue turnover.[7] For example, in healthy resting articular cartilage, the in vitro effects of the locally produced cytokine growth factors suggest a possible function in maintaining normal matrix turnover.[24] Furthermore, both bFGF and IGF-1 stimulate proliferation and proteoglycan synthesis in cartilage cell cultures. TGF-β, however, appears to have a variable effect on cartilage metabolism with both growth and stimulatory as well as inhibitory influences having been reported. It is also noteworthy that articular cartilage is responsive to various cytokine growth factors produced by other cell types.[24]

McIlwraith and Steadman have taken advantage of this understanding of how these biochemical modulators influence healing of articular cartilage defects in both equine and human athletes.[25, 26] By making small puncture holes through the underlying subchondral bone plate, access is gained to a source of mesenchymal stem cells as well as these various biochemical compounds that influence the development and turnover of the cells.[26] This example is but one of many situations in which tissue repair and regeneration can be influenced by these modulators of healing.

While at present it is necessary to rely upon the naturally occurring endogenous factors, we believe that in the future orthopedic sports medicine surgeons will have the ability to supply exogenously produced factors to influence the healing processes positively; that is, these biochemical modulators of healing may actually speed the healing process and may further encourage tissues to heal by regeneration rather than by a fibrotic response. As a result, the orthopedic sports medicine specialist will be able to reduce significantly the morbidity and rehabilitation time following injuries and surgical procedures and return the patient athlete back to the pre-injury level of performance at a much accelerated pace.

COMPUTER TECHNOLOGY

New uses for emerging computer technological advancements are also being described and placed into practical application almost as quickly as the technology can be developed. Two such practical applications that we believe will be of great benefit to the orthopedic sports medicine specialist are in the areas of computer modeling of both normal and abnormal musculoskeletal structures and in the area of surgical planning and decision making. Other important pertinent uses of computer technology for sports medicine include data acquisition, telemedicine, patient database management, and "virtual" surgery.

Data acquisition, an important computer capability, has been used extensively by musculoskeletal research scientists to quantify tissue properties, muscle activity, motion, forces, accelerations, and metabolic responses for various activities and patient populations. Results of such studies have profoundly affected surgical techniques, athletic performance, and rehabilitation and training.

The computer is vital to modeling, one important area of ortho-

pedic research. Mathematical models have been developed to estimate the roles of static and dynamic structures as well as forces and strains on internal structures during specific athletic activities. Modeling has improved the design of prosthetic devices as well as surgical instrumentation. With more research, interfaces for modeling anatomy will be simplified for both input and for the end-user. Computer modeling coupled with improved MR techniques has greatly enhanced the ability for finite element analyses (FEA). As this technology becomes more accessible, the increased use of FEA should be helpful to understand better the role of tissue subjected to complex biomechanical loads such as the meniscal cartilage of the knees. In addition to providing better understanding for normal tissue, FEA might also provide insight into the cause and effects of disease processes, such as the osteoarthritic changes that occur in many athletes due to the cumulative effect of microtrauma and macrotrauma.

We believe that in the near future we will witness increased use of telemedicine, virtual surgery, and on-line patient information and profiles that will provide immediate laboratory results and imaging data to the orthopedic sports medicine specialist. Telemedicine may provide medical care and expertise in more remote locations where such services were not previously available. Virtual surgery will be used to help train surgeons in techniques and instrumentation. In the near future this type of training will require only a simple computer and a modem to connect to a central teaching facility. We believe that the many present uses of the computer will be increased and greatly facilitated as this technology continues to develop.

CONCLUSIONS

In summary, we believe that the horizon is very bright for comparative orthopedic sports medicine. While we have attempted to focus on a selected number of areas that we believe may hold the greatest significance, we emphasize that by no means is this list complete. The information presented is very dynamic, and of all the chapters in this textbook, this one is the most likely to become obsolete. Although our crystal ball remains hazy, clearly we are very excited about the future.

References

1. Teitz CC: Scientific Foundations of Sports Medicine. Philadelphia, BC Decker, 1989.
2. Leadbetter WB, Buckwalter JA, Gordon SL: Sports-Induced Inflammation: Clinical and Basic Science Concepts. Park Ridge, Ill, American Academy of Orthopaedic Surgeons, 1990.
3. Kellert J: Acute soft tissue injuries—A review of the literature. Med Sci Sports Exerc 18:489–500, 1986.
4. Herring SA, Nilson KL: Introduction to overuse injuries. Clin Sports Med 6:225–239, 1987.
5. Woo SL-Y, Buckwalter JA: Injury and Repair of the Musculoskeletal Soft Tissues. Park Ridge, Ill, American Academy of Orthopaedic Surgeons, 1988.
6. Slocum DB, James SL: Biomechanics of running. JAMA 205:721–728, 1968.
7. Clark RAF, Henson PM: The Molecular and Cellular Biology of Wound Repair. New York, Plenum Press, 1988.
8. van der Meulen JC: Present state of knowledge on processes of healing in collagen structures. Int J Sports Med 3(suppl 1):4–8, 1982.
9. Knezevic PF, Wruhs O: Arthroscopy of the horse, ox, pig and dog. Vet Med Rev 1:53–63, 1977.
10. Siemering GH: Arthroscopy of dogs. JAVMA 172:575–577, 1978.
11. Van Ryssen B, van Bree H, Simoens P: Elbow arthroscopy in clinically normal dogs. Am J Vet Res 54:191–198, 1993.
12. Miller CW, Presnell KR: Examination of the canine stifle: Arthroscopy versus arthrotomy. J Am Anim Hosp Assoc 21:623–629, 1985.

13. Person MW: Arthroscopy of the canine shoulder joint. Compend Contin Educ Pract Vet 8:537–546, 1986.
14. Person MW: Arthroscopy of the canine coxofemoral joint. Compend Contin Educ Pract Vet 11:930–935, 1989.
15. Person MW: Arthroscopic treatment of osteochondritis dissecans of the canine shoulder. Vet Surg 18:175–189, 1989.
16. Taylor RA (ed): Proc First National Canine Arthroscopy Seminar, Colorado State University, May 21, 1994.
17. European College of Veterinary Surgeons Course in Canine Arthroscopy, Tutlingen, Germany, June 1995.
18. Skalak R, Fox CF: Tissue Engineering. New York, Alan R Liss, 1988.
19. Heineken FG, Skalak R: Tissue engineering: A brief overview. J Biomech Eng 113:111–112, 1991.
20. Yannas IV: Regeneration of skin and nerve by use of collagen templates. In Nimni ME (ed): Collagen: Biotechnology vol 3. Boca Raton, Fla, CRC Press, 1988, pp 87–115.
21. Stone KR, Rodkey WG, Webber RJ, et al: Future directions: Collagen based prosthesis for meniscal regeneration. Clin Orthop 252:129–135, 1990.
22. Stone KR, Rodkey WG, Webber RJ, et al: Meniscal regeneration with copolymeric collagen scaffolds: In vitro and in vivo studies evaluated clinically, histologically, and biochemically. Am J Sports Med 20:104–111, 1992.
23. Rodkey WG, Stone KR, Steadman JR: Replacement of the irreparably injured meniscus. Sports Med Arthrosc Rev 1:168–176, 1993.
24. Rodrigo JJ, Steadman JR, Syftestad G, et al: Effects of human knee synovial fluid on chondrogenesis in vitro. Am J Knee Surg 8:124–129, 1995.
25. Vachon AM, McIlwraith CW, Powers BE: Morphologic and biochemical study of sternal cartilage autografts for resurfacing induced osteochondral defects in horses. Am J Vet Res 53:1038–1047, 1992.
26. Rodrigo JJ, Steadman JR, Silliman JF, Fulstone AH: Improvement of full thickness chondral defect healing in the human knee after debridement and microfracture using continuous passive motion. Am J Knee Surg 7:109–116, 1994.

CHAPTER 54

RACING GREYHOUND ADOPTION PROGRAMS

LARRY G. DEE

In the past 10 years there has been a dramatic increase in the number of racing greyhounds placed as pets. Although the principal effort has come from greyhound-loving volunteers in the public sector, significant strides have been made by the greyhound racing industry and the veterinary profession. The public perception of the greyhound as an athlete that is too high strung to be a companion animal has changed to a more realistic one—that the greyhound, while having the unique personality of a sight hound, is a warm, loving companion that can be placed in most homes. In addition, the dissemination of knowledge to the veterinary community about greyhound medicine and surgery has increased the level of their care as pets.

INDUSTRY SUPPORT

As more volunteer groups have developed nationwide and internationally, the greyhound racing industry has responded with important support. The American Greyhound Council (AGC), a nonprofit corporation funded jointly by the American Greyhound Track Operators Association (AGTOA) and the National Greyhound Association (NGA) was formed in 1987 to provide for the welfare of racing greyhounds and the betterment of the greyhound racing industry. The AGC accepts and reviews proposals from individuals and organizations requesting funding for research and other activities that meet the goals of the council. The AGC has supported greyhound placement in several ways.

The AGC joined with the American Society for the Prevention of Cruelty to Animals (ASPCA) to increase the number of retired greyhounds that are adopted as pets by establishing the Greyhound Adoption Fund (GAF) and by promoting greyhounds as pets. The GAF is funded by the AGC and administered by the ASPCA. Following an initial grant of $100,000, the AGC continues to be the primary supporter of the GAF, with annual grants supplementing the initial funding. Following criteria developed jointly by the ASPCA and the AGC, grant applications are reviewed and approved solely by the ASPCA. The GAF is a financial resource for greyhound adoption agencies. Monies are available for two specific purposes—emergency funding (for example, for food or veterinary care) and funding for limited capital improvements but not for general operating expenses.

The AGC funds a toll-free number to assist the Greyhound Pets of America (GPA) in finding homes for retired racers. GPA is a national nonprofit volunteer organization that has chapters throughout the country working to place retired greyhounds. Calls to their toll-free number (1-800-366-1472) will direct the caller to their closest local chapter or to the closest greyhound adoption organization. In 1993, more than 42,000 calls were received.

An electronic bulletin board has been established by the AGC in the office of the NGA to assist in placing, caring for, and transporting retired greyhounds. This database service lists greyhound pet organizations, racetracks, haulers, greyhounds available for adoption, and adoption groups in need of greyhounds. The database can be contacted at 913-263-2266(BBS), 913-263-4684(Voice), or NGA@Access-one.com.

The AGC has developed two videos promoting greyhounds as pets—one to be shown at racetracks, the other an instructional video for prospective greyhound pet owners to learn more about their new pet.

The AGC has funded investigations to evaluate and to train

greyhounds through the Canine Working Companions program as animal aids for the hearing impaired or physically disabled.

The AGC provides annual grants of up to $1000 to greyhound adoption groups working with individual tracks. The AGC has supported the International Greyhound Sports Symposium for many years to increase and disseminate information about the breed. In addition, most greyhound tracks have active greyhound adoption programs at the local level.

VOLUNTEER SUPPORT

Although a tremendous amount of financial and organizational support comes from the greyhound industry, the backbone of greyhound adoptions is composed of the hundreds of volunteers who have committed themselves to assisting greyhounds. Two national networks refer inquiries about greyhound adoption to organizations based on the location of the inquirer. They are Greyhound Pets of America (1-800-366-1472) and National Greyhound Adoption Network (1-800-446-8637). The following can be contacted on the Internet:

Adopt a Greyhound Page on the World Wide Web at http://pasture.ecn.purdue.edu/~laird/Dogs/Greyhound
A Breed Apart an on-line magazine dedicated to greyhound adoption at http://www.pcix.com/abap/index.html
The *National Greyhound Adoption Program* at http://www2.pcix.com/~moser/ngap.html

These groups can be contacted by anyone interested in adopting a greyhound, finding a home for a greyhound, or volunteering to help place greyhounds.

Most greyhound adoption groups have an adoption application or agreement that they use to screen potential greyhound owners. Many require a fenced yard, an agreement to neuter, veterinary references, and the like. Some do not permit adoption if young children, cats, or stairs are in the home. Some require visual inspection of the home. Most adoption groups will provide health care and husbandry instructions, inoculations, and a preplacement veterinary examination. Others may also provide neutering services, heart-worm examinations, and dentistry before adoption. Ideally, a greyhound should be checked for occult heartworms, babesiosis, and ehrlichiosis, and intestinal and ectoparasites before adoption. Some groups cannot afford the capital or volunteer time to neuter, to provide dental prophylaxis, or to test for babesiosis or ehrlichiosis and must request or require the new owner to provide these services.

Adoption groups that have enough volunteers to provide a fostering service can significantly ease the transition from the track to the home. Fostering groups introduce and accustom greyhounds to many routine household distractions—stairs, television, furniture, children, and other dogs as well as cats. The alpha behavior and pack behavior of a greyhound can affect its integration into a household and should be evaluated before adoption. The amount of "prey drive" of a candidate will determine if a cat will be safe around that individual greyhound. House training, crate training,

and separation anxiety are all topics that should be addressed when adopting a greyhound. Anyone adopting a greyhound for the first time should have access to a local support group or hot line for advice in the event of a problem.

Most adoption groups charge between $50 and $200 for an adoption, depending on what services are provided by the agency before the pet is placed in the home.

VETERINARY SUPPORT

Veterinarians who examine greyhounds for adoption should:

Be knowledgeable about routine injuries of racing greyhounds and their prognosis in order to evaluate their individual potential as a pet.
Verify or provide basic vaccinations.
Perform an occult heartworm test as well as testing for babesiosis and ehrlichiosis if funds will permit.
Perform routine deworming, including whipworms.
Be able to perform anesthesia in a safe and predictable manner.
Be knowledgable and be available to discuss the idiosyncrasies of the breed.

Other sources of information about greyhound adoption and greyhounds as pets are the following:

The Greyhound Project, Inc., a volunteer, nonprofit organization dedicated to promoting the welfare of racing and retired greyhounds. It seeks to identify and circulate nationally information about greyhound adoption facilities and organizations and coordinate efforts to increase the number of greyhounds adopted. The Greyhound Project, Inc., is not affiliated with any greyhound adoption agency but provides *The Directory of Greyhound Adoption Resources,* which is updated annually, and the newsletter, *Speaking of Greyhounds,* which is published bimonthly. The Greyhound Project, Inc., may be contacted at 261 Robbins St, Milton, MA 02186, or at 617-333-4982, 617-527-8843.
Adopting the Racing Greyhound, by Cynthia Branigan, Macmillan Publishing Co, 1992. This text reviews selection of a greyhound as a pet, feeding, grooming, preparing the home, etc.
Veterinary Advice for Greyhound Owners, edited by J. Kohnke, 1993. Published by Ringpress. Written by veterinary researchers at Oregon State University.
Greyhound Club of America Newsletter, edited by Dani Edgerton, 7115 Wesdt Calla Road, Canfield, OH 44406; (330) 533-6576. This newsletter deals mostly with show greyhounds and their breeders.
The Greyhound Gazette, published by the CSRA Greyhound Adoption, 415 Brookside Dr., Augusta, GA 30904-4597; (706) 736-6335.
Greyhounds Today, Jeanette Steiner, editor/publisher, 936 Cornwall Avenue, Waterloo, IA 50702; (319) 235-9161.
Off Track Greyhound, newsletter published by Greyhound Pets of America/California, P.O. Box 2433, La Mesa, CA 91943-2433. No subscription; send donation.

CHAPTER 55

BANDAGES AND SPLINTS

MARK S. BLOOMBERG† \ ROBERT A. TAYLOR

Bandaging wounds and applying splints are common in animal care, and few things done as commonly have the potential for doing more harm than good. The art of bandaging requires scientific knowledge of normal anatomy and the temporal events associated with wound healing. What was a minor skin abrasion can be converted into a limb- or life-threatening problem for the animal, owner, and veterinarian. Animals poorly communicate their concerns regarding a painful bandage, and owners and inexperienced veterinary personnel may discount excessive licking or chewing at a bandage or splint as a behavioral problem instead of a manifestation of pain.

The purposes of the application of bandages, casts, or splints are to:

Protect wounds from bacterial environmental bacteria
Protect the wound from wound exudate and blood
Provide wound treatment and debridement
Serve as a vehicle for antibiotics and antiseptics
Immobilize a wound and support the limb
Provide compression to control and minimize hemorrhage and tissue swelling
Discourage licking and grooming
Secure splints or cast
Hold wound dressings in place
Serve as an indicator of wound secretions and to absorb wound drainage
Modulate wound contraction and speed epithelization
Keep a wound open to allow for adequate debridement and subsequent delayed closure

Proper bandaging requires melding scientific knowledge and artful application of the material. Establishing and utilizing certain principles will help minimize problems and provide standardization of care.

One should be aware of the anatomical structures of the body part to be bandaged. It is possible to damage the peroneal nerve or radial nerve with improperly applied bandages. Awareness of their location and appropriate padding can prevent this. The body part to be bandaged should be clean and free of coagulated blood and tissue debris. Any foreign material such as grass, dirt, and hair is best removed prior to bandaging.

There should be a purpose for the bandage and a goal for what is to be accomplished; given the risk associated with bandaging it is important to determine if it is necessary. The type of bandage needed may change as the wound heals—for example, with a contaminated open wound a wet-to-wet bandage may be indicated for the first 5 to 7 days and then as the wound matures a nonadherent semiocclusive bandage may be appropriate.

It is crucial to bandage the limb or body part in a functional and anatomical position. This ensures a well-fitted bandage without the

likelihood of the bandage material kinking or wrinkling and producing pressure sores, and it is comfortable for the animal as well. When possible, anatomical bandaging is best accomplished while the animal is still anesthetized following surgery or with the use of short-acting chemical restraining agents.

The bandage should be removed immediately at the first sign of animal discomfort; excessive biting and chewing are the animal's way of displaying its discomfort. It is usually not advisable to "wait until the next morning" but to address these problems as they occur (Fig. 55–1). Wet or soiled bandages must be immediately removed. It is helpful to instruct the owner in the care of the bandage and show how to keep it clean and dry. Plastic bags, socks, plastic wrapping used for newspaper, or other material can be used to keep the bandage dry. The use of adhesive tape to animal skin should be minimized; if subsequently it needs to be removed, tape solvent will facilitate its removal. Tape stirrups or double pieces of adhesive tape can be used to keep bandages secure.

The bandage or splint should be matched to the injury. A support wrap with a lateral splint made of casting material is not suited as a primary means of fracture immobilization. When the limbs are being bandaged, the bandage should be placed distally to and

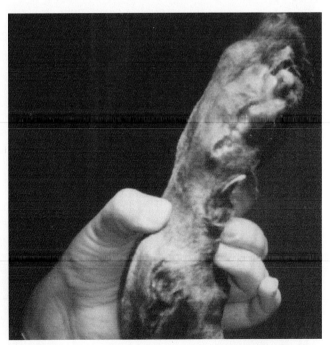

FIGURE 55–1. Gangrene is present in this leg and was the result of a tight bandage that was allowed to become soiled. The owner waited for 5 days before returning to have the soiled and partially chewed bandage removed.

†Deceased.

449

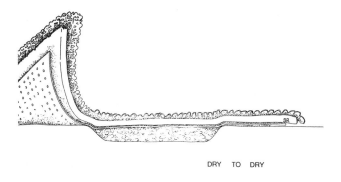

DRY TO DRY

FIGURE 55–2. An adherent bandage is used for mechanical debridement.

include the toes; merely placing a bandage over the carpus or tarsus should be avoided because there will be significant swelling distal to the bandage. As a general rule, one finger should be able to fit beneath a bandage at its proximal and distal end. This is a convenient way to make sure that it is not too tight. Bandage pads on bony protuberances should be placed around, not over them, effectively avoiding pressure necrosis beneath a bandage.

The owner is provided with specific written instructions regarding the care of the bandage, making him or her aware of the need to keep it clean and dry. A recheck office visit is scheduled for 1 week or sooner. A person who has never worn a bandage should have a colleague apply one to his or her arm and wear it for several hours to experience how it feels. The experience will help acquire some of the technique needed for proper bandaging.

Components of a Bandage. There are three layers to most bandages: the primary or contact layer, the secondary layer (which serves to absorb wound fluids and provide support and immobilization), and the tertiary layer (which protects and supports the previous layers).

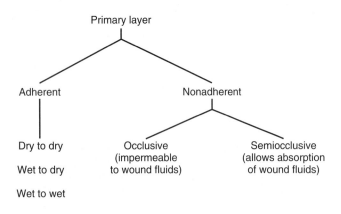

Adherent bandages are indicated when there is significant contamination and mechanical debridement is needed. Adherent layers are referred to as dry-to-dry, wet-to-dry (Fig. 55–2), or wet-to-wet. The nomenclature refers to the condition of the adherent layer when applied to the secondary layer, for example, dry-to-dry dressings imply dry adherent layer bandage and dry secondary layer, while wet-to-dry refers to saline or water-soluble antibiotic-moistened adherent bandages placed beneath a dry secondary layer. The absorbent secondary layer absorbs the wound fluid.

A suggested bandaging algorithm for a full-thickness unsutured skin wound is shown at the top of column 2.

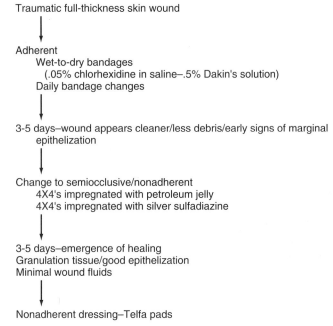

The most common adherent bandage is the wet-to-dry configuration and is commonly utilized for removal of thick exudate and loose debris requiring debridement. Wet-to-dry bandages must be changed daily or more frequently and can impede wound healing if used improperly. Sterile starch or dextranomer may be utilized with this type of bandage to absorb microorganisms, tissue breakdown products, and debris. While expensive, they have proven efficacious. Nonadherent bandages are designed to produce less damage to the wound during movement and removal since they do not adhere to the healing tissues.

Occlusive Bandages. This type of bandage is impermeable to wound fluids, and individual types of occlusive bandages vary in their permeability to gases (Fig. 55–3). Their use and development originated from the need to better treat burns and partial thickness skin injuries in man. There is good clinical and research evidence that occlusive bandages speed epithelization of partial thickness wounds. In studies of acute full thickness skin wounds of the dog, there was no difference in the healing parameters when occlusive and nonocclusive dressings were compared. In fact, wounds treated with semi-occlusive dressings had faster reepithelization and lower bacterial counts.

Occlusive bandages are useful in wounds with established granulation and may help speed epithelization and minimize contraction. The material is usually adhesive to the wound and skin margins, but even this is problematic in the dog and cat because of their hirsute nature.

Occlusive bandages may consist of foams, thin film, hydrocol-

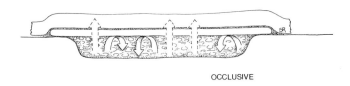

OCCLUSIVE

FIGURE 55–3. Occlusive bandages are impermeable to wound fluids and vary in their permeability to gases.

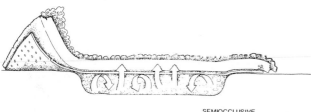

SEMIOCCLUSIVE
NONADHERENT

FIGURE 55–4. Nonadherent semi-occlusive bandages retain wound moisture but allow for some wound fluid to be absorbed.

lolds, or hydrogels. Hydrocolloid dressings have been utilized most frequently in dogs and cats to enhance wound healing. The material may be left in contact with the wound for days or even weeks, reducing the need for bandage changes as the wound matures. These materials are costly, and this should be weighed against possible advantages.

Nonadherent Semi-occlusive Bandages. Nonadherent semi-occlusive dressings allow for excessive wound fluid to move through the bandage but retain sufficient moisture for the wound (Fig. 55–4). These dressings also are less likely to disrupt healing tissue. Some nonadherent semi-occlusive dressings have a layer of absorbent material next to the nonadherent layer. This further facilitates excess tissue fluid removal. Gauze impregnated with petroleum jelly or silver sulfadiazine functions as a nonadherent semi-occlusive dressing.

Secondary Layer. This layer is added to provide a padded, absorbent layer to the bandage. The ideal material is some type of conforming cotton or synthetic fiber. The use of bulk cotton or synthetics should be avoided as they may apply unequal pressure on the extremity. The secondary layer provides a storage area to wick blood, serum tissue fluid, and necrotic debris away from the wound. The layer should have capillarity in addition to absorbent properties and be applied in sufficient layers to collect absorbed fluid and support the wound.

Tertiary Layer. This layer is composed of a gauze adhesive bandage roll or other material and is designed to hold the primary and secondary layers in place. Using elastic adhesive tapes in the tertiary layer provides pressure, conformation, and immobilization. The use of waterproof tape should be avoided as it causes excessive retention of fluid in the bandage. Whenever possible, placement of adhesive products on denuded or intact skin should be avoided.

BANDAGES

A wide variety of bandages is applicable to orthopedic surgery. These include the Velpeau sling, Robert Jones and modified Robert Jones bandages, Ehmer or "figure-of-8" sling, carpal flexion bandage, and pelvic limb sling.

Soft Padded Bandage. This type of bandage, depending upon the amount of material utilized, may also be described as a modified Robert "Bobby" Jones bandage. It is a very versatile type of dressing that can also be reinforced with a splint rod and the like to provide additional support. The basic materials utilized include tape stirrups, cast padding, roll cotton or combine roll, elastic or conforming roll gauze, and elastic tape or some type of elastic wrap. It is important to note that this type of bandage is more of a compressive wound dressing bandage than one that immobilizes joints. The degree of immobilization depends on how thick the layers of padding are and if the bandage is reinforced. Application of a soft padded bandage:

1. Tape stirrups are applied to lateral and medial or anterior and posterior aspects of the distal limb.
2. As with any limb bandage, one begins at the digits and works proximally
3. The toes of digits 3 and 4 should be partially exposed.
4. If a wound is present, proper primary covering is applied.
5. Cast padding, roll cotton, or combine roll is applied.
6. As bandage material is rolled on, it should always be applied by rolling from outward to inward so that the limb can be rotated into a varus position rather than valgus.
7. Padding is wrapped proximally to the desired level and continued back distally, overlapping half the width of material each time.
8. The number of layers of material varies with the purpose of the bandage.
9. Roll or conforming gauze is applied in a similar fashion.
10. All material should be applied with suitable tension.
11. Prominences should be padded.
12. The limb should be bandaged while held in the position desired; it should not be bandaged in an extended position and then flexed afterward.
13. Prior to final application of the elastic wrap or bandage, the stirrups are turned up and then secured.
14. Elastic tape or wrap is applied as the final layer, again from distal to proximal, overlapping by one-half the width of the material and in the same direction as other materials. It can be applied anywhere on the body. Indications for this type of bandage include wound dressing, compression of limb following injury preoperatively or postoperatively to minimize swelling of limb, and prevention of self-mutilation of limb by patient during convalescence.

Robert Jones Bandage. The Robert "Bobby" Jones bandage is a heavily padded support bandage that is utilized to support fractures or immobilize joints below the elbow and stifle (Fig. 55–5). Its objective is to apply even compression throughout the limb and immobilize it as well. It is usually applied for temporary situations preoperatively or postoperatively. Its bulk and even pressure minimize pain and swelling of the bandaged limb. It can be reinforced by application of wood or metal splints within the outer layers. The technique for applying the Bobby Jones bandage follows:

1. Exposed wounds are covered.
2. Tape stirrups (I use ether to make tape sticky) are applied.
3. Six-inch widths of roll cotton or combine roll are wrapped circumferentially up and down the limb beginning distally and working proximally, applying even tension.

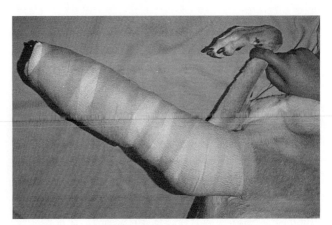

FIGURE 55–5. A properly applied Robert Jones bandage should be of anatomical shape and comfortable for the animal.

4. Extend limb so you can continue the bandage as far proximal as possible.
5. A medium-sized dog will require 2 pounds of roll cotton.
6. Elastic conforming gauze is applied circumferentially from distal to proximal and pulled as tight as possible.
7. The tape stirrups are reflected back.
8. Elastic wrap or adhesive wrap is applied the entire length of the bandage, again using tension.
9. The finished Bobby Jones bandages should be uniform in width and sound like a ripe watermelon when tapped.

Ehmer Sling. The Ehmer or figure-of-8 sling is designed to prevent weight bearing of the pelvic limb. In addition, the Ehmer sling has the advantage of providing abduction and internal rotation of the limb when properly applied. This results in maximizing acetabular coverage of the femoral head (Fig. 55–6).

The primary indications for application of the Ehmer sling are: reduction of the femoral head on the neck of fractures and acetabular fractures; after open or closed reduction of coxofemoral luxations; and prevention of weight bearing of rear limb.

The Ehmer sling is applied in the following manner:

1. Cast padding is applied to the metatarsal area.
2. The sling is applied with stifle and hock flexed.
3. 2- to 3-inch conforming gauze or tape is used.
4. The tape or gauze is wrapped in figure-of-8 fashion, starting on the medial or plantar surface of the metatarsal area, and wrapped toward the lateral surface.
5. The bandage material is brought over the lateral surface of the metatarsus, then around the inside of the thigh and behind the stifle, then over the lateral surface of the metatarsals, and up the medial side of the leg.
6. To place the limb in abduction, a band of tape is placed in bellyband fashion in the caudal lumbar area. Next, tape from the metatarsus and calcaneus is continued across the lateral aspect of the limb and over the top of the lumbar spine and held in place by the bellyband.

As with any bandage, the owner should be instructed to monitor the positioning of the bandage daily and return the animal to the veterinarian at least weekly for checks. Pressure sores can develop on the thigh just proximal to the patella and on the metatarsal area. If a bellyband is used, care must be taken to avoid the prepuce.

Carpal Flexion Bandage. The carpal flexion bandage functions to prevent weight bearing of the front leg. In addition, it flexes the carpus, thus relaxing the tendons while allowing movement of the

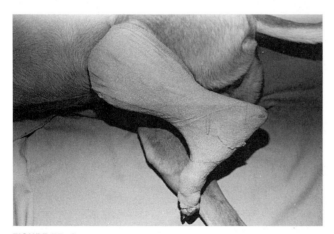

FIGURE 55–6. Ehmer slings are used to limit weight bearing of the pelvic limb. Pressure sores, tape burn, and in the male damage to the prepuce may occur.

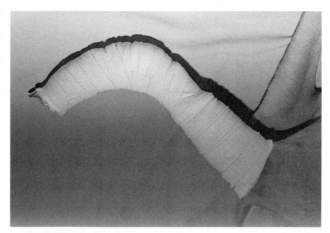

FIGURE 55–7. Flexion of the carpus has relaxed the flexor tendons.

elbow and shoulder (Fig. 55–7). This type of bandage is indicated for treatment of sprained ligaments of the carpus, for immobilization following flexor tendon repair, following reconstructive surgery of the elbow, and following reconstruction or conservative treatment of scapular fractures.

The materials needed for the carpal flexion bandage are identical to those for the Ehmer sling. The bandage is applied in the following manner:

1. The carpus is flexed to desired position and wrapped with two or three layers of cast padding or soft roll.
2. Padding is carried from the toes to midshaft of radius and ulna.
3. Conforming gauze is applied over the padding.
4. An outer layer of elastic or adhesive tape is applied over the gauze.
5. One-inch adhesive tape is then applied in a figure-of-8 fashion, spanning the flexed limb

The major complication arises when the carpus is bandaged in an extended position and then flexed to apply the adhesive tape. This can result in a tourniquet effect of the distal limb.

Velpeau Sling. The Velpeau bandage is used to prevent weight bearing of the front limb. It utilizes the same materials as the Ehmer sling. The velpeau sling is indicated (Fig. 55–8) in scapula fractures not requiring surgical repair, postoperative splinting of scapula fractures and shoulder luxation, following closed reduction of shoulder luxations (this is for medial luxation of the humeral head, which is contraindicated when the humeral head is luxated laterally).

The Velpeau sling is applied as follows:

1. The elbow is flexed.
2. The carpus is partially flexed and drawn upward across the ventral thorax to touch the opposite shoulder.
3. With the limb in this position, it is wrapped next to the body with wide, conforming gauze.
4. The wrap is crossed proximal to the carpus and posterior to the digits to keep the patient from stepping out of the bandage.
5. The gauze encircles the thorax, passing alternately from in front and behind the opposite thoracic limb.
6. Elastic tape or wrap is placed over the gauze.

A modification of this procedure involves placing a soft roll wrap over the distal limb prior to securing the limb to the chest. The paw may be left exposed to monitor for swelling, and the like, or be completely covered by the bandage. In the case of lateral shoulder luxation the Velpeau sling can be modified into a shoulder sling that allows immobilization of the shoulder, but the carpus

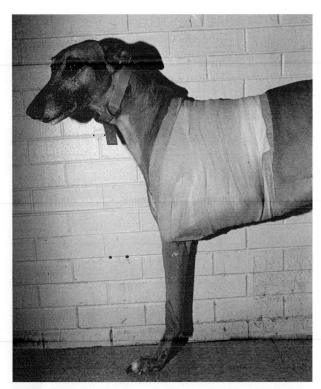

FIGURE 55–8. Velpeau slings are used to prevent weight bearing of the front leg.

extends out the front of the bandage perpendicular to the radius and ulna. A further modification involves application of the bandage materials to the shoulder area in a similar fashion, but allowing the elbow and remaining forearm to extend out of the bandage.

Pelvic Limb Sling. The pelvic limb or Robinson sling prevents weight bearing of the pelvic limb but allows flexion and extension of the hip, stifle, and hock (Fig. 55–9), the primary indication following surgery of the pelvis, hip, stifle, or femur when weight bearing is undesirable. Application of the pelvic limb sling is as follows:

1. A circular bellyband of 2-inch tape is applied around the lower abdomen; in the male the bellyband is applied to the caudal thorax.
2. A 10-foot strip of 3-inch adhesive tape is doubled on itself with the adhesive surfaces together.
3. The animal is placed in lateral recumbency.
4. The strip of tape is passed around the plantar surface of the metatarsus.
5. The limb is placed in slight flexion.
6. The two ends of the tape are passed, one on each side of the limb.
7. The free ends of tape are passed over the dorsal aspect of the bellyband.
8. The two arms of the sling are taped together at the metatarsus and midshaft of the tibia.
9. The ends of the tape sling are secured to the bellyband with adhesive tape.

EXTERNAL COAPTATION SPLINTS

Coaptation splints are supports that are applied in proximity to the limb to immobilize soft tissues, joints, or bones. They can be divided into metal shoe or spoon, Schroeder-Thomas (S-T), lateral, phalangeal, splint, and modified spica splints. The types of casts that are commonly used are full-cylinder long-leg and short casts and half casts.

The application of external coaptation must be based on knowledge of sound orthopedic principles. When utilized for immobilization of fractures, coaptation splints should be reserved for those fractures that fall into the following categories: (1) fractures below the elbow and stifle, (2) closed, minimally displaced fractures, (3) highly comminuted minimally displaced fractures. Spica splints and S-T splints can be used to immobilize fractures of the femur and humerus, but only temporarily while more definitive repair is awaited. Numerous forces acting upon a fracture include angular or bending, torsional or rotational, compressive, and tension or distractive. It is important to remember that coaptation devices, when properly applied, can neutralize angular or bending forces and, to a lesser extent, rotational forces, but they do not do an effective job of neutralizing compressive and tension forces. The veterinarian *must* know the limitations of coaptation devices.

Spoon Splint. The spoon splint is commonly referred to as the Mason metasplint. It is usually made of aluminum, but various materials, including plastic, are available. The splint may be obtained with a foam padding on the contact surface, or this padding can be added at application. Application of a spoon splint (Fig. 55–10) is indicated in (1) fracture/luxation of metacarpus, metatarsus, and digits; (2) fractures of carpus and tarsus; (3) nondisplaced fractures in the distal radius and ulna in young animals, ie, greenstick fractures; (4) solitary fractures of the radius or ulna. *A spoon splint should not be used in hyperextension injuries of the carpus.*

To apply the spoon splint:

1. Tape stirrups to the caudal aspect of the limb.
2. Prominences of the limb are padded, especially the metacarpal pad and accessory carpal bone.
3. Soft padded bandage is applied to the limb.
4. The thickness of the padded bandage should be adjusted so the limb fits snugly into the splint.
5. Once the limb is placed in the splint, the tape stirrup is twisted and pulled up along the posterior aspect of the splint so it sticks to the splint surface.
6. The limb is secured to the splint with encircling conforming gauze.

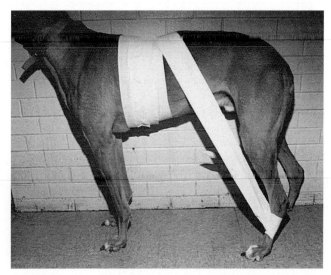

FIGURE 55–9. The pelvic limb sling allows for flexion-extension of the hip, stifle, and hock. (*Editor's Note*: This sling often includes a medial and lateral strip that goes behind the knee.)

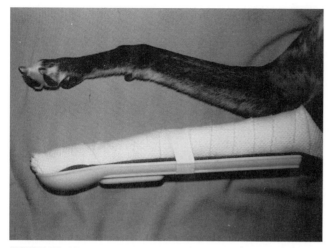

FIGURE 55–10. The spoon splint is quick and easy to apply and is best for fractures distal to the carpus and tarsus.

7. The splint must lie directly posterior on the limb.
8. The digits should be barely visible at the distal end of the splint.
9. An outer wrap of elastic or adhesive tape is then applied.

In the front limb the spoon extends from the digits as far proximally as the elbow, depending on the injury. When applied to the rear limb the splint extends just proximal to the calcaneus.

Schroeder-Thomas Splint. The Schroeder-Thomas (S-T) splint (Fig. 55–11) may be utilized to immobilize a joint or apply traction to immobilize fracture fragments. The S-T splint consists of the

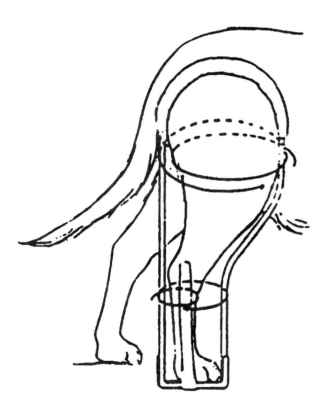

FIGURE 55–11. The Schroeder-Thomas splint can be used to apply traction for fracture immobilization. It does not work well for fractures of the humerus or femur.

combination of bandage materials and splint rods (aluminum, coat hangers, custom-made splints) fashioned to conform to the limb and particular injury. The S-T splint is indicated for (1) immobilization of the stifle and elbow joints, (2) minimally displaced fractures of the radius and ulna and tibia and fibula, (3) temporary traction immobilization of fractures of knee and tibia. *S-T splints and intramedullary pin fixation of humeral and femoral fractures* should not be combined.

The aluminum rods utilized for S-T splints come in sizes of 1/8, 3/16, and 3/8 inch. Wooden or plastic ring blocks and a vise are necessary adjuncts in shaping the splints. The aluminum rods are easily cut with a hacksaw or small pin cutter. Although premade S-T splints are available, custom-made splints are preferable.

Application of the S-T splint:

1. The patient should be heavily sedated, preferably anesthetized.
2. An assistant is needed.
3. The appropriate size splint rod is selected.
4. With rubber rings or the thumb and forefinger of each hand formed into a circle, the circumference of the axillary or inguinal area is measured.
5. The rod is bent around the appropriate sized template one and a half times.
6. The ring diameter is secured with adhesive tape and the ring then padded.
7. The ring is bent over the edge of the table to form a 30–45° angle.
8. The limb is placed in the desired position, whether for traction for a fracture or immobilization of a joint.
9. The front and back rods are bent to conform to the contour of the limb.
10. At the joint, the rods are bent around the bottom and up the other side to lie against the opposite rod (larger dogs may require extra lengths of rod taped to the original rod).
11. Once the splint is formed, the overlapping rods are secured to each other with adhesive tape.
12. Tape stirrups are applied to the foot.
13. With an assistant holding the S-T splint securely in the inguinal or axillary region, the tape stirrups are wrapped around the distal bar of the splint.
14. The distal portion of the limb is secured to the splint with 1-inch tape. At the metatarsal area the tape encircles the posterior rod and anterior portion of the limb; at the tarsal area it encircles both bars as it stabilizes the tarsus laterally and medially.
15. Combine roll or roll cotton is used next to provide the necessary traction in addition to medial and lateral stability.
16. The strip of combine roll is started on the side of the splint that is in the direction of the desired pull.
17. Usually two pieces of combine roll are applied with one placed around the distal limb (tibia) and one around the proximal limb (femur).
18. The strip should then pass medial to the limb and up between the limb and opposite rod.
19. The strip goes back around the first rod, and again medially up between the limb and second rod.
20. Pulling on the combine roll results in the desired traction.
21. The strip of combine roll is passed around both loops and pulled snugly.
22. Remaining strips of combine roll are applied in the same fashion.
23. The splint may be covered with tape or stockinette.
24. A second aluminum or rubber stirrup can be applied to the distal limb.

Postoperative management of the S-T splint is essential to avoid complications. It must be kept clean and dry as well as checked closely for signs of loosening or pressure sores.

Lateral Splint. Indications for lateral splints are the same as for the S-T splint. The splints neutralize angular or bending forces (Fig. 55–12). The lateral splint may be long or short, depending whether it is to be used to immobilize from the elbow or stifle distally or the distal limb. It consists of a padded or modified Robert Jones bandage to which has been added a lateral reinforcing splint of cast material, wood, or metal rod.

The lateral splint is applied as follows:

1. The padded bandage is applied.
2. Splint material is placed on the lateral surface of the bandage.
3. The splint should extend from just above the digits to just below the proximal cast padding
4. If cast material is being used it can be pinched into a vertical ridge to strengthen it against bending forces.
5. The reinforcing splint material should be shaped to conform to the limb.
6. An aluminum rod can be incorporated into the cast material.
7. The cast material is allowed to dry.
8. Conforming gauze is applied to encircle the limb.
9. Tape stirrups are reflected.
10. Once the cast material is dry, the limb is encircled with adhesive or elastic wrap.

As with any coaptation device, the patient should be hospitalized for 24 hours and the splint checked for slippage, discomfort, or swollen toes.

Modified Spica Splint. The spica splint can be applied to the foreleg or rear leg. It is basically a lateral splint that is extended over the shoulder or hip (Fig. 55–13). This type of splint can be used to immobilize the elbow, shoulder, hip, and stifle. This spica does a better job of neutralizing rotational and bending forces than other splints. A spica splint is indicated as an adjunct to internal fixation of femur, humerus, tibia and fibula, and radius and ulna; and for temporary immobilization of forelimb and rear limb.

Application of the spica splint:

1. The principles for applying a spica splint are the same as for the lateral splint.
2. At midshaft of humerus or femur, the padding is continued up over the shoulder.
3. Six to eight layers of cast padding are applied.
4. Lengths of cast material are measured from the toes to just beyond the dorsal midline.

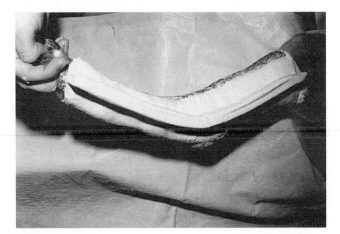

FIGURE 55–12. Lateral splints are ideal for immobilization distal to the elbow or stifle.

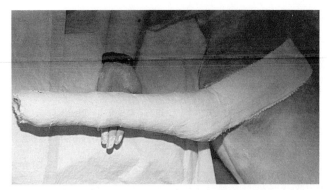

FIGURE 55–13. A spica splint can be used to augment immobilization of the femur or humerus.

5. The cast material is conformed to the lateral surface of the limb and allowed to dry.
6. The lateral splint is then secured to the limb and trunk of the body with conforming gauze.
7. Adhesive or elastic wrap is taped over the limb and trunk.

When the splint is properly applied, elevation of the limb should move the entire fore or hind quarter.

CASTS

The application of casts to the limb of the orthopedic patient should follow the basic principles described previously for bandages and splints. Cast application should be limited to conditions below the elbow and stifle. The types of casts that will be described include full-cylinder long-leg and short-leg casts and half-casts. Full-cylinder casts should not be applied over wounds and the wounds treated through a window in the cast. The removal of a portion of the cast to make a window greatly weakens the cast. A better alternative is to bivalve the cast so that it can easily be removed, the wound treated, and the cast reapplied.

Many varieties of cast material are available today, including the old standby plaster of Paris, and thermoplastic (Orthoplast, Hexcelite) and polyurethane resins (Vetcast, K-Cast, Delta-lite). The veterinarian should choose a material that he or she is comfortable with as concerns application and cost. These materials have limited shelf-lives, and rotation of cast material is crucial. Plaster of Paris is inexpensive and easy to work with but is not waterproof. The polyurethane resins are lighter in weight, easier to apply, much less messy in their application, and need replacing less often.

Long-Leg Cylindrical Cast. Application of the long-leg cylindrical cast will be described using polyurethane resin material (Fig. 55–14). Application of the short-leg cast is identical except that it extends from the digits to the distal one third of the forelimb or rear limb. The long-leg (full-length) cast should extend from the digits to the distal third of the femur or humerus. This type of cast is not appropriate for short, stubby legged animals. The materials needed include adhesive tape stirrups, cast padding (preferably synthetic), stockinette (polypropylene is desirable) cast padding, stockinette cast material, and splint rod.

The long-leg cylindrical cast is applied as follows:

1. Patient should be under general anesthesia.
2. The patient should be positioned in lateral or dorsal recumbency (I prefer lateral recumbency for short-leg and dorsal recumbency for long-leg casts).
3. Stockinette is applied to limb—it should be long enough to

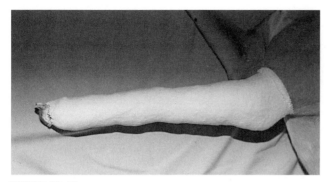

FIGURE 55–14. A long-leg cylindrical cast extends from the digits to the distal third of the femur or humerus.

extend 2 to 3 inches above and below the cast (the stockinette should fit snugly).

4. The distal portion of stockinette is rolled up and tape stirrups applied.

5. Padding is placed around any bony prominences, ie, accessory carpal bone, calcaneus, olecranon.

6. The limb should be positioned at the desired angle prior to application of bandage and cast materials.

7. Two layers of cast padding are added, starting at the toes and extending proximally to end 1 inch proximal to the proposed cast.

8. The cast padding should be wrapped as tightly as possible to the limb (the cast padding will break before it becomes too tight).

9. Plastic gloves should be worn.

10. The package of cast material is opened (only one package of cast material should be opened at a time or it will be ruined; cast material should be examined closely to be sure the resin has not settled to one area).

11. Cast material is immersed in water at room temperature for 15 to 20 seconds and the roll squeezed 3 to 4 times.

12. Lubricating lotion is applied to gloves.

13. Starting at the distal limb, material is rolled on smoothly with even pressure, ie, 3 to 4 inches are unrolled at a time before the limb is encircled.

14. The distal limb is encircled two to three times; the veterinarian then works proximally, overlapping each time by one-half the width of the roll (proximally the cast should be thicker also).

15. Following application of the first two layers of cast material, lateral-medial or cranial-caudal strips of cast material can be added for extra strength; this is followed by application of another two layers of cast material.

16. During application the material should be applied with even tension, avoiding pressure with fingertips and using the flat of the hand.

17. More tension should be applied on the cast material proximally as it has a tendency to loosen after application.

18. Following application of the cast material, the cast is smoothed with a lubricated glove, making certain that the limb is in the desired position (usually slight flexion of elbow and carpus or stifle and tarsus).

19. The cast material must be applied rapidly as it will harden in 4 to 5 minutes.

20. The stockinette and tape stirrups are reflected back on themselves and secured with adhesive tape or additional cast material.

21. Portions of digits 3 and 4 should be exposed at the distal end of the cast.

22. A walking bar of aluminum rod is contoured to the distal portion of the cast and secured with adhesive tape or cast material.

Post-application management of a full cylinder cast is critical. The patient should be hospitalized for 24 hours and the cast checked prior to discharge to determine if there is excessive swelling, discomfort, or damage to the cast. A water container should not be placed in the cage or used in post-cast application as the patient will undoubtedly step in it or spill it, necessitating reapplication of the cast.

The patient should be returned for reevaluation of the cast every 1 to 2 weeks, depending on the veterinarian's evaluation of the client. Animals under 9 months of age should be observed every 2 weeks, as rapid growth may necessitate application of a new cast. At the time of discharge, the veterinarian should explain in detail to the client how to check the cast for complications. He or she should be alert for usual discharges, mutilation of the cast by the patient, change of shape of the cast, and unusual odors. A written set of instructions for care that emphasizes keeping the cast clean and dry is an excellent idea. The most common complications of long-term cast application are pressure sores, soiled cast—wet, outgrowing the cast, failure to return for rechecks, breakdown of distal portion of cast, self-mutilation of cast, muscle atrophy resulting in loosening of the cast.

If at all possible, the original cast should remain in place until the fracture has healed. An advantage of the resin cast materials is that they allow for excellent radiographic follow-up with the cast in place. By all means, if complications do arise, there should be no hesitation to remove the cast and apply a new cast or choose an alternative means of external or internal support. Removal of the cast requires a cast cutter (oscillatory circular saw blade and cast spreader). Usually casts can be removed with little or no sedation. Care must be used so as not to traumatize the skin with the cast cutter. The underlying bandage material will prevent this from happening except over prominences. Possible re-application of a portion or all of the cast should be anticipated, and it should be bivalved in an appropriate direction. One should be prepared for surprises that await under the cast.

Half-Casts. The half-cast (Fig. 55–15) is utilized similarly to the lateral splint. A long-leg cylindrical cast is applied to the limb. After the cast is "set" it is bivalved in a cranial to caudal direction. The medial portion of the cast is discarded. The lateral portion of the cast is secured to the limb with conforming gauze and an adhesive or elastic wrap. The advantages of the half-cast are light weight, allowance for easier changes, ie, can be used over open

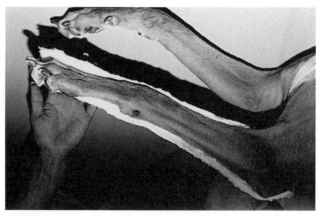

FIGURE 55–15. A half-cast allows for periodic inspection of the soft tissues.

wounds, allowance for cast material to be applied more proximal on the limb without pressure on axillary or inguinal area, fewer complications, better toleration by patient. The half-cast may be used any time a lateral splint is needed. It is especially applicable for immobilization of the stifle following anterior cruciate ligament reconstructions.

After application of any coaptation device and prior to discharge of the patient from the hospital, the owner should receive detailed verbal and written instructions on how to care for the splint or cast as well as what type of complications should alert him or her that there is a problem. A few minutes spent with the pet owner discussing these instructions is time well spent.

GLOSSARY

COMPILED BY ROBERT A. TAYLOR, JON F. DEE, JAMES R. GANNON

Achilles tendon: The tendon between the calf muscle and the point of the hock, composed of the tendons of the gastrocnemius and superficial digital flexor muscles, which are joined by the tendons of the biceps femoris and semitendinosus muscles.

AI (artificial insemination): Involves introduction of fresh, chilled, or frozen semen into the vagina or uterus of a female.

Ankle/wrist: Refers to the carpal area of the forelimb, the carpus.

Arthrodesis: Surgical fusion of a mobile joint.

Back muscle: Gracilis muscle located at the "back" or posterior aspect of the medial thigh.

Backside: Back stretch of a race track.

Bald-thigh syndrome: Refers to the bilateral posterior lateral alopecia seen on the thighs of racing greyhounds.

Biley throat: Accumulation of saliva and respiratory tree mucus containing small air bubbles.

Biscuits: Dry dog food; kibbles.

Bite-back lure: Mechanical device emitting sound and mild electrical stimulus when bitten.

Blade muscle: Deltoid muscle.

Blowout: Sudden development of loose, watery diarrhea.

Blue eye: Pigmentary keratitis secondary to antigen-antibody reaction associated with adenovirus (hepatitis) vaccine.

Bone flake: Lamella stress fracture of cortical bone.

Bone hormone: Trophobolene (progesterone-based mineralizing anabolic drug) and Reepair.

Book-a-Bitch: Reservation to a stud dog.

Bowed tendons: Enlargement of the digital flexor tendons, or the abductor digiti quinti tendon of the front foot due to strain or tearing.

Box: Container that holds the dogs just before the race and from which they are released to chase the lure.

Breaking-in: Educational program for adolescent greyhounds before racing.

Brown stain: Discoloration of hairs of upper lip where tongue sweeps over the area.

Bursa: Protective envelope of fluid located between a bony prominence and the skin; an adventitious bursa is one that gradually forms as a result of repeated trauma to a bony prominence.

Buttock pain: Pain in the area of the hip.

Calf muscles: Medial and lateral (gastrocnemius and superficial digital) flexor muscles.

Camber: Banking of racetrack on the turns (bends).

Catching pen: Collection or run-off area for dogs at the conclusion of a race.

Chest or brisket: Pectoral muscles.

Chest muscles: Pectoral muscles.

Chilblains: Inflammation and erosion of the tips of the ear.

Comes home; bottom: Greyhound that closes ground near race end.

Corn: Common term for either fibrous scar tissue or a wart (papilloma) in a digital or main pad.

Coupling: Lumbar area over the back between the last rib and the hip bone.

Cow hocks: Medial rotation of the lower aspect of the hind limbs leading to an approximation of the hocks when standing at rest. The hocks converge (point medially) whereas the toes diverge (point laterally).

Cramping: Prolonged painful spasm or contraction of a muscle or group of muscles.

Double: Two greyhounds sharing the same kennel.

Drift out: Running pattern in which the dog moves out toward the outer rail either on the curves or the straightaway.

Dropped hip: Downward displacement of the crest of the ilium; may be unilateral or bilateral.

Dropped toe: Toe with loss of either superficial digital flexor tendon function or both the superficial and deep digital flexor tendon functions.

Dropped wrist: Overextension of the wrist when standing.

Dry pads: Loss of flexibility with hyperkeratinization of footpads.

Early foot: Starts very fast out of the starting box.

Egg muscle (see also *Pin Muscle* and *Monkey Muscle*): Upper portion of the long head of the triceps muscle.

Fan muscle: Latissimus dorsi muscle; also called rib muscle.

Fatigue fractures: Incomplete disintegration of cortical bone; caused by repetitive stresses.

Fibula pain: Discomfort associated with fractures of fibula shaft or partial detachment of head of fibula from tibia.

Field-shy chaser: Voluntary avoidance of close contact with other race contestants.

Fighter: A dog that turns its head on the racetrack to fight another.

Flatfeet: Loss of angulation of toes.

Flat toe: See *Dropped toe.*

Fly worry: Irritation to the tips of the ears secondary to flies.

Fungous nail: See *Sand toe.*

Gaskin: Area between stifle and hock joint.

GC/MS: Gas chromatography/mass spectrometry.

GC/MS/MS: Gas chromatography/mass spectrometery/mass spectrometry.

Greenstick fracture: Partial break in the shaft of a bone, without complete fracture; seen in the young.

Greyhound asthma: Exercise-induced bronchoconstriction.

Groin muscle: Pectineus muscle.

Hairline fracture: Small crack in the shaft of a bone, but not extending the full depth of the bone cortex.

Hamstrings: Caudal thigh muscles and associated tendons.

Handslip: Releasing of racing greyhound by hand at the start of race or trial.

Hip support: Tensor fasciae latae muscle laterally; vastus lateralis muscle medially.

Hole: Small space with door in a trailer or starting box, also called the first hole.

Hot blood: Term indicating enthusiasm in a greyhound to run or chase the lure.

Hot spot: Area of acute moist erythematous dermatitis.

HPLC: High-performance liquid chromatography.

"Husk," post-exercise: Subdued cough or clearing of the throat after races and trials.

Interval training: Training consisting of short sprints alternating with rest used to develop anaerobic energy metabolism in muscle.

Jacks (see also *Track Leg*): Swelling of the skin on the inside of the leg over the mid-tibia. Periostitis and hematoma on medial aspect of tibia resulting from trauma when running.

Joint mice: Fragments of detached bone or cartilage inside a joint.

Kibble: Broken biscuit used as a carbohydrate source in the diet.

Kicked-up flat toe: Elevation of nail and loss of mid-toe angulation due to disruption of both flexor tendons.

Kicked-up toe: Elevation of nail due to disruption of deep flexor tendon.

Knocked-down hip: See *Dropped hip.*

Knocked-up flat toe: Flattening of the central toe joint and upward displacement of the nail and toe pad due to disruption of the superficial and deep digital flexor tendons.

Knocked-up toe: Upward displacement of the nail and toe pad due to disruption of the deep digital flexor tendon function.

Laser: Soft form of physical therapy of musculoskeletal injuries using a hand-held source of amplified light.

Load: Place dog into starting box or "box greyhound" (Australian term), also termed boxing.

Loin (also called The Coupling): Mass of muscle from the last rib to the hip and from the spine to the bottom of the flank; includes longissimus lumborum, iliocostalis, iliopsoas, and obliquus externus abdominis muscles.

Loose lip: Dog that does not attack training lure aggressively.

Lure drive: Manner in which the artificial hare is driven as an inducement for the greyhounds to chase to their maximum during a race or trial.

Maiden: Greyhound that has never won a race.

Mechanical fault: Refers to muscle pain syndromes (cervicothoracic or lumbar/sacral) that are thought to be secondary to spinal mechanical faults.

"Milk": Any type of secretion from the mammary glands.

Mobility faults: Spinal mechanical faults.

Monkey muscle: Long head of the triceps.

Muscle man: Layman offering physiotherapy and manipulation service for musculoskeletal injuries.

Muzzle: Wire or plastic cage applied to the head to enclose the mouth (upper and lower jaws).

Needling: Any kind of injection; usually associated with musculoskeletal injuries.

Nervy: Anxious, tense temperament in an animal.

Non-chaser: Poorly motivated race contender; one that loses concentration during a race.

OCD (osteochondritis dissecans): Loose osteochondral (bone and cartilage) fragment found associated with osteochondrosis (a disease of young developing bone).

Offal: Abdominal or chest contents of a beast used as a food source.

Onychogryposis: Deformed overgrowth of the nails, often seen with fungal infections of nail bed.

Outbreed: Introduction of a totally unrelated gene pool, of the same breed, to existing breeding stock.

Overshot jaw: Genetic defect in which the lower jaw is longer than the upper jaw.

Phony: Animal that (1) quits if racing conditions are not just right or (2) quits running at the racetrack altogether (see *Non-chaser*).

Pick up: At race end, to get a dog off the track.

Pin bones: Ilium bones; also refers to the crest of the ilium.

Pin-firing: Induction of acute inflammatory reaction by applying a pattern of lines or spots using a hot iron or heating device as a means of generating fibrous scar tissue. Procedure is largely discarded and illegal in some countries.

Pin muscle: Long head of the triceps.

"Plumpton" racing: Australian term for coursing, using an artificial drag lure on a straight grass track.

Poll injuries: Trauma to parietal crest; a forehead injury.

Proven cross: Bloodlines that have produced good track dogs having been previously bred to each other.

Proven female: Her pups have already won races.

Pulled nail: Complete loss of the horny covering of the nail bone.

Quarter bones: American term for the metatarsal bones of the hind feet (including metatarsal/metacarpal bones).

Quick: Highly sensitive soft tissue between the nail bone and the nail.

Racing thirst (see also *Water diabetes*): American term for post-race polydipsia (excessive water intake).

Rib muscle: Latissimus dorsi.

Roach back: Pronounced flexion (arching) of the spinal column when at rest.

Router: Racing greyhound that performs best in distance races; also called a distance runner.

Run back off: Overheating of a greyhound by running too hard for a long time, causing muscle damage.

Run its back off; ricked back: Dog that has suffered many episodes of "tying up" or rhabdomyolysis resulting in fibrosis and shrinkage of muscles along back and spine.

Saddle area: Thoracic area or area over the top of the chest.

Sand in the throat: Often an "explanation" for exercise-induced bronchoconstriction.

Sand rash (also Sand burns): Trauma, ranging from abrasion to complete disruption of the full thickness of skin of the ventral webbing, directly under the digital flexor tendons.

Sand toe: Mechanical trauma from sand in the nail bed with secondary infection of the Skin-Nail Junction (paronychia).

Schooling (also Breaking-in): Process of teaching the dog all the protocols of race conduct.

Scratched: Withdrawn from a race; the cancellation of a race entry.

She missed: Did not become pregnant when last bred.

She took: Is pregnant from last breeding.

Shin soreness: Metacarpal periostitis, an inflammatory tenderness of the metacarpals of one or both front feet; a stage preceding stress fracture.

Short: One that gets caught before race end or is losing ground.

Sickle hocks: The outward rotation of the lower aspect of the hind limb, leading to a pronounced separation of the hocks when standing at rest.

"Spare rib": An extranumerary rib; one at the rear of the rib cage not forming part of the costal arch.

Spinal manipulation: A chiropractic procedure conducted on the vertebral column.

Splayed toes: Flattening and excessive separating of the toes when standing, often associated with dropped wrist.

Split web: Tearing or disruption of the webbing, ranging from small splitting of the anterior margin to complete separation along the entire length between the toes.

Sprain: Inflammation due to overextension (overstretching).

Sprung toe: Sprain of the collateral ligament of a toe.

Stopper bone: Accessory carpal bone.

Stopper pad: Accessory carpal pad.

Stopper tendon: Tendon of insertion of the flexor carpi ulnaris muscle.

Strain: Overuse or overextension of a muscle or tendon.

Stress fracture: Partial or complete break in a bone as a result of excessive workload.

Stretch: Flank muscles.

TENS (Transcutaneous Electrical Nerve Stimulation): A form of physical therapy employing faradic (electrical) stimulation of muscle fibers.

Thigh: Biceps femoris.

"Throw" a leg: Excessive abduction (outward movement) of a hind limb during its forward motion when running.

Tin hare: Colloquialism for any artificial lure.

TLC: Thin-layer chromatography.

Track crossfall: The banking of the track on the turns.

Track leg: Swelling of the skin on the inside of the leg over the tibia.

Trailing: Another term for schooling. Australian term for assessing the ability and fitness of a dog prior to entering a race.

Trained off: Prolonged fatigue state; inability to cope with the workload; excessively trained.

Tucked up: Excessive tension of the abdominal muscles—often associated with roaching of the back.

Turnout: Period (varies) of time kennel dogs are let outside into a small pen called a turnout pen.

Types of lure: Bramish: Lure is mounted on a linear electric motor moving along a metal rail. Cable: Lure is attached to a wire cable encircling the track. Inside: Lure moves along the inside rail of the track. Outside: Lure moves along the outside rail of the track.

Undershot jaw: Genetic defect in which the lower jaw is shorter than the upper jaw.

$\dot{V}O_2$ max: A measure of oxygen consumption at maximal workload; a quantitative measure of aerobic capacity and degree of fitness.

Wasted calf: Disuse atrophy of the gastrocnemius.

Water diabetes: Excessive thirst and urine output (polydipsia and polyuria) consequent to the stress of a hard run or in response to corticosteroid administration.

Whip muscle: Sartorius muscle.

Withering: Loss of size of a muscle due to atrophy.

Work fast: Running behind a lure as an inducement to greater effort or speed.

Work slow: Walking exercise and/or voluntary running in an enclosure.

Wrist: The carpal joint, located between the forelimb and the foot of the front limb.

INDEX

Note: Page numbers in *italics* refer to illustrations; numbers followed by t indicate tables.

Fish, in racing greyhound diet, 332
Fish hydrolysate, in nutritional supplement for racing dog, 346t
Fish oil, in racing greyhound diet, 330
Fistula, perianal, in German shepherd, 440
Flat feet, defined, 458
Flat toe, defined, 459
    kicked-up, defined, 459
Flea(s), control of, in greyhound kennel, 78–79
    distribution and life cycle of, 77–78
Flea allergy dermatitis (FAD), 78
Flexion, in racing sled dog, 8–9
Flexor carpi radialis muscle, innervation of, *278*
Flexor carpi ulnaris muscle, *108*
    injury to insertion of, 97–98
    innervation of, *278*
Flexor carpi ulnaris tendon, *114*
    tear of, 432–433
Flexor reflex, 278–279
Flexor tendon(s), cross-section of, *256*
    laceration of, 98
    stretching of, 98
Flunixin meglumine, chromatogram of, *386*
    clearance of, 385
    for exertional rhabdomyolysis, 70
    gastrointestinal ulceration due to, 32–34
Fly worry, 20
    defined, 458
Folic acid, in racing greyhound diet, 333t
    limits and optimal daily intake of, 345t
Follicle-stimulating hormone (FSH), 305
    in normal male dog, 307
Follicular cysts, natural breeding and, 315–316
Folliculitis, 42
Food. See also *Diet; Nutrition.*
    digestibility of, 339, 339t
    energy equivalents for, 329
    for racing greyhound, aims of, 328
        common constituents of, 331–333, 332t
        energy requirements for, 328–329
        energy sources in, 329–331
        ergogenic aids and, 333–334, 334t
        feeding of, 334–336, 334t
    for working dog, 438
    refusal of. See also *Anorexia.*
        during pregnancy, 322, 323
Foot. See also *Paw(s).*
    examination of, 24–25, *25–26*
    injury to, in racing greyhound, track surveys of, 412t
        in racing sled dog, 377, 415–419, *416–419*
    radiography of, 405, *406–407*
    valgus deformity of, 102
Foreign body, tracheobronchial, 58
Foreleg, muscle injuries to, 85–86
    of racing greyhound, track surveys of injuries to, 414t
Forelimb, contracture of, 70
    examination of, 23–24, *23*
Forepaw, radiography of, 405, *406–407*
Four-wheelers, training sled dogs with, 375, *375*, 380
Fovea capitis, 175
Fracture, types of, fatigue, 458
    greenstick, 459
    hairline, 459
    stress, 460
Fragmented coronoid process (FCP), 242–244, *243–244*
Free fatty acids (FFAs), 337
    high-fat diet and, 351
Free-radical scavengers, for degenerative joint disease, *211*, 212–213, 212t
Freezing, in racing sled dog, 421, *421*
Friar's Balsam, 171
Friction massage, 3, 275
Front foot, examination of, 24–25, *26*
    radiography of, 405, *406–407*
Frostbite, in racing sled dog, 421, *421*
FSH (follicle-stimulating hormone), 305, 307

Fucosidosis, 53
Full-length cylindrical cast, 455–456, *456*
Functional compensation, 277
Functional return, 272–273
    documentation of, *272, 273*
Fungal arthritis, 219
Fungous nail, defined, 460

GAF (Greyhound Adoption Fund), 447
GAGPS (glycosaminoglycan polysulfate), for degenerative joint disease, *211–212*, 212t, 213–214
Gait, examination of, 22–23
Galactostasis, 326
Gallop, double-suspension, 426, *427–428*
    of greyhound puppy, 371
Game-bird dogs, 9–12, 11t
Gangliosidosis, 53
Gangrene, due to tight bandage, 449, *449*
Gas chromatograph/mass spectrometer, schematic of, *386*
Gas chromatography (GC), for drug identification, 385, *386*
Gaskin, defined, 459
Gastric blowout, avoidance of, 335
Gastric dilatation-volvulus (GDV), in working dog, 437–438
Gastric transit time, 339
Gastrocnemius muscle and tendon, contracture of, 70
    injuries to, 91, *91*, 112
    innervation of, *279*
Gastrointestinal epithelium, dietary fiber and, 354
Gastrointestinal parasites, in greyhound, anthelmintics for, 75–76
        resistance to, 74–75
    epidemiology of, 73–74
    public health aspects of, 76
    transmammary and transplacental transmission of, 74
Gastrointestinal system, problems of, in working dog, 437–443
Gastrointestinal transit time, 339
Gastropexy, 438
Gastrostomy, 438
Gazehound, 1
GC (gas chromatography), for drug identification, 385, *386*
GDV (gastric dilatation-volvulus), in working dog, 437–438
Gee (command), 377
Genetic muscle disorders, 70–71. See also specific disease.
Genetic neurological diseases, 50–53. See also specific disease.
Genitourinary diseases, in female, 46. See also specific disease.
    in male, 44–46. See also specific disease.
    racing-related, 46–47. See also specific disease.
Gentamicin, for mycoplasmal arthritis, 219
    for tracheobronchitis, 62
Geofabrics, 394, 395
German shepherd, acquired lumbosacral stenosis in, 196
    as military dog, 18
    as working dog, 14, 434
    hip dysplasia in, 182, 183
    lumbosacral stenosis in, 198
    perianal fistula in, 440
Gestation, timing of, 324
Giant axonal neuropathy, 52
Giardia canis, eggs and larvae of, in greyhound runs and pens, 74
Giardia lamblia, 29–30
Gingival disease, in working dog, 436, *437*
Global balance, of racing sled dog, 8
Glomerular vasculopathy, cutaneous and renal idiopathic, clinical
        laboratory findings in, 40
    clinical signs of, 39–40, *39*
    early cases of, 38–39
    prognosis in, 41
    treatment of, 41
Glossitis, in military dog, 437
Glucagon, as function of exercise, 340, *340*
Glucocorticoids, for chronic stress, 29
    for degenerative joint disease, *211*, 212, 212t
    for idiopathic polyarthritis, 215

Leishmaniasis, polyarthritis due to, 220
Leptospira icterohaemorrhagiae, nephritis due to, 47
Levothyroxine, for hypothyroidism, 316
LFAs (long-chain fatty acids), optimal intake of, in racing husky, *342*
LH. See *Luteinizing hormone (LH).*
Ligaments, injury to, 100
   repair of, 100–101
   shortened, chiropractic manipulation for, 275
Limber tail, 55
Limbs. See also *Foreleg; Forelimb; Hindlimb.*
   examination of, 20, 22–23
   mobilization of, 290–294, *291–294*
Linoleic acids, *352*
Lip, loose, defined, 458
Lipids. See also *Fats; Fatty acids; Omega–3 fatty acids.*
   digestibility of, 339t, 340
   for racing dog, sources of, 345
   in racing greyhound diet, 330–331
   in racing husky diet, 341–342, *342*
   oxidation of, 337
Lipofuscinosis, ceroid, 53
Lips, examination of, 20
Live lure, for greyhound racing, 372
LMN (lower motor neuron) disease, clinical signs of, 49t
Load, defined, 458
Loam, for track, 394–396, 394t, *395–396*
Local anesthetics, as performance-modifying drugs, 389
Locking loop suture, 95
Lofentanil, as performance-modifying drug, 390
Loin, defined, 458
Long bones, of racing greyhound, fractures of, 202–209
      track surveys of, 413t–414t
Long digital extensor (LDE) muscle, innervation of, *279*
Long digital extensor (LDE) tendon, avulsion of, 98, 142, 148
   osteochondritis of, 142
Long-chain fatty acids (LFAs), optimal intake of, in racing husky, *342*
Long-distance racing, 375
   energy metabolism in, 341
   energy requirements for, 338–339, 338t
Long-distance sled dog races, 415
Long-leg cylindrical cast, 455–456, *456*
Loose lip, defined, 458
Loperamide, for diahrrea-dehydration-stress syndrome, 424
Lordotic stance, in greyhound, 282
Lower motor neuron (LMN) disease, clinical signs of, 49t
LS (lumbosacral) disease, as contraindication to total hip replacement, 192
Lufenuron, for flea control, 79
Lumbar nerves, *279*
Lumbar spinal cord segments, in relation to muscles of hind limb, *279*
Lumbar spine, chiropractic manipulation of, 281–282, *282*
Lumbosacral canal, 196, *197*
Lumbosacral disease. See also *Lumbosacral stenosis.*
   as contraindication to total hip replacement, 192
Lumbosacral instability, 56. See also *Lumbosacral stenosis.*
Lumbosacral junction, normal vs. unstable, *197*
Lumbosacral nerve root compression. See *Lumbosacral stenosis.*
Lumbosacral pain, chiropractic manipulation for, 281
Lumbosacral plexus, *279, 280*
Lumbosacral stenosis, 196–202
   advanced imaging techniques in, 200, *201*
   degenerative, 197, *197*
   idiopathic, 198, *198*
   in German shepherd, 198
   pathophysiology of, 196–198, *197–198*
   physical examination in, 198–199, *198–199*
   radiographic examination in, 199–200, *200*
   treatment of, 200–201
Lung infections, parasitic, 60
Lupus erythematosus, systemic, 215–216
Lure, bite-back, defined, 458
   coyote hide for, 365
   for greyhound racing, 372–374, *373–374*
   types of, 460
Lure coursing, defined, 426

Lure coursing *(Continued)*
   greyhound breeding and, 328
Lure drive, defined, 458
Lure rail, *395*
Luteal cysts, natural breeding and, 315–316
Luteinizing hormone (LH), 302, 305
   in estrous cycle, *302,* 305, 313, 323t
   in male, 307
Luteolysis, prepartum, *323,* 323t
Luxation, of superficial digital flexor tendon, 99
Lyme disease, 30, 219
Lymphosarcoma, in working dog, 441

MA (megestrol acetate), for estrus control, 310–311, 311t
Magnesium, in nutritional supplement for racing dog, 346t
   in racing greyhound diet, 333t
   in racing husky diet, 343
Magnesium ions, in muscular contraction, 69
Magnetic field therapy, 269
Magnetic resonance imaging (MRI), in diagnosis of lumbosacral stenosis, 200, *201*
   in orthopedic sports medicine, 445
   of appendages, 402–404, *404*
Maiden, defined, 458
Maintenance diet, for racing dog, 329, 346
Maintenance energy requirement (MER), formula for, 338, 339
Malamute, 8
Malignant hyperthermia, 52, 71
Malinois. See *Belgian malinois.*
Malleolus, fracture of, 122–124, *123–124*
Manganese, in nutritional supplement for racing dog, 346t
   in racing greyhound diet, 333t
   limits and optimal daily intake of, 345t
Mange, otodectic, 81
   red, 80–81
   sarcoptic, 79–80
Manipulation, 269–271. See also *Passive range-of-motion (PROM) exercises.*
   defined, 460
Manners, teaching of, in sled dog, 377
Masking agents, for illicit drugs, 387
Mason metasplint, 453–454, *454*
Mass spectrometer, *386*
Mass spectrometry (MS), for drug identification, 385, *386*
Massage, for muscle spasm, 276
   types of, 3, 269, 275
Mastitis, 326
Maternal dystocia, 325
Mating(s), estimated time of, during estrous cycle, *323,* 323t
Mattress suture, *95*
Maximum Stress Diet, Medicated, 438
MDMA (methylenedioxymethamphetamine), as performance-modifying drug, 390
Meat(s), defined, 349
   drugs and other contaminants in, 335–336
   in racing greyhound diet, 331–332
Mechanical fault, defined, 458
Meclofenamic acid, for hip dysplasia, 189
   gastrointestinal ulceration due to, 32–34
Medial circumflex femoral artery, 175
Medial collateral ligament(s), tarsal, 120, *122*
Medial intertarsal subluxation/luxation, 135–137
Median nerve, *278*
Medroxyprogesterone acetate (MPA), for estrus control, 310, 311t
Megaesophagus, associated with myasthenia gravis, 71
   congenital, 52
Megestrol acetate (MA), for estrus control, 310–311, 311t
Meglumine antimonate, for leishmaniasis, 220
Melanoma, of pad, hyperkeratosis vs., 37, *38*
Meningoencephalitis, due to migrating plant awn, 53
Meningomyelitis, due to migrating plant awn, 53
Meniscal injury, 141